THE PRACTICE OF INTERVENTIONAL CARDIOLOGY

Second Edition

The Practice of Interventional Cardiology

Second Edition

John H.K. Vogel, M.D.
Cardiovascular Pulmonary Medicine Group
Santa Barbara, California

Spencer B. King III, M.D.
Professor of Medicine
Director of Interventional Cardiology
Department of Medicine (Cardiology)
Emory University
Atlanta, Georgia

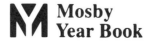

Mosby
Year Book

St. Louis   Baltimore   Boston   Chicago   London   Philadelphia   Sydney   Toronto

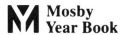
Mosby
Year Book

Dedicated to Publishing Excellence

Sponsoring Editor: Stephanie Manning
Associate Managing Editor, Manuscript Services: Deborah Thorp
Production Supervisor: Karen Halm
Proofroom Manager: Barbara M. Kelly

1 2 3 4 5 6 7 8 9 0 CL MV 97 96 95 94 93

Library of Congress Cataloging-in-Publication Data
The Practice of interventional cardiology / [edited by] John H.K.
  Vogel, Spencer B. King, III. — 2nd ed.
      p. cm.
    Rev. ed. of: Interventional cardiology. 1989.
    Includes bibliographical references and index.
    ISBN 0-8016-6694-5
    1. Heart — Diseases — Treatment. 2. Heart — Surgery. I. Vogel,
John H. K., 1932- . II. King, Spencer B., 1937-
III. Interventional cardiology.
    [DNLM: 1. Cardiovascular Diseases — therapy.   WG 166 P895]
RC683.8.P73 1992
617.4′ 12059 — dc20   92-18764
DNLM/DLC   CIP
for Library of Congress

Childhood Disappearances

*It's hard to know
if his footsteps were echos,
or if they were constantly changing,
time after time.
She'd see a shadow depart down the stairs,
to help others find a tomorrow or just a dawn.
Those unlucky ones would just see
the sunrise,
but if he disappeared into the night,
faster than the beat of a heart,
he could capture them from the glittering clouds
and bring them back so they could
push the sun behind the curtains
of the horizon,
to go play amongst the stars in their dreams.
He would come home,
tired,
satisfied,
and she saw his footsteps,
and wondered whom he helped,
as she heard his shadow pass.*

Kristen Marie Richmond Vogel

Dedicated to my Dad and all physicians devoted to their patients.

CONTRIBUTORS

Douglas Albagli, B.A.
Department of Physics
Massachusetts Institute of Technology
Cambridge, Massachusetts

John W. Allen, M.D.
Clinical Associate Professor of Medicine
Department of Medicine/Cardiology
University of Southern California School of Medicine
Los Angeles, California

Paolo Angelini, M.D.
Associate Professor of Internal Medicine
Baylor College of Medicine
Staff Cardiologist
Texas Heart Institute
St. Lukes Episcopal Hospital
Houston, Texas

Rosa M. Avolio, R.N.
Nurse Manager Cardiology
Ceoleta Valley Community Hospital
Santa Barbara, California

Juan J. Badimon, Ph.D.
Director, Cardiovascular Biology Research Laboratories
Cardiac Unit
Massachusetts General Hospital
Boston, Massachusetts

Lina Badimon, Ph.D.
Director, Cardiovascular Biology Research Laboratories
Cardiac Unit
Massachusetts General Hospital
Boston, Massachusetts

Pascal Barraud, M.D.
Department of Cardiology
Clermont Ferrand University
Clermont Ferrand, France

Christophe Bauters, M.D.
Department of Cardiology
Uniiversity of Lille II
Lille, France

George A. Beller, M.D.
Head, Division of Cardiology
Donald C. Barnes Professor of Medicine
Department of Medicine
University of Virginia Health Sciences Center
Charlottesville, Virginia

Bradford C. Berk, M.D., Ph.D.
Associate Professor of Medicine
Department of Medicine (Cardiology)
Emory University School of Medicine
Atlanta, Georgia

Martin R. Berk, M.D.
Cardiology and Internal Medicine Associates
Dallas, Texas

Michel E. Bertrand, M.D.
Professor of Medicine (Cardiology)
Head, Division of Cardiology
University of Lille
Lille, France

Giancarlo Biamino, M.D.
Professor of Medicine and Cardiology
Universitatsklinikum Rudolf-Virchow/Wedding
Berlin, Germany

John A. Bittl, M.D.
Assistant Professor of Medicine
Harvard Medical School
Co-Director of Interventional Cardiology
Brigham and Women's Hospital
Boston, Massachusetts

Peter C. Block, M.D.
Associate Director
St. Vincent's Heart Institute
Portland, Oregon

Raoul Bonan, M.D.
Director, Cardiac Catheterization Laboratory
Assistance Professor of Medicine
Department of Medicine
University of Montreal
Montreal, Canada

Tassilo R. Bonzel, M.D.
Director of Internal Medicine and Cardiology
Medical Clinic I
Fulda General Hospital
Fulda, Germany

Corrinne Bott-Silverman, M.D.
Department of Cardiology
Cleveland Clinic Foundation
Cleveland, Ohio

Barry Bravette, M.D.
Clinical Assistant Professor of Medicine
Department of Cardiology
Thomas Jefferson University Hospital
Philadelphia, Pennsylvania

Jeffrey A. Brinker, M.D.
Texas Heart Institute
St. Luke's Hospital
Houston, Texas

Cristopher E. Buller, M.D.
Division of Cardiology
Duke University Medical Center
Durham, North Carolina

James H. Chesebro, M.D.
Professor of Medicine
Mayo Medical School
Consultant in Cardiovascular Diseases and Internal Medicine
Mayo Clinic
Rochester, Minnesota

Thomas J. Clement
Director of Engineering
Heart Technology, Inc.
Bellevue, Washington

Robert M. Cothren, Ph.D.
Staff Scientist
Biomedical Engineering and Applied Therapeutics
The Cleveland Clinic Foundation
Cleveland, Ohio

Barry J. Coughlin, M.D.
Cardiologist, Medical Director
Non-Invasive Diagnostic Laboratory
Valley Medical Group
Lompoc, California

Michael J. Cowley, M.D.
Texas Heart Institute
St. Luke's Hospital
Houston, Texas

John R. Crew, M.D.
Director of Cardiovascular Research
San Francisco Heart Institute
Seton Medical Center
Daly City, California

Alain Cribier, M.D.
Professor, University of Rouen
Department of Cardiology
University of Rouen
Rouen, France

David C. Cumberland, M.D.
Consultant Radiologist
Department of Radiology
Northern General Hospital
Sheffield, England

Ramachandra R. Dasari, Ph.D.
Assistant Director
Spectroscopy Laboratory
Massachusetts Institute of Technology
Cambridge, Massachusetts

Marilyn Dean, R.V.T.
Vascular Laboratory
San Francisco Heart Institute
Seton Medical Center
Daly City, California

Anthony N. Demaria, M.D.
Professor of Medicine
Cardiology Division
University of California at San Diego Medical Center
San Diego, California

Timothy A. Dewhurst, M.D.
Senior Fellow
Division of Cardiology
University of Washington
Seattle, Washington

Germano DiSciascio, M.D.
Associate Professor of Internal Medicine
Department of Cardiology
Medical College of Virginia
Richmond, Virginia

Kathleen M. Donovan, R.N.
Research Nurse Coordinator
Interventional Devices
Washington Cardiology Center
Washington, D.C.

John S. Douglas, Jr., M.D.
Associate Professor of Medicine
Emory University School of Medicine
Co-Director
Cardiovascular Laboratory
Emory University Hospital
Atlanta, Georgia

Neal L. Eigler, M.D.
Associate Professor
Department of Medicine
University of California at Los Angeles
Los Angeles, California

James Fagin, M.D.
Assistant Professor of Medicine
Cedars-Sinai Medical Center
Department of Medicine
University of California at Los Angeles
Los Angeles, California

Michael S. Feld, Ph.D.
Professor of Physics
Director of Spectroscopy Laboratory
George Harrison Spectroscopy Laboratory
Massachusetts Institute of Technology
Cambridge, Massachusetts

Pim de Feyter, M.D., Ph.D.
Catheterization Laboratory
Erasmus University Rotterdam
Rotterdam, Netherlands

Michael Fishbein, M.D.
Adjunct Professor of Pathology
University of California at Los Angeles
Associate Pathologist
Cedars-Sinai Medical Center
Los Angeles, California

Peter J. Fitzgerald, M.D., Ph.D.
Senior Cardiology Fellows
Department of Cardiology
University of California at San Francisco
San Francisco, California

James S. Forrester, M.D.
Director, Division of Cardiology
Burns and Allen Chair in Cardiology
Department of Cardiology
Professor of Medicine
University of California at Los Angeles
Los Angeles, California

George I. Frank, M.D.
Department of Invasive Cardiology
Royal Brompton National Heart and Lung Hospital
London, England

Valentin Fuster, M.D.
Chief of Cardiology
Department of Cardiology
Massachusetts General Hospital
Boston, Massachusetts

Habib Gamra, M.D.
Interventional Cardiology Fellow
The Heart Institute
The Hospital of the Good Samaritan
Department of Medicine — Cardiology
Loma Linda University
Loma Linda, California

Lowell Gerber, M.D.
Salt Lake City, Utah

Robert Ginsburg, M.D.
Professor of Medicine
Director, Unit for Cardiovascular Interventions
University of Colorado Health Sciences Center
Denver, Colorado

Kenton W. Gregory, M.D.
Assistant Professor of Medicine
Oregon Health Sciences
St. Vincent Hospital Medical Center
Portland, Oregon

Cindy L. Grines, M.D.
Director, Cardiac Catheterization Laboratory
William Beaumont Hospital
Royal Oak, Michigan

Gary B. Hayes, B.A.
Research Engineer
George R. Harrison Spectroscopy Laboratory
Massachusetts Institute of Technology
Cambridge, Massachusetts

Richard Helfant, M.D.
Department of Cardiology
UCLA
Los Angeles, California

Walter R. M. Hermans, M.D.
Department of Interventional Cardiology
Erasmus University
Rotterdam, Netherlands

Tomoaki Hinohara, M.D.
Staff Cardiologist
Sequia Hospital
Redwood City, California

Paul Hirst
Principal Engineer
Heart Technology, Inc.
Bellevue, Washington

Kiyoshi Inoue, M.D.
Cardiovascular Disease Center
Tokyo Metropolitan Police Hospital
Tokyo, Japan

Irving Itzkan, Ph.D.
Senior Scientist
Laser Biomecial Research Center
George R. Harrison Spectroscopy Laboratory
Massachusetts Institute of Technology
Cambridge, Massachusetts

Joseph A. Izatt, Ph.D.
Postdoctoral Associate
Research Laboratory of Elect
Department of Electronic Engineering and Computer Science
Massachusetts Institute of Technology
Cambridge, Massachusetts

G. Sargent Janes, Ph.D.
Research Affiliate
George R. Harrison Spectroscopy Laboratory
Massachusetts Institute of Technology
Cambridge, Massachusetts

Ronald D. Jenkins, M.D.
Wayne State University School of Medicine
Detroit, Michigan

Hanjorg Just, M.D.
Department of Cardiology
University of Freiburg
Freiburg, Germany

Martin Katlenbach, M.D.
Chief Professor of Cardiology
Clinic Nordhein
University of Frankfurt
Bad Nauheim, Germany

W. Michael Kavanaugh, M.D.
Adjunct Assistant Professor in Medicine
Cardiovascular Research Institute
Department of Medicine
University of California at San Francisco
San Francisco, California

Kenneth M. Kent, M.D.
Cardiologist
Washington Cardiology Center
Washington, D.C.

Mehran J. Khorsandi, M.D.
Fellow in Cardiology
Department of Cardiology
Cedars-Sinai Medical Center
University of California at Los Angeles
Los Angeles, California

Spencer B. King III, M.D.
Professor of Medicine
Director of Interventional Cardiology
Department of Medicine (Cardiology)
Emory University
Atlanta, Georgia

Carter Kittrell, B.S.
Senior Research Scientist
Department of Chemistry
William Marsh Rice University
Houston, Texas

Gisbert Kober, M.D.
Professor of Internal Medicine and Cardiology
Clinic Nordrhein
University of Frankfurt
Bad Nauheim, Germany

John R. Kramer, M.D.
Staff Cardiologist
Department of Cardiology
Cleveland Clinic Foundation
Cleveland, Ohio

Keiichi Kuwaki, M.D.
Cardiovascular Disease Center
Tokyo Metropolitan Police Hospital
Tokyo, Japan

Jean M. Lablanche, M.D.
Professor of Medicine
Department of Cardiology
University of Lille II
Lille, France

Francis Y.K. Lau, M.D.
Professor of Medicine
Department of Medicine and Cardiology
Loma Linda University
Loma Linda, California

D. Richard Leachman, M.D.
Texas Heart Institute
St. Luke Hospital
Houston, Texas

Martin B. Leon, M.D.
Director, Investigational Angioplasty Program
Washington Cardiology Center
Department of Cardiology
Washington Hospital Center
Washington, D.C.

Fabrice Leroy, M.D.
Department of Cardiology
University of Lille II
Lille, France

Brice Letac, M.D.
Professor, Department of Cardiology
University of Rouen
Rouen, France

Vladilen S. Letokhov, M.D.
Department of Laser Spectroscopy
Institute of Spectroscopy
Russian Academy of Sciences
Troitzk, Russia

Frank Litvack, M.D.
Co-Director, Cardiovascular Intervention Center
Associate Professor of Medicine
Department of Cardiology
University of California at Los Angeles
Los Angeles, California

Floyd D. Loop, M.D.
Chief Executive Officer
Cleveland Clinic Foundation
Cleveland, Ohio

Bruce W. Lytle, M.D.
Surgeon, Department of Thoracic and Cardiovascular Surgery
The Cleveland Clinic Foundation
Cleveland, Ohio

Keith L. March, M.D., Ph.D.
Assistant Professor of Medicine
Department of Medicine
Krannert Institute of Cardiology
Indiana University
Indianapolis, Indiana

Antonio Martinez-Hernandez, M.D.
Professor of Pathology
University of Tennessee
Chief, Pathology and Laboratory Medicine Service
Department of Pathology
University of Tennessee
Memphis, Tennessee

Bruce J. McAuley, M.D.
Associate Clinical Professor of Medicine (Cardiology)
Stanford University
Stanford, California
Staff Cardiologist
Sequoia Hospital
Redwood City, California

Euguene P. McFadden, M.B., M.R.C.P. (I.R.E.L.)
Department of Cardiology
University of Lille II
Lille, France

R. Bruce McFadden, M.D.
Clinical Associate Professor of Medicine
Department of Medicine
University of Southern California
Los Angeles, California

R. Hardwin Mead, M.D.
Co-Director, Cardiac Surveillance Unit and Electophysiology
* Laboratory*
Sequoia Hospital
Redwood City, California

Bernhard Meier, M.D.
Chief of Cardiology
University Hospital
Bern, Switzerland

Anthony Don Michael, M.D.
Clinical Professor
Department of Cardiology
University of California at Los Angeles
Los Angeles, California

Hisatoshi Minato, M.T.
Cardiovascular Disease Center
Tokyo Metropolitan Police Hospital
Tokyo, Japan

Yoshio Mukaiyama, M.D.
Cardiovascular Disease Center
Tokyo Metropolitan Police Hospital
Tokyo, Japan

Charles E. Mullins, M.D.
Professor of Clinical Pediatrics
Department of Pediatric Cardiology
Baylor College of Medicine
Houston, Texas

Richard K. Myler, M.D.
Clinical Professor of Medicine
Executive Director
San Francisco Heart Institute
Seton Medical Center
Department of Cardiology
University of California at San Francisco
San Francisco, California

Donald T. Nardone, M.D.
Division of Cardiology
Thomas Jefferson University Hospital
Philadelphia, Pennsylvania

Michael R. Nihill, M.B., B.S., M.R.C.P.
Associate Professor of Pediatrics
Department of Pediatrics
Baylor College of Medicine
Houston, Texas

Leonard A. Nordstrom, M.D.
Assistant Professor of Clinical Medicine
University of Minnesota
Chairman, Department of Cardiology
Park Nicollet Medical Center
Minneapolis, Minnesota

Hidenobu Ochial, M.D.
Cardiovascular Disease Center
Tokyo Metropolitan Police Hospital
Tokyo, Japan

William W. O'Neill, M.D.
Director of Cardiology
William Beaumont Hospital
Royal Oak, Michigan

Alexander A. Oraevsky, M.D.
Department of Laser Spetroscopy
Institute of Spectroscopy
Russian Academy of Sciences
Troitzk, Russia

Igor F. Palacios, M.D.
Massachusetts General Hospital
Boston, Massachusetts

Russell Pflueger, B.S.
Laguna Nigeul, California

Harry R. Phillips, M.D.
Associate Professor of Medicine
Director, Interventional Cardiac
Catheterization Laboratory
Department of Cardiology
Duke University Medical Center
Durham, North Carolina

Augusto D. Pichard, M.D.
Director, Cardiac Catheterization Laboratory
Washington Cardiology Center
Washington, D.C.

Jeffrey J. Popma, M.D.
Cardiology Division
Washington Hospital Center
Washington, D.C.

Johann Christof Ragg, M.D.
Universitatsklinikum Rudolf-Virchow/Wedding
Berlin, Germany

Stephen R. Ramee, M.D.
Director, Interventional Cardiology
Department of Cardiology
Ochsner Medical Institutions
New Orleans, Louisiana

Richard P. Rava, Ph.D.
Principal Research Scientist
G.R. Harrison Spectroscopy Laboratory
Massachusetts Institute of Technology
Cambridge, Massachusetts

Benno J. Rensing, M.D.
Department of Interventional Cardiology
Erasmus University
Rotterdam, Netherlands

Rebecca Richards-Kortum, M.D.
Assistant Professor
Department of Electrical and Computer Engineering
University of Texas at Austin
Austin, Texas

James L. Ritchie, M.D.
Chief, Cardiovascular Disease Section
Veterans Administration Medical Center
University of Washington
Seattle, Washington

Gregory C. Robertson, M.D.
Staff Cardiologist
Sequoia Hospital
Redwood City, California

Arye Rosen, M.D.
Center Professor
Center for Microwave/Lightwave Engineering
Department of Electrical and Computer Engineering
Drexel University
Philadelphia, Pennsylvania

Allan Ross, M.D.
Professor of Medicine
Director, Division of Cardiology
Department of Medicine
The George Washington University
Washington, D.C.

Michael A. Ruder, M.D.
Attending Cardiologist
Sequoia Hospital
Redwood City, California

Carlos E. Ruiz, M.D., Ph.D.
Professor of Medicine and Pediatrics
Director of Cardiac Catheterization Laboratories and
*   Interventional Cardiology*
Loma Linda University
Loma Linda, California

Lowell F. Satler, M.D.
Director, High Risk Angioplasty Program
Washington Cardiology Center
Washington, D.C.

Richard A. Schatz, M.D.
Research Director
Cardiovascular Interventions
Heart Lung and Vascular Center
Scripps Clinic and Research Foundation
La Jolla, California

Gerhard Schreiner, M.D.
Medical Clinic I
Cardiology Department
Fulda General Hospital
Fulda, Germany

Doria Scortichini, M.D.
Fellow in Angioplasty and Hemodynamics
Montreal Heart Institute
Montreal, Canada

Jerome Segal, M.D.
Associate Professor of Medicine
Director, Cardiac Catheterization Laboratory
Department of Medicine
George Washington University
Washington, D.C.

Matthew R. Selmon, M.D.
Staff Cardiologist
Sequoia Hospital
Redwood City, California
Instructor of Cardiology
Stanford University Clinical
Stanford, California

Patrick W. Serruys, M.D., Ph.D.
Professor Interventional Cardiology
Erasmus University
Rotterdam, Netherlands

Ramachandra K. Setty, M.D.
Cardiologist, Marion Hospital
Santa Maria, California

Alexander Shaknovich, M.D.
Assistant Chief
Interventional Cardiology
Lenox Hill Hospital
New York, New York

Fayaz A. Shawl, M.D.
Director, Interventional Cardiology
Washington Adventist Hospital
Takoma Park, Maryland
Clinical Associate Professor of Medicine (Cardiology)
George Washington University School of Medicine
Washington, D.C.

Dennis J. Sheehan, M.D.
Staff Cardiologist
Sequoia Hospital
Assistant Clinical Medical Professor
Department of Internal Medicine (Cardiology)
Stanford University Medical Center
Stanford, California

Arie Shefer, M.D.
Visiting Assistant Professor of Medicine
Department of Cardiology
University of California at Los Angeles
Los Angeles, California

Tetsuro Shirai, M.D.
Cardiovascular Disease Center
Tokyo Metropolitan Police Hospital
Tokyo, Japan

Pamela A. Shotts, R.N., B.S.N.
Director of Research Nurse Services
Washington Cardiology Center
Washington, D.C.

Robert J. Siegel, M.D.
Staff Cardiologist
Cedars-Sinai Medical Center
Associate Professor of Medicine
Department of Medicine
University of California
Los Angeles, California

Ulrich Sigwart, M.D.
Department of Invasive Cardiology
Royal Bromptom National Heart and Lung Hospital
London, England

John B. Simpson, M.D.
Staff Cardiologist
Sequoia Hospital
Clinical Assistant Professor of Medicine
Department of Internal Medicine (Cardiology)
Stanford University School of Medicine
Stanford, California

Jai Pal Singh, M.D.
Lilly Research Lab
Cardiovascular Research
Indianapolis, Indiana

Pia Skarabis, M.D.
Universitatsklinikum Rudolf-Virchow/Wedding
Berlin, Germany

Michael H. Sketch, Jr., M.D.
Associate in Medicine
Interventional Cardiovascular Program
Division of Cardiology
Department of Medicine
Duke University Medical Center
Durham, North Carolina

Richard W. Smalling, M.D., Ph.D.
Associate Professor of Medicine
Chief of Cardiology
Hermann Hospital
The University of Texas Medical School at Houston
Houston, Texas

David L. Smith, M.D.
Department of Medicine
Thomas Jefferson University
Philadelphia, Pennsylvania

Mikel D. Smith, M.D.
Professor of Medicine
Director, Adult Echocardiography Laboratory
Division of Cardiology
University of Kentucky College of Medicine
Lexington, Kentucky

Nellis A. Smith, M.D.
Attending Cardiologist
Sequoia Hospital
Redwood City, California

J. Richard Spears, M.D.
Professor of Medicine
Director, Cardiac Laser Laboratory
Division of Cardiology
Harper Hospital
Wayne State University School of Medicine
Detroit, Michigan

William H. Spencer III, M.D.
Clinical Professor of Medicine
Department of Medicine
Baylor College of Medicine
Houston, Texas

Alexander A. Stratienko, M.D.
Lenox Hill Hospital
New York, New York

Bradley Strauss, M.D., Ph.D.
Assistant Professor
Department of Medicine
University of Toronto
Toronto, Canada

Gerhard Strupp, M.D.
Medical Clinic I
Cardiology Department
Fulda General Hospital
Fulda, Germany

Krishnankutty Sudhir, M.D.
C.J. Martin Fellow
Cardiology Division
Cardiovascular Research Institute
University of California at San Francisco
San Francisco, California

Kazuhiko Sugimoto, M.D.
Cardiovascular Disease Center
Tokyo Metropolitan Police Hospital
Tokyo, Japan

Etsuko Takano, M.T.
Cardiovascular Disease Center
Tokyo Metropolitan Police Hospital
Tokyo, Japan

Paul S. Teirstein, M.D.
Director, Interventional Cardiology
Scripps Clinic and Research Foundation
Division of Cardiovascular Diseases
La Jolla, California

Alan N. Tenaglia, M.D.
Division of Cardiology
Duke University Medical Center
Durham, North Carolina

Bradley Titus, M.D.
Medical Director
Cardiac Catheterization Laboratory
Portland Adventist Medical Center
Portland, Oregon

Christian Vallbracht, M.D.
Clinic Nordrhein
University of Frankfurt
Bad Nauheim, Germany

James W. Vetter, M.D.
Interventional Cardiologist
Sequoia Hospital
Redwood City, California

John H.K. Vogel, M.D.
Cardiovascular Pulmonary Medicine Group
Santa Barbara, California

Robert A. Vogel, M.D.
Herbert Berger Professor of Medicine
Head, Division of Cardiology
University of Maryland Hospital
Baltimore, Maryland

Rudolf Vracko, M.D.
Professor of Pathology
Chief, Laboratory Service
Department of Pathology
University of Wisconsin
Veterans Administration Medical Center
Seattle, Washington

Paul Walinsky, M.D.
Professor of Medicine
Department of Medicine
Thomas Jefferson University
Philadelphia, Pennsylvania

Christopher J. White, M.D.
Director, Cardiac Catheterization Laboratory
Department of Cardiology
Ochsner Medical Institutions
New Orleans, Louisiana

Roger A. Winkle, M.D.
Director, Cardiac Surveillance Unit and Electrophysiology
  Laboratory
Sequoia Hospital
Redwood City, California

Helmut Wollschlager, M.D.
Department of Cardiology
University of Freiburg
Freiburg, Germany

Paul G. Yock, M.D.
Assistant Professor of Medicine
Associate Director
Cardiac Catheterization Laboratory
University of California, San Francisco
San Francisco, California

Andreas Zeiher, M.D.
Department of Cardiology
University of Freiburg
Freiburg, Germany

He Ping Zhang, M.D.
Research Associate
The Heart Institute
Department of Medicine (Cardiology)
Loma Linda University
Loma Linda, California

FOREWORD

Seven years ago, following the tragic death of Andreas Gruentzig, Jack Vogel proposed bringing together many of the developers of new ideas in interventional cardiology to a symposium in Santa Barbara, California. Six such workshops have now been held, giving a forum to new, innovative, and sometimes uninhibited ideas in interventional cardiology. This volume is an outgrowth of those meetings and brings together in a single volume much of the recent progress and promise in the field.

My involvement in the workshops and this book have been largely advisory and editorial. Jack has really done the work of intimidating all of the authors into producing their manuscripts. Little effort has been directed at forcing the authors into a structured editorial position. The views expressed are often those of the developers of the techniques, and as often are those of interested skeptics.

This extensive volume is composed of 60 chapters divided into ten parts covering cardiac interventions. Diagnostic modalities necessary for evaluating coronary structure, lesion composition, and results of interventions leads off. Next, balloon angioplasty is explored, from its practical application, through new methods, to its comparison with bypass surgery. Atherectomy in its many forms from directional to rotary ablative consti-

tutes Part III. Part IV concerns the ups and downs of the use of laser techniques. The role of various stent devices completes the evaluation of new angioplasty techniques. Discussion of mechanical interventions for acute myocardial infarction is followed by the question of cardiac support during high-risk procedures. Part VIII, Restenosis, delves deeply into the component of restenosis that is determined by the biology of vascular healing. The book is completed with a discussion of interventional techniques applicable to congenital and valvular conditions and rhythm disturbances. For the cardiologist desiring an understanding of the breadth as well as the specifics of interventional cardiology, this volume is unparalleled. Jack's idea 7 years ago was a good one. Now we must apply a critical eye to the newly acquired techniques to evaluate which ones will be of service to our patients now and which may lead to the next important breakthrough in cardiology. Dr. Swan's introduction is appropriate in admonishing us not to become so enthralled by new technology itself that we forget the reasons for this technology: to improve the welfare of our patients.

Spencer B. King III, M.D.

PREFACE

The second edition of this book provides not only future and current directions of interventional cardiology, but important long-term observations with these new techniques. Applications have been refined and a broad interaction between the various approaches relating to aggressive interventional therapy is presented, with particular emphasis on a coordinated, individualized approach to a given patient. Specific therapies are discussed, including techniques and results of major cardiologists, both adult and pediatric, from around the world who are involved in the development of balloon valvuloplasty, laser angioplasty, balloon angioplasty, and mechanical devices, both microwave and ultrasound. An extensive experience with stents, both permanent and temporary, is presented. Restenosis and potential therapies for this problem are presented in detail. Direct angioplasty is compared to thrombolytic regimens for the treatment of acute myocardial infarction. New guidelines for surgical standby during PTCA are suggested.

New management approaches to rhythm disorders, including pacemaker therapy, implantable defibrillators, and ablation therapy, are presented in detail.

Major advances in myocardial support and protection utilizing active and passive perfusion, balloon pumping, and cardiopulmonary support are compared.

Methodology for the interpretation and evaluation of structural pathology, hemodynamics, and metabolic function is reviewed with particular attention to the role of observational studies utilizing angioscopy, and intravascular ultrasound as well as transthoracic ultrasound.

A major emphasis is placed on technique, with extensive illustrations.

The editors emphasize that no randomized studies of new techniques vs. plain old balloon angioplasty have been completed, that the future of some is uncertain, and no endorsement of a specific technique is intended.

I would like to offer my appreciation to my friend and co-editor, Spencer B. King III, M.D. I am deeply grateful for the continued help and understanding of my loving wife, Cynthia Marie, and my daughter, Kristen Marie Richmond, for their understanding of the time necessary to make this book a reality, as it was pursued during my continued active private practice of medicine and, to Mark O'Brien, M.D., whose surgical skills with the heart have given me a new life.

JOHN H.K. VOGEL, M.D.

INTRODUCTION

In my foreword to the first edition of *The Practice of Interventional Cardiology*, I addressed what was a prime issue at that time: post angioplasty restenosis. In spite of many innovative interventions, restenosis still remains the Achilles' heel of angioplasty. This second edition now includes extensive consideration of the fundamental biology of restenosis. Current understanding of the roles of injury, thrombosis, and growth factors for smooth muscle and collagen and their modification are discussed. However, as yet, no specific techniques have altered the excessive incidence of restenosis.

In the earlier forword I commented on the absence of controlled trials to provide objective demonstrations of the efficacy of balloon angioplasty (PTCA) in the relief of cardiac ischemia due to coronary atherosclerosis. At present, careful comparisons of PTCA to the results of coronary artery bypass grafting (CABG) in patients with multivessel disease are nearing completion. The strong clinical impression of benefit in symptomatic patients with one- or two-vessel disease appears well founded, although the timing or urgency of the intervention may be questioned. In the intervening years, only one small trial (ACME) has been published.[1] All of the patients in this trial had single-vessel coronary artery disease and significant symptoms, that is, angina pectoris, exercise-induced myocardial ischemia, or recent myocardial infarction. The authors concluded that angioplasty was "superior" to medical therapy in relieving angina and improving exercise performance. This benefit however, came at a considerable cost: a quarter of the angioplasty patients required major additional procedures within the observation period. Among the patients randomized to medical treatment, a small proportion "crossed over" to PTCA because of symptom worsening. The "natural history" of these medically treated patients is strikingly similar to those in the CASS trial, in which an increasing number of patients did require CABG with time, but a greater proportion did not receive operative intervention over the 5- to 7-year follow-up. It is equally reasonable to interpret the ACME data to indicate that of patients with angiographically significantly single-vessel coronary artery disease and a moderate symptom state, somewhat under 20% will require angioplasty within one year of initial presentation.

While testing of the efficacy of PTCA is admittedly incomplete, the assessment of new and costly mechanical devices is sadly deficient. There is no evidence to date that the incidence or severity of restenosis is less; indeed, it may be even greater with some devices. This raises a particularly thorny issue. The medical practitioners and engineers who collaborate as developers of such devices may have not only an ego stake in success, but also a major financial position that can seriously blunt objectivity. The resulting "conflict of interest" of the new physician/scientist/business entrepreneur cannot be ignored. The climate for unlimited growth in costly, unproven procedures is clearly unfavorable. Practitioners have to separate enthusiasm from concealment, truth from hyperbole, and science from marketing.

The Annual Symposium on Invasive Cardiology in the 1990s[2] considered clinical trials, new devices, and proliferation of data. It was concluded that balloon angioplasty per se still remained the standard of practice and that newer technology might find "niche" application. Serious difficulties were predicted for the implementation of truly randomized trials for evaluation of the multitude of new techniques and technologies. Without question, the current enthusiasm for angioplasty (sometimes described as the "occulodilatory response") and the large number of younger cardiologists with training in this procedure has resulted in inappropriate angioplasty in many patients. The dictum of the ACC/AHA Committee on Coronary Angioplasty that "not every cardiologist wishing to perform angioplasty . . . should"[3] has been completely ignored. Of the greatest concern is angioplasty in patients with no or minimal symptoms or lack of clear objective evidence of important myocardial ischemia. The "market" for such procedures is attractive to hospital administrators, as well as to cardiologists. Restenosis in these patients is a tragedy and is a striking departure from the high calling of our profession. Hence, it seems mandatory that the community of cardiologists who practice invasive procedures collectively support appropriate trials and comparative studies. The development of multicenter collaborative data-sharing programs and of extensive data bases for clinical use offers the possibility of an objecive solution to the dilemma of demonstration of efficacy. Carefully and accurately collected information relevant to the specific issues, centrally managed by an effective staff, offers the best possibility to answer and issues of safety, efficiency, and efficacy. The value of unusual interventions or novel approaches could be assessed in a relatively short time by pooling relevant objective data for comparison with untreated matched controls, or in patients matched to receive an alternate or competing treatment. Criteria for outcome analysis have not yet been established, but will be developed progressively during the coming decade and may determine economic reward. This issue remains and must be a high priority of all individuals concerned with the practice of interventional cardiology.

H.J.C. SWAN, M.D., PH.D.
Professor of Medicine
UCLA School of Medicine
Los Angeles, California

REFERENCES

1. Parisi AF, Folland ED, Hartigan P: For the Veterans Affairs ACME Investigators: A comparison of angioplasty with medical therapy in the treatment of single vessel coronary artery disease. *N Engl J Med* 1992; 326:10.
2. Shaw RE: Clinical Trials, New Devices and the Proliferation of Data. Where we are and Where we are going, the First Annual Symposium on Invasive Cardiology in the 1990s. *J Invasive Cardiol* 1992; 4:1–130.
3. Ryan TJ, Faxon DF, Gunnar RP: ACC/AHA Task Force: Guidelines for percutaneous coronary angioplasty. *J Am Coll Cardiol* 1988; 12:529–545.

CONTENTS

Foreword   xv
Preface   xvii
Introduction   xix
Color Plates   Chapter 5

PART I: APPLICATIONS OF DIAGNOSTIC MODALITIES IN INTERVENTIONAL CARDIOLOGY   1

1 / Use of Nuclear Cardiology Techniques for Assessment of Myocardial Viability   3
George A. Beller

2 / Transcatheter Assessment of Coronary Blood Flow and Velocity   19
Robert A. Vogel

3 / The Doppler Guidewire: A New Method to Evaluate Coronary Artery Flow During Percutaneous Transluminal Coronary Angioplasty   27
Jerome Segal and Allan Ross

4 / Clinical Experience With a New Angioscopic System   33
Giancarlo Biamino and J.C. Ragg

5 / Technical Feasibility and Clinical Benefits of Percutaneous Coronary Angioscopy: Valuable Lessons on In Vivo Coronary Atherosclerosis Based on 50 Consecutive Observations in Patient With Acute Coronary Syndrome   41
Kiyoshi Inoue, Keiichi Kuwaki, Tetsuro Shirai, Hidenobu Ochial, Yoshio Mukaiyama, Kazuhiko Sugimoto, Etsuko Takano, and Hisatoshi Minato

6 / Intravascular Ultrasound Imaging: Clinical Applications and Technical Advances   53
Paul G. Yock, Peter J. Fitzgerald, and Krishnankutty Sudhir

7 / Application of Echocardiography to Catheter Balloon Valvuloplasty   67
Martin R. Berk, Anthony N. Demaria, and Mikel D. Smith

PART II: BALLOON ANGIOPLASTY   77

8 / Balloon Angioplasty: Matching Technology to Lesions   79
John S. Douglas, Jr.

9 / Role of the Long-Wire Technique in Percutaneous Transluminal Coronary Angioplasty: The Frankfurt Experience   89
Gisbert Kober, Christian Vallbracht, and Martin Kaltenbach

10 / Magnum System for Coronary Angioplasty   101
Bernhard Meier

11 / Seven Years' Development and Application of the Sliding Rail System (Monorail) for PTCA   113
Tassilo Bonzel, Helmut Wollschlager, Andreas Zeiher, Hanjorg Just, Gerhard Strupp, and Gerhard Schreiner

12 / Comparison of Angioplasty and Coronary Bypass Surgery: The Emory Angioplasty vs. Surgery Trial   133
Spencer B. King, III

PART III: ATHERECTOMY   139

13 / Percutaneous Transluminal Coronary Rotary Ablation With the Rotablator   141
Michel E. Bertrand, Jean M. Lablanche, Fabrice Leroy, Christophe Bauters, Eugene McFadden

14 / Coronary Atherectomy With the TEC Device   149
Michael H. Sketch, Jr. and Harry R. Philips

15 / Directional Coronary Atherectomy   157
Matthew R. Selmon, Tomoaki Hinohara, Gregory C. Robertson, James W. Vetter, Dennis J. Sheehan, Bruce J. McAuley, John B. Simpson

16 / Percutaneous Rotational Thrombectomy: An Alternative Approach to Thrombolysis   171
Timothy A. Dewhurst, Paul Hirst, Thomas J. Clement, Rudolph Vracko, Bradley Titus, and James L. Ritchie

PART IV: LASER AND RELATED PROCEDURES   *177*

17 / Laser Angiosurgery: A Biomedical System Using Photons to Diagnose and Treat Atherosclerosis   *179*

John R. Kramer, Michael S. Feld, Floyd D. Loop, Robert M. Cothren, Gary B. Hayes, Rebecca Richards-Kortum, Bruce W. Lytle, Carter Kittrell, Corrine Bott-Silverman

18 / LAS II: An Integrated System for Spectral Diagnosis, Guidance, and Ablation in Laser Angiosurgery   *189*

Michael S. Feld, John R. Kramer, Douglas Albagli, Rim Cothren, Jr., Ramachandra R. Dasari, Gary B. Hayes, Joseph A. Izatt, Irving Itzkan, G. Sargent Janes, Richard P. Rava

19 / Pulsed Laser Ablation of Atherosclerotic Plaque in Blood Vessels   *203*

Alexander A. Oraevsky and Vladilen S. Letokhov

20 / Infrared Laser Angioplasty: Clinical Experience With the Holmium: YAG Laser   *215*

Christopher J. White and Stephen R. Ramee

21 / Excimer Laser Coronary Angioplasty   *223*

Arie Shefer and Frank Litvack

22 / Excimer Laser Coronary Angioplasty: Wire-Guided Techniques and Results From a Multicenter Trial   *233*

John A. Bittl

23 / Experience in Peripheral Laser Angioplasty   *243*

Giancarlo Biamino and Pia Skarabis

24 / Direct Argon Laser Angioplasty for the Treatment of Peripheral and Coronary Vascular Lesions: A Progress Report   *255*

Leonard A. Nordstrom

25 / Laser Balloon Angioplasty: Therapeutic Mechanisms and Clinical Correlations   *263*

Ronald D. Jenkins and J. Richard Spears

26 / Laser Thrombolysis   *273*

Kenton W. Gregory

27 / Microwave Balloon Angioplasty   *281*

Paul Walinsky, Arye Rosen, Antonio Martinez-Hernandez, David L. Smith, Donald T. Nardone, Barry Bravette

28 / Ultrasound Angioplasty   *287*

Robert J. Siegel, John R. Crew, Russell Pfleuger, Anthony Don Michael, Marilyn Dean, Richard K. Myler, David C. Cumberland

PART V: STENTS   *299*

29 / Stents for Bailout and Restenosis   *301*

Spencer B. King III

30 / Nonsurgical Implantation of a Self-Expanding Intravascular Stent Prosthesis   *307*

George I. Frank and Ulrich Sigwart

31 / The Palmaz-Schatz Coronary Stent   *319*

Alexander Shaknovich, Alexander A. Stratienko, Paul S. Teirstein, and Richard A. Schatz

32 / The Wallstent Experience: 1986–1990   *333*

Patrick W. Serruys and Bradley Strauss

33 / Temporary Coronary Stenting: Preliminary Experience With a Heat-Activated Recoverable Temporary Stent   *349*

Neal L. Eigler and Mehran J. Khorsandi

PART VI: INTERVENTIONAL PROCEDURES FOR ACUTE MYOCARDIAL INFARCTION   *357*

34 / Angioplasty Therapy for Acute Myocardial Infarction: Current Status and Future Directions   *359*

William W. O'Neill

35 / The Role of Angioplasty in the Treatment of Acute Myocardial Infarction   *367*

Allan M. Ross

36 / Thrombolytic Therapy for Acute Myocardial Infarction: Implications of the Randomized Trials   *375*

Cindy L. Grines

37 / Thrombolysis in Acute Myocardial Infarction in the Community Hospital   *387*

John H.K. Vogel, Barry J. Coughlin, Ramachandra K. Setty, Rosa M. Avolio, R. Bruce McFadden

PART VII: CIRCULATORY SUPPORT DURING BALLOON ANGIOPLASTY   *413*

38 / Guidelines for Surgical Standby in Patients Undergoing Percutaneous Transluminal Coronary Angioplasty   *415*

John H.K. Vogel

39 / Use of Prophylactic and Standby Circulatory Support During High-Risk Coronary Angioplasty   *425*

Robert A. Vogel

40 / Percutaneous Cardiopulmonary Bypass Support: Current Technique and Future Directions   *435*

Fayaz A. Shawl

41 / Myocardial Protection During Coronary Angioplasty   *457*

Paolo Angelini, D. Richard Leachman, Germano DiSciascio, Michael J. Cowley, Jeffrey A. Brinker

42 / Autoperfusion Balloon Angioplasty *471*
Alan N. Tenaglia, Christopher E. Buller, and Harry R. Phillips

43 / Left Ventricular Assist Devices Available to the Cardiologist: Indications, Techniques, and Early and Later Results *479*
Richard W. Smalling

PART VIII: MECHANISMS OF RESTENOSIS *493*

44 / A Paradigm for Restenosis Based on Cell Biology: Clues for the Development of New Preventive Therapies *495*
James S. Forrester, Michael Fishbein, Richard Helfant, and James Fagin

45 / Arterial Angioplasty: Injury, Mural Thrombus, and Restenosis *509*
James H. Chesebro, Juan J. Badimon, Lina Badimon, and Valentin Fuster

46 / Platelet-Derived Growth Factor: Future Directions in the Prevention of Restenosis *521*
W. Michael Kavanaugh

47 / Cell Biology of Restenosis: Role of Angiotensin II in Neointimal Cell Proliferation *527*
Bradford C. Berk

48 / Inhibitors of Vascular Smooth Muscle Cell Proliferation as Therapy for Restenosis Following Percutaneous Transluminal Coronary Angioplasty: Current Agents and Approaches *535*
Jai Pal Singh and Keith L. March

49 / Pharmacologic Therapy in the Prevention of Restenosis After Percutaneous Transluminal Coronary Angioplasty *547*
Walter R.M. Hermans, Benno J. Rensing, Pim de Feyter, and Patrick W. Serruys

PART IX: PROCEDURES FOR VALVULAR AND CONGENITAL DEFECTS *573*

50 / Percutaneous Balloon Aortic Valvuloplasty: Update of Techniques, Results, and Indications in the Rouen Experience *575*
Alain Cribier, Lowell Gerber, and Brice Letac

51 / Percutaneous Balloon Mitral Valvotomy *583*
Peter C. Block

52 / Percutaneous Double-Balloon Valvotomy for Patients With Severe Mitral Stenosis: Five Years' Follow-up Experience *589*
Carlos E. Ruiz, He Ping Zhang, Habib Gamra, John W. Allen, and Francis Y.K. Lau

53 / Long-Term Follow-up of Balloon Mitral Valvotomy: The Montreal Heart Institute Experience *609*
Doria Scortichini, Pascal Barraud, and Raoul Bonan

54 / Interventional Catheterization in the Treatment of Congenital Lesions *625*
Michael R. Nihill and Charles E. Mullins

PART X: PACING AND ABLATION *649*

55 / Optimal Pacing Therapy: Hemodynamics, Modes, and Devices *651*
William H. Spencer III

56 / Recent Advances in Implantable Defibrillator Therapy *665*
Roger A. Winkle

57 / Transvenous Catheter Ablation of Cardiac Arrhythmias *671*
Michael A. Ruder, Roger A. Winkle, Nellis A. Smith, and R. Hardwin Mead

58 / Percutaneous Balloon Pericardial Window *687*
Peter C. Block and Igor F. Palacios

59 / Overview of New Technologies: The Bottom Line *691*
Robert Ginsburg

60 / A Multidevice, Lesion-Specific Treatment Strategy for Unfavorable Coronary Lesions *695*
Martin B. Leon, Augusto D. Pichard, Kenneth M. Kent, Lowell F. Satler, Jeffrey J. Popma, Pamela A. Shotts, and Kathleen M. Donovan

Index *705*

PART I

Applications of Diagnostic Modalities in Interventional Cardiology

Use of Nuclear Cardiology Techniques for Assessment of Myocardial Viability

George A. Beller, M.D.

The noninvasive determination of myocardial viability is becoming increasingly more important for clinical decision making in identifying which patients with coronary artery disease (CAD) and left ventricular dysfunction will most benefit from revascularization. In recent years, there has been a greater appreciation among clinicians for recognizing the phenomena of "stunned" or "hibernating" myocardium.[1, 2] Both of these pathophysiologic states may result in profound regional left ventricular dysfunction in the absence of necrosis. Thus, mere assessment of regional systolic function by either echocardiography, radionuclide angiography, or contrast ventriculography is insufficient to distinguish between irreversibly injured and viable but dysfunctional myocardium. The purpose of this review is to summarize both experimental and clinical data suggesting that radionuclide imaging of perfusion and metabolism can provide clinically relevant information pertaining to the status of myocardial viability in the presence of regional and global myocardial systolic dysfunction. This ability to differentiate between acute necrosis and scarring in viable but asynergic myocardium can assist the clinician in identifying those patients with CAD who might benefit most from coronary bypass surgery or coronary angioplasty. Evidence from noninvasive techniques of preserved myocardial viability is summarized in Table 1–1.

STUNNED MYOCARDIUM

Evidence has accumulated that demonstrates that under various experimental conditions and in certain clinical syndromes, postischemic myocardial dysfunction (stunning) can be observed. This myocardial dysfunction may be prolonged despite restoration of blood flow

following brief periods of coronary occlusion. The precise pathophysiology of the stunning phenomenon is not entirely understood. Some mechanisms proposed have included impairment of myocardial energy production,[3] disruption or inefficient transfer of energy into myocyte contraction,[4, 5] impairment of sympathetic nerve activity due to ischemic damage,[6] altered calcium sensitivity at the myofilament level,[7] calcium overload, microvascular capillary obstruction by neutrophils, ischemic damage to the extracellular collagen matrix,[8] and detrimental effects of oxygen-free radicals liberated during reperfusion that cause membrane lipid peroxidation.[9, 10]

Clinically, myocardial stunning probably occurs after reperfusion in acute myocardial infarction since regional and global left ventricular function demonstrate delayed improvement during days or weeks after restoration of blood flow.[11, 12] Stunning might also be manifested in some patients with unstable angina who experience repeated episodes of coronary flow diminution caused by coronary vasospasm or cyclical obstruction by intraluminal thrombi.

Anderson and coworkers serially assessed regional wall motion by two-dimensional echocardiography in patients who were treated with intracoronary streptokinase for acute myocardial infarction.[13] Gradual improvement in regional wall motion as compared with prethrombolysis assessment was seen between 1 and 10 days after thrombolytic therapy. Similarly, Stack et al., employing serial left ventricular angiography in patients undergoing thrombolytic therapy, found that the percent radial shortening of segments in the infarct zone showed no significant change on day 1 but significant improvement 2 weeks following reperfusion.[11] Touchstone et al. from the University of Virginia evaluated re-

TABLE 1–1

Noninvasive Evidence of Preserved Myocardial Viability

Symptomatic angina in the setting of severe left ventricular asynergy

Akinetic wall motion on radionuclide angiography or echocardiography with a lack of corresponding electrocardiographic (ECG) Q waves

Extensive asynergy in the distribution of infarct-related vessels in association with only small rise in creatine kinase concentration

Preserved systolic thickening on echocardiography

Preserved ^{201}Tl uptake either on redistribution imaging or after reinjection at rest

Preserved uptake of ^{99m}Tc sestamibi after reperfusion for acute myocardial infarction or in chronic CAD

Preserved ^{18}F-2-deoxyglucose uptake on positron emission tomography (PET) imaging in zones of myocardial asynergy

Small area of necrosis on antimyosin antibody imaging but large perfusion defect on ^{201}Tl images after myocardial infarction

Preservation of myocardial systolic thickening on gated magnetic resonance imaging (MRI).

---

gional systolic function by two-dimensional echocardiography in a group of myocardial infarction patients receiving intravenous streptokinase.[12] All patients were treated within 4 hours of the onset of symptoms. Improvement in wall motion was observed in approximately half of the patients, but this functional recovery was not evident on days 1 to 3. By day 10, improvement was noted in patients with a patent vessel, with continued enhancement of systolic function by 6 weeks after discharge.

Thus, studies conducted in patients with acute myocardial infarction treated early with thrombolytic therapy show that soon after flow restoration, myocardial systolic function in the infarct zone remains depressed. Such patients may manifest hemodynamic instability or even cardiogenic shock in the early postreperfusion period as a consequence of postischemic cardiac dysfunction. It may be important to determine at that time whether the dysfunction in the infarct zone indeed represents "stunning" or is a manifestation of irreversible cellular injury. Urgent revascularization with the former state would most likely be beneficial, whereas with the latter situation of extensive necrosis, revascularization may not prove beneficial. If one had an accurate and cost-effective noninvasive approach to distinguish stunned from necrotic myocardium in postthrombolytic patients with hemodynamic compromise, selection of patients for revascularization could be made on a more rational basis.

HIBERNATING MYOCARDIUM

Hibernating myocardium is a term describing a state of persistently impaired left ventricular dysfunction in the resting basal state that is attributed to a chronic reduction in coronary blood flow.[2] It represents a state of reduced blood flow where neither ischemic pain nor myocardial necrosis are exhibited but myocardial function is substantially "downregulated." Hibernating myocardium implies that if regional flow is enhanced, then function will improve. Patients with chronic ischemic dysfunction may present with clinical symptoms and signs of ischemic cardiomyopathy with a depressed left ventricular ejection fraction and multiple regional wall motion abnormalities that correspond to severe and extensive multivessel underlying CAD.[14] As with the "stunned" myocardial state, the demonstration of viability in "hibernating" myocardial segments by noninvasive means in such patients would suggest that coronary revascularization would be of benefit for enhancing cardiac performance. Additionally, revascularization in patients whose myocardial dysfunction is due to chronic underperfusion rather than extensive scarring should experience enhancement of exercise tolerance with improvement in functional class following revascularization. Thus, as with patients who exhibit the stunned myocardium phenomena, radionuclide imaging might be useful if myocardial viability could be accurately determined in patients with left ventricular dysfunction secondary to hibernation.

MYOCARDIAL THALLIUM 201 IMAGING FOR DETECTION OF VIABLE MYOCARDIUM

Experimental Validation

After intravenous injection, the early myocardial uptake of thallium 201 (^{201}Tl) is proportional to regional blood flow and extraction by the myocardium.[15–18] The extraction fraction, which is defined as the percentage of the dose of ^{201}Tl extracted by the myocardium in the first pass through the heart after intracoronary injection, is in the range of 85%.[16] As with all other diffusible radionuclide agents, the extraction of ^{201}Tl diminishes at high myocardial blood flow. There is a slight diminution in the cellular extraction of ^{201}Tl with acidosis and hypoxemia.[16] In a recent study, the extraction and permeability × surface area (PS) product for ^{201}Tl was not affected by cellular hypoxia severe enough to cause cardiac hemodynamic dysfunction.[19] In another study by Leppo and colleagues, myocardial uptake of ^{201}Tl during a constant infusion into an isolated rabbit heart was unaffected by hypoxia when coronary flow was held constant.[20] Our group reported that the uptake and subsequent intracellular washout of ^{201}Tl was unaltered in stunned myocardium characterized by severe postischemic dysfunction following repetitive brief periods of flow reduction in an anesthetized canine model.[21] To produce myocardial stunning, open-chested dogs with a critical left anterior descending (LAD) coronary artery stenosis underwent ten 5-minute periods of total LAD occlusion, each interspersed with 10 minutes of reperfusion by reflow through the critical stenosis. This myocardial stunning protocol resulted in a reduction of systolic thickening in the LAD zone to 0.4% ± 2.4% as compared with 32% ± 2% thickening in control dogs. Despite this virtual akinesis in the LAD zone, the first-pass extraction fraction of ^{201}Tl was 0.78, a value identical to that measured in control animals (Fig 1–1). The half-life for the intracellular ^{201}Tl washout was also not significantly different in stunned (60 ± 13 minutes) vs. control (53 ± 14 minutes) dogs. In another study from our group by Sinusas et al., ^{201}Tl uptake was not affected by postischemic dysfunction produced by stunning the myocardium with 15 minutes of total LAD occlusion followed by reperfusion.[22] Thus, these experimental data from our laboratory are consistent with normal myocardial ^{201}Tl extraction and washout kinetics in canine models of severe postischemic stunning.

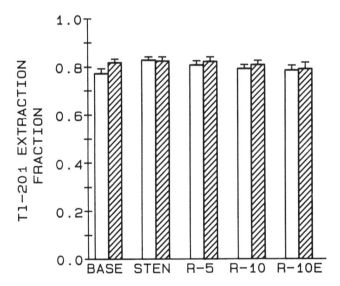

FIG 1–1.
First-pass myocardial ^{201}Tl extraction fraction in control *(open bars)* and stunned *(crosshatched bars)* dogs. Myocardial stunning was accomplished by repetitive 5-minute LAD occlusions, each interspersed by 10 minutes of reflow. Control dogs had a sustained LAD stenosis throughout. Measurements are made at baseline *(BASE),* after creation of a critical LAD stenosis *(STEN),* and following the fifth and tenth reflow *(R-5* and *R-10)* in the stunned group. The bars on the extreme right indicate measurements made 40 minutes after the tenth reflow *(R-10E).* (From Moore CA, Cannon J, Watson DD, et al: *Circulation* 1990; 81:1622–1632. Used by permission.)

[201]Tl uptake was also examined in a canine model of "hibernating myocardium."[22] In this study, myocardial ^{201}Tl uptake was not impaired out of proportion to the flow diminution in anesthetized dogs with a sustained reduction in regional blood flow resulting in systolic dysfunction. This experimental model was designed to mimic a "chronic ischemic" state that is the presumed pathogenesis of hibernating myocardium. Resting flow was reduced by approximately 40% in these experiments.

Irreversibly damaged myocardial tissue cannot concentrate ^{201}Tl intracellularly. Goldhaber et al., in a cultured fetal mouse heart preparation, found that accumulation of ^{201}Tl in hearts subjected to ischemia-like myocardial injury was related in a decreasing fashion to the loss of lactic dehydrogenase.[23] In a study performed in intact animals, necrotic myocardium did not concentrate ^{201}Tl intracellularly when administered after reperfusion preceded by a prolonged period of prior sustained coronary occlusion.[24]

Taken together, this experimental work suggests that the intracellular extraction of ^{201}Tl via transport across the sarcolemmal membrane is not altered unless irreversible membrane injury is present. Chronic underperfusion alone and postischemic dysfunction after brief periods of coronary occlusion do not inhibit thallium extraction as long as some blood flow is preserved to ensure adequate delivery of the radionuclide to the myocardial cell.

Following the initial myocardial uptake phase after intravenous injection, there is a continuous exchange of myocardial ^{201}Tl and ^{201}Tl in the blood pool.[25] [201]Tl is continually washing out of normally perfused myocardium and replaced by recirculating ^{201}Tl from the residual activity in the vascular compartment. This process of continuous exchange forms the basis of [201]Tl "redistribution." Redistribution or delayed defect resolution is observed when ^{201}Tl is administered during transient underperfusion of the myocardium[5, 25] or with a chronic reduction in myocardial blood flow ("rest redistribution").[26] With respect to myocardial ^{201}Tl scintigraphy, redistribution refers to the total or partial resolution of initial defects when assessed by repeat imaging at 2½ to 4 hours after ^{201}Tl administration.[5] The degree of resolution of an ischemic defect over time reflects the amount of redistribution. For example, when ^{201}Tl is injected during peak exercise or with peak vasodilation after intravenous dipyridamole or adenosine administration, the disparity of flow will be marked if one compares ^{201}Tl uptake between normal myocardium and myocardium that was relatively underperfused. With cessation of exercise stress or reversal of dipyridamole-induced vasodilation, there is restoration of relatively homogeneous flow to normal myocardium and to regions perfused by stenotic vessels. Delayed ^{201}Tl redistribution occurs under these conditions as ^{201}Tl washes out of the normal region and exhibits late accumulation or flat washout in the ischemic segment perfused by the stenotic artery. However, this redistribution can only occur if myocardium perfused by the stenotic artery is viable. Figure 1–2 shows the "filling in" of a septal defect on delayed ^{201}Tl imaging that is characteristic of the redistribution phenomenon in a patient who underwent exercise scintigraphy.

Experimental studies have shown that when myocardial necrosis is present, no delayed ^{201}Tl redistribution is seen in the zone of irreversibly injured myocardial tissue.[27] Partial redistribution is seen when there is a mixture of necrosis and ischemic myocardium in the presence of preserved antegrade flow or physiologically relevant collateral flow.

^{201}Tl redistribution over time when the tracer is injected in the resting state can be observed in patients with unstable angina or severe stable angina because of a preserved reduction in regional flow consequent to severe CAD.[28, 29] Patients with such "resting" ischemia and no myocardial scarring often demonstrate initial defects at rest that show subsequent delayed redistribution when repeat rest images are obtained 3 to 4 hours after tracer administration. The mechanism for this "rest redistribution" during chronic ischemia is both a diminution in the initial uptake of ^{201}Tl and a subsequent decrease in the intrinsic efflux rate of the tracer.[25] There is

a substantially slower washout of ^{201}Tl over time from the stenosis region as compared with thallium washout from nonischemic regions. These disparate washout rates from hypoperfused and normal myocardium result in ultimate normalization of ^{201}Tl activity between nonischemic and stenotic regions by 4 hours.

When ^{201}Tl is administered intravenously under conditions of a myocardial scar or acute necrosis, a "persistent" defect in the supply region of the irreversibly damaged area is observed. That is, in the presence of infarction or scarring, a defect is noted both soon after ^{201}Tl administration and several hours later when repeat imaging is performed. In this situation, no delayed redistribution can be detected. Figure 1–3 shows an example of a patient demonstrating a persistent decrease in ^{201}Tl uptake on the delayed images.

As will subsequently be discussed in greater detail, some persistent ^{201}Tl defects in which no redistribution is visually observed on images obtained 4 hours after tracer injection show improved ^{201}Tl uptake following revascularization.[30] Thus, in the clinical setting not all persistent defects represent myocardial scarring or acute myocardial damage.

Exercise Thallium Scintigraphy and Myocardial Viability

Currently, myocardial ^{201}Tl scintigraphy is most often performed in conjunction with exercise stress in pa-

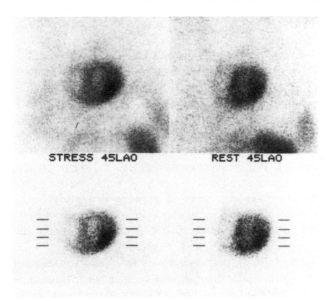

FIG 1–2.
An example of an initial postexercise ^{201}Tl defect in the intraventricular septum that demonstrates delayed redistribution (relative "filling in"). This indicates an ischemic response to stress.

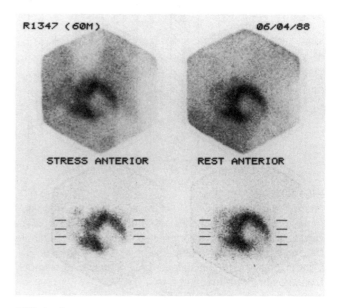

FIG 1–3.
Example of a patient demonstrating a persistent apical ^{201}Tl defect when initial and delayed postexercise images are compared. This finding suggests diminished or a lack of viable myocardium in the risk area of the LAD coronary artery.

tients with suspected or known CAD. The sensitivity and specificity for detection of physiologically significant stenosis employing quantitative planar or single-photon emission computed tomography (SPECT) ^{201}Tl scintigraphy are in the range of 85% to 90%.[31] Perfusion defects observed on the initial postexercise images can be indicative of either transient exercise-induced ischemia or scarring. To differentiate between the two, delayed images are obtained to assess whether redistribution is evident or not. As described in the previous section, an initial defect showing delayed redistribution implies ischemia and viability, whereas defects that remain persistent from the initial to the delayed images are suggestive of scars. Detection of redistribution is enhanced by utilizing quantitative image analysis where regional thallium uptake and washout are quantitated after appropriate background subtraction.[32-35] Partial redistribution may reflect the presence of a mixture of scarring and viable myocardium.[30]

Some persistent ^{201}Tl defects may represent significant ischemia rather than scars. These persistent defects most often are mild and exhibit no more than a 25% to 50% reduction in ^{201}Tl activity relative to activity in the normally perfused zone.[30-36] In contrast, few severe persistent defects demonstrating more than 50% reduction in ^{201}Tl counts as compared with a nonischemic region on initial images will show improvement in thallium uptake after revascularization.[30] Such severe persistent defects are usually associated with evidence of transmural myocardial infarction (Q wave) on the ECG.

Late redistribution imaging at 18 to 24 hours[37-39] or reinjection of ^{201}Tl in the resting state following acquisition of 3- to 4-hour redistribution images[36,40] has been undertaken to distinguish those persistent defects that represent viable but ischemic myocardium from those that represent scars. Cloninger et al. obtained 8- to 24-hour delayed images in 40 patients who demonstrated "incomplete" redistribution at 4 hours with exercise SPECT scintigraphy.[37] The late imaging studies showed further redistribution in approximately 45% of patients with prior infarction and 92% of patients without prior infarction. Kiat et al. reported that the presence or absence of late redistribution at 18 to 24 hours predicted the post–coronary bypass or postangioplasty effect on enhancing regional blood flow.[38] Ninety-five percent of segments showing late redistribution improved after revascularization, whereas only 37% of the segments that remained persistent at 18 to 24 hours showed improvement after intervention. Yang et al. prospectively assessed the frequency of late redistribution in 118 patients who underwent SPECT exercise ^{201}Tl scintigraphy.[39] Fifty-three percent of patients in this study were found to have late redistribution in one or more segments that appeared as persistent defects on the 4-hour images (Fig 1–4). Thirty-five percent of patients had late redistribution in two or more segments that appeared persistent on redistribution imaging. A total of 22% of 762 segments in these 118 patients showed late reversibility (Fig 1–4). These authors concluded that late redistribution imaging should be considered when 4-hour persistent defects are present. A potential limitation of 24-hour imaging in detecting late redistribution is the suboptimum count statistics. If one is undertaking this approach to differentiate between ischemia and scarring, an initial dose of 3 to 4 mCi of ^{201}Tl should be administered at peak exercise stress, and

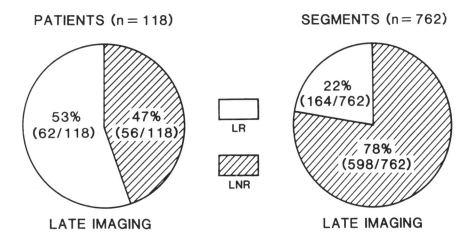

FIG 1–4.
Frequency of late reversibility *(LR)* and late nonreversibility *(LNR)* in patients undergoing 18- to 24-hour ^{201}Tl imaging after exercise stress. Findings related to the number of patients are shown on the *left,* and findings relative to the number of segments are shown on the *right.* Note that 53% of the patients studied had evidence of late redistribution on 18- to 24-hour images, whereas early images at 4 hours showed only persistent defects. (From Yang LD, Berman DS, Kiat H, et al: *J Am Coll Cardiol* 1990; 15:334–340. Used by permission.)

at least a 50% longer imaging time should be employed to enhance the quality of the 24-hour images. In our experience utilizing quantitative ^{201}Tl scintigraphy, few defects show redistribution only on the 24-hour images. Most defects exhibiting late redistribution at 24 hours have evidence of some redistribution on the 4-hour images as assessed by quantitative analysis.

An alternative to 24-hour delayed redistribution imaging for detection of viable myocardium is reinjection of ^{201}Tl at rest following the acquisition of the 2½- to 4-hour redistribution images (Fig 1–5). Dilsizian et al. studied 100 patients with CAD by using SPECT ^{201}Tl scintigraphy.[40] The protocol employed was that patients received 2 mCi of ^{201}Tl intravenously during exercise, with acquisition of immediate postexercise and 3- to 4-hour delayed images. Then, after obtaining the redistribution images, a second dose of 1 mCi of ^{201}Tl was injected at rest. Thirty-three percent of the abnormal segments in these patients showed persistent defects on the 3- to 4-hour redistribution images. Approximately half of these persistent ^{201}Tl defects demonstrated improved or normal ^{201}Tl uptake after reinjection of the second ^{201}Tl dose. The data from this study are summarized in Figure 1–6. Eighty-seven percent of regions that showed enhanced ^{201}Tl uptake on reinjection studies showed normal ^{201}Tl uptake and improved regional wall motion after coronary angioplasty. In contrast, among patients undergoing angioplasty with persistent defects identified on reinjection ^{201}Tl imaging, all had abnormal ^{201}Tl uptake and abnormal regional wall motion after dilatation. These authors concluded that reinjection of ^{201}Tl at rest after acquisition of redistribution images significantly enhances the detection of viable myocardium.

Tamaki et al. reported a series of 60 patients with CAD who showed improved thallium uptake following ^{201}Tl reinjection in 32% of segments with fixed defects on SPECT redistribution images.[41] In this study, 29% of patients with persistent defects and who had no evidence of redistribution in any segment on 3- to 4-hour delayed images showed enhanced ^{201}Tl uptake after reinjection. Thus, in this subgroup the ^{201}Tl reinjection protocol was the only manner in which myocardial viability was demonstrated.

In another study by Bonow and coworkers,[36] [201]Tl scintigraphy with reinjection was compared with PET imaging with ^{18}F-2-deoxyglucose (FDG). In this study, 38% of 432 myocardial segments in 16 patients with chronic CAD demonstrated persistent ^{201}Tl defects on redistribution images before reinjection. FDG uptake suggesting preserved metabolic integrity was present in 51% of segments showing marked persistent defects. In these defects, an identical number of segments (51%)

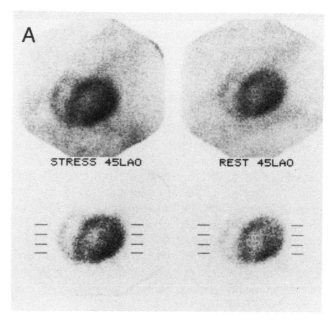

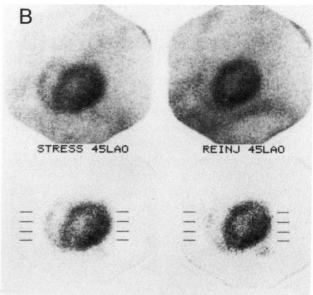

FIG 1–5.
A, initial postexercise stress and 2.5-hour delayed rest images in a patient with diminished ^{201}Tl uptake in the interventricular septum. **B,** initial stress image in the same patient as shown in **A** but compared with the image obtained after reinjection of 1.0 mCi of ^{201}Tl after the redistribution image in **A** was obtained. Note that the uptake of ^{201}Tl in the septal defect after ^{201}Tl reinjection appears more prominent.

demonstrated enhanced ^{201}Tl uptake after reinjection. Detection of myocardial viability by the two techniques was concordant in 88% of segments in these severe persistent defects. The conclusion derived from this study showed that the ^{201}Tl reinjection protocol was as pre-

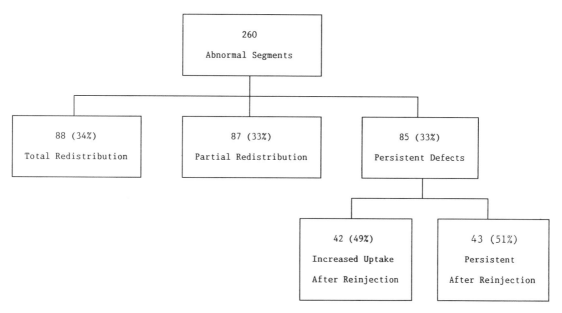

FIG 1–6.
Of 260 abnormal myocardial regions identified by SPECT stress ^{201}Tl imaging, 85 (33%) were persistent defects on 3- to 4-hour redistribution images. After reinjection of a second dose of ^{201}Tl, 49% of the persistent defects showed increased thallium uptake suggestive of viability. (From Dilsizian V, Rocco TP, Freeman NMT, et al: *N Engl J Med* 1990; 323:141–146. Used by permission.)

dictive as FDG imaging with PET for detecting viable myocardium in patients with chronic CAD and left ventricular dysfunction.

Interestingly, in this study from the National Institutes of Health (NIH) group,[36] most mild persistent defects showed evidence of myocardial viability as assessed by FDG uptake. This finding is consistent with those of Gibson et al.[30] who showed that most preoperative mild persistent ^{201}Tl defects (<50% reduction in ^{201}Tl uptake) exhibit improvement in ^{201}Tl uptake after bypass surgery. A conclusion that can be derived from all these studies is that a mild reduction in ^{201}Tl uptake on serial images (mild persistent defect) indicates preserved viability even if "redistribution" is not evident. The mere demonstration of preserved ^{201}Tl uptake, albeit reduced, identifies some myocardium that is viable in zones of hypoperfusion. Thus, reinjection of a second dose of ^{201}Tl is perhaps not required in such patients. The ^{201}Tl reinjection protocol appears most useful in detecting viability in those segments demonstrating a marked diminution in ^{201}Tl uptake on serial images. Furthermore, the "reinjection" protocol is preferred to 18- to 24-hour late redistribution imaging to detect viable myocardium in defects that remain persistent on 4-hour images. Finally, when quantitative ^{201}Tl imaging is employed, most segments showing enhanced ^{201}Tl uptake after reinjection do show at least some partial redistribution on the 2½- to 4-hour images. Visually,

however, such defects may appear to be persistent before reinjection of the second dose of thallium.

Dipyridamole Thallium 201 Scintigraphy

Ischemia can be distinguished from scarring with pharmacologic stress imaging employing dipyridamole infusion similar to what was described for exercise scintigraphy in the previous section.

Leppo et al. reported that 74% of myocardial scan segments demonstrating complete redistribution of an initial dipyridamole perfusion defect exhibited normal wall motion on ventriculography.[42] Conversely, 71% of scan segments demonstrating persistent ^{201}Tl defects were associated with akinetic or dyskinetic wall motion. Thus, segmental ^{201}Tl defect patterns on dipyridamole imaging predict normal or abnormal wall motion by ventriculography comparable to what has been reported for exercise scintigraphy. Okada and coworkers also compared various dipyridamole ^{201}Tl scan patterns with global and regional left ventricular function changes on exercise radionuclide angiography.[43] Redistribution defects on dipyridamole scans were associated with normal rest and exercise left ventricular ejection fractions and preserved regional wall motion. Mild persistent ^{201}Tl defects were associated with a normal ejection fraction and normal regional wall motion at rest but with a deterioration during exercise. As would be expected, severe persistent ^{201}Tl defects on dipyridamole scans were associated with a reduced ejection fraction and normal wall motion at rest but without further deterioration during exercise.

As with exercise imaging, dipyridamole perfusion scintigraphy can be used for distinguishing between ischemic and nonischemic cardiomyopathy. Eichhorn et al. were able to correctly classify 91% of patients with dipyridamole imaging when a perfusion defect of 15% or greater was used as a cutoff for nonischemic cardiomyopathy.[44] In this study, the mean perfusion defect was 25% ± 11% in patients with ischemic cardiomyopathy and 6% ± 6% in those with idiopathic dilated cardiomyopathy.

Resting Thallium 201 Imaging

Resting thallium scintigraphy has been successfully employed in patients with severe chronic stable angina or unstable angina to assess myocardial viability prior to and following revascularization.[28, 29] Berger et al. reported that 80% of patients showing initial resting defects with delayed "rest redistribution" preoperatively demonstrated a 5% or greater increase in left ventricular ejection fraction postoperatively.[29] In that study, only 22% of patients with persistent defects preoperatively on rest imaging showed a comparable improvement. Recent preliminary data reported from our group indicate that resting ^{201}Tl scintigraphy can assist in the selection of patients who might benefit from revascularization surgery and have severe depression of left ventricular systolic function.[45] In that study, approximately two thirds of akinetic/dyskinetic segments showed some preservation of myocardial viability by resting scintigraphy. The greater the number of viable scan segments observed preoperatively, the greater the improvement in left ventricular ejection fraction after bypass surgery.

Resting ^{201}Tl scintigraphy can be employed to assess the extent of reflow and myocardial salvage after coronary reperfusion. Several investigators have administered ^{201}Tl intravenously before infusing a thrombolytic agent and obtained post-thrombolysis images several hours later.[46–48] These studies demonstrated that patients exhibiting successful thrombolysis had more ^{201}Tl redistribution and smaller final ^{201}Tl defect sizes as compared with patients with persistently occluded infarct-related vessels. Patients who demonstrated redistribution 4 hours after institution of thrombolytic therapy may show even further improvement in ^{201}Tl uptake when imaging is repeated several weeks later.[46]

There are some significant limitations to the use of serial resting ^{201}Tl redistribution imaging in the early evaluation of patients receiving thrombolytic therapy. It may take up to 40 minutes to obtain pretreatment images, which would delay institution of thrombolytic therapy. On the other hand, if ^{201}Tl is injected for the first time immediately after establishment of reflow, the degree of salvage might be overestimated because ^{201}Tl may be taken up out of proportion to viable myocardium because of hyperemia.[49]

Resting ^{201}Tl scintigraphy may be useful when performed 24 hours or later after thrombolytic therapy to determine the success of reflow and to estimate the degree of salvage.[50] By delaying this injection of ^{201}Tl for 24 hours after thrombolytic therapy, the trapping of ^{201}Tl in the infarct region during the hyperemic flow phase that immediately follows reperfusion might be avoided. In the Western Washington Intravenous Thrombolytic Trial, patients who received streptokinase had significantly more ^{201}Tl uptake in the infarct zone as compared with controls.[51] It appears that the degree of regional thallium uptake in the infarct zone is proportional to the mass of viable myocytes.

Use of Thallium 201 Scintigraphy in Patients Undergoing Coronary Angioplasty

Exercise ^{201}Tl scintigraphy can be utilized to predict the efficacy of percutaneous coronary angioplasty.[52–55] Patients who are most suitable for angioplasty are those with symptomatic angina or silent ischemia who demonstrate significant ^{201}Tl redistribution or only mild persistent defects before the procedure. Following successful balloon dilatation of a stenotic vessel, there is usually substantial improvement in regional ^{201}Tl uptake when exercise scintigraphy is repeated after the procedure. This is not unlike the response to coronary bypass surgery in patients demonstrating preoperative ischemic responses on serial ^{201}Tl scans.

[201]Tl scintigraphy can also be performed following balloon dilatation to assess the presence or absence of restenosis.[53, 56] [201]Tl defects with redistribution following percutaneous transluminal coronary angioplasty (PTCA) is predictive of early recurrence of angina and implies that there was either incomplete dilatation or early restenosis. Data reported by Stuckey et al. demonstrate that ^{201}Tl scintigraphy performed in asymptomatic patients several weeks after PTCA has prognostic value in predicting angina recurrence that occurs secondary to restenosis.[53] In that study, ^{201}Tl redistribution was the only independent predictor of recurrent angina in asymptomatic patients undergoing routine exercise scintigraphy several weeks after successful balloon dilatation.

TECHNETIUM 99m MYOCARDIAL PERFUSION AGENTS

In recent years, new technetium 99m (^{99m}Tc)-labeled perfusion agents have undergone clinical testing for their efficacy in detecting myocardial ischemia and distinguishing viable from nonviable myocardium. The ^{99m}Tc isonitriles appear to be the most promising of this new group of agents for determination of myocardial viability.[57] ^{99m}Tc is an ideal radioisotope for clinical imaging with a gamma scintillation camera because of its peak voltage of 140 keV, ease of production from a generator, and favorable patient dosimetry permitting 10 to 20 times higher doses than feasible with ^{201}Tl.

^{99m}Tc Sestamibi is probably the most clinically applicable of the ^{99m}Tc isonitrile agents for human myocardial imaging. The myocardial uptake kinetics of ^{99m}Tc Sestamibi have been evaluated experimentally, and results of recent clinical trials with this agent have recently been reported.[59–63] Like ^{201}Tl, the myocardial uptake of ^{99m}Tc Sestamibi after intravenous injection is proportional to myocardial blood flow.[59] As expected, there is an inverse relationship between coronary blood flow and the extraction fraction for ^{99m}Tc Sestamibi.[61] Hypoxia and the administration of ouabain show minor effects on cellular extraction of ^{99m}Tc Sestamibi.[64] In cultured rat myocardial cells, Maublant et al. demonstrated that ^{99m}Tc Sestamibi uptake and washout were not affected by metabolic inhibitors such as cyanide and iodoacetate, which profoundly inhibit the respiratory chain and glycolysis, respectively.[65] In that preparation, ouabain did not affect ^{99m}Tc sestamibi uptake but did inhibit ^{201}Tl uptake. Thus, it appears that intracellular transport processes for ^{99m}Tc Sestamibi are less dependent on active transport mechanisms than ^{201}Tl is.

^{99m}Tc Sestamibi shows negligible "delayed redistribution" after initial intravenous injection.[59] The myocardial distribution of ^{99m}Tc Sestamibi with experimental myocardial ischemia in dogs shows an excellent correlation with radioactive microsphere uptake.[66] Myocardial stunning produced by 15 minutes of transient coronary occlusion followed by total reperfusion does not affect ^{99m}Tc Sestamibi uptake. The uptake of ^{99m}Tc Sestamibi in stunned myocardium was shown to be proportional to regional flow after reperfusion. This finding suggests that metabolic disturbances that contribute to the stunning process do not affect ^{99m}Tc Sestamibi uptake. It further suggests that like ^{201}Tl, this tracer can be employed for assessment of myocardial viability.

We assessed the myocardial uptake of ^{99m}Tc Sestamibi under conditions of a chronic low-flow state intended to simulate myocardial hibernation.[66] As reported for ^{201}Tl in this canine model, ^{99m}Tc Sestamibi activity was preserved and proportional to blood flow. Even though significant myocardial asynergy was produced, ^{99m}Tc Sestamibi uptake reflected the degree of viability.

Since ^{99m}Tc Sestamibi demonstrates almost no redistribution, separate injections of the radionuclide must be administered during stress and rest. Imaging with ^{99m}Tc Sestamibi has been utilized for detection, localizing, and sizing of myocardial perfusion defects in patients presenting with acute myocardial infarction.[67, 68] The agent may be particularly useful in assessing the efficacy of thrombolytic therapy. The first dose of ^{99m}Tc Sestamibi is administered just before thrombolytic therapy, but imaging can be postponed until several hours later following the complete infusion of a thrombolytic agent. In this way, institution of thrombolysis during the acute phase of infarction is not delayed. A "snapshot" of the perfusion pattern at the time of admission prior to reperfusion is obtained with this first injection of ^{99m}Tc Sestamibi. Even if one waits 4 to 6 hours after injection for obtaining the prethrombolysis images, one can still clearly observe the perfusion pattern that existed at the time of presentation during acute coronary occlusion. A second injection of ^{99m}Tc Sestamibi is administered some time after the first images are acquired, and this will delineate the degree of improvement in regional flow and extent of salvage.

Several experimental and clinical studies have been completed that validate the approach described above.[67–70] Wackers et al.[68] and Gibbons et al.,[67] with the assistance of several collaborating institutions, successfully applied serial ^{99m}Tc Sestamibi imaging in patients presenting with acute myocardial infarction who received thrombolytic therapy. Patients with a patent infarct vessel had a significantly greater decrease in defect size on repeat images performed 18 to 48 hours after thrombolytic therapy than did patients with persistently occluded vessels (Fig 1–7). A relative decrease of more than 30% in the size of ^{99m}Tc Sestamibi perfusion defects on planar images predicted the patency of the infarct-related vessel. These observations are of clinical significance since presently there are few reliable nonangiographic methods that predict successful reperfusion. ^{99m}Tc Sestamibi imaging could become a useful technique to incorporate into future clinical research trials aimed at evaluating the efficacy of pharmacologic approaches to reperfusion.

Infarct size may also be estimated from resting ^{99m}Tc Sestamibi images. Verani et al., in an experimental canine model, reported that the scintigraphic perfusion

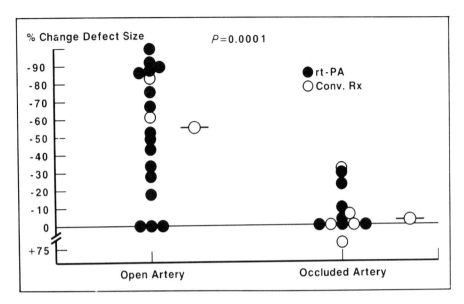

FIG 1–7.
Percent change in ^{99m}Tc Sestamibi defect size in patients with an open infarct artery vs. a closed infarct artery who underwent either thrombolytic therapy with recombinant tissue-type plasminogen activator *(rt-Pa) (solid circles)* or conventional therapy *(open circles)*. ^{99m}Tc Sestamibi was administered prior to and 24 hours after thrombolytic therapy or conventional treatment. All patients with a reduction in ^{99m}Tc Sestamibi defect size of 30% or greater on serial images before and after thrombolytic therapy had a patent infarct vessel. (From Wackers FJTh, Gibbons RJ, Verani MS, et al: *J Am Coll Cardiol* 1989; 14:861–873. Used by permission.)

defect size after reflow correlated well with pathologic infarct size.[69] Sinusas et al. from our institution confirmed these findings and found that the ^{99m}Tc defect area as defined by autoradiography correlated closely with postmortem infarct area ($r = 0.98$).[70] Figure 1–8 depicts this high correlation in the anesthetized canine model.

One feature of ^{99m}Tc Sestamibi imaging is that one can simultaneously assess regional blood flow and regional myocardial wall motion. This may be a unique feature applicable to assessment of myocardial viability in chronic CAD or in acute ischemic syndromes. One assesses regional wall motion by gating the perfusion images and viewing the end-systolic and end-diastolic images derived from the perfusion scans. Regions that show preserved ^{99m}Tc Sestamibi uptake as well as systolic thickening would be considered zones of viable myocardium. Regions that demonstrate abnormal systolic thickening but preserved ^{99m}Tc Sestamibi uptake would suggest viable but stunned or hibernating myocardium. A marked reduction in ^{99m}Tc Sestamibi imaging with a total absence of systolic thickening would indicate a zone of predominant irreversible myocardial injury. Further clinical studies are warranted to evaluate the clinical utility of gated perfusion imaging with ^{99m}Tc Sestamibi to enhance detection of viable myocardial segments.

^{99m}Tc Sestamibi imaging can be utilized to evaluate the efficacy of primary coronary angioplasty in acute myocardial infarction. Behrenbeck et al. reported a significant decrease in ^{99m}Tc Sestamibi defect size (48% ± 17% to 29% ± 19% of the left ventricle) after angioplasty in 17 patients experiencing their first transmural infarction.[71]

INFARCT-AVID IMAGING WITH RADIOLABELED MYOSIN-SPECIFIC ANTIBODY

Infarct-avid imaging has been available for many years to identify zones of myocardial necrosis in patients with acute myocardial infarction. In this nuclear cardiology technique, the radiopharmaceutical that is administered is selectively bound in myocardial regions of recent necrosis to yield a "hot spot" of radioactivity that can be detected and localized on myocardial scintigraphy. Initially, ^{99m}Tc stannous pyrophosphate was the agent most commonly utilized in this approach. More recently, a new infarct-avid imaging technique has emerged that involves the scintigraphic detection and quantification of myocardial necrosis after intravenous administration of radiolabeled myosin-specific antibody.[72] This approach is based on the principle that an-

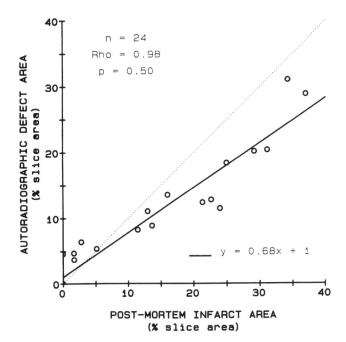

FIG 1–8.
Correlation of ^{99m}Tc-labeled methyoxyisobutyl isonitrile (MIBI) defect area on autoradiography and postmortem infarct area by histochemical staining in dogs receiving ^{99m}Tc Sestamibi intravenously after reperfusion preceded by 3 hours of sustained LAD coronary occlusion. (From Sinusas AJ, Trautman KA, Bergin JD, et al: *Circulation* 1990; 82:1424–1437. Used by permission.)

tibody specific for cardiac myosin will bind to the intracellular protein when sarcolemmal membrane integrity has been altered by ischemic myocardial injury. Experimental studies have shown that the location of antimyosin antibody uptake correlates to the region of necrosis as determined by histologic techniques.[73] As with ^{99m}Tc pyrophosphate, one has to wait at least 24 hours after the administration of radiolabeled antimyosin antibody before imaging can be performed. This delay permits clearance of the agent from the blood pool. To detect myocardial necrosis, a discrete "hot spot" of antimyosin uptake should be demonstrated.

Jain et al. sought to determine whether antimyosin antibody imaging was useful for establishing the diagnosis of myocardial infarction in patients presenting without diagnostic ECG changes.[74] In 75 patients with suspected infarction, 7 had no diagnostic ECG changes despite normal conduction patterns. Antimyosin antibody scans were positive in all 7 and were localized to regions supplied by diseased coronary vessels. All had abnormal wall motion at the site of antibody uptake.

Antimyosin antibody imaging has yielded a 92% sensitivity for identifying acute transmural myocardial infarction.[72] Faint tracer uptake can sometimes be ob-

served in patients with a persistently occluded infarct vessel and absence of collateral flow. Volpini and co-workers demonstrated that a myocardial scar from a previous old infarction did not demonstrate antimyosin antibody uptake.[75] The specificity of this radionuclide technique is high, with virtually no focal uptake observed in healthy volunteers. Some patients with the clinical syndrome of unstable angina pectoris will show antimyosin uptake. It is felt that these patients actually experienced some myocardial necrosis that was not detected by conventional ECG and enzyme criteria.

Assessment of myocardial viability can be undertaken with the dual imaging technique where both indium 111 antimyosin antibody and ^{201}Tl are administered to patients with acute infarction. Johnson et al. showed a significant correlation between subsequent ischemic events and mismatching ^{201}Tl/^{111}In antimyosin activity.[76] The identification of abnormal perfusion in myocardial zones outside the area of antimyosin uptake could be potentially useful for risk stratification. This would indicate that areas of ischemic and jeopardized myocardium were present in addition to the zone of myocardium that was rendered necrotic.

There are limitations of antimyosin antibody imaging that deserve mention. The actual role this imaging technique will take in the clinical setting has not yet been ascertained. Since one cannot accurately image very soon after the onset of infarction to detect necrosis, those situations requiring urgent early decision making cannot be aided by this imaging approach. Small inferior infarcts may not easily be detected, and there is decreased sensitivity in localizing regions of necrosis associated with closed infarct-related vessels and the absence of collateral flow. With respect to risk stratification and prognostication, the relative benefit of this technique vs. mere quantification of the global ejection fraction or solely performing ^{201}Tl scintigraphy has not been ascertained. Myocardial viability can be determined after myocardial infarction solely with the use of ^{201}Tl rest scintigraphy and assessment of regional wall motion. The addition of antimyosin imaging to the combination of evaluating perfusion and function may be of additional value in assessing viability and assisting in risk stratification. However, further clinical investigation is warranted in this regard.

POSITRON EMISSION TOMOGRAPHY TO ASSESS MYOCARDIAL VIABILITY

More sophisticated imaging techniques such as PET may be even more sensitive in identifying zones of myocardial viability than are conventional single-photon imaging approaches. Increased regional uptake of FDG in a zone of myocardial asynergy identifies myocardial tissue that is metabolically active and hence is viable.

In one study, ^{201}Tl and FDG were compared in an open-chest canine model in which 2 hours of coronary occlusion were followed by 4 hours of reflow.[77] [201]Tl was injected before reperfusion, and FDG was administered 3 hours after reflow. Both normal FDG uptake and delayed thallium redistribution reflected myocardial viability after reperfusion. A lack of redistribution and depressed FDG uptake were observed in irreversibly injured myocardial zones.

PET with [13]NH$_3$ and FDG has been used to assess regional myocardial perfusion and viability in patients with chronic CAD and ECG Q waves.[78] Infarcted regions were identified by a matched reduction in regional [13]NH$_3$ activity and glucose utilization, whereas regions of ischemia were identified by enhanced FDG uptake in regions of diminished [13]NH$_3$ activity (Fig 1–9). This is designated as a "mismatch" and suggests viability in regions of abnormal perfusion. In this study, PET with FDG revealed evidence of persistent tissue metabolism in a high proportion of myocardial regions that correlated with chronic ECG Q waves, thereby identifying viable myocardium not easily detected by conventional evaluation.

In a subsequent study by Brunken et al., PET demonstrated evidence of preserved glucose uptake in many segments demonstrating only partial ^{201}Tl redistribution or in zones corresponding to fixed ^{201}Tl defects.[79] In this study, 58% of segments showing no ^{201}Tl redistribution at 4 hours demonstrated some preservation of regional FDG uptake. These authors concluded that markers of perfusion alone would underestimate the extent of viable myocardium, particularly in regions supplied by severely stenotic vessels. Reinjection of a second dose of ^{201}Tl at 4 hours to enhance the sensitivity of ^{201}Tl scintigraphy for distinguishing viable from nonviable myocardium was not undertaken in this study.

Tillisch et al. monitored the functional outcome of segmental wall motion abnormalities after bypass surgery relative to the preoperative FDG findings on PET.[80] Systolic function was enhanced in 85% of myocardial segments showing a mismatch between blood flow and FDG uptake, whereas no improvement was noted in 92% of patients who had a matched diminution in blood flow and metabolism.

From such studies in the literature, one can conclude that PET imaging of blood flow and metabolism is useful for the preoperative evaluation of patients with markedly depressed left ventricular function. Many patients with chronic CAD have severe regional wall motion abnormalities, and myocardial viability is an important factor with respect to consideration of surgery.

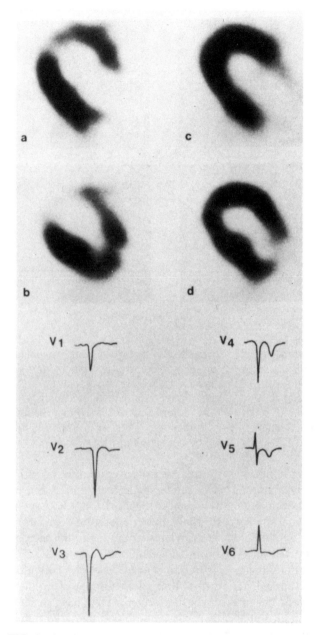

FIG 1–9.
ECG and tomographic PET images in a 59-year-old man with a previous myocardial infarction. The left ventricular ejection fraction was 26%, and multiple wall motion abnormalities were noted on ventriculography. Perfusion defects are noted on the ^{13}N-ammonia study in the anterior and septal regions (panels *a* and *b*). Glucose metabolism is well preserved in these regions as indicated by preserved uptake of ^{18}F-2-deoxyglucose (panels *c* and *d*). The preservation of glucose metabolism is indicative of myocardial viability.

More recently, PET imaging of ^{11}C-acetate has been evaluated to assess myocardial oxygen consumption.[81, 82] Measurement of the oxidation of acetate could provide an indirect noninvasive measure of regional oxygen utilization. This new PET technique could also prove useful for detecting viable myocardium in zones of regional asynergy.

CLINICAL DECISION MAKING IN RADIONUCLIDE ASSESSMENT OF MYOCARDIAL VIABILITY

There is no doubt that radionuclide imaging of myocardial perfusion, function, and metabolism for assessment of myocardial viability can assist in clinical decision making in certain subsets of patients with CAD. As described in this review, the sole measurement of regional myocardial systolic function may not be adequate to distinguish viable from irreversibly injured myocardium in patients who have recently undergone coronary reperfusion or in patients with severe chronic CAD who manifest "hibernating" myocardium as the cause of left ventricular dysfunction. In these clinical situations, stress-rest or solely resting ^{201}Tl imaging will aid in distinguishing ischemic from infarcted myocardium. With exercise imaging, one may have to administer a second dose of ^{201}Tl following the "reinjection" protocol described in this review to best differentiate reversible ischemia from a myocardial scar.

In patients who are unable to exercise, resting ^{201}Tl scintigraphy alone should be highly accurate in identifying those asynergic regions that are still viable. In both situations, demonstration of preserved ^{201}Tl uptake, albeit reduced, would suggest that following revascularization regional function should improve. Those patients with severe CAD and depressed function most likely to benefit from revascularization will demonstrate evidence of thallium uptake with standard stress and 4-hour redistribution imaging, with stress and delayed 18- to 24-hour imaging, or by enhanced thallium uptake with reinjection. [201]Tl uptake in the resting state alone indicates viability and also predicts improvement in function after revascularization. Patients with no evidence of viable myocardium in the distribution of severely obstructed vessels by ^{201}Tl scan criteria would be spared the risk of surgery and the potential lack of benefit even if revascularization surgery or angioplasty were technically successful.

It is somewhat premature to predict whether or not [99m]Tc Sestamibi imaging will prove more beneficial than ^{201}Tl scintigraphy for identifying viable myocardium after coronary reperfusion. Certainly, the results of clinical studies in which regional function and perfusion are simultaneously assessed by gated [99m]Tc Sestamibi imaging will be of interest. It is quite likely that [99m]Tc Sestamibi imaging in patients with acute myocardial infarcts who are undergoing thrombolytic therapy will prove more useful than ^{201}Tl imaging in this patient population for the early assessment of success of reflow and extent of myocardial salvage. The preliminary clinical studies reported to date are certainly encouraging in this regard. Acute infarction patients who do not exhibit a significant reduction in [99m]Tc Sestamibi defect size on serial imaging after thrombolysis might be candidates for "rescue angioplasty." A lack of defect size reduction would suggest a failure to reperfuse with pharmacologic therapy alone. In the future, perhaps dual simultaneous imaging of [99m]Tc Sestamibi and ^{201}Tl when both radionuclides are administered together under various clinical situations will be undertaken. [99m]Tc Sestamibi would be injected prior to thrombolytic therapy and ^{201}Tl administered after drug infusion. Only one set of images would be obtained. The uptake of [99m]Tc Sestamibi would delineate the "area at risk," and the ^{201}Tl uptake pattern would reflect viability.

It is unclear whether or not infarct-avid imaging with antimyosin antibody will gain popularity in clinical practice for evaluation of viability after acute infarction. Perhaps a limited diagnostic role for this imaging approach will emerge in those presumed infarct patients with uninterpretable ECG findings (e.g., bundle-branch blocks) whose creatine kinase enzyme values are nondiagnostic (e.g., admission more than 48 hours after the onset of symptoms).

The cost-effectiveness of the more expensive PET imaging techniques for assessment of viability have not yet been adequately ascertained. To date, evidence is lacking that shows the superiority of PET imaging of myocardial metabolism with FDG to conventional imaging techniques for the detection of CAD and determination of myocardial viability. The studies reported from the NIH and cited in this review seem to indicate a comparable sensitivity of SPECT ^{201}Tl imaging using the reinjection protocol and PET imaging with FDG for distinguishing viable from nonviable myocardium. However, further studies in a larger number of patients in which the gold standard for viability is enhanced regional function after revascularization should be conducted.

Finally, nuclear cardiology techniques can be of assistance in evaluating results of interventional cardiology techniques such as coronary angioplasty, laser angioplasty, atherectomy, and the like. All of these techniques are aimed at enhancing coronary blood flow and improving function in regions that have been acutely or chronically underperfused. When performed in high-quality nuclear cardiology laboratories with significant attention paid to quality control and meticulous imaging techniques, perfusion imaging with ^{201}Tl or [99m]Tc Sestamibi should be a useful adjunct to angiographic assessment of patients undergoing these new interventional techniques. SPECT or planar ^{201}Tl imaging is quite demanding from the technical standpoint, and knowledge of image artifacts is mandatory for minimizing false-positive interpretations. Quantitation of ^{201}Tl uptake and clearance may certainly enhance the capability of detecting viable myocardium in zones of myocardial asynergy.

REFERENCES

1. Braunwald E, Kloner RA: The stunned myocardium: Prolonged postischemic ventricular dysfunction. *Circulation* 1982; 66:1146–1149.
2. Rahimtoola SH: The hibernating myocardium. *Am Heart J* 1989; 117:211–221.
3. Swain JL, Sabina RL, McHale PA, et al: Prolonged myocardial nucleotide depletion after brief ischemia in the open-chest dog. *Am J Physiol* 1982; 242:818–826.
4. Greenfield RA, Swain JL: Disruption of myofibrillar energy use: Dual mechanisms that may contribute to postischemic dysfunction in stunned myocardium. *Circ Res* 1987; 60:283–289.
5. Stahl LD, Weiss HR, Becker LC: Myocardial oxygen consumption, oxygen supply/demand heterogeneity and microvascular patency in regionally stunned myocardium. *Circulation* 1988; 77:865–872.
6. Ciuffo AA, Ouyang P, Becker LC, et al: Reduction of sympathetic inotropic response after ischemia in dogs: Contributor to stunned myocardium. *J Clin Invest* 1985; 75:1504–1509.
7. Kusuoka H, Porterfield JK, Weisman HF, et al: Pathophysiology and pathogenesis of stunned myocardium: Depressed Ca^{2+} activation of contraction as a consequence of reperfusion-induced cellular calcium overload in ferret hearts. *J Clin Invest* 1987; 79:950–961.
8. Zhao M, Zhang H, Robinson TF, et al: Profound structural alterations of the extracellular collagen matrix postischemic dysfunctional ("stunned") but viable myocardium. *J Am Coll Cardiol* 1987; 10:1322–1334.
9. Bolli R: Oxygen-derived free radicals in postischemic myocardial dysfunction ("stunned myocardium"). *J Am Coll Cardiol* 1988; 12:239–249.
10. Hess ML, Manson NH: Molecular oxygen: Friend and foe. The role of oxygen free radical system in the calcium paradox, the oxygen paradox and ischemia/reperfusion injury. *J Mol Cell Cardiol* 1984; 16:969–985.
11. Stack RS, Phillips HR III, Grierson DS, et al: Functional improvement of jeopardized myocardium following intracoronary streptokinase infusion in acute myocardial infarction. *J Clin Invest* 1983; 72:84–95.
12. Touchstone DA, Beller GA, Nygaard TW, et al: Effects of successful intravenous reperfusion therapy on regional myocardial function and geometry in humans: A tomographic assessment using two-dimensional echocardiography. *J Am Coll Cardiol* 1989; 13:1506–1513.
13. Anderson JL, Marshall HW, Bray BE, et al: A randomized trial of intracoronary streptokinase in the treatment of acute myocardial infarction. *N Engl J Med* 1983; 308:1312–1318.
14. Brill DA, Deckelbaum LI, Remetz MS, et al: Recovery of severe ischemic left ventricular dysfunction after coronary bypass grafting. *Am J Cardiol* 1988; 61:650–651.
15. Strauss HW, Harrison K, Langan JK, et al: Thallium-201 for myocardial imaging. Relation of thallium-201 to regional myocardial perfusion. *Circulation* 1975; 51:641–645.
16. Weich HF, Strauss HW, Pitt B: The extraction of thallium-201 by the myocardium. *Circulation* 1977; 56:188–191.
17. Pohost GM, Zir LM, Moore RH, et al: Differentiation of transiently ischemic from infarcted myocardium by serial imaging after a single dose of thallium-201. *Circulation* 1977; 55:294–302.
18. Nielson AT, Morris KG, Murdock R, et al: Linear relationship between the distribution of thallium-201 and blood flow in ischemic and non-ischemic myocardium during exercise. *Circulation* 1980; 61:797–801.
19. Leppo JA: Myocardial uptake of thallium and rubidium during alterations in perfusion and oxygenation in isolated rabbit hearts. *J Nucl Med* 1987; 28:878–885.
20. Leppo JA, Macneil PB, Moring AF, et al: Separate effects of ischemia, hypoxia, and contractility on thallium-201 kinetics in rabbit myocardium. *J Nucl Med* 1986; 27:66–74.
21. Moore CA, Cannon J, Watson DD, et al: Thallium 201 kinetics in stunned myocardium characterized by severe postischemic systolic dysfunction. *Circulation* 1990; 81:1622–1632.
22. Sinusas AJ, Watson DD, Cannon JM Jr, et al: Effect of ischemia and postischemic dysfunction on myocardial uptake of technetium-99m–labeled methoxyisobutyl isonitrile and thallium-201. *J Am Coll Cardiol* 1989; 14:1785–1793.
23. Goldhaber SZ, Newell JB, Alpert NM, et al: Effects of ischemia-like insult on myocardial thallium-201 accumulation. *Circulation* 1983; 67:778–786.
24. Granato JE, Watson DD, Flanagan TL, et al: Myocardial thallium-201 kinetics and regional flow alterations with 3 hours of coronary occlusion and either rapid reperfusion through a totally patent vessel or slow reperfusion through a critical stenosis. *J Am Coll Cardiol* 1987; 9:109–118.
25. Grunwald AM, Watson DD, Holzgrefe HH Jr, et al: Myocardial thallium-201 kinetics in normal and ischemic myocardium. *Circulation* 1981; 64:610–618.
26. Pohost GM, Okada RD, O'Keefe DD, et al: Thallium redistribution in dogs with severe coronary artery stenosis of fixed caliber. *Circ Res* 1981; 48:439–446.
27. Khaw BA, Strauss HW, Pohost GM, et al: Relation of immediate and delayed thallium-201 distribution to localization of iodine-125 antimyosin antibody in acute experimental myocardial infarction. *Am J Cardiol* 1983; 51:1428–1432.
28. Gewirtz H, Beller GA, Strauss HW, et al: Transient defects of resting thallium scans in patients with coronary artery disease. *Circulation* 1979; 59:707–713.
29. Berger BC, Watson DD, Burwell LR, et al: Redistribution of thallium at rest in patients with stable and unsta-

ble angina and the effect of coronary artery bypass graft surgery. *Circulation* 1979; 60:1114–1125.

30. Gibson RS, Watson DD, Taylor GJ, et al: Prospective assessment of regional myocardial perfusion before and after coronary revascularization surgery by quantitative thallium-201 scintigraphy. *J Am Coll Cardiol* 1983; 1:804–815.

31. Kotler TS, Diamond GA: Exercise thallium-201 scintigraphy in the diagnosis and prognosis of coronary artery disease. *Ann Intern Med* 1990; 113:684–702.

32. Wackers FJT, Fetterman RC, Mattera JA, et al: Quantitative planar thallium-201 stress scintigraphy: A critical evaluation of the method. *Semin Nucl Med* 1985; 15:46–66.

33. Berger BC, Watson DD, Taylor GJ, et al: Quantitative thallium-201 exercise scintigraphy for detection of coronary artery disease. *J Nucl Med* 1981; 22:585–593.

34. Watson DD, Campbell NP, Read EK, et al: Spatial and temporal quantitation of plane thallium myocardial images. *J Nucl Med* 1981; 22:577–584.

35. Maddahi J, Garcia EV, Berman DS, et al: Improved noninvasive assessment of coronary artery disease by quantitative analysis of regional stress myocardial distribution and washout of thallium-201. *Circulation* 1981; 64:924–935.

36. Bonow RO, Dilsizian V, Cuocolo A, et al: Identification of viable myocardium in patients with chronic coronary artery disease and left ventricular dysfunction. Comparison of thallium scintigraphy with reinjection and PET imaging with ^{18}F-fluorodeoxyglucose. *Circulation* 1991; 83:26–37.

37. Cloninger KG, DePuey EG, Garcia EV, et al: Incomplete redistribution in delayed thallium-201 single photon emission computed tomographic (SPECT) images: An overestimation of myocardial scarring. *J Am Coll Cardiol* 1988; 12:955–963.

38. Kiat H, Berman DS, Maddahi J, et al: Late reversibility of tomographic myocardial thallium-201 defects: An accurate marker of myocardial viability. *J Am Coll Cardiol* 1988; 12:1456–1463.

39. Yang LD, Berman DS, Kiat H, et al: The frequency of late reversibility in SPECT thallium-201 stress-redistribution studies. *J Am Coll Cardiol* 1990; 15:334–340.

40. Dilsizian V, Rocco TP, Freeman NMT, et al: Enhanced detection of ischemic but viable myocardium by the reinjection of thallium after stress-redistribution imaging. *N Engl J Med* 1990; 323:141–146.

41. Tamaki N, Ohtani H, Yonekura Y, et al: Significance of fill-in after thallium-201 reinjection following delayed imaging: Comparison with regional wall motion and angiographic findings. *J Nucl Med* 1990; 31:1617–1623.

42. Leppo J, Boucher CA, Okada RD, et al: Serial thallium-201 myocardial imaging after dipyridamole infusion: Diagnostic utility in detecting coronary stenoses and relationship to regional wall motion. *Circulation* 1982; 66:649–657.

43. Okada RD, Dai Y, Boucher CA, et al: Serial thallium-201 imaging after dipyridmamole for coronary disease detection: Quantitative analysis using myocardial clearance. *Am Heart J* 1984; 107:475–480.

44. Eichhorn EJ, Kosinski EJ, Lewis SM, et al: Usefulness of dipyridamole–thallium-201 perfusion scanning for distinguishing ischemic from nonischemic cardiomyopathy. *Am J Cardiol* 1988; 62:945–951.

45. Ragosta M, Gimple LW, Kron IL, et al: Preoperative assessment of myocardial viability by rest–thallium-201 imaging in patients with reduced ventricular function (abstract). *Circulation* 1990; 82(suppl 3):294.

46. DeCoster PM, Melin JA, Detry JMR, et al: Coronary artery reperfusion in acute myocardial infarction: Assessment by pre- and postintervention thallium-201 myocardial perfusion imaging. *Am J Cardiol* 1985; 55:889–895.

47. Reduto LA, Freund GC, Gaeta JM, et al: Coronary artery reperfusion in acute myocardial infarction: Beneficial effects of intracoronary streptokinase on left ventricular salvage and performance. *Am Heart J* 1981; 102:1168–1177.

48. Simoons ML, Wijns W, Balakumaran K, et al: The effect of intracoronary thrombolysis with streptokinase on myocardial thallium distribution and left ventricular function assessed by blood-pool scintigraphy. *Eur Heart J* 1982; 3:433–440.

49. Granato JE, Watson DD, Flanagan TL, et al: Myocardial thallium-201 kinetics during coronary occlusion and reperfusion: Influence of method of reflow and timing of thallium-201 administration. *Circulation* 1986; 73:150–160.

50. Schwarz F, Hofmann M, Schuler G, et al: Thrombolysis in acute myocardial infarction: Effect of intravenous followed by intracoronary streptokinase application on estimates of infarct size. *Am J Cardiol* 1984; 53:1505–1510.

51. Ritchie JL, Cerqueira M, Maynard C, et al: Ventricular function and infarct size: The Western Washington Intravenous Streptokinase in Myocardial Infarction Trial. *J Am Coll Cardiol* 1988; 11:689–697.

52. Hirzel HO, Nuesch K, Grüntzig AR, et al: Short- and long-term changes in myocardial perfusion after percutaneous transluminal coronary angioplasty assessed by thallium-201 exercise scintigraphy. *Circulation* 1981; 63:1001–1007.

53. Stuckey TD, Burwell LR, Nygaard TW, et al: Quantitative exercise thallium-201 scintigraphy for predicting angina recurrence after percutaneous transluminal coronary angioplasty. *Am J Cardiol* 1989; 63:517–521.

54. Wijns W, Serruys PW, Simoons ML, et al: Predictive value of early maximal exercise test and thallium scintigraphy after successful percutaneous transluminal coronary angioplasty. *Br Heart J* 1985; 53:194–200.

55. Wijns W, Serruys PW, Reiber JH, et al: Early detection of restenosis after successful percutaneous transluminal coronary angioplasty by exercise-redistribution thallium scintigraphy. *Am J Cardiol* 1985; 55:357–361.

56. Breisblatt WM, Weiland FL, Spaccavento LJ: Stress thallium-201 imaging after coronary angioplasty predicts restenosis and recurrent symptoms. *J Am Coll Cardiol* 1988; 12:1199–1204.

57. Sinusas AJ, Beller GA, Watson DD: Cardiac imaging with technetium 99m–labeled isonitriles. *J Thorac Imaging* 1990; 5:20–30.

58. Wackers FJTh, Berman DS, Maddahi J, et al: Technetium-99m hexakis 2-methoxyisobutyl isonitrile: Human biodistribution, dosimetry, safety, and preliminary comparison to thallium-201 for myocardial perfusion imaging. *J Nucl Med* 1989; 30:301–311.

59. Okada RD, Glover D, Gaffney T, et al: Myocardial kinetics of technetium-99m-hexakis-2-methoxy-2-methylpropyl isonitrile. *Circulation* 1988; 77:491–498.

60. Li QS, Frank TL, Franceschi D, et al: Technetium-99m

methoxyisobutyl isonitrile (RP-30) for quantification of myocardial ischemia and reperfusion in dogs. *J Nucl Med* 1988; 29:1539–1548.

61. Leppo JA, Meerdink DJ: Comparison of the myocardial uptake of a technetium-labeled isonitrile analogue and thallium. *Circ Res* 1989; 65:632–639.

62. Kiat H, Maddahi J, Roy LT, et al: Comparison of technetium 99m methoxy isobutyl isonitrile and thallium 201 for evaluation of coronary artery disease by planar and tomographic methods. *Am Heart J* 1989; 117:1–11.

63. Sinusas AJ, Beller GA, Smith WH, et al: Quantitative planar imaging with technetium-99m methoxyisobutyl isonitrile: Comparison of uptake patterns with thallium-201. *J Nucl Med* 1989; 30:1456–1463.

64. Meerdink DJ, Leppo JA: Comparison of hypoxia and ouabain effects on the myocardial uptake kinetics of technetium-99m hexakis 2-methoxyisobutyl isonitrile and thallium-201. *J Nucl Med* 1989; 30:1500–1506.

65. Maublant JC, Gachon P, Moins N: Hexakis (2-methoxy isobutylisonitrile) technetium-99m and thallium-201 chloride: Uptake and release in cultured myocardial cells. *J Nucl Med* 1988; 29:48–54.

66. Sinusas AJ, Watson DD, Cannon JM Jr, et al: Effect of ischemia and postischemic dysfunction on myocardial uptake of technetium-99m–labeled methoxyisobutyl isonitrile and thallium-201. *J Am Coll Cardiol* 1989; 14:1785–1793.

67. Gibbons RJ, Verani MS, Behrenbeck T, et al: Feasibility of tomographic ⁹⁹ᵐTc-hexakis-2-methoxy-2-methylpropyl-isonitrile imaging for the assessment of myocardial area at risk and the effect of treatment in acute myocardial infarction. *Circulation* 1989; 80:1277–1286.

68. Wackers FJTh, Gibbons RJ, Verani MS, et al: Serial quantitative planar technetium-99m isonitrile imaging in acute myocardial infarction: Efficacy for noninvasive assessment of thrombolytic therapy. *J Am Coll Cardiol* 1989; 14:861–873.

69. Verani MS, Jeroudi MO, Mahmarian JJ, et al: Quantification of myocardial infarction during coronary occlusion and myocardial salvage after reperfusion using cardiac imaging with technetium-99m hexakis 2-methoxyisobutyl isonitrile. *J Am Coll Cardiol* 1988; 12:1573–1581.

70. Sinusas AJ, Trautman KA, Bergin JD, et al: Quantification of area at risk during coronary occlusion and degree of myocardial salvage after reperfusion with technetium-99m methoxyisobutyl isonitrile. *Circulation* 1990; 82:1424–1437.

71. Behrenbeck T, Pellikka PA, Huber KC, et al: Primary

angioplasty in myocardial infarction: Assessment of improved myocardial perfusion with technetium-99m isonitrile. *J Am Coll Cardiol* 1991; 17:365–372.

72. Johnson LL, Seldin DW, Becker LC, et al: Antimyosin imaging in acute transmural myocardial infarctions: Results of a multicenter clinical trial. *J Am Coll Cardiol* 1989; 13:27–35.

73. Khaw BA, Yasuda T, Gold HK, et al: Acute myocardial infarct imaging with indium-111–labeled monoclonal antimyosin Fab. *J Nucl Med* 1987; 28:1671–1678.

74. Jain D, Lahiri A, Raftery EB: Immunoscintigraphy for detecting acute myocardial infarction without electrocardiographic changes. *Br Med J* 1990; 300:151–153.

75. Volpini M, Giubbini R, Gei P, et al: Diagnosis of acute myocardial infarction by indium-111 antimyosin antibodies and correlation with the traditional techniques for the evaluation of extent and localization. *Am J Cardiol* 1989; 63:7–13.

76. Johnson LL, Seldin DW, Keller AM, et al: Dual isotope thallium and indium antimyosin SPECT imaging to identify acute infarct patients at further ischemic risk. *Circulation* 1990; 81:37–45.

77. Melin JA, Wijns W, Keyeux A, et al: Assessment of thallium-201 redistribution versus glucose uptake as predictors of viability after coronary occlusion and reperfusion. *Circulation* 1988; 77:927–934.

78. Brunken R, Tillisch J, Schwaiger M, et al: Regional perfusion, glucose metabolism, and wall motion in patients with chronic electrocardiographic Q wave infarctions: Evidence for persistence of viable tissue in some infarct regions by positron emission tomography. *Circulation* 1986; 73:951–963.

79. Brunken R, Schwaiger M, Grover-McKay M, et al: Positron emission tomography detects tissue metabolic activity in myocardial segments with persistent thallium perfusion defects. *J Am Coll Cardiol* 1987; 10:557–567.

80. Tillisch J, Brunken R, Marshall R, et al: Reversibility of cardiac wall-motion abnormalities predicted by positron tomography. *N Engl J Med* 1986; 314:884–888.

81. Henes CG, Bergmann SR, Walsh MN, et al: Assessment of myocardial oxidative metabolic reserve with positron emission tomography and carbon-11 acetate. *J Nucl Med* 1989; 30:1489–1499.

82. Armbrecht JJ, Buxton DB, Schelbert HR: Validation of [1-¹¹C] acetate as a tracer for noninvasive assessment of oxidative metabolism with positron emission tomography in normal, ischemic, postischemic, and hyperemic canine myocardium. *Circulation* 1990; 81:1594–1605.

Transcatheter Assessment of Coronary Blood Flow and Velocity

Robert A. Vogel, M.D.

Despite its clinical importance for patients with coronary ischemia and myocardial infarction, the measurement of regional coronary blood flow remains clinically difficult. This is especially problematic in the catheterization laboratory where interventional procedures often require precise assessment of coronary anatomy and physiology. Improved diagnostic accuracy in these areas has been accomplished through the recent development of automated quantitative coronary arteriography and digital radiographic assessment of coronary flow reserve.[1-3] The former technique substantially reduces the observer variability associated with the visual assessment of stenosis severity and provides absolute dimensions of arterial segments. Quantitation of "normal" arterial diameter has proved helpful for sizing angioplasty catheters.[4] Digital radiography provides regional information on coronary flow reserve measured following pharmacologic vasodilatation.[4] Considerable debate continues on the relative clinical value of percent stenosis vs. absolute parameters of stenosis geometry (e.g., minimal lesion diameter), the effects of a stenosis on coronary blood flow, and the accuracy of blood flow measurements.[5-16] Both coronary anatomy and flow physiology change substantially in the immediate postangioplasty period, thus making predictions of long-term success difficult.[17-22] Additionally, despite the help provided by quantitative arteriography and digital radiographic blood flow analysis in assessing the need for coronary angioplasty in individual instances, these techniques cannot be performed during the actual dilatation. Along with the technological explosion that has taken place over the past 10 years in coronary interventional equipment, numerous new catheter diagnostic techniques have been developed for use during this critical period.[23] These included angioscopy and ultrasonography for assessing coronary anatomy and Doppler and impedance catheter determinations of coronary blood velocity and flow. This chapter summarizes the principles and clinical applications and limitations of transcatheter blood flow measurement.

THERMODILUTION CORONARY SINUS CATHETER

In 1971, Ganz et al. introduced a thermodilution method for measuring coronary sinus flow in humans that uses the indicator dilution principle.[24] A catheter is introduced retrogradely into the coronary sinus through which is infused room-temperature saline at a constant rate. Adequate mixing is achieved despite a relatively short distance between the indicator port and thermistor by injecting the saline through a small side hole perpendicular to the blood flow. Although this technique is simple and inexpensive, it has two major problems.[25] First, the position of the catheter in the coronary sinus is often unstable, which makes repeated determinations variable. This was not evident in initial validation studies that employed fixation of the catheter and/or cannulation of the coronary sinus for timed collection measurements. Subsequently, however, comparisons of thermodilution catheter and electromagnetic flow probe determinations with the catheter left unrestrained in the coronary sinus have shown poor correlations.[26] Second, regional specificity, even with the catheter positioned in the great cardiac vein, is often problematic, so measurements can only be considered estimates of overall coronary blood flow. Additional doubt as to the accuracy of thermodilution coronary sinus measurements comes from the finding that normal coronary flow reserve measurements have been found to be only approximately 2, in comparison with determinations greater than 3 to 4 with numerous other methodologies.[22, 26] Due to these problems, coronary sinus thermodilution catheter assessment of flow physiology is rarely clinically used to assess the clinical efficacy of coronary artery interventions.

DOPPLER CATHETER AND GUIDEWIRE

In an attempt to increase the regional specificity of flow measurements, subselective dedicated and balloon catheters have been developed that allow measurement of coronary blood flow velocity by using Doppler techniques.[27] In 1971, Benchimol et al. first reported the measurement of coronary artery blood velocity in patients by using a continuous-wave Doppler probe.[28] Initial studies were limited by the catheter's diameter and absence of a lumen through which hyperemia-inducing agents could be injected or through which a guidewire could be passed. Catheter diameter was subsequently reduced by using pulsed Doppler instrumentation. Since pulse generation and reception are done at different times, the same crystal can be used for both purposes. In 1974, Hartley and Cole described a pulsed Doppler catheter that was modified from a Sones coronary catheter.[29] Although the catheter was used clinically by Cole and Hartley for experimental studies, its relatively large size (5 F) and absence of a steerable guidewire prevented widespread clinical application.[30] Wilson et al. described the first 3 F diameter subselective Doppler catheter for clinical studies in 1985,[31] and Sibley et al. reported on the first clinical catheter that utilized a separate steerable guidewire in 1986.[32] More recently, Doppler crystals have been mounted on the tip of angioplasty balloon catheters to eliminate the need for separate diagnostic and interventional devices.[33]

All current clinically utilized Doppler flow velocity catheters utilize range-gated instrumentation that samples the velocity of blood flow a short distance from the crystal. Crystal frequency has generally been 20 MHz. Red cell reflectivity increases substantially with sound frequency, but sound absorption also increases. Two of the most commonly utilized designs employ a front-facing catheter tipped with a circular crystal through which can be passed a 0.014-in. guidewire and a side-mounted angulated crystal catheter with a separate guidewire lumen exiting at the catheter's tip.

Neither of these approaches allow assessment of absolute coronary blood flow, but simply sense velocity within a small arterial volume remote from the transducer. Excellent correlations have been found between Doppler shift assessment of flow velocity and relative volumetric flow changes in both arterial phantom and animal validation tests. Flow velocity changes increase linearly to a level at least ten times the resting blood flow. Although absolute coronary blood flow cannot be measured by this approach, coronary flow reserve can be determined by comparing blood velocities under pharmacologically induced hyperemic and baseline conditions. Intracoronary-injected papaverine has proved especially useful for this purpose because it provides both near-maximal vasodilation and short duration of action.[34] Intravenous dipyridamole and intracoronary adenosine have also been used for this purpose. Major advantages of the Doppler catheter approach are that both phasic and mean blood flow data are provided continuously and that injection of an indicator substance is not required. Therefore, there is no interference with intrinsic blood flow. Blood flow velocity can be monitored during the actual coronary artery intervention through the use of a crystal-tipped balloon catheter[29] (Fig 2–1).

Specific limitations of this approach are that blood flow velocity measurements are extremely sensitive to catheter position and varied by changes in coronary artery diameter. Both hyperemic and baseline measurements are also significantly altered when the catheter is located translesionally.[15]

A general problem is that coronary flow reserve can be reduced by many factors other than epicardial coronary stenosis, including myocardial hypertrophy, hypertension, prior myocardial infarction, collateralization, coronary spasm and intrinsic vasoactivity, syndrome X, prolonged ischemia, angioplasty, and vasoactive drugs. Arterial, ventricular end-diastolic, and intrathoracic pressures, which can vary during arteriographic procedures, also affect flow reserve.[3] Changes in coronary flow in one artery may affect flow in another artery. Finally, as a relative parameter, flow reserve ratios are altered by changes in resting blood flow. This latter issue is especially problematic immediately following angioplasty, which has often been found to be associated with reduced determinations of flow reserve despite adequate dilatation.[17–22] This is thought to be likely due to increases in resting blood flow occurring during this period. These factors need to be considered in using flow reserve to clinically determine the physiologic severity of lesions and may explain, in part, conflicting anatomic and physiologic data. Specifically, flow reserve measurements obtained immediately following angioplasty do

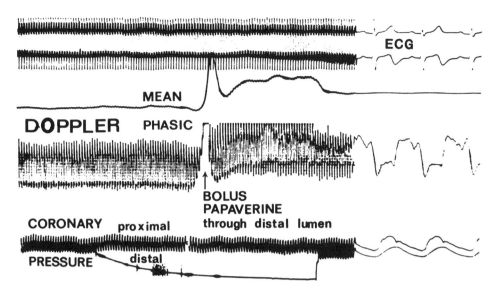

FIG 2–1.
Mean and phasic Doppler balloon catheter coronary artery blood velocity tracings obtained before and after papaverine administration. (Courtesy of P.W. Serruys, Rotterdam, The Netherlands.)

not appear to predict those individuals who will develop restenosis.[19] To reduce interference with intrinsic blood flow and to make blood flow assessment during use of any over-the-wire balloon catheter, Segal et al. have developed a flexible 0.018-in. steerable guidewire with a Doppler crystal mounted at the tip.[35, 36] A broad-beam 12-MHz transducer is utilized, and signals are analyzed by fast Fourier transformation. Flow velocity has been shown to correlate closely with phantom flow ($r = 0.92$ to 0.99), with validation being performed in vessels from 1.2 to 3.3 mm in diameter.[35] This method also has the advantage of accurately measuring absolute blood flow by multiplication of mean flow velocity and quantitative arteriographic cross-sectional area. Mean velocity is estimated at 0.5 times the peak velocity by assumption of a parabolic velocity profile.

The Doppler guidewire appears to be compatible with standard angioplasty technique, with 11 of 12 successful lesional crossings in its initial clinical trial.[36] As was previously demonstrated by other methods, coronary flow measured by Doppler guidewire was found to be inconsistently improved following successful (by lesion appearance) angioplasty, although measurements made distal to the lesion correlated best.[36] Phasic flow profiles, however, appear to be very clinically helpful. Normal vessels consistently show diastolic-to-systolic flow ratios greater than 2.0, whereas diseased vessels have been found to have ratios between 1.0 and 1.5. Following successful angiplasty, phasic flow ratios return to normal in 5 to 20 minutes. This observation may have significant clinical impact on the decision whether to proceed with further dilatation.

IMPEDANCE CATHETER AND GUIDEWIRE

Our laboratory has recently developed a method for measuring absolute coronary blood flow by using either a standard angioplasty catheter or a guidewire and the indicator-dilution principle.[23, 37, 38] The initial intraluminal device employed was a standard angioplasty catheter modified with the addition of a third lumen that terminates in a small side hole located just proximal to the balloon[37, 38] (Fig 2–2). Impedance measurements are made at the catheter's tip by two pairs of microelectrodes. Impedance is measured at a frequency of 50 kHz and a constant current of approximately 10 μA between the two proximal and distal microelectrodes spaced 2

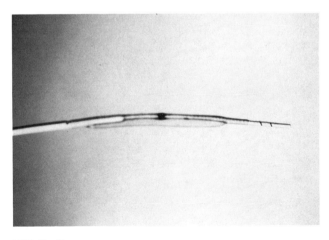

FIG 2–2.
Impedance catheter: Note the side infusion port proximal and the two electrodes distal to the balloon.

mm apart. One-half milliliter of a 5% glucose-in-water solution (D_5W) is injected over a 3- to 6-second period through the proximal port. The solution is hypertonic relative to blood, thereby causing an increase in impedance measurable at the microelectrodes. Absolute coronary blood flow is determined by inverse proportionality to the area under the impedance curve in a manner analogous to the determination of cardiac output with thermodilution catheters. Absolute blood flow is calculated by the following equation: flow = $K_s\, I/A$, where K_s is a sensitivity constant expressing the slope of the impedance D_5W concentration relationship, I is amount of D_5W indicator, and A is the area under the first-pass transit curve. By the indicator-dilution principle, blood flow is determined at the site of introduction of the indicator substance. Subsequent arterial branching does not affect this determination as long as adequate mixing is achieved. The impedance catheter utilizes two factors to ensure adequate indicator mixing. First, the D_5W indicator is sprayed out the side hole in a direction perpendicular to blood flow. Second, the presence of the dilatation balloon causes turbulence, further increasing mixing. Experimental studies have shown that mixing is essentially complete within 1 to 2 cm from the point of ejection. While coronary artery irregularities may further increase mixing, it is unlikely that the impedance catheter could accurately measure absolute blood flow due to partial occlusion of the lumen by the catheter. This is especially problematic for maximal hyperemic blood flow and for both resting and hyperemic flow when the catheter is positioned translesionally. In practice, this necessitates that the catheter be withdrawn proximally in the coronary vessel in order to assess maximal blood flow or coronary flow reserve.

The necessity of withdrawing the impedance catheter proximal to the stenosis led us to develop an impedance guidewire capable of measuring blood flow by using the same principles.[37] We are currently studying a 0.014-in.-diameter guidewire that has a 1-mm electrode gap located 3.5 cm from its tip (Fig 2–3). The tip of the electrode is composed of a spring wire with characteristics analogous to standard angioplasty guidewires. We employ the guidewire through a 2 F "monorail"-type infusion catheter that ejects the D_5W indicator through the catheter's distal side port. This allows the indicator to be infused at a point immediately proximal to the coronary stenosis, with sufficient distance to achieve mixing being provided by the guidewire extending distally across the stenosis. In contrast to the impedance catheter, this much smaller-diameter guidewire has not been found to reduce even hyperemic flow substantially. The guidewire system allows a determination of blood flow through very proximal stenoses, which would not be possible with the catheter system because the point of ejection would be in the aorta or guiding catheter. Attempts to inject the indicator bolus through an end-hole catheter have not proved successful due to incomplete mixing.

Impedance measurements are affected by blood conductivity, vessel volume, and parallel conduction. The unwanted contribution to impedance measurements of parallel conduction is reduced by minimizing the electrode gap. Preliminary studies suggest that vessel cross-sectional area varies inversely with baseline impedance.[38] Although this may enable the catheter and guidewire systems to assess vessel dimensions, this is a complicating feature for the measurement of blood flood. This effect is partially negated by the larger component of parallel conduction contributing to measured impedance that occurs in small vessels, which have decreased intrinsic conductivity. Additionally, partial correction of the effect of vessel diameter is achieved in practice by normalizing the sensitivity constant K_s to baseline impedance values.

Validation of these approaches to measuring absolute coronary blood flow was performed in four phases. In vitro studies in arterial phantoms, experimental studies in canine femoral arteries, experimental studies in canine coronary arteries, and clinical studies during coronary angioplasty have been performed. The catheter

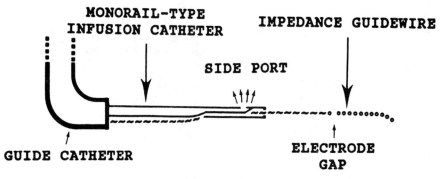

FIG 2–3.
Schematic of an impedance guidewire–infusion catheter system.

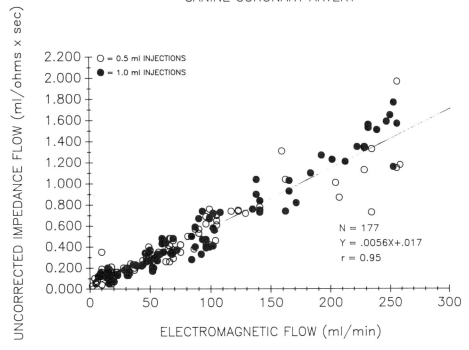

FIG 2–4.
Correlation between the impedance guidewire inverse of the first-pass curve area and electromagnetic flowmeter determinations.

and guidewire systems were found to accurately measure saline flow in plastic tube phantoms ranging from 2 to 4 mm in diameter by employing baseline impedance-corrected sensitivity constants. These data verify that the two basic requirements for application of the indicator-dilution principle are met by this technique, namely, adequacy of mixing and linearity of indicator detection. The latter was additionally validated by direct measure-ment of the linearity of the area under first-pass curves that results from injection of from 0.1- to 2.0-mL indicator boluses.

Due to intrinsic limitations of measuring absolute coronary blood flow, validation of the catheter and guidewire systems was performed in canine femoral arteries by using timed arterial collection as the standard. Blood flow was varied over a wide range from 5 to 300

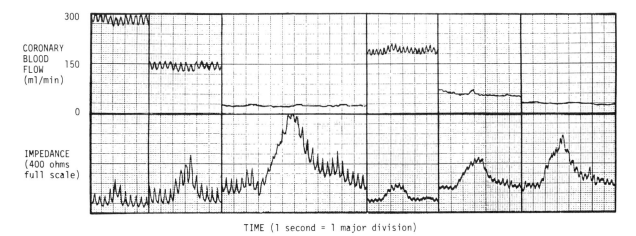

FIG 2–5.
Examples of coronary blood flow and first-pass impedance catheter curves from which absolute coronary blood flow is calculated in a canine coronary artery model.

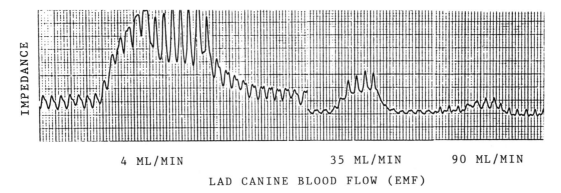

FIG 2–6.
Examples of first-pass, impedance guidewire curves in a canine coronary artery model. *LAD* = left anterior descending; *EMF* = electromagnetic flowmeter.

mL/min by using vessel constriction and vasodilating drugs. Close correlations between catheter and guidewire calculated and timed arterial collection data were found ($r = 0.96$).

Blood flow measurements were also studied in canine coronary vessels ranging in diameter from 2.3 to 3.3 mm by using stenosis and pharmacologically varied blood flow. Again, close correlations were found between impedance catheter and guidewire and electromagnetic flowmeter determinations over a wide range of

flow. A slightly lower correlation coefficient ($r = 0.95$) was found, likely due to intrinsic inaccuracies in electromagnetic flowmeter determination (Fig 2–4). Guidewire measurements were found to be more accurate when a 1.0-mL D_5W bolus was used. Of importance, the injection of the indicator bolus was found to affect intrinsic blood flow minimally. Examples of first-pass impedance catheter and guidewire curves are shown in Figures 2–5 and 2–6, respectively. Injection of the D_5W bolus is seen to cause little change in intrinsic

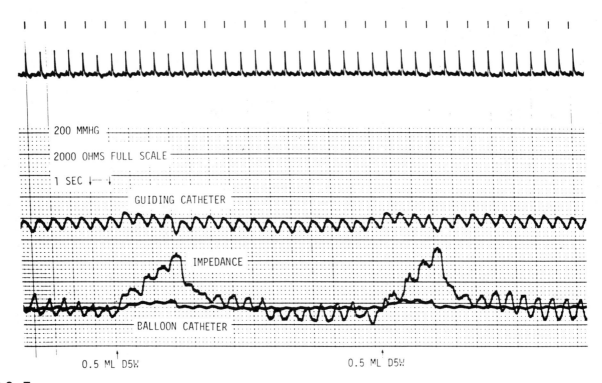

FIG 2–7.
Examples of first-pass impedance catheter tracings obtained during clinical angioplasty of the left anterior descending coronary artery.

coronary blood flow (top panels, Fig 2–5). The inverse relationship between blood flow and area under the first-pass curves is seen in the lower panels (Fig 2–5).

Following successful validation of the impedance catheter in experimental situations, we have started to employ it during clinical angioplasty. Repeated first-pass curves obtained during angioplasty of a mid–left anterior descending coronary stenosis are shown in Figure 2–7. Coronary blood flow was calculated to be approximately 30 mL/min. These findings suggest that it will be clinically possible to measure absolute coronary blood flow in interventional situations by using standard catheter and guidewire systems. It is likely that the impedance guidewire will have the greatest clinical application because it produces the least compromise of the vessel lumen.[39,40]

The major advantages of the impedance guidewire system are that it allows a measurement of absolute coronary blood flow, thus reducing the uncertainty over baseline blood flow that is intrinsic in coronary flow reserve calculations, and interferes minimally with intrinsic flow due to its very small cross-sectional area. Disadvantages are that blood flow cannot be monitored continuously due to the necessity for indicator injection, potential problems with inadequate mixing caused by indicator injection at points of arterial branching, and variability of determinations caused by varying vessel size affecting parallel conduction.

Technological advantages in catheter systems now allow the measurement of relative and absolute coronary blood flow in the catheterization laboratory during interventional procedures. It remains to be proved that these measurements affect interventional and clinical patient outcome. This is likely to occur, however, as techniques become simpler and flow physiology more defined.

REFERENCES

1. Brown BG, Bolson E, Frimer M, et al: Quantitative coronary arteriography: Estimation of dimension, hemodynamic resistance, and atheroma mass of coronary artery lesions using the arteriogram and digital computer. *Circulation* 1977; 55:329.
2. Mancini GBJ, Simon SB, McGillem MJ, et al: Automated quantitative coronary arteriography: In-vivo morphologic and physiologic validation of a rapid method utilizing digital angiography. *Circulation* 1987; 75:452–460.
3. Vogel RA: The radiographic assessment of coronary blood flow parameters. *Circulation* 1985; 72:460–465.
4. Beauman GJ, Vogel RA: Accuracy of individual and panel visual interpretations of coronary arteriograms: Implications for clinical decision. *J Am Coll Cardiol* 1990; 16:108–113.
5. Klocke FJ: Measurements of coronary blood flow and degree of stenosis: Current clinical implications and continuing uncertainties. *J Am Coll Cardiol* 1983; 1:31–42.
6. Wilson RF, Marcus ML, White CW: Prediction of the physiologic significance of coronary artery lesions by quantitative lesion geometry in patients with limited coronary artery disease. *Circulation* 1987; 75:723–732.
7. Zijlstra F, van Ommeren J, Reiber JHC, et al: Does the quantitative assessment of coronary artery dimensions predict the physiologic significance of a coronary stenosis? *Circulation* 1987; 75:1154–1161.
8. Vogel RA: Assessing stenosis significance by coronary arteriography: Are the best variables good enough? *J Am Coll Cardiol* 1988; 12:692–693.
9. LeGrand V, Mancini GBJ, Bates ER, et al: A comparative study of coronary flow reserve, coronary anatomy and the results of radionuclide exercise tests in patients with coronary heart disease. *J Am Coll Cardiol* 1986; 8:1022–1032.
10. Gould KL: Pressure-flow characteristics of coronary stenoses in unsedated dogs at rest and during coronary vasodilation. *Circ Res* 1978; 43:242–248.
11. Harrison DG, White CW, Hiratzka LF, et al: The value of lesion cross-sectional area determined by quantitative coronary angiography in assessing the physiological significance of proximal left anterior descending coronary arterial stenoses. *Circulation* 1984; 69:1111–1119.
12. Marcus ML, Shorton DJ, Johnson MR, et al: Visual estimates of percent diameter coronary stenosis: "A battered gold standard." *J Am Coll Cardiol* 1988; 11:882–885.
13. Gould KL: Percent coronary stenosis: Battered gold standard, pernicious relic or clinical practicality? *J Am Coll Cardiol* 1988; 11:886–888.
14. Zijlstra F, Fioretti P, Reiber JHC, et al: Which cineangiographically assessed anatomic variables correlate best with functional measurements of stenosis severity? A comparison of quantitative analysis of the coronary cineangiogram with measured coronary flow reserve and exercise/redistribution thallium-201 scintigraphy. *J Am Coll Cardiol* 1988; 12:686–691.
15. Serruys PW, Zijlstra F, Reiber HHC, et al: Intracoronary blood flow velocity, reactive hyperemia and coronary blood flow reserve during and following PTCA, in Serruys PW, Simon R, Keatt (eds): *PTCA: An Investigational Tool and a Non-operative Treatment of Acute Ischemia.* Durdrecht, Kluwer, 1990, pp 93–120.
16. Hess OM, McGillem MJ, DeBoe SF, et al: Determination of coronary flow reserve by parametric imaging. *Circulation* 1990; 82:1438–1448.
17. Bates E, Aueron FM, LeGrand V, et al: Comparative long-term effects of coronary artery bypass graft surgery and percutaneous transluminal coronary angioplasty on regional flow reserve. *Circulation* 1985; 72:833–839.
18. Smalling RW: Can the immediate efficacy of coronary angioplasty be adequately assessed? *J Am Coll Cardiol* 1987; 10:261–263.
19. Wilson RF, Johnson MR, Marcus ML, et al: The effect of coronary angioplasty on coronary flow reserve. *Circulation* 1988; 77:873–885.
20. Zijlstra F, den Boer A, Reiber JHC, et al: Assessment of immediate and long-term functional results of percutaneous transluminal coronary angioplasty. *Circulation* 1988; 78:15–24.

21. Ultstra F, Reiber JC, Juilliere Y, et al: Normalization of coronary flow reserve by percutaneous transluminal coronary angiplasty. *Am J Cardiol* 1988; 61:55–60.
22. Kern MJ, Deligonal U, Vandormael M, et al: Impaired coronary vasodilator reserve in the immediate post-coronary angioplasty period: Analysis of coronary flow velocity indexes and regional cardiac venous efflux. *J Am Coll Cardiol* 1989; 13:860–872.
23. Vogel RA: Transcatheter assessment of coronary artery anatomy and blood flow, in Vogel JHK, King SB III (eds): *Interventional Cardiology: Future Directions.* St Louis, Mosby–Year Book, 1989, pp 487–498.
24. Ganz W, Tamura K, Marcus HS, et al: Measurement of coronary sinus blood flow by continuous thermodilution in man. *Circulation* 1971; 44:181.
25. Marcus ML: *The Coronary Circulation in Health and Disease.* New York, McGraw-Hill, 1983, pp 47–50.
26. Kurita A, Azorin J, Granier A, et al: Estimation of coronary reserve in left anterior descending and circumflex coronary arteries by regional thermodilution technique. *Jpn Circ J* 1982; 46:964–973.
27. Hartley CJ: Review of intracoronary Doppler catheters, in Bom N, Roelandt J (eds): *Intravascular Ultrasound: Techniques, Developments, Clinical Perspectives.* Dordrecht, Kluwer, 1989, pp 159–168.
28. Benchimol A, Stegall HF, Gartlan JL: New method to measure phasic coronary blood velocity in man. *Am Heart J* 1971; 81:93–101.
29. Hartley CJ, Cole JS: A single-crystal ultrasonic catheter-tip velocity probe. *Med Instrum* 1974; 8:241–243.
30. Cole JS, Hartley CJ: The pulsed Doppler coronary catheter: Preliminary report of a new technique for measuring rapid changes in coronary artery flow velocity in man. *Circulation* 1977; 56:18–25.
31. Wilson RF, Laughlin DE, Ackell PH, et al: Transluminal, subselective measurement of coronary artery blood flow velocity and vasodilator reserve in man. *Circulation* 1985; 72:82–92.
32. Sibley DH, Millar HD, Hartley CJ, et al: Subselective measurement of coronary blood flow velocity using a steerable Doppler catheter. *J Am Coll Cardiol* 1986; 8:1332–1340.
33. Serruys PW, Jullier EY, Zijlstra F, et al: Coronary blood flow velocity during percutaneous coronary angioplasty as a guide for assessment of the functional results. *Am J Cardiol* 1988; 61:253–259.
34. Wilson RF, White CW: Intracoronary papaverine: An ideal coronary vasodilator for studies of the coronary circulation in conscious humans. *Circulation* 1986; 73:444.
35. Doucette JW, Corl PD, Payne HM, et al: Validation of a Doppler guidewire for assessment of coronary arterial flow (abstract). *Circulation* 1990; 82(suppl 3):621.
36. Segal J, Sheehan D, Corl PD, et al: A Doppler guidewire used to assess coronary flow during PTCA in humans (abstract). *Circulation* 1990; 82(supp 3):622.
37. Vogel RA, Martin LW: Transcatheter coronary artery diagnostic techniques including impedance-catheter and impedance guidewire measurement of absolute coronary blood flow. *Tex Heart J* 1989; 16:195–203.
38. Martin LW, Johnson RA, Scott H, et al: Impedance measurement of absolute coronary blood flow using an angioplasty catheter: A validation study. *Am Heart J* 1990, in press.
39. Martin LW, Vogel RA, Johnson RA, et al: Impedance measurement of absolute blood flow using an angioplasty guidewire (abstract). *J Am Coll Cardiol* 1989; 13:194.
40. Vogel RA, Martin LW, Johnson RA: Impedance measurement of absolute arterial diameter using a standard angioplasty catheter (abstract). *J Am Coll Cardiol* 1988; 11:130.

3

The Doppler Guidewire: A New Method to Evaluate Coronary Artery Flow During Percutaneous Transluminal Coronary Angioplasty

Jerome Segal, M.D.

Allan Ross, M.D.

An easy-to-use and highly reliable method for measuring coronary artery flow (velocity, volume, and pattern) has long been the goal of investigators and clinicians alike. The current assessment of coronary artery disease in man relies primarily on angiographic determination of the severity of stenosis. The accuracy of angiography has been questioned due to significant intraobserver and interobserver variability[1-4] and a lack of correlation to postmortem studies.[5-7] Clearly, a means of accurately measuring coronary artery flow would provide additional information concerning the physiologic impact of a coronary stenosis and the results of pharmacologic or mechanical interventions such as balloon angioplasty, laser angioplasty, atherectomy, and stent placement.

The most commonly utilized methods of measuring coronary artery blood flow have included coronary sinus thermodilution, indicator dilution including impedance measurement, digital subtraction angiography, angiographic contrast transit time measurement, xenon 133 scintigraphy, and positron emission tomography. None of these approaches have gained widespread acceptance due to problems with accuracy or reproducibility and because of the cumbersome nature of the systems that limits their use during routine angiography.

Recently catheter-based Doppler ultrasound systems have been extensively investigated as a practical, simple, and relatively inexpensive method of obtaining subselective coronary artery flow measurements. However,

problems exist with the use of these Doppler catheters. Doppler catheters provide measurement of flow velocity only in the proximal coronary artery and are sensitive to any changes in vessel cross-sectional area, flow profile, angulation, or position. Additionally, the size of these Doppler catheters (3 F or 1 mm outside diameter) relative to the size of the coronary arteries and stenoses can cause significant disturbance of flow that extends well beyond the location of the Doppler sample volume[8] and results in an underestimation of true flow velocity. Also, the use of zero–cross frequency techniques to estimate blood flow velocity with Doppler catheters has been shown to be inaccurate in disturbed flow fields such as those beyond a coronary stenosis.[9-11]

Despite these shortcomings, Doppler catheters continue to be the primary method of measuring subselective flow and hyperemic response in humans during cardiac catheterization and angioplasty procedures. Clearly, better methods of evaluating changes in phasic coronary artery flow before and after revascularization would contribute significantly to our understanding of the physiologic response of the coronary circulation to various interventions.

In animals, studies of phasic coronary artery flow have revealed changes in the normal diastolic predominant pattern to a less diastolic predominant pattern, with greater systolic flow contribution occurring with increasing severity of the epicardial coronary artery

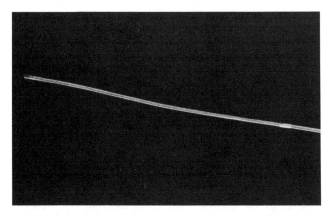

FIG 3–1.
Doppler coronary artery guidewire.

stenosis.[12-14] This decrease in the diastolic/systolic flow ratio (DSVR) with increasing epicardial stenosis may be explained by the increased influence of an epicardial stenosis on flow during periods of low vascular resistance (diastole) as compared with periods of high vascular resistance (systole).[15] Alternative explanations using the intramyocardial "pump" model of Spaan et al.[16] suggest that epicardial resistance will become the limiting factor for antegrade coronary flow during periods of no reverse intramyocardial flow and low distal arterial and venous resistance (diastole). However, during systole, reverse coronary flow from the intramyocardial pump continues to "charge" the epicardial coronary capacitance at the expense of increasing the transstenotic (aortic-intramyocardial) pressure difference. The influence

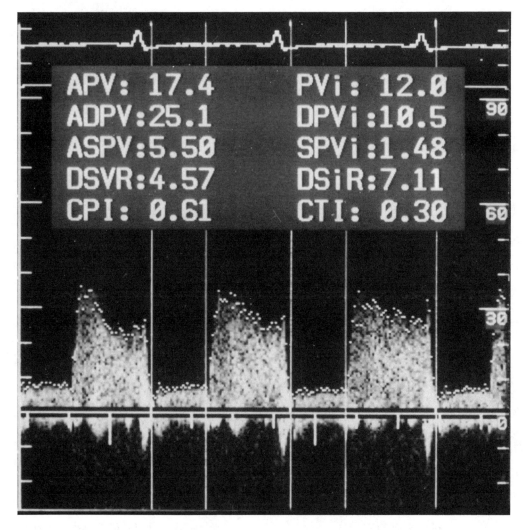

FIG 3–2.
Doppler velocity spectral display. The *dotted line* represents instantaneous peak velocity tracking. *APV* = time average peak velocity; *PVi* = peak velocity integral; *ADPV* = average diastolic peak velocity; *DPVi* = diastolic peak velocity integral; *ASPV* = average systolic peak velocity; *SPVi* = systolic peak velocity integral; *DSVR* = diastolic/systolic velocity ratio; *DSiR* = diastolic/systolic velocity integral ratio; CPI = pulsatility index; CTI = tracking index.

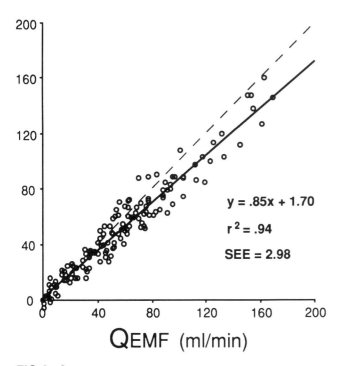

FIG 3–3.
Plot of Doppler-determined flow vs. electromagnetic flow in the proximal segment of the left circumflex coronary artery in four dogs. Doppler flow was estimated as half the spectral peak velocity times the area. This assumes a parabolic velocity profile with the space average mean velocity equal to half the spectral peak velocity. The area was determined by using quantitative angiography. *SEE* = standard error of the estimate. (From Doucette JW, Corl PD, Payne HM, et al: *Circulation* 1992; 85:1899–1911. Used with permission.)

of increasing forward flow resistance due to the epicardial stenosis and increasing transstenotic pressure drop tend to cancel each other and result in little flow change during systole.

Recently, similar observations have been obtained in man through the use of an 80-channel pulsed Doppler velocimeter and surgically placed epicardial coronary artery probe.[9, 10] Intraoperative measurement of poststenotic velocities revealed high systolic flow components and reduced diastolic flow components. After bypass grafting, the velocity patterns distal to the graft insertion returned to a normal diastolic predominant flow pattern with relatively little flow during systole. These changes in diastolic-systolic flow pattern appear to parallel similar changes noted in the acute animal models tested. These changes in the diastolic-systolic flow patterns may provide important information concerning the physiologic significance of a coronary artery stenosis and the hemodynamic result of a revascularization procedure such as angioplasty.

Recently, a low-profile Doppler angioplasty guidewire

with a spectral analysis flow velocimeter (Cardiometrics, Inc., Mountain View, Calif) has been developed for use during percutaneous transluminal coronary angioplasty (PTCA). The Doppler guidewire is constructed of a 175-cm-long, 0.018-in.-diameter, flexible, steerable guidewire with a 12-MHz piezoelectric ultrasound transducer integrated onto its tip (Fig 3–1). The transducer produces a relatively broad-beam ultrasound signal (25-degree divergence angle) with an estimated sample volume size of 2.25 mm (diameter) at a range gate depth of 5 mm.

The Doppler velocimeter consists of a real-time spectral analysis system with a scrolling gray-scale display (Fig 3–2). The Doppler system has the capacity to compute a variety of on-line spectral parameters including peak velocity, time average peak velocity, diastolic and systolic velocity integrals, and DSVRs (see below).

The Doppler guidewire system was validated in both in vitro and in vivo models of coronary artery flow,[17] and Doppler-derived volume flow was shown to be highly correlated with electromagnetic flow (Fig 3–3). Doppler flow was calculated by using the product of the mean Doppler velocity (estimated as half the spectral peak velocity) and the vessel area, obtained from quantitative angiography.

A recent multicenter clinical trial of the Doppler guidewire has been completed.[18] Blood flow velocity, phasic diastolic/systolic velocity patterns, DSVRs, and coronary flow reserve were measured, both proximal

Distal Average Peak Velocity

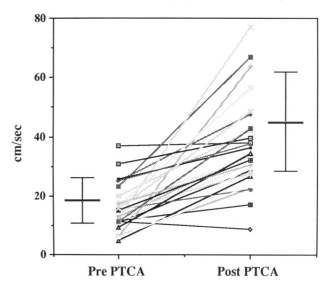

FIG 3–4.
Time average peak velocity measured distal to a coronary stenosis pre- and post-PTCA. ± = Mean of the time average peak velocity in the distal coronary artery, ± standard deviation (*P* < .01).

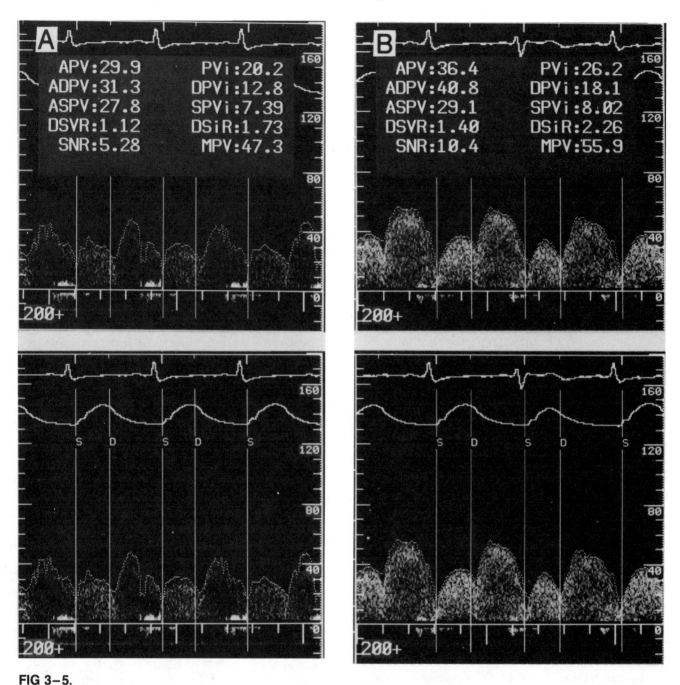

FIG 3–5.
A, Doppler velocity measurement in the left anterior descending coronary artery (LAD) distal to a 90% stenosis. **B,** Doppler velocity measurements in the distal portion of the LAD 2 minutes following PTCA. *(Continued.)*

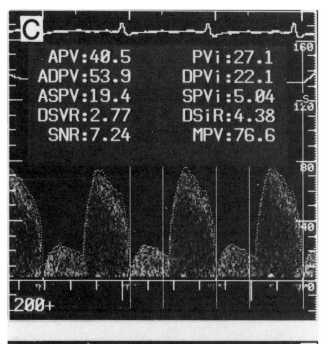

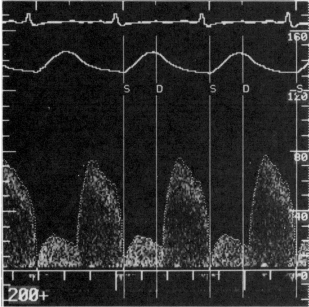

FIG 3–5 (cont.).
C, Doppler velocity measurements in the distal segment of the LAD coronary artery 12 minutes following PTCA. Acronym definitions are as in Figure 3–2.

Distal Diastolic/Systolic Velocity Ratio

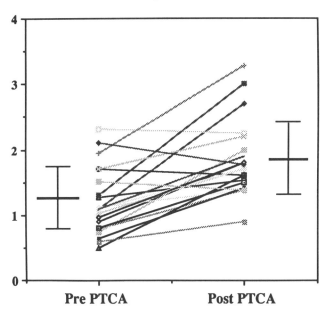

Pre PTCA   **Post PTCA**

FIG 3–6.
Diastolic/systolic velocity ratio (DSVR) pre- and post-PTCA as measured in distal coronary arteries. + = mean distal DSVR, ± standard deviation ($P < .01$).

and distal to significant coronary artery stenoses in 38 patients undergoing PTCA of the left anterior descending and/or left circumflex coronary arteries.

Significant improvement in mean time–average peak velocity was noted in distal coronary arteries following PTCA (pre-PTCA, 19 ± 12 cm/sec; post-PTCA, 35 ± 16 cm/sec; $P < .01$) (Fig 3–4). As noted in previous studies, the mean coronary flow reserve remained unchanged following PTCA (1.6 ± 1.0 vs. 1.5 ± 0.5; $P > .10$), with some patients showing improvement while others demonstrated no change or even a decrease in coronary flow reserve. Before angioplasty, phasic flow velocity patterns distal to a stenosis were noted to be abnormal with increased systolic flow components and decreased diastolic components (Fig 3–5). Following PTCA, abnormal phasic velocity patterns in the distal coronary arteries generally returned to normal with significant increases in mean DSVR (1.3 ± 0.5 vs. 1.9 ± 0.6; $P < .01$) (Fig 3–6). Normalization of these phasic velocity patterns often required up to 10 minutes following PTCA to reach maximum DSVR values (Fig 3–5,B and C).

The Doppler guidewire appears capable of characterizing phasic diastolic and systolic flow velocity patterns in distal coronary arteries and was easily incorporated into the clinical angioplasty procedure. As previously demonstrated, coronary flow reserve measurements made immediately following angioplasty were of limited utility in assessing the hemodynamic effects of the procedure. Alternative measurements made in the distal coronary arteries such as a change in absolute distal velocity or DSVR following coronary angioplasty were more important in assessing the clinical outcome of the procedure.

Volumetric flow measurements may also be performed by using Doppler guidewire–determined spectral peak velocity and vessel area obtained from any of a number of available on-line, quantitative angiographic systems.

Additional studies are currently under way to evaluate these various hemodynamic measurements obtained by using the Doppler guidewire. The information derived from these studies should improve our understanding of the physiologic effects of various coronary interventions.

REFERENCES

1. Detre KM, Wright E, Murphy MC, et al: Observer agreement in evaluating coronary angiograms. *Circulation* 1975; 52:979–986.
2. Zir LM, Miller SW, Dinsomore RE, et al: Interobserver variability in coronary angiography. *Circulation* 1978; 53:627–632.
3. DeRouen TA, Murray JA, Owen W: Variability analysis of coronary arteriograms. *Circulation* 1979; 55:324–328.
4. Galbraith JE, Murphy ML, DeSoyza N: Coronary angiogram interpretation: Interobserver variability. *JAMA* 1978; 240:2053–2056.
5. Hutchins GM, et al: Correlation of coronary arteriograms and left ventriculograms with postmortem studies. *Circulation* 1977; 53:32–37.
6. Grondin CM, Dyrda I, Pasternac A, et al: Discrepancies between cineangiographic and postmortem findings in patients with coronary artery disease and recent myocardial revascularization. *Circulation* 1974; 49:703–708.
7. Arnett EN, et al: Coronary artery narrowing in coronary heart disease: Comparison of cineangiographic and necropsy findings. *Ann Intern Med* 1979; 91:350–356.
8. Tadaoka S, Kagiyama M, Hiramatsu O, et al: Accuracy of a 20 MHz Doppler catheter coronary velocimeter for measurement of coronary blood flow velocity. *Cathet Cardiovasc Diagn* 1990; 12:205.
9. Kajiya F, Ogasawara Y, Tsujioka K, et al: Evaluation of human coronary blood flow with an 80 channel 20 MHz pulsed Doppler velocimeter and zero-cross and Fourier transform methods during cardiac surgery. *Circulation* 1986; 74(Suppl 3):53.
10. Kajiya F, Ogasawara Y, Tsujioka K, et al: Analysis of flow characteristics in post-stenotic regions of the human coronary artery during bypass graft surgery. *Circulation* 1987; 76:1092.
11. Johnson EL, Yock PG, Hargrave VK, et al: Assessment of severity of coronary stenoses using a Doppler catheter: Validation of a method based on the continuity equation. *Circulation* 1989; 80:625.
12. Gould KL, Lipscomb K, Hamilton GW: Physiologic basis for assessing critical coronary stenosis. *Am J Cardiol* 1974; 33:87.
13. Furuse A, Klopp EH, Brawley RK, et al: Hemodynamic determinations in the assessment of distal coronary artery disease. *J Surg Res* 1975; 19:25.
14. Wiesner TF, Levesque MJ, Rooz E, et al: Epicardial coronary blood flow including the presence of stenoses and aortocoronary bypasses — II. Experimental comparison and parametric investigations. *Trans Am Soc Mech Engineering* 1988; 110:144.
15. Logan SE: On the fluid mechanics of human coronary artery stenosis. *IEEE Trans Biomed Eng* 1975; 22:327.
16. Spaan JAE, Breuls NPW, Laird JD: Diastolic-systolic coronary flow differences are caused by intramyocardial pump action in the anesthetized dog. *Circ Res* 1981; 49:584.
17. Doucette JW, Corl PD, Payne HM, et al: Validation of a Doppler guidewire for intravascular measurement of coronary artery flow velocity. *Circulation* 1992; 85:1899–1911.
18. Segal J, Kern MJ, Scott NA, et al: Alterations of phasic coronary artery flow velocity in man during percutaneous coronary angioplasty. *J Am Coll Cardiol* (in press).

4

Clinical Experience With a New Angioscopic System

Giancarlo Biamino, M.D.

Johann C. Ragg, M.D.

In the last few years in addition to balloon angioplasty, a wide variety of transcutaneous revascularization procedures have been developed to intervene in patients with peripheral or coronary artery disease.

Whether the intervention is intended to reduce the obstructing sclerotic or thrombotic material by laser ablation, by mechanical atherectomy, or by dilating the artery with conventional percutaneous transluminal angioplasty, it is increasingly thought that additional information is needed to better visualize and perhaps to quantitate the blocking atherosclerotic plaque before, during, and after treatment.

In fact, the conventional or computer-assisted "gold standard" angiography permits an approximate assessment of the narrowing of the lumen but only limited information about the extent of the atheroma and very poor indication regarding size, composition, and interluminal location of the obstructing material. The first experiments using rigid endoscopes during vascular surgery[1-3] indicated that intraluminal examination may partially overcome the angiographic limitations.[4-14] Further development of thinner, more flexible fiber-optic systems led to increased application in vascular surgery and opened the possibility of transcutaneous inspection of the vascular lumen.[11, 15-33]

Initial limitations of the general application of angioscopy were the quality of the color image and the size and the stiffness of the optical probes. The major problem restricting the transcutaneous use of angioscopic systems, however, remained the displacement of blood necessary to have a clear view of the obstructing material or the endovascular structures.

Technological advances in the form of a new microangioscopy system and the development of disposable guiding catheters with an inflatable cuff permitting the blockage of blood flow intermittently were regarded as prerequisites for a systematic clinical comparison of these techniques during peripheral intervention with uniplanar angiography.

The present study was conducted to validate this new system in peripheral vessel and to compare angiography performed routinely before, during, and after excimer laser angioplasty with angioscopic findings.

TECHNICAL ASPECTS

The angioscope system used is a modular angioscope system (MASY, A.D. Krauth, Hamburg, Germany) (Fig 4–1). One of the main components is a 23-g, light, miniature CCD color camera (AngioCam) (see Table 4–1). The camera is 17.5 mm in diameter and 43 mm in length. The pictures are composed of 360,000 pixels with a resolution of 360 lines horizontally and 420 lines vertically.

A minimum illumination of 3 lux is needed. Via a TV adapter (PAL or NTSC) the camera is connected to an ocular system focusing from 1 mm to infinity. If required, an additional zoom function permits magnification of intravascular structures during intervention.

A special high-power light source (SHL 1000 W) with electronic regulation provides a light intensity 10 to 15 times higher than the usual halogen lamps. The color temperature is 5800 K and corresponds to the spectrum of sunlight.

A flexible light guide consisting of 25,000 single glass

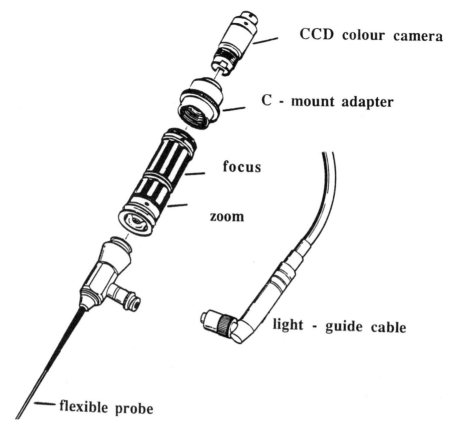

FIG 4−1.
Components of the microangioscope system (MASY).

fibers about 5 μm in diameter and 3.0 m in length (outside diameter, 8.0 mm; active diameter, 3.5 mm) connects the light source with the optical probe. The steerable highly flexible probes (AngioFlex) have a large amount of very thin fibers (2.0 to 3.0 μm). They are available in several sizes (0.5 to 1.4 mm) and incorporate 5,000 to 12,000 fibers glued together in a special procedure that prevents them from breaking and permits a bending radius between 20 and 40 mm. A highly sophisticated lens system (SELFOC) is mounted to the tip of the probe, so that different angle views can be achieved that range from 50 degrees to the standard of 70 degrees and to the fish-eye view of 140 degrees.

The displacement of blood that is needed during inspection is achieved by using specially developed guiding catheters (7 or 9 F) supplied with a silicone balloon. The cuff is mounted just at the end of a 2.5-mm metal tip marker, is 10 mm long, and is inflatable up to 12 mm with a mixture of saline and contrast medium. After the blood flow is blocked by intermittently inflating the balloon, the optical probe is positioned just at the tip of the guiding catheter, and heparinized saline is flushed through the Y connector, a direct observation of the en-

dovascular structures on a high-resolution monitor (Sony, PVM 1440-QM) becomes possible simultaneous with storage of the images on a U-matic video recorder (Sony, VO 9600 SP). By using a high-quality color printer (Sony, UP 5000 P), on-line documentation of the observed endovascular structures is also possible. Because an exact anatomic correlation of parallelly recorded angioscopic and angiographic images is very time-consuming and almost impossible, the use of a video production system (FOR.A VPS-500) seems to be mandatory for an adequate documentation. The video mixer permits the screen to be split into different patterns so that simultaneous evaluation and storage of angioscopic insights and fluoroscopic or angiographic findings become possible.

PATIENTS

Seventy-six of 204 patients undergoing percutaneous excimer laser−assisted angioplasty (functional class III and IV) had angioscopic evaluation of the affected artery.

TABLE 4–1.

Components of the Modular Angioscopy System (MASY)

Miniature CCD—color video camera (AngioCam)
  PAL or NTSC system
  Pixels: 360,000
  Resolution: 360 lines horizontal, 420 lines vertical
  Minimal illumination, 3 lux; operating voltage, 12 V (4 W); electronic shutter, 1/1,000 sec
  Ocular: luminous intensity, 1:1.6; focus, 1 mm to infinity
  Weight: 23 g
  Length: 43.0 mm
  Diameter: 17.5 mm
  Length: 67.0 mm
  Diameter: 27.0 mm
Illumination
  High-power light source (1,000 W): color temperature 5,800 K; white light corresponding to the
    spectrum of sunlight
  Flexible light conductor: 25,000 single glass fibers of 5-μm diameter; length, 3.0 m; outside
    diameter, 8.0 mm; active diameter, 3.5 mm

Flexible Probes (AngioFlex)

		Glass Fibers			
		Imaging		Illumination	Angle View (SELFOC Lens System)
Diameter (mm)	Length (m)	Diameter (mm)	n	(n)	(degrees)
1.4	0.5–1.5	2.0–3.0	12,000	6,000	70 (opt., 140)
0.96	0.5–1.5	2.0–3.0	10,000	4,000	70 (opt., 50)
0.7	0.5–1.5	2.0–3.0	7,000	2,500	70 (opt., 50)
0.5	1.0–1.5	2.0–3.0	5,000	2,500	70

Guiding Catheters

		Diameter		Balloon	
Type	Length (cm)	Outside (F)	Inside (mm)	Length (mm)	Max. Inflatable Diameter (mm)
Peripheral	60	9	1.6	10	8
	80	7	1.3	10	12

Imaging/Documentation
  High-resolution color monitor (Sony PVM 1440-QM)
  U-matic video recorder (Sony VO 9600 P)
  Video printer (Sony UP-5000 P), PAL, 256 color steps
  Video production system (FOR.A VPS-500)

All patients were informed of and accepted the additional investigation. This group included 52 men and 24 women whose mean age was 65.5 years. In 56 cases the major region of interest was the distal part of the superficial femoral artery (SFA), in 15 cases the popliteal and trifurcation areas were inspected, and in 5 cases a retrograde observation of totally occluded pelvic arteries was possible.

In the majority of patients the region of interest was inspected before intervention, after lasering, and after final balloon dilatation.

In 25 cases an endovascular ultrasound examination was performed.

ANGIOSCOPIC PROTOCOL

After local anesthesia a hemostatic sheath (8 or 9 F) is introduced via the antegrade puncture of the ipsilateral common artery into the SFA.

Preliminary characterization of the obstructed segment is obtained with baseline angiography. After road mapping and storage of the vascular area to be inspected, the angioscope guiding catheter is first positioned in front of the obstruction. Heparin (5,000 IU) is injected through the guiding catheter. The optical probe is then introduced into the guiding catheter via a conventional Y connector used for PTCA (Advanced

Cardiovascular Systems [ACS]) and advanced under fluoroscopic control to the tip of the catheter.

After the cuff of the guiding catheter is inflated and saline is flushed through one arm of the Y connector, displacement of blood is achieved and permits undisturbed analysis and documentation of the intravascular structures simultaneously with angiographic or fluoroscopic correlation in 85% of cases.

The same procedure is repeated after each relevant step of the intervention.

Both the introduction of the guiding catheter and the inflation of the silicone balloon are completely pain free. Clear angiography-related complications have not been observed in this preliminary study.

Each transcutaneous excimer laser angioplasty is prolonged about 20 to 30 minutes by angioscopy. Furthermore, it must be remembered that the simultaneous recording of fluoroscopic images increases the irradiation time at least 10 minutes per intervention.

OBSERVATIONS

In all but six cases the angioscopic system could be advanced to the lesion. The six failed cases showed multiple proximal stenoses blocking safe advance of the guiding catheter so that the major region of interest could not be approached. In five cases it was not possible to sufficiently replace blood with saline solution because of intensive retrograde blood flow.

In the case of a total occlusion or a subtotal stenosis prior to the intervention the guiding catheter wedged the artery so that inflation of the silicone balloon was not necessary.

Visualization was obtained by injecting a few milliliters of saline with a hand-controlled syringe. A clear view of a few seconds to 45 seconds was maintained, depending on the collateral or retrograde flow.

The degree of visualization of the target was excellent or good in the majority of cases.

Because of the 70-degree view of the 0.96- or 1.4-mm optical probes the entire lumen of the vessel could be observed. Only in a few cases was coaxial alignment of the probe not achieved after inflation of the cuff.

The intimal surface of a normal peripheral artery is smooth and whitish gray (Fig 4–2). Yellowish areas indicate infiltration of atheromatous material (Plate 1).

A yellowish intima in combination with helix-like, irregularly undulating folds has to be considered a lipomatous-sclerotic, nonobstructing adhesion of the vessel wall. These changes are often observed in the proximal segments of distally obstructed femoral arter-

ies. Angiographically such arteries frequently show "mural calcification."

Independently of stenotic or occlusive lesions, parietal thrombus is a very common finding with small atheromatous plaques (Plate 2).

It was extremely surprising to find that spontaneous floating structures are a frequent phenomenon in the arterial system. However, such floating or apparently loose structures as intimal flaps, atheromatous material partly detached from the vessel wall, or thrombotic material were never observed in a normal artery segment.

The surface of the more or less craglike atheroma is in the majority of the cases smooth and yellowish. Only in the case of a quite marked calcification is surface disruption observed, and the obstruction assumes a florid, sometimes coral cliff–like aspect. Hemorrhagic or thrombotic infiltrations of the atheroma are regular findings.

The position, configuration, and extension of the obstructing sclerotic material show an impressive variability. Consequently, it is not possible at this time to classify the different types of atheroma. It is important to stress the fact that relevant atheroma was observed in angiographically normal vessels.

The situation in the case of a complete occlusion of the artery seems to be different. In our experience it is possible to classify the type and to estimate the age of the occlusion. It is easy to recognize when a thrombotic or predominantly thrombotic occlusion has occurred. In the case of a mixed obstruction, angioscopy clearly permits one to identify whether the thrombotic material was the definitive factor in obstructive blockage of the vessel.

In line with a history of claudication symptoms, we could observe that 3- to 6-month old obstructions assume a light red, partially whitish discoloration. Fibrotic occlusions show a whitish gray surface. Older occlusions are frequently characterized by a tissue-like brownish structure (Figs 4–3 to 4–5; Plates 3 and 4). In such cases a discontinuity of the vessel structures, often observed in conventional ultrasound analysis, is a sign for potential perforation during laser recanalization.[34]

In 26 cases we could perform angioscopic analysis after excimer laser recanalization. In the majority of successful procedures a relatively smooth channel could be observed, without signs of "dottering" or thermic or mechanical damage. In contrast, after final balloon dilatation, it was found that serious wall injuries may occur independently of type, location, and extension of the obstruction.

A consistent finding was the presence of intimal flaps after intervention. Particularly in cases with relevant laceration of the intimal and subintimal layers, with re-

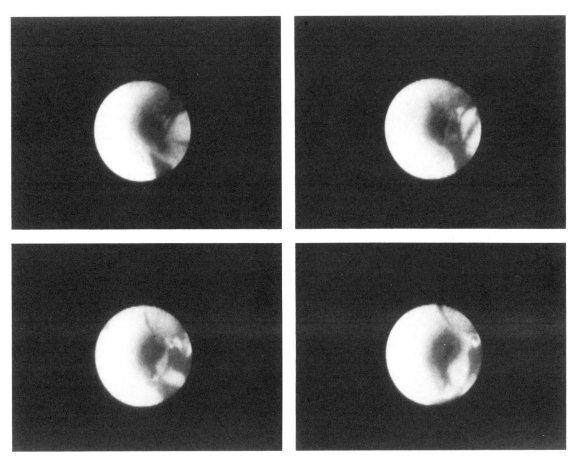

FIG 4–2.
Normal whitish gray intimal surface.

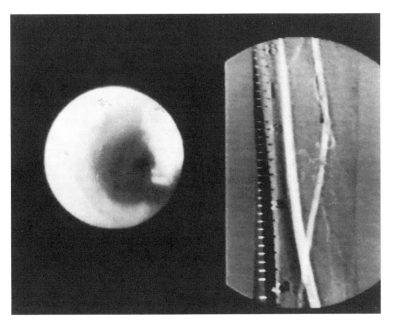

FIG 4–3.
Simultaneous recording of the "roadmapping" and arterioscopic views. The optical probe has reached cm 30 in the mid SFA. A calcified rugged plaque (1 to 3 o'clock) is observed around a floating fresh thrombus in a moderately sclerotic SFA.

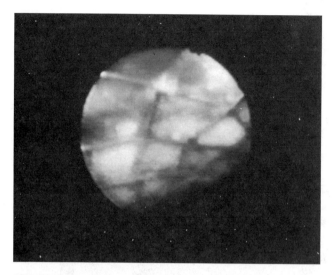

FIG 4–4.
Angioscopic view of a Strecker stent implanted in the left common iliacal artery after a PTCA-induced split and consequent instability of the vessel wall.

maining extensive parietal thrombi, or with a longitudinal cleft or dissection of the fractured plaque, the final angioscopy shows to what extent this new intravascular imaging technique revealed lesions that had been either nonvisualized or underrated by angiography.

DISCUSSION

During the last few years diagnostic procedures and percutaneous treatment of vascular obstructive disease have undergone a unique technological development: replacement of old and the introduction of new concepts and limits in cardioangiology.

The interventionist demands more and more exact information about the endovascular structures from modern imaging systems in order to improve the primary success rate and to ameliorate the long-term results. The long list of demands for improvement of imaging systems indicates that illuminating shadows of pathologic changes by the "gold standard" angiography no longer fulfills the expectations in interventional cardioangiology.[1, 16, 30]

On the basis of the results presented in this paper and our clinical impression, the angioscopic system used is a technological step permitting high-quality endovascular evaluation of diseased atheromatous arteries.

Operating in the spectrum of sunlight the MASY angioscopy system allows direct visualization of anatomic details previously not identifiable by angiography.

One potential hazard of angioscopy is trauma to the artery[20, 26] even when introducing the angioscopy sys-

tem or inflating the cuff of the guiding catheter and intermittently blocking blood flow.

The risk of injury to the vessel wall might be higher after overlapping balloon dilatations in the peripheral bed. In fact, after looking at ruptured plaques, dissections, or floating thrombotic material, in some areas we decided not to inspect the artery extensively after intervention.

Nevertheless, as previous experience has confirmed,[14, 30, 31, 33] angioscopy seems to be safe and should be routinely used as a diagnostic tool without complications. One of the major problems limiting the acceptance of this technique was the difficulty in using such instruments in flowing blood.[26, 31] In the past, a relatively large volume of infusate was necessary to displace blood,[19, 20, 26, 30, 31] but this only permitted an observation time of few seconds. The guiding catheter used in this study permits one to minimize the amount of saline infusion to a few milliliters per intervention and simultaneously prolong the inspection time. Furthermore, a relevant technological step permitting the continuous simultaneous correlation of angiographic and angioscopic findings was the incorporation of a video mixer in the system.

These video angiographic-angioscopic recordings will permit one to exactly evaluate the pathophysiologic history of intimal flaps or shredding, deep cracking of plaque, stenoses, or dissections in follow-up studies and contribute to solving problems concerning restenosis or pharmacologic effects.

Furthermore, video angioscopy yields information not demonstrated by angiography[11, 18, 22, 24, 26, 27, 31] and expands our understanding particularly with regard to pathologic changes induced by mechanical intervention in chronic vessel occlusion. It also may provide a new insight into the progression or regression process of vascular atherosclerotic disease.

Particularly for the diagnosis of intravascular thrombi, dissections, and nonobstructing atheroma, this study has further documented the lack of sensitivity of single-plane angiography, normally used in routine peripheral interventions. On the other hand, the actual sensitivity and specifity of angioscopy in the diagnosis of intravascular pathology remains unknown because the number of peripheral segments examined in this study is relatively small and thus statistically inconclusive.

Although the angioscopic findings demonstrate that angiography underestimated the extent of atheroma,[26] the problem of quantification of the degree of stenosis before and after intervention remains an unsolved problem for this new technique. As a consequence, only after an angioscopic calibration method has been established[31] that permits a real quantitative analysis of coronary and

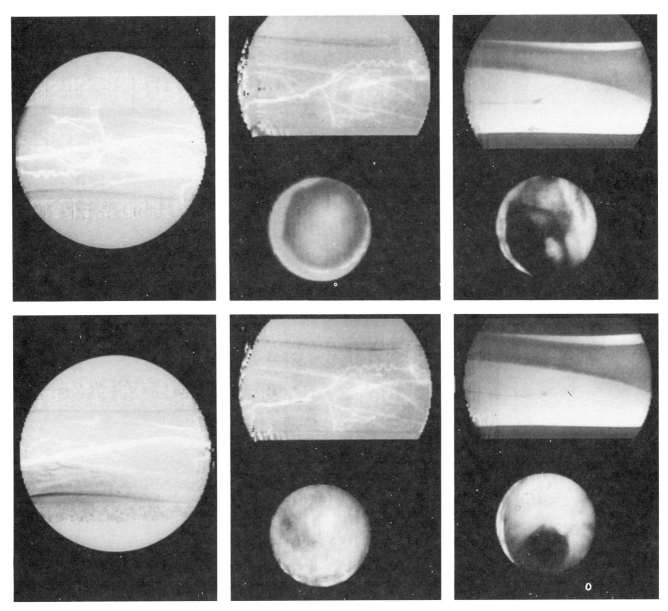

FIG 4–5.
Laser-assisted recanalization of an occluded SFA. The *left upper frame* shows the severe atherosclerosis of the mid SFA 1 cm in front of the occlusion. Corresponding to the angiographic picture at 12 o'clock the origin of the side branch is observed. The *right upper frame* shows the smooth fibrotic surface of the total occlusion. It was possible to pass the obstruction with a 7 F AIS (American Interventional Systems) catheter. Observe the smooth entrance of the channel achieved without signs of thermal or mechanical damage *(left below).* After final PTCA an excellent angiographic result was achieved. The angioscopic views indicate a laceration of the subintimal layer after balloon dilatation.

peripheral vessel obstructions can angioscopy be accepted as a new gold standard.

Novelty is not enough to replace well-established techniques. It is our opinion that angiography will remain superior for visualizing the entire vascular bed; video angioscopy, after some technical limitations are overcome, will be routinely used for assessing the vascu-lar interior and surface, and ultrasound could be of relevance for evaluating the blood vessel wall.

REFERENCES

1. Looking inside arteries (editorial). *Lancet,* 1987; 2:374–375.

2. Towne J: Vascular endoscopy: Useful tool or interesting toy. *Surgery* 1977; 82:415–419.

3. Vollmar J, Junghanns K: Die Arterioskopie. *Langenbecks Arch Klin Chir* 1969; 325:1201.

4. Baxter BT, Rizzo RJ, Flinn WR, et al: A comparative study of intraoperative angioscopy and completion arteriography following femorodistal bypass. *Arch Surg* 1990; 125:997–1003.

5. Chaux A, Lee M, Blanche C, et al: Intraoperative coronary angioscopy: Technique and results in initial 58 patients. *J Cardiovasc Surg* 1986; 92:972–976.

6. Fleisher HL, Thompson BW, McGowan T: Angioscopically monitored saphenous vein valvulotomy. *J Vasc Surg* 1986; 4:360–364.

7. Miller A, Jepsen SJ, Stonebridge PA, et al: New angioscopic findings in graft failure after infrainguinal bypass. *Arch Surg* 1990; 125:749–753.

8. Miller A, Campbell DR, Gibbons GW, et al: Routine intraoperative angioscopy in lower extremity revascularisation.

9. Seeger JM, Abela GS: Angioscopy as an adjunct to arterial reconstructive surgery: A preliminary report. *J Vasc Surg* 1986; 5:315–320.

10. Segalowitz J, Grundfest WS, Treiman EL, et al: Angioscopy for intraoperative management of thrombolectomy. *Arch Surg* 1990; 125:1357–1362.

11. Sherman CT, Litvack F, Grundfest W, et al: Coronary angioscopy in patients with unstable angina pectoris. *N Engl J Med* 1986; 315:913–919.

12. Tanabe T, Yokota A, Sugic S: Cardiovascular fiberoptic endoscopy: Development and clinical application. *Surgery* 1980; 87:375–379.

13. White GH, White RA, Kopchok GE, et al: Intraoperative video angioscopy compared with arteriography during peripheral vascular operations. *J Vasc Surg* 1987; 6:488–495.

14. White GH, Sigel SB, Colman PD, et al: Intraoperative coronary angioscopy: Development of practical techniques. *Angiology* 1990; 41:793–800.

15. Bauriedel GB, Höfling B: Adjunctive angioscopy during percutaneous atherectomy. *Eur Heart J* 1988; 9(suppl A):132.

16. Forrester JS, Litvack F, Grundfest W, et al: A perspective of coronary disease seen through the arteries of living man. *Circulation* 1987; 75:505–513.

17. Forrester JS, Jakubowski A, Hickey A, et al: Coronary and peripheral vascular angioscopy, in Vogel J, King S (eds): *Interventional Cardiology: Future Directions.* St Louis, Mosby–Year Book, 1989, pp 36–53.

18. Gehani AA, Ball SG, Latif AB, et al: Experimental and clinical percutaneous angioscopy experience with dynamic angioplasty. *Angiology* 1990; 41:809–816.

19. Hombach V, Höher M, Hannekum A, et al: Erste klinische Erfahrungen mit der Koronarendoskopie. *Dtsch Med Wochenschr* 1986; 111:1135–1140.

20. Konishi T, Inden M, Nakano T: Clinical experience of percutaneous angioscopy in cases with coronary artery disease. *Angiology* 1989; 40:18–23.

21. Lee G, Garcia HJ, Corso P, et al: Correlation of coronary angioscopic to angiographic findings in coronary artery disease. *Am J Cardiol* 1986; 58:238–241.

22. Mizuno K, Arai T, Satomura K, et al: New percutaneous transluminal coronary angioscope. *J Am Coll Cardiol* 1989; 13:363–368.

23. Ramee SR, White CJ: Percutaneous coronary angioscopy, in White GH, White RA (eds): *Angioscopy: Vascular and Coronary Applications.* Chicago, Mosby–Year Book, 1989, pp 161–169.

24. Ramee SR, White CJ, Collins TJ, et al: Percutaneous angioscopy during coronary angioplasty using a steerable microangioscope. *J Am Coll Cardiol* 1991; 17:100–105.

25. Rees MR, Gehani A, Richens D, et al: Use of angioscopy as an aid to laser angioplasty. *Lasers Med Sci* 1988; 327.

26. Rees MR, Gehani AA, Ashley S, et al: Percutaneous video angioscopy in peripheral vascular diseases. *Clin Radiol* 1989; 40:347–351.

27. Siegel RJ, Chae JS, Forrester JS, et al: Angiography, angioscopy, and ultrasound imaging before and after percutaneous balloon angioplasty. *Am Heart J* 1990; 120:1086–1090.

28. Uchida Y, Masuo M, Tomaru T, et al: Fiberoptic observation of coronary luminal changes caused by transluminal coronary angioplasty. *Circulation* 1985; 72(suppl 3):218.

29. Uchida Y, Tomaru T, Nakamura F, et al: Percutaneous coronary angioscopy in patients with ischemic heart disease. *Am Heart J* 1987; 114:1222.

30. Uchida Y: Percutaneous coronary angioscopy by means of a fiberscope with steerable guidewire. *Am Heart J* 1989; 117:1153–1155.

31. Uchida Y, Hasegawa K, Kawamura K, et al: Angioscopic observation of the coronary luminal changes induced by percutaneous transluminal coronary angioplasty. *Am Heart J* 1989; 117:769–776.

32. Wendt TH, Bettinger R, Kober G: Angioskopie der Herzkranzgefäße. *Versicherungsmedizin* 1990; 42:83–88.

33. White GH, White RA: Percutaneous angioscopy as adjunct to laser angioplasty in peripheral arteries. *Lancet* 1989, 1:99.

34. Biamino G, Skarabis P, Böttcher H, et al: *Excimer Laser Assisted Angioplasty of Peripheral Vessels.* Kluwer 1991, in press.

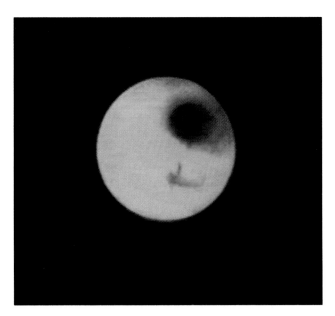

PLATE 1.—Yellowish surface discoloration already indicating lipomatous-atherosclerotic infiltration.

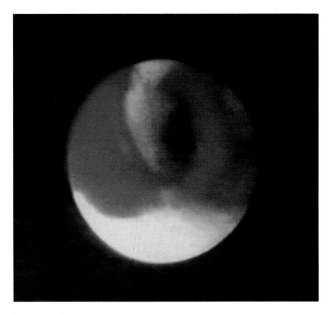

PLATE 2.—Partially floating parietal thrombi are relatively often observed in atherosclerotic arteries.

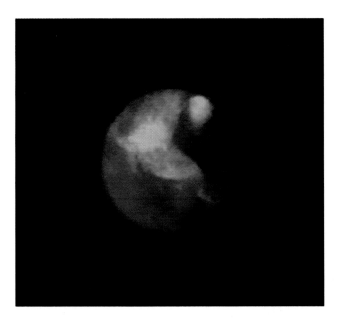

PLATE 3.—Severe hemorrhagic subintimal dissection of the SFA after PTCA.

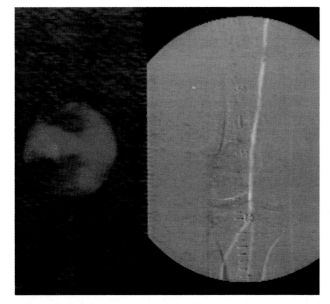

PLATE 4.—The occluded SFA and the first part of the popliteal artery were successfully recanalized. An ulcerated stenosis was dilated (cm 47 in "road mapping"). The angioscopic picture shows a severe hemorrhagic intimal edema with partial dissection. Thirty minutes later the artery occluded, and a bypass intervention became necessary.

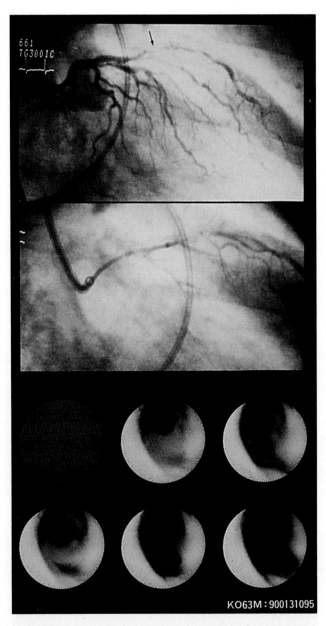

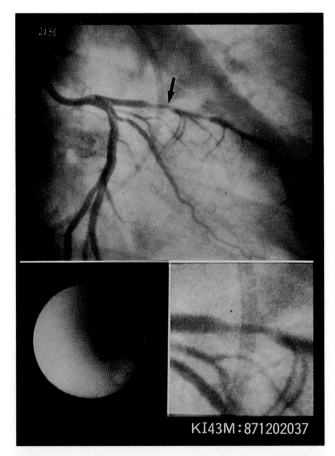

PLATE 6.—Recanalization following PTCR by t-PA (*arrow* in the contrast arteriograph) and the dissolved thrombus (teared thin, red mass in the *bottom left* panel) in the same patient as in Figure 5–9.

PLATE 5.—Contrast arteriogram of the PTCA double-catheter system. *Top frame:* left coronary segment; the *arrow* indicates the culprit lesion as the observational target for angioscopy. *Middle frame:* distinction of the 8 F guiding catheter within the aorta and the inner guiding catheter wedged at the culprit lesion. *Bottom frame:* flushing of the saline solution for clear viewing. The *top left* was just prior to flushing. The pressurized solution instantly clears the field for 5 to 6 seconds. The white section filling the lower left portion of the circles is the wall of the guiding catheter. The 90% stenosis from atheromatous plaque can be clearly seen in the third and fourth frames. The image is then lost as backflow clouds the solution.

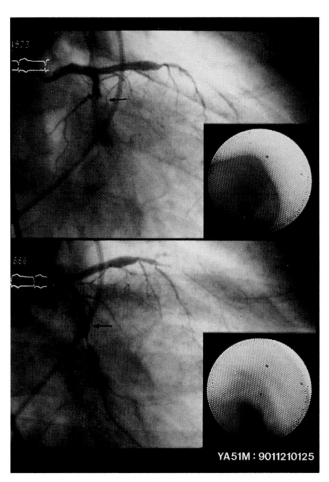

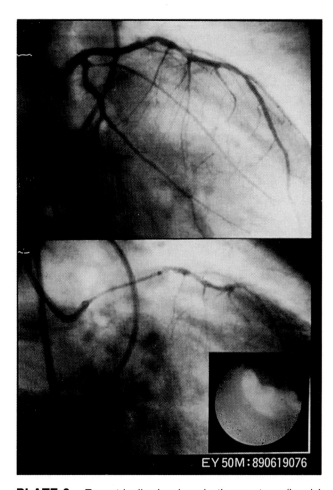

PLATE 7.—Before *(upper panel)* and immediately after *(bottom panel)* PTCR by t-PA in a 51-year-old male AMI patient. Thrombolysis produced recanalization and left 99% residual stenosis *(arrow* in the contrast arteriograph). Angioscopy demonstrates the dissolution of thrombus and uncovered a fairly large amount of eccentrically developed atheromatous plaque.

PLATE 8.—Eccentrically developed atheromatous (level I atheroma of Table 5–3) plaque covered by a fibrous cap *(bottom right)* at a mildly stenotic lesion of the proximal segment of the LAD artery following thrombolysis in a 50-year-old male AMI patient.

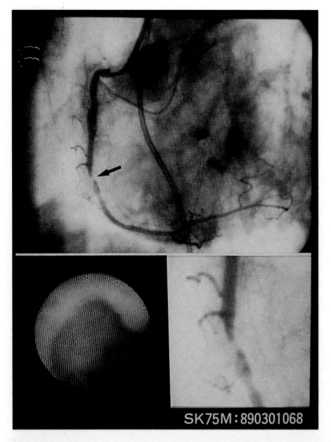

PLATE 9.—Eccentrically developed atheromatous plaque (level III atheroma of Table 5–3) of fairly large amounts narrowed the lumen of the RCA (*arrow* in the contrast arteriograph and angioscopy in the bottom left panel). Lipoidosis is prominent in the proximal area in this 75-year-old male AMI patient, who was photographed immediately after thrombolysis by t-PA.

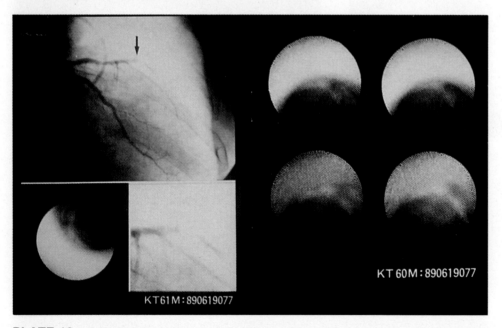

PLATE 10.—Following thrombolysis, 99% stenosis with a filling delay (*arrow* in the contrast arteriograph) and voluminous atheromatous plaque with its marginal tear (level V atheroma in Table 5–3) were demonstrated in this 60-year-old male AMI patient.

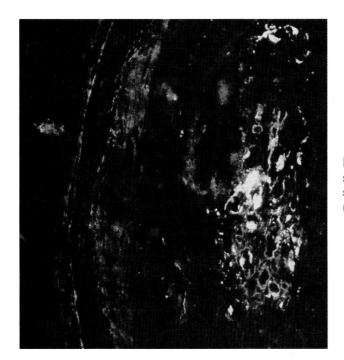

PLATE 11.—A photomicrograph of a section of an atherosclerotic plaque excited with 476-nm blue laser light and observed through a 515-nm barrier filter shows the autofluorescent ceroid "target."

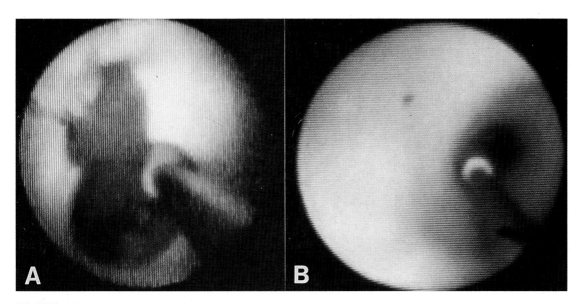

PLATE 12.—**A,** angioscopy demonstrates a thrombotic occlusion of a canine superficial femoral artery in vivo. **B,** after 3 minutes of exposure to ultrasound ablation the clot has been completely disrupted. Note that the arterial surface remains intact.

5

Technical Feasibility and Clinical Benefits of Percutaneous Coronary Angioscopy: Valuable Lessons on In Vivo Coronary Atherosclerosis Based on 50 Consecutive Observations in Patients With Acute Coronary Syndrome

Kiyoshi Inoue, M.D.

Keiichi Kuwaki, M.D.

Tetsuro Shirai, M.D.

Hidenobu Ochial, M.D.

Yoshio Mukaiyama, M.D.

Kazuhiko Sugimoto, M.D.

Etsuko Takano, M.T.

Hisatoshi Minato, M.T.

Angioscopy is a technique that provides tomographic views of the vascular lumen and allows identification of the various stages of atherosclerosis.[1-3] For this reason, there is growing interest in its clinical application as a guiding tool for use in coronary interventions (Chapters 5 and 53).[4-13] Theoretically, this technique could offer direct visual evidence that would enable the differentiation of thrombotic from atherosclerotic occlusions and support a decision for or against intracoronary thrombolysis and balloon angioplasty. It would therefore be advantageous if angioscopy could be combined with routine diagnostic contrast arteriography to describe the macropathologic nature of an obstructive coronary lesion prior to and immediately after the implementation of recanalizing procedures.[14-16] However, the technique of clinical angioscopy that has been developed to date is unsatisfactory for practical use due to the persistence of several technical barriers,[17, 18] namely, (1) lack of a pliable angioscopic catheter that is able to pass through the tortuous coronary artery without causing endothelial injury, (2) targeting difficulties, (3) blood opacity, and (4) lack of an optical system that can produce high-resolution images. These factors describe the minimal criteria for a practically usable angioscope and are requirements that had not been satisfactorily met.

Since 1983, we have been working on the technique of percutaneous transluminal coronary angioscopy (PTCAS) (Chapter 5).[9, 10, 18, 19] This report documents the technical feasibility of meeting such criteria by using the procedure that has been developed in our laboratory and describes how much and exactly what we can learn from our procedure about in vivo coronary atherosclerosis in patients with acute coronary syndrome.

METHOD

Study Patients

The study group consisted of 50 patients with acute coronary syndrome and included 20 subjects with unstable angina and 30 subjects with acute myocardial infarction (AMI). The diagnosis of these conditions followed the American Heart Association criteria. Emergency contrast arteriography was performed on all patients in the early hours after the initial onset of AMI or soon after the last episode of clusters of chest pain in unstable angina. Emergency coronary arteriography revealed obstructions of greater than 90% at the offending sites of these coronary arteries, and these sites were considered to be responsible for the immediate ischemic event based on electrocardiographic findings. All candidates were considered eligible for emergency percutaneous thrombolytic coronary revascularization (PTCR) and/or percutaneous transluminal coronary angioplasty (PTCA) on the basis of clinical evidence of ongoing ischemia and hemodynamic compromise. Informed consent to perform angioscopy was obtained from each patient. PTCAS was first undertaken in combination with emergency coronary arteriography and then repeated during the subsequent recanalizing intervention. In total, we examined 50 offending sites within the coronary artery by this technique.

Indication for Angioscopy

In order to decide whether PTCR or PTCA is indicated for the recanalization, it must first be determined whether the occlusion is thrombotic or atherosclerotic in nature. For this differentiation, angioscopy is far superior to arteriography.[16–18, 21] Despite this, the only tool currently available to determine the indications for or against PTCR and/or PTCA and to assess the completeness of recanalization is contrast arteriography, which alone cannot show the detailed intraluminal morphology of the lesion. From our past experiences (Chapter 44),[9, 19–21] we know that angioscopy can demonstrate the exact nature of such lesions under direct vision and thus, if used successfully in combination with emergency contrast arteriography, would be an invaluable tool in supporting the decision for or against PTCR and/or PTCA. The indication for angioscopy in this study was patients with acute coronary syndrome in

need of recanalizing interventions and in whom it had been conclusively established that the offending site identified within the coronary artery was responsible for the ongoing ischemia.

Coronary Angioscopy Catheter

Two models of ultrathin, flexible, disposable, sterile coronary angioscopy catheters that we developed (Fig 5–1) were used to perform the coronary angioscopy in this study. The coronary angioscopic catheters consist of an image guide containing either 3,000 or 1,800 pixels of extremely fine quartz fiber and a light guide containing either 13 or 45 multicomponent glass fibers, respectively. These two optic bundles are concentrically arranged and covered by a coating of a fluorine-containing polymer. The catheter is 300 cm in length and 0.68 mm (regular type) or 0.5 mm (thin type) in outer diameter and has a bend radius of 8 mm. A rod-type focusing lens built into the tip end of catheter is able to resolve a pair of lines separated by 0.1 mm to an object distance of 0.8 to 13 mm and has an 80-degree field of vision.

Light and Imaging Units

A 75-W xenon lamp is used to provide intraluminal illumination. The white light, which is condensed at the light guide connector and passed through the light guide, is projected toward the observational target. The image is reflected through the image guide, divided into two by a half mirror, and then directed into both a VTR unit and a still photography unit. The image received by the CCD color video camera head is displayed on a 6-in. television monitor.

The compact unit (Fig 5–2) that we developed for exclusive use in percutaneous coronary angioscopy con-

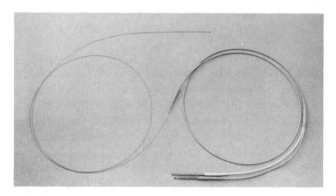

FIG 5–1.
Coronary angioscopy catheter. On the *left* is the catheter itself. The coil on the *right* splits to a connection to the camera (*top* of split, coil) called the "image guide," and to a xenon light source (*bottom* of split coil) called the "light guide."

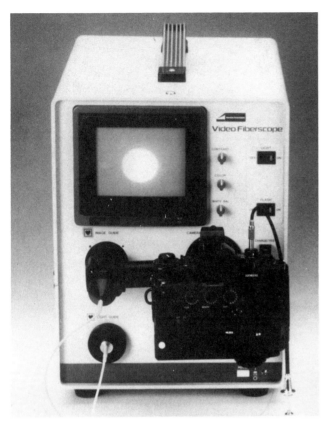

FIG 5–2.
This compact imaging unit for angioscopy includes a monitor, camera, and connectors for the image and light guides.

tains image and light guide connectors, a video coupler, video camera head, light source, TV monitor, and a still photograph unit. This system allows the reflected images to be either stored or displayed on a high-resolution video monitor. In addition, 35-mm still photographs can be taken. This unit also contains a flash synchronizing device that functions to synchronize the camera's shutter speed with that of the flashing light.

Angioscopy Guiding Catheter

Three types of flexible, thin-walled, soft-tipped guiding catheters were developed for exclusive use in PT-CAS: a balloon type, a bent type, and a straight type (Figs 5–3 and 5–4). Each is used to guide the angioscopic catheter toward the observational site and aid in manipulating the catheter into the target site. They are also used to deliver the transparent solution needed to flush the blood. The distal 20 cm of the guiding catheter is composed of polyurethane and is designed to be softer and more flexible than the rest of the catheter, which is composed of two layers of a combination of polyurethane and nylon so as to allow the catheter pas-

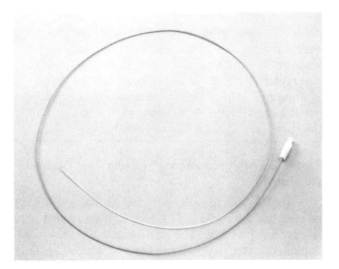

FIG 5–3.
Guiding catheter exclusively for use with coronary angioscopy. The darker section is rigid while the white, distal section is soft and pliable.

sage through the tortuous coronary tree. A radiopaque gold ring marker is attached to the tip end of the catheter to enable identification of the catheter's position under fluoroscopy. The guiding catheter has a length of 1,250 mm, an outer diameter of 4.3 and 5 F, and an inner diameter of 1.2 mm. The outer diameter of the tip end portion is 4.3 F, and the inner diameter is 0.9 mm. The detached portion of the inflatable balloon is 1.7 mm in outer diameter. Guiding catheters without the balloon attachment were generally used, but in those

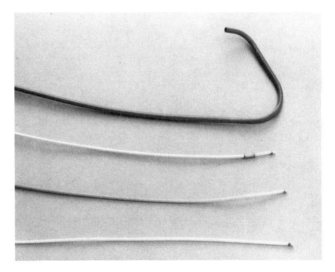

FIG 5–4.
Lineup of the catheter system. From top to bottom, 8 F guiding catheter as used for PTCA and 4.3 to 4.5 F guide catheters for PTCAs: balloon type, bent type, and straight type.

rare cases where the culprit lesion had less that 75% stenosis and high blood flow, the balloon was needed to curb the rapid flow. Examination of intraluminal morphology following angioplasty, PTCR, and/or PTCA also required the attachment to control rapid flow.

Figure 5–5 shows a distal lineup of the catheters prepared for percutaneous coronary angioscopy, including the three guiding catheters: balloon, bent, and straight.

Technique of Percutaneous Transluminal Coronary Angioscopy

A double guiding catheter system that we developed is used for angioscopy. The system is composed of a regular 8 F PTCA guiding catheter and the angioscopy guiding catheter (Fig 5–6 and Plate 5). The 8 F guiding catheter is first introduced into the coronary artery via the femoral artery by using Judkin's technique. Then, the angioscopy guiding catheter is delivered into the proximal site of the offended coronary artery through the 8 F guiding catheter by using a guidewire. The 8 F guiding catheter is then removed from the coronary artery and held within the aorta. Next, the angioscopy guiding catheter is advanced toward the observational target so as to position the radiopaque marker of the tip end just proximal to the offended site of the coronary artery. The guidewire is then removed and the angioscopy guiding catheter left in place.

The angioscopic catheter is then inserted through the guiding catheter. Before insertion of the angioscopic catheter, an adjustment of visual focus and lighting is made. In addition, the surface and tip of the angioscopic catheter are wiped with heparin gauze to prevent clot-

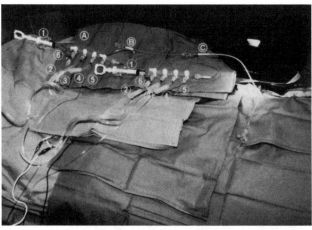

DOUBLE GUIDING CATHETER SYSTEM

- Ⓐ Coronary Angioscopic Catheter Guide Wire
- Ⓑ Inner Guiding Catheter
- Ⓒ Outer Guiding Catheter
- ① Syringe
- ② Infusion line (Compression Bag)
- ③ Saline Solution
- ④ Radiopaque solution
- ⑤ Pressure Monitoring
- ⑥ (Open)

FIG 5–6.
Lineup of catheters for the double guiding catheter system. Numbers and letters correspond with the equipment in the photograph.

ting. The angioscopic catheter is inserted toward the tip end of the guiding catheter, and its tip is positioned just slightly within the tip end of the guiding catheter. This is confirmed by adjusting the radiopaque silhouette of the tip-end lens portion of the angioscopic catheter to the radiopaque gold marker on the guide catheter. By ensuring that the tip end of the angioscopic catheter is always kept within the shell of the guiding catheter, manipulation of the guiding catheter with torque to bring the observational target into sight can be done without causing unnecessary endothelial injury.

Flushing with a warm 5% dextrose solution is performed by manual injection or through a compression bag with a Y connector. The rate of flushing needed to create a transient blood-free viewing field for angioscopy is 1 to 3 mL/sec for total amounts of 5 to 9 mL. However, these values may vary depending upon the rate and amount of flow within the offended coronary artery. If the flow of the coronary circulation exceeds those levels facilitated by flushing, the balloon attached to the angioscopy guiding catheter is inflated so that a optimal bloodless visual field is created.

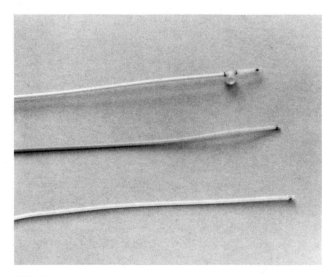

FIG 5–5.
Inflated balloon-type, bent-type, and straight-type angioscopic catheters.

After insertion of the catheter, routine contrast arteriography is repeated via the guiding catheter and Y connector to confirm the distance between the tip end of the guiding catheter and the offended site. During the procedure, the electrocardiogram and pulmonary and coronary pressures are continuously monitored. If any appreciable changes appear in these parameters during angioscopy, subsequent procedures are postponed until they return to baseline levels.

Variables for the Assessment of Angioscopy

In order to test the technical feasibility of our method and its ability to visualize the intraluminal lesion responsible for ongoing ischemia, a semiquantitative analysis was performed. The following variables were taken into consideration: (1) ability to deliver the angioscopy guiding catheter directly toward the target lesion; (2) ability to deliver the angioscopic catheter toward the tip end of the guiding catheter; (3) ability to create a transient but clear bloodless visual field by flushing fluid through the guiding catheter; (4) ability to bring the observational target into sight by manipulating the angioscopy guiding catheter; (5) ability to see the intraluminal aspects of the culprit lesion so that greater than half of the visual image, excluding the unavoidable image of a portion of the interior of the guiding catheter, is occupied by the observational target; and (6) diagnostic value of images obtained by angioscopy as compared with those of accompanying contrast arteriography in differentiating intracoronary thrombus from atheromatous plaque.

RESULTS

A total of 50 sites considered responsible for ongoing ischemic events were examined before and immediately after PTCR and/or PTCA by contrast arteriography with our current techniques (Fig 5–7). Thirty-seven of 50 attempts (74%) were successful. None of these patients had serious complications during endoscopy that required the procedure to be stopped. Transient and mild chest pain, without significant ischemic changes in the electrocardiogram, were encountered in 3 patients during the maneuver.

Catheter Insertion and Flushing

In all cases, we attempted to deliver the angioscopic catheter just proximal to the offended site in a direct fashion, and the catheter was kept within the tip end of the guiding catheter just proximal to the observational target in 86%. Of those, insertion of the angioscopic

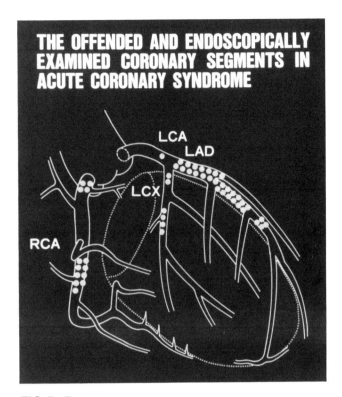

FIG 5–7.
The *dots* indicate the number of attempts at PTCAs in each coronary segment. (*LCA* = left coronary artery; *LAD* = left anterior descending; *LCX* = left circumflex; *RCA* = right coronary artery.

catheter toward the tip end of the guiding catheter and the observational target was achieved in 94%. A transient bloodless visual field needed for endoscopy was created by flushing with a warm dextrose solution at an approximate rate of 0.5 to 3.0 mL/sec for total amounts of 3.0 to 9.0 mL. This was achieved in 90% of those successfully targeted. Since the majority of the lesions that underwent endoscopy had greater than 90% stenosis, the rate and amount of flushing used were sufficient to create the transient bloodless visual field necessary for endoscopy in all attempts.

Success of Angioscopy

The success rate of our attempts at endoscopy and the proposed reasons for failed attempts are summarized in Table 5–1. Of the two series of 50 attempts made, we were successful in 37 (74%) before and 33 (66%) after recanalizing interventions were undertaken. Out of the 33 successes obtained following recanalizing interventions, 28 were achieved out of 42 attempts immediately after PTCR, and 5 successes were achieved out of 8 attempts made immediately after PTCA. Thus, we were successful at angioscopy in 74% before recanaliz-

TABLE 5–1

Success Rate of Percutaneous Angioplasty in 50 Consecutive Cases of Acute Coronary Syndrome

Artery	Attempts	Success	Percentage
LMT*	1	1	100
LAD*			
No. 6	14	11	79
No. 7	12	10	83
No. 8	4	3	75
Total	30	24	80
LCx*			
No. 11	2	1	50
No. 13	4	3	75
Total	6	4	67
RCA*			
No. 1	4	3	75
No. 2	9	5	55
Total	13	8	62
Total	50	37	74

*LMT = left main trunk; LAD = left anterior descending; LCx = left circumflex; RCA = right coronary artery.

ing interventions and 66% after the recanalizing interventions. Within the four major coronary branches, 1 out of 1 attempt made in the left main trunk (LMT), 4 out of 6 attempts made in the left circumflex (LCx), 8 out of 13 attempts made in the right coronary artery (RCA), and 24 out of 30 attempts made in the left anterior descending (LAD) artery were successful.

Angioscopic Findings in Acute Coronary Syndrome

Figure 5–8 summarizes the major endoscopic findings at the 37 offended sites of the coronary artery

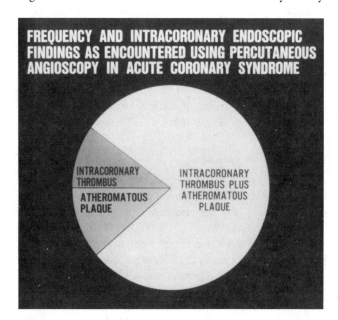

FIG 5–8.
Frequency of endoscopic findings.

in 50 consecutive cases of acute coronary syndrome just prior to recanalizing interventions. Among 37 successful angioscopic examinations, atheromatous plaque (10%), thrombus (14%), or atheromatous plaque together with thrombus (76%) were encountered at the offended coronary sites. These consisted of 22 cases of acute myocardial infarction (AMI) and 15 cases of unstable angina. Either partially or totally occlusive thrombi were a common finding shared by the patients with AMI. The thrombi in those lesions appeared mixed and mural in nature (Fig 5–9) and were partially torn by intracoronary thrombolysis with tissue-type plasminogen activator (t-PA) (Plate 6). This uncovered matured atheromatous plaque in fairly large amounts that were hidden behind the thrombi (Figs 5–10 and 5–11). Matured atherosclerotic plaque occupying a large part of the lumen and partially covered by thrombus was also observed at the offended site of the coronary segment in the group with unstable angina. Ulcers, focal hemorrhage, mural thrombi, and fibrin

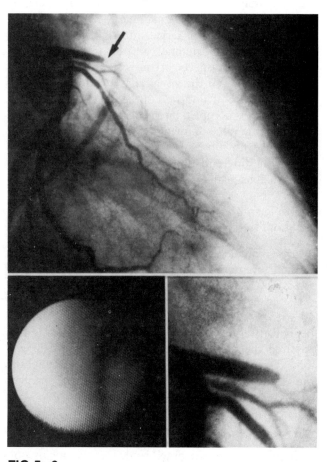

FIG 5–9.
Complete obstruction (*arrow* in the contrast arteriograph) of the proximal segment of the LAD artery in a 43-year-old male AMI patient and intracoronary thrombus of a soft spongy nature (thin darker mass in the *bottom left* panel) obliterating the lumen.

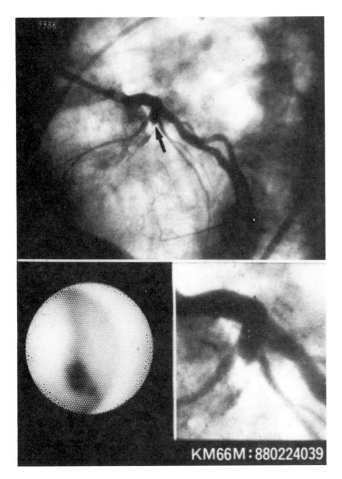

FIG 5–10.
Complete obstruction (*arrow* in the contrast arteriograph) of the proximal segment of the LAD artery in a 66-year-old male AMI patient and intracoronary thrombus obliterating the central position of the narrowed lumen by the presence of a fairly large amount of atheromatous plaque *(bottom left panel).*

TABLE 5–2

Angioscopic Definition of Coronary Endothelium

Intact endothelium:
   Systolic narrowing and diastolic dilation
   Flat, smooth, and silky texture
   Shiny, grayish white color
Atherosclerotic endothelium:
   Atheromatous plaque
     Reduced systolic and diastolic motion
     Convex mass with irregular margins
     Surface: coarse, rough, or rugged
     Shape: wavelike, stemmed (polypoid), or torn
     Color: white, yellow, brown
   Intracoronary thrombus
     Flowing with the fluid stream; attached or floating
     Color: white, yellow, brown, or red

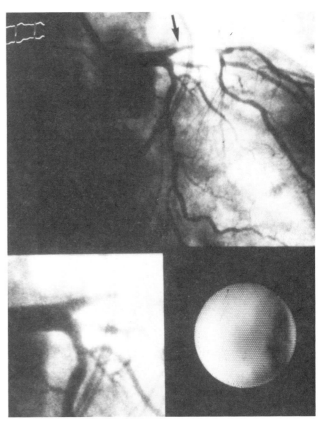

FIG 5–11.
Recanalization following t-PA (*arrow* in the contrast arteriograph) with 99% residual stenosis left in a 69-year-old male AMI patient and mural thrombus adhering to the well-developed atheromatous plaque (*bottom left* angioscopy image).

netting were frequently seen on the surface of those plaques.

Angioscopy Following PTCR and/or PTCA

Satisfactory angioscopy following recanalizing interventions was achieved in 20 lesions from the patient group with AMI and in 5 lesions from patients with unstable angina in which thrombus was angioscopically identified in advance of the recanalizing interventions. These atheromatous changes were angioscopically defined to differentiate between thrombus and atheromatous plaque (Table 5–2). Following PTCR, the thrombi were dissolved (see Plate 7), and atheromatous plaques of varying morphology were identified. On the surface of the atheromatous plaques, ulcers, focal hemorrhage, and residual thrombi were seen. These observations indicate that the presence of thrombus has a strong link with the occurrence of acute coronary events and that the frequency of stage III and IV atheroma was high in this study population (Fig 5–12). Additionally, stages

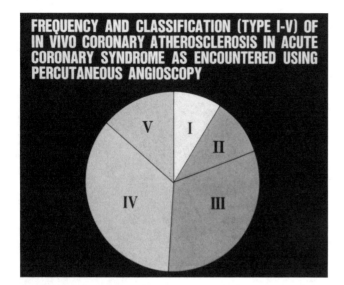

FIG 5–12.
Frequency of plaque types (see Table 5–3).

TABLE 5–3

Angioscopic Classification of Coronary Plaque

Type	Shape	Surface	Color
I	Flat	Smooth/shining	Grayish white
II	Uneven	Coarse/dim	Yellow, grayish white
III	Undulated	Rough	Grayish yellow
IV	Stemmed	Rugged	Patchy; white, gray, yellow, brown
V	Torn/ulcerated	Rugged	Mixed; white, gray, yellow, brown, red

matous plaque was identified before PTCA. Following PTCA, coarse endothelial surfaces composed of intimal flaps, focal hemorrhage, mural thrombi, and fibrin netting were seen around the plaque, which was cracked as a result of the balloon inflation. Part of the disease-free wall could be seen in contrast as well (Fig 5–13).

DISCUSSION

Since the mid-1980s research into the development of coronary angioscopy has taken place.[14–16, 18, 19–23] The results accumulated during this period have suggested the following three areas in which coronary angioscopy could play a contributory role: (1) diagnosis of the macropathology of the coronary segment responsible for the ongoing ischemia[14, 19, 21]; (2) inspection of the culprit lesion before, during, and immediately after coronary recanalizing interventions (Chapter 5)[24]; and (3) study of the pathophysiology and mechanism of restenosis following angioplasty.[8, 19, 25]

III to V were classified by their distinct appearance as follows: III has a corrugated surface, IV has stalagmite-like protrusions, and V represents serious endothelial disruption. The stages seem to be linked developmentally. Therefore, intracoronary thrombus and stage III to V atheromatous plaques play important roles in the mechanism of acute coronary syndrome. The atheromatous plaques were classified progressively into stages I to V based on severity and frequency (Table 5–3).

Angioscopy following PTCA was successful in two cases of AMI and three cases of unstable angina in which high-grade intraluminal narrowing by an athero-

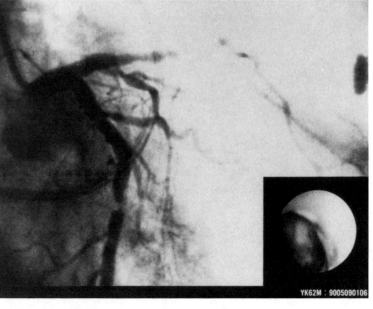

FIG 5–13.
Contrast arteriography and coronary angioscopy immediately after balloon angioplasty in a 62-year-old male unstable angina patient.

However, the technique of PTCAS developed to date has not been able to be put to practical use in the above-mentioned areas due to several technical barriers. A major setback to its general use has been the technical difficulty experienced in delivering, directing, and positioning the angioscopic catheter toward the site responsible for the immediate coronary event within the tortuous and beating coronary arterial trees. Another obstacle confronted is the limitation on the time available for endoscopy due to the use of a nonoxygenated fluid such as saline or dextrose solution for the flushing needed to create a transient bloodless visual field. Criticism that the passage of the angioscope and the directing or the positioning of the lens-bearing tip of the angioscope toward the observational target may cause serious sloughing of the endothelial lining and that the endoscopic information obtained from this brief glance at the culprit lesion may be incomplete and could lead to some errors in diagnosis has also arisen (Chapter 44).[16-18]

In recognition of these problems we propose the following eight criteria as general requirements for performing simple and effective percutaneous angioscopy in combination with routine contrast arteriography:

1. The angioscopic catheter should be disposable and delivered into the coronary artery by using Judkin's technique.

2. The catheter should be advanced to the culprit lesion by using a guiding catheter in order to avoid sloughing of the endothelial lining, which could be caused by the lens-bearing tip of the angioscope. This procedure should be quickly and easily performed to enable its routine usage in combination with contrast arteriography.

3. The lens-bearing tip of the angioscope must be manipulated by using the guiding catheter so that it directly approaches the observational target and is positioned in front of the target to provide maximum viewing capacity within the tortuous and rapidly beating coronary artery.

4. A flushing system should be incorporated into and developed in combination with the technique of angioscopy. Flushing with fluid should produce an appropriate transient bloodless visual field without causing serious ischemia within the offended myocardium or without detaching atherosclerotic intraluminal flaps.

5. The limitations on viewing time imposed by the flushing of the coronary artery with deoxygenated fluid necessitate that some proof of observation be recorded for diagnosis. Therefore, two means of imaging are required, i.e., a video tape recording system and 35-mm still photographs.

6. Coronary angioscopy should not only be limited to observation and diagnosis but should also be used simultaneously and in combination with the therapeutic methods of PTCA/PTCR to provide visual assistance.

7. The system in its entirety should be able to be used quickly as a simple routine procedure that is safe and efficient.

8. The system should contain the facilities necessary to make measurements of the precise size and location of the observational target.

If any method of angioscope is able to satisfy these criteria, it will take its place alongside coronary arteriography and fulfill the role within the areas of use to which it has been assigned.

The ability of our technique to produce satisfactory endoscopic images in approximately two thirds of the cases examined is sufficient to justify and promote the practical use of our technique in diagnosing severely stenotic coronary lesions and assisting in the three areas listed.

In this study, we were successful in performing PTCAS in 74% before and 66% after intracoronary thrombolysis and/or balloon angioplasty in a consecutive series of patients with acute coronary syndrome. We have defined the success of angioscopy as the ability to obtain satisfactory endoscopic images that allow visualization of the interior of the coronary segment responsible for ongoing ischemia such that the endoscopic image occupies greater than half of the total field of vision. The production of what we currently describe as a satisfactory endoscopic image is obviously the minimum requirement necessary for clinically practical coronary endoscopy. Previous researchers emphasized the ability to make even the briefest of glances at the culprit lesion without paying much attention to either their success rates or the possibility that their targeted lesion might not be the lesion responsible for the ongoing ischemia. Such cases may support the possibility of errors in the efficacy of clinical coronary angioscopy. Success rates were also quoted without providing the criteria upon which their definition of success was based.

Although the general rate for obtaining satisfactory angioscopic images, in our series, exceeded half of the total lesions examined, individual success rates varied from 33% to 100% depending upon their location in the coronary artery. The success of percutaneous coronary angioscopy obviously depends on completing the following three maneuvers: (1) delivery of the angioscopic catheter to the site responsible for ongoing ischemia, (2) positioning of the lens-bearing tip of the angioscopic catheter so that it directly faces the observational target, and (3) creation of a bloodless visual field with the aid of optimal flushing and an illuminating system. The rate of success in our series was higher for lesions located in the LAD coronary artery as compared with those in the LCx and RCA arteries. The lowest success rates were made when the observational target was in segments 2, 3, or 11. Major factors contributing to the low success rate in examining lesions located in segments 2, 3, and 11 were as follows:

1. Difficulty in passing the angioscopic catheter through coronary portions having some anatomic bend (Fig 5–14) such as a "shepherd's crook" in the RCA.

2. Lack of correspondence in size between the angioscopy guiding catheter and the vessel being examined. For example, when the size of the vessel being examined was much larger than that of the guiding catheter, it was difficult to position the catheter in the center of the lumen and manipulate the guiding catheter to position the lens-bearing tip of the angioscopic catheter so that it directly faced the observational target.

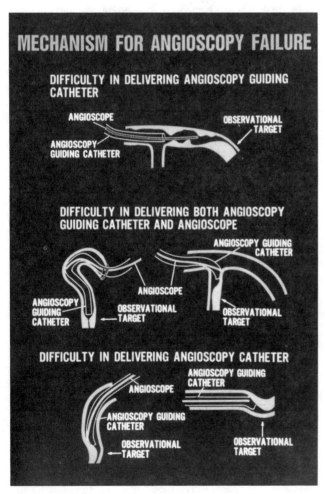

FIG 5–14.
Reasons for failed angioscopy.

3. Blood flow at the culprit lesion exceeding that produced by flushing the clear solution, primarily experienced during angioscopy immediately after balloon dilatation.

The latter two factors could for the most part be resolved by using a balloon-tipped guiding catheter, which we developed and used in this study. Hence, the first factor was the principal limitation of our current procedure.

The angioscopic catheter used in this study was designed to be extremely thin and flexible, but we did in fact encounter some difficulties and found a few breaks in the quartz fibers after attempts made in lesions located in the right and the left circumflex arteries. At the current stage of development of fiber optics, a fiber-optic bundle containing 3,000 pixels of quartz fibers is the minimum required to produce tolerable image resolution. However, we felt that even the use of this minimal number of fibers would result in an angioscope that would still be somewhat rigid and not allow a smooth, easy entrance into the RCA and adjustment of the catheter tip so that it directly faces the observational target. The number of quartz fibers could be reduced to enhance flexibility, but as a consequence the resolution of the image would also be reduced. Thus the present level of fiber-optic technology is a major dilemma. Our compromise to this problem, which was included in the current model of our angioscopic catheter, was to reduce the outer diameter to 0.68 mm and to add more flexibility to the angioscope by using a polyurethane and nylon mixture for the cover. In addition, we made a 0.5-mm model that has 1,800 pixels of imaging fibers but has larger numbers of optic plastic bundles for augmented illumination.

Our current results with these angioscopic catheters and a double guiding catheter system indicate that PTCAS in combination with routine diagnostic contrast arteriography can successfully be performed in lesions located within coronary segments 1, 6, 7, 8, and 9. In other words, percutaneous coronary angioscopy, using our technique, is technically feasible for the endoscopy of all lesions within the proximal segment of the left coronary artery. Lesions located in the distal segments of the right and the left circumflex arteries at its junction are within a range subject to some technical difficulty due to the lack of tip angulation technology, thus presenting a limitation to our current procedure.

Both a 35-mm still photograph and videotape of the image visualized by the angioscope are obviously needed to make an exact macropathologic diagnosis of the culprit lesion. In addition, more than two pictures of the lesion taken at different catheter positions may be re-

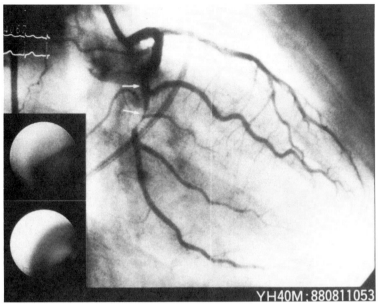

FIG 5-15.
Intact vs. atheromatous plaque (type III atheroma in Table 5-3), producing 99% luminal narrowing (indicated by the *arrows* in the contrast arteriograph) and their intraluminal images by angioscopy *(left panel).*

quired to identify its entire proximal aspect. For example, photographs were taken at positions 1.5 to 2.0 cm and 0.5 to 1.0 cm proximal to the observational target. Photographs must be taken from multiple positions in cases where the offended site is located within a fast-moving and tortuous portion of the coronary artery because it is often difficult to visualize the entire proximal aspect of the lesion from one catheter position due to poor positioning of the catheter tip and as a result of the relatively narrow field of vision of the lens assembly system.

Percutaneous coronary angioscopy by our method has allowed us to differentiate between intact and ath-

erosclerotic endothelium (Fig 5-15) and identify lipid stains, atheromatous plaque of varying pathology (see Figs 5-16 to 5-18 and Plates 8 to 10), ulcers, focal hemorrhage, and intimal flaps on the surface of the atherosclerotic lumen. The differentiation between thrombotic and atherosclerotic occlusions was also successfully made. A rapidly appearing thrombus of fairly large proportions at a section undergoing vasospasm within a disease-free coronary segment and its disappearance following the administration of intracoronary nitroglycerine were, for the first time, clearly observed. Marginal tears of atheromatous plaque (Plate 10) seen by angioscopy immediately after intracoronary thrombolysis in

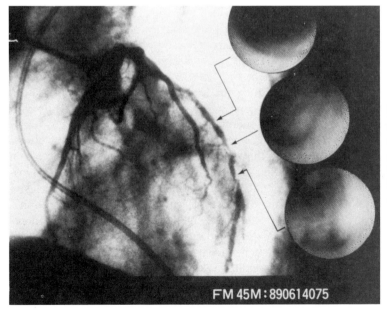

FIG 5-16.
Atheromatous plaques of varying angioscopic morphology through the proximal to distal portions of the LAD artery in a 45-year-old patient with unstable angina. The coronary site responsible for the recent episodes of angina is in the bottom right atheroma (type II atheroma in Table 5-3).

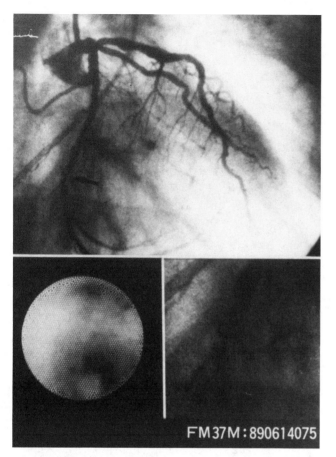

FIG 5–17.
An eccentric mass (type IV atheroma of Table 5–3) observed by angioscopy *(bottom left)* at the proximal site of the LCx was responsible for the ongoing ischemia in a 37-year-old male AMI patient following thrombolysis.

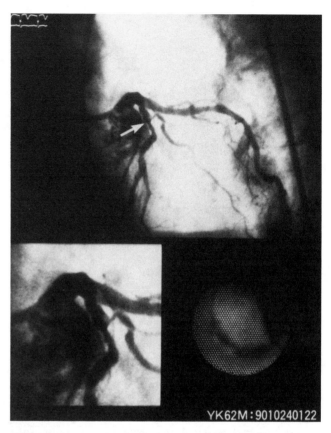

FIG 5–18.
A voluminous eccentric mass with lipoidosis (type IV atheroma in Table 5–3) is shown by the *arrow* and is the coronary site responsible for the recent episode of clusters of angina in a 62-year-old male patient with unstable angina.

AMI patients provide a window of opportunity for understanding the mechanism of both sudden thrombotic occlusion and reocclusion following PTCR. Evidence of tearing or fracturing of the atheromatous plaque, focal hemorrhage around its margins, and the plaque-free wall seen by angioscopy immediately after balloon dilatation, as well as the large amount of lipid staining around the balloon-injured plaque tissue in association with organized thrombus as visualized by angioscopy undertaken a month after PTCA, all offer a unique opportunity for the preventive study of restenosis following balloon angioplasty in patients with acute coronary syndrome. These findings, made at the time a patient was experiencing symptoms and seen by angioscopy within the coronary segment responsible for the ongoing ischemia, were far more specific than those that could have been recognized by contrast arteriography alone. The findings of PTCAS included specific information concerning the severity of coronary atherosclerosis not seen by coronary angiography. However, the broad scope provided by coronary angiography in examining the rate of flow, severity of stenosis, and view of the entire coronary tree can by no means be replaced by PTCAS. Hence, both procedures are needed for maximum benefit.

Concerning the safety of our methods, possible endothelial injury, which could have been caused by contact of the endothelium and both tip ends of the angioscopic and the guiding catheters, was avoided by always ensuring that the angioscopic catheter was kept within the guiding catheter and by using a soft-tipped angioscopy guiding catheter, which we developed for exclusive use in angioscopy. Mild chest pain was experienced in 3 of the 50 study patients, but electrocardiographic monitoring in these patients during the symptoms did not show any ischemic changes and therefore did not pose a hazard necessitating that angioscopy be stopped.

Since the study group had greater than 90% stenosis

TABLE 5–4

Categories of Angioscopy Classified According to the Level of Technical Development

1. First-generation angioscopy: Simple use of a thin fiber-optic device developed for endoscopic purposes within the biliary, bronchial, or urethral tracts in combination with a routine catheterization maneuver
2. Second-generation angioscopy: Use of a thin, flexible fiber-optic device developed for exclusive use in vascular endoscopy
3. Third-generation angioscope: Use of a total angioscopy system consisting of a disposable angioscopic catheter, a guiding catheter for exclusive use in angioscopy, and an imaging system
4. Fourth-generation angioscopy: Same as the third category, but with additional facilities for measuring the location and size of the observational target and with devices for assistance in angioplasty.

at the offended site before PTCR and/or PTCA and greater than 75% after PTCR, we did not have any difficulty in obtaining a transient clear visual field by manual flushing. But after PTCA, we experienced difficulties in producing a clear bloodless visual field due to the increase in flow in the circulation, poor fixation of the tip of the angioscope toward the observational target, and trembling of the image due to fast-moving flow within the vessels. We could have adjusted the rate and amount of flushing to accommodate these factors, but this was avoided because it might have produced unnecessary detachment of the intraluminal residue following PTCA and caused myocardial ischemia, both of with could have produced life-threatening arrhythmias. As a solution, an inflatable balloon guiding catheter that we developed was applied in the series and was found to be helpful in achieving successful angioscopy.

From a review of our and other researchers' efforts to date, we propose that angioscopy be classified into four categories according to the level of its technical development as listed in Table 5–4. The angioscopy used in this series belongs to the category of the third generation, and an encouragingly high success rate was achieved by our current technique of PTCAS.

Our experience and the results accumulated in this study have led us to the conclusion that a clinically practical method of coronary angioscopy should (1) be made by a percutaneous transluminal approach, (2) be able to be performed during or in combination with routine diagnostic coronary arteriography, (3) provide diagnostic visual information, (4) be technically simple to perform, (5) be carried out in a relatively short period of time, and (6) be of low cost. The system that we have developed and tested in this series satisfies these factors.

CONCLUSION

This study suggests new capabilities for the use of PTCAS in identification and assessment of obstructive coronary lesions. Greater technical feasibility and decreased risks make practical application of this procedure a reality. When this procedure is used in combination with routine diagnostic contrast arteriography, we conclude that it contributes to the study of in vivo coronary atherosclerosis at severely stenotic coronary lesions and may assist in the performance of recanalizing interventions in patients with acute coronary syndrome.

REFERENCES

1. Greenstone SM, et al: Arterial endoscopy (arterioscopy). *Arch Surg* 1966; 93:811.
2. Vollmar JF, Storz WL: Vascular endoscopy. *Surg Clin North Am* 1974; 54:111–122.
3. Litvack F, Grundfest WS, Lee ME, et al: Angioscopic visualization of blood vessels interior in animals and humans. *Clin Cardiol* 1986; 8:65.
4. Lee G, Reis RL, Chan MC, et al: Clinical laser recanalization of coronary obstruction. Angioscopic and angiographic documentation. *Chest* 1986; 90:770–772.
5. Abela GS, Seeger JM, Barbieri E, et al: Laser angiography with angioscopic guidance in man. *J Am Coll Cardiol* 1986; 8:184–192.
6. Van Steigman G, Bartle EJ, Pearce WH, et al: Vascular endoscopy with a new laser capable angioscope. *Lasers Surg Med* 1985; 5:170.
7. Ritchie JL, Nanses DD, Vracko R, et al: In vivo rotational thrombectomy — evaluation by angioscopy. *Circulation* 1986; 74:457.
8. Forrester JS, Litvack F, Grundfest W, et al: A perspective of coronary disease seen through the arteries of living man. *Circulation* 1987; 75:505.
9. Inoue K, Kuwaki K, Ueda K, et al: Angioscopy guided coronary thrombolysis (abstract): *J Am Coll Cardiol* 1987; 9:62.
10. Uchida Y, Hasegawa K, Kawamura K, et al: Angioscopic observation of the coronary luminal changes induced by percutaneous transluminal coronary angioplasty. *Am Heart J* 1989; 117:769–776.
11. Hofing GA, Bauridel G, Backa D, et al: Use of angioscopy to assess the results of percutaneous atherectomy. *Am J Cardiac Imaging* 1989; 3:20–26.
12. Siegel RJ, Chae JS, Forrester JS, et al: Angiography, angioscopy, and ultrasound imaging before and after percutaneous balloon angioplasty. *Am Heart J* 1990; 120:1086.
13. Ramee SR, White CJ, Collins TJ, et al: Percutaneous angioscopy during coronary angioplasty using a steerable microangioscope. *J Am Coll Cardiol* 1991; 17:100.
14. Sherman CT, Litvack F, Grundfest WS, et al: Demonstration of thrombus and complex atheroma by in vivo angioscopy in patients with unstable angina pectoris. *N Engl J Med* 1986; 315:913.
15. Lee G, Garcia JM, Carso PJ, et al: Correlation of coronary angioscopic to angiographic findings in coronary artery disease. *Am J Cardiol* 1986; 57:238.

16. Spears JR, Spokojny AM, Marais J: Coronary angioscopy during cardiac catheterization. *J Am Coll Cardiol* 1985; 6:93–97.

17. Towne JB, Berngard VM: Vascular endoscopy: Useful tool or interesting toy. *Surgery* 1977; 82:415–419.

18. Lee G, Beerline D, Lee MH, et al: Hazard of angioscopic examination: Documentation of damage to the arterial intima. *Am Heart J* 1988; 11:1530.

19. Inoue K, Kuwaki K, Takahashi M: Transluminal cardioangioscopy. *Circulation* 1983; 68(suppl 3):7.

20. Inoue K, Kuwaki K, Takahashi M: In vivo transluminal angioscopy. *Circulation* 1984; 70(suppl 2):6.

21. Inoue K, Kuwaki K: Observation in vivo de al structure interieure des vaisseaux bu chien utilisant un angioscope ultrafine fibre optique. *Lett Commun Med*, May 14, 1986.

22. Spears JR, Marais HJ, Serur J, et al: In vivo coronary angioscopy. *J Am Coll Cardiol* 1983; 1:1311.

23. Lee G, Ikeda RM, Stobbe D, et al: Laser irradiation of human atherosclerotic obstructive disease: Simultaneous visualization and vaporization achieved by a dual fiberoptic catheter. *Am Heart J* 1983; 105:163–164.

24. Lee G, Ikeda RM, Stobbe D, et al: Intraoperative use of dual fiberoptic catheter for simultaneous in-vivo visualization and laser vaporization of peripheral atherosclerotic obstructive disease. *Cathet Cardiovasc Diagn* 1984; 10:11–16.

25. Grundfest WS, Litvack F, Sherman T, et al: Delineation of peripheral and coronary detail by intraoperative angioscopy. *Am Surg* 1985; 202:394–400.

26. Nanto S, Mishima M, Hirayama A: Monorail angioscopy with movable guide wire. *Circulation* 1988; 78:11–84.

6

Intravascular Ultrasound Imaging: Clinical Applications and Technical Advances

Paul G. Yock, M.D.

Peter J. Fitzgerald, M.D., Ph.D.

Krishnankutty Sudhir, M.D., Ph.D.

In the past year catheter ultrasound imaging has come of age technically for coronary applications. Ultrasound catheters can now be routinely delivered to most proximal and midvessel locations by using standard angioplasty guiding catheters and wires. Image quality has improved substantially, so interpretable pictures of the extent and distribution of the plaque can be obtained at most catheter positions. A productive phase of clinical research is under way in which the significance of different morphologic features of diseased vessels is beginning to be understood. Technical advances are continuing at a brisk pace, with emphasis being placed on improving catheter size and function and the development of combined imaging and therapeutic catheters.

FEATURES OF CATHETER DESIGN; NEW ADVANCES

There are two basic approaches to catheter ultrasound imaging: utilization of mechanical or solid-state transducers (Fig 6-1). The majority of companies involved in intravascular imaging have chosen the mechanical transducer approach in the anticipation of superior image quality, given the size constraints on the transducer.[1-3] Mechanical transducers in turn can be categorized into two major types. One design involves direct rotation of the transducer itself, with the transducer oriented generally perpendicular to the long axis of the catheter.[3] This is the more straightforward design and potentially minimizes the length of the stiff portion

at the catheter tip due to the transducer. A disadvantage of this approach arises from the fact that the portion of the beam immediately adjacent to the transducer has a zone of "ring-down" in which any image is obscured by reverberations from the transducer. As the transducer is rotated, this creates a bright artifact resembling a halo around the catheter. This region around the catheter is generally not wide enough to cause concern if the catheter is free in the vessel, but it may be a problem if the catheter is against the wall or wedged in a tight stenosis. A second basic design addresses this issue by mounting the transducer in the long axis of the catheter and reflecting the ultrasound signal from a rotating mirror.[1,2] This configuration results in a longer beam path within the catheter so that in effect the ring-down zone is consumed within the catheter. The resulting image has little or no ring-down artifact, with good resolution beginning at the surface around the catheter. This configuration also allows for better focusing of the beam, both because of the extra beam path length within the catheter and the opportunity to focus the beam at the reflector. A potential disadvantage of this design is that it can result in a longer zone of stiffness in the transducer region.

The mechanical systems in general benefit from some basic acoustic properties that are particularly relevant in the setting of extreme transducer miniaturization. For a start, the mechanical catheters are able to use transducers made of a piezoelectric ceramic that is similar to that used in the noninvasive echocardiographic transducers. This material provides excellent

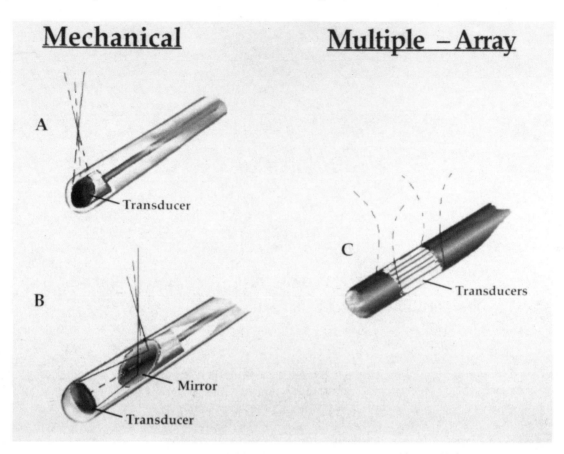

FIG 6–1.
Schematics for different basic ultrasound catheter designs. **A,** mechanical system with direct rotation of the transducer. **B,** mechanical system with a rotating reflector. **C,** multiple-array system. See the text for a more detailed description.

signal strength, which translates into the ability to achieve good penetration even from a tiny transducer. The mechanical transducers can also be focused in all three dimensions to achieve an image with relatively high resolution. The use of a circular transducer in the mechanical catheters also reduces side lobe artifacts, thus leading to an enhanced dynamic range (better gray-scale image).

Although basic acoustics favor the mechanical approach to miniature transducers, the engineering challenge in designing the catheters has been formidable. The most difficult and critical feature of the mechanical catheter design is the smooth and uniform rotation of the transducer. Any significant deviation from precise rotation can cause image distortion.[4] The industry has responded to this problem with the development of sophisticated torque cables, generally involving special winding technologies, that transmit the rotational torque accurately through a tortuous path. Miniaturization of the catheters for coronary applications has also been a technical challenge. The first generation of mechanical imaging catheters had an effective crossing

profile of 5.5 to 6 F (1.7- to 1.9-mm diameter) and required the use of high-flow 8 or 9 F guiding catheters.[5] Recently catheters have been released with lower profiles, with tips ranging between 4.3 and 4.8 F at the imaging plane, including the guidewire. This size range is comparable to the original coronary over-the-wire balloon catheters and can be used with regular 8 F or, in some cases, high-flow 7 F guides.

Two different delivery strategies for the mechanical catheters relative to the guidewire have been developed by the industry. Two of the currently Food and Drug Administration (FDA)-approved catheters use a sleeve-type guidewire lumen that is short relative to the entire catheter, similar to the Rx or Piccolino balloon catheters. This design has the same advantage as for these balloon catheters, namely, the ability to make rapid exchanges with a standard-length guidewire. This has been touted as a particularly desirable approach for an imaging device, where exchange is a fundamental aspect of the use of the catheter. A disadvantage of this approach is that the guidewire runs parallel to and outside the transducer region, so the shadow of the guidewire shows up as an artifact on the image. The second basic approach to delivery features a sheath that is advanced deeply into the artery of interest before imaging. The guidewire is then completely removed and the transducer and drive cable introduced in its place into the sheath. One potential advantage of this configuration is that the artery is protected from direct exposure to repeated passage of the imaging catheter over the area of interest. On the other hand, there is potential for trauma from the sheath in the distal segment of the artery as well as the possibility of ischemia from the deep fixed placement of the sheath. In addition, use of the sheath requires an extra step when the the guidewire is removed.

The second major category of imaging catheter design is solid-state, in which there are no moving parts to the catheter.[6, 7] The transducer consists of multiple elements in a cylindrical array at the catheter tip. The elements transmit and receive in a timed sequence to produce a beam that is swept out in a circle perpendicular to the catheter tip, just as in the mechanical systems. One approach to multielement imaging is a "dynamic aperture" method, which uses different groupings of elements both to change the position in the sweep where information is collected and to change the numbers of elements involved as a function of the distance from the target to the catheter. In the one FDA-approved implementation of this approach, tiny integrated circuits are mounted in the tip of the catheter to perform the appropriate sequencing of elements. The resulting signals are then collected in a relatively powerful image-processing computer and the images reconstructed rapidly and displayed. Development of a different solid-state catheter system has been announced recently. This system is said to involve a true "phased-array" approach similar to that used in noninvasive ultrasound scanners. In vivo studies have not been reported, so it is too early to attempt to assess the relative advantages and limits of this system vs. mechanical catheters.

Sufficient experience has accumulated with the dynamic aperture system, however, to make some initial comparisons with the other FDA-approved catheters. The catheter is coaxial for its entire length, similar to the most commonly employed balloon configuration. This may improve the tracking of the catheter in comparison to the offset guidewire lumen used in the mechanical catheters. In addition, the radial array of the imaging elements around the central guidewire lumen means that there is no external guidewire artifact to shadow a portion of the vessel wall. Connection to the system electronics is straightforward, without the need for a motor drive unit as in the mechanical catheter systems.

The major limitation of the dynamic aperture system is the quality of the images. The catheter has both a ring-down artifact around the transducer and a zone of limited quality of image due to "near-field" distortions. One approach to reducing the impact of the ring-down artifact has been employed recently and involves creating a "mask" of the ring-down artifact before cannulating the artery and then subtracting this mask digitally. This strategy improves the appearance of the image and allows some degree of tissue resolution close to the catheter. In practice, the near-zone problems are partially camouflaged in the presentation of the image by a circular mask larger than the true dimension of the catheter (2.0 mm for the 1.7-mm catheter). Resolution of the dynamic aperture system is also limited, particularly in the dimension parallel to the long axis of the catheter where there is no focusing of the beam. The current dynamic aperture system also has a comparatively "bistable" or black-and-white image that limits the amount of gray scale available for tissue differentiation. The catheter also uses a film transducer, which has limited ability to penetrate relative to the mechanical transducers, so imaging in tight stenoses or larger vessels can be problematic. Finally, because of the need to reconstruct the dynamic aperture images, the frame rate of the images is lower than for the mechanical systems. This last feature does not appear to be a significant detriment clinically.

Clinical studies using the dynamic aperture catheter have employed a 5.5 F catheter compatible with a 0.014-in. guidewire and a high-flow 8 F guiding catheter.[6, 7] Recently, in vitro tests have been conducted with a catheter in the 3.5 F size range. As with any attempt at continued miniaturization of transducers, further degradation of image quality will be a significant issue with these smaller catheters.

IMAGE INTERPRETATION

The basis of image interpretation of the intravascular scans is the ability to recognize the contour of the lumen, the extent and distribution of plaque, and the presence of any other significant morphologic features such as dissections. The appearance of normal vessel wall on an ultrasound scan is fairly straightforward (Fig 6–2). In muscular arteries such as the coronary system, the medial layer frequently stands out as a dark band sandwiched between two brighter layers.[8] The media is relatively echo poor (dark) relative to the other layers because it contains more muscle, which is weakly reflective of ultrasound as compared with the collagen and elastin found in the other layers. The bright inner layer is caused by a combination of the intima and internal elastic lamina.[5] In normal, young coronary arteries these layers may not be thick enough to generate a distinct band on the ultrasound image (Fig 6–2, left).[9] Most adults have sufficient intimal thickening of the coronary arteries, however, that the bright inner layer is present on at least some level in the coronary tree. As significant atherosclerotic plaque develops in an area, the three-layered appearance of the vessel becomes more prominent (Fig 6–2, right). The dark band of the media serves as a very useful reference point to define the outer border of the plaque accumulation. In the case of advanced plaque deposition, there is frequently significant thinning of the media underlying the plaque.[10] In these cases a clearly defined medial layer may not be detectable on the ultrasound scan, although it is usually possible to identify the plaque–vessel wall interface based on the differing appearance of plaque from the normal wall structures. Scanning adjacent regions by advancing or retracting the catheter a short distance can

also be very useful in identifying the level of the media.

Catheter ultrasound images can also provide information on different types of plaque and plaque components. Calcification is prominent in the scans as a very brightly reflective area, with shadowing of all of the deeper tissue structures.[11] Densely fibrotic material can also cause shadowing, so the presence of this finding is not diagnostic for calcification. Discrete lipid accumulations are weakly echo reflective and so show up as dark regions within the body of a plaque.[11, 12] At its current level of development catheter ultrasound is not highly sensitive for the detection of lipid accumulations, however. False-positive identification of lipid pools is also possible: a similar appearance can be caused by false lumina within the plaque or potentially by shadowing due to a region of calcification or fibrosis outside of the major imaging plane. Catheters with poor dynamic range (poor gray-scale discrimination) can also create the false impression of lipid pools within homogeneous, fibrous plaque.

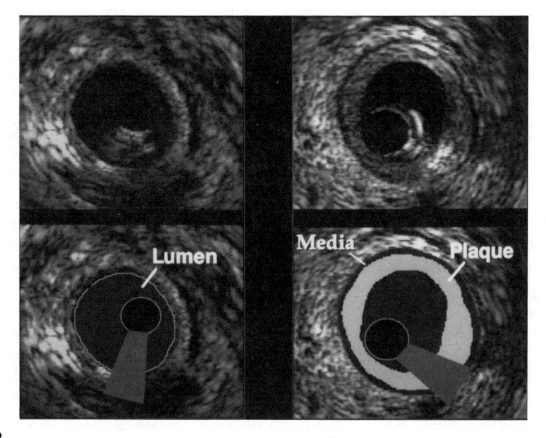

FIG 6–2.
Essentials of coronary image interpretation. The image on the *left* (with a schematic overlay below) shows a normal coronary artery from a young person without significant plaque deposition. The lumen is clearly defined, but there is no three-layered appearance. The ray extending between 6 and 7 o'clock is the positioning vector. The scan on the *right* is from a left anterior descending artery with circumferential plaque. The media shows up clearly as a thin dark band marking the outer boundary of plaque accumulation.

One significant imaging limitation for catheter ultrasound at present is in attempting to differentiate between thrombus and soft plaque.[13] The overall intensity of the ultrasound signal from these two tissues may be quite similar. Some clues can be of help, however, in suggesting the presence of thrombus. An undulating motion of the material with the pulse cycle is more characteristic of thrombus than plaque. Fresh thrombus may also have a finely granular or "scintillating" appearance, which in our early experience appears to be characteristic. More often than not, however, the discrimination between thrombus and soft plaque remains ambiguous from the image alone. This is an area where new technical developments may be of use (see below).

COMPARISON WITH ANGIOSCOPY

The basic format of the angioscopic image is fundamentally and obviously different from catheter ultrasound. The angioscopic image is three-dimensional in a direction forward from the catheter tip. Intravascular ultrasound is intrinsically two-dimensional, with the current catheters having a side-looking format. Angioscopy provides a very high-resolution picture of the endoluminal surface that is extremely sensitive for the detection of thrombus, even in small amounts.[14, 15] Angioscopy is also capable of resolving intimal tears occurring at the surface of the vessel in great detail.[15] The major limitation of angioscopy, however, is that it is unable to provide information about pathology below the luminal surface. Catheter ultrasound, by contrast, reveals information about the depth of plaque in any given direction. Ultrasound also does not require clearing of blood from the lumen in order to image — in fact, the blood provides an effective coupling medium between the transducer and the vessel wall.

Both angioscopy and ultrasound catheters can be used over the wire with conventional guiding catheter technologies. Although the fiber-optic bundles used to create images in the angioscopes are quite small (less than 1 mm in diameter), the actual catheter diameters may be substantially larger due to the requirement for a flushing lumen and/or an inflation lumen for the occlusion balloon. As a result, the caliber of the current angioscopic catheters approaches that of the ultrasound catheters. Positioning of an angioscope for obtaining optimal images in the coronary system can be a challenging and time-consuming undertaking. By contrast, once an ultrasound catheter is set up, imaging can be performed at essentially any position without attempting to specifically direct the catheter.

QUANTITATION BY CATHETER ULTRASOUND

In addition to providing information about tissue types within the vessel wall, catheter ultrasound provides an accurate quantative assessment of lumen and plaque areas. In vitro validation studies have demonstrated generally good accuracy in lumen area determinations.[12] Angulation of the imaging plane with respect to the long axis of the vessel causes the cross section of the vessel to be elliptical in appearance and can lead to an "overestimation" of cross-sectional area (although the area is in fact correct for the portion of vessel intersected by the angled plane of the beam). Precision of area measurements from the in vitro studies averages in the 5 to 8% range. In vivo comparisons of dimensions and areas between ultrasound and angiography have also demonstrated generally close correlations in normal vessels or in segments with concentric plaque. Higher rates of discordance are seen in the presence of eccentric plaque, perhaps reflecting errors in the angiographic cross-sectional area determination due to the asymmetrical shape of the lumen.[16] The lack of correlation between catheter ultrasound and angiography is even more pronounced in the postangioplasty setting, where there can be significant luminal irregularities due to dissection. The area measured by ultrasound may exceed the angiographic cross-sectional area because the ultrasound measurement takes into account the irregular lumen channels created by dissections.

In vitro studies comparing quantitative estimates of plaque volume by ultrasound and histologic sectioning have shown correlations that are generally close but not as strong as the lumen area correlations.[2] In part this is due to the problem of defining the plaque-media interface at all locations in the vessel. As a practical matter, it is generally possible in the clinical setting to move the catheter a short distance forward or backward to establish the level of the media in an immediately neighboring segment.

GUIDANCE FOR CATHETER THERAPIES

Although catheter ultrasound imaging is a diagnostic procedure, its major initial application will be to serve as an enabling modality for various vascular interventions. As clinical experience with the imaging catheters accumulates, a much clearer picture is emerging concerning the effects of different catheter technologies on the vessel wall.

Intravascular ultrasound used in the context of balloon angioplasty has confirmed the results of prior pathologic studies suggesting that the major mechanism of lumen enlargement involves stretching of normal vessel wall, fracture of plaque, and tearing of the plaque free from the vessel wall in limited dissection planes at the level of the media (Fig 6–3). Ultrasound imaging could potentially be effective in differentiating stable dissections from more severe dissections associated with a greater likelihood of progression to abrupt closure.[17, 18] Whether or not ultrasound will be more useful than conventional angiography (or angioscopy) in this respect remains to be clarified. One technical problem in imaging dissections with catheter ultrasound is the tendency of the catheter to "prop up" the dissected portion of plaque against the vessel wall, potentially masking the true extent of the dissection.

Perhaps the most impressive finding from catheter ultrasound imaging in the context of angioplasty is the degree of elastic rebound following balloon deflation. It is not uncommon to see the lumen return to 50% or less of the inflated balloon diameter. Angiography appears to underestimate the extent of recoil, in part because contrast entering into dissection planes exaggerates the apparent lumen dimension. The combined balloon ultrasound imaging catheter *(BUIC)* tested by Isner et al.[19] (see below) has shown dramatic, real-time images of the rebound following balloon angioplasty in peripheral lesions.

At present there is limited understanding of the effects of different plaque types on the outcome of balloon angioplasty. Pathologic studies have suggested that calcification in a lesion may influence the likelihood of a successful and sustained angioplasty effect. The presence of severe calcification can of course inhibit full balloon inflation, but it may also predispose to severe dissection. On the other hand, a complete lack of calcium or fibrous tissue in a plaque may make it relatively elastic and thereby more likely to rebound extensively postinflation. Plaque eccentricity may also influence the outcome of balloon inflation, and it has been suggested that optimal balloon sizing might be different for eccentric vs. concentric plaque. These are issues that are now beginning to be addressed as better-quality intracoronary images are being obtained routinely. With the current-size catheters, scanning of a vessel prior to any balloon inflation is not practical in many cases because of the necessity to cross the lesion in order to obtain the images. As with any catheter, however, it is difficult to predict a priori whether or not it will be possible to cross a given lesion.

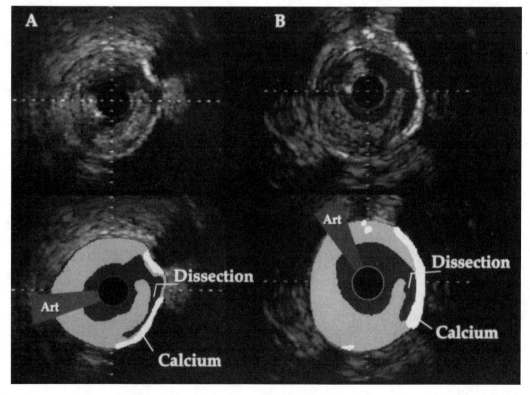

FIG 6–3.
Two examples of plaque fracture following balloon angioplasty. In both cases the dissection plane is seen to track along a rim of calcification and lift up an arm of plaque into the lumen. (**B,** courtesy of Ray Matthews, M.D., Good Samaritan Hospital, Los Angeles.)

To date, there are no data relating morphologic features of a lesion postangioplasty to the likelihood of restenosis. One plausible predictor of restenosis is the extent of dissection, specifically, whether or not the dissection invades the media.[20] A recent clinicopathologic study suggested that restenosis rates with medial dissection were double those involving tears limited to the intima only.[21] It is also likely that an accurate measure of the cross-sectional area of the vessel (as can be provided by catheter ultrasound) will prove to correlate with the risk of restenosis. Clinical studies designed to evaluate potential morphologic predictors of restenosis are now under way.

Catheter ultrasound has also been applied to monitoring the results of plaque removal strategies, including atherectomy and laser ablation. In the case of directional atherectomy with the Simpson Atherocath, preliminary studies have helped to clarify the mechanism of action and have suggested some possibilities for procedural improvement.[22] In both the periphery and in the

coronary arteries, ultrasound imaging demonstrates a significant residual plaque burden following successful atherectomy. In one report, the mean angiographic percent stenosis following directional coronary atherectomy was 11%, but the percentage of lumen area still occupied by plaque averaged 61%.[23] This discrepancy demonstrates several important features of directional atherectomy. First, the improvement in lumen area suggested by the angiogram following the procedure is generally valid. However, areas of intimal tearing and dissection can be seen with atherectomy, as well as regions of trough-like cuts — all of which lead to an exaggerated concept of lumen area by angiography (Fig 6–4). It is important to note that these luminal irregularities are in general less than what is seen with balloon angioplasty (which correlates with the clearer, less hazy appearance of many atherectomy lesions on angiography). Despite the significant improvement in lumen area, however, there is a significant plaque burden left following the procedure. Part of this burden is due to

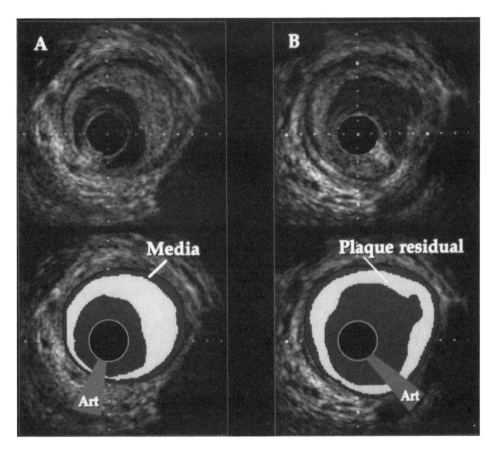

FIG 6–4.
Directional atherectomy (superficial femoral artery). The preatherectomy image **(A)** shows eccentric plaque accumulation, most significant between 12 and 5 o'clock. Atherectomy cuts were concentrated in this region and resulted in a significantly larger lumen **(B)** without any cuts into the media. A typical atherectomy trough is seen at 2 o'clock. (Courtesy of Mark Wholey, M.D., Pittsburgh Vascular Institute.)

the fact that the extent of plaque present in the first place is greatly underestimated by the angiogram; part is due to an angioplasty effect caused by a combination of the relatively stiff housing of the device and the balloon inflation. An ultrasound study by Smucker et al.[24] suggested that approximately a third of the luminal dimension improvement with directional atherectomy is due to tissue removal and two thirds is due to an angioplasty effect. These numbers are very similar to previously published estimates of the same phenomenon based on angiographic data.[25, 26]

Composition of the plaque – in particular, the amount and distribution of calcium — appears to have a significant influence on the amount of tissue removed by the atherectomy device. The most common pattern of calcification seen by ultrasound imaging is a thin crescent occurring deep within the plaque at the plaque-media interface. Occasionally deposits of calcium occur midway within the substance of the plaque. Superficial calcification at the luminal border can also be seen relatively frequently. It is this superficial calcification pattern that correlates with a reduction in the mass of plaque removed by atherectomy.[27]

Potentially the most important question to be approached with catheter ultrasound monitoring of directional atherectomy is whether there are morphologic predictors of restenosis. In a preliminary report with small numbers of patients, the best predictor of restenosis following directional coronary atherectomy was the minimal cross-sectional area of the lumen as determined by ultrasound.[27] In patients with restenosis, the mean postprocedure luminal cross-sectional area was 4.6 mm^2; in patients with no restenosis at an average of 6 months of follow-up, the mean postprocedure area was 9.2 mm^2. The results of this study are in line with a current dogma concerning restenosis with various devices[28]: the larger the lumen created by the procedure, the less likely that angiographically significant restenosis will occur. In the context of directional atherectomy this suggests that more aggressive debulking of plaque may be desirable. One obvious liability to this approach is vessel perforation. It is very difficult in some cases to have a clear concept of which portion of the vessel wall may be thin and vulnerable based on the angiogram. In addition, it appears that restenosis rates increase when normal vessel wall is sampled (that is, media or adventitia is present in the specimens). Data from several groups suggest that in peripheral vessels, in coronary bypass grafts, and in vessels that have previously restenosed, the risk of postatherectomy restenosis is increased when media is sampled. The data are presently conflicting from different groups concerning the relation of media and restenosis in de novo coronary artery lesions.[29, 30]

Because of its ability to gauge plaque thickness, ultrasound imaging appears to be an excellent guidance modality for directional atherectomy. One limitation to this approach in practice is the need to correlate the orientation of the atherectomy device with the plaque accumulations detected by ultrasound. In the coronary arteries this can be accomplished to a reasonable degree by careful attention to the branching pattern on the ultrasound scan. For example, the origin of circumflex, diagonal, and septal vessels can be defined from a catheter position in the left anterior descending artery and the appropriate orientation for atherectomy deduced accordingly. The catheter used by our group has an "orientation vector" that is visible both on the ultrasound scan and fluoroscopically, theoretically allowing more rapid orientation of the ultrasound images. This system works well in the periphery but is limited in the coronary circulation at present due to difficulty in precisely torquing the imaging catheters. A more elegant (but technically demanding) solution to this problem is to combine imaging with atherectomy in a single catheter, as described below.

There is less experience at present with imaging in association with coaxial atherectomy devices, i.e., the Rotablator[31] and the transluminal extraction or TEC[32] catheters. Anecdotal experience suggests that the lumen caliber created by these devices is the same or slightly smaller than the outer diameter of the catheters. A recent preliminary report indicates that the lumen created by the Rotablator has a smoother, more rounded appearance than with either the directional or extraction atherectomy devices.[33] Use of a stand-alone imaging catheter in association with the coaxial atherectomy procedures may be useful in attempting to decide whether to "size up" to a larger-diameter device. The presence of a concentric plaque distribution with reasonable margins would favor the use of the larger catheter.

Essentially the same logic applies for the current generation of over-the-wire laser catheters. Again, the lumen created by the catheters appears to be approximately the same caliber as the device. Inspection of a laser-treated segment of vessel may help the operator to decide whether a larger-diameter catheter can be used safely. Accurate lumen area determinations may also help determine whether adjunctive balloon angioplasty is indicated.

One of the most fascinating applications of ultrasound imaging technology recently has been in the assessment of stent placement.[34] Because of the intense echogenicity of the metallic struts of the currently available stents, ultrasound images of the stents are fairly dramatic (Fig 6–5). Stent restenosis can be gauged with reasonable accuracy since the struts can be seen clearly

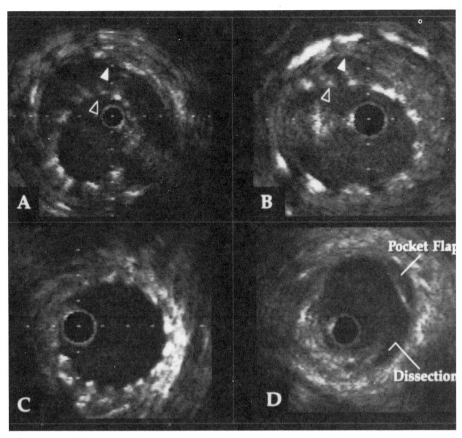

FIG 6–5.
Sequential levels of images from a freshly implanted Palmaz stent in an iliac artery. Panel **A** demonstrates an area of incomplete apposition of the stent *(open arrow)* to the vessel wall *(closed arrow).* In panel **B** the stent is well apposed to the vessel except for a small area at 12 o'clock *(arrows).* Panel **C** shows complete apposition of the stent for the entire circumference of the vessel. In panel **D** two areas of dissection are detected just adjacent to the caudal margin of the stent. (Courtesy of Richard Schatz, M.D., Scripps Clinic, San Diego.)

embedded within the material of the restenosis lesion. Perhaps a more important application of ultrasound imaging, however, will be assessment of the adequacy of deployment of stents at the time of implantation.[35] Incomplete apposition of the stent to the vessel wall may lead to enhanced thrombosis by virtue of increased exposure of the metal of the stent to the bloodstream and by means of local flow disturbances. Portions of the stent that are free of the vessel wall may also fail to endothelialize, with potentially significant late consequences. Imaging with catheter ultrasound at the time of stent implantation allows the operator to redilate any sections of the stent that are incompletely expanded.

ANTICIPATED DEVELOPMENTS

The catheter ultrasound industry is very young, and advances in both image quality and catheter performance characteristics are continuing at a brisk pace. There is still considerable room for refinement in the images, including improved resolution and dynamic range, minimization of catheter artifacts, and consistency of good-quality scans. There is also impetus in catheter development to continue to reduce the size of the catheters and improve delivery characteristics, including tip flexibility.

One of the most exciting areas of advanced technical development is in the area of combined imaging and therapeutic catheters. Several groups have shown prototypes of combined balloon–ultrasound imaging catheters,[19, 36, 37] and two groups have initiated clinical trials. Hodgson and colleagues have reported on a combined dynamic aperture–imaging catheter where the transducer is placed behind the balloon, in the proximal part of the shoulder.[37] This allows the deflated balloon profile ahead of the transducer to be minimized in order to facilitate crossing tight stenoses. Once the lesion is dilated, the balloon can be advanced distal to the lesion to allow inspection by the imaging element. Clinical studies have been performed in human coronary arteries, and the images have proved useful in making decisions about repeat inflations or upsizing of the balloon. Isner et al. have reported a combined balloon-imaging catheter with a mechanical catheter mounted in the center of the balloon.[19] This configuration allows inspection of one plane of the lesion as the balloon is expanded, potentially providing information about the mechanism of angioplasty. This catheter has undergone clinical testing in peripheral vessels and has given graphic demonstrations of the extent of elastic recoil in these vessels following deflation of the balloon.

A prototype combined imagining–directional atherectomy device has also been developed and tested in vitro.[38] This device generates images from a transducer mounted in association with the cutter to allow a segment of interest to be scanned before cutting. Ultrasound imaging guidance has also been proposed as a method for guiding laser debulking. In one system, an imaging element is mounted in the same catheter as a side-directed laser fiber.[39] A three-dimensional representation of the vessel wall is built up by moving the catheter within the region of interest in the vessel. This image then provides a map for plaque ablation with the laser. Clinical trials have not yet begun for either the combined atheterectomy or laser devices.

Another promising area of development is three-dimensional image reconstruction of the ultrasound images.[40, 41] Catheter ultrasound imaging lends itself extremely well to three-dimensional imaging since the tomographic, two-dimensional slices obtained from a series of catheter positions can be "stacked" directly to build the three-dimensional representation (Fig 6–6). In practice, images recorded during a steady pullback of the catheter are sent to an external computer that generates the three-dimensional reconstruction within a period of a minute or less. Once assembled, the images can be displayed in a variety of formats and projections. One useful display is a computer "hemisection" of the vessel in the long axis, effectively opening up the vessel lengthwise (Fig 6–6). With current systems, some degradation of image resolution occurs in forming the three-dimensional images. This is not an intrinsic limitation with the technology but reflects the need for higher processing speeds and memory. The full range of applications of three-dimensional reconstruction of the vessel images remains to be fully appreciated. Preliminary experience suggests, however, that display of the information in three dimensions gives a more accurate concept of complex vessel morphologies — for example, dissections and false channels — than is available from two-dimensional imaging alone.

Potential for image enhancement exists in another

direction of technical advance called "tissue characterization."[42–44] In general, tissue characterization refers to a set of computer-based methods for extracting information about tissue types from the raw, backscattered ultrasound signal before it is processed into an image. Although there has been a series of important research studies on potential applications of ultrasonic tissue characterization to the heart, practical applications have been extremely limited. In large part this is due to the fact that the pure backscattered signals returning from myocardium are adulterated as they pass through the tissues of the chest wall on the way out to the transducer on the skin. With catheter ultrasound, by contrast, the transducer is closely adjacent to the tissue of interest (plaque), with a relatively homogeneous coupling material between (blood). The relatively high frequencies of catheter ultrasound also increase the discriminating power for tissue characterization methods. There are several potential applications of tissue characterization for intravascular ultrasound that might have important clinical benefit. As has been mentioned above, discrimination of thrombus from soft plaque may be difficult by imaging alone. A preliminary report suggests that statistical analysis of the backscattered ultrasound signal may allow for differentiation of these two tissue types.[45] Potentially an even more important application is enhancing the ability to detect lipid-laden plaques. Although the appearance of lipid can be characteristic on the two-dimensional images, sensitivity for detecting lipid pools is by no means high. This is a critical issue clinically since it appears that lipid-rich plaque is relatively unstable and susceptible to rupture with subsequent myocardial infarction.[46]

SUMMARY

Intravascular ultrasound is a promising new technology for directly imaging the extent and distribution of plaque within the vessel wall. Rapid technical advances over the last several years have yielded a first generation of coronary catheters that can be used to image proximal and midrange vessels with relative ease. Further improvement in catheter profiles, performance, and image quality are ongoing, along with the development of combined imaging and therapeutic devices. Clinical studies are now being launched to help identify the appropriate and cost-effective applications of this powerful new technology.

Acknowledgment

Images presented in this chapter were obtained by using the Insight system from Cardivascular Imaging

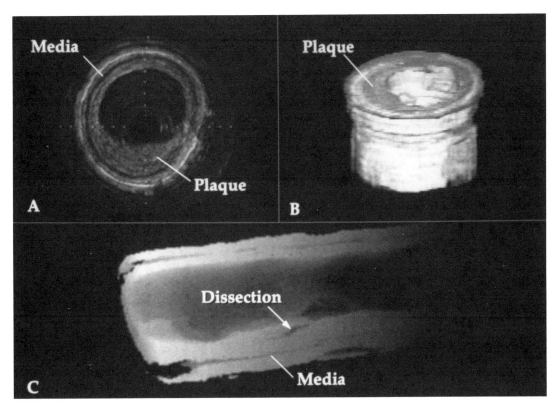

FIG 6–6.
Three-dimensional reconstruction of a diseased iliac vessel. **A,** single two-dimensional cross-sectional image from one level within the segment of interest. **B,** three-dimensional representation of the entire reconstructed segment shows plaque and lumen. **C,** computer-generated hemisection of the vessel shows the level of the media and a small dissection within the plaque substance. (**B** courtesy of Terry Laas , Santa Clara, Calif.)

Systems (Cvis) of Sunnyvale, Calif. All images are single-frame excerpts from real-time videotape without postprocessing (overall contrast and brightness may be adjusted for publication). We gratefully acknowledge the skilled editorial assistance of Barbara Herz.

REFERENCES

1. Yock PG, Johnson EL, Linker DT: Intravascular ultrasound: Development and clinical potential. *Am J Card Imaging* 1988; 2:185–193.
2. Tobis JM, Mallery JA, Gessert J, et al: Intravascular ultrasound cross-section imaging before and after balloon angioplasty in vitro. *Circulation* 1989; 80:873–882.
3. Pandian NG, Kreis A, Brockway B, et al: Ultrasound angioscopy: Real-time two-dimensional, intraluminal ultrasound imaging of blood vessels. *Am J Cardiol* 1988; 62:493–494.
4. ten Hoff H, Korbijn A, Smit TH, et al: Imaging artifacts in mechanically driven ultrasound catheters. *Int J Card Imaging* 1989; 4:195–199.
5. Yock PG, Linker DT, Angelsen BA: Two-dimensional intravascular ultrasound: Technical development and initial clinical experience. *J Am Soc Echocardiogr* 1989; 2:296–304.
6. Hodgson JM, Graham SP, Savakus AD, et al: Clinical percutaneous imaging of coronary anatomy using an over-the-wire ultrasound catheter system. *Am J Card Imaging* 1989; 4:186–193.
7. Nissen SE, Grimes CL, Gurley JC, et al: Application of a new phased-array ultrasound imaging catheter in the assessment of vascular dimensions. *Circulation* 1990; 81:2007–2012.
8. Meyer CR, Chiang EH, Fechner KP, et al: Feasibility of high-resolution intravascular ultrasonic imaging catheters. *Radiology* 1988; 168:113–116.
9. Fitzgerald PJ, St. Goar FG, Kao AD, et al: Intravascular ultrasound imaging of coronary arteries: Is three layers the norm? (abstract). *J Am Coll Cardiol* 1991; 17:217.
10. Isner JM, Donaldson BS, Fortin AH, et al: Attenuation of the media of coronary arteries in advanced atherosclerosis. *Am J Cardiol* 1986; 58:937–939.
11. Gussenhoven EJ, Essed CE, Lancee CT, et al: Arterial wall characteristics determined by intravascular ultrasound imaging: An in vitro study. *J Am Coll Cardiol* 1989; 14:957–962.
12. Potkin BN, Bartorelli AL, Gessert JM, et al: Coronary artery imaging with intravascular high-frequency ultrasound. *Circulation* 1990; 81:1575–1585.
13. Pandian NG, Kreis A, Brockway B: Detection of intraarterial thrombus by intravascular high frequency two-

dimensional ultrasound imaging in in vitro and in vivo studies. *Am J Cardiol* 1990; 15:1280–1283.

14. Sherman CT, Litvack F, Grundfest W, et al: Coronary angioscopy in patients with unstable angina pectoris. *N Engl J Med* 1986; 315:912–919.

15. Ramee SR, White CJ, Collins TJ, et al: Percutaneous angioscopy during coronary angioplasty using a steerable microangioscope. *J Am Coll Cardiol* 1991; 17:100–105.

16. Nissen SE, Gurley JC, Grimes CL, et al: Comparison of intravascular ultrasound and angiography in quantitation of coronary dimensions and stenosis in man: Impact of lumen eccentricity (abstract). *Circulation* 1990; 82(suppl 3):440.

17. Tobis JM, Mahon D, Lehmann K, et al: Intracoronary ultrasound imaging after balloon angioplasty (abstract). *Circulation* 1990; 82(suppl 3):676.

18. Leon M, Keren G, Pichard A, et al: Intravascular ultrasound assessment of plaque responses to PTCA helps to explain angiographic findings (abstract). *J Am Coll Cardiol* 1991; 17:47.

19. Isner JM, Rosenfield K, Mosseri M, et al: How reliable are images obtained by intravascular ultrasound for making decisions during percutaneous interventions? Experience with intravascular ultrasound employed in lieu of contrast angiography to guide peripheral balloon angioplasty in 16 patients (abstract). *Circulation* 1990; 78(suppl 3):17.

20. Steele PM, Chesebro JGH, Stanson AW, et al: Balloon angioplasty: Natural history of the pathophysiological response to injury in pig model. *Circ Res* 1985; 57:105–112.

21. Nobuyoshi M, Kimura T, Ohishi H, et al: Restenosis after percutaneous transluminal coronary angioplasty: Pathologic observations in 20 patients. *J Am Coll Cardiol* 1991; 17:433–439.

22. Yock PG, Linker DT, White NW, et al: Clinical applications of intravascular ultrasound imaging in atherectomy. *Int J Card Imaging* 1989; 4:117–125.

23. Yock PG, Fitzgerald PJ, Sykes C, et al: Morphologic features of successful coronary atherectomy determined by intravascular ultrasound imaging (abstract). *Circulation* 1990; 82(suppl 3):676.

24. Smucker ML, Scherb DE, Howard PF, et al: Intracoronary ultrasound: How much "angioplasty effect" in atherectomy (abstract). *Circulation* 1990; 82(suppl 3):676.

25. Safian RD, Gelbfish JS, Erny RE, et al: Coronary atherectomy: Clinical angiographic and histological findings and observations regarding potential mechanisms. *Circulation* 1990; 82:69–79.

26. Sharaf BL, Williams DO: "Dotter effect" contributes to angiographic improvement following directional coronary atherectomy (abstract). *Circulation* 1990; 82(suppl 3):310.

27. Yock PG, Fitzgerald PJ, Sykes C, et al: Morphologic features of successful coronary atherectomy determined by intravascular ultrasound imaging (abstract). *Circulation* 1990; 82(suppl 3):676.

28. Kuntz RE, Safian RD, Schmidt DA, et al: Restenosis following new coronary devices: The influence of postprocedure luminal diameter (abstract). *J Am Coll Cardiol* 1991; 17:2.

29. Garrett KN, Holmes DR, Bell MR, et al: Restenosis af-

ter directional coronary atherectomy: Difference between primary atheromatous and restenosis lesions and influence of subintimal tissue resection. *J Am Coll Cardiol* 1990; 16:1665–1671.

30. Simpson JB, Robertson GC, Selmon MH, et al: Restenosis following successful directional coronary atherectomy (abstract). *Circulation* 1989; 80(suppl 2):582.

31. Hansen DD, Auth DC, Hall M, et al: Rotational endarterectomy in normal canine coronary arteries: Preliminary report. *J Am Coll Cardiol* 1988; 11:1073–1077.

32. Stack RS, Quigley PJ, Sketch MH, et al: Extraction atherectomy, in Topol EJ (ed): *Interventional Cardiology*. Philadelphia, WB Saunders, 1990, pp 590–602.

33. Keren G, Pichard AD, Satler LF, et al: Intravascular ultrasound of coronary atherectomy (abstract). *J Am Coll Cardiol* 1991; 17:157.

34. Chokshi SK, Hogan J, Desai V, et al: Intravascular ultrasound assessment of implanted endovascular stents (abstract). *J Am Coll Cardiol* 1990; 15:29.

35. Slepian MJ, White NW, Rowe MH, et al: Intravascular two-dimensional US: Sensitive imaging modality for detection of complete versus partial stent expansion (abstract). *Radiology* 1989; 173:106.

36. Mallery JA, Gregory K, Morcos NC, et al: Evaluation of an ultrasound balloon dilatation imaging catheter (abstract). *Circulation* 1987; 76(suppl 4):371.

37. Hodgson JM, Cacchione JG, Berry J, et al: Combined intracoronary ultrasound imaging and angioplasty catheter: Initial in-vivo studies (abstract). *Circulation* 1990; 82(suppl 3):676.

38. Yock PG, Fitzgerald PJ, Jang YT, et al: Initial trials of combined ultrasound imaging/mechanical atherectomy catheter (abstract). *J Am Coll Cardiol* 1990; 15:17.

39. Aretz HT, Martinelli MA, LeDet EG: Intraluminal ultrasound guidance of transverse laser coronary atherectomy. *Int J Card Imaging* 1989; 4:153–157.

40. Kitney RI, Moura L, Straughan K: 3-D visualization of arterial structures using ultrasound and voxel modelling. *Int J Card Imaging* 1989; 4:135–143.

41. Losordo DW, Chokshi SK, Harding M, et al: Three-dimensional intravascular ultrasonic imaging of intraarterial stents: Validation of technique by histologic morphology (abstract). *Circulation* 1990; 82(suppl 3):103.

42. Landini L, Sarnelli R, Picano E, et al: Evaluation of frequency dependence of backscatter coefficient in normal and atherosclerotic aortic walls. *Ultrasound Med Biol* 1986; 12:397–401.

43. Barzilai B, Saffitz JE, Miller JG, et al: Quantitative ultrasonic characterization of the nature of atherosclerotic plaques in human aorta. *Circ Res* 1987; 60:459–463.

44. Linker DT, Yock PG, Groenningsaether A, et al: Analysis of backscattered ultrasound from normal and diseased arterial wall. *Int J Card Imaging* 1989; 4:177–185.

45. Fitzgerald PJ, Connolly AJ, Watkins RD, et al: Distinction between soft plaque and thrombus by intravascular tissue characterization (abstract). *J Am Coll Cardiol* 1991; 17:111.

46. Richardson PD, Davies MJ, Born GVR: Influence of plaque configuration and stress distribution on fissuring of coronary atherosclerotic plaques. *Lancet* 1989; 2:941–944.

7

Application of Echocardiography to Catheter Balloon Valvuloplasty

Martin R. Berk, M.B., B.Ch.

Anthony N. Demaria, M.D.

Mikel D. Smith, M.D.

The increasing use of the invasive interventional technique of catheter balloon valvuloplasty has resulted in a proportional reliance on the noninvasive method of echocardiography. Thus the ability to perform valvuloplasty has increased the interventional cardiologist's interest in and reliance on the findings in the noninvasive laboratory. The contribution of echocardiography to valvuloplasty has taken several forms (Table 7–1). Echocardiography provides the first method to confirm the diagnosis and quantify the lesions of mitral and aortic stenosis. Echocardiography also allows the diagnosis of associated lesions that may determine the suitability of patients for catheter valvuloplasty. More importantly, particularly in regard to the mitral valve, morphologic characteristics of the echocardiogram relate quite well to the potential for an excellent hemodynamic result following valvuloplasty. In addition, transesophageal echocardiography is extremely sensitive in detecting left atrial thrombus, especially in the appendage. Echocardiography has been advocated and utilized by some to guide the valvuloplasty procedure by means of localizing the balloon itself and assessing the degree of mitral regurgitation in the catheterization laboratory. Of greater significance, echocardiography has provided an important tool for the detection of complications following valvuloplasty, as well as assessment of the effects in both the long and short term following the procedure. Therefore echocardiography now plays an integral role in the assessment of patients undergoing balloon valvuloplasty.

QUANTITATION OF VALVE STENOSIS

Echocardiography has been demonstrated during the past several years to provide an excellent modality to quantify the severity of valvular stenosis.[1] A variety of echocardiographic imaging and Doppler velocity measurements can be performed that enable quantitation of both valvular gradient and cross-sectional area.[2] Although all echocardiographic maneuvers are potentially applicable to both mitral and aortic valves, certain assessments have been found to be of greater value with respect to specific valves.

Several methods exist to quantify the severity of mitral stenosis by echocardiography. The oldest method is based on the ability to visualize the cross-sectional area of the mitral valve. When images of the mitral valve leaflets are obtained in short-axis views, the area of the orifice can be easily planimetered, and these values have been shown to correlate well to either catheter or surgical measurements of the mitral valve area.[3] Such measurements are influenced by a variety of technical factors: the smallest orifice of the funnel-shaped mitral leaflets must be located and visualized, an excessive gain setting may obliterate some portion of the orifice by ul-

TABLE 7–1

Echocardiography in Catheter Balloon Valvuloplasty

Diagnosis and quantitation of lesion
Detection of associated abnormalities (regurgitation)
Evaluation of suitability for valvuloplasty
Guiding procedure
Detection of complications
Assessment of results
Long-term follow-up

trasound reflectances, and angulation of the ultrasound beam to traverse the orifice tangentially may result in false estimates of its size. Therefore utilization of echocardiographic imaging techniques may not be suitable in some patients with mitral stenosis. Nevertheless they provide an excellent modality for quantitation in the majority of patients with this lesion.

An alternate method for assessing the severity of both mitral and aortic stenosis is Doppler velocity measurements. Based on the Bernoulli equation, pressure gradient = $4(velocity)^2$, the transvalvular flow velocity can be related to both the mean and the maximal gradient across the mitral valve during diastole.[4] For transaortic gradients, both maximal and mean gradients have been found to predict catheterization results well.[5] For transmitral gradients simultaneous measurements of the mean gradient, in particular, have shown a good correlation with catheterization pressure measurements. However, owing to influences of heart rate and cardiac output, a much superior estimate of the severity of mitral stenosis is the mitral valve area. An estimate of mitral valve area can be obtained with Doppler techniques by means of the pressure half-time approach.[6] Specifically, the time interval required for the velocity to fall to one half of the pressure equivalent is measured from the transmitral Doppler recording and then divided into the empirical constant of 220 to achieve an estimate of mitral valve area (Fig 7–1). Studies in several laboratories have demonstrated that the mitral pressure half-time method provides values of mitral valve area that correlate well with those derived by cardiac catheterization.[2, 6] Studies performed in our laboratory have demonstrated that both planed measurements of the mitral valve orifice from two-dimensional echocardiographic images and estimates of mitral valve area derived by the pressure half-time Doppler method yield values that correlate equivalently with catheterization-derived measures of mitral valve area in patients with native mitral valves.[2] However, of potential relevance to catheter balloon valvuloplasty, these studies have demonstrated that Doppler values are superior to those derived from planed echocardiographic images in patients who have

undergone previous mitral commissurotomy. The apparent explanation for this relates to scarring and distortion of the mitral valve leaflets following the commissurotomy procedure.

As compared with the mitral valve leaflets, the aortic valve orifice is quite difficult to define by echocardiographic imaging because of multiple reflectances and the triangular shape of the valve.[7] Therefore the quantitation of aortic stenosis has focused on calculation of the transvalvular gradient by the Bernoulli equation and continuous-wave Doppler echocardiography (Fig 7–2). Studies have demonstrated that the continuity equation may be utilized to estimate aortic valve area.[8] This equation is based on the fact that the volume of blood flow through the left ventricular outflow tract must equal the volume of blood flow through the aortic valve orifice. Since volumetric blood flow equals the product of velocity and cross-sectional area and since the velocity in the cross-sectional area of the left ventricular outflow tract as well as the velocity of blood through the aortic valve orifice can be measured, one can therefore calculate the cross-sectional area of the aortic valve. Numerous studies have demonstrated the ability of Doppler echocardiography measurements of aortic valve severity to correlate well with catheterization determinations.

DETECTION OF ASSOCIATED LESIONS

A variety of lesions associated with the primary stenotic process may be detected by echocardiography (Table 7–2). Predominant among these defects, of course, is the presence of valvular regurgitation. Since valvulotomy may result in the appearance of exacerbation of regurgitation, the determination that valvular insufficiency as well as stenosis is present is an important finding. The primary modality utilized to detect valvular regurgitation is Doppler recordings. Although both pulsed and continuous-wave Doppler recordings can yield evidence of the lesion, as well as some indirect information about the relative hemodynamic consequences, the primary quantitative modality utilized at

TABLE 7–2

Detection of Associated Abnormalities by Doppler Echocardiography in Catheter Balloon Valvuloplasty

Regurgitation
Additional lesions
Cardiac thrombi
Pulmonary hypertension
Left ventricular size and function

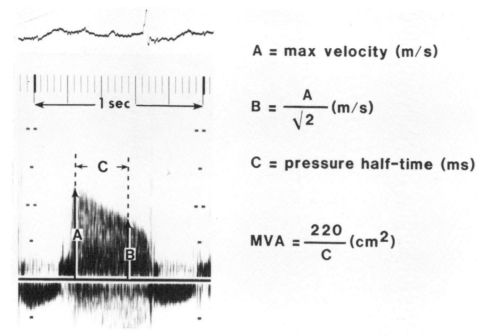

$$A = max \ velocity \ (m/s)$$

$$B = \frac{A}{\sqrt{2}} \ (m/s)$$

$$C = pressure \ half\text{-}time \ (ms)$$

$$MVA = \frac{220}{C} \ (cm^2)$$

FIG 7–1.
Shown is the transmitral velocity trace obtained by continuous-wave Doppler echocardiography in a patient with mitral stenosis. Velocity is plotted on the vertical axis, while time is on the horizontal axis. Pressure half-time is defined as the interval required for the maximal velocity (point *A*) to fall to half of the pressure equivalent (velocity *B*). Mitral valve area can be obtained by dividing this interval in milliseconds into the empirical constant of 220.

present is color-flow mapping. Thus, by utilizing color Doppler flow imaging the regurgitant jet may be visualized, as well as the area of the jet plane determined. Several studies have demonstrated that the size of regurgitant jets visualized in this fashion relates in a general way to the quantitative severity of the lesion as assessed by cineangiography.[9, 10] Echocardiographic images can also detect abnormalities of additional valves other than the primary stenotic lesion. Of greater significance, however, is the detection of intracardiac thrombi. Echocardiography has proved to be an effective method for the recognition of intra-atrial thrombi when these masses have been centrally located with major intracavitary projection. However, transthoracic echocardiography has thus far been less successful with thrombi involving the left atrial appendage. Recent studies have demonstrated that transesophageal echocardiography provides superior sensitivity in the recognition of left atrial thrombi, and it is likely that this procedure may well play an important role in evaluation of the patient with mitral stenosis who is being considered for catheter balloon mitral valvuloplasty. In regard to left ventricular thrombi, echocardiography provides an excellent modality for identification and assessment. Echocardiography can, in addition to the above abnormalities, be utilized to assess left ventricular and left atrial size and function. Simple dimensional measurements of chamber size may be made in a variety of projections in the patient with a nongeometrically distorted left ventricle. In addition, two-dimensional echocardiography, particularly from the apical window, can enable visualization of the entire outline of the left ventricle in most patients. Measurements derived from such echocardiographic images by utilizing either area-length or Simpson's approach may then be employed to derive measurements of left ventricular size and ejection fraction. In regard to cardiac function and hemodynamics, Doppler echocardiography can be employed to assess diastolic function and estimate pulmonary artery pressures. Thus, by utilizing the Bernoulli approach in the patient with tricuspid regurgitation or by measuring the acceleration time of the pulmonary artery flow trace, Doppler can be employed to evaluate pulmonary artery pressures.

SUITABILITY FOR VALVULOPLASTY

Having identified a patient with mitral or aortic stenosis who does not have another lesion contraindicating catheter balloon valvuloplasty, one now turns to an assessment of the likelihood of a beneficial effect from this

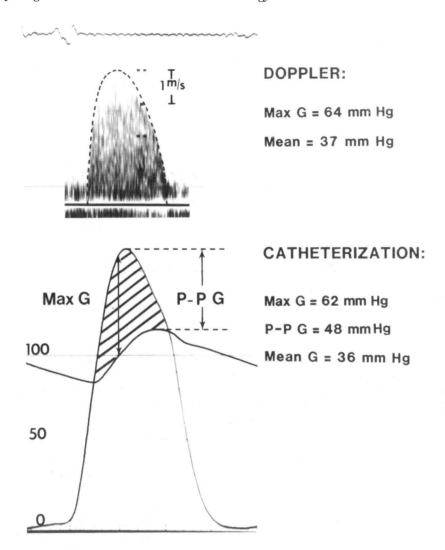

FIG 7–2.
Shown is the Doppler trace *(top)* and the pressure tracings at catheterization *(bottom)* in a patient with aortic stenosis. The aortic stenosis jet was recorded by continuous-wave Doppler echocardiography in the ascending aorta with the transducer in the suprasternal notch. The maximal velocity is measured in meters per second at the greatest magnitude of the jet (here 4 m/sec), while the mean gradient is taken as the average of gradients obtained at multiple intervals during systole. The maximal Doppler gradient correlates well with the instantaneous catheterization gradient *(max G)*, but tends to overestimate the peak-to-peak gradient *(P-PG)* by catheterization. Mean gradients correlate best.

procedure. Echocardiography has been valuable in this regard, particularly as applied to the mitral valve. Thus a variety of morphologic criteria have been utilized to determine the likelihood of a favorable response to catheter balloon valvuloplasty in the patient with mitral stenosis (Table 7–3). Four criteria have primarily been assessed: (1) mitral valve leaflet pliability, (2) leaflet thickness, (3) calcification of the leaflets, and (4) thickening and distortion of the subvalvular mitral apparatus. In regard to pliability of the mitral valve leaflets, motion of the midportion of the anterior leaflet has been primarily studied. The highly flexible leaflet will, in middiastole, exhibit considerable angulation of the midleaflet moving anteriorly and apically in the area that is not tethered at the base or tips. An estimate of flexibility has been attempted as the ratio of the height of such angulation to the length of the leaflet.[11] The thickness of the mitral valve leaflet has also been assessed in a semiquantitative fashion. Increased thickening of greater than 5 mm or greater than 8 mm has been applied. In addition, a distinction has been drawn between the presence of thickening involving a portion of the mitral valve leaflets and that involving the entire mitral valve leaflets. Calcification has proved to be a more ellusive criterion. The presence of highly dense reflectances within the mitral valve leaflets have suggested calcification and

TABLE 7–3

Suitability of Doppler Echocardiography in Catheter Balloon Valvuloplasty

---

Morphologic characteristics
  Mitral
    Valvular mobility
    Leaflet thickening
    Calcification
        Leaflets
        Commissures
    Subvalvular apparatus thickening and distortion
  Aortic
    Bicuspid Valve

---

have again been semiquantitatively assessed in terms of the amount of the mitral valve apparatus involved. Finally, thickening, shortening, and fusion of the subvalvular apparatus have been visualized by echocardiography and indicate a poor prognosis for valvuloplasty. These four criteria have been assigned values from 1 to 4+, indicative of greater degrees of abnormality.[12] Existing data have demonstrated that the higher the grade of morphologic distortion, the less likely one is to achieve an excellent hemodynamic result with valvuloplasty.[12] In general a good result can be expected with a score of 8 or less, while an unsatisfactory result often occurs with a score of 12 or more. The assessment of mitral valve morphology as an indicator of the suitability for valvuloplasty continues to be evaluated. As with all other echocardiographic measurements, the tomographic nature of the technique makes it imperative that the entire mitral valve apparatus be scanned. The experience to date, however, has indicated that patients with heavily thickened, calcified, immobile mitral valve leaflets with substantial subvalvular apparatus thickening and shortening are less likely to achieve good results with catheter valvuloplasty,[12, 13] although this has recently been challenged when the Inoue baloon has been used in a controlled fashion.[14] Current data suggest that leaflet score is the strongest predictor of postvalvotomy valve area[12, 13, 15] and confirm that better results can be expected if the mitral valve is less calcified, although data from Lin et al. showed calcium not to be predictive.[16] Other authors mention additional variables that influence the results of valvuloplasty like balloon size[17, 18] as well as age, gender, left atrial size, and pulmonary artery pressure.[15]

The aortic valve leaflets have been more difficult to visualize by echocardiography, although aortic valve area can often be planimetered directly by employing the transesophageal approach. In addition, an assessment can be made as to whether the valve is bicuspid or tricuspid (if the anatomy is not too distorted) since bi-

cuspid valves may be more liable to restenosis postvalvuloplasty.

DOPPLER ECHOCARDIOGRAPHY IN GUIDING CATHETER VALVULOPLASTY

It has been proposed that Doppler echocardiographic studies may be useful in the actual performance of catheter balloon valvuloplasty. Specifically, it has been suggested that the ability of echocardiography to visualize the mitral valve apparatus might be useful in positioning of the balloons, determining whether or not movement occurs during inflation, and ensuring that the balloon occupies the entire valve orifice. In addition, evaluation of the degree of mitral regurgitation by color-flow imaging has also been performed during the procedure in an attempt to maximize the valve area and minimize the amount of regurgitation.[19] However, additional information will be required on the utility of intraprocedural imaging.

Echocardiography clearly has a role in detecting the complications of balloon valvuloplasty. Four specific complications can be considered: (1) valvular regurgitation, (2) torn leaflet apparatus, (3) pericardial effusion, and (4) atrial septal defects. Doppler echocardiography has been shown to be of value in detecting each of these abnormalities. The performance of color-flow mapping not only can detect the presence of regurgitation[20] but can also help to localize the lesion. Torn leaflets or leaflet apparatus can be well visualized by echocardiographic imaging techniques. In regard to tearing of the valvular apparatus, this may be determined by either valvular regurgitation or multiple forward jets. We have observed several patients with severe mitral regurgitation in whom two separate flow jets were seen to emanate from the mitral leaflets in diastole following catheter balloon valvuloplasty. In these cases, clearly a disruption of the valve apparatus had taken place and resulted in flow occurring through some area other than the central orifice. Pericardial effusion may occur with perforation of the heart, and again echocardiography provides the best technique for the recognition of this abnormality. A specific word might be said in regard to atrial septal defect. The dilation of the foramen ovale was initially feared to have the potential of creating atrial septal defects. Indeed, most patients have been observed to have at least some intra-atrial flow following valvuloplasty. However, the flow as visualized by Doppler echocardiography has consisted of a very narrow stream in most patients, and there is little evidence that significant shunting persists long-term in the majority of patients. The potential for larger defects, however, can be well assessed by Doppler echocardiographic techniques.[21, 22]

EVALUATION OF THE EFFICACY OF BALLOON VALVULOPLASTY

Doppler echocardiography techniques provide the best and most practicable method for assessing the efficacy of catheter balloon valvuloplasty. Direct invasive measurements may be performed immediately after the procedure, but they may be influenced by factors attendant to the procedure itself such as alterations in cardiac output, changes in loading, and perhaps the production of myocardial ischemia. Importantly, only Doppler echocardiography enables an assessment of the results of valvuloplasty following stabilization of the patient and in repeat assessments during long-term follow-up. It is not surprising, therefore, that Doppler echocardiography constitutes the major evidence for long-term success of valvuloplasty in the Catheter Balloon Valvuloplasty Registry sponsored by the National Institutes of Health.

As in the assessment of the severity of stenosis, Doppler echocardiographic techniques can be applied in a similar manner to assess the reduction in stenosis (Fig 7–3). Accordingly, calculations of the transvalvular gradient and valve area can be performed for both mitral and aortic valves in the usual fashion. Studies performed in our laboratory on patients who have undergone open surgical commissurotomy as treatment for mitral stenosis have demonstrated that although echocardiographic imaging and Doppler echocardiography are similar in their assessment of mitral stenosis in the native valve, Doppler measures of the transvalvular gradient may actually be slightly superior in patients following commissurotomy.[2] The explanation for this seemed to reside in the scarring and distortion of the mitral valve leaflets in the long term following commissurotomy. Whether similar findings would be present in the short term is uncertain. Indeed, current data suggest that Doppler assessment of the transmitral gradient is less reliable after balloon valvuloplasty than is echocardiographic assessment of the planed mitral valve area.[11, 23, 24] This may be due to acute alterations in loading[25] as well as acute changes in left atrial and left ventricular compliance since 48 hours postvalvotomy the accuracy improves.[24]

In regard to the aortic valve, data by Come and associates have indicated that Doppler assessment of the severity of aortic stenosis remains reasonably accurate in comparison with catheterization after and before valvuloplasty.[26, 27]

As has been stated previously, Doppler echocardiography techniques provide an excellent modality for assessing the presence of valvular regurgitation. Such assessment can be performed not only immediately after the procedure but also during long-term follow-up. In addition, echocardiographic imaging can provide important information in regard to pulmonary hypertension by virtue of measurements of pulmonary artery systolic pressure obtained by the Bernoulli approach. Finally, echocardiography can provide additional important information regarding the status of systolic and diastolic ventricular function and left atrial size.[28-31]

MECHANISM OF BENEFIT

Doppler echocardiographic studies may play an important role in assessing the mechanism of efficacy of catheter balloon valvuloplasty. Thus, in important studies by Reid and associates a variety of measures of the mitral valve orifice were made from the short-axis projection on echocardiograms.[11] The width of the mitral valve leaflets as well as the angle formed at the junction of the two commissures of the anterior and posterior leaflets was assessed both before and after valvuloplasty. The data from this study documented that the width of the mitral valve orifice increased following valvuloplasty, as did the angles for both commissures. An in vitro study by Kaplan et al. has confirmed the above observations.[32] Thus it is clear that catheter balloon valvuloplasty induces a freeing of fusion of the leaflets at the periphery that increases orifice width as well as the opening angles of the mitral valve. These data were important in verifying that catheter balloon techniques were capable of splitting fused commissures as the mechanism of increasing the orifice rather than merely inducing stretching of the leaflets or even tearing or breaking of the apparatus.

CONCLUSIONS

Doppler echocardiography continues to play a central role in the diagnosis and quantitation of valvular heart disease and will certainly continue to do so in the future. In addition, Doppler echocardiography measures are of value in determining the suitability for balloon valvuloplasty as well as in assessing contraindications such as left atrial thrombi. Doppler echocardiography will likely continue to be the major method to assess the long-term results of the procedure. It appears certain, therefore, that whatever the role of catheter balloon val-

BALLOON VALVULOPLASTY

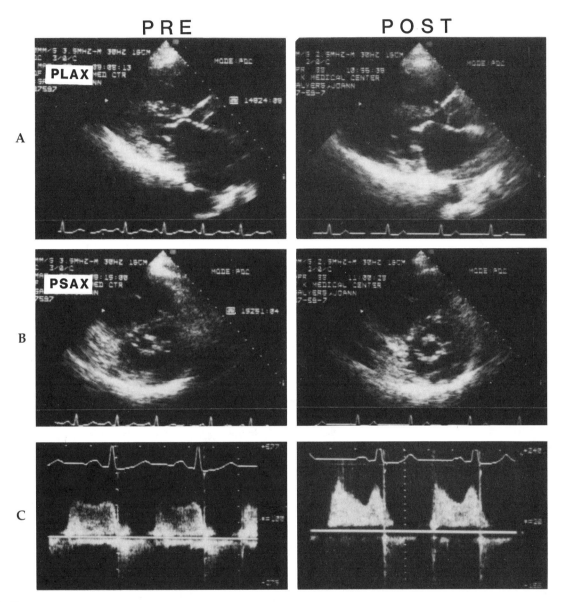

FIG 7–3.
A, the preprocedure echocardiogram and the echocardiogram after balloon valvuloplasty obtained in the parasternal long-axis view *(PLAX)* in a patient with mitral stenosis. The left ventricle is bigger and the mitral valve leaflet separation increased following valvuloplasty. **B,** shown is the short-axis view of the mitral valve leaflets before *(left)* and after *(right)* balloon valvuloplasty. The mitral valve orifice is clearly larger after valvuloplasty. Importantly, an increase in the medial collateral diameter is indicative of separation along the commissures. **C,** shown are the preprocedure and postprocedure continuous-wave Doppler transmitral velocity recordings in the same patient with mitral stenosis as seen in **A** and **B.** The prevalvuloplasty Doppler recording *(left)* shows a markedly reduced deceleration phase with velocities in excess of 2 m/sec. Following balloon valvuloplasty *(right)* the deceleration phase is much more rapid, consistent with a decrease in pressure half-time and an increase in mitral valve area.

vuloplasty is in the future, it will be intimately intertwined with Doppler echocardiographic techniques.

REFERENCES

1. Smith MD, Kwan OL, DeMaria AN: Value and limitations of continuous-wave Doppler echocardiography in estimating severity of valvular stenosis. *JAMA* 1986; 255:3145–3151.
2. Smith MD, Handshoe R, Handshoe S, et al: Comparative accuracy of two-dimensional echocardiography and Doppler pressure half-time methods in assessing severity of mitral stenosis in patients with and without prior commissurotomy. *Circulation* 1986; 73:100–107.
3. Henry WL, Griffith J, Michaelis LL, et al: Measurement of mitral orifice area in patients with mitral valve disease by real-time two-dimensional echocardiography. *Circulation* 1975; 51:827.
4. Holen J, Aasled R, Landmark K, et al: Determination of pressure gradient in mitral stenosis with a non-invasive ultrasound Doppler technique. *Acta Med Scand* 1976; 199:455–460.
5. Hatle L, Angelsen BA, Tromsdal A: Noninvasive assessment of aortic stenosis by Doppler ultrasound. *Br Heart J* 1980; 43:284–292.
6. Hatle L, Angelsen B, Tromsdal A: Noninvasive assessment of atrioventricular pressure half-time by Doppler ultrasound. *Circulation* 1979; 60:1096–1104.
7. DeMaria AN, Bommer W, Joye J, et al: Value and limitations of cross-sectional echocardiography of the aortic valve in the diagnoses and quantification of valvular aortic stenosis. *Circulation* 1980; 62:304–312.
8. Skjaerpe T, Hegrenaes L, Hatle L: Noninvasive estimation of valve area in patients with aortic stenosis by Doppler ultrasound and two-dimensional echocardiography. *Circulation* 1985; 72:810–818.
9. Perry GJ, Nanda NC: Recent advances in color Doppler evaluation of valvular regurgitation. *Echocardiography* 1987; 4:503–513.
10. Spain MG, Smith MD, Grayburn PA, et al: Quantitative assessment of mitral regurgitation by Doppler color flow imaging: Angiographic and hemodynamic correlations. *J Am Coll Cardiol* 1989; 13:585–590.
11. Reid CC, McKay, CR, Chandrarathna PAN, et al: Mechanisms of increase in mitral valve area and influence of anatomic features in catheter balloon valvuloplasty in adults with mitral stenosis. *Circulation* 1987; 76:628.
12. Herman HC, Wilkins GT, Abascal VM, et al: Percutaneous balloon mitral valvotomy for patients with mitral stenosis. *J Thorac Cardiovasc Surg* 1988; 96:33–38.
13. Abascal VM, Wilkins GT, Choong CY, et al: Echocardiographic evaluation of mitral valve structure and function in patients followed for at least 6 months after percutaneous balloon mitral valvuloplasty. *J Am Coll Cardiol* 1988; 12:606–615.
14. Dietz WA, Waters JB, Ramaswamy K, et al: Adverse echocardiographic score does not preclude successful outcome in patients undergoing mitral valvuloplasty with Inoue balloon (abstract). *J Am Coll Cardiol* 1991; 17:155.
15. Reid C, Otto C, Davis K, for NHLBI Balloon Valvulo-
plasty Registry: Influence of mitral valve morphology on valve area after mitral balloon commissurotomy. *Circulation* 1990; 82(suppl 3):46.
16. Lin SL, Chang MS, Lee GW, et al: Usefulness of echocardiography in the prediction of the early results of catheter balloon valvuloplasty. *Jpn Heart J* 1990; 31:161–174.
17. Chen CY, Lin SL, Pan JP, et al: Minimal requirement of effective dilation diameter of balloon(s) in percutaneous transluminal mitral valvotomy. Chung Hua i Hsueh TSA Chih. *Chin Med J* 1989; 44:287–292.
18. Chen CB, Wang X, Wang Y, et al: Value of 2D echocardiography in selecting patients and baloon sizes for percutaneous balloon mitral valvuloplasty. *J Am Coll Cardiol* 1989; 14:165–168.
19. Dietz WA, Waters JB, Ramaswamy K, et al: Use of Inoue balloon catheter to perform staged balloon inflations in combination with serial evaluation by color-flow Doppler minimizes mitral regurgitation as a complication of percutaneous mitral valvuloplasty (abstract). *J Am Coll Cardiol* 1991; 17:82.
20. Abascal VM, Wilkins GT, Choong C, et al: Mitral regurgitation after percutaneous mitral valvuloplasty in adults: Evaluation by pulsed Doppler echocardiography. *J Am Coll Cardiol* 1988; 11:257–263.
21. Legvier A, Bonan R, Serra A, et al: Left to right atrial shunting after percutaneous mitral valvuloplasty: Incidence and long term hemodynamic follow-up. *Circulation* 1990; 81:1190–1197.
22. Kronzone I, Tunick PA, Goldfarb A, et al: Echocardiographic and hemodynamic characteristics of atrial septal defects created by percutaneous valvuloplasty. *J Am Soc Echocardiogr* 1990; 3:64–71.
23. Thomas JD, Wilkins GT, Choong CYP, et al: Inaccuracy of mitral pressure half-time immediately after percutaneous mitral valvotomy. *Circulation* 1988; 78:980–993.
24. Chen CG, Wang YP, Guo BL, et al: Reliability of the Doppler pressure half-time method for assessing effects of percutaneous mitral balloon valvuloplasty. *J Am Coll Cardiol* 1989; 13:1309–1313.
25. Wisenbaugh T, Berk M, Essop R, et al: Effect of mitral regurgitation and volume loading on pressure half-time before and after balloon valvotomy in mitral stenosis. *Am J Cardiol* 1991; 67:162–168.
26. Come PC, Riley MF, McKay RG, et al: Echocardiographic assessment of aortic valve area in elderly patients with aortic stenosis and changes in valve area after percutaneous balloon valvuloplasty. *J Am Coll Cardiol* 1987; 10:115–125.
27. Come PC, Riley MF, Safian RD, et al: Usefulness of non-invasive assessment of aortic stenosis before and after percutaneous aortic valvuloplasty. *Am J Cardiol* 1988; 61:1300–1306.
28. Ferguson JJ, Bush HS, Riuli FP: Doppler echocardiography assessment of the effect of balloon aortic valvuloplasty on left ventricular systolic function. *Am Heart J* 1989; 117:18–24.
29. Harpole DH, Davidson CJ, Skelton TN, et al: Changes in left ventricular systolic performance immediately after percutaneous aortic balloon valvuloplasty. *Am J Cardiol* 1990; 65:1213–1218.
30. Stoddard MF, Vandormael MG, Pearson AC, et al: Im-

mediate and short-term effects of aortic balloon valvuloplasty on left ventricular diastolic function and filling in humans. *J Am Coll Cardiol* 1989; 14:1218–1228.

31. Vermilion RP, Snider AR, Meliones JN, et al: Pulsed Doppler evaluation of right ventricular diastolic filling in children with pulmonary valve stenosis before and after balloon valvuloplasty. *Am J Cardiol* 1990; 66:78–84.

32. Kaplan JD, Isner JM, Karas RH, et al: In vitro analysis of mechanisms of balloon valvuloplasty of stenotic mitral valves. *Am J Cardiol* 1987; 59:318–323.

PART II

Balloon Angioplasty

8

Balloon Angioplasty: Matching Technology to Lesions

John S. Douglas, Jr., M.D.

Since the landmark initial procedure by Grüntzig, coronary angioplasty has evolved rapidly to become the most commonly applied myocardial revascularization technique of the 1990s. Although coronary artery balloon angioplasty has many limitations, it is the success of the technique even more than its limitations that has led to the staggering array of new intracoronary devices and strategies. Which will replace the balloon? Only with time will this become clear. In the early 1990s, however, the simplicity, broad applicability, and reasonable predictability of balloon angioplasty has led this author and most percutaneous transluminal coronary angioplasty (PTCA) operators to continue to favor plain old balloon angioplasty (POBA) for most percutaneous coronary revascularization procedures. In 1,002 consecutive recent PTCA procedures involving 1,376 arterial sites, balloon angioplasty alone was utilized in 91% of patients (Fig 8–1). One half of the remainder were treated with a new device as primary therapy and one half for balloon angioplasty failure. Thus, while relying heavily on balloon angioplasty, success rates were quite acceptable (96% for subtotal occlusion and 80% for total occlusion) in spite of a largely referral clientele made up predominantly of patients with multivessel disease. Urgent bypass surgery and Q wave infarction were infrequent (1.7% and 1.1%, respectively), and all deaths occurred in salvage situations. The total in-hospital mortality rate was 0.5%. It is clear, however, that the outcome of balloon angioplasty remains somewhat dependent on the equipment selected and operator experience. Assuming that the ideal lesion (type A) can be managed with almost any balloon catheter and guidewire (and some of the new devices), this chapter will focus on problems in PTCA and potential solutions including new strategies where appropriate (Fig 8–2).

BIFURCATIONS

When atherosclerotic lesions involve bifurcations, angioplasty is associated with an increased complication rate and reduced success.[1, 2] This is in part attributable to the more extensive disease present and the heightened probability of dissection and occlusion. In addition, ostial bifurcation lesions frequently yield a suboptimal angiographic outcome due to elastic recoil. Keys to success in this anatomic subgroup include provisions for protection of important jeopardized branches (Fig 8–3), precise balloon sizing to each leg of the bifurcation, and a two-balloon approach whenever this is justified by discrepant size requirements of each leg or anatomy favoring simultaneous balloon inflation (such as heavy involvement of the carina of a bifurcation). Although a two-wire, single-balloon approach is frequently effective in the younger, less severely involved patient, angioplasty in advanced disease, particularly in the elderly, is best initiated with two balloon catheters (Fig 8–4). Radiolucent guidewires are generally preferred for this anatomy to enhance lesion visualization during the procedure. A large-lumen, 8 F guide catheter (0.080-in. internal diameter) will accommodate an over-the-wire system and a balloon-on-a-wire setup easily, and the combination is "user friendly" and highly recommended. If exquisite guidewire performance is necessary for crossing, two (or even three) wires and two low-profile over-the-wire balloons can be accommodated in an 8 F guide catheter. In general, the more difficult vessel is wired first, care is taken to avoid wrapping the wires, and the first balloon inflation is made in the most important artery. Simultaneous balloon inflations are favored if the parent vessel is large enough. If the parent vessel is too small for full inflation of both balloons, si-

PERCUTANEOUS CORONARY REVASCULARIZATION STRATEGIES IN 1002 CONSECUTIVE PATIENTS

1990

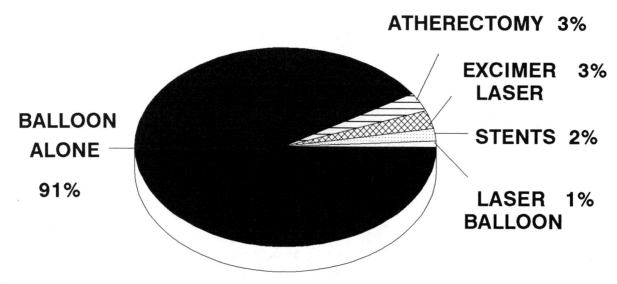

ATHERECTOMY 3%

EXCIMER 3%
LASER

BALLOON
ALONE

STENTS 2%

91%

LASER 1%
BALLOON

FIG 8–1.
The author's choice of strategies in 1,002 consecutive PTCA procedures during which 1,376 arterial sites were treated in calendar year 1990. Over half had multivessel disease, and 21% had prior coronary bypass surgery; 122 had total occlusion, and there were 99 saphenous vein graft lesions. In the same time period, 1,863 PTCA procedures were performed at Emory University Hospital, 88% with balloon angioplasty alone.

multaneous inflation to 2 or 3 atm is still employed if alternating balloon inflations have yielded an inadequate angiographic result. If balloon inflations to patient tolerance (determined by symptoms and evidence of ischemia) fail to produce an adequate result, options include the use of a perfusion balloon or a stent in the dominant vessel (not recommended when the side branch is large). It is worth noting that side branches encompassed by a Cook (Gianturco-Roubin) stent can be dilated through the stent wires whereas branches encompassed by the Johnson & Johnson (Palmaz-Schatz) stent cannot. Directional coronary atherectomy (DCA) may be used to remove focal projections of tissue into the lumen that remain in spite of multiple balloon inflations. This strategy has proved invaluable in selected patients; however, DCA has not been widely applied in bifurcations as primary therapy.

THROMBUS, LENGTH, AND BEND POINT

Of the other lesion characteristics noted in the American College of Cardiology/American Heart Association (ACC/AHA) classification, three appear to be more important predictors to this author and others; these are thrombus, lesion length, and bend point location of the lesion.[1, 3–7] The best strategy for lesion-associated thrombi is intravenous heparin therapy until the clot has diminished before PTCA is attempted. Even large thrombi resolve in about a week, and PTCA at that time is usually successful even if there is some residual clot.[3] If waiting is not possible due to clinical instability, an intracoronary infusion of a thrombolytic agent for several hours may reduce the clot burden. Aggressive balloon sizing[4] with or without intracoronary thrombolytic therapy has also been reported to yield favorable results.

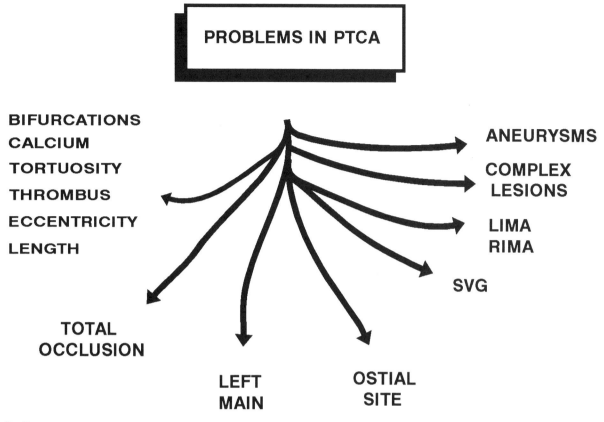

FIG 8–2.
Factors that predict reduced success, complications, or technical difficulty during conventional balloon angioplasty. (*LIMA/RIMA* = left/right internal mammary artery; *SVG* = saphenous vein graft.)

Lesions with a length of 15 to 20 mm or even longer may respond well to prolonged inflations with a long (30-mm) balloon, and this strategy is usually preferred (Fig 8–5). Patients with multiple sites in tandem may also do well with a 30-mm-long balloon inflated for 1 to 2 minutes (Fig 8–6). In our experience with 181 patients with lesion length ≥2 cm, angiographic success was obtained in 86%, and in-laboratory acute closure occurred in 4%, Q wave infarction in 1.7%, and emergency coronary artery bypass grafting (CABG) in 7.7% without in-hospital deaths. Among the 59% of patients who underwent recatheterization, restenosis was noted in 51%.[8] Occasionally, debulking or stand-alone excimer laser therapy is applied, even in the presence of diffuse disease and calcification.[9] Long lesions may represent a nitch for the excimer laser.

Lesions on bend points have increased complications[5, 7] and restenosis.[6] Theoretically and experimentally, polyethylene terephthalate (PET) balloons produce less arterial straightening and should be preferred in this situation. However, at the practical level, slight undersizing of the balloon seems equally important.

CALCIFICATION

Lesion and arterial calcification are associated with more frequent dissection[10] and, in some reports[11] but not others,[5, 7] are predictors of failure and complications. In the presence of significant calcification we prefer a noncompliant balloon that is capable of a high-pressure inflation (greater than 14 atm). This can be accomplished with PET (USCI, Schneider), with Duralyn (CORDIS), and recently with polyethylene (Advanced Cardiovascular Systems [ACS]). For rigid distal lesions in older patients, a balloon-on-a-wire system with high pressure capability is preferred (Orion by CORDIS or Probe by USCI). Calcification is a predictor of failure for directional atherectomy, but in our hands with mild or moderate calcification, directional atherectomy is frequently successful as primary therapy or as a bailout in PTCA failure.[12] Calcium is less of a problem for the excimer laser and the Rotablator.[13, 14]

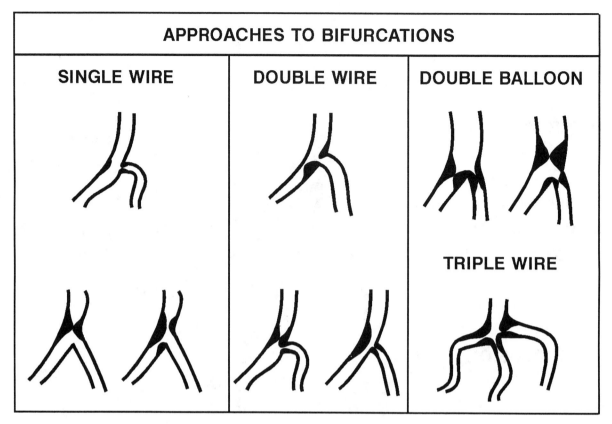

FIG 8–3.
Strategies in PTCA of bifurcation lesions.

ECCENTRICITY

In general, eccentricity is a weak predictor of poor PTCA outcome,[5, 7, 11] and PTCA can usually be successfully performed. However, in this author's experience the presence of marked eccentricity and a mature, fibrotic plaque tends to yield suboptimal results. With this type of lesion, there is little alteration of the plaque itself; rather, PTCA results in tearing of the normal arc of the vessel, and in some cases, the plaque is avulsed from the wall resulting in a type of PTCA failure for which directional atherectomy or stenting is an effective bailout. When marked eccentricity is encountered in the proximal portions of large vessels (Fig 8–7), directional atherectomy is a reasonable initial strategy as an alternative to PTCA.[15] If conventional PTCA is performed with suboptimal outcome, a perfusion balloon may be effective and is an excellent strategy for patients in whom atherectomy is inappropriate or unavailable.

TOTAL OCCLUSION

Chronic total occlusions constitute about 10% of our experience. Success is highly dependent on the duration of occlusion, with recent occlusions having success rates of about 75% to 85% and occlusions in place over 3 months having success rates of less than 50%. Predictors of success in our experience include tapering at the site of occlusion, short-segment occlusion, and proximal location. We begin with a soft guidewire, stiffen it by placing the balloon catheter immediately proximal to the lesion, and progress to stiffer wires as needed. The use of hydrophilic coatings may enhance wire crossing, and this is currently being evaluated. If a balloon-on-a-wire setup has already been selected for another vessel but will not cross the total occlusion, we use a stiff wire (0.014 to 0.018 in. intermediate or standard USCI or ACS) to punch across the lesion and then remove the stiff wire and recross with the balloon-on-a-wire system. Others have based their routine approach to total occlusions on the use of a balloon-on-a-wire strategy.[16] After crossing the lesion with a guidewire, a 4 F polyethylene sheath is positioned immediately proximal to the lesion, and it serves as a conduit to deliver the balloon-on-a-wire system to the lesion, where it is then advanced through the tract created by the guidewire. The use of a sheath may be especially advantageous when anatomy is difficult or fluoroscopic visualization is poor. If the dis-

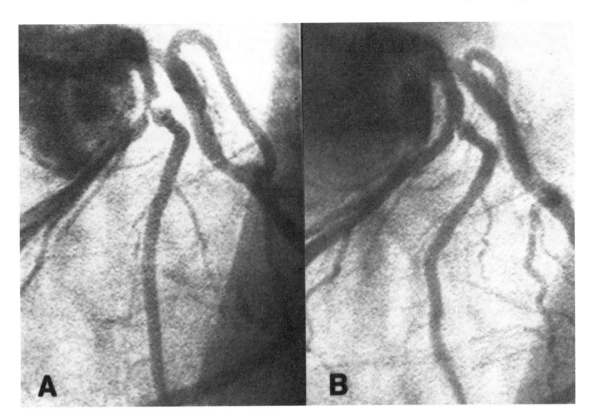

FIG 8–4.
A and **B,** complex lesions of the left anterior descending diagonal bifurcation treated with double balloon approach.

tal portion of the vessel is "uncharted territory" owing to poor collaterals, we cross with a wire, then "Dotter" the lesion with a deflated balloon to permit some antegrade flow or inject contrast distally via the balloon catheter itself, or if necessary, perform a low-pressure inflation to permit some distal visualization prior to a definitive inflation. This allows one to confirm that the balloon is properly placed and not grossly oversized or malpositioned in a side branch. Patience, incremental progression to more aggressive strategies, and the use of long balloons for long occlusions and prolonged inflations are keys to success in our view. New devices have not had a significant impact on success rates in this difficult subgroup.[17–20] In our experience and that of others, successful recanalization of total occlusions, by maintaining interventional options, permits avoidance of coronary bypass surgery during long-term follow-up.[21] However, complications (especially abrupt reclosure and distal thromboembolism) are more common than many appreciate, and emergency surgery is required in about 1% of patients overall. Given restenosis rates of about 50%, selection criteria should remain narrow until a technological breakthrough occurs. We believe that attempts at recanalization of occluded vein grafts[22] are seldom indicated due to the even higher rate

of thromboembolism and restenosis. In a few patients short-segment occlusions of internal mammary grafts have been successfully recanalized with favorable long-term outcome.

LEFT MAIN DISEASE

Unfortunately, balloon angioplasty of left main coronary disease has yielded disappointing results due to an increased rate of early reclosure and late restenosis.[23, 24] Although occasional patients with protected left main stenosis have experienced quite favorable outcome from PTCA, the majority of patients with obstruction at this location have dense fibrocalcific disease, and attempts at balloon dilatation yield suboptimal results. In carefully selected patients we have found atherectomy to be quite helpful even in the presence of moderate calcification, although predilating with a 2-mm high-pressure balloon is usually necessary. (See Figure 8–8 and the discussion of ostial lesions below.) In a few patients with apparent catheter-induced left main disease (prior circumflex or LAD PTCA) routine balloon angioplasty has proved effective.

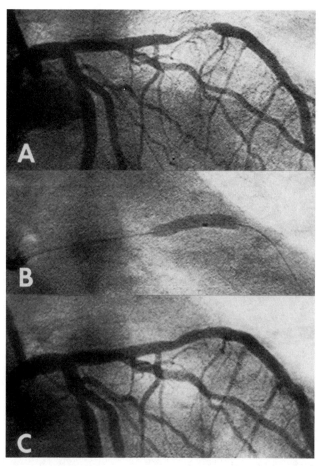

FIG 8–5.
A–C, 54-year-old male with prolonged ischemic pain and a 17-mm-long LAD lesion was successfully treated with a 30-mm-long balloon catheter.

OSTIAL LESIONS

Most but not all PTCA operators have been dissatisfied with the results obtained with balloon dilatation of aorto-ostial lesions, both native coronary artery and graft.[25, 26] Elastic tissue elements favor early recoil. Lesion calcification and the need for aggressive guide catheter maneuvers have resulted in more frequent dissection, early abrupt closure, and equally important, high restenosis rates. Our conservative approach to aorto-ostial lesions, tempered by earlier experiences, has been considerably altered by the relative effectiveness of excimer laser and directional atherectomy and by the ability to stent unfavorable initial results and avoid ischemic complications and emergency bypass surgery.[27–30] Whenever possible, we apply nonballoon strategies to aorto-ostial lesions primarily and favor the excimer laser for calcified stenoses in older patients and directional atherectomy for noncalcified lesions. When the lumen created by the excimer laser is simply not large enough, adjunctive atherectomy is frequently successful (Fig 8–9). So-called ostial lesions of the origin of the LAD artery can be dilated with conventional balloon angioplasty with high initial success rates and few complications, but restenosis is common. Many currently favor directional atherectomy for this site, but a clear-cut long-term advantage has not been documented.

PRIOR BYPASS SURGERY

Patients who have already had coronary bypass surgery make up over 20% of our experience at Emory University Hospital, and the proportion attributable to this patient subgroup is growing. Although disease in ungrafted vessels is sometimes the target, more commonly the interventionalist finds the culprit lesion(s) within or beyond saphenous vein or internal mammary artery grafts. Negotiating grafts to reach distal native coronary sites is not usually difficult unless the location of the lesion(s) requires retrograde passage of the dilatation catheter from the graft into the more proximal portions of the native coronary artery (Fig 8–10). In this case, the graft–native coronary artery angle is frequently acute, which places unusual demands on equipment performance. Keys to success here are good guide catheter backup, optimal dilatation catheter performance, the use of guidewires without transition points, and progression to stiffer wires during balloon catheter passage.[31] An over-the-wire dilatation system is usually preferred and, for optimal guide catheter support, an Amplatz shape for left-sided venous grafts, multipurpose shape for right-sided grafts, and 8 F size for internal mammary artery guide catheters. When passage must occur through a redundant or long internal mammary graft to reach a distal site (right internal mammary artery [RIMA] to the RCA, for example), an extra long (150 cm) balloon catheter or short internal mammary guide catheter may be required.

Initial and long-term results with balloon angioplasty of insertion site stenoses of vein and mammary artery grafts that occur within a year or so of bypass surgery are excellent,[32–34] and the use of nonballoon interventional strategies for these lesions is not warranted. Recurrence rates are about 20%, and the 5-year survival rate exceeds 90% in our experience. However, the best strategy for lesions within the body or shaft portion of these grafts is less clear. There is virtually no data on long-term outcome in PTCA of the shaft portion of internal mammary artery grafts. Restenosis following PTCA of mid saphenous vein graft sites occurs in about

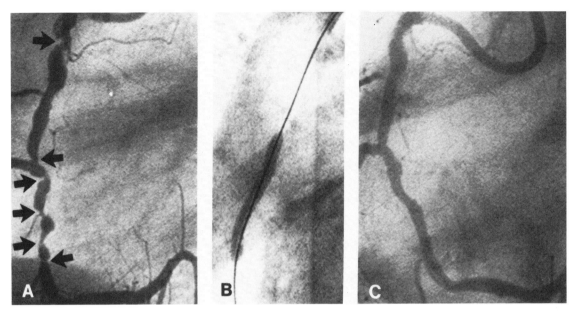

FIG 8–6.

A–C, 48-year-old man with unstable angina and multiple stenoses *(arrows)* in the proximal segment of the right coronary artery (RCA) that were dilated with a 30-mm-long balloon catheter.

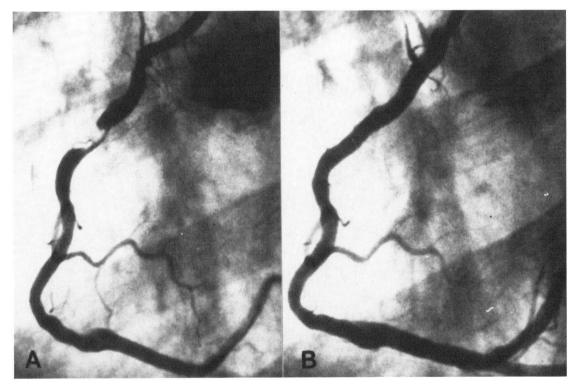

FIG 8–7.

Extremely eccentric stenosis in the proximal segment of the RCA of a 47-year-old male. Use of prolonged inflation or directional atherectomy (DCA) was considered the best option. DCA was performed.

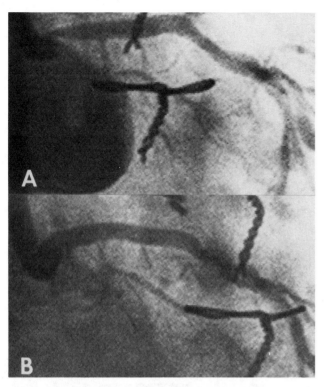

FIG 8–8.
Results of PTCA plus directional atherectomy of a long-standing left main coronary stenosis 2 years after coronary bypass surgery resulted in graft occlusion. **A,** angiogram before intervention. **B,** angiogram after PTCA and DCA.

a third of patients at 6 months, but in contrast to native-vessel PTCA, there is continued attrition, with restenosis occurring in over two thirds of those recatheterized at 2 years.[34] Periprocedural atheroembolism occurs rarely in vein grafts in place for less than 3 years but appears to occur in about a quarter of conservatively selected patients undergoing PTCA of vein grafts in place for over 5 years.[33] Predictors of embolism include the presence of diffuse disease, thrombus, and bulky lesions.[35] We continue to perform PTCA on these lesions when reoperation is not indicated or desired and by doing this buy the patient symptomatic relief, time for collateral recruitment, and in a minority of patients long-term patency. When attempting vein graft PTCA, we reserve balloon oversizing for situations where suboptimal initial results have been obtained and prefer a high-pressure balloon capability (greater than 14 atm). Use of the Palmaz-Schatz stent for primary therapy of mid vein graft lesions appears promising.[36] However, longer follow-up is needed to determine restenosis rates following vein graft stenting. In the presence of shelflike proximal lesions or vein graft lesions with thrombus unresponsive to prolonged heparin infusion, we favor directional atherectomy; others have used extraction atherectomy or the excimer laser.

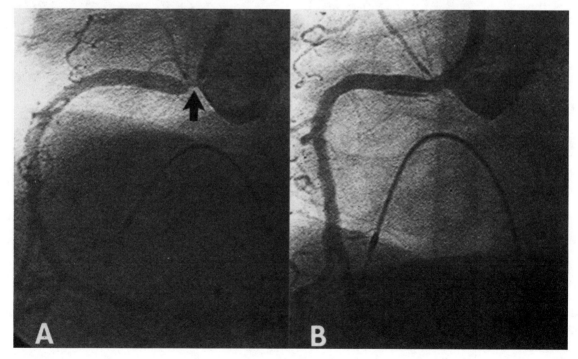

FIG 8–9.
Calcified stenosis of the right coronary ostium *(arrow)* of an 85-year-old male with disabling angina treated with the excimer laser plus DCA. **A,** prior to intervention. **B,** after excimer laser plus DCA.

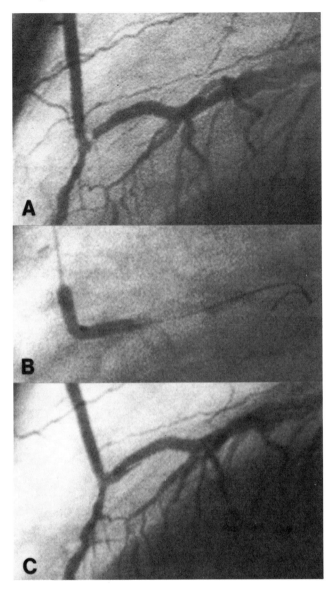

FIG 8–10.
PTCA of the LAD proximal to the left internal mammary artery (LIMA) insertion required retrograde passage of a balloon catheter 4 months following bypass surgery. **A,** left lateral view prior to intervention. **B,** balloon inflation. **C,** post-PTCA.

COMPLEX LESIONS

Lesions with multiple angiographic predictors of poor outcome, so-called complex lesions, require special planning with an eye toward avoidance of PTCA complications. It is in this subgroup of patients that initial dilatation with a perfusion balloon or primary use of stents, DCA, or other investigational strategies may be considered.[37] Although it is difficult to generalize, we use DCA for many such patients as a backup to conventional balloon angioplasty and reserve stent placement for PTCA or DCA failures who develop lengthy dissections or evidence of elastic recoil. Development of a nonthrombogenic stent would probably shift the pendulum in the favor of primary stent placement for many complex lesions.

ANEURYSM

There is no large reported experience with PTCA in the presence of coronary aneurysms. In our experience the most common cause of lesion-associated aneurysms is previous balloon dilatation. PTCA can be safely performed in most patients with a lesion-associated aneurysm as long as balloon sizing is conservative and the wall of the aneurysm is not stretched by the balloon. When the neck of the aneurysm is narrow, stent placement may result in complete or partial aneurysm obliteration due to occlusion of the neck of the aneurysm.

CONCLUSION

In the current climate of medical cost containment, it is apparent that treatment strategies that are simple and cost-effective will prevail. Since none of the new interventional strategies are either simple or cheap and given the difficulty of demonstrating superior effectiveness in a heterogeneous coronary population, it would appear that POBA will be the dominant interventional strategy for the foreseeable future.

REFERENCES

1. Ryan TJ, Faxon DP, Gunnar RM, et al: Guidelines for percutaneous transluminal coronary angioplasty. *J Am Coll Cardiol* 1988; 12:529–545.
2. Mathias DW, Mooney JF, Lange HW, et al: Frequency of success and complications of coronary angioplasty of a stenosis at the ostium of a branch vessel. *Am J Cardiol* 1991; 67:491–495.
3. Douglas JS Jr, Lutz JF, Clements SD, et al: Therapy of large intracoronary thrombi in candidates for percutaneous transluminal coronary angioplasty (abstract). *J Am Coll Cardiol* 1988; 11:238.
4. Mooney MR, Mooney JF, Goldenberg IF, et al: Percutaneous transluminal coronary angioplasty in the setting of large intracoronary thrombi. *Am J Cardiol* 1990; 65:427–431.
5. Ellis SG, Roubin GS, King SB III, et al: Angiographic and clinical predictors of acute closure after native vessel coronary angioplasty. *Circulation* 1988; 77:372–379.
6. Ellis SG, Roubin GS, King SB III, et al: Importance of stenosis morphology in the estimation of restenosis risk after elective percutaneous transluminal coronary angioplasty. *Am J Cardiol* 1989; 63:30–34.
7. Tenaglia AN, Fortin DF, Nelson CL, et al: Predicting the risk of angioplasty abrupt closure using lesion morphology. *Circulation* 1991; 84(Suppl 2):517.

8. Ghazzal ZMB, Weintraub WS, Ba'albaki HA, et al: PTCA of lesions longer than 20 mm: Initial outcome and restenosis. *Circulation* 1990; 82(suppl 2):509.

9. Raizner A, Litvack F, Goldenberg T, et al: Improved results in patients with long coronary stenoses using excimer laser angioplasty. *Circulation* 1990; 82(suppl 3):671.

10. Fitzgerald PJ, Sudhir K, Sykes CM, et al: Localized calcium is a major risk for arterial dissection during angioplasty: A catheter ultrasound study. *Circulation* 1991; 84(suppl 2):722.

11. Savage MP, Goldberg S, Hirshfeld JW, et al: Clinical and angiographic determinants of primary coronary angioplasty success. *J Am Coll Cardiol* 1991; 17:22–28.

12. Robertson GC, Vetter JW, Selmon MR, et al: Directional coronary atherectomy is less effective for calcified primary lesions. *Circulation* 1991; 84(suppl 2):520.

13. Leon MB, Kent KM, Pichard AD, et al: Percutaneous transluminal coronary rotational angioplasty of calcified lesions. *Circulation* 1991; 84(suppl 2):521.

14. Levine S, Mehta S, Krauthamer D, et al: Excimer laser coronary angioplasty of calcified lesions (abstract). *J Am Coll Cardiol* 1991; 17:207.

15. Hinohara T, Vetter JW, Selmon MR, et al: Directional coronary atherectomy is effective treatment for extremely eccentric lesions. *Circulation* 1991; 84(suppl 2):520.

16. Little T, Rosenberg J, Seides S, et al: Probe angioplasty of total coronary occlusion using the probing catheter technique. *Cathet Cardiovasc Diagn* 1990; 21:124–127.

17. Meier B, Carlier M, Finci L, et al: Magnum wire for balloon recanalization of chronic total coronary occlusions. *Am J Cardiol* 1989; 64:148–154.

18. Kaltenbach M, Vallbracht C, Hartmann A: Chronic coronary occlusions — reopening with low speed rotational angioplasty. *Circulation* 1991; 84(suppl 2):250.

19. Rothbaum DA, Linnemeier TJ, Krauthamer D, et al: Excimer laser angioplasty in total coronary occlusions: A registry report. *Circulation* 1991; 84(suppl 2):744.

20. Hamm CW, Kupper W, Kuck KH, et al: Recanalization of chronic, totally occluded coronary arteries by new angioplasty systems. *Am J Cardiol* 1990; 66:1459–1463.

21. Bell MR, Berger PB, Reeder GS, et al: Successful PTCA of chronic total coronary occlusions reduces the need for coronary artery bypass surgery. *Circulation* 1991; 84(suppl 2):250.

22. Hartmann JR, McKeever LS, Stamato NJ, et al: Recanalization of chronically occluded aortocoronary saphenous vein bypass grafts by extended infusion of urokinase: Initial results and short-term clinical follow-up. *J Am Coll Cardiol* 1991; 18:1517–1523.

23. O'Keefe JH Jr, Hartzler GO, Rutherford BD, et al: Left main coronary angioplasty: Early and late results in 127 acute and elective procedures. *Am J Cardiol* 1989; 64:144–147.

24. Vogel RA, Shawl F, Tommaso C, et al: Initial report of the national registry of elective cardiopulmonary bypass supported coronary angioplasty. *J Am Coll Cardiol* 1990; 15:23–29.

25. Topol EJ, Ellis SG, Fishman J, et al: Multicenter study of percutaneous transluminal angioplasty for right coronary ostial stenosis. *J Am Coll Cardiol* 1987; 9:1214–1218.

26. Bedotto JB, McConahay DR, Rutherford BD, et al: Balloon angioplasty of aorta coronary ostial stenoses revisited. *Circulation* 1991; 84(suppl 2):251.

27. Douglas JS Jr, Ghazzal ZMB, Ba'albaki HA, et al: Excimer laser coronary angioplasty of ostial lesions. *Cathet Cardiovasc Diagn* 1991; 23:74.

28. Eigler NL, Douglas JS Jr, Margolis JR, et al: Excimer laser coronary angioplasty of aorto-ostial stenosis: Results of the ELCA registry. *Circulation* 1991; 84(suppl 2):251.

29. Robertson GC, Simpson JB, Vetter JW, et al: Directional coronary atherectomy for ostial lesions. *Circulation* 1991; 84(suppl 2):251.

30. Teirstein P, Stratienko AA, Schatz RA: Coronary stenting for ostial stenosis: Initial results and six month follow-up. *Circulation* 1991; 84(suppl 2):250.

31. Kahn JK, Hartzler GO: Retrograde coronary angioplasty of isolated arterial segments through saphenous vein bypass grafts. *Cathet Cardiovasc Diagn* 1990; 20:88–93.

32. Douglas JS Jr, Grüntzig AR, King SB III, et al: Percutaneous transluminal coronary angioplasty in patients with prior coronary bypass surgery. *J Am Coll Cardiol* 1983; 2:745–754.

33. Douglas JS Jr: Angioplasty of saphenous vein and internal mammary artery bypass grafts, in Topol EJ (ed): *Textbook of Interventional Cardiology.* Philadelphia, WB Saunders, 1990, pp 327–343.

34. Douglas JS Jr, Weintraub WS, Liberman HA, et al: Update of saphenous graft (SVG) angioplasty: Restenosis and long term outcome. *Circulation* 1991; 84(suppl 2):249.

35. Liu MW, Douglas JS Jr, King SB III: Angiographic predictors of coronary embolization in the PTCA of vein graft lesions. *Circulation* 1989; 80(suppl 2):172.

36. Leon MB, Ellis SG, Pichard AD, et al: Stents may be the preferred treatment for focal aortocoronary vein graft disease. *Circulation* 1991; 84(suppl 2):249.

37. Robertson GC, Rowe MH, Selmon MR, et al: Directional coronary atherectomy for lesions with complex morphology. *Circulation* 1990; 82(suppl 3):312.

9

Role of the Long-Wire Technique in Percutaneous Transluminal Coronary Angioplasty: The Frankfurt Experience

Gisbert Kober, M.D.

Christian Vallbracht, M.D.

Martin Kaltenbach, M.D.

Since 1982, percutaneous transluminal coronary angioplasty (PTCA) has been performed nearly exclusively with the aid of wire-guided steerable balloon catheters, a technical development that had originally been promoted by Simpson et al.[1] With this technique, a movable guidewire passing through the balloon catheter and coming out at its tip is introduced together with the balloon catheter into the guiding catheter and the respective coronary vessel.

DISADVANTAGES OF THE CONVENTIONAL STEERABLE TECHNIQUE

When balloon catheters are introduced into the commonly used 8 F guiding catheter, sufficient vessel opacification is rarely achieved, and thus probing is impeded, especially in the case of lesions extremely difficult to access. This results in a marked reduction in the degree of safety. Once the tip of the wire has passed the lesion, no further exchange of the balloon catheter for a smaller or larger balloon is possible. An exchange can only be achieved by withdrawing the existing equipment and subsequently reprobing the lesion with the exchanged instruments, which is often time-consuming and involves further procedural risks. Emergency measures undertaken when dissection and subsequent vessel occlusion occur, such as redilatation of the occluded segment or perfusion of the ischemic area to either bridge

waiting times before emergency bypass operations or serve as a curative procedure by applying perfusion balloon catheters[2] or introducing coronary stents as a bailout procedure, are clearly limited since probing of the occlusion through a dissected area can be difficult, not always possible, and possibly risky.

LONG-WIRE TECHNIQUE

Further technical improvement was desirable to facilitate the PTCA procedure and to reduce the risk of complications. For this purpose, the long-wire technique was introduced in March 1983[3] and has been applied virtually exclusively in a total number of 4,200 interventions since June 1984. Figure 9–1 shows statistics for angioplasties performed over the past 13 years in Frankfurt. Commencing in 1977, the frequency of interventions rose steadily until reaching a capacity of approximately 1,100 cases per year. The success rate rose to nearly 95%, whereas the percentage of emergency operations decreased to 0.6%.[13]

In most cases we start the PTCA procedure with a Medtronic guiding catheter with side holes by using the brachial or femoral approach; an ACS, Datascope, or Schneider 3-m-long wire; and a Mansfield, Datascope, Medtronic, or Advanced Cardiovascular Systems (ACS) balloon catheter.

With the long-wire technique, the arterial stenosis is

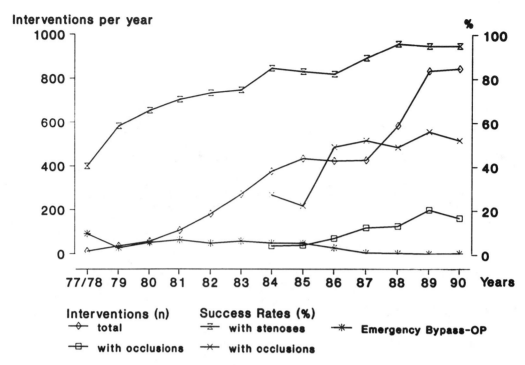

FIG 9–1.
Development of transluminal coronary angioplasty in stenoses and occlusions in Frankfurt, starting in 1977. With time a remarkable increase in the frequency of interventions and success rates can be seen while emergency operations decreased to 0.6%.

initially passed with a special wire only. This 3-m Teflon-coated wire with a diameter of 0.014 in. (rarely 0.012 or 0.010 in.) is introduced into the guiding catheter through a valve and advanced through the stenosis into the distal segment of the diseased coronary vessel (Fig 9–2). To reduce the danger of intimal injuries, the wire is tipped with a 0.45-mm hemisphere. The larger outer part of the wire is protected in a cochleate plastic tube. A small plastic torque clipped onto the wire sideways enables rotating, longitudinal maneuvering of the wire, thus preventing damage to the Teflon coating and allowing it to be removed without having to pull the entire wire out of its tube. After positioning the guidewire, the selected balloon catheter is threaded across the exterior part of the wire and then advanced through the hemostatic valve into the guiding catheter and stenosis, respectively. The wire tip has to be consistently followed fluoroscopically and held in place while gradually retracting the wire back into the tubing and simultaneously advancing the balloon catheter. With a 0.014-in. wire, almost all balloon catheters currently available can be applied, even low-profile ones. After dilatation, the balloon catheter is pulled into the guiding catheter or entirely back out of the guiding catheter, consequently allowing optimum angiographic visualization of the results of angioplasty. The guidewire is held in place for some minutes until good procedural results are confirmed.

To prevent thrombus formation, especially at the site of the dilated coronary segment as well as inside the guiding catheter and on the surface of the Teflon-coated guidewire, 200 units/kg body weight of heparin was administered as a bolus at the beginning of the procedure followed by a constant infusion of 2,000 units/hr of heparin diluted in a 200-mL saline solution via the guiding catheter. On account of this treatment, minimization of fibrin deposits and thrombus formations was evident through microscopic evaluation of the wire surface.[4]

In addition, patients were treated with salicylates (0.5 to 1.5 g/day) calcium antagonists (verapamil, 80 mg three times daily, or gallopamil, 50 mg twice daily), and isosorbide dinitrate (20 mg three times daily) at least 24 hours before commencement of the procedure. This treatment was continued over the next 4 months following successful intervention.

OPTIMUM STENOSIS OPACIFICATION DURING PROBING AND JUDGMENT OF DILATATION RESULTS

The sole introduction of the guidewire into the guiding catheter does not create any resistance to contrast material flow. Thus, opacification of the large coronary

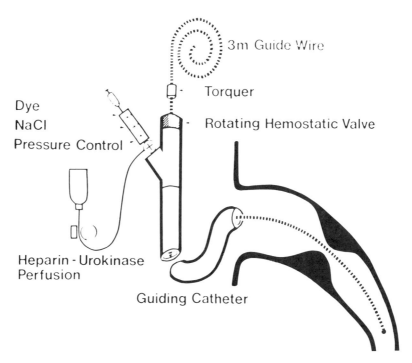

FIG 9–2.
Schematic diagram of the long-wire technique. The wire is advanced via a hemostatic valve through the guiding catheter and lesion into the poststenotic coronary vessel. The balloon catheter is then introduced through the valve into the stenosis under fluoroscopic control.

vessels and all their side branches, the shape of the stenosis, and the position of the guidewire tip can be achieved optimally (Fig 9–3).

After dilatation, an angiogram permits the observation of not only the runoff of the contrast medium into the distal segment of the vessel but also the dilatation results regarding stenosis reduction, residual stenosis, dissections, or the sudden occurrence of an occlusion.

Further therapeutic consequences can also be derived from this angiogram. Figure 9–4 shows a left anterior descending (LAD) coronary artery stenosis not yet adequately dilated after using a 2.5-mm balloon; good results were achieved after the successive use of a 3.7-mm balloon. Both angiograms were taken after dilatation with the wire still in place.

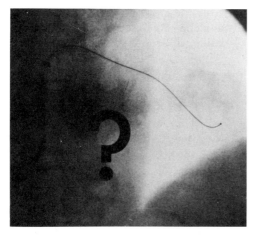 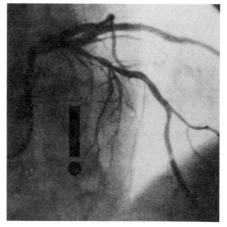

FIG 9–3.
Guidewire tip in the periphery of the coronary system *(left)*. Optimum opacification *(right)* enables safe confirmation of its position.

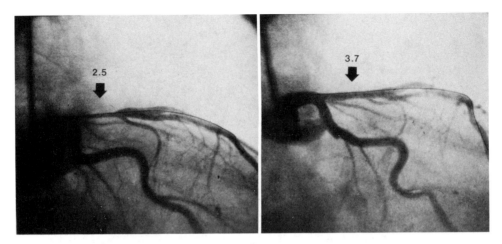

FIG 9–4.
Angiograms obtained with the wire still in place confirm the results of proximal LAD coronary artery angioplasty after successive use of 2.5- and 3.7-mm balloons (*left* and *right,* respectively).

EXCHANGE OF BALLOON CATHETERS

With the wire placed in the distal coronary segment, it is often not possible to pass the stenosis with the balloon catheter selected on account of the balloon diameter or the catheter stiffness. In this case, changing to a smaller balloon catheter presents no problem. Following unsatisfactory dilatation results, wider balloon catheters can be easily introduced with the guidewire still in place without having to reprobe the stenotic area, thus saving time and diminishing procedural risks (Fig 9–4.) Exchanging balloon catheters for smaller or larger ones proved necessary in about 20% of the procedures performed. Whenever passage was only achieved with the wire but not with a balloon catheter, the ROTAC system introduced over the wire often helped to first widen the obstructed segment.[5, 6]

TREATMENT OF BRANCHING STENOSES

The dilatation of a large vessel bears a certain risk of sudden occlusion of the side branches originating within the stenosis.[7] Thus, dilatation of the main vessel and side branch origin or the protection of the side branch may prove desirable in the case of branching stenoses with larger perfusion areas of the side branches. Usually, probing the side branch is only feasible before main vessel dilatation. Thus, wires have to be placed into both vessels before the first dilatation. Two long wires can be advanced simultaneously into both vessels through the same 8 F lumen guiding catheter, once again under optimum opacification of the anatomy. As a result, it is no longer necessary with this technique to introduce two guiding catheters via two different pe-

ripheral arteries. Stenosis dilatation is subsequently performed by changing the balloon catheter from one wire to the other (Fig 9–5).[8]

It is neither possible nor essential to simultaneously dilate both stenoses as is done with the kissing balloon technique.[7, 9] In many cases, placement of the wire in the side branch is merely a precaution, and dilatation is rendered unnecessary if the flow into the branching vessel is not impeded after dilating the mainstem stenosis. To avoid the impending risk of side branch occlusions, this technique has been applied in 1.5% of the interventions performed.

TREATMENT OF CHRONIC OCCLUSIONS

Occlusions of unknown age that are not caused by a recent acute infarction can be reopened successfully by using the long-wire technique. It is especially important to identify the exact site of the occlusion, which is again provided by the long-wire technique. First, the wire alone is tried. Once the occlusion has been passed, balloons of different sizes can be subsequently introduced. About 20% of the chronic occlusions tried were reopened. If the wire alone fails to pass the lesion, a recanalization catheter[10] can be introduced via the 3-m wire. It is equipped with a 4 F shaft and an extremely tapered distal end. The inner lumen allows pressure to be measured and dye injected with the wire still inside the catheter. This catheter is pushed along the wire to the obstruction. On contact with the occlusion, proximal pressure drops to zero, and phasic pressure raises again when the catheter has passed the occlusion and found the distal vessel lumen. The wire can be pushed through the recanalization catheter downward in the

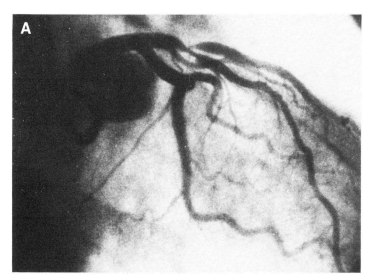

RAO

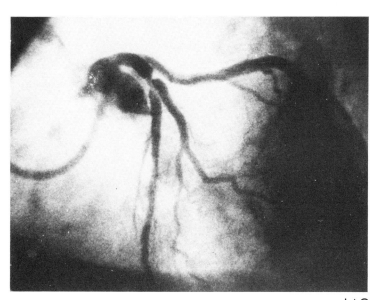

LAO

FIG 9–5.
Treatment of a branching stenosis **(A)** with the double-wire technique. *(Continued.)*

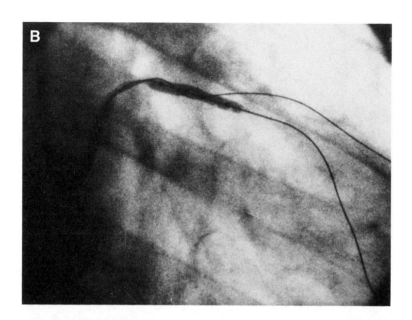

Dilatation 2

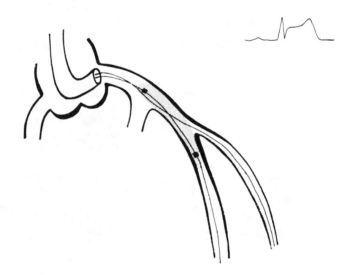

FIG 9–5 (cont.).
After positioning both wires, the balloon catheter is successively introduced into each vessel and inflated (**B** and **C**).

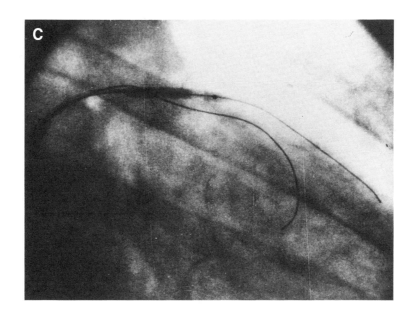

Dilatation 3

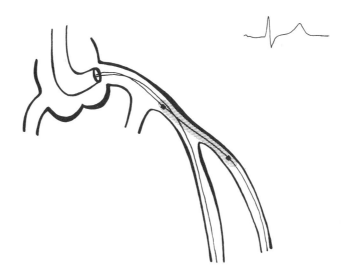

FIG 9–5   (cont.).

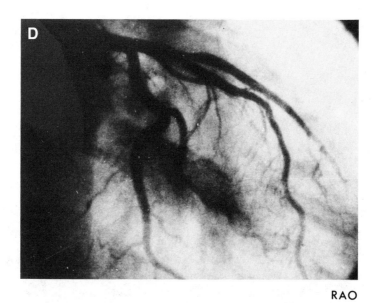

RAO

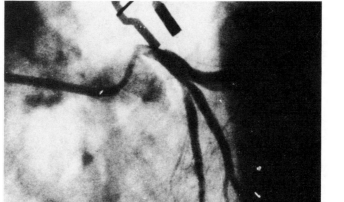

LAO

FIG 9–5 (cont.).
The control angiogram shows the success achieved acutely **(D).**

vessel and the catheter subsequently easily exchanged for an appropriate balloon catheter. With this technique an additional 30% of the occlusion can be recanalized (total, 50%). When recanalization catheters fail to create a channel or in case of a primarily unsuitable occlusion, a ROTAC catheter can be advanced to the occlusion and the tip rotated through it and exchanged for a balloon catheter once the distal end of the lumen is reached.[5, 6, 11, 12] This technique increased the overall recanalization rate to a total of 60% to 70% of all attempted occlusions.

The ROTAC system, a new technique to reopen chronic coronary artery occlusions, uses low-speed rotating, blunt, flexible catheters with a suitably rounded, relatively big tip (1.2 to 1.6 mm). Once the tip has touched the cross-sectional area of the occlusion it starts to search the way of least resistance. The last real section of lumen occluded by a thrombus remains the softest part of the obstruction, sometimes for a long period of time (with coronary arteries up to 1 year), and the ro-

tating catheter will consequently reopen the last real segment of lumen (transluminal recanalization).

TREATMENT OF ACUTE CORONARY OCCLUSIONS FOLLOWING ANGIOPLASTY

In the event of an occlusion of the dilated vessel mainly attributable to a large dissection at the site of the stenosis, an emergency bypass operation may become necessary. The need for emergency operations recently dropped from 5% to 0.6% (see Fig 9–1). It is often possible to avoid such an intervention through repeat introduction of a larger balloon catheter over the still inserted guidewire by using long inflation times. A perfusion catheter can also be introduced easily via the long wire still in place. It may, however, be inevitable to refer the patient for bypass surgery if redilatation of the occluded segment does not result in a stable reopening of

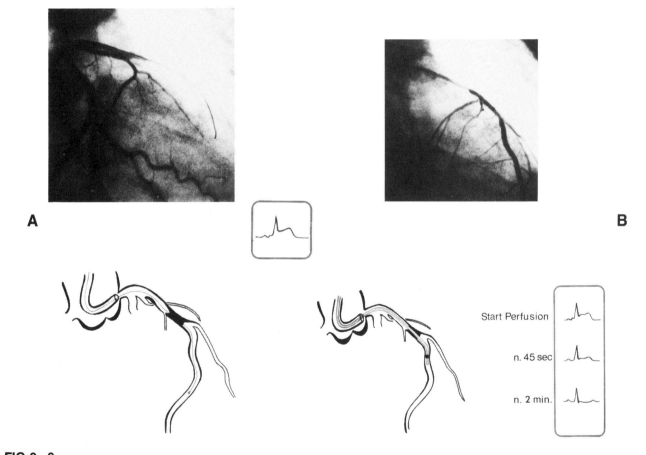

A

B

FIG 9–6.
A, the long wire is still in place with occlusion of the LAD coronary artery after PTCA causing angina and ischemic electrocardiographic (ECG) changes. **B,** distal perfusion using a 5 F perfusion catheter by means of the long wire immediately minimized symptoms and ECG changes.

the vessel to satisfactorily perfuse the myocardium.

The period of ischemia before operative revascularization of the endangered myocardium is one of the most important determinants of the degree of irreversible damage to the heart muscle.[13] The severity and duration of ischemia can be reduced by perfusing the ischemic area with a Stack perfusion balloon catheter. If with the help of this device ischemia cannot be completely eliminated, a 5 F perfusion catheter (Schneider-Medintag, Zurich, Switzerland) can easily be introduced with the aid of the long wire still in place (Fig 9–6). Oxygenated blood from the femoral artery is then injected manually.[14] Model experiments[15] demonstrated the possibility of appropriate perfusion of the ischemic myocardium by using perfusion catheters at a rather low perfusion pressure. The above-mentioned perfusion technique was used in 16 cases. Its clinical value can easily be seen from the favorable response of anginal symptoms and the effect on ischemic changes in the ECG.

Coronary stents have now been in place for more than 1 year in an investigational phase for recurrent restenosis and acute occlusion mostly caused by vessel dissection during dilatation. These stents were also easily inserted by exchanging the angioplasty catheter with the stent introduction device along the track of the long wire (Fig 9–7).[16, 17]

MEASUREMENT OF PERIPHERAL CORONARY PRESSURES

Peripheral pressures can be easily measured by means of the long-wire technique. Whereas it is known that intracoronary pressure gradient measurements provide no reliable diagnostic indications of either the severity of stenoses or the results of angioplasty,[18, 19] measurements of occlusion pressure, on the other hand, are of some diagnostic and prognostic value. Patients with high occlusion pressures (>20 mm Hg) are less prone to severe ischemia or ischemic damage to the myocardium in the event of acute occlusion of the treated vessel. Restenosis, however, tends to occur less often in patients with low occlusion pressures (<20 mm Hg).

CONCLUSION

The long-wire technique, first introduced in 1983 and applied virtually exclusively in 4,200 interventions

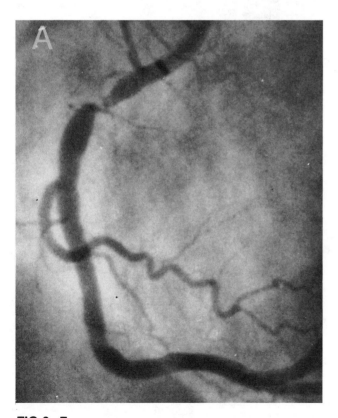
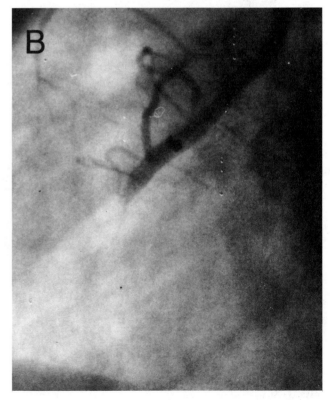

FIG 9–7.
When a stenosis in the proximal segment of the right coronary artery **(A)** was treated by angioplasty, an occlusion occured **(B)** and could not be reopened by repeat angioplasty.

(Continued.)

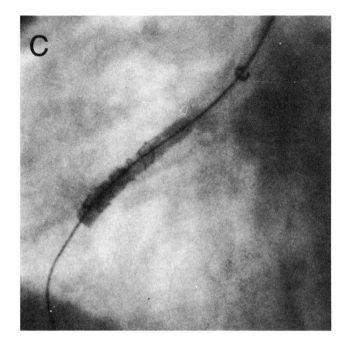

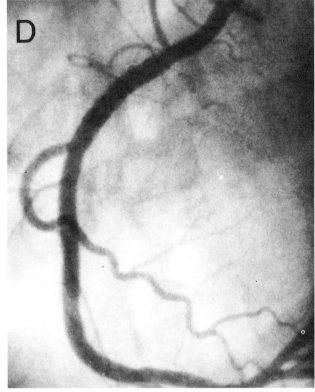

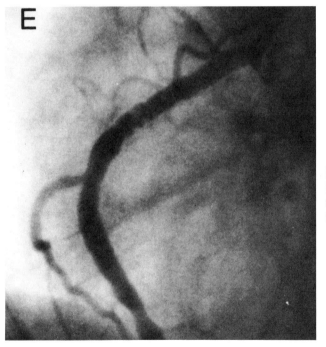

FIG 9-7 (cont.).
Implantation of a Wiktor stent with the balloon and the long wire still in place **(C)**, after removal of the balloon **(D)**, and 6 months following implantation **(E)**.

since June 1984, has effected a slight additional increase in the acute success rate of coronary angioplasty and has reduced the number of emergency operations despite the treatment of more and more complicated cases.

One of the most important advantages of this technique vs. the conventional steerable technique is optimum visualization of the coronary vessels (including side branches and stenoses) during lesion probing and reangiography following angioplasty. Balloon catheters can, if necessary, be exchanged for those with smaller or larger diameters without having to recross the stenosis with the wire, thus improving the procedural safety factor. Branching stenoses can also be treated by using two wires introduced with the same 8.0 F lumen guiding catheter. In case of emergency, distal coronary perfusion can be easily achieved by inserting a perfusion catheter or a stent.

Maneuvering the long wire, 170 cm of which is encased in plastic cochleate tubing outside the patient, becomes familiar after only a few interventions. The extra fluoroscopy time for introducing the catheter into the lesion from outside and removing it after the procedure is relatively short in comparison with the total fluoroscopy time and is compensated for in many interventions by faster and safer probing of the coronary vessels and stenoses. Thus, the long-wire technique makes angioplasty easier and more successful and improves the safety both with routine interventions and in the event of complications.

REFERENCES

1. Simpson JB, Baim DS, Robert E, et al: A new catheter system for coronary angioplasty. *Am J Cardiol* 1982; 49:1216–1222.
2. Stack RS, Quigley PJ, Collins G, et al: Perfusion balloon catheter. *Am J Cardiol* 1988; 61:776–806.
3. Kaltenbach M: The long wire technique: A new technique for steerable balloon catheter dilatation of coronary artery stenoses. *Eur Heart J* 1984; 5:1004–1009.
4. Kadel C, Jonczyk C, Kaltenbach M: Thrombotic deposits on angioplasty guide wires. *Eur Heart J* 1987; 8:248.
5. Kaltenbach M, Vallbracht C: Reopening of chronic coronary artery occlusions by low speed rotational angioplasty. *J Intervent Cardiol* 1989; 2:137–145.
6. Kaltenbach M, Vallbracht C: Rotationsangioplastik – ein neues Katheterverfahren für die nichtoperative Gefäßeröffnung. *Fortschr Med* 1987; 105:36–38.
7. Meier B, Grüntzig AR, Kind SB, et al: Risk of side branch occlusion during coronary angioplasty. *Am J Cardiol* 1984; 53:10.
8. Vallbracht C, Kaltenbach M, Kober G: Doppel-Langdrahttechnik zur Ballondilatation von Verzweigungsstenosen. *Herz/Kreis* 1986; 8:378–382.
9. Grüntzig AR: The technique of percutaneous transluminal coronary angioplasty, in Hurst JW, Hogue RB, Rackley CE, et al (eds): *The Heart*. New York, McGraw-Hill, 1984.
10. Sievert H, Kober G, Kaltenbach M: Katheter-Rekanalisation langstreckig verschlossener aortokoronarer Venenbypasses (abstract). *Z Kardiol* 1987; 76(suppl 2):28.
11. Vallbracht C, Liermann D, Prignitz I, et al: Results of low speed rotational angioplasty for chronic peripheral occlusions. *Am J Cardiol* 1988; 62:935–940.
12. Vallbracht C, Kress I, Schweitzer M, et al: Rotationsangioplastik – ein neues Verfahren zur Gefäßwiedereröffnung und -erweiterung. Experimentelle Befunde. *Z Kardiol* 1987; 76:608–611.
13. Klepzig H Jr, Schraub J, Huber H, et al: Aortokoronare Bypassoperation als Notfalleingriff nach transluminaler koronarer Angioplastik: Welche Faktoren verhindern das Auftreten eines großen Infarktes? *Dtsch Med Wochenschr* 1986; 111:737–741.
14. Hopf R, Kunkel B, Schneider M, et al: Koronarperfusion bei akutem Gefäßverschluß im Rahmen der transluminalen Koronarangioplastik (TCA). *Z Kardiol* 1985; 74:580–584.
15. Busch UW: Selective coronary perfusion via angioplasty catheters: Technical and physiological aspects, in Höfling B (ed): *Current Problems in PTCA*. New York, Springer-Verlag, 1986.
16. Serruys PW, Strauss BH, Beatt KJ, et al: Angiographic follow-up after placement of a self-expanding coronary artery stent. *N Engl J Med* 1991; 324:13–17.
17. Burger W, Hartmann A, Kandyba I, et al: Angiographic and histologic course after implantation of balloon expandable stents in miniswine coronary arteries: Short- and mid-term observations. *J Intervent Cardiol* 1990; 3:87–98.
18. Sievert H, Kaltenbach M: Intrakoronare Druckgradientenmessung: Wert und methodische Grenzen. *Z Kardiol* 1987; 76:323–325.
19. Sievert H, Kober G, Kaltenbach M: Pressure measurements during coronary angioplasty. *Eur Heart J* 1987; 8(suppl 2):245.

10

Magnum System for Coronary Angioplasty

Bernhard Meier, M.D., F.E.S.C.

The Magnum wire was developed in 1987 to improve the unsatisfactory performance of conventional coronary guidewires in terms of passing chronic total occlusions.[1] Its initial version was a 0.035-in. (0.89-mm) wire with a blunt tip that proved efficacious in recanalizing occlusions in proximal straight vessel segments (Fig 10–1). However, this prototype was not appealing. First, it required substantial backup by the guiding catheter to advance the wire around bends. Second, there was no possibility of distal contrast medium injections. Third, the wire had to be removed after successful recanalization to complete angioplasty with a conventional balloon catheter after renegotiating the lesion with a standard coronary guidewire.

In its current form, the Magnum wire features a Teflonized solid-steel shaft with a diameter of 0.021 in. (0.53 mm), a flexible, shapable distal part, and an olive tip 1 mm in diameter (Fig 10–2). It is compatible with Magnum, Magnarail, and Mega Balloons of Schneider that are made of polyethylene terephthalate (low balloon compliance) or nylon (high balloon compliance) and certain balloon models of other manufacturers. Although the Magnum wire has been especially designed for angioplasty of chronic total occlusions in coronary arteries, it may be useful for peripheral occlusions[2] or routine angioplasty of nontotal lesions as well.

TECHNIQUE

There is only one significant difference in technique between the Magnum and a conventional system for coronary balloon angioplasty. In conventional coronary angioplasty, subtle use of the guidewire is recommended. Tight stenoses are passed by gently "floating" the wire past the lesion. The Magnum wire has to be advanced with more firmness and determination. Not only total occlusions but also tight lesions with a diameter less than 1 mm can only be passed forcefully. This frequently requires stiffening of the distal part of the Magnum wire with the balloon or a bracing catheter.[3] Such a technique is safe because the ball tip of the Magnum wire prevents perforation and minimizes the risk of subintimal passage.

MAGNUM SYSTEM FOR CHRONIC TOTAL CORONARY OCCLUSIONS

Balloon recanalizations of chronic total coronary occlusions with conventional angioplasty techniques and materials may be virtually free of serious complications related to the occluded site itself, such as death, Q wave infarctions, and need for emergency bypass surgery. Yet they are afflicted by a low success rate. Primary success rates ranged from 42% to 72% with a mean of 67% in roughly 2,000 patients of ten major reports.[4-14] They are even lower if functional occlusions are excluded and only anatomically total occlusions are considered.

The Magnum wire was designed to overcome some of the major shortcomings of conventional wires when dealing with total occlusions. Used unsupported, they exhibit insufficient pushability, and when stiffened by a bracing catheter, they have a tendency to create subintimal pathways. Since 1990, we have used the Magnum wire exclusively in its Monorail[15] version (Fig 10–3). This precludes selective distal contrast medium injections since the only lumen in the catheter shaft is reserved for balloon inflation. However, guiding catheter injections opacify the distal part of the vessel sufficiently well if the balloon catheter is advanced maximally. The contrast medium enters the guidewire lumen jointly

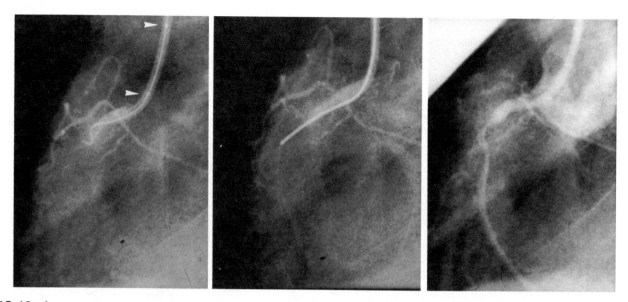

FIG 10–1.
Successful recanalization in 1987 of a chronic total occlusion of the right coronary artery of a 66-year-old man by using a first-generation 0.035-in. (0.89-mm) Magnum wire *(middle panel)* after failure of a 0.014-in. (0.36-mm) standard coronary guidewire braced by a balloon catheter *(left panel, arrowheads* indicate the balloon markers). Note the lumen created mechanically by passage of the wire alone *(right panel)*. The result was subsequently improved by using the standard guidewire and balloon catheter of the left panel again.

with the guidewire about 15 cm proximal to the balloon and leaves it at the tip to outline the position of the olive of the Magnum wire and the distal lumen once it has been reached (Fig 10–4).

Step-by-Step Instruction for Magnum Recanalization

Advancement of the Magnum wire through the coronary artery proximal to the occlusion is done as with ordinary coronary guidewires. Most turns and bifurcations can be negotiated with a small J bend just proximal to the olive. Once the occlusion is reached, the wire rarely passes through it without being braced since its distal portion is floppy and the ball tip increases resistance. To splint the flexible portion of the Magnum wire, the balloon catheter or, to save money in case of a failure, a Magnarail probing catheter[3] is advanced close to the olive. This not only supports the wire but also provides for distal contrast medium injections to ascertain the correct position of the olive in the vessel stump as explained above. The Magnum wire is then thrust forward with half turns in either direction if progression is halted. The backup for the Magnum wire advancement is provided by the balloon or probing catheter held in place just proximal to the occlusion and the guiding catheter kept in a power position in the coronary orifice or the proximal portion of the vessel. Alternatively, the

balloon or probing catheter and the Magnum wire can be advanced en bloc. Injections of contrast medium through the guiding catheter inform about a subintimal pathway or, in case of successful passage through the occlusion, about first antegrade flow. Frequently, it is obvious that the patent distal segment of the vessel has been reached when the Magnum wire suddenly progresses effortlessly. Antegrade flow may still be absent with the wire obstructing the newly created passage, and the distal portion of the vessel entered may not be the major one to recanalize (Fig 10–4). While the Magnum wire tip is far in the distal part of the coronary artery, the balloon or probing catheter is cautiously advanced. As soon as its tip reaches the lumen distal to the occlusion, the correct position of the Magnum wire in the largest vessel distal to the occlusion (commensurate with the balloon diameter selected) is confirmed by contrast medium injection. Finally, the balloon is placed across the occlusion, and the lesion is dilated in the usual fashion. If a Magnarail Probing catheter had been used for wire splinting, it is exchanged for an appropriate balloon catheter. This exchange is facilitated by the Monorail design.[15] The angiographic result is first filmed with the Magnum wire across the lesion without the ball tip wedging the distal part of the vessel and then after withdrawal of the Magnum wire from the coronary artery. Unless the Magnum wire is completely withdrawn from the guiding

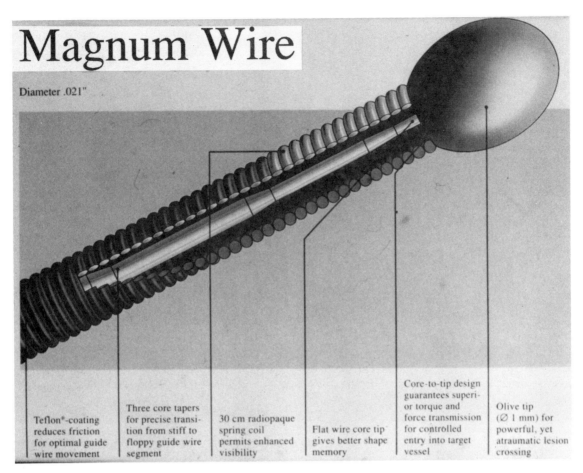

Magnum Wire

Diameter .021"

Teflon®-coating reduces friction for optimal guide wire movement	Three core tapers for precise transition from stiff to floppy guide wire segment	30 cm radiopaque spring coil permits enhanced visibility	Flat wire core tip gives better shape memory	Core-to-tip design guarantees superior torque and force transmission for controlled entry into target vessel	Olive tip (⌀ 1 mm) for powerful, yet atraumatic lesion crossing

FIG 10–2.
Schematic diagram of the current model of the Magnum wire. (Courtesy of Schneider Europe.)

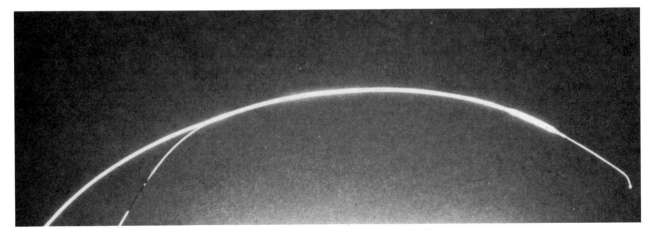

FIG 10–3.
Magnarail system consisting of a Magnum wire (0.021 in./0.053 mm; olive tip, 1 mm) and a balloon catheter featuring a single lumen shaft (*left,* 3 F) except for the distal portion, where there is a second lumen for the guidewire communicating with the balloon tip.

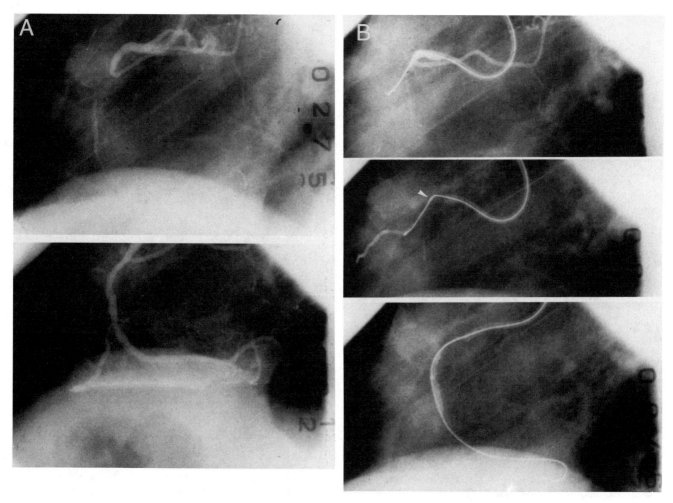

FIG 10–4.
Faked distal contrast medium injection with the Magnarail system during recanalization (**A**) of the right coronary artery of a 58-year-old man. A contrast medium injection through the guiding catheter fails to opacify the vessel distal to the tip of the bare Magnum wire (**B**, *top*). After advancing the Magnarail balloon catheter to the tip of the Magnum wire (central balloon marker indicated by an *arrowhead*), a repeat injection through the guiding catheter results in opacification of the distal portion of the vessel, which happens to be a marginal branch of the right ventricle rather than the main right coronary artery (**B**, *central*). The contrast medium traveled through the short guidewire lumen of the Magnarail catheter and was helpful for the final correct placement of the balloon catheter (**B**, *bottom*) and a satisfactory result (**A**, *bottom*).

catheter, it has to be secured in place to prevent inadvertent reinjection of the wire by the flow of contrast medium during the final angiogram.

Results of Magnum Recanalization

In the initial 50 consecutive recanalization attempts with a Magnum wire using 12 first-generation (0.035-in./0.89-mm) and 38 second-generation (0.021-in./0.53-mm) wires in 23 right, 18 left anterior descending, 8 left circumflex coronary arteries, and 1 diagonal branch,[1] the Magnum wires reached the occlusion in all cases. Technical success (correct balloon positioning) was achieved for 30 occlusions (60%). In 2 cases, a 0.035-in.

(0.89-mm) and in 1 case a 0.021-in. (0.53-mm) Magnum wire did not cross the occlusion completely but enabled the previously impossible passage of a conventional 0.014-in. (0.36-mm) or 0.012-in. (0.30-mm) coronary guidewire. Angiographic success was obtained in only 29 cases (58%) since 1 vessel reoccluded during the procedure. Of the 17 cases with prior failure of a conventional attempt, 8 (47%) could be recanalized with the Magnum wire. In the 33 cases with the Magnum wire as the initial instrument, success was achieved in 22 (67%). Conventional wires were subsequently employed in 9 of the 11 failures but succeeded in none. Of the 38 cases attempted with the 0.021-in. (0.53-mm) Magnum wire, angiographic success was attained in 26 (68%). Finally, if only the 31 cases of this last group with the Magnum wire as the initial instrument are considered, angiographic success was achieved in 22 (71%).

In all instances where a Magnum wire could be placed in the distal segment of the coronary artery, a balloon selected according to the diameter of the segment to be dilated could be correctly positioned without a need for predilatation with a smaller balloon. Impossibility to reach the lumen distal to the occlusion with the Magnum wire accounted for all 20 technical failures. A significant subintimal passage of the Magnum wire causing the failure of the procedure was observed in 3 cases (6%). It was extensive in 2 cases but did not cause relevant adverse effects. In 2 of the 3 cases with subintimal passage of the Magnum wire, subsequent attempts to find the correct lumen with a conventional coronary guidewire were done, but they were unsuccessful. Of the 17 cases that were initially attempted with conventional coronary guidewires, significant false pathways were created in 3 (18%), which invariably prevented subsequent passage with a Magnum wire.

No relevant proximal dissections occurred during Magnum wire manipulations, but three did during utilization of conventional coronary guidewires. In two of them, proximal side branches occluded. In one, a rise of the creatine kinase level to less than twice the normal value was observed. In the other, the side branch was reopened by balloon dilatation but reoccluded the next day after the intravenous heparin therapy had been discontinued. It was reopened immediately by repeat angioplasty, and a stent was implanted with an uneventful clinical course and good patency at control angiography 5 months later. There were no major complications such as coronary perforation, Q wave myocardial infarction, a need for emergency bypass surgery, or death.

Subsequently, a randomized study was performed to compare the advantages and disadvantages of Magnum/Magnarail and conventional systems.[16] The study population consisted of 100 consecutive unselected patients accepted for balloon angioplasty for chronic total coronary occlusion without antegrade flow. The baseline characteristics of the patients are depicted in Table 10–1.

Indications for the balloon recanalization attempt were angina and/or positive stress test findings. Additional angiographic selection criteria included a visible stump and opacification of the distal segment of the artery by collaterals. The age of the occlusion was estimated when possible on the basis of a documented myocardial infarction in the respective territory, a marked change in clinical symptoms, or the date of a prior angiogram showing the occlusion. The length of the occluded segment was assessed on the angiogram by measuring the distance between the proximal end of the stump and the closest distal opacification by collaterals in the least foreshortened view.

TABLE 10–1

Baseline Characteristics of Patients With Chronic Total Coronary Occlusion Randomized to the Magnum/Magnarail System or Conventional Systems*

Characteristic	Magnum/Magnarail	Conventional
Patients/lesions	50/52	50/51
Age (yr, mean ± SD, range)	58 ± 11, 33–76	58 ± 10, 35–82
Mean angina class†	1.8 ± 1.3	2.2 ± 1.4
Positive stress test	17/28 (61%)	19/27 (70%)
Previous myocardial infarction	40 (80%)	38 (76%)
Q wave	27 (54%)	29 (58%)
Non–Q wave	13 (26%)	9 (18%)
Ejection fraction (%)	56 ± 12	57 ± 13
Age of occlusion (mon)	(N = 40)	(N = 45)
Mean	1.4 ± 1.9	1.4 ± 1.8
Range	<1–8	<1–7
Length of occlusion (cm)	(N = 39)	(N = 42)
Mean	1.4 ± 1.3	1.6 ± 1.7
Range	0.2–5.2	0.2–8.5
Coronary artery with occlusion		
Left anterior descending	19 (37%)	21 (41%)
Left circumflex	9 (17%)	11 (22%)
Right coronary	24 (46%)	19 (37%)
Proximal/mid/distal	9/42/1	15/35/1
Balloon size (mm)	3.0 ± 0.3, 2.5–3.5	3.0 ± 0.3, 2.5–4.0

*Corresponding values not significantly different.
†According to the classification of the New York Heart Association.

Success with the allocated system was defined as correct balloon placement within 20 minutes of fluoroscopy time. A crossover to the nonallocated system was imposed if this goal was not attained. Crossover success was defined as correct balloon placement within 20 minutes of fluoroscopy time after crossover.

The Magnum/Magnarail system as a primary tool was successful in 35 lesions (67%), and conventional systems were successful in 23 lesions (45%) ($P < .05$). Consequently, there were 17 crossovers (33%) from the Magnum/Magnarail group and 28 (55%) from the conventional group. As second tool, the Magnum/Magnarail system was also more successful, with 29% (11/28 cases) vs. 12% (2/17 cases) ($P < .05$). The Magnum/Magnarail system was significantly more successful than conventional systems for recanalization of right coronary arteries ($P < .05$). For left anterior descending and circumflex coronary arteries, the differences were in its favor as well but did not reach statistical significance due to small numbers.

The complications observed in both groups were comparable and occurred only in patients with technical failures. Thus clinical success rates of both groups were identical with technical success rates. Myocardial infarction with a rise of creatine kinase concentrations to more than twice normal was seen in one patient (2%) in the Magnum/Magnarail group. Coronary perforations were not seen, and emergency bypass surgery was not required in either group. There was one in-hospital death in the conventionally treated group due to an anaphylactic reaction to protamine administered prior to sheath removal.

There were no significant differences regarding the numbers and sizes of guiding and balloon catheters used. The expected difference in guiding catheter size was blunted by the fact that 8 F guiding catheters were used in the conventional group because a crossover to a Magnum wire was anticipated. Although the Magnum/Magnarail system was already compatible with the 7 F guiding catheters commercialized at that time, this combination was not ideal. A single guidewire per case was used in the Magnum/Magnarail group vs. 1.4 ± 0.7 in the conventionally treated group ($P < .001$). In the successful cases of the Magnum/Magnarail group, the fluoroscopy time to cross the lesion with the guidewire was 5.3 ± 3.9 vs. 4.2 ± 3.2 minutes in the conventionally treated group, the fluoroscopy time to position the balloon once the guidewire was in place was 1.0 ± 1.4 vs. 1.5 ± 2.1 minutes, the fluoroscopy time for the actual dilatation was 6.2 ± 3.9 vs. 5.3 ± 3.2 minutes, and the total fluoroscopy time was 12.5 ± 5.8 vs. 10.9 ± 5.3 minutes. These differences were not statistically significant.

Hence, this randomized study concerning chronic total coronary occlusions revealed significantly higher success rates with the Magnum/Magnarail system as compared with conventional systems be it as a primary or a crossover tool. The low success rates observed with conventional systems can be attributed to the fact that only complete occlusions without antegrade flow were included and only 20 minutes of fluoroscopy time were allowed. Fewer guidewires per case were used in the Magnum/Magnarail group, which in itself does not make this system cost-efficient since a Magnum wire is twice as expensive as a standard wire. However, Magnum wires may be reused if local policies permit. Conventional wires are usually considered too fragile for cleaning and resterilization. Operators accustomed to predilate lesions for an easier passage may achieve substantial savings by using the Magnum wire because it obviates the need for predilatation with a small balloon.

For economic reasons, it is appealing to try to cross an occlusion with a bare Magnum wire and to unwrap a balloon catheter only if the lesion has been passed. Yet since it is premature to give up on a case without having reinforced the distal part of the Magnum wire with a catheter, such an approach is a waste of time. As described above, a simple splinting catheter, called a Magnarail probing catheter,[3] can be employed to save the cost of a balloon catheter should even the rigidified Magnum wire fail to pass. In case of successful crossing of the occlusion, however, this increases cost because the probing catheter has to be exchanged for a balloon catheter to perform the dilatation. When indications are restricted to cases projecting success rates of 70% or more, it is more economical, regarding time and money, to use a balloon catheter from the start.

Failure to pass the occlusion with the wire despite increased pushing power and creation of subintimal pathways remain problems even with the Magnum system. The blunt tip of the Magnum wire should, however, get underneath plaque less often than the sharp tip of a conventional wire. The current olive diameter (1 mm) emerged as a compromise between larger diameters with too much resistance to cross the occlusion and smaller diameters with an increased risk of creating a subintimal pathway. Once a subintimal entry is created by an initially used conventional wire or the Magnum wire, the Magnum wire will readily reenter such a false channel and may powerfully advance in it. Even if the distal part of the lumen can be found with the Magnum wire or a conventional wire, there is only hope for long-term patency if the subintimal channel is short. In addition, balloon inflation in a subintimal position harbors some risk of vessel rupture.

MAGNUM SYSTEM FOR ROUTINE CORONARY ANGIOPLASTY

The Magnum wire may well be the most steerable coronary guidewire currently available. It provides an extremely stable track for the balloon catheter. Acute-angle takeoffs sometimes render angioplasty with conventional systems impossible. The conventional wire may be able to negotiate the angle, but it gets crimped by the more rigid balloon, which tends to follow the straight path and drags the doubled-over wire along (Fig 10–5), or it may even fold over together with the wire (Fig 10–6). Tight lesions may require substantial backup during balloon crossing. The more rigid wire already improves backup, which probably more than makes up for the larger profile of the Magnum-compatible balloons. Furthermore, it allows for deep advancement of the guiding catheter (Fig 10–7). Finally, the ball tip may avoid subintimal passage in subtotal and eccentric lesions (Fig 10–8).

A randomized study with an identical protocol as the one concerning chronic total occlusions was performed to assess the comparative performance of Magnum/Magnarail and conventional systems for routine coronary angioplasty.[17] The study population consisted of 200 consecutive unselected patients undergoing balloon angioplasty. The baseline characteristics of the patients were well balanced (Table 10–2). Fixed wire balloons accounted for 14% of the conventional systems.

Primary success per vessel (as initial tools) was achieved in 91% with the Magnum/Magnarail system

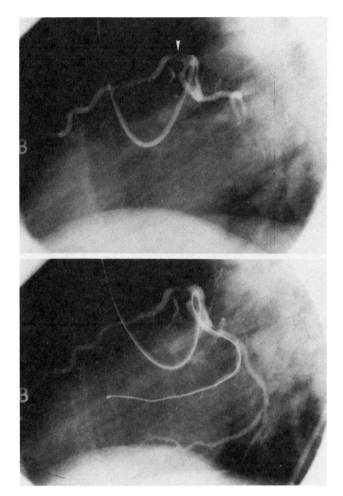

FIG 10–5.
Impossibility to negotiate an acute-angle takeoff of the left circumflex coronary artery of a 56-year-old man with a balloon catheter tracking over a 0.014-in. (0.36-mm) conventional coronary guidewire (Schneider). The advancing balloon folds over the wire and drags it along the straight left anterior descending coronary artery *(arrowhead)* rather than following it into the left circumflex coronary artery *(top)*. The problem is solved by substituting a 0.021-in. (0.53-mm) Magnum wire *(bottom)*.

TABLE 10–2

Baseline Characteristics of Routine Coronary Angioplasty Patients Randomized to the Magnum/Magnarail System or Conventional Systems

Characteristic	Magnum/Magnarail	Conventional
Patients/vessels	100/115	100/118
Age (yr, mean ± SD)	60 ± 10	60 ± 11
Angina class III/IV*	25 (25%)	34 (34%)
Positive stress test	40/61 (66%)	28/48 (58%)
Previous myocardial infarction	56 (56%)	64 (64%)
Ejection fraction (%)	63 ± 13	62 ± 12
Chronic total occlusion	18 (16%)	22 (19%)
Diameter stenosis (%)	83 ± 12	86 ± 11†
Coronary artery attempted		
Left anterior descending	47 (41%)	51 (43%)
Left circumflex	26 (23%)	30 (26%)
Right	39 (34%)	32 (27%)
Bypass graft	3 (2%)	5 (4%)
Proximal/mid/distal	25/78/12	34/76/8
Balloon size (mm)	3.0 ± 0.3	3.0 ± 0.3

*According to the classification of the Canadian Cardiovascular Society.
†*P* = .02.

and in 86% with conventional systems. After crossover for failure with the allocated system, the Magnum/Magnarail system was significantly superior with a 39% success rate (7/19) as compared with 9% (1/11) with conventional systems (*P* < .05)

The complications observed in both groups were comparable. Myocardial infarction with a rise in creatine kinase concentration to more than twice normal was seen in 5% of both groups and Q wave infarctions in 2% (Magnum/Magnarail) and 1% (conventional), respectively. Emergency bypass surgery was not required in either group. There was one in-hospital death in the

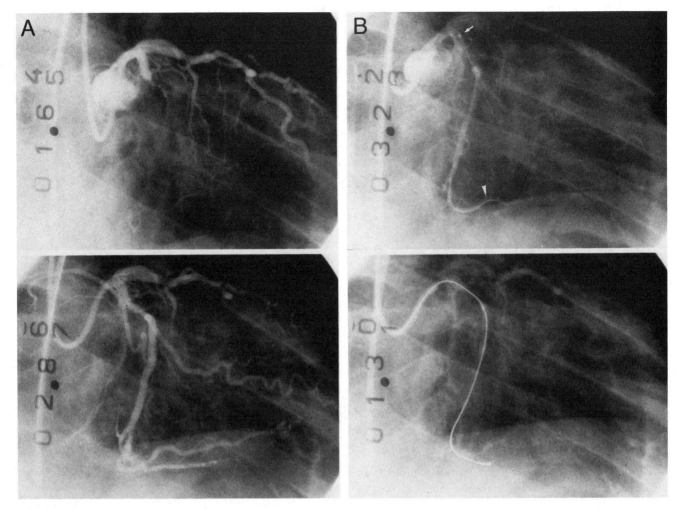

FIG 10–6.
Impossibility to advance a balloon across a tight lesion (**A**, *top*) in the left circumflex coronary artery of a 73-year-old man while it is tracking over a 0.014-in. (0.36-mm) standard coronary guidewire (Advanced Cardiovascular Systems) (**B**, *top*). The balloon marker is indicated by an *arrow* and the guidewire by an *arrowhead*. The advancing balloon folds over together with the wire into the left anterior descending coronary artery because of the resistance exerted by the lesion in the proximal left circumflex coronary artery. The problem is solved by substituting a 0.021-in. (0.53-mm) Magnum wire (**B**, *bottom*), which led to a satisfactory angiographic result (**A**, *bottom*).

conventionally treated group due to an acute stent occlusion 3 weeks after angioplasty with elective stent implantation.

The only procedure variable discrediting the Magnum/Magnarail system was the size of the guiding catheters used, with 66% 8 F and only 34% 7 F catheters vs. 42% 8 F, 56% 7 F, and 2% 6 F catheters[18] in the conventionally treated group ($P < .05$). Moreover, all use of 8 F catheters in the group treated by conventional wires was in anticipation of or secondary to a crossover to a Magnum wire. Had the second-generation 7 F guiding catheters with internal diameters of >0.070 in. (1.78 mm) been available at that time, no 8 F catheters would have been used in either group. On the other hand, the

availability of modern 6 F catheters featuring internal diameters of ≥0.055 in. (1.40 mm) would have increased the use of 6 F catheters in the conventional group, thus reinstating an advantage for conventional systems.

The procedure variables significantly in favor of the Magnum/Magnarail system were a shorter fluoroscopy time to place the balloon once the wire was in place and the number of wires used per artery. There was a tendency to use fewer balloons per lesion as well in the Magnum/Magnarail group.

This randomized study concerning routine angioplasty cases thus demonstrated some advantages of the Magnum/Magnarail system over conventional systems

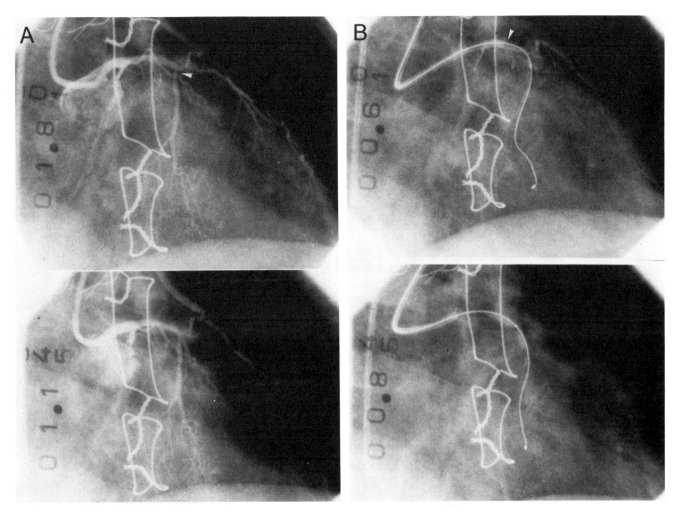

FIG 10–7.
Impossibility to dilate, with conventional angioplasty material, a tight lesion (**A,** *top*) at the orifice of a large septal branch of the left anterior descending coronary artery *(arrowhead)* of a 63-year-old man. After substituting a 0.021-in. (0.53-mm) Magnum wire, the balloon can be placed correctly because the sturdy wire enables deep intubation of the coronary artery with the 8 F guiding catheter (tip of the guiding catheter pointed out by an *arrowhead*) (**B,** *top*). The stenosis only yields to an inflation pressure of 12 bar (**B,** *bottom*), which, in addition to the acute-angle takeoff is a second explanation for the difficulties in passing the lesions. The angiographic result is satisfactory (**A,** *bottom*).

in terms of success in difficult cases, ease of balloon advancement once the wire is in place, and reduced consumption of disposable material.

OVERALL RESULTS OF MAGNUM CORONARY ANGIOPLASTY

Among the first 474 vessels (398 patients) with Magnum coronary balloon angioplasty at our institution, the Magnum wire was used as the initial tool in 402 vessels (329 patients) and as a bailout instrument after failure of one or several conventional wires in 72 vessels (69 patients). Chronic total occlusions accounted for 47% of the Magnum utilization as the initial instrument and

60% as the bailout instrument. The success and complication rates are summarized in Table 10–3.

GENERAL ASSESSMENT OF THE MAGNUM/MAGNARAIL SYSTEM AND OUTLOOK

An additional line of balloon catheters has to be stocked with the Magnum wires when this device is added to the armamentarium of a laboratory. These items are used instead and not in addition to conventional balloons and do not necessarily increase cost. The higher price of the Magnum wire vs. conventional wires can be compensated in part by a reduced need for wire

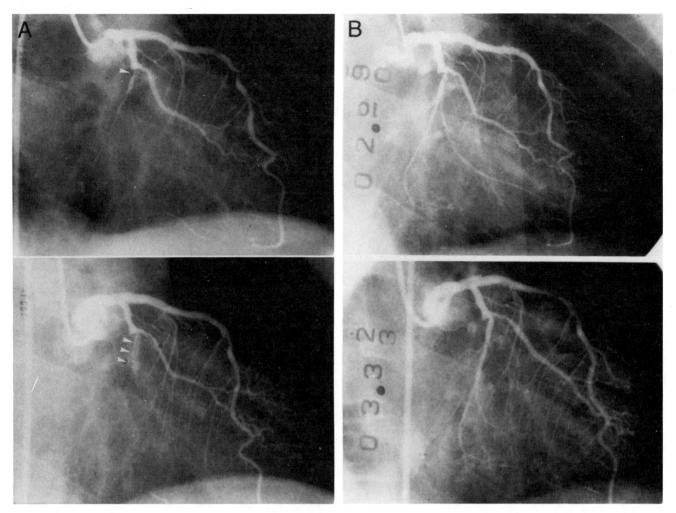

FIG 10–8.
A failed attempt to pass a subtotal eccentric lesion *(arrowhead)* in the left circumflex coronary artery of a 45-year-old man (**A,** *top*) resulted in a total occlusion due to a subintimal pathway *(arrowheads)* of the conventional coronary guidewire used (**A,** *bottom*). One month later, the lesion had recanalized spontaneously (**B,** *top*) and was successfully dilated by using a 0.021-in. (0.53-mm) Magnum wire to find the correct path (**B,** *bottom*).

replacement during the case and by reutilization if such is consistent with local policies. In addition, the initial passage of the 1-mm olive tip and the sturdy rail provided by the Magnum wire obviate the need for predilatation with small balloons in the vast majority of cases, which may amount to substantial savings for operators used to predilate tight lesions. The Magnum wire requires little special training. It proved universally applicable with advantages over conventional wires for total occlusions (particularly those a few months old) and difficult cases. The blunt tip also reduces the risk of vessel damage by inadvertent movements of the wire. The relative stiffness of the wire is advantageous in cases where the balloon does not track properly over a conventional wire around a sharp bend or into an acute-angle takeoff.

Retraction of the guiding catheter from a wedging position or deep intubation of the coronary artery for backup also appears easier and safer with the Magnum wire.

The following disadvantages of the Magnum system are of note: first, it requires balloons with a large central lumen and thus a less ideal deflated profile. This problem is largely overcome by the increased pushability of the system. Second, the presence and high radiopacity of the Magnum wire and particularly the olive tip occasionally hamper the distal runoff or its assessment in small vessels. This may require partial or complete withdrawal of the wire from small arteries. Readvancing the wire, if necessary, is rarely a problem since the Magnum wire is unsurpassed in terms of steerability and ma-

TABLE 10-3

Overall Results of Cases Involving a Magnum Wire

Result	Magnum as the First Wire (402 Vessels/329 Patients)	Magnum as the Second or Greater Wire (72 Vessels/69 Patients)
Success		
Stenoses	91% (202/211)	64% (18/28)
Occlusions	73% (140/191)	43% (19/44)
≤1 mo*	80% (20/25)	40% (4/10)
≤3 mo*	89% (8/9)	38% (3/8)
≤6 mo*	40% (2/5)	50% (3/6)
>6 mo*	0% (0/1)	0% (0/1)
Complications		
Infarction†	4% (14)	1% (1)
Emergency CABG‡	1% (3)	0% (0)
In-hospital death	1% (5)§	1% (1)

*Only patients with a reasonably reliable identification of occlusion date included.
†Creatine kinase more than twice the norm.
‡CABG = coronary artery bypass grafting.
§Three with angioplasty for cardiogenic shock after infarction.

neuverability. Third, the use of the Magnum system with ≤6 F guiding catheters is impossible. It can be used with all 7 F guiding catheters, although its use is comfortable only in conjunction with newer 7 F guiding catheters providing an internal lumen of ≥0.070 in. (1.78 mm).

Overall, the Magnum system is a helpful adjunct not only for angioplasty of chronic total occlusions but also for routine cases. It necessitates minor adjustments to conventional techniques but facilitates several basic maneuvers such as wire steering, guiding catheter placement and stabilization for backup, and balloon advancement.

Its primary use will remain restricted to chronic total occlusions, particularly in light of the tendency to use 6 F or smaller guiding catheters for routine coronary angioplasty of stenoses.[18] For total-occlusion angioplasty, it stands a good chance to prove superior to comparable systems currently tested against it in randomized studies, such as the Omniflex balloon catheter (Medtronic), which is a fixed wire balloon lacking free wire movement and distal contrast medium delivery,[19] and the Rotac system (Osypka), which requires a conventional coronary guidewire and a balloon catheter in addition to the dedicated recanalization device and is only compatible with 8 F guiding catheters.[20] It has to be reiterated that even if the primary success of angioplasty of chronic total coronary occlusions can be improved by new technologies and skills, the clinical yield will never compare with that of coronary angioplasty of stenoses. Since recanalization angioplasty is a low-yield procedure, it has to remain low risk and low cost. This sets limits to new tools and techniques. Laser technology,[21]

which has the highest potential for passing old occlusions, is disqualified for risk and cost reasons.

For routine angioplasty, the Magnum wire may find supporters among operators still employing 7 F or larger guiding catheters for routine cases. Once they have accustomed themselves to the unfamiliar technique of using power to pass total occlusions and tight lesions alike, they may prefer the Magnum system for its easy handling and stability in facilitating guiding catheter and balloon movements. This may be particularly handy if a Palmaz Schatz stent[22] needs to be implanted. It can be crimped on the Magnarail balloon (preferably nylon balloons) used for the initial dilatation. The excellent trackability and pushing stability of the system should facilitate precise stent placement even through tortuous coronary arteries.

REFERENCES

1. Meier B, Carlier M, Finci L, et al: Magnum wire for balloon recanalization of chronic total coronary occlusions. *Am J Cardiol* 1989; 64:148–154.
2. Villavicencio R, Meier B: Left axillary approach for balloon recanalization of an occlusion of the right common femoral artery. *Vasa* 1991; 20:186–187.
3. Meier B: Magnarail Probing catheter: New tool for balloon recanalization of chronic total coronary occlusions. *J Invasive Cardiol* 1991; 2:227–229.
4. Meier B: Total coronary occlusion: A different animal? *J Am Coll Cardiol* 1991; 17:50–57.
5. Dervan JP, Baim DS, Cherniles J, et al: Transluminal angioplasty of occluded coronary arteries: Use of a movable guide wire system. *Circulation* 1983; 68:776–784.
6. Serruys PW, Umans V, Heyndrickx GR, et al: Elective PTCA of totally occluded coronary arteries not associ-

ated with acute myocardial infarction: Short-term and long-term results. *Eur Heart J* 1985; 6:2–12.

7. Holmes DR Jr, Vlietstra RE: Angioplasty in total coronary arterial occlusion. *Herz* 1985; 10:292–297.

8. Kereiakes DJ, Selmon MR, McAuley BJ, et al: Angioplasty in total coronary artery occlusion: Experience in 76 consecutive patients. *J Am Coll Cardiol* 1985; 6:526–533.

9. Kober G, Hopf R, Reinemer H, et al: Langzeitergebnisse der transluminalen koronaren Angioplastie von chronischen Herzkranzgefässverschlüssen. *Z Kardiol* 1985; 74:309–316.

10. DiSciascio G, Vetrovec GW, Cowley MJ, et al: Early and late outcome of percutaneous transluminal coronary angioplasty of subacute and chronic total coronary occlusion. *Am Heart J* 1986; 111:833–839.

11. Melchior JP, Meier B, Urban P, et al: Percutaneous transluminal coronary angioplasty for chronic total coronary arterial occlusions. *Am J Cardiol* 1987; 59:535–538.

12. Safian RD, McCabe CH, Sipperly ME, et al: Initial success and long-term follow-up of percutaneous transluminal coronary angioplasty in chronic total occlusions versus conventional stenoses. *Am J Cardiol* 1988; 61:23–28.

13. Ellis SG, Shaw RE, Gershony G, et al: Risk factors, time course and treatment effect for restenosis after successful percutaneous transluminal coronary angioplasty of chronic total occlusion. *Am J Cardiol* 1989; 63:897–901.

14. Stone GW, Rutherford BD, McConahay DR, et al: Procedural outcome of angioplasty for total coronary artery occlusion: An analysis of 971 lesions in 905 patients. *J Am Coll Cardiol* 1990; 15:849–856.

15. Finci L, Meier B, Roy P, et al: Clinical experience with the Monorail balloon catheter for coronary angioplasty. *Cathet Cardiovasc Diagn* 1988; 14:206–212.

16. Pande AK, Meier B, Urban P, et al: Magnum/Magnarail versus conventional systems for recanalization of chronic total coronary occlusions: A randomized comparison. *Am Heart J*, in press.

17. Nukta ED, Meier B, Urban P, et al: Magnum system for routine coronary angioplasty: A randomized study. *Cathet Cardiovasc Diagn*, in press.

18. Villavicencio R, Urban P, Muller T, et al: Coronary balloon angioplasty through diagnostic 6 French catheters. *Cathet Cardiovasc Diagn* 1991; 22:56–59.

19. Hamm CW, Kupper W, Kuck KH, et al: Recanalization of chronic, totally occluded coronary arteries by new angioplasty systems. *Am J Cardiol* 1990; 66:1459–1463.

20. Kaltenbach M, Vallbracht C: Reopening of chronic coronary artery occlusions by low speed rotational angioplasty. *J Intervent Cardiol* 1989; 2:137–145.

21. Mast EG, Plokker HWM, Ernst JMPG, et al: Percutaneous recanalization of chronic total coronary occlusions: Experience with the direct argon laser assisted angioplasty system (LASTAC). *Herz* 1990; 15:241–244.

22. Schatz RA, Baim DS, Leon M: Clinical experience with the Palmaz Schatz coronary stent: Initial results of a multi-center study. *Circulation* 1991; 83:148–161.

Seven Years' Development and Application of the Sliding Rail System (Monorail) for PTCA

Tassilo Bonzel, M.D.

Helmut Wollschläger, M.D.

Andreas Zeiher, M.D.

Hanjörg Just, M.D.

Gerhard Strupp, M.D.

Gerhard Schreiner, M.D.

With the establishment and general acceptance of PTCA in about 1980, efforts have focused on technical improvements to facilitate PTCA, to reach and to pass any stenosis, and to obtain acceptable results in well-defined discrete stenoses. In later years, with improvement in technology and increasing experience, indications have broadened and expectations for results have escalated.

The original hardly steerable Grüntzig catheter[1-3] was replaced in 1982 by steerable systems, such as that described by Simpson et al.[4] In 1984, the exchangeability of balloons was addressed by Kaltenbach, who described a rational approach to the long-wire technique.[5, 6] With these techniques, it was finally possible to place balloons in practically any segment of the coronary system and to pass most of the stenoses, even extremely narrow ones, where a low-profile balloon could be used first and then exchanged for larger-sized ones.

Though saving of time then was not of prime importance, the complicated exchange procedure with two or three physicians or nurses seemed to be impractical. The long-wire technique also significantly increased the risk of inadvertent guidewire withdrawal, so fluoroscopy time had to be extended to secure the guidewire tip distal to the stenosis during exchange procedures.

The rapid and reliable exchange of balloons of different diameters was the predominant objective of sliding rail ("monorail") dilatation catheters when they were conceived in 1983. Other objectives were improved steerability and unimpaired contrast flow for optimal visualization of coronary arteries and of stenoses during PTCA, as well as a general simplification of intracoronary instrumentation.[7-10] The idea was therefore extended to the exchange of different diagnostic, bailout, and therapeutic devices for routine and research procedures.

DESCRIPTION OF THE MONORAIL PTCA SYSTEM

The sliding rail, or monorail, system (Schneider)* consists of two parts: (1) a stationary part (the

*Bülach, Switzerland, and Minneapolis. The author has patents on monorail catheters licensed to Schneider.

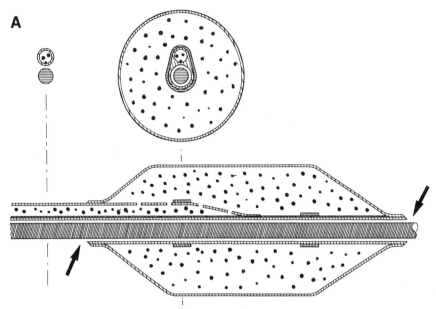

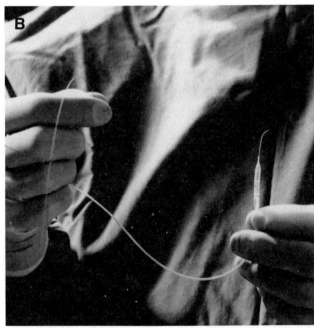

FIG 11–1.
A, axial section (below) and cross-sections (above) of the monorail catheter balloon part. Note central coaxial tube (arrows) fitting the guidewire. Over most of the shaft distance, the shaft and the guidewire run parallel to each other. Once the guidewire has passed the stenosis it remains stationary for the rest of the procedure, and the balloon can be moved independently over the whole of the distance or can be exchanged. **B,** monorail Piccolino balloon PTCA catheter. The relatively short guidewire lumen typical for monorail catheters exits the catheter shaft 17 cm proximal to the distal tip.

guidewire) and (2) an exchangeable part to hold the diagnostic or therapeutic devices. The functional unit formed by the two parts was primarily called the "sliding rail" system. The idea was first fabricated as an intracoronary balloon dilatation catheter, for which B. Meier, Geneva, suggested the name "monorail" catheter. This name has been widely accepted and its use has been expanded to the terms "monorail system," "monorail principle," and "monorail technique."[†]

> [†]*The term "monorail" catheter is often used synonymously with the terms "sliding rail," "rail type," or "monorail type" catheter. Monorail is a trademark of Scheider/Pfizer.*

The balloon catheter consists of three main parts: (1) the shaft, (2) the balloon and (3) a relatively short distal tube fitting the guidewire (Fig 11–1A). The shaft is made of elastic material of sufficient strength and contains a single lumen. The shaft serves to impart axial load to the distal balloon tip for axial pushability and to transmit pressure to the balloon interior, the balloon member, and to the vessel wall. The diameter of the longest part of the shaft is size 3 F, leaving sufficient space within standard size 7 F or 8 F guiding catheters for contrast injections (Table 11–1). The balloon is a typical coronary dilatation balloon. The distal tube is

TABLE 11–1

Relation of Balloon Catheter Shaft Sizes and Luminal Space Within Standard Guiding Catheters*

Guiding Catheter				
	Internal Diameter		Balloon Catheter Shaft	Remaining Luminal Space
Size (F)	(in.)	(mm)	Diameter (F)	(mm^2)
8	.079	2.00	3.6	1.88
8	.077	1.95	3.4	1.86
8	.075	1.90	3.2	1.83
7/8	.073	1.85	3.0	1.81
7/8	.071	1.80	2.8	1.76
7	.068	1.75	2.6	1.80
7	.067	1.70	2.4	1.77
7	.065	1.65	2.2	1.71
6	.051	1.30	2.0	1.00

*Guiding catheters of 7 and 8 F and balloon catheter shafts are coordinated with respect to optimal contrast flow. A remaining luminal space of about 1.8^2 (with balloon catheter within guiding catheter) allows for unimpaired contrast flow by hand injection with a 10 cc syringe. Monorail catheters with 3 F shafts have optimal conditions in all 8 F and in high-flow 7 F guiding catheters (but can also be used in standard 7 F and 6 F guiding catheters).

the most characteristic feature of the monorail catheter. It is delimited by an endhole forming the balloon tip (as in conventional catheters) and by a more or less eccentrically placed sidehole proximal to the balloon. The length of the tube was between 4 and 9 cm in early models and is now about 17 cm in monorail catheters (Fig 11–1B; Tables 11–2 and 11–3). When the

guidewire is fitted into the central tube, the catheter is suspended with its distal end on the wire and can be pushed forward or pulled backward on the guidewire as on a sliding rail. The guidewire may be principally any standard length guidewire of appropriate diameter.

As the guidewire tube is relatively short as compared to over-the-wire systems, and is not extended to the

TABLE 11–2

Sliding Rail System PTCA Catheters, Basic Shaft Characteristics

Type	Manufacturer	Proximal Single-Lumen Shaft		Distal Double-Lumen Shaft			Guidewire (in.)
		Material	φ (F)	Material	φ (F)	Tube Length (cm)	
Monorail							
Generation 1/2[1]	S/E[2]	PVC[3,4]	3.0	PVC	3.6	4/9	.012
Piccolino[1]	S/E	PVC[4]	3.0	PVC	3.6	17	.014
Piccolino forte	S/E	Polyester[4]	3.3	PVC	3.6	17	.014
Piccolino	S/US[5]	Polyester[4]	3.0	Polyester	3.0	17	.014
Speedy/Speedy plus	S/E	PM[6]300[4]	3.0	PM 200[4]	3.3	17	.018
Others							
Rx	ACS[7]	PE[8]	3.3/3.7	PE	3.3	30[9]	.014/.018
Rx Alpha/Streak	ACS	Stainless steel[10]	2.3/3.3	PE	3.3	30[9]	.014
Express	Sci-Med[11]	Stainless steel[10]	1.8	PE	2.7	35	.014
Solitaire	USCI[12]	Stainless steel[10]	1.7	PE	3.0	40	.014
Quick 14	Baxter[13]	PE	.9	PE	2.7–2.9	28	.014

1. Out of production.
2. Schneider Europe, Bülach, Switzerland.
3. Polyvinyl chloride.
4. Wire reinforced.
5. Schneider USA, Minneapolis.
6. Modified nylon.
7. Advanced Cardiovascular Systems, St Clara, Calif.
8. Polyethylene.
9. Peel away.
10. Polymer coated.
11. Sci-Med Life Systems, Minneapolis.
12. USCI, Billerica, Mass.
13. Baxter, Irvine, Calif (preliminary information).

TABLE 11–3
Sliding Rail System PTCA Catheters: Balloons (Examples With Balloon Diameter 3 mm, Length 20 mm)*

	Manufacturer	Material	Deflated or Crossing Profile (in.)	Burst Pressure (atm)	Compliance
Monorail					
Generation 1/2	S/E	PVC	>.04	10†	+ +
Piccolino	S/E	PET‡	.036	10†/>18§	(+)
Piccolino forte	S/E	PET	.036	10†/>18§	(+)
Piccolino	S/US	PET	.031	16‖	(+)
Speedy	S/E	PM300	.034	12†/>16§	+ +
Others					
Rx .014/.018	ACS	PE600	.037/.040	8‖	+ +
Rx Alpha/Streak	ACS	PE600	.033	8‖	+ +
Express	Scimed	POC¶	.035	9‖	+ + +
Solitaire	USCI	PET	.032	12‖	(+)
Quick 14	Baxter	POC	.035	9‖	+ + +

*For abbreviations see Table 11–2.
†Maximum recommended pressure.
‡Polyethyleneteraphtalate.
§Authors' own experience (unpublished results).
‖Rated burst pressure.
¶Modified polyolefine

proximal end of the catheter, sliding rail systems do not provide distal pressure measurement. A temporarily available monorail pressure balloon catheter with a third catheter-long lumen[10] was not further developed when the general interest in routinely measured transstenotic pressure gradients dropped.

DESCRIPTION OF THE PROCEDURE

In using the monorail system the PTCA procedure is essentially modified as compared to over-the-wire systems (Fig 11–2).

1. First, the standard length guidewire alone, without the balloon catheter, is advanced through the Y-connector, the guiding catheter, and across the stenosis. The large remaining space within the guiding catheter has two consequences: (1) motion of the wire is hardly impeded by friction and (2) contrast flow is unimpaired. These two factors allow for controlled steerability of the guidewire through the fully visualized coronary pathway and stenosis instead of the previously often observed trial-and-error passage. If necessary, guidewires with different properties in stiffness or tip shape can be rapidly exchanged. After passing the stenosis, the guidewire becomes the stationary part and at the same time the "rail" for the entire procedure.

2. Next, the proper balloon catheter is selected and pushed up onto the guidewire and, sliding on the guidewire as on a sliding rail, advanced through the guiding catheter and across the stenosis while the guidewire is fixed at the outside. Depending on the situation, selection and unwrapping of the balloon can be delayed until the successful placement of the guidewire is completed.

3. In case of need for another balloon size, the exchange of balloons can be performed in the same way. An example is shown in Fig 11–3. Fluoroscopic control of the guidewire tip distal to the stenoses is not necessary when the balloon passes through the guiding catheter because the guidewire can be fixed at the outside. This can contribute essentially to the reduction of fluoroscopy time, especially in exchange procedures. The time required for a balloon exchange measured in 20 cases was 2 minutes, on average. This time included withdrawal of the primary balloon from the distal guiding catheter, unwrapping and preparation of the new balloon, and advancing the balloon across the stenosis.

4. To control the dilatation result, but also to position the balloon within the stenosis, a sufficient flow of dye ensures optimal visualization with standard size 8 F, but also with newer size 7 F guiding catheters. This even holds for the use of nondiluted contrast media of standard viscosities and for the balloon part of the catheter being positioned in the coronary system.

5. To reduce staff hours, a monorail PTCA can be performed as a "single operator" procedure. This means that a single experienced physician can perform an uncomplicated coronary balloon dilatation only with the help of one circulating nurse and without the additional

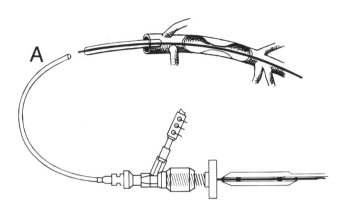

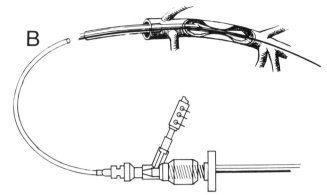

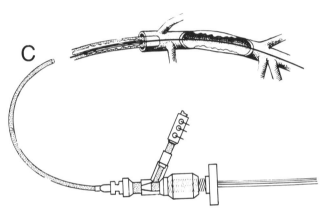

FIG 11–2.
Monorail procedure. **A,** the bare wire is pushed through the Y-connector and guiding catheter nearly free of friction and is guided across the stenosis under fluoroscopy with unimpaired contrast visualization of branches, plaques, etc. Next, the balloon is pushed onto the guidewire. **B,** the balloon is advanced across the stenosis and is exactly positioned under unimpaired contrast flow. **C,** the balloon is retracted into the distal 8 F guiding catheter (in 7 F catheters, more proximally) while the guidewire tip remains distal to the stenosis. The result is checked again with unimpaired contrast flow for detailed analysis of stenosis diameter and possible dissections or thrombosis before the guidewire is removed.

help of a second scrubbed assistant. A second person would then scrub only as required for difficult procedures or for limited stages of a procedure. A second physician-operator would remain in a problem-oriented standby capacity.

TECHNICAL DEVELOPMENT OF MONORAIL PTCA CATHETERS

Monorail catheters (as other catheters) have been developed continuously since 1985 according to evolving balloon catheter technology and following users' needs. Changes have concerned mainly balloon and shaft materials, surface properties, shaft stiffness, and dimensions of the typical guidewire tube. The combined modifications resulted specifically in improved pushability and trackability (Table 11–4).

Pushability is achieved by adding stiffness to the shaft, so that axial load is imparted without essential loss to the balloon tip and is not used up by friction within the guide catheter and within proximal coronary segments. Stiffness can be increased by three ways in monorail systems: (1) by shaft material selection (e.g.,

by special polymers or metal or by implementing a stiffening wire into the shaft); the more stiff part should have a gradual transition to a more flexible distal shaft part; (2) in the distal shaft and in the balloon segment stiffness is also increased by material selection or more easily when the guidewire runs within the guidewire tube; thus, stiffness and pushability of the distal balloon catheter can also be influenced by modifying the dimensions of the guidewire tube; (3) use of stiffer or thicker guidewires, as in some Rx models (Advanced Cardiovascular Systems, St. Clara, Calif) (.018-in.), the Speedy and Speedy plus (Bülach, Switzerland and Minneapolis) (.018-in.), and especially in the Magnum and Magnarail (Bülach, Switzerland and Minneapolis) (.021-in.) (see Table 11–2).

Trackability depends largely on the optimal balance of flexibility and stiffness of the distal shaft and balloon, on the deflated balloon profile, on the gliding characteristics of the polymer surface or coating, and, finally, of the catheter tip design.

In typical monorail catheters optimal pushability and trackability have to be obtained without compromising ease of catheter exchange and safety. This is guaranteed in our experience as long as balloon catheters can be

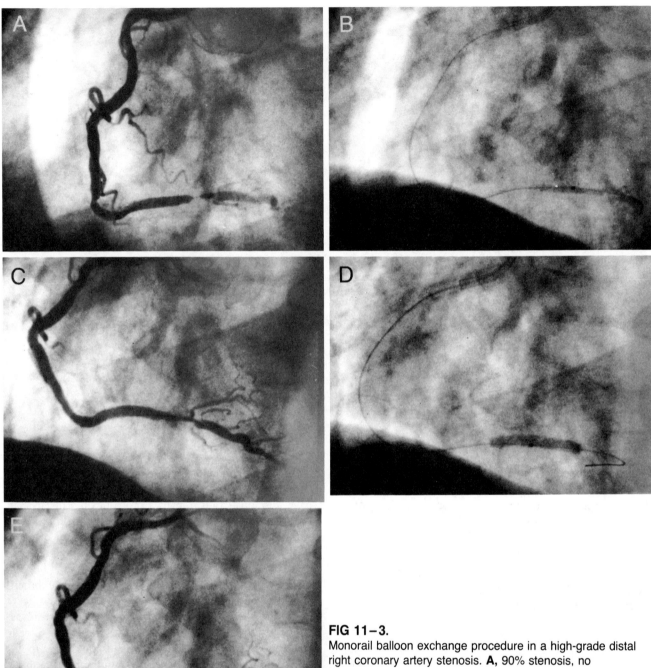

FIG 11–3.
Monorail balloon exchange procedure in a high-grade distal right coronary artery stenosis. **A,** 90% stenosis, no passage with a 3-mm monorail Piccolino balloon. **B,** monorail balloon exchange for a 1.5 mm Piccolino balloon, passage of the stenosis, and dilatation. **C,** 50% stenosis after first dilatation. **D,** balloon re-exchange for the 3-mm Piccolino balloon, passage of the stenosis and dilatation. **E,** result: no residual stenosis.

routinely exchanged over standard length guidewires without extension wires.

With the first polyvinyl chloride (PVC) monorail catheter with a 4-cm guidewire lumen and also the second PVC snake version with a 9-cm guidewire lumen

(generations 1 and 2) we could prove that rapid balloon exchange was easily realized in relatively proximal stenoses and that the access to these stenoses was facilitated by this device.[7–9] The Piccolino catheter (Bülach, Switzerland and Minneapolis) has been substantially im-

TABLE 11–4

Typical Balloon Catheter Characteristics in Regard to Standard Routine Balloon PTCA of High-Grade Stenoses in Single- and Multivessel Disease: Catheter Exchange Included

	Steerability	Pushability	Trackability	Stenosis Passage	Occlusion Passage	Balloon Exchange	Contrast Flow "Imaging"	Investigation Speed	Short Fluoroscopy	Single Operator	Distal Pressure
Monorail Generation 1 and 2*	++	+	+	+	+	+++	+++	++	++	+++	−
Monorail Piccolino forte	+++	+++	++	++	+	+++	+++	+++	+++	+++	−
Monorail Speedy/Speedy plus	+++	+++	++	++	+	+++	+++	+++	+++	+++	−
Magnarail	+++	+++	+++	++	+++	+++	+	+++	+++	+++	−
Rx Alpha/Streak	+++	+++	++	++	+	+++	+++	+++	+++	+++	−
Express	+++	+++	++	++	+	++	+++	++	++	++	−
Solitaire	+++	+++	++	++	+	++	+++	++	++	++	−
Over-the-wire systems (newer ones)	++	+++	++	++	++	++	++	+	+	−	++
Fixed wire systems	+	+++	+++	+++	+	−	+++	++	++	+	−

*Out of production.

proved due to several technological changes. These include specifically selected materials with better surface properties, more shaft stiffness, a thinner balloon material (PET) for small deflated balloon profiles, and a dimensional change of the distal guidewire tube, which was elongated to 17 cm. The changes added pushability and trackability to monorail catheters (see Fig 11–1).[12] Finally the latest versions, the Speedy and Speedy plus catheters, refine these elements in combination with a moderately compliant however thin balloon material (see Tables 11–2 and 11–3).

Magnum catheters (Bülach, Switzerland, and Minneapolis) have been primarily designed by B. Meier for recanalization of complete occlusions,[13] but they have also been used for standard PTCA.[14] The idea is to increase pushability by use of a very stiff but distally flexible guidewire, which has an ovally shaped blunt tip. When additionally reinforced by an economic probing catheter without balloon, the system can transmit enormous penetrating force to the occluding material. This system has been combined with monorail characteristics without substantial loss of pushability under the name Magnarail.[15, 16] In this version, the rapid exchange of probing and balloon catheters is especially useful. In our experience, the catheters combination of stiffness, pushability, and a blunt tip allow it to find its way through a variety of soft materials with low risk of vessel perforation.

OTHER SLIDING RAIL BALLOON CATHETER SYSTEMS

The monorail concept has stimulated other companies to produce similar catheters operating according to the sliding rail principle. Some of these companies have taken advantage of investigator experience and technological progress and have produced catheters with very good performance (see Tables 11–2 and 11–3). When discussing these catheters it should be kept in mind that the overall performance of catheters depends on a large variety of factors, including investigator habits, and that categories such as "sliding rail," "coaxial," or "over-the-wire," and "fixed wire" characterize different categories and do not describe individual construction and material properties.

Advanced Cardiovascular Systems (St Clara, Calif) has produced the Rx catheter with a 30-cm guidewire lumen. This resulted in improved pushability. The main purpose of this catheter also was rapid exchange, as the name indicates. The "peel-away" function of the distal tube underlined this purpose. In later versions of this catheter polyethylene-coated stainless steel was chosen for the main part of the shaft. The Rx catheter has a moderately compliable polyester balloon (PE600).

Sci-Med (Minneapolis) emphasized the reinforcement of the proximal shaft part in the Express catheter by using a polymer-coated stainless steel tube instead of polymer reinforced by a stainless steel wire. This decreased the shaft diameter but also the flexibility, thus the distal part including the guidewire lumen was made of flexible polymer and extended to 35 cm. As an individual feature, the Express has a more compliant polyolefine (POM) balloon with a rather linear diameter increase, but with also a significant increase in balloon length with pressure. In our tests, a 3-mm balloon increased by 15% in length when inflated from 2 to 12 atm.

United States Catheter Inc (Billerica, Mass) produces the Solitaire catheter, which has also a thin polymer-coated stainless steel shaft (1.7 F), very similar to the balloon-on-the-wire catheter, and a guidewire tube of 40 cm. In this catheter, the balloon is made from non-compliant (or minimally compliant) polyethyleneteraphtalat (PET). Pushability and trackability are excellent in this catheter; however, in our experience, the ease of balloon catheter exchange — though still considerably better than in over-the-wire systems — is reduced as compared to monorail catheters. In exchange procedures, at least short fluoroscopy is often needed to secure the guidewire tip distal to the stenosis.

FURTHER APPLICATIONS OF THE MONORAIL TECHNIQUE

The ease of exchange of intracoronary devices along a stationary guidewire offered itself for devices for clinical and scientific purposes. Besides the simplified guidewire access to the coronary segment of choice, the rapid exchange of devices helps to implement scientific studies into routine dilatation (see Table 11–5).

Autotransfusion Catheter

A large-diameter single-lumen active "transfusion" catheter for autologous transfusion of blood was designed to overcome acute ischemia in acute coronary occlusion.[17, 18] This transfusion catheter has a 4.3 F thin-walled shaft, a 1-cm soft distal tip with a radiopaque marker, and one or two large sideholes approximately 1 cm from the endhole. The guidewire enters through the endhole and exits through the sidehole. In case of coronary occlusion, the transfusion catheter is

TABLE 11–5

Monorail and Monorail-Type Catheters, Special Design*

Type	Shaft (F)	Tip	Wire (in.)	Specialty
Magnarail, S/E	3.0	PET balloon	.021†	Recanalization of occluded arteries
Magnarail probing S/E	3.4	Tapered, no balloon	.021†	Recanalization, stiffening, backup
Monorail mega S/E	3.3	4.5/5.0 mm balloon	.021*	Large balloon, bypass, renal artery
Speedflow, S/E	3.0/3.7/4.6‡	PET balloon	.018	Continuous perfusion, prolonged inflation
Rx Perfusion, ACS	3.7/4.2§	PE 600 balloon	.018	Continuous perfusion, prolonged inflation
Monorail transfusion S/E.	4.0	Tapered, no balloon	.016	Femorocoronary bailout autotransfusion
Monorail pressure catheter S/E	3.0	Tip φ 3.0 F	.014	Transstenotic pressure, intracoronary drug application
Monorail Doppler catheter S/E	3.0/3.6§	20 MHz Doppler	.014	Intracoronary Flow velocity

*For abbreviations see Table 11–2.
†Recommended wire: magnum φ .021-in., 1 mm spheric tip, S/E.
‡Proximal/middle/distal.
§Proximal/distal.

exchanged for the balloon catheter and advanced across the stenosis along the guidewire. The proximal end is connected via a three-way stopcock with a second large-diameter single-lumen catheter (8 F), the distal end of which is inserted into the contralateral femoral artery with standard techniques. Heparin is added up to a cumulative dose of 30,000 or 40,000 units, and after venting of the system, blood is withdrawn by hand from the femoral artery through the stopcock into a tight sealing 10-cc syringe and transfused into the coronary segment distal to the obstruction. In our experience, a flow rate of 40 to 60 mL/min can be maintained over 60 to 90 minutes when injections are continuously repeated. The device is not intended for longer treatment periods but only to prevent ischemia during transfer to the operating room in a bailout fashion.

Perfusion Catheter

Clinical results with passive coronary perfusion balloon catheters, already described in 1984,[19] were first reported by Erbel et al.[20] and later by Stack et al. with a similar device (ACS, St Clara, Calif). The Stack device and the CPC Mainz catheter described by Erbel were modified to adopt monorail characteristics and were then called Rx perfusion catheter and Speedflow catheter, respectively. Limited experience with this type of catheter shows favorable performance when special care in handling of the guidewire is taken.

Intracoronary Diagnostic (Pressure Monitoring) Catheter

An intracoronary catheter with a flexible low-profile tip that is suspendable on a guidewire was designed to be used largely atraumatically within the coronary system. The catheter serves mainly for selective drug injection and for transstenotic pressure gradients. For example, it has been used successfully to inject papaverine into distal coronary segments to test flow-dependent dilatation of the proximal segments.[21] Transstenotic gradients have been helpful in cases of inadequate visual or digital stenosis quantification or for scientific purposes.

Intracoronary Doppler Catheters

Intracoronary monorail Doppler catheters have been designed as Doppler balloon catheters and as stand-alone Dopplers for scientific purposes; they have been used for several studies (Fig 11–4).[21, 22]

Hot Balloon

A radiofrequency hot balloon is under development for monorail use and has been tested to date in animal studies.[23, 24] The primary goal of this development is a bailout device that can be used rapidly and economically to reopen and stabilize occluding dissections after PTCA.

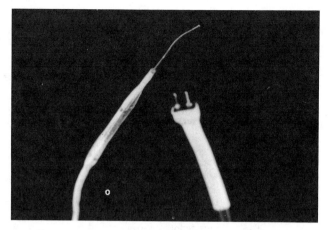

FIG 11–4.
Monorail Doppler balloon catheter. Axial arrangements of crystals at distal catheter tip.

Other Diagnostic and Therapeutic Devices

In past years the sliding rail technique has been applied by several investigators for a number of different devices for intracoronary diagnosis and therapy. Among these are two-dimensional and Doppler ultrasound devices, glass-fiber angioscopes, and laser probes. These devices have in common a relatively short tube or bore at the tip connected in some way with the distally located "active" diagnostic or therapeutic part. With the help of this tube they can slide along a stationary, standard length guidewire into the remote coronary system from the outside.

CLINICAL EXPERIENCE WITH THE MONORAIL SYSTEM

Routine PTCA with the monorail balloon catheter system was performed under the responsibility of one of the authors (T.B.) from 1985 to 1988 at the University Medical Clinic of Freiburg (Germany) and since April 1988 at the Fulda General Hospital (Germany) in a total of about 1,200 cases. The most often used catheters between 1985 and 1987 were generation 1 and 2 monorail PVC catheters; from 1988 to 1990, Piccolino; and from 1990 to 1992, monorail Speedy catheters. The following experiences and results are limited to elective balloon PTCA in stable and unstable ischemia and in single-vessel as well as in multivessel disease. Results do not include PTCA in acute myocardial infarction, special research procedures, combined balloon and nonballoon procedures (e.g., rotablation), and recanalization procedures.

Clinical Results With Monorail Balloons

For better comparison we have studied two series of patients. Group 1 consisted of the first 131 consecutive attempted monorail dilatations in Freiburg performed with generation 1 and 2 PVC catheters. Group II consisted of 132 consecutive monorail dilatations in 1989 in Fulda with Piccolino catheters.

In group 1 the primary success rate (or gain of at least 20% of vessel diameter) with monorail catheters alone was 82%. Eight distal stenoses could only be reached and passed with fixed-wire Hartzler catheters (ACS, St Clara, Calif), increasing the overall success rate to 89%. In 2/8 Hartzler dilatations the final result was improved by an additional monorail catheter; in these two cases the bare wire for the monorail catheter was easily passed across the predilated stenosis, with the Hartzler catheter staying in place as a "road" marker. Vessel distribution was as follows: left anterior descending, (LAD), 65.6%; left circumflex, 21.4%; right coronary artery (RCA), 9.2%; and bypass, 3.8%. The mean stenosis severity of successful dilated stenoses before PTCA was 77%; the average stenosis improvement was 51% of the vessel diameter with monorail catheters alone (and 46% with Hartzler catheters alone). Complications were 3% emergency ACVB and two myocardial infarctions (one with ACVB, one not operated on), with no deaths.

In group 2, the primary success rate (also 20%) was 123/132 stenoses or 93% with monorail Piccolino catheters alone; one stenosis required an additional angled balloon and another stenosis an additional monorail snake balloon, increasing the overall success rate to 95%. A Hartzler catheter was used in one stenosis without effect; in six unsuccessful attempts no other catheter was tried. Vessel distribution was as follows: LAD, 37.1%; RCA, 34.1%; left circumflex, 22.6%; and bypass, 6.1%. The mean stenosis severity of successful dilated stenoses before PTCA was 86%; the average improvement was 59%. Complications were one emergency coronary artery bypass graft (CABG) (.8%) and one myocardial infarction (.8%), with no deaths. Piccolino catheters have improved the primary success rate, presumably because of increased pushability and trackability, resulting in improved stenosis passage ability.

Transfusion Catheters in Acute Coronary Occlusion

Between 1986 and 1989, transfusion catheters were used in five patients undergoing emergency coronary artery bypass graft (CABG).[18] Transfusion catheters were only used in acute LAD occlusion with severe ischemia, following extended intimal dissection during PTCA. Flow rates maintained with intermittent (8 to 10 cc injections about 5 to 6 times per minute), manually controlled femorocoronary autotransfusion were 40 and 60 mL/min over a period of up to 60 minutes starting in the cardiac laboratory and ending with the institution of cardiopulmonary bypass. After 45 to 60 minutes, the flow resistence within the transfusion catheter increased and flow could drop to less than 40 mL/min. In all patients, initial ischemia was at least temporarily completely reverted during transfer to the operating room in the same building. In 4/5 patients, cardiopulmonary bypass was initiated without complications, one patient had redevelopment of ischemia before bypass and suffered a major infarction; another patient had a postoperative infarction, probably not related to the autotransfusion. This patient was not restudied. In three patients Q-wave infarction could be ruled out, and control left ventricular angiograms showed normal anterior wall motion. One problem is that with reversal of ischemia the patient appears to be stable and asymptomatic, which may "mask" the urgency of the situation and slow the speed with which anesthesia is initiated and surgical action taken. Since 1990 stents or perfusion catheters with prolonged inflation were preferred to stabilize severe ischemia.

Monorail Stenting With the Palmaz-Schatz Stent

From early 1990 Palmaz-Schatz stents[25, 26] were implanted in 64 (11.8%) of PTCA patients aged 37 to 79 years (65 stenoses), mainly after failed PTCA, for persisting diameter reduction of more then 50% (n=33) or acute occluding dissection (n=21), but also as primary treatment for restenosis (n=6) and for bypass stenoses (n=5). We used a monorail Piccolino catheter with PVC balloon (Fig 11–5) in connection with Palmaz-Schatz coronary stents (Johnson & Johnson, New Brunswick, NJ).[27, 28] In a few patients, monorail Speedy balloons were used.

Procedure

In case of acute intractable obstruction with flow reduction (TIMI 1 and 2), the used balloon was left in the stenosis, dilatation was repeated as needed, and a Piccolino PVC was unwrapped and loaded with the stent, following standard rules. Medication was given as recommended by Schatz with minor modifications (e.g., starch was used instead of dextran in most patients). Then the first balloon was withdrawn and the balloon and stent were carefully advanced to the stenosis. Stents were meticulously positioned under fluoroscopic control and with repeated dye injections, especially when side branch covering was to be avoided or when half stents

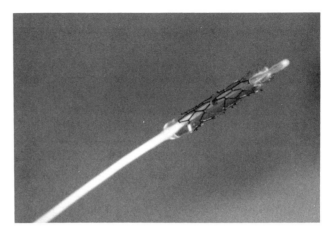

FIG 11–5.
Monorail Piccolino catheter with PVC balloon, inflated, with Palmaz-Schatz stent. The irregular stent appearance is in part due to the fact that the membrane does not straighten out simultaneously in all regions.

were preferred in short occlusions. With our fluoroscopy system (Siemens Digicor) stents were usually visible for positioning as long as they were squeezed onto the balloon, but visualization was limited after widening of the stent. In less acute obstruction, the last used balloon was often removed, deflated, loaded with the stent, and reinserted. In proximal stenoses it was usually decided before dilatation, if monorail stenting or stenting with the Johnson & Johnson catheter would be attempted in case of PTCA failure. Proximal coronary kinking and angles were regarded as contraindications for monorail stenting. The Johnson & Johnson preloaded catheter was available in 1991 and was successfully used in two occasions with strongly bent coronary arteries; however, contrast flow was strongly impeded with this catheter. After stenting, patients were treated according to standard protocols with special respect to checking prothrombin time (every 4 hours during the first two days) and overlapping warfarin treatment, combined with acetyl salicylic acid. All patients stayed in the coronary care unit for at least four days.

Two stents were placed into the protected left main stem; 26 into the LAD; 7 into the left circumflex; 22 into the RCA; and 8 into bypasses. Twenty four patients had single-vessel, 23 double-vessel, and 17 triple-vessel disease. One stent was implanted in 54 cases; 2 in 3 cases; 1.5 in 1 case, and a half in 7 cases.

Primary Results

Stents were successfully placed in 63 of 65 attempted stenoses (96.9%). Two patients with stent misplacements in angled arteries were operated on within 48 hours. There were 3/63 in-hospital and 1 late thrombotic stent occlusion (6.5%), each recanalized, one with Q-wave infarction (the only infarction in the group). There were no deaths, but a significant number of bleeding complications occurred. The restenosis rate after three months was 19.4%; redilatation was always possible with monorail catheters, sometimes with pressures up to 16 atm and more.

Logistical Developments Related to the Monorail Technique

In an early study in 1985 and 1986, fluoroscopy time could be reduced by 27% with the use of monorail catheters and patient laboratory time by 10%. Besides x-ray protection, this allows a savings of about 20 minutes of staff time per PTCA, or more than 3 hours per day assuming 4 staff members per procedure and 10 procedures per day.

In the past years, PTCA during a first diagnostic coronary angiogram (termed "Prima-vista-PTCA") was systematically included into the cardiac laboratory routine in our hospital for patients with stable and unstable angina. Prima-vista-PTCA was performed in 10% of patients in 1988, in 29% in 1989, and in 40% in 1990. The following criteria had to be fulfilled: (1) adequate diagnostic fluoroscopic coronary image, (2) standard positive indications for PTCA, (3) written consent (including for possible emergency surgery or stenting), signed in advance, and (4) acute surgical standby available if judged necessary. Typical reasons for elective PTCA or deferring PTCA were complex coronary anatomy and/or uncertain PTCA indications. The success rates were between 86% and 91% for prima-vista-PTCA and between 88% and 94% for electively scheduled PTCA in the different years; the in-laboratory times were between 81 and 99 minutes for prima-vista-PTCA and between 147 and 152 minutes for the added diagnostic and PTCA procedure times in elective PTCA; the fluoroscopy times were between 19 and 16 minutes for prima-vista-PTCA and between 34 and 25 minutes for the added diagnostic and PTCA procedures in elective PTCA. Complication rates were not significantly different for prima-vista-PTCA and elective PTCA, with .4% to 1.7% emergency CABG and .6% to 1% myocardial infarction. There was one death in elective PTCA and none in prima-vista-PTCA. The percentage of multivessel disease was between 49% and 52% for both prima-vista-PTCA and elective PTCA.

In our opinion the monorail technique has supported the establishment of the prima-vista-PTCA as a standard procedure. The transition from a diagnostic to a therapeutic procedure is simplified with a reduced number of equipment parts and connections, and the ease of exchange of balloons and bailout devices shortens the overall procedure time, may improve safety, and reduces the need for immediate surgical standby. It may be even more important that the number of staff need not be increased when changing a diagnostic into a therapeutic procedure.

Acceptance

The acceptance of monorail or sliding rail catheters for rapid exchange has continuously increased in Europe. In Europe, for balloon dilatation, preference is clearly given to monorail systems (which are used more than 50% of the time) compared to over-the-wire systems. In the United States the share of monorail systems is significantly lower, but is also increasing. With good results obtainable with nearly all systems, acceptance will strongly depend on material and production characteristics and the performance in critical situations or noncritical situations. It is also supposed that numbers of staff members in U.S. hospital cardiac laboratories are, despite rising health care costs, on average, still higher than in most European laboratories.

DISCUSSION

The discussion will be restricted to the main areas of monorail PTCA or to those areas in which the authors have personal experience.

Rationale of Balloon Catheter Exchange

When the monorail concept was conceived, balloon exchange was a major issue. Deflated balloon profiles often did not allow stenosis passage. For predilatation in tight stenoses, a small (1.5 or 2 mm) balloon was used first, which had then to be replaced by the correctly sized balloon for the vessel diameter. This still applies in some cases today (see Fig 11–3). An additional oversized balloon is still commonly tried in case of inadequate results, especially in cases of threatening occlusion, where bailout devices may also be needed. In these cases, a reliable rail traversing the dissected stenosis can be essential. In case of branching stenosis with the double-wire technique, a single balloon can be quickly removed from the first branch and wire to be reinserted into the second branch over the other wire[29,30] (Fig 11–6). When two stenoses requiring different balloon sizes are to be dilated through the same guide catheter, both in the left or in the right coronary, balloon exchange over the same wire is fast and easy; if necessary,

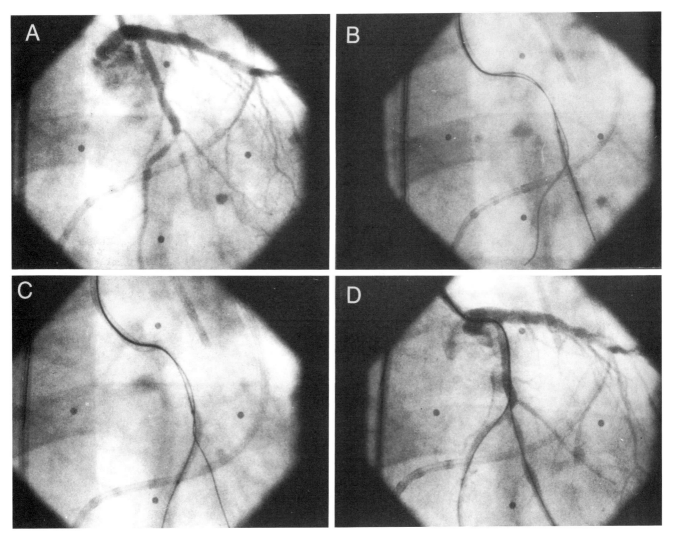

FIG 11-6.
Monorail PTCA of a left circumflex artery branching stenosis with the double-wire technique. **A,** the two bare wires were first placed across the stenosis. **B,** a monorail generation 1 2.5-mm balloon catheter was advanced across the subtotal posterolateral branch stenosis and inflated. **C,** the same balloon was removed, switched to the second wire, and advanced to dilate the left circumflex stenosis. **D,** result.

the wire can be replaced in between the exchange across the second stenosis into another vessel or branch. In case of PTCA failure because of elastic recoil or nonoccluding or occluding dissection, exchange may be useful for oversized balloons, for perfusion balloon catheters, for bailout perfusion or transfusion catheters, or for stented balloon catheters. Exchange can be useful for a number of nonballoon devices, mentioned earlier. As it does not seem appropriate or feasible to attach several different tools to the tip of a single coronary catheter, the possibility of rapid exchange allows the consecutive use of such tools within minutes.

For some devices, however, a coaxial over-the-wire

design is an integral part of the system, so that sliding rail systems with normal length wires may not be compatible. In these cases, extension wires are used as effective bridges to the over-the-wire technique.

Steerability and Contrast Flow

Steerability in sliding rail systems is equivalent with guidewire steerability. This means that the steerability of the system is as good as the steerability of the wire and depends on wire properties, friction, and lumen visibility. The bare wire approach offers unimpaired contrast flow, low friction, and wire exchange: wires can be easily, safely, and quickly removed, reshaped, or replaced as needed. There has been an objection that this is not possible when the balloon has already entered the coronary system, as occasionally is done with over-the-wire systems to cross complicated stenoses. It should be emphasized that stenoses are passed initially with bare wires, and that the bare wire steerability is superior to that of wires running in a dilatation catheter. In our experience stenosis passage with modern steerable wires is not an issue, and permits fast and controlled stenosis passage in nearly every nontotal lesion. In rare instances, a monorail balloon catheter on the wire adds push to the guidewire tip, but is normally not needed for steering purposes.

In the early and the mid-1980s, dilatation catheter shafts and guiding catheter dimensions did not permit adequate contrast flow into the coronaries during or after dilatation. In addition, fluoroscopic x-ray images did not meet the requirements for PTCA, i.e., optimal information for correct decisions. With traditional equipment it was often hardly possible to see what was really going on. As a consequence, at least up to 1987, distal pressure measurements were required in many institutions. With thinner shafts of monorail and fixed-wire catheters and with the development of x-ray technology, coronary visualization finally yielded more information than distal pressure. The wire could be controlled, the balloon could be located precisely, and the result of dilatation could be monitored with contrast injections after dilatation—with or without balloon catheter in place. As opposed to this, transstenotic pressure monitoring is limited to the short period during which the balloon remains within the stenosis. Also, transstenotic pressures yield no information on the type or cause of a possible obstruction.

For Schneider monorail catheters, optimal contrast flow and visualization can also be obtained with high-flow 7 F catheters, which currently is not the case for 6 F guiding catheters. Other sliding rail catheters with thinner shafts may be used with reasonable contrast flow in 6 and 5 F catheters. Thinner dilatation and guide catheters will often go together with a loss of pushability—but there may be more backup when the small guide catheter is inserted more deeply into the proximal coronary artery.[31] A major drawback of smaller guide catheters is that they lack the exchange advantages of sliding rail systems; many other devices require 8 F (or larger) guide catheters.

Clinical Results of Balloon Angioplasty

In our two prospectively studied groups with consecutive dilatations, results with monorail catheters have shown primary success rates of 82% in 1986 with generation 1 and 2 catheters alone and of 93% in 1989 with Piccolino catheters alone. The mean stenosis diameter increase as estimated from visual interpretation was 51% in group 1 and 59% in group 2 with a predilatation stenosis severity of 77% and 86%. The complication rate was low, with an emergency bypass rate of 3.1% in 1986 and .8% in 1989, and infarction rates of 1.5% and .8%, respectively. There were no deaths (Table 11–6). There were clearly better results with improved technology in the Piccolino catheter.

In 1988, Finci et al.[32] studied the primary PTCA success rate in 73 stenoses (including 9 total occlusions) of 61 patients using generation 1 monorail balloon catheters. Primary success was obtained in 85% of lesions with monorail catheters alone, and total success rate was 90%. In 1989 de Feyter et al.[33] evaluated 1,014 patients who underwent dilatation with monorail catheters. The average success rate in this study was 92% of lesions in patients with stable angina and 95% of lesions in patients with unstable angina; bypass rates were 2% and 2.3%; infarction rates were 1.6% and 3.0%; and death rates were 0% and .6%. This group also noted the insufficient performance of the generation 1 monorail catheters in some cases, which was "substantially improved" in the Piccolino version, and they underlined the advantages of catheter exchange, wire steerability, and contrast flow.

Currently available data for PTCA show general suc-

TABLE 11–6

PTCA Results With Monorail Catheters in High-Grade Stenoses Without Total Obstruction*

		Primary Success (%)		Vessel Distribution† (%)					Complications (%)		
		Monorail Alone	Total	LAD	LCx	RCA	Pre-PTCA Obstruction	Diameter Gain	Emergency Bypass	Infarct	Death
Group 1	(n=131)	82	89	65.6	21.4	9.2	77	51	3.1	1.5	0
Group 2	(n=132)	93	95	37.1	22.7	34.1	86	59	0.8	0.8	0

*Group 1: 131 consecutive stenoses dilated with generation 1 PVC catheters in 1985 and 1986; group 2: 130 consecutive stenoses dilated with Piccolino catheters in 1989.

†LAD = left anterior descending; LCx = left circumflex; RCA = right coronary artery.

cess rates above 80% to 90%. In the earlier NHLBI registry study of 1985 to 1986,[34] probably comparable with our group 1 patients, the overall success rates were 85% for 1,234 stenoses in patients with stable angina and 90% for 1,519 stenoses in patients with unstable angina, the mean stenosis improvement was 56% and 57%, the emergency bypass rate 2.2% and 4.4%, and the infarction rate 2.0% and 3.3%, respectively. In the M-Heart trial in 1,000 lesions in patients who underwent dilatation between 1985 and 1987, the average success rate was 88.6% using steerable guidewire catheter systems.[35] The reported emergency bypass rate was .3%, one patient suffered a myocardial infarction, and two patients (.2%) died. In another multicenter registry of dilatations performed from 1988 to 1989 (in the same years as our group 2 patients), the overall success rate was 90% of 734 lesions for which dilatation was attempted.[36] In this study, monorail Piccolino or Rx catheters were used for complex stenoses, which made up 69% of all lesions, whereas Hartzler microdilatation catheters were used in "classic" noncomplex lesions. The emergency bypass rate was 1.8%, the infarction rate was 1.8%, and the death rate was .4%.

We conclude that our success rates with monorail generation 1 catheters alone (limited to one device in group 1 in 1985 to 1986) were lower (82%) than success rates of a comparable study of the same period (85% to 90%),[34] which was not restricted to a certain device. However, when taking our total success rate of group 1 into account (89%), the comparison was more favorable. With Piccolino catheters alone in group 2, our success rates seemed to be better (93%) than those of major multicenter trials usually including the use of a variety of devices (88% to 90%).[35,36] Our results were confirmed by the success rates of 92% to 95% in monorail studies of Finci et al.[32] and de Feyter et al.[33] Good or excellent results can be achieved with different catheter systems and depend on a large number of factors beyond catheter technology. Nevertheless, good results may be attributable to some characteristics of monorail catheters. In our opinion these are steerability, contrast flow, and rapid balloon exchange (combined with optimal pushability in the Piccolino and Speedy versions). Easier exchange may encourage the willingness of the investigator to try to achieve optimal results by using additional balloon sizes.

Stenting With Monorail Catheters

Clinical experience in stenting with monorail Piccolino PVC and Speedy catheters demonstrated several advantages. Loading of the balloon with the stent—after some training—was fast and reliable; advancing of the balloon and stent was easy in rather straight and wide proximal coronary segments, positioning of the stent by millimeter increments with repeated and unimpaired dye injections was shown to be possible, and, often, only one balloon was needed for the complete dilatation procedure. The typical advantage of monorail catheters, however, was the fast placement of stents, especially in high-risk patients (Fig 11–7) and in patients with critical ischemia. In our experience, the time between decision making and flow restoration by stenting was between 2 and 12 minutes, and a reasonable time span seems to be 5 minutes. Another advantage was the precision achieved in stent positioning, which was due to unimpaired contrast imaging. The major disadvantage was the inability to cross angled coronary segments, and special care and experience are required to avoid errors, including underestimation of coronary obstacles.

Our primary success rate of 97% correctly placed stents with monorail catheters in 65 stenoses was comparable to the findings of Haude et al. with 100% of 22 stents,[37] and of Schatz et al.,[38] with success in 94% of patients. Their stent delivery success rate has increased to 99%, with use of a sheath to protect the stent during placement.[38] This could be shown in our study group as well, in 2 of the 65 stenoses. The disadvantage of the sheath technique, however, is the limited contrast flow through the guiding catheter alongside the sheath, so that a precise placement of the stent is strongly hampered.

Other Devices

The use of the monorail technique in other devices has steadily increased. This holds for diagnostic or therapeutic stand-alone systems or for the combination in a consecutive application. The latter particularly offers an accessible variety of therapeutic attempts in high-grade or complex stenoses, but also facilitates the implementation of scientific studies into standard diagnostic or therapeutic procedures. One example is the use of monorail systems in the study of the endothelially mediated coronary vasodilating response to various stimuli in humans.[21,22] A disadvantage is the lack of compatibility with non-monorail devices designed for over-the-wire or long wire use. Extending standard length guidewires with "extension wires" can overcome this problem.

Comments on Logistics

With increasing numbers of PTCA procedures and increasing health care costs, logistic data are becoming more and more important. In Germany, especially large

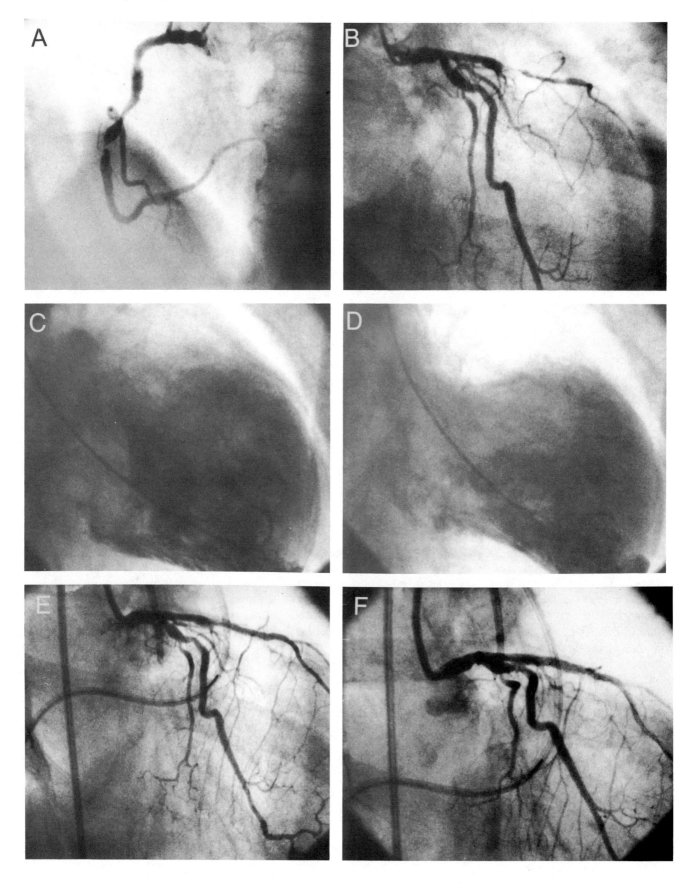

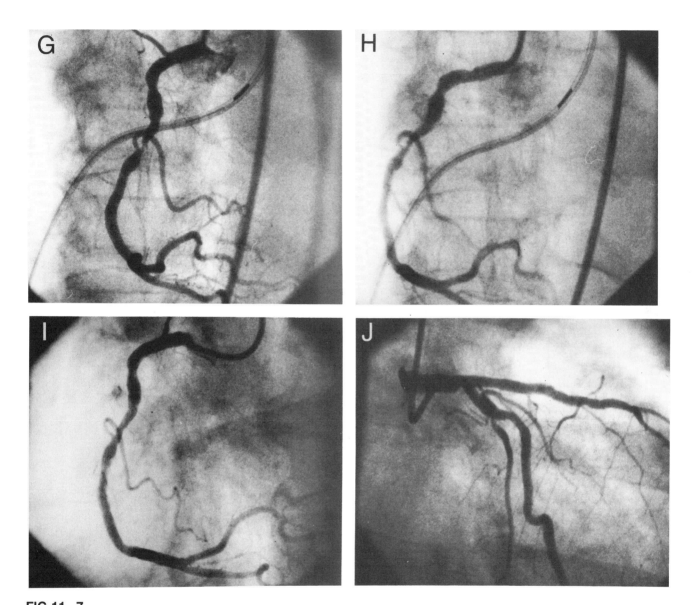

FIG 11–7.

PTCA with monorail Piccolino polyethyleneteraphtalate and stenting with monorail Piccolino PVC balloons and Palmaz-Schatz stents in a 72-year-old woman with double-vessel disease, left ventricular aneurysm, angina with minimal activity, and high CABG risk. **A,** 90% right coronary artery (RCA) stenosis distal to right ventricular branch. **B,** functional occlusion of the left anterior descending (LAD) **C,** left ventricle, diastole. **D,** systole with aneurysm. **E,** obstructive dissection after PTCA of LAD. **F,** widely patent LAD after stenting to provide collaterals to the RCA. **G,** widely patent RCA stenosis distal to right ventricular branch after stenting for major dissection, new obstruction proximally. **H,** 30% residual stenosis after redilatation of the proximal portion. **I,** control angiogram 6 weeks later without restenosis in RCA. **J,** same, no restenosis in the LAD. The RCA had to months after stenting because of symptomatic late restenosis, the last control angiogram 1 year after stenting showed no restenosis. Rapid balloon exchange for stenting after RCA dissection was felt to be essential in this high-risk patient.

centers with 2,000 or 3,000 procedures per year favor the ease and simplicity of use of monorail systems. The strongest argument of groups in these centers are reduced investigation time and, thus, reduced staff hours. Staff hours are also reduced by single-operator dilatations. In our experience, the balloon exchange can easily be performed by a single operator (without an additional scrubbed assistant) within 2 to 5 minutes. The short exchange times claimed by experienced investigators for the long-wire technique are usually obtained with the cooperation of at least two, often three, scrubbed staff members. Even if the frequency of exchange procedures is reduced due to advanced catheter technology, the ease and speed of sliding rail systems will be an increasingly important economic factor. This is underlined by a tendency to perform PTCA immediately after a diagnostic procedure, an approach that is strongly supported by the reduced equipment and staff requirements. In our institution, this "prima-vista-PTCA" accounts for more than 50% of all cases of dilatation after a first diagnostic coronary angiogram and is currently requested by most patients. In patients with new angina pectoris after previous dilatation or bypass interventions, immediate PTCA is also becoming the procedure of choice, even in complex pathological-anatomical situations. In many of these patients the number of repeated interventions can be limited when PTCA is performed in combination with the diagnostic study. Prima-vista-PTCA again is facilitated by the ready availability of monorail-supported bailout devices, such as perfusion or transfusion catheters and stents.

SUMMARY

Monorail catheters have been designed to facilitate PTCA procedures. Seven years experience have shown this to be an achievable goal. At first, rapid exchangeability, optimal steerability, and improved contrast flow in monorail systems could be proved with monorail generations 1 and 2. Piccolino and Speedy catheters, as well as similar products from different manufacturers with technological improvements, have added adequate pushability and trackability to sliding rail systems.

The clinical success rates with monorail catheters alone are at least as good as general success rates of large studies in which the successful treatment of a stenosis is not limited to the use of one device alone.

Monorail or sliding rail systems offer logistical advantages. With appropriate use, investigation time and staff hours can be reduced significantly. In particular, it is possible, if required, to perform a complete standard PTCA procedure with two persons, e.g., one scrubbed

physician and a circulating nurse. After a first diagnostic coronary angiogram or in repeated studies, making a decision about immediate PTCA is facilitated with monorail catheters. With increasing numbers of patients treated, the effect on reducing PTCA costs with the help of sliding rail systems will become increasingly important. Though less frequently performed in routine PTCA at this time, balloon exchange remains imperative in case of failed PTCA or vessel occlusion for stabilizing procedures. Moreover, exchange helps in the consecutive use of nonballoon therapeutic devices and in intracoronary diagnostic studies, especially in research procedures.

REFERENCES

1. Grüntzig A: Die perkutane Rekanalisation chronischer arterieller Verschlüsse (Dotter Prinzip) mit einem neuen doppellumigen Dilatationskatheter. *Fortschr Rontgenstr* 1976; 124:80–86.
2. Grüntzig A: Perkutane Dilatation von Koronarstenosen — Beschreibung eines neuen Kathetersystems. *Klin Woschr* 1976; 54:534–545.
3. Grüntzig A, Senning A, Siegenthaler WE: Nonoperative dilatation of coronary artery stenosis: Percutaneous transluminal coronary angioplasty. *N Engl J Med* 1979; 301:61–68.
4. Simpson JB, Baim DS, Robert EW, et al: A new catheter system for coronary angioplasty. *Am J Cardiol* 1982; 49:1216–1222.
5. Kaltenbach M: Neue Technik zur steuerbaren Ballondilatation von Kranzgefäßverengungen. *Z Kardiol* 1984; 73:669–673.
6. Kaltenbach M: The long-wire technique — a new technique for steerable balloon catheter dilatation of coronary artery stenoses. *Eur Heart J* 1984; 5:1004–1009.
7. Bonzel T, Wollschläger H, Just H: Ein neues Kethetersystem zur mechanischen Dilatation von Koronarstenosen mit austauschbaren intrakoronaren Kathetern, höherem Kontrastmittelfluß und verbesserter Steuerbarkeit [A new catheter system for coronary angioplasty (PTCA) with exchangeable intracoronary catheters, high flow of contrast agent, and improved steerability]. *Biomed Tech* 1986; 31:195–200.
8. Bonzel T, Wollschläger H, Meinertz T, et al: The steerable monorail catheter system — a new device for PTCA (abstract), Circulation 74 (supp II): II-459,1986
9. Bonzel T, Wollschläger H, Kasper W, et al: The sliding rail system (monorail): Description of a new technique for intravascular instrumentation and its application to coronary angioplasty. *Z Kardiol* 1987; 76 (suppl 6:119–122.
10. Meier B, *Coronary Angioplasty; Technique, Special Balloon Catheters.* Orlando, Fla, Grune & Stratton, 1987, pp 13–15.
11. Deleted in proof.
12. Mooney MR, Douglas JS Jr, Mooney JF, et al: Monorail Piccolino catheter: A new rapid exchange/ultra low profile coronary angioplasty system. *Cathet Cardiovasc Diagn* 1990; 20:114–119.

13. Meier B, Carlier M, Finci L, et al: Magnum wire for balloon recanalization of total coronary occlusions. *Am J Cardiol* 1989; 64:148–154.

14. Meier B: Magnum system for routine coronary angioplasty: A randomized study. *Cathet Cardiovasc Diagn* (in press).

15. Meier B: Magnarail probing catheter: New tool for balloon recanalization of chronic total coronary occlusions. *J Invasive Cardiol* 1990; 2:227–229.

16. Pande AK, Meier B, Urban P, et al: Magnum/Magnarail versus conventional systems for recanalization of chronic total coronary occlusions: A randomized comparison. *Am Heart J* (in press).

17. Meier B: *Coronary Angioplasty: Occlusive Dissection.* Orlando, Fla, Grune & Stratton, 1987, pp 122–123.

18. Bonzel T, Wollschläger H, Kasper W, et al: Myokardprotektion mit dem Monorailsystem bei akutem Koronarverschluß während PTCA (abstract). *Z Kardiol* 1987; 76 (suppl 1):223.

19. Clas W, Erbel R, von Seelen W, et al: Ein neuentwickelter Ballonkatheter zur Reduzierung der myokardialen Ischämie während transluminaler Angioplastie. *Biomed Technik* 1984; 29:195–196.

20. Erbel R, Clas W, Busch U, et al: New balloon catheter for prolonged percutaneous transluminal coronary angioplasty and bypass flow in occluded vessels. *Cathet Cardiovasc Diagn* 1986; 12:116–123.

21. Drexler H, Zeiher AM, Wollschläger H, et al: Flowdependent coronary artery dilatation in humans. *Circulation* 1989; 80:466–474.

22. Zeiher AM, Drexler H, Wollschläger H, et al: Modulation of coronary vascular tone in humans: Progressive endothelial dysfunction with different early stages of coronary atherosclerosis. *Circulation* 1991; 83:391–401.

23. Zeiher AM, Bonzel T: A prototype RF-heated "hot balloon" PTCA catheter: Design parameters and in vitro tissue studies (abstract). *Circulation* 1988; 78 (suppl II):II–296.

24. Zeiher AM, Bonzel T, Just H: "Hot balloon"-Angioplastie mithilfe eines Radiofrequenz-PTCA-Katheters: Entwicklung und erste experimentelle Ergebnisse eines neuen Konzepts (abstract). *Z Kardiol* 1989; 78 (suppl I):58.

25. Palmaz JC, Sibbitt RR, Reuter SR, et al: Expandable intraluminal graft: Preliminary study. *Radiology* 1985; 156:73–77.

26. Schatz RA: A view of vascular stents. *Circulation* 1989; 79:1–13.

27. Strupp G, Bonzel T, Schreiner G, et al: Stenting mit Hilfe von Monorailkathetern (abstract). *Z Kardiol* 1991; 80 (suppl III):29.

28. Strupp G, Bonzel T, Schreiner G, et al: Angiographisch kontrollierte akute und mittelfristige Ergebnisse 6 and 12 Wochen nach koronarer Stentimplantation. *Z Kardiol* (submitted for publication).

29. Finci L, Meier B, Divernois J: Percutaneous transluminal coronary angioplasty of a bifurcation narrowing using the kissing wire monorail balloon technique. *Am J Cardiol* 1987; 60:375–376.

30. Renkin J, Wijns W, Hanet C, et al: Angioplasty of coronary bifurcation stenoses: Immediate and long-term results of the protecting branch technique. *Cathet Cardiovasc Diagn* 1991; 22:167–173.

31. Feldman R, Glemser E, Kaizer J, et al: Coronary angioplasty using new 6 French guiding catheters. *Cathet Cardiovasc Diagn* 1991; 23:93–99.

32. Finci L, Meier B, Roy P, et al: Clinical experience with the monorail balloon catheter for coronary angioplasty. *Cathet Cardiovasc Diagn* 1988; 14:206–212.

33. de Feyter PJ, Serruys PW, van den Brand M et al: Short term results of percutaneous transluminal coronary angioplasty with the monorail technique: Experience in the first thousand patients. *Br Heart J* 1990; 63:253–259.

34. Bentivoglio LG, Holubkov R, Kelsey SF, et al: Short and long term outcome of percutaneous angioplasty in unstable versus stable angina pectoris: A report of the 1985-1986 NHLBI PTCA registry. *Cathet Cardiovasc Diagn* 1991; 23:227–238.

35. Savage PM, M-Heart investigators: Clinical and angiographic determinants of primary coronary angioplasty success. *JACC* 1991; 17:22–28.

36. Stammen F, Piessens J, Vrolix M, et al: Immediate and short-term results of a 1988–1989 coronary angioplasty registry. *Am J Cardiol* 1991; 67:253–258.

37. Haude M, Erbel R, Straub U, et al: Results of intracoronary stents for management of intracoronary dissection after balloon angioplasty. *Am J Cardiol* 1991; 67:691–696.

38. Schatz RA, Goldberg S, Leon M, et al: Clinical experience with the Palmaz-Schatz coronary stent. *JACC* 1991; 17:155B–159B.

12

Comparison of Angioplasty and Coronary Bypass Surgery: The Emory Angioplasty vs. Surgery Trial

Spencer B. King III, M.D.

When angioplasty was first envisioned by Grüntzig, it was intended for patients with single obstructions. Although the initial group of patients treated in Zurich contained 40% with more than single-vessel disease, all but two received angioplasty of only the one lesion that was judged the culprit. The results in those patients has been well characterized and shows that with long-term follow-up, the overall survival is excellent, as is the improvement in exercise performance and freedom from cardiac events.[1] Similarly, the first patients treated at Emory exhibited a 5-year cardiac survival rate of 98% with an overall survival rate of 97%, and 80% of those patients were free from cardiac death, myocardial infarction, or the need for bypass surgery.[2]

Over the years with the development of more sophisticated equipment, it has been possible to expand angioplasty to more complex lesions and therefore treat patients with multivessel disease. The percentage of angioplasty patients with multivessel disease had gradually increased at Emory so that by the year 1966, half the patients had multivessel disease. This figure is somewhat misleading since most post–bypass surgery patients are classified as having multivessel disease but many of them have only one culprit site involved. The 1985–1986 registry of the National Heart, Lung and Blood Institute (NHLBI) also showed that half the patients treated in that registry had multivessel disease.[3] Many centers have applied angioplasty in multivessel disease as a substitute for bypass surgery, and this practice continues to increase.[4–11] As early as 1982 there were calls for randomized trials comparing angioplasty with bypass surgery. In the early days of angioplasty

there was little opportunity to perform the procedure in comparable patients going for bypass surgery; however, once the equipment improved and experience was gained, such trials became possible. In 1984 such a trial was proposed by Grüntzig and was submitted to the NHLBI for consideration. Although this trial was approved, it was not funded; following Grüntzig's death, an amended proposal was submitted in 1986, and in June of 1987 final National Institutes of Health (NIH) funding was obtained.

Much had been learned from previous trials of coronary bypass surgery vs. medical therapy in the 1970s.[12–16] The Coronary Artery Surgery Study (CASS) and the Veterans Administration coronary bypass surgery cooperative study group in the United States and the European coronary surgery study group in Europe all provided valuable data in making selections between surgery and medical therapy.[17–19] Whereas each study showed some groups of patients who benefited from the point of view of survival, they also showed groups who did not benefit. All the studies showed that bypass surgery reduces angina when compared with medical therapy; however none showed improved survival in single-vessel disease.

STRUCTURE OF THE EMORY ANGIOPLASTY VS. SURGERY TRIAL

The Emory trial was designed to address only patients with multivessel disease. The rationale was that these patients with multivessel disease and without prior bypass surgery represent the group in which the current dilemma exists. Despite extensive observational reports in the past regarding the outcome of angioplasty in multivessel disease, there has always been a great deal of selection in the type of patients with multivessel disease going to angioplasty and those going for surgery. It has therefore been impossible to compare these very different cohorts in order to learn the true value of angioplasty vs. bypass surgery in this group in whom there is a dilemma. The Emory Angioplasty vs. Surgery Trial (EAST) is a single-institution study being conducted at Emory University Hospital, Crawford W. Long Hospital of Emory University, and the Emory-affiliated Veterans Administration Hospital. Eligible patients are those who have a greater than 50% diameter stenosis of at least two of the major coronary artery systems and are judged on clinical grounds to be in need of revascularization. Since the treatment options are entirely revascularization, the decision made by the attending clinicians and patient himself must be for either bypass surgery or angioplasty, and therefore the judgment must have been made that medical therapy is no longer adequate management for that patient. This decision is made by clinicians other than the investigators in the trial and is based on symptoms, objective evidence of ischemia, and the coronary pathoanatomy that the patient exhibits. During the period of enrollment in the trial, July 13, 1977, through April 15, 1990, all patients presenting to the three Emory University hospitals mentioned were screened for the presence of multivessel disease and the absence of prior angioplasty or bypass surgery. All such patients with multivessel disease and no prior procedure were evaluated whether they underwent catheterization at the Emory hospitals or underwent angiography at other facilities and were subsequently referred to Emory. All patients were screened regardless of whether they were referred directly for bypass surgery, referred for angioplasty or medical therapy, or referred with no treatment assignment recommended.

All such patients underwent scrutiny for the presence of certain clinical and angiographic features that excluded them from further participation in the EAST trial. Clinical exclusions included (1) revascularization not needed, (2) the presence of a noncardiac illness influencing survival, (3) myocardial infarction within the past 5 days, (4) class III or IV congestive heart failure on the New York Heart Association classification, and (5) unavailability for follow-up. Criteria for exclusion on angiographic grounds included (1) left main coronary stenosis greater than 30%; (2) total occlusion of a major vessel that supplies viable myocardium and is judged to have occurred more than 8 weeks prior to the evaluation, (3) total occlusion of two or more major coronary

vessels regardless of left ventricular wall motion abnormalities, (4) left ventricular ejection fraction less than 25%, (5) coronary artery lesions longer than standard balloons (20 mm), (6) coronary lesions with large filling defects judged to be thrombi, and (7) a need for other cardiac surgery such as mitral valve replacement or aneurysmectomy. The rationale for excluding patients with total occlusions was based on the projected success rate in chronic total occlusions greater than 2 months in age at the time the application was written in 1986. It was felt at that time that angioplasty results would be significantly hindered if a success rate for dilating the total occlusions was in the 60% to 70% range, which was anticipated. Even though patients with total occlusion continue to undergo angioplasty with better success rates, these types of lesions continued to exclude patients from the EAST randomization. If patients are not excluded because of the angiographic or clinical exclusion criteria listed, the film is reviewed by the EAST surgeons and the EAST angioplasty operators. Each independently makes a judgment as to whether the respective procedure can be safely and reasonably carried out in the patient under consideration. If the operators feel that the procedure they are asked to perform could not be carried out safely, then the patient is excluded.

Patients who satisfy the clinical and angiographic requirements and are not excluded by the angioplasty operators or surgeons are eligible for the trial. Discussions were then initiated with the patient's physician, and if all parties were in agreement, the patient was approached and invited to participate in the EAST trial.

PURPOSE AND END POINTS

The EAST trial is a moderate-sized, intermediate-term trial designed to evaluate the relative value of the strategy of selecting angioplasty or bypass surgery for the patient with multivessel disease. Because of the scope of this trial and the follow-up period planned, it was not anticipated that survival would be significantly different between treatment groups. Other adverse events, however, strongly influence the selection strategy, and therefore a composite end point that would reflect the outcome of the patient was selected. The primary end point of EAST is a combined end point that includes freedom from the following events: (1) death from any cause, (2) new Q wave myocardial infarction, and (3) a large ischemic thallium defect. The purpose of this end point is to reflect an adverse outcome that, if found to be dramatically more prevalent in one group or the other, would strongly influence the selection of patients for angioplasty or surgery. A large thallium ischemic defect is defined as a perfusion deficit as large as one third the left anterior descending distribution or one half the right or circumflex artery redistribution. That defect must on reinject thallium imaging at rest show complete or nearly complete redistribution. The methodology of this thallium scan is that partly developed at Emory University by using thallium single-photon emission computed tomography (SPECT).

This composite primary end point will be analyzed by the intention-to-treat method. The goal is to show that angioplasty is not a materially worse choice than surgery. Assumptions must be made about the possible event rates in order to select the levels of type I or type II errors that need to be excluded. For example, if the type I error rate (α) is 0.05 and the type II error rate (β) is 0.20 and if the true event rates for coronary bypass surgery are between 10% and 20% and the event rates for angioplasty are greater than 10 percentage points higher, then 176 to 250 patients would be required in each treatment group to show this magnitude of difference.

OTHER END POINTS

The status of the angiographic revascularization is of obvious interest. However, because the strategy applied with angioplasty differs significantly from that applied with bypass surgery, this cannot be chosen as the primary end point. Patients assigned to bypass surgery usually have all lesions bypassed. Patients undergoing angioplasty frequently have only the more severe lesions dilated, with less severe lesions felt not to be hemodynamically threatening left alone for future interventions should that need arise. Nonetheless, the degree of revascularization in the late follow-up period will be very interesting, and because of the single-center nature of this trial, it was decided to have an independent quantitative assessment of the coronary anatomy made at the University of Washington by Dr. Greg Brown's laboratory. The degree of revascularization will be categorized by the initial index obstructive segments identified at the time the patient was entered into the trial and the success at revascularizing those segments as judged by the follow-up angiograms. The clinical status of the patient as regards the presence or absence of angina and congestive heart failure will be evaluated. Functional status judged by exercise duration and the timing of electrocardiographic (ECG) changes, as well as maximum exercise performed, will be measured. An important secondary end point that will have great impact on the selection process will be the number of subsequent procedures required relative to the group to which the patient was assigned. It will be interesting to know whether a high percentage of angioplasty patients re-

quire bypass surgery in the follow-up period as well as how many surgical patients require additional procedures. This will dramatically influence the economic comparisons that are being carefully tabulated, not only for medical costs but also to reflect the economic condition of the patient and his family. Various quality-of-life measures are also being evaluated between the groups.

In some respects the secondary end points may be of more interest than the primary end point. One should remember that even though the reports of the results of this trial may take on the appearance of a consumer report with some end points favoring one therapy and some another, these will be helpful in influencing patients and physicians as they struggle with the decision of which procedure to select.

BASELINE SCREENING

During the 3-year, 9-month entry period of the trial, 16,499 patients' films were evaluated in the Emory University system. Five thousand one hundred eighteen of these patients had multivessel coronary artery disease without having had prior angioplasty or prior bypass surgery. The angiographic exclusions previously mentioned totaled 3,371 patients, clinical exclusions amounted to 714 patients, and the operator exclusions totaled 191 patients, which left 842 patients who were eligible for the EAST trial, that is, they met the definition of patients in whom there is a significant dilemma between the choice of angioplasty or surgery (Fig 12–1). Most of the not randomized but eligible patients were excluded by their own referring physicians. Of the 842 eligible patients, 353 were not approached because the referring physician had a bias toward one procedure or the other. Many of these exclusions came about because the patient had been previously referred to Emory for bypass surgery. Of the 489 patients available to be approached for the trial, only 97 refused to participate, which left 392 patients (or 80% of the ones approached) who actually enrolled.

In order to ensure that adequate representation of various degrees of multivessel disease was achieved in the two treatment arms, the patients were divided by angiographic strata prior to randomization. The four strata are A, single lesions in two of the major artery systems; B, involvement of two major artery systems but with multiple lesions in at least one of those systems; C, single lesions in all three major artery systems; and D, involvement of all three major artery systems but with multiple lesions in at least one system. Randomized patients were evenly distributed between these four strata: 113 patients in stratum A, 123 in B, 51 in C, and 105 in D. Whereas the distribution of patients was even be-

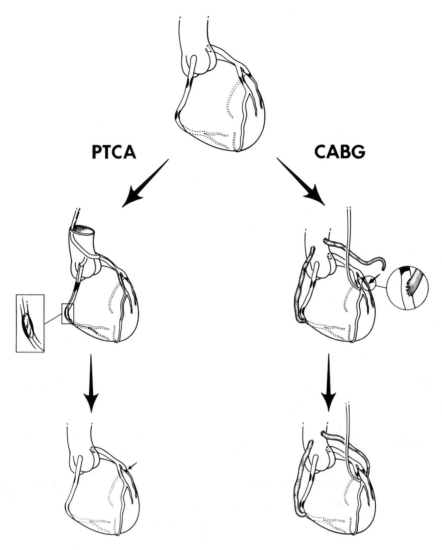

FIG 12–1.
Schematic representation of the choice between coronary angioplasty (PTCA) and coronary bypass surgery (CABG).

tween the treatment arms because of randomization, in the eligible but not randomized group there was an obvious bias by the attending physician that influenced the selection of therapy. In the two-vessel single-lesion group, 82 patients underwent angioplasty, and 37 patients had bypass surgery. At the opposite end of the spectrum in those patients with triple-vessel diffuse disease, 17 patients underwent angioplasty, and 126 patients underwent surgery. Although surgery was more commonly performed in the other two strata as well, the difference was less striking.

The baseline characteristics of the 198 randomized patients undergoing angioplasty and the 194 patients undergoing bypass surgery were not different in any category and were as follows: age, 62 years; gender, 74% males; and angina class (Canadian Cardiovascular Society classification): no angina, 7%; class I, 5%; class II, 10%; class III, 17%; and class IV, 60%. Con-

gestive heart failure was absent in 96% of the patients, prior myocardial infarction was present in 41%, the left ventricular ejection fraction was 61% ± 12%, the proportion of patients with double-vessel disease was 60%, and those with triple-vessel disease amounted to 40%. Seventy-two percent of the patients had involvement of the proximal segment of the anterior descending coronary artery.

COMPARISON OF RANDOMIZED AND ELIGIBLE BUT NOT RANDOMIZED PATIENTS

The EAST patients have been compared against those eligible but not randomized patients, and a few differences have been identified. The education and employment level is somewhat different, with 33% of the randomized patients having some college education or higher and 50% of the eligible but not randomized patients having this level of education. Similarly, more patients in the eligible but not randomized group had professional executive or self-employed status than in the randomized group. Importantly, items such as duration of the angina, time since last pain, the presence of rest pain, angina class, history of congestive heart failure, smoking history, presence of carotid or peripheral vascular disease, hypertension, diabetes, activity level, family history of coronary artery disease, number of previous myocardial infarctions, hypercholesterolemia, obesity, body weight, ejection fraction, end-diastolic pressure, and ventricular wall motion did not show significant differences between the randomized and eligible patients. As indicated earlier, in the eligible but not randomized group, there was a difference in the distribution of coronary disease, with more diffusely diseased patients going for bypass surgery and more discrete-lesion cases going for angioplasty.

STATUS OF THE FOLLOW-UP IN THE EMORY ANGIOPLASTY VS. SURGERY TRIAL

The patient entry phase of the EAST trial ended in April 1990. At the present time all the patients have passed the 1-year window for follow-up. Clinical follow-up has been obtained in greater than 99% of the randomized patients and in greater than 98% of the eligible but not randomized patients. Ninety-one percent of the randomized patients who were eligible have undergone the 12-month thallium testing and 91% have undergone the 12-month coronary angiogram programs. By mid-1991 approximately half the patients had become eligible for the 3-year follow-up examination. Greater than 99% of the randomized patients had clinical follow-ups, and greater than 97% of the eligible but not randomized patients have been similarly followed. Of the randomized patients eligible for the 36-month angiogram and thallium scan, 80% have had these examinations.

The investigators remain blinded to the results of the EAST trial and will remain so until the completion of the follow-up studies, which will occur in spring 1993.

WHAT SHOULD BE EXPECTED FROM THE EMORY ANGIOPLASTY VS. SURGERY TRIAL?

There are several reasonable expectations from a trial of this scope: (1) an improved understanding of the outcome of patients with multivessel disease in whom angioplasty or surgery is a viable option, (2) the quality of life of patients 3 years following initial therapy analyzed by intention to treat, (3) the requirement for further interventional therapy or surgery in these patients, and (4) the relative cost of the two strategies.

There are also some things that cannot reasonably be expected to be identified in this trial. We will not establish definitively whether percutaneous transluminal coronary angioplasty (PTCA) or surgery is superior regarding survival. The study is about balloon angioplasty and therefore does not measure whether new technologies will affect the outcome of angioplasty or not. We will also not be able to expand these results to all patients with multivessel disease because many subsets are not included in this trial.

OTHER TRIALS ADDRESSING THE PROBLEM OF SELECTION FOR ANGIOPLASTY OR SURGERY IN MULTIVESSEL DISEASE

The Bypass Angioplasty Revascularization Investigation (BARI) is a large multicenter study funded by the NHLBI as well. This trial, headed by Dr. Robert Frye, is a collaborative effort among 16 centers. Randomization occurred over a 3-year period and was terminated in August 1991. Approximately 1,800 patients have been entered into that trial and will be followed for a 5-year period, with mortality the primary end point. Although there are differences in the selection and exclusion criteria, this study is very similar to the EAST trial. Several differences will emerge, however. Being a multicenter trial, BARI may give a better indication of the practice of surgery and angioplasty as reflected across the country. EAST, on the other hand, being a single-center trial, will reflect the complete experience in one center, whereas the BARI trial reflects the patients undergoing diagnostic catheterization at those hospitals only. Patients with prior catheterization are not included. It is interesting that the number of eligible patients out of the total multivessel disease population is essentially equal for both trials (16%). The primary end point of BARI is to evaluate whether the strategy of PTCA is as safe regarding mortality as the strategy of starting with bypass surgery. The mortality end point will be examined in 5 years.

The Randomized Intervention Treatment of Angina (RITA) is a trial sponsored jointly by the British Cardiac Society, the British Heart Foundation, and the Department of Health and is performed in the United Kingdom under the direction of Dr. Edgar Souten. This trial differs from EAST and BARI in that each lesion the patient has must be suitable for both angioplasty and surgery. The operators must agree on the suitability prior to the procedure, and revascularization is to be attempted on all lesions so identified. The goal of both strategies in this trial will be to provide complete revascularization and will measure the ability of each procedure to do that in this subset of patients rather than attempt to evaluate the strategy of angioplasty or surgery in a broader segment of patients.

The Coronary Artery Bypass Revascularization Investigation (CABRI) is another multicenter trial in Europe under the direction of Dr. Michele Bertrand, Patrick Serruys, Tony Rickards, and Paul Hugenholtz. This trial resembles the EAST and BARI trials very much in the selection process. This trial will include follow-up angiography and stress thallium testing as well. End points include subjective improvement in angina, objective assessment of ischemia on exercise testing, and quality of life.

The German Angioplasty Bypass Intervention (GABI) trial is a multicenter trial taking place in West Germany under the direction of Dr. Blifeld. This trial will also include coronary angiography and thallium stress testing in its final evaluation.

Whereas angioplasty has become a mainstay in the management of some patients with multivessel disease, the true value of this approach vs. bypass surgery has not been established. Practice patterns change based on local experience, which may vary widely. These trials, which for the first time address patients randomly assigned, should go a long way in providing some objective guidance to the selection for angioplasty or surgery in experienced centers.

REFERENCES

1. Grüntzig AR, King SB, Schlumpf M, et al: Long-term follow-up after percutaneous transluminal coronary angioplasty: The early Zurich experience. *N Engl J Med* 1987; 316:1127–1132.
2. Talley JD, Hurst JW, King SB, et al: Clinical outcome 5 years after attempted percutaneous transluminal coronary angioplasty in 427 patients. *Circulation* 1988; 77:820–829.
3. Detre KI, Hulobkov R, Kelsey S, et al: Percutaneous transluminal coronary angioplasty in 1985–1986 and 1977–1981. The National Heart, Lung and Blood Institute Registry. *N Engl J Med* 1988; 318:265–270.
4. Finci L, Meier B, DeBrugal B, et al: Angiographic followup after multivessel percutaneous transluminal coronary angioplasty. *Am J Cardiol* 1987; 60:467–470.
5. Thomas FS, Most AS, Wilburn DO: Coronary angioplasty for patients with multivessel coronary artery disease: Follow-up clinical status. *Am Heart J* 1988; 115:8–13.
6. Deligonul V, Vandormael MG, Kern MJ, et al: Coronary angioplasty: A therapeutic option for symptomatic patients with two and three vessel coronary disease. *J Am Coll Cordiol* 1988; 11:1173–1179.
7. Reeder GS, Holmes DR, Detre K, et al: Degree of revascularization in patients with multivessel coronary disease: A report from the National Heart, Lung, and Blood Institute Percutaneous Transluminal Coronary Angioplasty Registry. *Circulation* 1988; 77:638–644.
8. Vandormael MB, Deligonul V, Kern MJ, et al: Multilesion coronary angioplasty: Clinical and angiographic followup. *J Am Coll Cardiol* 1987; 10:246–252.
9. Mata LA, Osch X, David PR, et al: Clinical and angiographic assessment 6 months after double vessel percutaneous coronary angioplasty. *J Am Coll Cardiol* 1985; 6:1239–1244.
10. Cowley MJ, Vetrovec GW, DiSciasio G, et al: Coronary angioplasty of multiple vessels: Short-term outcome and long-term results. *Circulation* 1985; 72:1314–1320.
11. OKeefe JH Jr, Rutherford BD, McConahay DR, et al: Multivessel coronary angioplasty from 1980 to 1989: Procedural results and long-term outcome. *J Am Coll Cardiol* 1990; 16:1097–1102.
12. Chatterjie K: Is there any long-term benefit from coronary artery bypass surgery? *J Am Coll Cardiol* 1988; 12:881–882.
13. Reduzzi P, Huttgren H, Thomsen J, et al: Ten year effect of medical and surgical therapy on quality of life: Veterans Administration cooperative study of coronary artery surgery. *Am J Cardiol* 1987; 59:1017–1023.
14. Loop F, Lytle B, Cosgrove D, et al: Influence of the internal mammary artery graft on 10 year survival and other cardiac events. *N Engl J Med* 1984; 314:1–6.
15. Cameron A, et al: Clinical implications of internal mammary artery bypass grafts: The coronary artery surgery study experience. *Circulation* 1988; 77:815–819.
16. Lytle BW, Loop FD, Cosgrove DM, et al: Long-term (5 to 12 years) serial studies of internal mammary artery and saphenous vein coronary bypass grafts. *J Thorac Cardiovasc Surg* 1985; 89:248–258.
17. Weintraub WS, Jones EL, King SB III, et al: Changing use of coronary angioplasty and coronary bypass surgery in the treatment of chronic coronary artery disease. *Am J Cardiol* 1990; 65:183–188.
18. The Veterans Administration Coronary Artery Bypass Surgery Cooperative Study Group: Eleven-year survival in the Veterans Administration randomized trial of coronary bypass surgery for stable angina. *N Engl J Med* 1984; 311:1333–1339.
19. Varnauskas E: The European Coronary Surgery Study Group: Survival, myocardial infarction, and employment status in a prospective randomized study of coronary bypass surgery. *Circulation* 1985; 72(suppl 5):90–101.

PART III

Atherectomy

13

Percutaneous Transluminal Coronary Rotary Ablation With the Rotablator

Michel E. Bertrand, M.D.

Jean M. Lablanche, M.D.

Fabrice Leroy, M.D.

Christophe Bauters, M.D.

Eugene McFadden, M.D.

Over the past 5 years, interventional cardiologists sought to develop new methods of recanalization to address the limitations of coronary balloon angioplasty. Several new methods have been described, but atherectomy is one of the most interesting. This term, now applied to any catheter-based mechanical device that removes atherosclerotic material from the vessel wall in situ, includes directional or excisional atherectomy,[1] transluminal extraction atherectomy,[2] and rotary ablation with the Rotablator. In this chapter we describe the different aspects of this technique of high-speed rotary ablation.

HISTORICAL AND EXPERIMENTAL STUDIES

The device was designed by D. Auth and has two main goals: The first is to grind atherosclerotic material into millions of small particles capable of passing through the capillaries without clogging these vessels. This was achieved with high-speed rotation. This latter characteristic explains the selective cutting effect: at high-speed rotation, the abrasive tip is unable to cut the elastic tissue, which is deflected beneath the knife while hard calcified tissue, unable to deflect, is cut as microfissures are generated at the contact zone of the burr and hard material. These concepts have been supported by different experimental studies.[3-5] Hansen et al.[3, 4] collected the perfusate of segments of aorta perfused during rotary ablation. On average, the particles were less than 5 μm, and fewer than 2% of them were greater than 10 μm. We made similar observations[6] when we studied the resected segments of iliac arteries treated by the Rotablator; scanning electronic microscopy showed that 75% of the debris was smaller than 10 μm. The abraded surface was smooth and polished; the endothelium of the adjacent normal vessel disappeared, but the media was not damaged.

The first human rotary ablation was performed by Zacca et al.[7] in 6 patients with femoropopliteal narrowing. We performed the first percutaneous coronary rotary ablation in January 1988 in man.[8, 9]

DESIGN OF THE ROTABLATOR

The Rotablator (Heart Technology, Inc., Bellevue, Wash) is shown in Figure 13–1. It consists of an abrasive tip welded to a long flexible drive shaft tracking along a central flexible guidewire. The ablation tip is an elliptically shaped burr of various sizes (1.0, 1.25, 1.50, 1.75, 2.00, 2.15, 2.25, and 2.5 mm in diameter). The front of the burr is coated with diamond chips 30 to 50

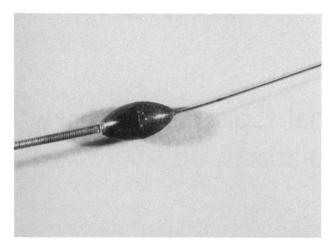

FIG 13–1.
Abrasive tip of the Rotablator.

μm in size. Rotational energy is transmitted by a disposable compressed air motor driving the flexible helical shaft at very high speeds up to 190,000 rpm. The number of revolutions per minute is measured by a fiber-optic light probe and displayed on a control panel. The speed of rotation is controlled by the air pressure, which itself is controlled by a pedal. During rotation a small volume of sterile saline solution irrigates the catheter sheath to lubricate and cool the rotating system. The burr and the drive shaft track along a central coaxial guidewire (0.09 in.) with a flexible radiopaque platinum distal part (20 mm). The central guidewire can be controlled and moved with a pin vise. The wire and abrasive tip can be advanced independently; thus, the wire can be placed in the selected artery and the burr di-rected safely into the diseased artery. The steerable guidewire does not rotate with the burr during abrasion.

PROCEDURE

After local anesthesia, a sheath is inserted into the femoral artery by using the standard Seldinger technique. A large guiding catheter (10 or 11 F) is placed into the ostium of the coronary artery, and 10,000 units of heparin is injected. The first step is to place the small guidewire across the lesion to a safe distal vessel location. Then the burr and the drive shaft are manually advanced over the guidewire to the lesion site. The motor is activated, and rotation starts. When an adequate speed of rotation is reached (>175,000 rpm), the abrasive tip is advanced gently over the guidewire. If resistance is encountered, the tip is successively pulled back and advanced to maintain high-speed rotation. Several slow passes are required to achieve maximal plaque removal. When residual stenosis remains significant after rotational atherectomy (>50%), percutaneous transluminal balloon angioplasty completes the procedure.

MEDICATIONS

All patients are pretreated with 100 to 300 mg of aspirin and a calcium channel blocker. After insertion of the sheath, 10,000 units of heparin is administered, with 5,000 units added every hour of the procedure. An intracoronary injection of 3 mg of isosorbide dinitrate is systematically administered to prevent coronary artery spasm.

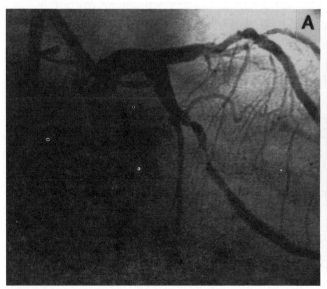
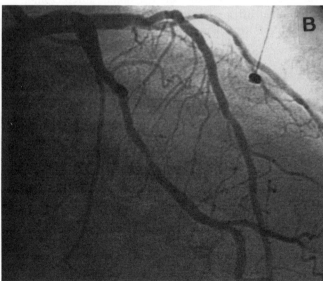

FIG 13–2.
Narrowing of obtuse marginal artery. **A,** before rotary ablation. **B,** After rotary ablation (stand-alone procedure)

Heparin injection is continued after the procedure if a dissection or a thrombus has been identified or if sheath removal should be postponed until the morning. Patients are usually discharged under a regimen of aspirin, 100 mg/day, and a calcium channel blocker.

ROTARY ABLATION EXPERIENCE— INTERNATIONAL REGISTRY

The results collected in 14 centers (4 European and 10 American centers) were included in an international registry.[9–15] The data bank includes 495 patients and 574 treated lesions. Seventy-eight percent of the patients were male, and the mean age was 61 years (range, 30 to 87). Fifty-two percent of the patients had stable angina, and 40% had unstable angina. Sixty-five percent

had multiple-vessel disease. The left anterior descending coronary artery was the most commonly treated vessel (47%), while right coronary artery and circumflex were treated in 33% and 19% of cases, respectively. Fifty-nine percent of the lesions were eccentric, 34% were calcified, 26% were located at bifurcations, and 31% were observed on tortuous vessels.

Primary success was defined as (1) an absolute reduction of 20% in the degree of stenosis and (2) residual nonsignificant (<50%) narrowing without major complications.

The primary success of Rotablator alone was 82%, and when adjunctive percutaneous transluminal coronary angioplasty (PTCA) was performed, the primary success rate was 94%. Figures 13–2 and 13–3 show typical examples.

Overall complications included 0.4% with perfora-

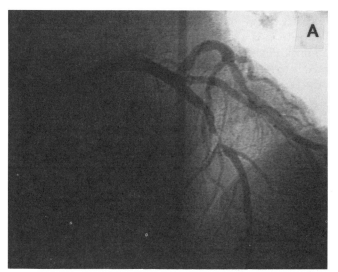
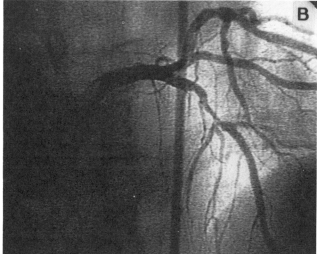
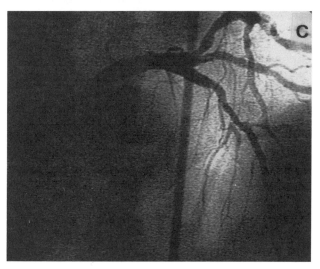

FIG 13–3.
Narrowing of the midsegment of the left anterior descending coronary artery. **A,** before rotary ablation. **B,** after rotary ablation: insufficient result. **C,** after adjunctive balloon angioplasty.

tion. Abrupt closure occurred in the catheterization laboratory in 5.6% of cases: 2.8% were transient, probably due to spasm, and were relieved by nitroglycerin, while 2.8% were persistent. Flap/dissection (non–flow limiting) was observed in 10.1% and thrombosis in 2.4%. A no-reflow phenomenon was seen in 1.8% of cases. A 0.8% rate of abrupt closure postcatheterization was observed. As a result of the events, 0.8% of patients had Q wave myocardial infarction, there was an increase in enzyme concentrations in 4.8%, and 2.4% of patients underwent emergency bypass surgery. One percent of the patients died within the hospitalization period.

Success Rate According the Type of Lesion

There was no significant difference in success rates according to lesion location, although the procedure was less successful in the right coronary artery than in the left anterior descending or circumflex arteries. The success rate in long, calcified, eccentric, bifurcated lesions and lesions on tortuous vessels was similar to the rate observed in other vessels. Interestingly, the success rate in calcified lesions was high: 86% with the Rotablator alone and 93% for the Rotablator followed by adjunctive balloon angioplasty.

Restenosis

Among 358 patients eligible for angiographic follow-up, 280 (78%) were studied angiographically at 6 months on average after the procedure. The restenosis rate was 38% in the cohort treated by the Rotablator as a stand-alone procedure and 40% when the patient had adjunctive PTCA.

QUANTITATIVE CORONARY ANGIOGRAPHY

Seventy-seven patients in the European series underwent quantitative coronary angiography analysis. Automatic edge detection and measurements were performed with the help of the CAESAR system (computerized assisted evaluation of stenosis and restenosis). These patients were subdivided in 2 groups.

Group A: Rotablator as a Stand-Alone Procedure

The results for this group are reported in Table 13–1. The reference diameter was measured at 2.84 ± 0.61 mm before the Rotablator and decreased slightly but nonsignificantly at 2.70 ± 0.62 mm after treatment. The size of the burr used in this group of patients was slightly less than the reference diameter of the vessel; the burr/reference diameter ratio was calculated at 0.70

TABLE 13–1.

Measurements of the Coronary Arteries Before and After the Procedure

Measurement	Before RA*	After RA	After RA + Balloon
Group A			
Reference diameter (mm)	2.84 ± 0.61	2.70 ± 0.62†	
MLD* (mm)	0.75 ± 0.28	1.54 ± 0.41†	
Stenosis (%)	72 ± 10	40 ± 13†	
Group B			
Reference diameter (mm)	2.74 ± 0.36	2.64 ± 0.36	2.69 ± 0.42
MLD (mm)	0.60 ± 0.25	1.19 ± 0.42†	2.04 ± 0.49†
Stenosis (%)	74 ± 9.2	57 ± 15†	30 ± 9.8†

*RA = rotary ablation; MLD = minimal luminal diameter.
† P < .001.

± 0.17. The minimal luminal diameter increased significantly from 0.75 ± 0.28 to 1.54 ± 0.41 mm (*P* <0.001). As a result, the percentage of reduction in luminal diameter significantly decreased from 72% ± 10% to 40% ± 13%.

Group B: Rotary Ablation Completed by Adjunctive Balloon Angioplasty (n = 30)

Before Rotablator treatment the reference vessel diameter measured 2.74 ± 0.54 mm, and the minimal luminal diameter reached 0.60 ± 0.25 mm. Thus, the treated narrowing was 74% ± 9.2%. The burr/reference diameter ratio was 0.69 ± 0.16.

After rotary ablation the reference diameter was unchanged (2.74 ± 0.36 before vs. 2.64 ± 0.36 mm after; not significant). The minimal luminal diameter significantly increased from 0.60 ± 0.25 to 1.19 ± 0.42 mm. However, residual stenosis, calculated at 57% ± 15%, was most often still significant (>50%). Due to this un-

TABLE 13–2.

Measurements of the Treated Segments Before, Immediately After, and the Following Day

Measurement	Before	After	Day After
Group A			
Reference diameter (mm)	3.00±0.46	3.04± 0.38	2.99±0.62
MLD* (mm)	0.87±0.32	1.76±0.48†	1.77±0.46
Stenosis (%)	69.8± 11	40± 16†	38± 15
Group B			
Reference diameter (mm)	2.68±0.42	2.81± 0.36	2.78±0.23
MLD (mm)	0.67±0.30	1.56±0.53†	1.89±0.31
Stenosis (%)	74± 13	41± 20†	31± 10

*MLD = minimal luminal diameter.
†*P* <.001.

satisfactory result, the procedure was completed by balloon angioplasty. Then the minimal luminal diameter increased to 2.04 ± 0.49 mm, and the residual stenosis was considered acceptable (30% ± 10%).

Quantitative Coronary Angiography 24 Hours After the Procedure

These results are reported in Table 13–2. In patients treated by the Rotablator alone there are no modifications the day after the procedure. The reference diameter is unchanged, but the most important observation is the absence of modification of the minimal luminal diameter: 1.76 ± 0.48 mm immediately after Rotablator treatment vs. 1.77 ± 0.46 mm (not significant) the day after. The residual stenosis was also unchanged (40% ± 16% vs. 38% ± 15%; not significant).

This observation can also be applied to the group of patients treated by the Rotablator and adjunctive PTCA.

Relationship Between the Burr Size and the Residual Luminal Diameter

We compared the size of the residual luminal diameter to the size of the burr. Figure 13–4 shows that in most of the cases the residual luminal diameter is under the identity line. The minimal residual luminal diameter/burr diameter ratio was on average 0.75 ± 0.19. This clearly demonstrates that the burr was unable to completely remove the atherosclerotic material.

COMMENTS

The mechanism of action of the Rotablator is abrasion of the occlusive material to allow restoration of lumen patency. The diamond chips of the burr remove material in millions of tiny particles. Previous experimental studies[3–5] and observations made on iliac segments treated by rotary ablation[6] showed that the resulting arterial lumen was smooth and polished.

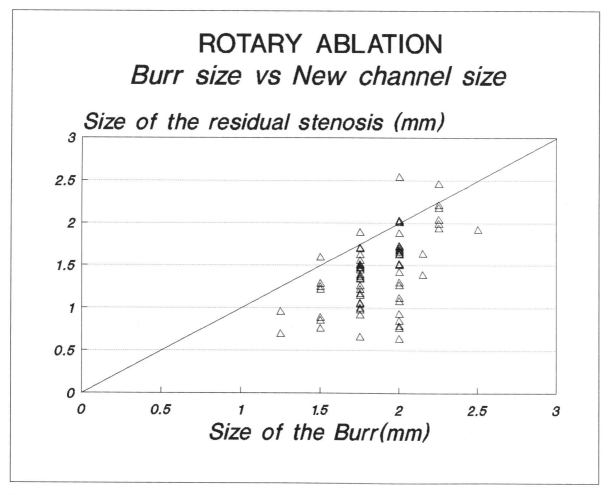

FIG 13–4.
Comparison of the burr size and the diameter of the residual stenosis.

Nevertheless, endothelium and different portions of the atherosclerotic tissue were missing. In most cases the media was not damaged.

Several problems related to this technique are of concern. It is well known that most atherosclerotic plaque is eccentric. Therefore, abrasion could cause severe injury to the normal part of the wall. Moreover, when the spinning burr is moving inside the vessel, some damage could occur in the adjacent part of the narrowing.

However, it has been shown that rotary micropulverization selectively removes firmer noncompliant material while normal elastic tissue, deflected beneath the burr, is only displaced.

Differential removal, limited to diseased surfaces, with particular affinity for harder materials including calcium is obviously clinically relevant.

It is indubitable that the endothelium of segments next to stenosis is removed. This could explain the vasospasm seen after rotational abrasion. However, in our experience, spasm can be observed 2 to 3 cm beyond the treated segment and could be related to some vibrations transmitted to the guidewire during the rotation. Similar spasms have been reported by Hansen et al.[3] in rabbit atherosclerotic arteries treated by rotational atherectomy.

Transient bradycardia and atrioventricular blocks may be related to microcavitation production. As a result of the high velocity, at the burr surface cavitations are produced according to the Bernoulli phenomenon and were documented in experimental studies.[16]

The second concern is related to the size of the particles created by rotary abrasion. Hansen et al.[3] collected the perfusate of segments of aorta treated by rotary ablation. The particles were sized and counted with a fluorescence-activated cell sorter (FACS) analyzer (Becton Dickinson), while standard-sized beads were analyzed for comparison. Large, macroscopically visible debris was not seen, and only 1.5% to 2% of particles generated by the device were larger than 10 μm. On average, the particle size was less than 5 μm. Similar observations were made by Ahn et al.[5] Furthermore, injection of technetium 99m–labeled particles into the femoral artery in dogs revealed that very few were lodged in the lower extremity and that most of them were found in the spleen, liver, etc.

Finally, scanning electronic microscopy of human iliac arteries treated by the Rotablator showed than 75% of the particles on the surface were less than 10 to 15 μm. Thus the debris is most often too small to clog capillaries.

The size of the burr is a limitation of the Rotablator: the abrasive tips are manufactured in various sizes up to 4.5 mm. To insert the device in coronary arteries we must use large guiding catheters. But even with a giant lumen guiding catheter, the inside luminal diameter is only 2.2 or 2.5 mm. In coronary arteries the size of the burr cannot exceed 2 to 2.5 mm. Therefore, for a coronary vessel of 3 to 3.5 mm, significant residual stenosis is frequently observed after treatment. Moreover, when one uses quantitative coronary angiography to compare the size of the burr and the diameter of the new channel resulting from coronary ablation, the size of this latter is only 75% of the size of the burr.

From these observations two types of strategy could be developed: one consists of starting with a small, intentionally undersized burr, with stepwise increments in abrasive tip sizes until the optimal result can be obtained. Another strategy includes the use of a small burr (1.75 to 2 mm) to "debulk" the vessel and achieve a smooth residual surface and to systematically complete the procedure with a balloon inflated at a very low pressure. Nevertheless, these strategies require further data and longer follow-up.

At present, high-speed rotary ablation appears to be most useful for (1) small vessels (2 to 2.5 mm in diameter), (2) distal locations of the lesions, (3) calcified or nondistensible lesions, and (4) eccentric lesions. More recently, Teirstein et al.[17] treated 42 patients with diffuse coronary artery disease. The procedure was very effective (success rate, 92%) in short (<1 cm) lesions, but longer lesions (>1 cm) had a decreased procedural success rate and a higher restenosis rate (75% vs. 22%).

Large coronary vessels (>3.7 mm), intracoronary thrombus, and degenerated saphenous vein grafts with friable atherosclerotic materials should be avoided.

REFERENCES

1. Simpson JB, Robertson GC, Selmon MR: Percutaneous coronary atherectomy (abstract). *J Am Coll Cardiol* 1988; 11:110.
2. Stack RS, Quigley PJ, Sketch MH: Treatment of coronary artery disease with the transluminal extraction-endarterectomy catheter: Initial results of a multicenter study (abstract). *Circulation* 1989; 80(suppl 2):852.
3. Hansen DD, Auth DC, Vrocko R, et al: Rotational atherectomy in atherosclerotic rabbit iliac arteries. *Am Heart J* 1988; 115:160–165.
4. Hansen DD, Auth DC, Hall M, et al: Rotational endarterectomy in normal canine coronary arteries. Preliminary report. *J Am Coll Cardiol* 1988; 11:1073–1077.
5. Ahn SS, Auth DC, Marcus DR, et al: Removal of focal atheromatous lesions by angioscopically guided high speed rotary atherectomy. *J Vasc Surg* 1988; 7:292–299.
6. Fourrier JL, Stankowiak C, Lablanche JM, et al: Histopathology after rotational angioplasty of peripheral arteries in human beings (abstract). *J Am Coll Cardiol* 1988; 11:109.
7. Zacca NM, Raizner AE, Noon GP, et al: Short term fol-

low up of patients treated with a recently developed rotational atherectomy device and in vivo assessment of the particles generated (abstract). *J Am Coll Cardiol* 1988; 11:109.

8. Fourrier JL, Auth DC, Lablanche JM, et al: Human percutaneous coronary rotational atherectomy: Preliminary results (abstract). *Circulation* 1988; 78(suppl 2):82.

9. Fourrier JL, Bertrand ME, Auth DC, et al: Percutaneous coronary rotational angioplasty in humans: Preliminary report. *J Am Coll Cardiol* 1989; 14:1278–1282.

10. Ginsburg R, Teirstein PS, Warth DC, et al: Percutaneous transluminal coronary rotational atheroablation: Clinical experience in 40 patients (abstract). *Circulation* 1989; 80(suppl 2):584.

11. Teirstein PS, Ginsburg R, Warth DC, et al: Complications of human coronary rotablation (abstract). *J Am Coll Cardiol* 1990; 15:57.

12. Bertrand ME, Lablanche JM, Fourrier JL, et al: Percutaneous rotary ablation. *Herz* 1990; 15:285–287.

13. Buchbinder M, O'Neill W, Warth D, et al: Percutaneous coronary rotational ablation using the Rotablator: Results of a multicenter study (abstract). *Circulation* 1990; 82(suppl 3):309.

14. Bertrand ME, Fourrier JL, Auth D, et al: Percutaneous coronary rotational angioplasty, in Topol EJ (ed): *Textbook of Interventional Cardiology*. Philadelphia, WB Saunders, 1990, pp 580–589.

15. Bertrand ME, Fourrier JL, Dietz U, et al: European experience with percutaneous transluminal coronary rotational ablation (abstract). *Circulation* 1990; 82(suppl 3):310.

16. Zotz R, Stahr P, Erbel R, et al: Analysis of high-frequency rotational angioplasty–induced echo contrast. *Cathet Cardiovasc Diagn* 1991; 22:137.

17. Teirstein PS, Warth DC, Haq N, et al: High speed rotational coronary atherectomy for patients with diffuse coronary artery disease. *J Am Coll Cardiol* 1991; 18:1694–1701.

14

Coronary Atherectomy With the TEC Device

Michael H. Sketch, Jr., M.D.

Harry R. Phillips, M.D.

The era of interventional cardiology began with the introduction of percutaneous transluminal coronary angioplasty (PTCA) by Andreas R. Grüntzig and associates in 1977.[1] Since its introduction, PTCA has gained widespread acceptance as the "gold standard" in the catheter-based treatment of acutely and chronically obstructed coronary arteries. Increased operator experience and advances in balloon catheter technology have resulted in a higher primary success rate (90% to 95%) and access to most lesions within the coronary vasculature.[2] Despite these advances, PTCA's mechanism of action results in several serious limitations. Plaque fracture with stretching of the intima and media may unpredictably result in acute occlusive dissection in 2% to 12% of patients undergoing balloon dilatation.[3] Furthermore, secondary sequelae of this disruptive process, such as thrombosis, elastic recoil, and neointimal hyperplasia, may contribute to the 30% to 45% incidence of restenosis.[4, 5] These limitations of PTCA and the desire to extend the indications for percutaneous revascularization have been the impetus behind the development of new interventional technologies.

One of these new technologies is atherectomy, which is the mechanical excision and removal of atheromatous plaque. The concept of atherectomy was introduced by John B. Simpson in an attempt to overcome some of the limitations of PTCA.[6] The hypothesis is that by excising and removing plaque a larger and smoother surface would be created with less trauma to the vessel wall than that created by balloon angioplasty, thereby reducing the potential for acute occlusion and restenosis.

HISTORICAL PERSPECTIVE

The transluminal extraction-endarterectomy catheter (TEC) is an atherectomy device designed by Interventional Technologies, Inc. (San Diego), and developed at Duke University Medical Center.

Initial success in using the TEC was demonstrated in both normal arterial segments (human cadaveric and in vivo canine) and atherosclerotic human cadaveric segments in 1987.[7, 8] These studies demonstrated that the TEC could be easily maneuvered percutaneously in canine peripheral and coronary arteries. In normal arterial segments, histologic analysis revealed focal intimal disruption with occasional excision limited to 25% of the medial thickness. In atherosclerotic arterial segments, the depth of the excision was typically limited to the media, although occasional disruption of the external elastic lamina was evident. There was no angiographic or histologic evidence of dissection or perforation. These studies led to Food and Drug Administration (FDA) approval for clinical investigation of this device in human peripheral arteries.

In December 1987, the first peripheral TEC procedure was performed in an iliac artery. The early peripheral TEC experience at Duke University Medical Center demonstrated a high success rate (94%) without perforation or distal embolization.[9] This preliminary experience demonstrated a lesion restenosis rate of 20% and a patient restenosis rate of 32%. Further analysis of these rates revealed several anatomic, clinical, and procedural variables associated with a trend toward a lower restenosis rate. These variables were subtotal occlusions (13% restenosis rate) and good distal runoff (21% restenosis rate). This initial study suggested that restenosis following this procedure may be lower than that associated with balloon angioplasty in peripheral vessels. In May 1989, this device was approved by the FDA for market release in the United States as a treatment modality for obstructive disease in peripheral vessels.

The first coronary TEC procedure was performed on a lesion in a right coronary artery in July 1988. Following the initial 50 cases at Duke University Medical Center, 18 additional investigational sites in the United States joined in the FDA multicenter investigation. Currently, over 700 coronary TEC procedures have been performed in the United States.

DESCRIPTION OF THE TEC

As previously described, the TEC device is a percutaneously introduced flexible torque tube (1.8 to 2.5 mm in diameter) designed to excise and extract atherosclerotic plaque (Fig 14–1).[8, 10] At the conical head of the catheter, there are two stainless steel blades that rotate at 750 rpm (Fig 14–2). The excised fragments are extracted through the central lumen of the catheter by vacuum suction. The proximal end of the TEC is connected to a catheter drive unit. This unit houses the motor and trigger with attachment sites for a remote battery power source and a glass reservoir to retrieve the excised debris (Fig 14–3). On top of the catheter drive unit, a lever controls both the antegrade and retrograde excursion of the cutter over a 0.014-in. guidewire in the coronary artery.

PROCEDURE

All patients are pretreated with 80 to 325 mg of aspirin, 75 mg of dipyridamole, and a calcium channel blocker. As with PTCA, the procedure is performed via a percutaneous transfemoral technique. A 10.5 F arterial sheath is used to permit insertion of a 10 F guide catheter. After insertion of the sheath, 10,000 units of heparin is administered with additional boluses hourly as necessary to maintain an activated clotting time greater than 300 seconds. The guide catheter is advanced to the ascending aorta over a 0.063-in. J wire to prevent trauma to the vessel wall. The catheter is torqued gently in a similar way to the angioplasty guiding catheter to engage into the coronary ostium. A 0.014-in. guidewire is advanced across the lesion to the distal portion of the vessel. By placing the wire as far distally as possible, the

cutter will be advanced over the more proximal stiffer portion of the wire, thus minimizing lateral movement. The torque tube cutter is then advanced over the wire proximal to the lesion and connected proximally to the catheter drive unit. Intracoronary nitroglycerin (0.1 to 0.3 mg) is administered prior to cutting to prevent coronary spasm. In addition, lactated Ringer's solution is infused through the guide catheter during periods of cutter activation.

The cutter sizes are 5.5 F (1.8 mm), 6 F (2.0 mm), 6.5 F (2.2 mm), 7 F (2.3 mm), and 7.5 F (2.5 mm). The selection of cutter size is a function of the severity of the stenosis and the adjacent normal arterial diameter. In severely stenotic lesions, a smaller cutter is initially utilized, with progression to larger cutters as necessary to achieve maximal resection of the lesion. One to three passes are made with each cutter across the lesion — each pass lasting 10 to 15 seconds. If the result remains visually unsatisfactory after treatment with the TEC (>25% luminal diameter narrowing by visual assessment), particularly in patients with large coronary vessels or saphenous vein grafts, adjunctive PTCA is performed to optimize the angiographic appearance.

Following the procedure, the heparin therapy can be discontinued if there is no evidence of dissection or thrombus, and the sheath can be removed. The patient is maintained on an aspirin regimen for an indefinite period of time. Prior to discharge, arrangements are made for 6-month clinical/angiographic follow-up.

CASE SELECTION

The selection criteria for transluminal extraction-endarterectomy have been altered by the evolution in the technology and growing operator experience. The initial criteria included patients meeting standard clinical criteria for angioplasty revascularization with proximal, discrete, concentric lesions in nontortuous vessels. The criteria have expanded to include more diffuse and complex lesions often unfavorable for PTCA, such as ostial lesions and bypass vein graft lesions with thrombus present. The current exclusion criteria are as follows:

1. Tortuous anatomy proximal to the target lesion
2. Major side branch (<2 mm) involvement at the target lesion
3. Severe eccentricity or angulation of the target lesion
4. Heavily calcified lesion
5. Total occlusion unable to be successfully recanalized with a guidewire
6. Coronary ectasia
7. Major dissection

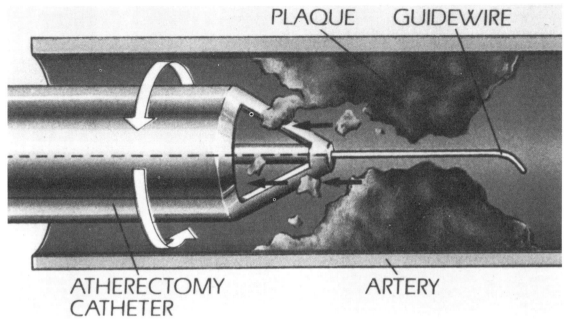

FIG 14–1.
Diagrammatic illustration of the transluminal extraction–endarterectomy catheter being advanced across an atherosclerotic plaque by tracking over a steerable 0.014-in. guidewire. (From Roto-rooter Artery Cleaner. *Popular Mechanics* 1988; 165:18. Used by permission.)

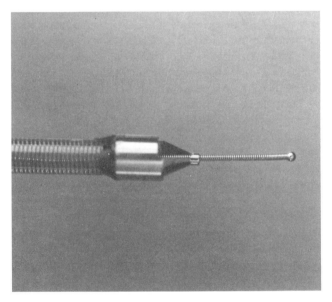

FIG 14–2.
A close-up of the torque tube and cutter head of the TEC over a 0.014-in. guidewire.

8. Severe peripheral vascular disease
9. Aspirin allergy
10. Bleeding diathesis including thrombolytic drug therapy

Lesions with marked angulation (>45 degrees) should be considered a contraindication because of the potential risk of vessel perforation by deep cuts due to the angulation of the vessel. Heavily calcified lesions often prevent the device from crossing the lesion. Treatment of lesions with major dissections should be avoided because of the risk of perforation due to the pre-existing poor integrity of the vessel wall. The need for a 10.5 F sheath excludes certain patients with extensive peripheral vascular disease.

There have been several reports of a favorable outcome with the use of the TEC in the presence of thrombus.[11, 12] In addition, several investigators have reported the TEC to be effective in treating ostial lesions. With continued operator experience and catheter refinements, the indications for the TEC should expand.

RESULTS

In July 1988, clinical investigation of the coronary TEC was begun at Duke University Medical Center.

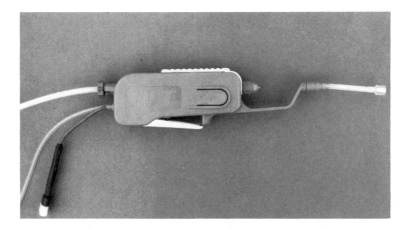

FIG 14–3.
The catheter drive unit of the TEC that houses the motor and trigger with sites for attachment of a remote battery power source and vacuum bottle for retrieval of excised material.

After an initial experience with 50 cases, the Duke Multicenter Coronary TEC Registry was initiated with five clinical sites. In addition to Duke, these sites include William Beaumont Hospital in Royal Oak, Michigan (William W. O'Neill, M.D.); Wichita Institute for Clinical Research in Wichita, Kansas (Joseph P. Galichia, M.D.); Samuel Merritt Hospital in Oakland, California (Robert C. Feldman, M.D.); and Cardiovascular Institute of the South in Houma, Louisiana (Craig M. Walker, M.D.).

In a preliminary series of patients from this registry, coronary transluminal extraction-endarterectomy was performed on 223 lesions in 201 patients.[13] The TEC was used exclusively in 76 (34%) lesions and in conjunction with balloon angioplasty in 147 (66%). The lesion distribution was protected left main, 8; left anterior descending, 53; circumflex, 23; right coronary, 55; and saphenous vein grafts, 84. Primary success (<50% residual diameter stenosis by digital analysis) was achieved in 94% (130/139) native coronary and 98% (82/84) vein graft lesions. The mean digital diameter stenosis of 76% was reduced to 36%.

In this initial series, the procedural complications included abrupt coronary reocclusion (2), major dissection (3), distal embolization (3), perforation (4), and thrombosis (1). These resulted in emergency coronary bypass surgery in seven patients. There were no procedural deaths. Distal embolization was not seen in any patient following transluminal extraction-endarterectomy.

Six-month angiographic follow-up (by digital analysis) was obtained in 95 of the 102 eligible patients (93%) in this series. The restenosis rate was 44% (42/95), with restenosis defined as <50% luminal diameter narrowing by quantitative digital analysis. In comparison, these results are similar to the restenosis rate of 43% recently reported in 2,191 consecutive PTCA patients at Duke University Medical Center during a similar time period with an 84% 6-month angiographic follow-up rate.[5]

The preliminary results of a study examining the safety and efficacy of the TEC in the management of patients with saphenous vein graft stenosis were presented at the 40th Annual Scientific Session of the American College of Cardiology in March 1991.[12] In this study, 125 vein graft lesions in 98 patients were treated with the TEC. The mean vein graft age was 8.8 years with a range of 1 to 18 years. Thirty percent of the lesions were considered unsuitable for PTCA due to diffuse disease or intraluminal thrombi. The procedural success rate (<50% residual stenosis) was 96% (120/125). There was no evidence of distal embolization with an acute myocardial infarction.

SUMMARY

The TEC is one of an array of new devices undergoing clinical investigation since the introduction of PTCA by Andreas Grüntzig in 1977. The device is still in the early phases of evaluation. Less than 2½ years have passed since the first transluminal extraction-endarterectomy was performed in a human coronary artery, and the majority of cases have been performed over the past year. In this time frame, the device has evolved significantly and become more reliable and functional.

The initial experience with the TEC in coronary arteries demonstrated that the device can be used to excise and remove atheromatous plaque percutaneously from a wide variety of sites in diseased coronary arteries, with resultant improvement in coronary luminal diameter in a high percentage of patients. Distal embolization was

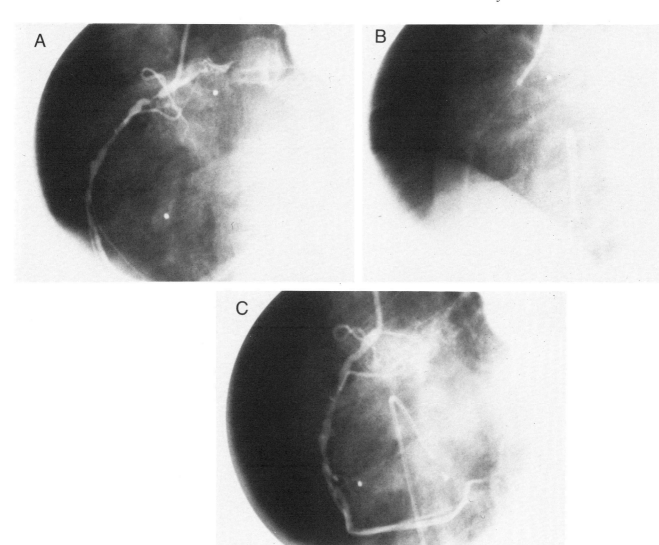

FIG 14–4.
A, a diffusely diseased right coronary artery with a proximal 95% stenosis. **B,** the rotating TEC being advanced over the guidewire into the occlusion. **C,** a residual 15% stenosis at the TEC site. (From Stack RS, et al: Extraction atherectomy, in Topol EJ (ed): *Textbook of Interventional Cardiology.* Philadelphia, WB Saunders, 1990, pp 590–602. Used by permission.)

not seen in any patient following TEC atherectomy. In this initial experience, the restenosis rate appears similar to PTCA; however these data are limited by the small number of patients.

While balloon angioplasty of diffusely diseased grafts is associated with a low success rate and a high acute complication rate including distal embolization and myocardial infarction, preliminary studies suggest that the TEC may have special utility in this situation. Although 30% of the graft lesions were considered unsuitable for PTCA due to diffuse disease or intraluminal thrombi, early studies with the TEC in vein bypass grafts have demonstrated a high procedural success rate (96%) without evidence of distal embolization or myo-

cardial infarction. The effect of the TEC on restenosis in saphenous vein grafts remains to be determined.

The major limitation of the current TEC design is that the maximum cutter size is only 7.5 F (2.5 mm). As a result, adjunctive balloon angioplasty is frequently needed to optimize the angiographic appearance, especially in patients with large coronary vessels or saphenous vein grafts. To overcome this limitation and enable the TEC to be used as a stand-alone treatment in the majority of coronary artery lesions, an expandable cutter and eccentric cutter are in the developmental phases.

Upon completion of the developmental phases of the TEC, further studies will be necessary to evaluate the

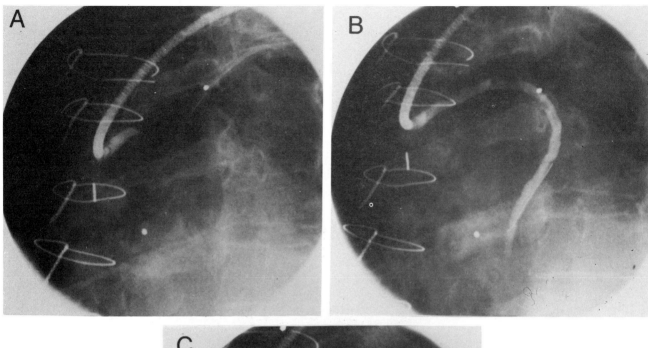

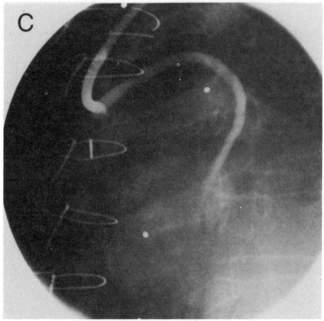

FIG 14–5.
A, a total occlusion of a saphenous vein graft to the left anterior descending artery. **B,** the result following treatment with the TEC above—a guidewire is present across the lesion. **C,** the final result after both the TEC and adjunctive balloon angioplasty.

efficacy of this device for both acute and long-term outcome, including randomized trials with PTCA and coronary artery bypass surgery. In addition, the TEC will need to be compared with other new devices undergoing clinical investigation for use in myocardial revascularization.

REFERENCES

1. Grüntzig AR, Senning A, Siegenthaler WE: Nonoperative dilatation of coronary artery stenosis: Percutaneous transluminal coronary angioplasty. *N Engl J Med* 1979; 301:61–68.
2. Baim DS (ed): A symposium: Interventional cardiology 1987. *Am J Cardiol* 1988; 61:1176.

3. Simpfendorfer C, Belardi J, Bellamy G, et al: Frequency, management and follow-up of patients with acute coronary occlusion after percutaneous transluminal angioplasty. *Am J Cardiol* 1987; 59:267–269.

4. Blackshear JL, O'Callaghan WG, Califf RM: Medical approaches to prevention of restenosis after coronary angioplasty. *J Am Coll Cardiol* 1987; 9:834–848.

5. Tcheng JE, Fortin DF, Frid DJ, et al: Conditional probabilities of restenosis following coronary angioplasty (abstract). *Circulation* 1990; 82(suppl 3):1.

6. Simpson JB: Future interventional techniques, in Califf RM (ed): *Acute Coronary Care in the Thrombolytic Era.* St Louis, Mosby–Year Book, 1988, pp 392–404.

7. Perez JA, Hinohara T, Quigley PJ, et al: In-vitro and in-vivo experimental results using new wire-guided concentric atherectomy device (abstract). *J Am Coll Cardiol* 1988; 11:109.

8. Stack RS, Califf RM, Phillips HR, et al: Advances in cardiovascular technologies: Interventional cardiac catheterization at Duke Medical Center. *Am J Cardiol* 1988; 62:1–44.

9. Sketch MH Jr, Newman GE, McCann L, et al: Transluminal extraction–endarterectomy in peripheral vascular disease: Late clinical and angiographic follow-up (abstract). *Circulation* 1989; 80(suppl 2):305

10. Sketch MH Jr, Phillips HR, Lee M, et al: Coronary transluminal extraction–endarterectomy. *J Intervent Cardiol* 1991; 3:23–28.

11. Rosenblum J, Pensabene JF, Kramer B: The TEC device: Distal atherectomy and removal of an intracoronary thrombus. *J Intervent Cardiol* 1991; 3:41–43.

12. O'Neill WW, Meany TB, Kramer B, et al: The role of atherectomy in the management of saphenous vein graft disease (abstract). *J Am Coll Cardiol* 1991; 17(suppl 4):384.

13. Sketch MH Jr, O'Neill WW, Galichia JP, et al: The Duke Multicenter Coronary Transluminal Extraction–Endarterectomy Registry: Acute and chronic results (abstract). *J Am Coll Cardiol* 1991; 17(suppl 4):31.

15

Directional Coronary Atherectomy

Matthew R. Selmon, M.D.

Tomoaki Hinohara, M.D.

Gregory C. Robertson, M.D.

James W. Vetter, M.D.

Dennis J. Sheehan, M.D.

Bruce J. McAuley, M.D.

John B. Simpson, M.D.

Coronary revascularization with percutaneous transluminal coronary angioplasty (PTCA) has become a widely accepted strategy for the management of atherosclerotic coronary artery disease, with over 400,000 procedures performed in the United States in 1990. Despite improved balloon technology and increased operator experience, abrupt closure, primary failure, and restenosis remain major limitations of PTCA.[1-4] As a response to these problems, the concept of atheroma removal was introduced by John B. Simpson, and the term *atherectomy* was coined.[5-7] It was postulated that atherectomy rather than dilatation may offer the following advantages:

1. Dissection may be avoided by "debulking" the atherosclerotic plaque and leaving the luminal borders smooth (with less residual stenosis).
2. By increasing lumen diameter and improving flow characteristics, platelet aggregation and thrombosis may be reduced (possibly avoiding acute closure).
3. Increased control and efficacy may allow percutaneous revascularization in lesions unfavorable for PTCA because of "high-risk" anatomy or subsets with known poor results such as eccentric and ostial lesions.

After extensive experience at Sequoia Hospital and a large multicenter trial demonstrating safety and efficacy, directional coronary atherectomy (DCA) was approved by the Food and Drug Administration (FDA) for general use in September 1990. Despite significant differences in equipment and technique from PTCA, DCA has become widespread in the United States. Over 25,000 procedures have now been performed in 500 centers. The Sequoia experience and multicenter data along with the technical aspects for the performance of DCA will be reviewed.

HISTORICAL PERSPECTIVE

By the early 1980s the limitations of angioplasty were well recognized, and alternative technologies became appealing.[8] The DCA catheter was conceived and designed to improve the safety and efficacy of revascularization by controlled plaque removal. The initial prototype catheters, similar in concept and design to the current peripheral catheter, were used in cadaver and rabbit iliac arteries in early 1985. After demonstrating that atheroma could be effectively removed transluminally without causing perforation or significant vessel wall disruption, the first peripheral atherectomy was performed in August 1985. As an intraoperative procedure, a midvessel superficial femoral artery stenosis was removed with an excellent angiographic result and retrieval of four small atherosclerotic specimens. Subsequently in 1985, a percutaneous application to iliac and superficial femoral arteries was demonstrated to be feasible and effective as well.[6] The peripheral experience continued at Sequoia Hospital and demonstrated its safety and efficacy with a low incidence of complications, specifically perforations and dissections.[9] Based on these data and early multicenter experience, atherectomy was approved by the FDA for the treatment of peripheral vascular disease in May 1987.

Subsequent follow-up angiographic studies of the Sequoia peripheral experience demonstrated that restenosis was significantly reduced when less than 30% residual stenosis was achieved as compared with 30% to 50% residual stenosis. This suggested that more complete atheroma removal was important to lower restenosis rates.[10] More recently, Graor and Whitlow have compared their peripheral DCA experience with angioplasty and have demonstrated both excellent acute results and restenosis rates lower than can be achieved with balloon dilatation.[11]

After the initial feasibility studies in 1985, work began on the application of atherectomy to the coronary arteries. The initial catheters were based in concept on the original peripheral device, with a tubular housing, a window, enclosed cutter, and balloon support member. A smaller housing was required along with a flexible nose cone and over-the-wire coaxial technology. A relatively large guiding catheter system was required to allow passage of the device and provide adequate support for traversing the coronary arteries.

By 1986 the first coronary devices were available and tested in cadaver arteries.[12] In October 1986 the first human coronary atherectomy was attempted but was unsuccessful because of the inability to advance the catheter to the lesion. Subsequent improvements in both guiding catheter and AtheroCath design led in February 1987 to the first successful DCA of a right coronary artery stenosis. The initial 50 DCA procedures were performed at Sequoia Hospital before investigational sites were selected across the United States and Europe.[10] Multicenter experience began in June 1988 and included St. Vincent's Hospital in Indianapolis (Cass Pinkerton); Beth Israel Hospital in Boston (Don Baim and Robert Safian); the University of Michigan (Eric Topol and Steve Ellis); Cleveland Clinic (Jay Holman and Pat Whitlow); Mayo Clinic in Rochester, Minnesota (Ron Vlietstra and David Holmes); Emory University in Atlanta (Spencer King, John Douglas, Gary Roubin, and Nicholas Lembo); and Christ Hospital in Cincinnati (Dean Kereiakes and Charles Abbot-Smith). After review by the FDA for safety and efficacy as well as restenosis in the first 1,000 patients, DCA was approved for the treatment of coronary atherosclerotic disease in September 1990.[13, 14]

Over the past 5 years catheters have evolved to provide a lower profile, safer nose cone, enhanced torque control, and improved quality to avoid technical failures. Experience gained through multicenter evaluation has led to current recommendations regarding case selection and procedural techniques. Our experience at Sequoia Hospital as well as the multicenter data demonstrate a learning curve even for experienced PTCA operators, with lower success rates and higher complications in the first 25 cases.[15] Training courses have been established to teach DCA techniques to minimize the effect of the learning curve as the technology is disseminated. It is important to maintain objective critical viewpoints regarding the efficacy and safety of any new technique. Trials have now begun in a prospective randomized fashion to compare DCA with standard conventional balloon angioplasty. The atherectomy procedure, however, will continue to evolve rapidly as design changes are available based on growing experience over the next several years.

ATHERECTOMY CATHETER DESIGN

The Simpson Coronary AtheroCath (Devices for Vascular Intervention, Redwood City, Calif) is composed of three functional units: the proximal control assembly, the midshaft, and the distal cut and retrieval mechanism (Fig 15–1). The proximal assembly includes the motor drive unit (MDU), ports for flushing and balloon inflation, and a rotator connection to the shaft. The MDU is a disposable, hand-held, battery-operated motor that spins the cutter drive cable at 2,500 rpm. A small lever operated with the thumb advances and retracts the cutter. The MDU attaches to the AtheroCath by a friction lock. Two Luer connections are located just distal to the MDU. The larger connection is a one-way valve for flushing the catheter around the cutter drive cable. Flush exits through the housing window. The other port is for balloon inflation and connects to any standard inflation device. A rotator connection is located just distal to the inflation and flush ports and allows nearly a 1:1 torque control of the distal catheter housing for directional alignment of the window. The catheter shaft is 130 mm long and designed coaxially with a cutter torque cable (CTC) and housing torque cable (HTC) over a 0.014-in. wire. It connects to the distal housing and cutter mechanism.

The distal cutter housing is made of gold-plated stainless steel and available in 5 F (1.66 mm), 6 F (2 mm), and 7 F (2.3 mm) sizes (Fig 15–2). The window is 10 mm long and opens over a 120-degree arch. A bal-

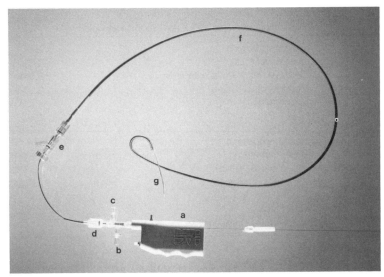

FIG 15–1.
Directional coronary atherectomy equipment. **A,** motor drive unit; **B,** flush port; **C,** inflation port; **D,** rotator; **E,** rotating hemostatic valve (RHV); **F,** guiding catheter; **G,** AtheroCath.

loon support member made of Surlyn is attached opposite the window. The balloon functions to anchor the device in position during cutting and is designed for relatively low-pressure inflations, less than 50 psi. A cup-shaped cutter is located inside the housing and coaxially over the 0.014-in. guidewire. It advances the length of the window and cuts any plaque that protrudes inside the housing window. The design attempts to prevent deep vascular wall structures from access to the cutter. The nose cone is attached distally to the housing and is made of a stainless steel braid covered with Surlyn. A safety ribbon and a vent are incorporated into the design for ease of use and safety. The nose cone is flexible and tapered to provide improved tracking and crossing profiles. After cutting, tissue is packed around the guidewire in the nose cone and retrieved after the catheter is removed from the artery.

A second-generation catheter is now available that incorporates improvements in overall profile and nose cone design. The balloon material, polyethylene terephthalate (PET), is thinner and allows a full 1 F size improvement over the standard catheters. The nose cone is a urethane-covered gold coil that is more flexible for better tracking and offers a larger lumen for tissue storage. The catheter overall allows access to smaller and more tortuous vessels and distal stenoses with less concern over nose cone trauma.

A guiding catheter system was required to allow passage of the large, relatively stiff catheters to the coronary ostium and provide backup support for entering and crossing coronary lesions. New shapes were designed that straightened the acute angles of conventional catheters into C-shaped configurations. Guiding catheters for the left coronary artery are available in 10 and 11 F sizes (JL 4 and JL 4.5) with internal dimensions of 8 and 9 F, respectively. The right coronary ar-

tery guiding catheters are available only in 9.5 and 10 F (JR 3.5 and JR 4) after an increased rate of guide catheter–induced dissections was seen with the 11 F size. Right and left graft guides are available for directional coronary atherectomy of saphenous vein grafts (JRG and JLG). All guiding catheters are constructed of stainless steel braid covered with urethane, with three distal side holes, a radiopaque tip marker, and a soft, 2-mm distal end for atraumatic engagement.

CLINICAL RESULTS

Experience at Sequoia Hospital and subsequently the multicenter data have documented the safety and efficacy of DCA.[15] Through June 1991, 1,092 lesions were treated in 939 patients at Sequoia Hospital. Success was

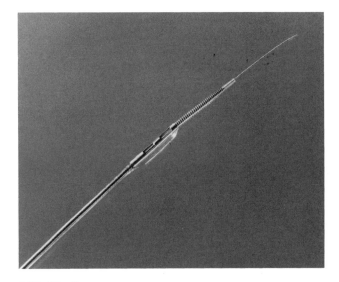

FIG 15–2.
Distal atherectomy catheter.

defined as less than 50% residual stenosis with tissue retrieval and absence of major complications. In 89% of the cases, DCA success was achieved. When combined with PTCA, 94% of cases were successful, with major complications occurring in 3.3%. An average of 14.9 mg of tissue was removed from each lesion with a residual stenosis of 17% by quantitative analysis. The average postprocedure luminal diameter was 2.7 mm. Success rates for various coronary arteries are shown in Table 15–1.

Complications related to DCA are summarized in Table 15–2. Major complications included death (0.3%), Q wave myocardial infarction (0.5%), and coronary events requiring emergency coronary bypass surgery (3.2%). Coronary perforation was an infrequent complication occurring in 4 patients (0.4%). None of the perforations resulted in hemopericardium in the Sequoia experience. Cardiac tamponade as a result of coronary perforation has been reported, however, in the multicenter experience. The risk of coronary perforation remains the single greatest difference between complications of conventional balloon angioplasty and DCA, and avoidance requires meticulous case selection and technique. Other less significant complications such as distal embolization occurred in 1.8% of native vessels, but more commonly in diffusely diseased saphenous vein grafts. This is probably due to the degenerated atheromatous material commonly seen in the older vein grafts. Guiding catheter–induced dissection occurred in 0.6%, primarily of the right coronary artery, before a decrease in the size of the guiding catheter from 11 F to 9.5 F occurred. In-hospital late occlusions were infrequent (0.8%) and probably related to dissections and thrombus. This apparent stable lumen following DCA has been an attractive advantage of the technique.

Data from the multicenter experience was collected from June 1988 to early 1990 and included the initial experience of 1,200 cases (at 25 centers in the United

TABLE 15–2.

Complications Related to DCA—Sequoia Hospital

Major complications	3.3%
In-hospital death	0.3%
Q wave myocardial infarction	0.5%
Emergency CABG*	3.2%
Perforation	0.4%
Guide dissection	0.2%
Occlusive complication	2.6%
Other complications	16.2%
Distal embolism	1.8%
CK* elevation (mild)	12.3%
In-hospital occlusion	0.8%
Stroke	0.3%
Groin repair	1.0%

*CABG = coronary artery bypass grafting; CK = creatine kinase.

States). The results were similar to the Sequoia experience, with an overall success rate of 86% and a major complication rate of 4.0%. Interestingly, the major complication rate fell from 5.3% in the first 600 cases to 2.3% in the latter 600 cases. This probably reflects operator experience, case selection, and improved equipment.[16]

Because of the stable lumen following plaque removal with DCA, the procedure has been applied to a variety of patients who were felt to be poor candidates or at high risk for conventional PTCA.[17] The effect of lesion characteristics on the outcome of DCA is summarized in Table 15–3. For eccentric and complex lesions, success remains high at 87%. Even for lengthy lesions, the success rate is 88%, although the incidence of major complications is as high as 6.3%. DCA also appears to be effective for intimal flaps, ulceration, dissections, and nonaorta ostial lesions. Calcification of the diseased artery either at the site or proximal to the stenosis remains a significant obstacle, with success falling to 70% when calcium is present (52% for primary lesions and 83% for restenosis lesions). When combined with PTCA, however, the overall success rate of calcified lesions reaches 87%. The reasons for failure include the inability to reach the lesion as well as the inability to cross or successfully remove the plaque.

When PTCA fails, DCA may be used as a salvage technique in certain circumstances. At Sequoia Hospital, 42 PTCA failures have been approached with DCA as a salvage technique.[18] Twenty-five were performed emergently and 17 electively following the failed angioplasty. Overall success was achieved in 86%, with a bypass surgical rate of 10%. High success was obtained when angioplasty was due to short focal elastic lesions that simply failed to dilate adequately (90%). Marginal success (70%) was achieved when large dissections were approached. This category of patients represents a

TABLE 15—1.

Vessel and DCA Outcome—Sequoia Hospital*

Vessel[†]	n	DCA Success (%)	Major Complication[‡] (%)
LM	45	80	0
LAD	528	92	2.6
RCA	277	85	5.1
Cx	62	86	3.3
Branch	21	90	0
SVG	158	92	1.9

*One thousand ninety-two consecutive lesions treated through June 1991.

[†]LM = left main; LAD = left anterior descending; Cx = circumflex; SVG = saphenous vein graft.

[‡]Death, Q wave myocardial infarction or emergency coronary artery bypass grafting.

TABLE 15–3.

Lesion Characteristics and Outcome of DCA*

Characteristic	No. of Lesions	DCA Success (%)	DCA & PTCA Success (%)[†]	Major Complications (%)
Single lesion	105	97	91	0
Complex	342	87	93	3.8
Eccentric	188	87	93	3.2
Lesion ≥ 10 mm	97	88	92	6.3
Calcification	70	70	87	5.7
Abnormal contour	54	93	94	5.6
Angulation	55	86	91	3.6

*From Hinohara T, Robertson GC, Selmon MR, et al: *J Am Coll Cardiol* 1991; 17:1112–1120. Used by permission.
[†]Combined success rate for DCA and PTCA for DCA failures.

highly selected population in which success was anticipated because of the anatomy proximal to the stenosis. Due to difficult logistic circumstances, the cases are more complex and should only be attempted by operators highly experienced with elective DCA. If extensive spiral dissection is present, DCA should be avoided because of the potentially high risk of perforation.

CASE SELECTION

Selection of cases for DCA differs from PTCA. Its application is limited in many patients because of the large, rigid catheter housing. In other circumstances, however, the side-cutting mechanism and predictable results may extend the indication for percutaneous revascularization. For consideration of DCA, the primary issue involves accessibility to the stenosis. Accessibility is determined by vessel size, location of the lesion, vessel curvature and tortuosity, vessel compliance, and guiding catheter alignment and support. Case selection issues are summarized in Table 15–4. The minimum vessel size of the referenced segment should be 2.5 mm. Lesions in the left main artery are easily approached as well as in the proximal and midsegments of the left anterior descending coronary artery. Lesions in the proximal and midsegments of the right coronary artery are also accessible in most patients. A significant "shepherd's crook" deformity of the proximal segment of the right coronary artery or an extremely anterior origin of the right coronary artery may limit accessibility. Lesions beyond the acute margin may also be difficult to reach unless the proximal length of the right coronary artery is large and relatively straight. Stenoses beyond the crux or in the posterior descending artery are not recommended for DCA. Circumflex stenoses remain challenging because of the angled origin from the left main artery. Most patients with a large, short left main and a large circumflex artery have favorable anatomy for access to the proximal and midportions of the circumflex artery. If the angle off the left main artery is greater than 45 degrees or if calcium is present in the bifurcation, DCA should be avoided. Saphenous vein grafts are typically large and straight and offer little resistance to passage of the AtheroCath. Difficulties may arise, however, if severe angulation is present proximally in the graft. Atherectomy of an aorta ostial lesion is also technically difficult, especially when guiding catheter alignment is not coaxial. Atherectomy of internal mammary grafts is not feasible with the current-generation catheter and guiding equipment.

The primary determinants of accessibility beyond vessel size and location involve tortuosity and vessel compliance. Because of the rigid nature of the AtherCath housing, the vessel proximal to the stenosis is required to "straighten out" to allow passage, except in very large arteries. This is easily achieved in most normal arterial segments. When diffuse atherosclerotic plaque is present or calcification of the vessel wall creates a noncompliant and inflexible artery, passage of the

TABLE 15–4.

Case Selection for DCA

Vessel size: ≥2.5 mm
Lesion type: Primary or restenosis
Accessibility:
    Location*:
        LM
        LAD: Ostial, proximal, mid
        RCA: Ostial, proximal, mid
        Cx: Ostial, proximal, mid, shallow takeoff
        SVG: Ostial, proximal, mid, distal anastomosis
        Large branch: Diagonal, marginal
    Tortuosity: None or mild
    Diffuse disease: Absent
    Peripheral vascular disease: Absent

*LM = left main; LAD = left anterior descending; RCA = right coronary artery; Cx = circumflex artery; SVG = saphenous vein graft.

AtheroCath may be very difficult or impossible. In large, diffusely diseased arteries, the catheter typically will pass without significant resistance. In a smaller artery, however, especially combined with some tortuosity, resistance may increase to the point at which the catheter may not pass successfully.

Another consideration in case selection is the 15- to 20-mm arterial segment immediately distal to the stenosis. This segment should be relatively large, straight, and disease free to accommodate the nose cone of the AtheroCath. If plaque is present, it may need to be treated either with DCA or PTCA if dissection or disruption occurs following trauma with the nose cone. When distal disease is present, a second-generation device with a more flexible and atraumatic nose cone should be chosen.

DIRECTIONAL CORONARY ATHERECTOMY PROCEDURE (TECHNICAL ASPECTS)

The procedure for DCA is based on standard PTCA technique, although significant differences in equipment make DCA generally more difficult. After initial angiography is performed to confirm anatomy, an 11 F sheath is introduced into the femoral artery. If tortuosity is present in the iliac system, a long sheath should be used. The guiding catheter is advanced over an introducer and a 0.038-in. guidewire to protect the guide catheter and avoid trauma to the walls of the aorta. The wire and introducer are held fixed after reaching the supravalvular area, and the guiding catheter is advanced over the introducer and wire until it is near the coronary ostium. The wire and introducer are removed, and the catheter is flushed. Engagement of the left guide is frequently achieved by a gentle clockwise rotation and advancement. If the anatomy is unusual, the guide may require other manipulation to engage. The right coronary guides are engaged in a manner similar to PTCA guides. Care should always be taken to not deeply seat the guide or vigorously torque after engagement. The atherectomy catheter is then introduced through the rotating hemostatic valve (RHV) and advanced to the distal end of the guide, just above the side holes. Care should be taken during insertion through the RHV to avoid damaging the nose cone. The 0.014-in. Hi-Torque Floppy (Advanced Cardiovascular Systems [ACS], Temecula, Calif) guidewire is then advanced across the stenosis and distally in the target artery. The AtheroCath is advanced over the wire, through the artery, and across the lesion. Significant resistance will be met as the AtheroCath nears the distal end of the guid-

ing catheter and enters the coronary. The resistance to entering the coronary artery may be minimized and guide position will be more stable if a coaxial alignment can be achieved between the guide and the coronary ostium. As the AtheroCath is advanced, constant forward pressure and gentle torque can be applied. "Jackhammering" to cross the lesion is rarely effective and should be avoided. If the lesion cannot be crossed, the catheter is removed and the lesion predilated with a 2-mm balloon, or a smaller AtheroCath is chosen. It is preferable to perform an exchange once crossing has been attempted so that wire position is maintained in case lesion trauma results in vessel closure. In de novo lesions with calcification, standard predilatation with a 2-mm balloon is advisable to minimize crossing time and vessel trauma.

After the AtheroCath is placed across the lesion, the position of the window should be confirmed with gentle contrast injection through the guiding catheter. The balloon is then inflated to low pressures (10 psi) to stabilize the catheter and "push" the plaque into the window (see Fig 15–3). The cutter is then withdrawn and the MDU activated. The cutter is advanced slowly forward over a period of 4 to 7 seconds until the cut is completed. A tactile sense of resistance can be appreci-

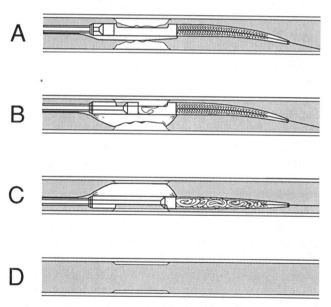

FIG 15–3.
Directional coronary atherectomy procedure. **A,** device is positioned across the stenosis. **B,** balloon is inflated to low pressure (10 psi), the cutter is retracted, then activated and advanced, excising any tissue that protrudes into the window. **C,** balloon is deflated and the catheter is rotated to another area, then the balloon-cutter sequence repeated, collecting excised atheroma in the nose cone. **D,** postatherectomy.

ated during cutting as experience is gained. If significant resistance is met, as with calcified lesions, the cutting rate and balloon pressures should be reduced sequentially as needed. After the cut is completed, the balloon is deflated and the catheter torqued 45 to 90 degrees to direct the window to another area of plaque on the vessel wall, and the sequence of balloon inflation and cutting is repeated. A series of four to eight cuts is completed, and the catheter is withdrawn to assess results. During the cutting sequence, wire position in the distal portion of the target vessel should be monitored and fixed by holding the wire to prevent movement. Additional passes are made until the catheter is filled or the desired angiographic result is obtained. Balloon pressures may be slowly increased to 20 to 30 psi if needed to remove plaque. If the AtheroCath is relatively small for the vessel, higher pressures may be needed to achieve an atherectomy result. If the device size-to-vessel ratio is appropriate or somewhat large, low pressure should suffice. When significant calcification is present, pressure up to 30 to 50 psi may be needed to successfully remove plaque. As the nose cone fills with atheroma, guidewire movement becomes "sticky" and ultimately fixed, and the nose cone must be removed with the catheter to empty it. Typically, repeat crossing with the guidewire can be accomplished safely and easily if needed after the initial series of cuts.

Determining an end point to complete the procedure is based primarily on the angiographic appearance. Intraluminal ultrasound or angioscopy may be helpful for operators experienced in the application of these new techniques. At Sequoia Hospital the goal is to achieve a 0% to 20% residual stenosis, with smooth luminal borders and retrieval of tissue. We try to avoid "overtreating" because deep arterial wall cuts risk perforation and possible pseudoaneurysm formation.

The recommended medication is similar to angioplasty methods. Sequoia Hospital patients receive premedication with aspirin, 80 to 325 mg at least 24 hours in advance of the procedure, and a calcium channel blocker. Heparin is administered prior to atherectomy as a bolus of 10,000 units with an additional 3,000 units/hr. The activated clotting time (ACT) is checked after the initial bolus, with additional heparin to achieve and maintain an ACT greater than 350 seconds. Intracoronary nitroglycerin is given frequently if coronary spasm is seen or suspected. In patients with unstable symptoms or visible intraluminal thrombus, intracoronary urokinase may be helpful prior to or after atherectomy. Following the procedure sheaths are removed approximately 3 hours after the heparin effect is diminished. The ACT is checked prior to sheath removal. If a suboptimal result is achieved or there has been intraluminal

thrombus, the heparin therapy is continued for an additional 18 to 24 hours before sheath removal. The patients subsequently remain on an aspirin regimen indefinitely and a calcium channel blocker for 1 to 3 weeks.

FAVORABLE AND UNFAVORABLE LESIONS FOR DIRECTIONAL CORONARY ATHERECTOMY

Focal, concentric, smooth lesions in a large, nontortuous vessel, which are ideal for PTCA, are also ideal lesions for DCA; a high success rate is achieved with a low complication rate (see Fig 15–4). In addition to these simple lesions, many types of lesions that are unfavorable for PTCA are often treated effectively by DCA. These favorable characteristics are summarized in Table 15–5.

Because of the nature of the side-cutting mechanism, eccentric lesions are often treated effectively by DCA.[17] The normal vessel wall can be avoided and the window directed toward the atheromatous side of the involved vessel. Frequently with angioplasty the normal vessel wall is simply stretched, and plaque recoils back into the lumen following dilatation, with significant dissection, although with continued high-grade residual stenosis (see Fig 15–5). Other types of abnormal contour such as flaplike lesions, ulcerations, or minor spontaneous dissections can also be treated effectively with DCA, which leaves a large angiographic lumen and smooth borders following the procedure (see Fig 15–6). Lesions less than 10 mm seem to be ideal for atherectomy since the length of the window is 10 mm. Longer lesions up to 20 mm, however, can be effectively treated by overlapping cuts. There may be a distinct advantage in longer lesions by removing plaque and preventing dissections where a large amount of atheromatous

TABLE 15–5.
Lesion Characteristics Favorable and Unfavorable for DCA

Favorable
  Eccentricity: Eccentric, concentric
  Contour: Normal, limited dissection, ulceration, flap
  Ostial involvement:
    Aorta ostial lesion (LM, RCA, SVG)
    Nonaorta ostial lesion (LAD, Cx, branches)
  Lesion Length: Discrete or tubular, <20 mm.
Unfavorable
  Vessel size: <2.5 mm
  Calcification: Moderate, heavy
  Angulation: >45 degrees
  Lesion length: >20 mm
  Dissection: Extensive or spiral
  Degenerative SVG

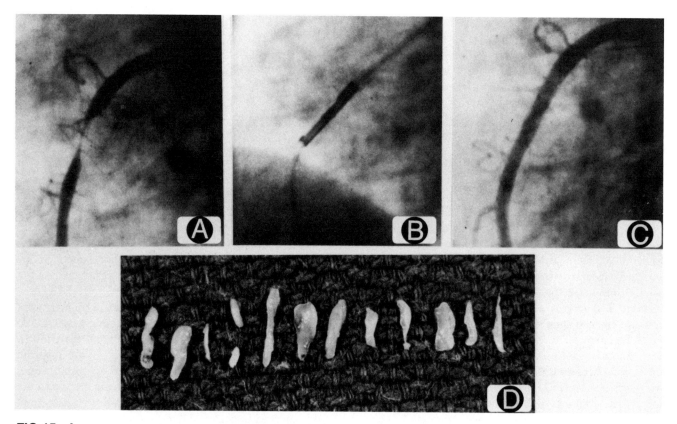

FIG 15–4.
A, proximal RCA stenosis favorable for DCA. **B,** AtheroCath in position; note window orientation "upward." **C,** postatherectomy result: large lumen with smooth borders. **D,** excised atheroma.

plaque exists. Atherectomy is generally not recommended for lesions greater than 2 cm because of the increasing risk of complications when a very large plaque mass is present.

Ostial lesions have also been treated effectively with DCA, particularly the ostium of the left anterior descending coronary artery (Fig 15–7). A high success rate with a low complication rate has been demonstrated. PTCA in the left anterior descending ostial location has traditionally yielded rather poor results because of a variety of problems including a tendency toward elastic recoil, dissections propagating proximally from the ostial left anterior descending and into the left main, and a known high incidence of restenosis. When plaque is predictably removed and a large and smooth residual lumen is left, elastic recoil is prevented. The predictability of this technique, especially in the left anterior descending ostial location, has made DCA the treatment of choice at this location. Somewhat more difficult ostial lesions include aorta ostial lesions of the left main and right coronary arteries. The aorta ostial location tends to be more technically difficult because of difficulty in guiding catheter manipulation. The procedure also tends to be less effective in removing tissue and achieving a large lumen. Treating the ostia of saphenous vein grafts is also technically more challenging. The results in the aorta ostial location, however, are better than can be achieved with angioplasty. In treating aorta ostial lesions it is important to obtain coaxial alignment of the guiding catheter in the coronary ostium and to position the middle of the window across the true ostium. Typically, higher pressures are also needed in the balloon, and the largest device that can be advanced into the area offers the best results. Often two experienced operators are required, one to manipulate the guide catheter and the second to advance the AtheroCath.

There are three lesion characteristics that make DCA unfavorable: (1) calcification, (2) small arteries, and (3) severe angulation or tortuosity (see Table 15–5). Calcification is the most significant determinant for the outcome of DCA, and in the presence of moderate-to-severe calcification, the success rate falls significantly in comparison to that of noncalcified vessels. The presence of calcification affects the performance of the device in several ways: (1) because of the rigidity of the vessel

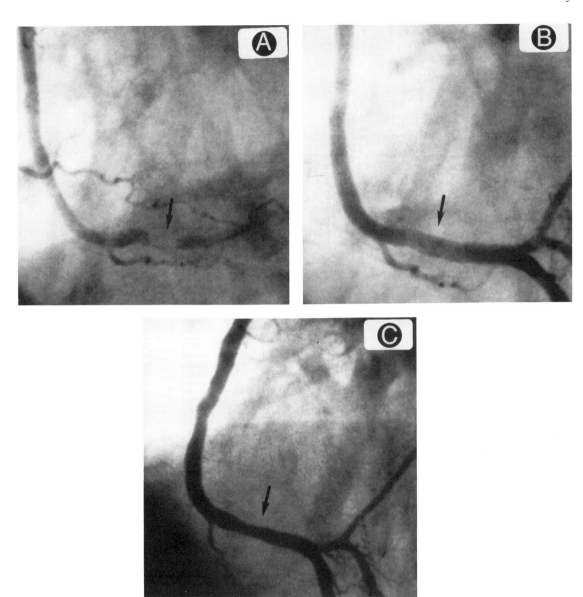

FIG 15–5.
Eccentric distal RCA stenosis. **A,** preatherectomy. **B,** immediately postatherectomy. **C,** 6-month follow-up.

walls when calcification is present before the lesion, there is increased resistance to catheter movement, and the device may fail to traverse the segment in front of the lesion and therefore fail to reach the lesion. (2) When calcification is present at the stenosis and creates an extremely hard lesion, the device may not be able to cross because of inelasticity. (3) Once the device is placed across the lesion, some calcified lesions cannot be excised because of an inability to cut the hard calcified plaque. When calcification is seen on angiograms or fluoroscopically, careful consideration should be given prior to undertaking atherectomy. Considerations include the size of the vessel, the curvature or bends that

must be traversed, and the segment distal to the vessel where the nose cone will be placed during cutting. If the vessels are relatively small with moderate tortuosity and calcification, atherectomy should not be considered.

Areas of severe angulation greater than 45 degrees are also considered unfavorable for DCA. When the window is placed across an area of significant angulation, there is a significant risk of deep cuts in the angulated segment and the potential for perforation. If the angulation is only modest and noncalcified, this segment will typically straighten as the device is placed across the area, and if balloon pressures are maintained at relatively low values, then deep wall cuts can be avoided.

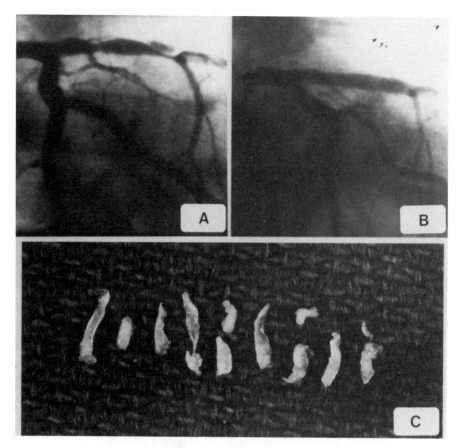

FIG 15–6.
A, ulcerated LAD stenosis. **B,** postatherectomy. **C,** excised tissue.

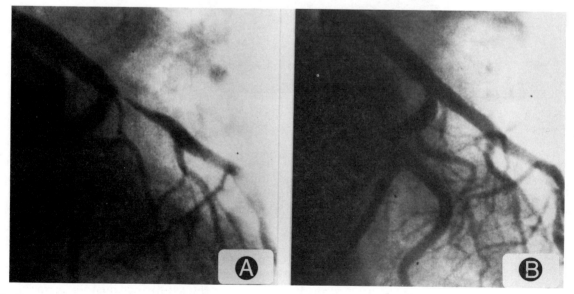

FIG 15–7.
Ostial LAD stenosis treated with DCA. Note large lumen with dissection at atherectomy site.

Again, the segment distal to the stenosis should be relatively straight to avoid nose cone trauma.

Bifurcation lesions have previously been felt not to be favorable for DCA; however, with the new short window device that traverses angled segments, large branch vessels may be treated effectively with atherectomy as well as the larger main branch. Side branch placement of a guidewire is not recommended during atherectomy of the main branch because of the risk of wire breakage. Frequently, however, if a side branch occludes during atherectomy, it can be relatively easily reopened with guidewire manipulation. For very small side branches, however, angioplasty is frequently a better option.

Diffusely diseased vessels are also considered poor candidates for atherectomy because of lower success rates and higher complication rates when diffuse plaque is present. In addition, diffusely diseased vessels are typically noncompliant and are therefore technically difficult to do because of device placement issues. With the rigid, relatively large profile and despite multiple cuts, an adequate result can rarely be achieved.

RESTENOSIS

Information on restenosis following DCA has been somewhat limited. Since the catheter as well as the technique continues to evolve, the restenosis rates may not reflect the current technology. Between October 1986 and December 1989 at Sequoia Hospital, 332 lesions in 289 patients were successfully treated with DCA and followed prospectively. The results are summarized in Table 15–6.[19] Ninety-eight percent had clinical follow-up information available, and angiographic follow-up information was obtained in 82% at 6 months, or earlier if symptoms recurred. Angiograms were quantitatively analyzed, and restenosis was defined as greater than 50% stenosis at the interventional site. Seventy-four percent of the patients remained asymptomatic or clinically improved following the procedure. The restenosis rate in native coronary arteries was 31% for primary lesions, 28% for lesions treated with one previous angioplasty, and 49% for lesions treated with two previous angioplasties. The restenosis rate for saphenous vein grafts was 53% for primary lesions, 58% for lesions treated with one previous angioplasty, and 82% for lesions treated with two previous angioplasties.[20] Restenosis occurred at a median of 133 days. There was no significant difference between restenosis rates in the left anterior descending, circumflex, or right coronary arteries. Restenosis was noted to be less frequent, however,

for larger vessels and for lesions with large post-DCA diameters. The restenosis rate of primary lesions in native arteries was 24% for vessels greater than or equal to 3 mm, 15% for those greater than or equal to 3 mm in diameter after DCA, and 12% when a 7 F device was used. The restenosis rate for lesions that occurred less than 120 days following prior angioplasty was significantly higher than those that occurred after 120 days, with restenosis rates of 55.8% for the shorter interval vs. 18.8% for the longer interval.

The incidence of restenosis in saphenous vein grafts is significantly higher than in native coronary artery lesions. For de novo lesions in saphenous vein grafts, the restenosis rate is 46%; however, in previously treated segments, the restenosis rates rise as high as 73%.

A comparison of restenosis rates between directional atherectomy and either conventional balloon angioplasty or other new interventional techniques is difficult because of significant differences in case selection. Prospective randomized trials (CAVEAT and CCAT) are under way to compare directional atherectomy and conventional PTCA with a target goal of 1,000 patients. The primary end point for this study will be angiographic restenosis.

HISTOLOGY

Unique to directional atherectomy is the biopsy mechanism that supplies tissue for histologic analysis (see Fig 15–8). As a research tool, this histologic information has helped in understanding the pathophysiology of not only restenosis but also the atherosclerotic process. Initial histologic evaluation of postangioplasty restenosis has confirmed the etiology of restenosis as primarily intimal hyperplasia of modified smooth muscle cells. Preliminary data suggest that histology may help identify patients at risk of restenosis following atherectomy.[21] In primary lesions, the restenosis rate is higher for those with high cellularity in the fibrous plaque as compared with those with more dense collagen and less cellularity suggestive of mature atherosclerotic plaque. Among the restenosis lesions, higher cellularity of the intimal hyperplasia excised was also associated with higher restenosis rates. It is not clear at this time whether the presence of deep wall components (media and adventitia) is important in predicting restenosis.[22] Future research with cell cultures, monoclonal antibody techniques, and in situ hybridization may provide genetic and biochemical clues to restenosis as well as the atherogenesis process.

TABLE 15-6.

Angiographic and Procedural Factors and Native Vessel Restenosis Following DCA*

Factor	Overall	Primary	Restenosis
Angiographic factors			
Lesion length			
<10 mm	29.3% (167)	26.0% (74)	31.9% (94)
≥10 mm	57.4% (47)	42.9% (14)	63.6% (33)
	P = .0007	P = .34	P = .003
Vessel diameter			
<3 mm	44.4% (90)	39.4% (33)	47.4% (57)
≥3 mm	29.6% (125)	23.6% (55)	34.3% (70)
	P = .03	P = .18	P = .18
Procedural factors			
Device			
≤6 F	42.5% (101)	56.4% (39)	43.5% (62)
7 F	27.6% (123)	12.0% (50)	38.4% (73)
	P = .002	P = < .0001	P = .66
Post-DCA diameter	41.4% (116)	38.5% (52)	43.7% (64)
<3 mm	27.7% (94)	14.7% (34)	35.0% (60)
≥3 mm	P = .054	P = .03	P = .42

*Adapted from Hinohara T, Robertson GC, Selmon MR, et al: *J Am Coll Cardiol* 1992, in press.

WHEN SHOULD DIRECTIONAL CORONARY ATHERECTOMY BE CONSIDERED?

For complex lesions that are easily accessible to the atherectomy device, DCA may provide improved safety and efficacy over conventional PTCA. Eccentric lesions, the presence of abnormal contour such as intimal flaps, ulceration, or localized dissections, as well as ostial lesions, particularly of the left anterior descending coronary artery, are effectively treated with DCA. For ideal PTCA lesions such as concentric stenoses in a proximal location, it is not clear whether DCA offers any advantage. In our experience, however, restenosis rates for de novo lesions in proximal locations, particularly in large vessels, are lower at approximately 20% when compared with conventional PTCA. If this observation holds in patients studied on a larger scale in randomized studies, it may be more appropriate to treat these ideal PTCA lesions in large proximal vessels with atherectomy because of the possibility of a lower incidence of restenosis.

Patients who have restenosis after prior angioplasties are also treated adequately with DCA. The success rate for DCA of restenosis lesions is higher than for de novo lesions. The restenosis rate following atherectomy for multiple PTCA restenosis lesions, however, is higher than for de novo lesions in our preliminary experience. Further evaluation is needed to determine how DCA compares with PTCA in treating these lesions. Those patients with restenosis after poor results with angioplasty may be good candidates for atherectomy since elastic recoil or localized dissection may have been a prominent feature of the restenosis process.

The use of DCA as a salvage procedure following failed PTCA is another alternative use for the technology. DCA appears particularly effective for failures due to ineffective dilatation, immediate elastic recoil, intimal flaps, and minor dissections. In contrast, DCA should probably be avoided in those patients with extensive spiral dissections from PTCA because of the potential risk of perforation. Because of technical challenges, attempts at salvage of poor PTCA results should only be undertaken by operators with substantial experience with elective DCA.

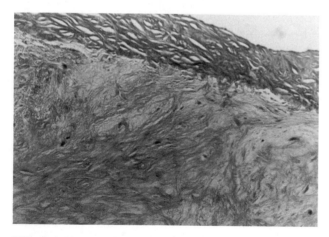

FIG 15-8.
Histology of tissue excised with DCA from a post-PTCA restenosis lesion. Note fibrous plaque over smooth muscle cell proliferation (intimal hyperplasia).

FUTURE DIRECTIONS

The goal of future catheter design is to provide more complete and effective atherectomy with improved safety and ease of use. Shorter windows will soon be available to traverse angles and access distal locations, as well as a wider variety of catheter and balloon sizes. Longer-term goals include guided directional coronary atherectomy (GDCA) using ultrasound guidance with a crystal embedded in the cutter to provide imaging of the stenosis on-line prior to excision. Flexible catheter housings also remain an attractive long-term goal. Cutters to improve the efficacy of cutting calcified lesions and faster and more powerful MDUs may also improve the efficacy in harder plaques.

SUMMARY

DCA has been shown to be an effective and safe method of percutaneous coronary revascularization. Initial experience with DCA suggests that certain types of lesions may be treated more safely and effectively with DCA, such as lesions in large vessels, ostial lesions, eccentric lesions, and stenoses with abnormal contour. Further conclusions, however, await results of ongoing randomized trials.

Acknowledgment

We would like to thank Connie Brooks for her assistance in the preparation of this manuscript.

REFERENCES

1. Ellis SG, Roubin GS, King SB, et al: Angiographic and clinical predictors of acute closure after native vessel coronary angioplasty. *Circulation* 1988; 77:372–379.
2. Cowley MJ, Dorros G, Kelsey SF, et al: Acute coronary events associated with percutaneous transluminal coronary angioplasty. *Am J Cardiol* 1984; 53:12–16.
3. Bredlau CE, Roubin GS, Leimgruber PP, et al: In-hospital morbidity and mortality in patients undergoing elective coronary angioplasty. *Circulation* 1985; 72:1044–1052.
4. Hirshfeld JW, Schwartz JS, Jugo R, et al: Restenosis after coronary angioplasty: A multivariate statistical model to relate lesion and procedure variables to restenosis. *J Am Coll Cardiol* 1991; 18:647–656.
5. Simpson JB, Johnson DE, Thapliyal HV, et al: Transluminal atherectomy: A new approach to the treatment of atherosclerotic vascular disease (abstract). *Circulation* 1985; 72(suppl 3):146.
6. Selmon MR, Robertson GC, Simpson JB: Transluminal atherectomy: Early results in the treatment of atherosclerosis (abstract). *J Am Coll Cardiol* 1988; 11:109.
7. Simpson JB, Robertson GC, Selmon MR: Percutaneous coronary atherectomy (abstract). *J Am Coll Cardiol* 1988; 11:110.
8. King SB: Role of new technology in balloon angioplasty. *Circulation* 1991; 84:000.
9. Simpson JB, Selmon MR, Robertson GC, et al: Transluminal atherectomy for occlusive peripheral vascular disease. *Am J Cardiol* 1988; 61:96–101.
10. Selmon MR, Robertson GC, Hinohara T, et al: Factors associated with restenosis following successful peripheral atherectomy (abstract). *J Am Coll Cardiol* 1989; 13:13.
11. Graor RA, Whitlow PL: Transluminal atherectomy for occlusive peripheral vascular disease. *J Am Coll Cardiol* 1990; 15:1551–1558.
12. Simpson JB, Johnson DE, Braden LJ, et al: Transluminal coronary atherectomy (TCA): Results in 21 human cadaver vascular segments (abstract). *Circulation* 1986; 72(suppl 2):202.
13. Pinkerton C, Simpson J, Selmon M, et al: Percutaneous coronary atherectomy: Early experiences of multicenter trial (abstract). *J Am Coll Cardiol* 1989; 13:108.
14. U.S. Directional Coronary Atherectomy Investigator Group: Directional coronary atherectomy: Multicenter experience (abstract). *Circulation* 1990; 82(suppl 3):71.
15. Simpson J, Hinohara T, Selmon M, et al: Comparison of early and recent experience in percutaneous coronary atherectomy (abstract). *J Am Coll Cardiol* 1989; 13:108.
16. U.S. Directional Coronary Atherectomy Investigator Group: Complications of directional coronary atherectomy in a multicenter experience (abstract). *Circulation* 1990; 82(suppl 3):311.
17. Hinohara T, Rowe MH, Robertson GC, et al: Effect of lesion characteristics on outcome of directional coronary atherectomy. *J Am Coll Cardiol* 1991; 17:1112–1120.
18. Vetter JW, Simpson JB, Robertson GC, et al: Rescue directional coronary atherectomy for failed balloon angioplasty. *J Am Coll Cardiol* 1991; 17:384.
19. Hinohara T, Robertson GC, Selmon MR, et al: Restenosis after directional coronary atherectomy. *J Am Coll Cardiol* 1992, in press.
20. Selmon MR, Hinohara T, Robertson GC, et al: Directional coronary atherectomy for saphenous vein graft stenosis (abstract). *J Am Coll Cardiol* 1991; 17:23.
21. Johnson D, Hinohara T, Selmon MR, et al: Histologic predictors of restenosis after directional coronary atherectomy (abstract). *J Am Coll Cardiol* 1991; 17:53.
22. Garratt KN, Holmes DR, Bell MR, et al: Restenosis after directional coronary atherectomy: Differences between primary atheromatous and restenosis lesions and influence of subintimal tissue resection. *J Am Coll Cardiol* 1990; 16:1665–1671.

16

Percutaneous Rotational Thrombectomy: An Alternative Approach to Thrombolysis

Timothy A. Dewhurst, M.D.

Paul Hirst

Thomas J. Clement, M.D.

Rudolph Vracko, M.D.

Bradley Titus, M.D.

James L. Ritchie, M.D.

Although thrombolysis has revolutionized care for many thrombotic disorders involving the coronary circulation, coronary thrombi continue to be a difficult clinical problem in a variety of settings. Residual thrombi are common after local or systemic thrombolytics, and these may be associated with early rethrombosis. Similarly, not all thrombi are successfully lysed with thrombolytics, and some thrombi cannot be treated with thrombolytics in the first place. Currently, the principal alternative approach is percutaneous transluminal coronary angioplasty (PTCA), which, although variably effective, obviously cannot remove thrombi per se. We describe herein ongoing experimental animal studies of an alternative mechanical approach to thrombolysis in which thrombi are removed from the circulation.

CONCEPT AND THEORY

The concept of rotational thrombectomy was initially described by our laboratory in 1986[1] and is briefly reviewed here. When a thin steel wire is rotated at 5,000 rpm within a fresh thrombus, the fibrin scaffold is extracted and wrapped around the wire shaft analogous to the wrapping of cotton candy around a paper cone. Since fibrin provides the scaffold in which other elements are embedded, the cellular elements are released into the circulation as the fibrin is removed. With in vitro testing, a fresh clot could be entirely liquified after about 10% of its wet weight was removed by rotation of our thrombectomy device. After this concept was successfully tested in vitro, a catheter was fabricated for intravascular use.

Theoretical advantages of this system of mechanical thrombolysis include the lack of a systemic lytic state (and therefore a potentially lowered risk of hemorrhagic complications) and the removal of a thrombus instead of its displacement and thus a potentially lowered risk of distal embolization. The removal of a clot, if completely accomplished, should lessen the risk of subsequent rethrombosis since one of the most potent stimuli to thrombosis, a thrombus itself, is removed. The preeminent disadvantages are the need for invasive diagnosis and treatment. However, patients with acute infarction and a variety of contraindications to thrombolytic therapy are often managed invasively.

CATHETER DESIGN AND USE

The first generation of catheters consisted of a thin, hollow, stainless steel wire with a 6- x 2-mm blunt platinum tip. This tip assists in radiographic visualization and protects the vessel from what would otherwise be a sharp and stiff catheter tip. The stainless steel wire was enclosed in a separate 4F Teflon sheath for longitudinal support and the entire device delivered via standard 8F angioplasty guide catheters.

The catheter has gone through a series of engineering modifications to enhance its facile and safe use. The present support catheter is a commercially available flexible 4F polyethylene catheter that is placed in the coronary artery with the aid of a standard 0.014-in. angioplasty guidewire. The guidewire is then removed and the percutaneous rotational thrombectomy (PRT) catheter inserted into the support catheter's lumen. The use of a guidewire is necessary because the distal shaft of the PRT used to extract the fibrin is too stiff to permit safe, accurate placement of the catheter in the delicate coronary vasculature. The general approach to placement of this device in the coronary artery is thus similar to that of most intracoronary interventional systems in that an atraumatic guidewire is used for initial steering and guidance and the stiffer treatment catheter is inserted directly via a guide (in this case an external support catheter) to the lesion of interest. Thus, the support catheter is positioned just proximal to the thrombus with the aid of the guidewire, and the PRT catheter is delivered precisely to the area of thrombosis as a replacement for the initial guidewire. The present catheter design is shown in Figure 16–1. Figure 16–2 illustrates the distal tip of the PRT after use on which fibrin has accumulated.

INITIAL WORK

The device was initially tested in a canine femoral arterial thrombosis model.[1] Twenty-seven arteries were occluded or subtotally occluded (Thrombolysis in Myocardial Infarction trial [TIMI] flow grade 1) by endothelial balloon denudation, followed by temporary ligature closure of the arterial segment and the injection of thrombin. This occlusion was approached either via a local arteriotomy in the occluded artery (n = 17) or remotely via the left carotid artery (n = 10). Twenty of 22 arteries were partially or completely recanalized after treatment with the PRT. Four of 5 control arteries that had the catheter passed through the thrombosed area without rotation remained totally occluded at 75 minutes, while the other opened subtotally at 20 minutes. Electron microscopy of the removed material from the catheter (Fig 16–3) showed fibrillar material consistent with fibrin. This material was largely free of cellular elements typical of a whole clot. This fibrinous material was very tightly adherent to the catheter shaft and appeared to be at low risk for embolization off the catheter shaft.

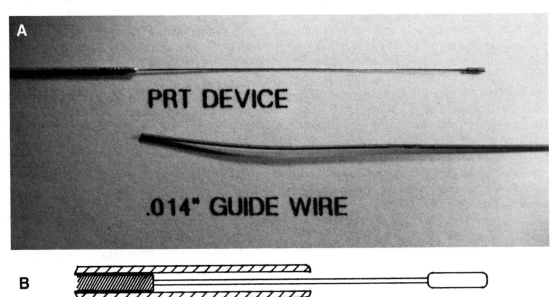

FIG 16–1.
A, distal, fibrin-removing end of the present device. This platinum tip is 0.16 mm in diameter (on the *right*), the central stainless steel wire core is in the *middle,* and the distal portion supporting a helical drive coil is shown proximally (to the *left*). **B,** this schematic drawing (not to scale) shows the PRT catheter partially enclosed within the support catheter *(black arrow).*

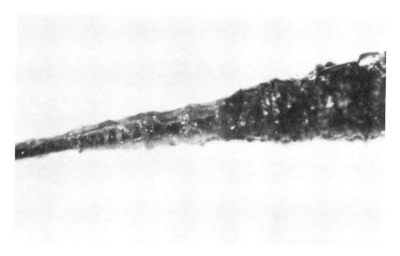

FIG 16–2.
The distal tip of the PRT is to the *right* and shows fibrin wrapped about the catheter shaft.

CORONARY STUDIES

After successful femoral use of the device, it was investigated in a canine coronary occlusion model.[2] Total coronary thrombosis was induced in 11 canine coronary arteries by external crush injury, temporary occlusion, and thrombin injection. Thirty minutes after injury, complete coronary occlusion was documented arteriographically and treatment then begun. The PRT was spun within its supporting catheter and slowly advanced

through the thrombus in 30-second passes. After each rotational pass, the catheter system was removed and examined for fibrin. These passes were repeated until complete relief of obstruction with normal distal coronary flow was demonstrated or until no more fibrin was accumulated on the tip. There was no evidence of coronary spasm or distal embolization. The angiographic coronary stenosis was reduced from 100% prior to treatment to 28% after treatment. Technical difficulties with the remote use of this device led to catheter rede-

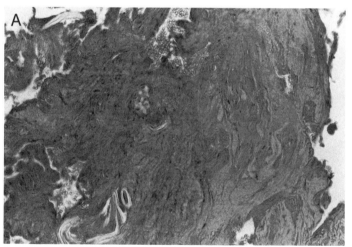
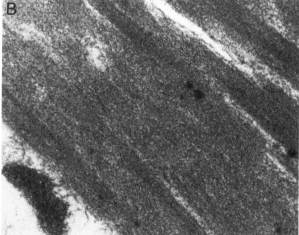

FIG 16–3.
A, histologic examination of the tissue attached to the tip of the catheter revealed interlaced homogeneous material containing occasional nuclear debris *(dark dots),* red blood cells (the clusters of *small open rings*), and a few strands of cotton fibers *(white loops).* Cotton gauze was used to remove the tightly adherent fibrin from the catheter. **B,** electron micrograph of the material at the catheter tip shows loosely structured fibrillar material and nuclear debris (the *very dark areas*). The fibrillar material does not stain for collagen or elastin. It is arranged in parallel arrays and has the ultrastructural appearance of fibrin strands that may have been pulled into parallel bundles by the rotation of the catheter tip. (From Ritchie JL, Hansen DD, Vracko R, et al: *Circulation* 1986; 73:1006–1012. Used by permission.)

sign, including the use of smaller-diameter shafts for the distal portion and the incorporation of a proximal helical coil section to accommodate the more acutely angled bends encountered in percutaneous coronary placement.

CORONARY THROMBOSIS AND REOCCLUSION

A closed-chest swine model of coronary thrombosis was developed by Titus and Ritchie for further testing of this device in simulated clinical conditions (unpublished observations). Swine hearts have a larger right coronary circulation than do canine hearts, as well as fewer intramyocardial collaterals. Coronary thrombosis in this model is created by repetitive oversized balloon angioplasty of the distal left anterior descending (LAD) coronary artery. The circumflex artery is generally the major epicardial artery in swine. Ninety percent of ani-

mals prepared in this manner develop complete occlusion within an hour. Histologic examination has shown that occlusion is secondary to thrombosis and not due to intimal flaps. The PRT device was used for treatment of the thrombotically occluded LAD arteries in half of the animals and results compared with PTCA treatment in identically prepared animals. After recanalization of the vessel was demonstrated, the animal was followed with serial angiograms up to 3 hours or until reocclusion was demonstrated. Figure 16–4 demonstrates a sequence of normal vessel, initial occlusion after oversized angioplasty, use of the PRT device being rotated, and the recanalized vessel. Histologic examination of the treated vessels shows extensive damage to all segments of the vessel wall from the oversized angioplasty used to induce the initial thrombosis. Examination of control vessels where only the PRT was rotated shows only minimal intimal disruption and no damage to the internal elastic lamina or media (Fig 16–5). That is, this device appears to create considerably less local vessel wall

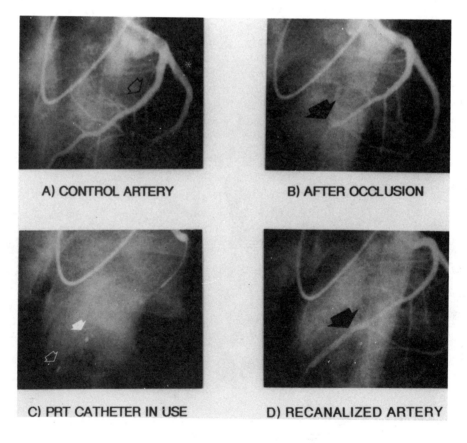

A) CONTROL ARTERY
B) AFTER OCCLUSION
C) PRT CATHETER IN USE
D) RECANALIZED ARTERY

FIG 16–4.
This series of photographs demonstrates the sequence of events in the swine coronary model of occlusion. **A,** initial view of a normal vessel. **B,** total thrombotic occlusion after oversized balloon angioplasty. **C,** the PRT system placed in the left anterior descending coronary artery. **D,** the recanalized artery, 2 hours after PRT treatment. *Open black arrow* = left anterior descending coronary artery; *white asterisk* = circumflex coronary artery; *solid black arrow* = point of total occlusion; *solid white arrow* = distal tip of the PRT support catheter; *open white arrow* = platinum tip of the PRT device.

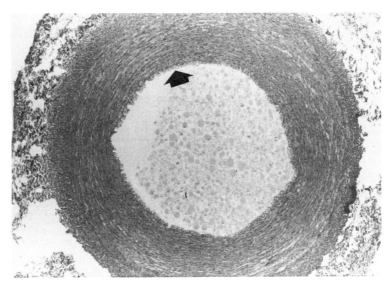

FIG 16–5.
A photomicrograph of a control vessel exposed only to rotation of the PRT device shows minimal disruption of the endothelium and the maintained integrity of the internal elastic membrane *(dark arrow)* and media.

trauma than would be anticipated from high-pressure balloon angioplasty inflations.

Two mechanical failures of the catheter have been associated with advancement of the rotating catheter into a small side branch which caused mechanical stress on the catheter wire and subsequent wire fracture. Our protocol has since been revised so as not to advance the rotating catheter and to rotate the PRT device only during the withdrawal phase. With this approach, no further fractures have occurred.

Work on this project is ongoing, but preliminary results suggest that the rate of reocclusion is lowered by PRT as compared with PTCA. We have also tested the PRT device in an exteriorized arterial segment model of thrombosis by comparing the weights (and angiographic presence) of residual thrombi between PRT and PTCA. The weights of residual thrombi were nonsignificantly lower for the PRT-treated group. The presence of angiographically visible thrombi was significantly lower in the PRT-treated arteries.[3]

POTENTIAL CLINICAL USE

Where might rotational thrombectomy fit in the clinical arena of human cardiovascular disease? Clearly it is not effective against atherosclerotic plaque as PTCA is. It also has less efficacy against older clots in an animal model, although this is of uncertain significance in clinical intra-arterial thrombi in patients, where the balance between thrombosis and thrombolysis is probably a dynamic one in most unstable clinical syndromes.[4] It has been shown that most acute ischemic syndromes (unstable angina and myocardial infarction) are related to the formation of thrombi on and about atherosclerotic plaque. Enzymatic thrombolytic therapy, aspirin, and heparin are all useful in this situation, but all cause a systemic lytic state favoring increased thrombolysis or reduced thrombosis. This systemic state can lead to hemorrhagic complications. The rotational thrombectomy catheter treats a clot by the selective removal of fibrin without the production of systemic anticoagulated states and thus might be suitable for use in patients where conventional antithrombotic agents are either contraindicated or have failed.

Since all intravascular failures of the device have occurred when the rotating catheter was advanced into side branches of the native coronary circulation, it is now clear that the device should be rotated only during withdrawal, thereby eliminating this possible complication.

A potential first site of human clinical investigation might be saphenous vein grafts, where no side branches are present and placement of the device may be facilitated by the lack of acute angles to be traversed. Saphenous vein grafts also have a higher tendency to have large thrombi that may be unsuitable for PTCA treatment because of the risk of embolization. Thrombolytic therapy has also had limited success in the setting of total, thrombotic graft occlusions.[5] This is presumably attributable to both the large volume of thrombi that can develop as well as the lack of side branches that promote delivery of the thrombolytic agent to the clot. The relatively low-profile PRT device penetrates thrombi with less force than is needed to penetrate a clot with a PTCA balloon, and thus a lesser risk of downstream embolization seems likely. Also PRT may reduce the likelihood of embolization as compared with PTCA by removing thrombi. This is in contrast to PTCA, which does not remove a thrombus, but displaces or remodels it with the attendant risk of embolization and causes damage to the media of almost all vessels treated. PRT, by contrast, does not damage the internal elastic membrane or the media of the artery. The PTCA balloon almost always causes some splits in the arterial elastica or media, thereby providing a potent surface for thrombogenesis. Experimentally, damage to the media appears to be a major stimulus to late restenosis from smooth muscle hyperplasia.[6] PRT may thus not lead to late restenosis, although this remains to be tested.

SUMMARY

The PRT catheter has been developed as a possible option for the treatment of acute intracoronary and/or intragraft thrombi in patients undergoing left heart catheterization for acute ischemic events. Possible applications may also exist in primary treatment of acute myocardial infarction in patients with contraindications

to or a failure of systemic lytic therapy. To date, studies in a variety of animal models show technical feasibility, and it is hoped that clinical studies can be initiated soon.

REFERENCES

1. Ritchie JL, Hansen DD, Vracko R, et al: Mechanical thrombolysis: A new rotational catheter approach for acute thrombi. *Circulation* 1986; 73:1006–1012.
2. Hansen DD, Auth DC, Vracko R, et al: Rotational thrombectomy in acute canine coronary thrombosis. *Int J Cardiol* 1988; 22:13–19.
3. Titus BG, Auth DC, Ritchie JL: Distal embolization during mechanical thrombolysis: Rotational thrombectomy vs. balloon angioplasty. *Cathet Cardiovasc Diagn* 1990; 19:279–285.
4. Hansen DD, Auth DC, Vracko R, et al: Mechanical thrombectomy: A comparison of two rotational devices and balloon angioplasty in subacute canine femoral thrombosis. *Am Heart J* 1987; 114:1223–1231.
5. Grines CL, Booth DC, Nissen SE, et al: Mechanism of acute myocardial infarction in patients with prior coronary artery bypass grafting and therapeutic implications. *Am J Cardiol* 1990; 65:1292–1296.
6. Schwartz RS, Murphy JG, Edwards WD, et al: Coronary artery restenosis and the "Virginal membrane": Smooth muscle cell proliferation and the intact internal elastic lamina *J Invasive Cardiol* 1991; 3:3–8.

PART IV

Laser and Related Procedures

17

Laser Angiosurgery: A Biomedical System Using Photons to Diagnose and Treat Atherosclerosis

John R. Kramer, M.D.

Michael S. Feld, Ph.D.

Floyd D. Loop, M.D.

Robert M. Cothren, Ph.D.

Gary B. Hayes, B.A.

Rebecca Richards-Kortum, Ph.D.

Bruce W. Lytle, M.D.

Carter Kittrell, B.S.

Corrine Bott-Silverman, M.D.

Laser angiosurgery[1-3] is an overall term used by colleagues at the Cleveland Clinic Foundation and the Massachusetts Institute of Technology to describe a large, ongoing research project aimed at the development of laser delivery systems that can recognize and ablate intra-arterial atherosclerotic obstructions with precisely controlled and aimed photon beams. Because the power of the ablation beam is immense and because the diseased arterial wall is thin and easily damaged by heat, there is little room for error, thus necessitating a sophisticated and complex delivery system.[4] This chapter describes our approach to the use of laser light in the vascular system, i.e., laser angiosurgery (LAS).

LASER CATHETER DESIGN

The LAS laser catheter is based on a multifiber approach in which the distal tip is formed of an array of optical fibers encased in a protective, transparent shield[5, 6] (Fig 17–1). As the lesion is contacted, blood is displaced, and this provides the light exiting the fibers with a clear path to the target. Each fiber produces a small light spot at the tip of the shield and irradiates a correspondingly small "field" of tissue. The fibers are arranged inside the shield so that the spots all overlap to provide coverage of the entire distal tip of the device. Tissue fields can be irradiated sequentially or simultaneously. Thus, with an array of small spots (typically 0.5

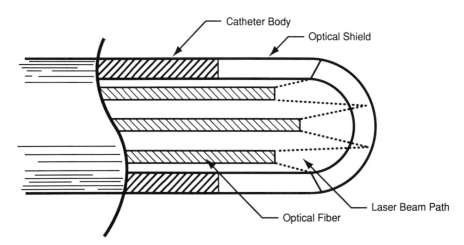

FIG 17–1.
Cross-sectional diagram of a multifiber laser catheter with an optical shield.

mm in diameter), a large-diameter arterial lumen (typically 2 to 3 mm in diameter) can be recanalized to allow advancement of the catheter.

There are two distinct aspects of the LAS removal process, target recognition and target ablation. Each tissue field is treated individually. A given field is first diagnosed, and then it can be ablated or spared, as indicated. The objective is to remove the diseased tissue causing the stenosis and leave healthy tissue and blood intact. In our past work the functions of recognition and ablation were studied separately. An integrated system is now being developed.

TARGET ABLATION

Strikwerda and colleagues[5, 7–9] have demonstrated that relatively char-free craters can be consistently produced in noncalcified atherosclerotic plaque with continuous-wave argon-ion laser light if the appropriate light intensity and exposure time are used. Once over a practical threshold (intensity, 25.5 W/mm^2; fluence, 3.2 J/mm^2), ablation depths are predictable even when aortic segments exhibit varying stages of disease and come from different patients.

By analyzing the data of Strikwerda, Partovi, and colleagues[10] we have been able to theoretically model the ablation process and mathematically predict crater depth in relation to the photon dose delivered:

$$l = v\,(t - t_0) = [f(x)/h_{abl}] \cdot (I - I_0) \cdot (t - t_0) \quad (1)$$

where

l = crater depth
v = ablation velocity

t = exposure time
t_0 = threshold time
$f(x)$ = fraction of light absorbed in the cylinder of the tissue being removed
x = d/D, with d being the diameter of the light spot and D the penetration depth of light in the tissue
I = laser intensity (power/unit area)
I_0 = threshold intensity
h_{abl} = amount of heat needed to reach the water–steam-phase transition temperature and then evaporate a unit volume of tissue

The parameter D is due to the interplay of scattering and absorption and is determined by the tissue properties and the wavelength of light used. Similarly, h_{abl} depends on the composition of the target tissue. However, the factors I and d and hence $f(x)$ can be controlled by the delivery system itself. This equation is derived to describe the ablation of soft tissues, which are largely composed of water and can be ablated at relatively low laser intensities. For hard tissue and/or use at higher intensities additional considerations are needed.

Experiments with samples of fresh cadaver arterial wall have established the laser light parameters required for a useful working range. In order to obtain reproducible tissue craters, the intensity I should be much larger than the threshold intensity I_0. With this limit Equation 1 reduces to

$$l = [f(x)/h_{abl}] \cdot (\phi - \phi_0) \quad (2)$$
$$= D(\phi/\phi)_0 - 1),$$

with $\phi = It$ being the fluence (J/mm^2) of the impinging light beam and $\phi_0 = h_{abl} \cdot D/f(x)$ being the threshold

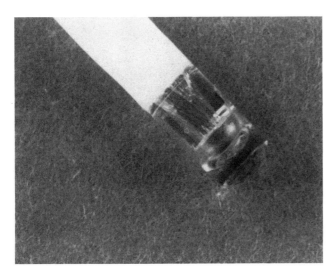

FIG 17–2.
Distal (output) end of the shielded laser angiosurgery catheter.

fluence. In this regimen the independent values of intensity and exposure time are not important; only their product is.

The LAS system has been designed to allow physicians to control the delivery of a predetermined photon dose:

$$\phi = [\text{power }(W) \times \text{time (sec)}] \text{ spot area (mm}^2) \quad (3)$$

The LAS catheter (Fig 17–2) is designed to control beam intensity by predetermining the spot diameter. Interfacing of the catheter and the delivery system therefore allows control of dosimetry (power, exposure time, and spot diameter). The delivery scheme is shown in Fig 17–3.

Additionally, the LAS catheter protects the optical fibers with an optical shield and is capable of producing a large new lumen by using an array of optical fibers with overlapping spots that can be fired sequentially (one round) and in series (many rounds, one after the other).[11, 12]

An interventional operating room incorporating an LAS system has been constructed at the Cleveland Clinic Foundation (Fig 17–4). A coherent Innova 100

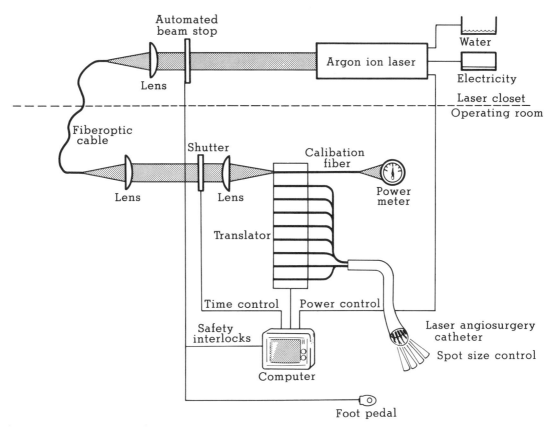

FIG 17–3.
Schematic of the delivery scheme.

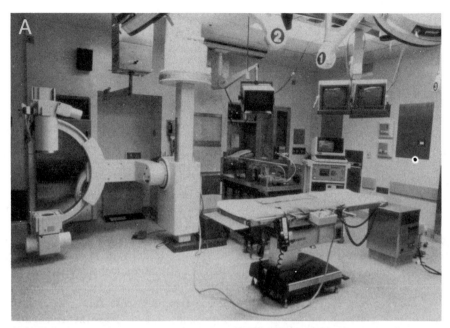

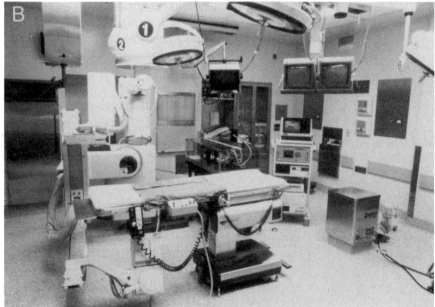

FIG 17–4.
Laser angiosurgery operating room. **A,** "operating room" configuration for intraoperative experiment. **B,** "catheterization laboratory" configuration for percutaneous experiments.

argon-ion (blue-green) laser is housed in a closet outside of the operating room so that surgeons are isolated from the noise of the power supply and cooling water. Light is transmitted to the operating room via a 50-μm fiber-optic cable strung through the ceiling. In the operating room the fiber-optic cable is connected to a small optical bench that sits near the patient and contains the hardware for timing exposures and focusing the beam into the LAS catheter.

A foot pedal allows the surgeon to control beam entry into the operating room. A computer controls laser power and exposure time.

The system has been tested extensively in vitro.[13] The catheter removes 0.16 mm^3 of tissue for each joule of energy delivered. This ablation yield is consistent over a range of operating parameters and does not change with repeated firing despite a gradual exfoliation of the outer surface of the quartz shield.

Kjellstrom and colleagues, using a canine model, have shown in vivo that the system allows removal of focal, noncalcified, fibrotic obstructions without vascular perforation.[14] Histologic evaluation of arterial segments from animals followed for up to 60 days after LAS showed reendothelialization of the treated area within 30 days, thus confirming the earlier work of Gerrity and colleagues where a different wavelength (one that could not be transmitted through a fiber) was used.[15]

Because of these encouraging results, the system was next tested in an intraoperative setting during open heart surgery in patients requiring multiple bypass grafts. Between August 1987 and October 1988, seven men aged 54 ± 11 years (range, 42 to 68 years) who were to undergo bypass grafting for significant, symptomatic obstructive coronary artery disease agreed to testing of the system during surgery. In each case, a severe, focal, angiographically noncalcified obstruction in either the right or left anterior descending coronary artery was identified as the target lesion. At the time of surgery, the lesion was examined with an Olympus angioscope to confirm lesion location and severity (Fig 17–5). The LAS catheter was then advanced through the arteriotomy retrograde to the lesion to make gentle contact with the obstruction, and laser light of a known fluence was delivered to the target lesion. Results are summarized in Table 17–1. Following treatment, the segment was again examined with the angioscope (Fig 17–6) and the vessel bypassed. Repeat cineangiography was performed 6 weeks after open heart surgery to determine whether the treated segment remained patent (Fig 17–7, Table 17–1).

This experience demonstrated that lumen diameter can be improved by using continuous-wave argon-ion laser light primarily by removing softer (noncalcified) portions of the atherosclerotic plaque. Six-week patency was also shown to occur in some cases. Clearly, calcified plaque was not removed with the continuous-wave laser light, which accounts for the inability to cross some lesions.[16] In addition, vessel perforation remained a problem despite very careful control of the dose.

Two important areas for further research were thus identified. First, target recognition will be necessary to entirely avoid perforation, and second, a new wavelength strategy will be required for the ablation of calcified plaque.

TARGET RECOGNITION

The purpose of target recognition is to determine the identity of a given tissue field. The field may be normal or diseased, or it may be filled with blood. The LAS recognition process is based on a process called "spectral diagnosis."[17] In the specific spectral diagnostic scheme used at present, called laser-induced fluorescence, 476-nm (blue) argon-ion laser light is conducted from a given fiber to a given tissue field to cause emission at longer visible wavelengths. Some of this fluorescence is collected by the same fiber and carried back to the proximal end of the catheter where it is analyzed with a spectrometer and an optical multichannel analyzer. The spectral pattern of this light is distinct for

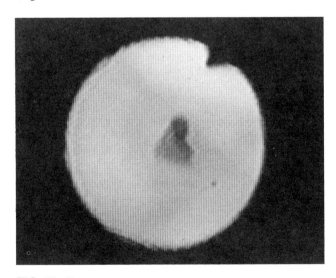

FIG 17–5.
Angioscopic appearance of an obstruction in the proximal segment of the left anterior descending artery prior to laser treatment (patient 6).

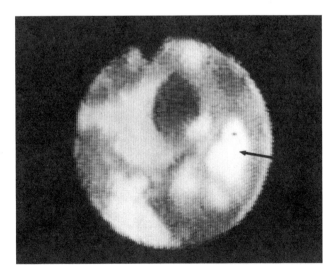

FIG 17–6.
Angioscopic appearance of the same segment following laser treatment. The fibrous and fatty portions of the obstruction have been removed, the lumen diameter is improved, but calcified disease *(arrow)* remains.

TABLE 17–1.

Summary of Results

Patient	Sex	Age (yr)	Artery*	Pretreatment Stenosis (%)	Firing Sequence	Total Energy (J)	Catheter Passed Lesion	Perforation	Angiographic Status at 6 wk (Stenosis)	Clinical Status at 1 yr
1	M	44	LAD	70	5 W, 0.03 sec 20 fibers 12 rounds	36	Yes	Yes, repaired surgically	40%	Alive, asymptomatic
2	M	60	LAD	90	5 W, 0.03 sec 20 fibers 10 rounds	30	No	No	50%	Alive, asymptomatic
3	M	42	Diag	60	5 W, 0.03 sec 20 fibers 22 rounds	66	No	No	Occluded	Alive, asymptomatic
4	M	68	Diag	80	5 W, 0.03 sec 20 fibers 38 rounds	96	No	No	Occluded	Alive, asymptomatic
5	M	42	LAD	70	5 W, 0.06 sec 20 fibers 8 rounds	48	Yes	No	60%	Alive, asymptomatic
6	M	59	LAD	90	5 W, 0.06 sec 20 fibers 20 rounds	120	Partial (see Fig 5–7)	No	70%	Alive, asymptomatic
7	M	64	RCA	95	5 W, 0.06 sec 20 fibers 7 rounds	42	No	Yes, repaired surgically	Not studied	Alive, asymptomatic

*LAD = left anterior descending coronary artery; Diag = diagonal; RCA = right coronary artery.

normal and atherosclerotic tissue (Fig 17–8), and these differences are exploited to make a diagnosis.[18] The individual morphologic structures contributing to the spectra ("morpholophores") have been identified[19, 20] and are correlated with features of the tissue spectra by using a model of tissue fluorescence (Plate 11).[21] The morpholophores of a normal artery include the struc-

tural proteins collagen and elastin, as well as hemoglobin. In an atherosclerotic artery, these same morpholophores are present (in different proportions), along with an additional substance, ceroid, which is an oxidation product of lipids (Fig 17–9).

The parameters of this model, which are proportional to the concentrations of the tissue morpholo-

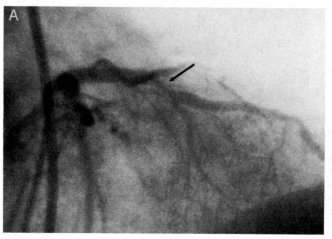
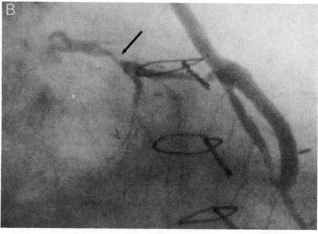

FIG 17–7.

A, a cineangiogram (patient 6) of the left coronary artery in the right anterior oblique projection prior to laser treatment shows focal obstruction *(arrow)* in the proximal segment of the left anterior descending artery. **B,** cineangiogram of the same vessel 6 weeks following laser angiosurgery and bypass surgery with a saphenous vein graft. The treated segment, visualized by retrograde filling during an injection into the saphenous vein graft *(arrow)*, remains patent.

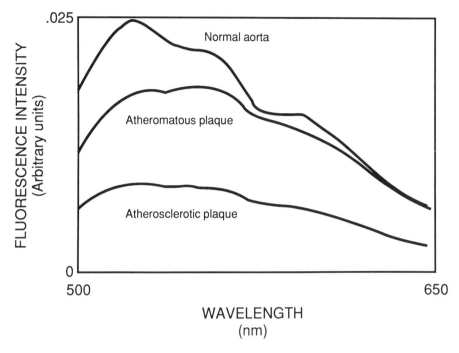

FIG 17–8.
Excited fluorescence spectra (476 nm) of normal aorta and aorta exhibiting atherosclerotic and atheromatous plaque.

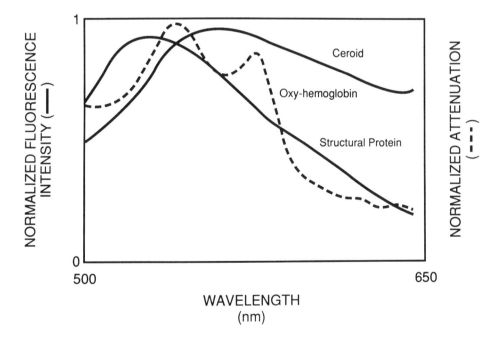

FIG 17–9.
Fluorescence line shapes of structural protein and ceroid and the attenuation line shape of oxyhemoglobin. The structural protein fluorescence is responsible for the tissue fluorescence peak observed at 520 nm. This is largest in normal tissue. Ceroid fluorescence is responsible for the peak at 560 nm, which, relative to the 520-nm peak, is largest in atherosclerotic and atheromatous plaques (see Fig 17–8). The attenuation of oxyhemoglobin creates the valleys observed between 540 and 580 nm.

phores, are used to make a spectroscopic diagnosis for each tissue field. The parameters for structural protein and ceroid are used in the diagnostic algorithm, as shown in Figure 17–10. This algorithm was chosen to maximize the number of samples correctly diagnosed in a group of 150 in vitro samples of human aorta. It has a specificity of 85%, a sensitivity of 91%, and a predictive value of 85%.

The process of spectral diagnosis can be performed rapidly, tissue field by tissue field, under computer control. Low-intensity exciting light sufficiently weak to ensure that the tissue is not damaged or its spectral response altered is used. Collected spectra are displayed on a computer screen to create a 20-pixel map of the vascular lumen.[22] Once target determination is accomplished, high-intensity light from the same laser source can be used to ablate the diseased tissue while sparing the structural integrity of the vessel.

FUTURE DIRECTIONS

Because continuous-wave argon-ion laser light does not effectively remove calcified materials, an intensive investigation of hard-tissue ablation was undertaken. A systematic in vitro study using laser light at a variety of wavelengths and pulse durations was conducted to elucidate the hard-tissue ablation mechanism and define the laser beam parameters for which calcified plaque can be ablated with a high degree of control. The results indicate that high-intensity pulsed radiation is most effective, and this is supported by theoretical modeling. Calcified plaque is a composite substance composed of micron-sized mineralized particles of mixed apatites suspended in a soft matrix of lipids and cross-linked proteins. An intense light pulse can rapidly vaporize the soft material, and the exiting vapor can entrain the hard microparticles and carry them away. In order to obtain a good biological effect, it is important to use a wavelength that is absorbed close to the tissue surface.

With deeply penetrating light, subsurface tissue can become the hottest, and ablation can begin below the surface and cause cracking and fissuring. Chips and large-sized particle debris can be produced. For this reason, strongly absorbing light should be used. Ultraviolet wavelengths below about 400 nm and infrared wavelengths at 2.5 to 3.0 μm are effective for this purpose.

Short-wavelength light is known to be mutagenic. Light in the ultraviolet B wavelength range, 280 to 320 nm, is the most toxic and should be avoided.[23] For these

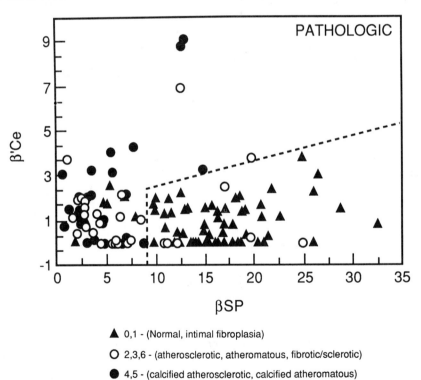

FIG 17–10.
Scatter plot indicating model parameters for 150 cadaver aorta specimens. β'Ce is plotted vs. βSP, where β is the parameter proportional to the fluorophore concentration. These parameters can be used diagnostically; the decision surface shown (two straight lines) correctly classifies 88% of the 150 samples as atherosclerotic or normal.

reasons we have selected tripled Nd: YAG laser light at 355 nm as an appropriate ablation source. Integration of this source and a low-power diagnostic laser in a multi-fiber shielded guidewire catheter within an interventional catheterization laboratory–operating room is under way.

REFERENCES

1. Kitrell C: Strategic plaque intiative. *Spectrograph* 1987; 6:1.
2. Goth PR, Kramer JR, Kittrell C, et al: Multifiber optically shielded catheter for laser angiosurgery, *Proc SPIE* 1987; 713:58–63.
3. Kjellstorm BT, Cothren RM, Kramer JR: The use of lasers in vascular and cardiac surgery: A review. *Acta Chir Scand* 1987; 153:493–499.
4. Kramer JR, Strikwerda S, Kittrell C, et al: Laser angiosurgery: A brief overview of tissue micromachining with spectral diagnostics, in Bruschke AVG, Spaan JAE, Gittenberger AC (eds): *Coronary Circulation, From Basic Mechanisms to Clinical Implications.* Boston, Martinus Nijhoff, 1987, pp 225–234.
5. Cothren RM, Kittrell C, Hayes GB, et al: Controlled light delivery for laser angiosurgery. *IEEF, J Quant Electron* 1986; 22:4–7.
6. Cothren RM, Hayes GB, Kramer JR, et al: A multifiber catheter with an optical shield for laser angiosurgery. *Lasers Life Sci* 1986; 1:1–12.
7. Strikwerda S, Bott-Silverman C, Ratliff NB, et al: Effects of varying argon ion laser intensity and exposure time on the ablation of atherosclerotic plaque. *Lasers Surg Med* 1988; 8:66–71.
8. Strikwerda S, Partovi F, Cothren RM, et al: Ablation thresholds of atheromatous tissue for argon ion laser light exposures. *Lasers Life Sci* 1989; 3:61–70.
9. Strikwerda S, Kramer JR, Partovi F, et al: Consideration of dosimetry for laser-tissue ablation, in Vogel JHK, King SB III (eds): *Interventional Cardiology, Future Directions.* St Louis, Mosby–Year Book, 1989, pp 54–66.
10. Partovi F, Izatt JA, Cothren RM, et al: A model for thermal ablation of biological tissue using laser radiation. *Laser Surg Med* 1987; 7:141–154.
11. Cothren RM, Kramer JR, Hayes GB, et al: Engineering of a multifiber catheter with an optical shield for laser angiosurgery. Proceedings of the Ninth Annual Conference, Boston, Massachusetts. *IEEE Eng Med Bio*, Nov 13–16, 1987, pp 200–201.
12. Kramer JR, Bott-Silverman C, Ratliff NB, et al: Removal of atherosclerotic plaque using multiple short exposures of argon ion laser light. *Am Heart J* 1987; 113:1038–1040.
13. Cothren RM, Costello B, Hoyt C, et al: Tissue removal using an 8F multifiber shielded laser angiosurgery catheter. *Lasers Life Sci* 1988; 2:75–90.
14. Kjellstrom BT, Bylock AL, Bott-Silverman C, et al: Removal of surgically induced fibrous arterial plaques by argon laser angiosurgery using a multifiber delivery system: An experimental study in the dog. *J Thorac Cardiovasc Surg* 1988; 96:925–929.
15. Gerrity RG, Loop FD, Golding LAR, et al: Arterial response to laser operation for removal of atherosclerotic plaques. *J Thorac Cardiovasc Surg* 1983; 85:409–421.
16. Litvak F: Pulsed laser angioplasty: Wavelength power and energy dependencies relevant to clinical application. *Lasers Surg Med* 1988; 8:60–65.
17. Richards-Kortum R, Mehta A, Hayes G, et al: Spectral diagnosis of atherosclerosis using an optical fiber laser catheter. *Am Heart J* 1989; 118:381–391.
18. Kittrell C, Willett RL, de Los Santos-Pacheo C, et al: Diagnosis of fibrous arterial atherosclerosis using fluorescence. *Appl Optics* 1985; 24:2280–2281.
19. Fitzmaurice M, Bordagaray JO, Englemann GL, et al: Argon ion laser–excited autofluorescence in normal and atherosclerotic aorta and coronary arteries: Morphologic studies. *Am Heart J* 1989; 118:1028–1038.
20. Verbunt RJ, Cothren RM, Fitzmaurice M, et al: Characterization of ultraviolet laser–induced autofluorescence of ceroid deposits and other structures in atherosclerotic plaques as a potential diagnostic for laser angiosurgery. *Am Heart J* 1992; 1:208–216.
21. Richards-Kortum RR, Rava R, Fitzmaurice R, et al: A one-layer model of laser induced fluorescence for diagnosis of disease in human tissue: Applications to atherosclerosis. *IEEE Trans Biomed Eng* 1989; 36:1222–1232.
22. Hoyt CC, Richards-Kortum RR, Costello B, et al: Remote biomedical spectroscopic imaging of human artery wall. *Lasers Surg Med* 1988; 8:1–9.
23. Tiphlova OA, Karu TI, Furzikov NP: Lethal and mutagenic action of XeCl laser radiation on *Escherichia coli*. *Lasers Life Sci* 1988; 2:155–159.

18

LAS II: An Integrated System for Spectral Diagnosis, Guidance, and Ablation in Laser Angiosurgery

Michael S. Feld, Ph.D.

John R. Kramer, M.D.

Douglas Albagli, B.A.

Rim Cothren, Jr., Ph.D.

Ramachandra R. Dasari, Ph.D.

Gary B. Hayes, B.A.

Joseph A. Izatt, Ph.D.

Irving Itzkan, Ph.D.

G. Sargent Janes, Ph.D.

Richard P. Rava, Ph.D.

Since the introduction of percutaneous transluminal balloon angioplasty (PTCA) by Grüntzig et al. in 1979,[1] there has been a dramatic growth in the use of this technique for the treatment of coronary atherosclerosis. Physicians and patients often elect this form of therapy because it is less invasive and less expensive and requires a shorter hospitalization than coronary artery bypass grafting.

Several recent studies, however, have shown late event-free survival to be significantly lower in patients having PTCA when compared with patients having coronary artery bypass grafting. Kramer and colleagues[2] compared 413 patients who had PTCA of an isolated obstruction in the left anterior descending artery with 368 patients who had either a left internal thoracic artery anastomosis or saphenous vein bypass graft to the left anterior descending artery. The 5-year actuarial event-free survival rate was 92.6% for the surgical patients as compared with 62.2% for the PTCA patients ($P = .0001$).

Henderson and colleagues[3] showed a similar low 5-year actuarial event-free survival rate in 412 patients undergoing PTCA for single-vessel disease, 60.2%, and suggested that the need for repeat interventions, either repeat PTCA or coronary artery bypass grafting, substantially reduced event-free survival in patients undergoing PTCA as an initial therapy.

Restenosis, an intimal proliferative process occurring in response to balloon-induced vascular injury,[4, 5] most likely accounts for the high incidence of repeat interventions. Nobuyoshi and colleagues[6] have shown that restenosis can occur in up to 50% of treated vessels within 1 to 3 months of the initial intervention. In a subset of 95 patients with a primary, single-vessel intervention, the actuarial patient rate of restenosis was 41.4% and 53.9% at 3 months and 1 year, respectively.

Attempts to prevent restenosis by the use of a variety of pharmacologic approaches before and after angioplasty have not been successful.[7, 8] Examples of agents tried, without success, include aspirin, dipryidamole, sulfinpyrazone, warfarin, (Coumadin), dextran, nifedipine, diltiazem, glucocorticosteroids, eicosapentanoic acid, and ciprostene.[8]

Because pharmacologic approaches have failed to reduce the frequency of restenosis significantly, interventionists have begun to explore nonpharmacologic, or mechanical, approaches to the problem. Initial efforts using laser light delivered through bare optical fibers and hot-tip laser angioplasty have been demonstrated to be of little value.[9] Other techniques such as intravascular stents, atherectomy devices, laser balloon angioplasty, and excimer laser angioplasty are being actively investigated, although none has yet been shown to be superior to PTCA in terms of a reduced incidence of restenosis.

There is, however, animal data to suggest that laser light that directly irradiates the artery wall in an atraumatic manner can remove arterial obstructions while leaving a surface compatible with healing by complete reendothelialization and no evidence of intimal proliferation. Gerrity and colleagues,[10] using continuous-wave carbon dioxide laser light in atherosclerotic swine, showed the feasibility of plaque removal with laser light irradiation. Follow-up studies showed that the ablated vascular surface healed by resurfacing with a neoendothelium and that, despite maintenance of a high lipid diet, no subsequent recurrence of the atherosclerotic plaque occurred at the treated site. Kjellstrom and colleagues,[11] using a canine model and continuous-wave argon-ion laser light delivered through a multifiber catheter, demonstrated similar healing characteristics with formation of a neointima within 30 days of laser treatment.

Whether laser light can be used in the human to treat coronary artery disease with a lower restenosis rate than in the case of PTCA remains to be seen. Preliminary experiments performed at the Cleveland Clinic,[12] described in Chapter 17, showed that a dose-controlled, continuous-wave argon-ion laser system was not sophisticated enough to test the hypothesis. Perforation and the inability to remove densely calcified plaque precluded an adequate evaluation of long-term restenosis rates following laser ablation of coronary atherosclerosis.

Intensive research focusing on ablation mechanisms and spectroscopy has led to the development of a new, more refined laser angiosurgery system, LAS II, that is capable of removing densely calcified plaque under the guidance of a laser-induced fluorescence feedback loop. The LAS II system is designed to produce a therapeutically significant increase in the lumen diameter of occluded arteries in an atraumatic manner. Diseased atherosclerotic tissue is selectively removed and healthy tissue and blood spared. Selective removal is achieved by means of multiple ablation fibers that are spectroscopically controlled. Thus, in addition to delivery of ablation light, the catheter transmits spectroscopic light to the tissue and collects the return fluorescence for spectral analysis. Spectroscopic control enables ablation light to be delivered at the outer edges of the catheter without the risk of perforation. The catheter is designed to completely recanalize a vessel without follow-up balloon angioplasty. These requirements necessitate precision in light delivery and place stringent conditions on system design.

Two key technical issues have dominated this program. The first entails the identification of a clinically effective combination of lasers and optics for the removal of calcified plaque whose output can be transmitted through the catheter without damaging the optical fibers and related components. The second entails the identification and experimental verification of a reliable spectroscopic scheme and related decision algorithms for diagnosing cardiovascular tissue that has the capability of looking into the tissue at a depth sufficient to ensure that the ablation energy initially directed onto diseased tissue will not inadvertently overstep itself and damage healthy tissue.

This article describes the elements of the LAS II system and the underlying scientific considerations that have led to its design. This system consists of five interconnected subsystems (Fig 18–1). The catheter subsystem is designed to couple light both into and out of a number of specifically identified tissue domains in contact with its distal tip. The diagnostic subsystem, which contains a small laser and spectroscopic apparatus, is coupled into the catheter. It obtains site-specific spectroscopic data that enable the analysis subsystem to make a determination regarding the nature of the tissue (or blood) in each domain. This information is, in turn, delivered to a control subsystem that contains the operator interface, selects and recommends the appropriate treatment for each domain, and controls the operation of the ablation subsystem. The ablation subsystem, which also includes optical switching capability for the spectroscopic subsystem, provides and regulates the high-power laser light that is focused into optical fibers corresponding to specifically selected domains at the distal end of the catheter.

The next section of this chapter discusses the physical basis of laser ablation of biological tissue, which re-

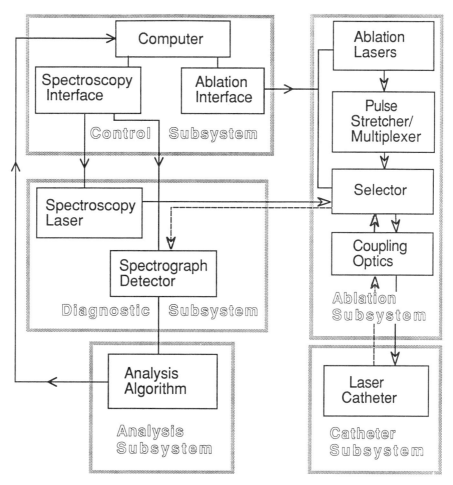

FIG 18–1.
LAS II block diagram.

sulted in the selection of frequency-tripled Nd:YAG as the ablation laser. The section "Optical Fiber Considerations and Pulse Stretching" presents our studies of optical fiber transmission, the requirements on laser pulse parameters to avoid fiber breakdown, and the development of a pulse stretching system to achieve pulses of the required duration. The next section discusses the LAS II catheter, a multifiber, optically shielded device for selective tissue removal. Then the section "Spectroscopy and Diagnostic Algorithm" discusses the use of laser-induced fluorescence to diagnose the tissue and control the laser ablation process. After this, control and operation of the system are discussed, followed by some conclusions.

SELECTION OF AN ABLATION LASER

Successful laser recanalization of coronary arteries containing advanced-stage atherosclerotic plaques requires a laser source capable of ablating densely calcified

tissue as well as softer fibrofatty tissue with a desirable clinical end point but without destroying the optical fibers in its own delivery system. Calcified tissue is far more difficult to ablate than are softer tissues, and delivery of high-energy pulses of laser light to the target is required. For this reason, understanding the mechanisms of both laser ablation of calcified tissue and laser-induced breakdown of optical fibers is a prerequisite to selecting a suitable ablation laser. This section discusses pulsed laser calcified tissue ablation and explains the choice of a frequency-tripled Nd: YAG laser for LAS II. The following section addresses the problem of optical fiber light delivery.

Ablation of biological tissue is governed by three basic laser parameters: irradiance, fluence, and wavelength. Irradiance, sometimes referred to as intensity, is the laser power per unit area delivered to the tissue and is measured in watts per square centimeter. Fluence, the energy per unit area in the laser pulse, is measured in joules per square centimeter. Wavelength determines the "color" of the light beam and is measured in nanometers. The visible wavelength range extends from about 400 nm (violet) to 700 nm (red). Ultraviolet (UV) light lies at shorter wavelengths and infrared (IR) light at longer wavelengths.

Irradiance

Irradiance is the laser parameter that determines the mechanism of ablation. Continuous-wave laser light with irradiance below $\sim 10^5$ W/cm^2 ablates noncalcified tissue and can be used to cut soft plaque.[13, 14] At irradiances greater than $\sim 10^9$ W/cm^2, plasma formation accompanies and contributes to tissue ablation.[5] In the irradiance range between these two limits, calcified tissue can be effectively ablated over a wide range of wavelengths without production of a plasma.[16] The mechanism for this is tied to the morphology of these particular tissues. Calcified plaque, bone, and other similar body tissues consist of hard microparticles composed of calcium salts embedded in a soft matrix of connective tissue. The soft component absorbs the laser light and explosively expands, dragging the hard material with it.[17] We refer to this as two-component ablation.

Some researchers have proposed an alternate mechanism for calcified tissue removal at UV wavelengths that is based on laser photochemistry, perhaps to account for the clean cutting and lack of thermal damage observed at the crater walls.[18, 19] The ablation mechanism in our two-component model is based solely on thermal heating, as determined by the penetration depth of the light in the tissue at a given wavelength. The crater walls are not significantly heated because the hot material is removed before the heat can diffuse to the surrounding tissue. This two-component picture is supported by strobe photographs of the blast wave and material ejected during ablation, and it explains why pulsed ablation with similar properties can occur at visible and IR wavelengths, as well as in the UV range.[17]

Fluence

Experimental studies in our laboratory have shown that within the irradiance range for which two-component ablation takes place, fluence (and not irradiance or pulse duration separately) determines the volume of tissue removed during ablation. Figure 18–2 shows plots of crater depth vs. fluence that were obtained with 355-nm light from a frequency-multiplied Nd:YAG laser incident on a sample of bovine cortical bone both in air and under a 2-mm layer of saline. The fluence dependence of ablation depth can be divided into three regions: (1) subthreshold fluences, at which no tissue removal is discernable under microscopic examination; (2) a region above threshold in which crater depth increases

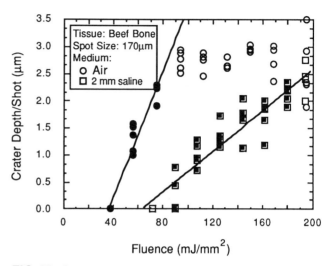

FIG 18–2.
Crater depth vs. $\lambda = 355$ nm laser fluence for beef bone in air and under 2 mm of saline. The filled-in data points indicate the data used for the linear data fit.

approximately linearly with fluence; and (3) the high-fluence regimen in which crater depth increases more slowly with increasing fluence. Two important parameters that characterize the fluence behavior are the fluence threshold ϕ_0, and the ablation yield Y, which is the slope of a plot of crater depth vs. fluence. Although, in general, the ablation yield varies with fluence, for practical applications only the threshold region of the curve is of interest. Thus, ϕ_0 (units, joules per square millimeter) and Y (units, cubic millimeters per joule) may be extracted from data of crater depth (l) vs. fluence (ϕ) by fitting to the linear equation $l = Y(\phi - \phi_0)$.

Wavelength

The wavelength of the laser light controls the scale of the ablation process by determining the depth to which light can penetrate into the tissue. In order to investigate the effects of wavelength on calcified tissue ablation and to judge the suitability of different wavelengths for laser angiosurgery, we studied ablation characteristics at several wavelengths in the near-UV visible, near-IR, and mid-IR regions of the spectrum. In this study, laser irradiances were on the order of megawatts per square millimeter, fluences ranged up to 1,000 mJ/mm^2, repetition rates varied between 0.3 and 10 Hz, and spot diameters on the tissue surface ranged from 150 to 850 μm. The primary tissue studied was bovine shank bone (as a model for the densest calcified tissue), while human arterial calcified plaque and normal human artery wall were studied at selected wavelengths for comparison.

The visual appearance of craters with similar diameters, produced with similar doses of ablating light (measured in terms of the number of times above ablation threshold), varied substantially with laser wavelength. Craters made by using laser wavelengths below about 400 nm and near 3 μm had sharp edges and closely followed the profile of the illuminating beam. There was no evidence of large debris particles or flakes in the vicinity of these craters. Histologic examination of craters in bone at λ = 308 nm and 2.8 μm showed that for both of these wavelengths the crater walls were smoothly cut to within a few tens of micrometers of surface roughness, with little or no thermal damage to underlying tissue. Debris produced during ablation of bone at 308-nm, 355-nm, and 2.8-μm wavelengths was captured in flight and examined with scanning electron microscopy. Debris particle sizes at all of these wavelengths ranged from a few hundred nanometers to a few tens of micrometers in diameter. Craters made with wavelengths between 450 nm and 590 nm had irregular shapes that were clearly dependent on the local morphology of the bone. In addition, large (> 500 μ) flakes of bone were found attached to the edges of the crater and scattered nearby. For the 530-nm and 590-nm wavelengths, many craters were substantially larger in diameter than that of the illuminating beam.

Fluence thresholds as a function of wavelength for all wavelengths studied are plotted in Figure 18–3. The fluence thresholds were obtained by straight-line fits to the threshold-region data of depth vs. fluence plots at each wavelength. The error bars in Figure 18–3 represent the standard error of the data fit and are a measure of the amount of scatter in the data. The steady increase in fluence threshold with wavelength from the near-UV to the visible and near-IR and the decrease again in the mid-IR correlate with the changes in attenuation depth over those wavelengths. This finding is consistent with

an explanation of fluence threshold as the the minimum amount of heat that must be deposited in the tissue before ablation can begin.[13]

Ablation results in different tissues and ablation conditions were also compared at several wavelengths. Figure 18–4 presents a comparison of ablation at 308 nm of fibrous soft plaque, calcified plaque, fresh bone in air, and fresh bone under a 1-mm layer of saline and a 1-mm-thick quartz slide (which acts as an optical shield; see the section "Spectroscopy and Diagnostic Algorithm"). Fluence thresholds measured with the tissue sample under a layer of saline and a shield were approximately twice the air thresholds, while ablation yields remained approximately equal. At all wavelengths for which different tissues and ablation conditions were compared, fluence thresholds under saline and a shield were approximately twice the air thresholds, while ablation yields were higher than in bone by a factor of 1 to 5 for calcified plaque and 2 to 10 for fibrous plaque.

The mutagenic potential of various wavelengths was also considered. In particular, laser wavelengths in the ultraviolet B (UVB) range (280 to 320 nm) are known to be very effective in inducing tumors.[20] The cytotoxic and mutagenic effects are due to photochemically induced DNA damage or error-prone repair mechanisms.[21] The potential for carcinogenesis has been demonstrated in cell line and in animal studies with both UV lamps and laser light. Several relevant cell line studies have been conducted with 308-nm light from a XeCl excimer laser.[22–24] At doses as low as 2 to 10 mJ/mm², cytotoxic and mutagenic effects were observed. Animal studies with UVB light have established that carcinoma, fibrosarcoma, and angiosarcoma can be produced at fluences of 1 to 16 mJ/mm² delivered in multiple doses.[25] More recently, it has been shown that tumors can be in-

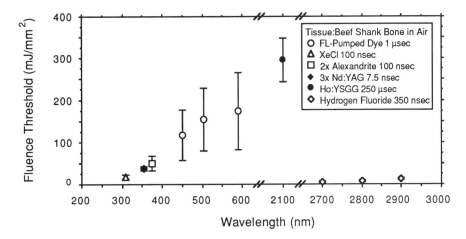

FIG 18–3.
Fluence thresholds in beef bone as a function of wavelength. Note the breaks in the fluence axis.

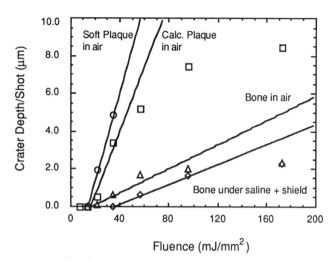

FIG 18–4.
Comparison of ablation at λ = 308 nm of soft plaque, calcified plaque, bovine shank bone in air, and bovine shank bone under 1 mm of saline and a 1-mm-thick quartz shield.

duced with a single dose of UVB light.[26, 27] Strickland studied squamous cell tumor induction in rats and mice and showed that at a wavelength approximately equivalent to that of XeCl laser, significant tumor production was achieved by using single doses of only 10 mJ/mm². These doses are comparable to the ablation parameters measured in our studies and to those used in laser angioplasty clinical studies employing XeCl excimer lasers. Clinical trials employ working fluences in the range of 35 to 50 mJ/mm², with hundreds to thousands of pulses being delivered in the course of a procedure.[28, 29] While ablated tissue is removed, nonablated adjacent tissue may be irradiated many times by significant doses of XeCl laser light, thus subjecting healthy tissue to levels of light known to be mutagenic.

The primary selection criteria for the laser source for the LAS II system were the sharpness of the laser cut in fibrous and calcified tissue, the size of ablation debris particles, removal dosimetry considerations (including fluence threshold and ablation yield), and the potential of the wavelength for mutagenicity. For the reasons discussed above, wavelengths below 320 nm, although excellent tissue cutters, were rejected because of their mutagenic potential. Wavelengths between 320 and 400 nm were also excellent tissue cutters, had low ablation thresholds and high yields, are not mutagenic, and were found to generate debris particles on the order of micrometers in dimension. (Debris characteristics for wavelengths below 320 nm were similar.) Debris particle sizes in this range have been judged satisfactory even for percutaneous applications. Visible wavelengths, above about 400 nm exhibited unsatisfactory cutting and debris along with substantial tissue cracking and fissuring. The

2.1-µm wavelength of the Ho:YSGG laser had good cutting qualities. However, it had a high fluence threshold and low ablation yield, which raises concerns about heat deposition and collateral damage effects. Wavelengths in the 3-µm region, available from Er:YAG and HF lasers, exhibited excellent ablation quality by all selection criteria.

Considerations related to the light delivery system further limited the choices for the ablation laser. No currently available fibers can deliver sufficient light in the 3-µm region to ablate tissue, which excludes that otherwise excellent wavelength range from consideration. Fiber breakdown considerations constrained the range of permissible irradiances usable in the remaining 320- to 400-nm wavelength region, as will be discussed in detail in the following section. Finally, good laser beam quality was necessary to implement the advanced features of LAS II, such as the ability to separately address each fiber or any group of fibers in the catheter tip. With all of these constraints in mind, the λ = 355 nm third harmonic of the Nd:YAG laser was chosen as a proven, reliable, and commercially available laser system that has sufficient beam quality to allow for external optical pulse stretching to satisfy fiber transmission requirements. The design catheter tip fluence was set at 140 mJ/mm², twice the fluence threshold of bone under saline. With this design fluence being delivered by a 3.5-W average power laser and with a catheter tip area of 1.5 mm², a catheter tip advancement rate in the densest calcified tissue of the order of 15 µm/sec was projected.

OPTICAL FIBER CONSIDERATIONS AND PULSE STRETCHING

In a laser angiosurgery system, one must deliver sufficient light to effectively ablate the target tissue without damaging the optical fiber delivery system. To estimate the required laser energy to be transmitted by each optical fiber, consider the 12-fiber laser catheter of Figure 18–6 with a catheter tip area of 1.5 mm². Taking into account the tissue dosimetry at 355 nm, the geometry of the catheter, and coupling and transmission losses, 30 mJ of light must be delivered into each optical fiber. Since the pulse width of the commercial Nd:YAG lasers that are currently available is typically 7.5 ns, this corresponds to a peak power of 4 MW and a peak irradiance of over 10 GW/cm². Since optical fibers cannot withstand these high peak powers and intensities, an understanding of fiber breakdown thresholds and fiber breakdown processes is important. Through an understanding of these, we have achieved the required 30-mJ optical fiber energy delivery by using a novel optical delay system to construct a 400-ns pulse. (Alternatively, an Nd:YAG laser with a 400-ns pulse could be used.) This long pulse lowers the peak intensity and peak power in the optical fiber to tolerable levels while maintaining the ability to effectively ablate the target tissue.

Two distinct mechanisms of optical fiber breakdown usually limit the amount of energy that can be coupled into a fiber: surface breakdown and self-focusing (which leads to bulk breakdown). Surface breakdown critically depends on surface defects, cleanliness, impurities, and the nature of the surrounding medium. If all these factors are controlled, the surface breakdown threshold can be made to approach the bulk breakdown threshold. Self-focusing is a nonlinear effect that causes the laser beam to focus while propagating through the fiber. Material damage to the fiber can occur at the focal point. Surface breakdown can occur at either the input or output faces of the fiber. Whereas the threshold for surface breakdown depends on the intensity of the incident light, breakdown due to self-focusing depends only on the peak power. Understanding both of these mechanisms and the interplay between intensity and peak power is essential.

Self-focusing is the focusing of a beam by itself as a result of the nonlinear change in refractive index induced by the beam. Since the beam is most intense at its center, a radial variation in refractive index is produced that acts as a lens. At a certain incident power, P_1, the focusing of the beam just cancels the spreading due to diffraction. At higher powers the focusing becomes stronger until at a certain critical power, P_2, the beam will focus to a singularity. Depending on the properties of the material, bulk damage will occur at a power between P_1 and P_2. Values for P_1 and P_2 for fused silica at 355 nm are 125 kW and 462 kW, respectively.[30] These values scale as the square of the wavelength, and thus self-focusing is more important at UV wavelengths than in the visible or IR range.

Surface breakdown is an intensity-dependent phenomenon that is not fully understood. Recent work by Reif[31] has classified wide band-gap transparent solids into two categories, each with its own breakdown mechanism. The solids with a high surface defect density, such as LiF and BaF_2, undergo a resonant enhancement of multiphoton processes. The absorbed energy is transferred to the lattice, and material damage occurs. Solids with a low surface defect density, such as CaF_2, MgF_2, and SiO_2, have very low multiphoton absorption cross sections. These materials have higher intensity breakdown thresholds. The breakdown mechanism for these materials may be surface-assisted dielectric air breakdown.[31]

Some previous experimental data relating the surface breakdown fluence threshold to the pulse width may be found in the literature. Taylor et al.[32] found that the surface fluence damage threshold for fused silica scaled as the square root of the pulse width in the nanosecond regime at 308 nm. Rainer et al.[33] also found a square root dependence at 248 nm for MgF_2 and CaF_2. Thus, by increasing the pulse width, one can increase the surface fluence damage threshold as well as decrease the peak power below the self-focusing threshold. This will lead to an increase in the energy that can be transmitted through the fiber.

In order to test this approach at 355 nm, an optical delay system was designed to extend a 7.5 ns tripled Nd:YAG pulse to variable widths of up to 200 ns. This passive system, which uses only mirrors, lenses, and beam splitters, has achieved an overall energy throughput efficiency of 60%. Pulse widths of 400 ns are produced by using a second laser triggered to fire 200 ns after the first one.

In the first stage of this system, the input pulse (Fig 18–5,A) is divided into four equal pulses by using beam splitters. Each pulse travels a successively longer distance before being recombined with the others. This produces a 30-ns pulse train as shown in Figure 18–5,B. All delay paths contain focusing elements that are used to reimage the beam from the beginning to the end of its path thus ensuring that the four pulses that make up the 30-ns profile maintain identical spatial distributions. It is important to note that this first stage actually has two identical 30-ns outputs, each with half the energy. Since we are interested in illuminating four fibers simultaneously, we make use of both of these outputs.

The second stage of the system, a commercially available device produced by Exitech, Inc., transforms an input pulse (in this case, a 30-ns pulse train) into six identical output pulses (followed by a train of exponentially decreasing pulses), each separated by 30 ns. This device contains six beam splitters spaced sequentially at 30-ns path length intervals, each of which reflects a portion of the beam back nearly parallel to the incoming beam. The reflectivities of the beam splitters are chosen to give six equal-amplitude output pulses. Focusing elements are used to equalize the apparent distance traveled by each pulse.

Through careful alignment of the system, one can achieve a series of collinear, identical pulses. By blocking various beam paths, one can obtain essentially a top-hat temporal profile of various pulse widths between 7.5 and 200 ns. A 400-ns pulse made up of 200-ns pulses from two different lasers is displayed in Figure 18–5,C.

With this optical delay system, experiments were performed on fused silica substrates to determine the functional dependence of pulse width on surface break-

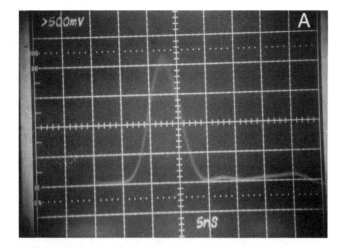

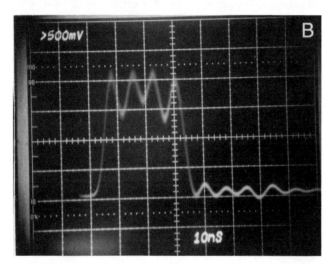

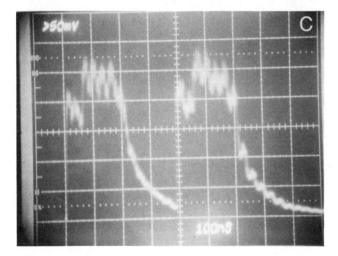

FIG 18–5.
Temporal pulse profile of the 7.5-ns laser output **(A)**, a 30-ns stretched pulse **(B)**, and the final pulse train consisting of two 200-ns pulses **(C)**.

down. It was found that the breakdown fluence threshold increased as the pulse width to the 0.8 power for pulse widths between 7.5 and 150 ns.[34] This scaling behavior is significantly stronger than the scaling found by Taylor and Rainer mentioned earlier.

Breakdown thresholds for 200-μm-core fused silica fibers appear to follow this scaling law, although the breakdown fluences are a factor of 4 below those of the substrate. This factor of 4 may be attributed to the nonuniform beam profile on the input face of the fiber and to the superior surface polish of the substrate. By stretching our pulses to 400 ns, significant increases in the amount of 355-nm light that can be transmitted through 200-μm-core optical fibers have been achieved, from 1 to 2 mJ at 7.5 ns to over 30 mJ at 400 ns.

Thus, by using two lasers and the optical delay system described above, a temporal profile was created that allowed the proper dose of 355-nm light to be delivered through 200-μm-core optical fibers.

LAS II CATHETER DESIGN

The LAS system employs an optically shielded, multifiber, spectroscopically guided laser catheter with guidewire capability.[14, 35] Its distal tip consists of a bundled array of optical fibers enclosed in a transparent "optical shield." Light rays emitted from each individual fiber diverge through the shield and exit at predetermined locations on the output surface to produce a pattern of spots of predetermined diameter. Individual light spots overlap to uniformly irradiate the entire output face of the catheter tip. The tip is designed to be brought into contact with the lesion to be removed. This displaces blood and other fluids to provide a clear field for light delivery. Further, because the diameter of the light spots is fixed, the fluence and intensity of the light irradiating the tissue can be precisely controlled, thus enabling dosimetry to be accurately specified. In addition, the controlled geometry enables the intensity of the collected fluorescence light to be calibrated. The shield also protects the polished optical fibers from the contents of the artery and the patient from the fibers should a malfunction occur and the fibers shatter.

The optical fibers in the catheter are arranged and oriented so that each output spot partially overlaps adjacent spots to enable light to completely cover the distal tip of the optical shield. This results in 100% coverage and permits all tissue with which the tip is in contact to be ablated. Care is taken to ensure that the ablation light fully fills the numerical aperture of each fiber and produces a "top-hat" output intensity profile across the fiber diameter. Incomplete filling of the optical fiber modes adversely affects the diameter and shapes of the craters. Uniform irradiation of the shield leads to uniform ablation and thus avoids creation of a "Swiss cheese" pattern of craters, and uniform illumination of the outer circumference of the shield prevents the creation of a composite hole with scalloped edges.

Laser catheter designs that do not utilize the optical shield concept and rely instead on direct optical fiber contact do not yield complete overlap and produce a Swiss cheese ablation pattern in the tissue. These laser catheters are also designed to *avoid* illuminating the outer circumference of the catheter tip in order to reduce the likelihood of perforation. As a result, tissue is not removed over the the entire cross section of the device, so in order to advance, the catheter must be forced through a narrow lumen with resultant trauma to the artery wall. This may result in dissection, thrombogenic surfaces, and distal emboli and is a likely cause of the high restenosis rates reported in these devices.[36–38] In contrast, in the LAS catheter the outer circumference of the output face can be fully illuminated because spectroscopic guidance is used to avoid tunneling into the artery wall. Complete illumination of the shield ensures ablation without leaving intervening residual tissue and produces a composite hole the same diameter as that of the catheter. Mechanical trauma (the Dotter effect), which is thought to contribute to restenosis, is thus minimized. The ability to produce a large increase in lumen diameter is another important factor in preventing restenosis of the recanalized vessel.

One current LAS catheter, a 12-fiber device constructed for intraoperative coronary use, is shown in Figure 18–6. It is 1.5 mm in diameter, has a quartz optical shield and a central lumen for passage of a 0.01-in. guidewire, and contains 12, 200-μm-core-diameter fused silica optical fibers. The numerical aperture of the fibers is 0.22. The fibers and shield readily transmit the 355-nm, UV radiation and are capable of withstanding the rigors of ablation. The overall distal stiff section is approximately 3 mm. A radiopaque marker is provided for fluoroscopic visualization.

A central lumen in the catheter is provided for insertion of a guidewire. The guidewire maintains coaxial positioning of the catheter as it advances through the lumen so that it cannot point directly at the wall of the artery. This also allows the catheter to safely track the tortuous coronary vessel without mechanical vascular perforation. The lumen can also be used for injection of contrast fluid and removal of debris.

At the input (proximal) end of the catheter, the 12 optical fibers are arranged in a line (Fig 18–7). Ablation light is delivered to the input array by means of a 4-fiber light transmission line mounted on a computer-controlled translator. An additional optical fiber, mounted with the transmission line, is used to conduct spectroscopic excitation light to the catheter and collect return fluorescence. A spectroscopic diagnostic image is acquired by successively stepping through the fibers one at a time. The spectroscopy module is described in the following section.

The 12 output spots of the catheter, each 500 μm in diameter, completely overlap the output face of the shield. Note that the spot of light emerging from each fiber expands in area by a factor of 6. The need to expand the spots to maintain overlap places stringent requirements on the light-carrying capacity of the optical fibers in the catheter body.

As mentioned above, a working fluence of 140 mJ/mm² has been selected, and each fiber can deliver up to 24 mJ into a 500-μm-diameter light spot on the output face of the optical shield. Individual craters produced are equal in diameter to the light spot diameters and have clean walls, and composite holes are approximately the same diameter as the catheter. In a 1.5-mm-diameter artery with a clinically significant stenosis of 90%, or

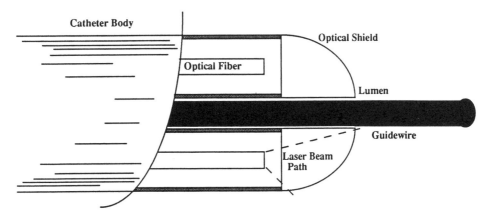

FIG 18–6.
LAS optically shielded, multifiber, spectroscopically guided laser catheter with a central lumen and guidewire—distal end.

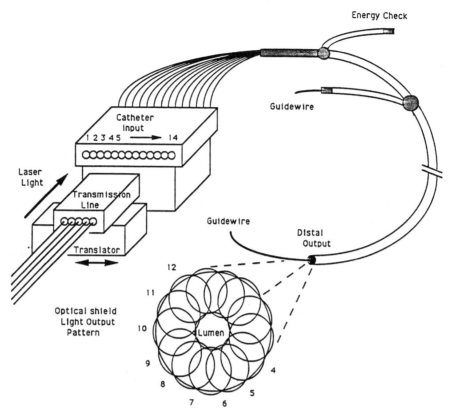

FIG 18–7.
LAS catheter, transmission line, linear input, and distal output.

a 0.5-mm-diameter opening, the catheter should be capable of full restoration of flow without postexposure balloon dilatation.

For percutaneous applications, smaller-diameter optical fibers, on the order of 50 to 100 μm, are preferred because of their increased flexibility. Although the total number of fibers required will increase as smaller-core fibers are utilized (in order to maintain delivery of adequate energy), flexibility and resolution increase. Catheters with a range of overall outer diameters have been constructed and are required for a variety of vessel dimensions, both coronary and peripheral. Devices with no guidewire for treating total occlusions have also been constructed. All configurations maintain the design criteria of controlled ablation through precise light delivery and selectivity in tissue removal.

SPECTROSCOPY AND DIAGNOSTIC ALGORITHM

Several authors have suggested that the technique of fluorescence spectroscopy may be used in a laser recanalization system for feedback control to prevent perforation.[35, 39, 40] For fluorescence spectroscopy to be effective as a guidance system for laser angiosurgery in the tortuous coronary arteries, it obviously must allow for removal of atherosclerosis while preventing arterial perforation. To avoid perforation, a fluorescence diagnostic system must be capable of identifying the area of interest in a coronary artery as normal, noncalcified atherosclerotic plaque or calcified atherosclerotic plaque, both before and after removal of tissue by laser ablation. Furthermore, it must do this at a depth sufficient to ensure that the ablation energy initially directed onto diseased tissue will not inadvertently overstep itself and damage healthy tissue.

A diagram of the LAS II diagnostic subsystem is shown in Figure 18–8. Short (2-ns) pulses of weak excitation light at 480 nm are provided by a small nitrogen-pumped dye laser (10 Hz). A single pulse of excitation light is transmitted via an optical fiber to a dichroic mirror, which reflects the beam and directs it through a focusing lens and into one of the optical fibers at the proximal end of the LAS catheter. This fiber conducts the excitation pulse to a particular tissue site, where it forms a circular spot 500 μm in diameter. The resulting fluorescence signal produced from this "pixel" of tissue

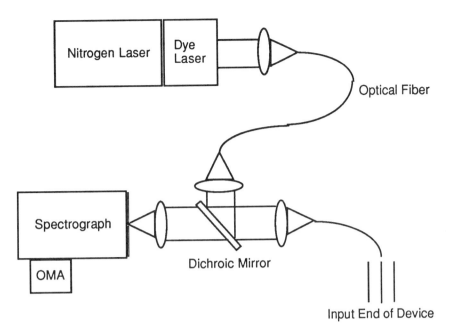

FIG 18–8.
Diagnostic subsystem.

is returned by this same fiber to the proximal end of the catheter, where it is collimated by the same lens, passes through the dichroic mirror, and is focused (f-matched) into a 0.25-m imaging spectrograph. The signal is detected at the output image plane of the spectrograph by using an optical multichannel analyzer (OMA). The signal-to-noise ratio of the fluorescence spectrum produced from a single pulse of excitation laser light is excellent, in excess of 30:1.

The system is calibrated at the start of each procedure. A wavelength calibration is performed through an auxiliary fiber on the catheter. The position of each fiber on the translator is checked and validated, and background fluorescence from individual fibers is determined and subtracted in subsequent scans. The intensity response of each fiber is calibrated against a fluorescence standard, and each succeeding spectrum is corrected.

Corrected fluorescence spectra from each of the individual tissue sites are fit to a one-layer model of tissue fluorescence, which has been described in detail previously.[41–43] Briefly, the model describes tissue fluorescence in terms of four parameters, two of which (βs) represent intrinsic tissue fluorescence contributions and two of which (xs) describe contributions due to attenuation of light. β_{SP}, which is proportional to the concentration and quantum yield of structural protein, describes the portion of tissue fluorescence that can be ascribed to chromophores in or associated with the structural proteins collagen and elastin. Similarly, β_{Ce} is

proportional to the concentration and quantum yield of ceroid and represents the portion of tissue fluorescence that is due to ceroid,[44] an oxidation product of lipids found in necrotic regions of atheromas. Finally, x_{Hb} describes the contribution of attenuation by oxyhemoglobin to the tissue fluorescence spectrum. Normalized fluorescence and attenuation line shapes corresponding to structural protein, ceroid, and hemoglobin were determined previously for aorta.[41–43] Here, we apply these same line shapes to fit data from coronary arteries.

Thus, our method of data analysis is to reduce individual tissue fluorescence spectra into a three-dimensional vector with components β_{SP}, β_{Ce}, and x_{Hb}. The components of this vector are proportional to the concentration and peak quantum yield or attenuation coefficient of the three arterial chromophores (structural proteins, ceroid, and hemoglobin) and can be used to calculate the likelihood that the area of interest in a human coronary artery is normal, noncalcified atherosclerotic plaque or calcified atherosclerotic plaque. Diagnostic algorithms for coronary artery atherosclerosis can be derived from this likelihood.

An example of the diagnostic algorithm for a coronary artery that utilizes the model parameters β_{SP} and β_{Ce} is shown in the contour plot of Figure 18–9. In this figure, the contour lines represent the probabilities that a particular β_{SP}, β_{Ce} pair of model parameters (determined from a coronary fluorescence spectrum) represents normal, soft plaque or calcified plaque in the tis-

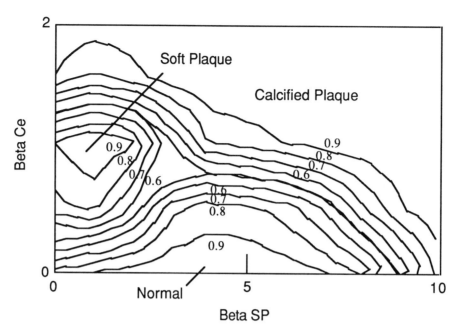

FIG 18–9.
Contour plot of diagnostic probabilities.

sue. The probabilities have been determined from a data set of over 100 in vitro specimens of coronary artery. The classification of tissue as atherosclerotic is considered correct if the probability is determined to be greater than 70% for diseased tissue.

SYSTEM CONTROL AND OPERATION

The LAS II system is controlled by an 80386 UNIX–based microcomputer. The modular software was developed for each of the subsystems, ablation and diagnostic individually, to allow flexibility and reliability in operation.

Each time a new catheter is placed in the system, the system is calibrated for optimal performance. System operation begins by moving the linear translator such that the optical fiber delivering spectroscopic light from the nitrogen-pumped dye laser is brought into alignment with fiber no. 1 of the LAS catheter (see Fig 18–7). A fluorescence spectrum is obtained, background and intensity response corrected, and model parameters calculated. In addition, the probability that the tissue pixel irradiated by this fiber is normal, soft atherosclerotic tissue or calcified atherosclerotic tissue is determined. The linear translator then automatically brings the spectroscopic delivery fiber into alignment with the next fiber at the proximal end of the catheter. This process is rapidly repeated for all 12 fibers.

Once the entire set of 12 pixels has been analyzed in this fashion, the resulting image is analyzed for contigu-

ity to determine which tissue pixels should be irradiated with ablation light. Three criteria must be fulfilled in order to label a single pixel as diseased: (1) the probability of disease (soft plaque and calcified plaque combined) is greater than 70%, (2) the model parameters are physically reasonable, and (3) the model adequately describes the data according to statistical criteria (condition on the χ-squared value). If three or more contiguous fibers are determined to be atherosclerotic in this fashion, the four-fiber transmission line that delivers the ablation light is moved into alignment with the proximal end of the catheter, and the the ablation sequence is activated.

Before applying ablation light to the tissue, the dosimetry for each contiguous region is computed. The same dose (number of light pulses of a given energy) is delivered to all of the pixels in a given contiguous region. This dose is a weighted average of the individual doses determined from the relative amounts of hard and soft atherosclerotic tissue present in the region. In the current algorithm the pulse energy is fixed, and the dose is adjusted by varying the number of pulses delivered to each fiber. The dosimetry selected advances the catheter approximately 100 μm in each ablation round. This ensures that the depth of tissue removed between diagnostic scans is significantly less than the penetration depth ($\approx$500 μm) of the diagnostic light.

In the current system ablation proceeds four fibers at a time, and a firing pattern must be specified before actually carrying out ablation. This pattern is decided by two simple rules: (1) fire on single fibers as infrequently as possible, and (2) break the image into equal parts if possible. As an example of the former, if the ablation image consists of five fibers, the system would fire on three of these and then two rather than four and one. As an example of the latter rule, if the ablation image consists of six fibers, the system would fire on three and three rather than four and two.

After all of these calculations are made, the system prepares itself by setting the transmission line shutters for the proper ablation sequence. The appropriate shutters are then opened to apply the correct number of laser pulses to provide the required dosimetry. Ablation energy is delivered as long as foot switches controlled by the clinician and computer operator are depressed. Upon completion of the ablation cycle, the proximal end of the catheter is moved back to the diagnostic subsystem and the process repeated.

Several "failure" conditions halt the ablation sequence before the specified dose has been delivered and return the catheter to the diagnostic subsystem: (1) raising a foot switch for any reason, (2) detection of a fiber failure, (3) detection of greater than a 20% decrease or increase in the ablation laser power, and (4) detection of inoperative laser shutters. The system continues to take spectroscopic data until the error is corrected.

A block diagram of the LAS II system is shown in Figure 18–1. The entire system is under computer control, with a touch screen acting as an interface to the operator. After the diagnostic cycle the touch screen displays a diagnostic image of the tip of the catheter that indicates which of the fibers will be activated for ablation, as well as a bar graph of the computed probabilities for noncalcified and calcified plaque that led to the ablation decisions. An example touch screen output display after the diagnostic step for a typical artery is shown in Figure 18–10. At this point, the fibers illuminating the diseased tissue are automatically selected to deliver high-energy pulses of ablation light at 355 nm. Approximately 100 µm of tissue is removed during an ablation sequence, and a new diagnostic image is generated and presented on the display. The diagnosis-ablation sequence is repeated until the lesion is removed and the lumen recanalized. Each diagnostic and ablation step in the process is designed to take 1.5 seconds. For a typical coronary lesion with a length of several millimeters, LAS recanalization should be completed in several minutes.

CONCLUSION

LAS II is a scientifically based laser angiosurgery system in which diagnosis and tissue removal are integrated. The system is designed to produce a therapeutically significant increase in lumen diameter of occluded

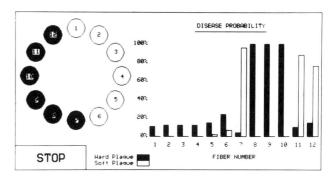

FIG 18–10.
Photograph of the touch screen display.

arteries in an atraumatic manner. It employs an optically shielded catheter whose fibers can be independently fired to selectively remove diseased tissue and a unique system for delivering therapeutic light to the target. The laser power, pulse duration, and wavelength have been carefully optimized. An FDA-approved trial is now under way to test the fully integrated system.

Acknowledgments

This research was supported by GV Medical, Inc., and the National Institutes of Health under grant no. RR02594. The research was performed at the MIT Laser Biomedical Research Center and the Cleveland Clinic Foundation.

REFERENCES

1. Grüntzig AR, Senning A, Sergenthaler WE: Nonoperative dilatation of coronary artery stenosis: Percutaneous transluminal coronary angioplasty. *N Engl J Med* 1979; 301:61.
2. Kramer JR, Proudfit WL, Loop FD, et al: Late follow-up of 781 patients undergoing transluminal coronary angioplasty or coronary artery bypass grafting for an isolated obstruction in the left anterior descending coronary artery. *Am Heart J* 1989; 118:1144–1153.
3. Henderson RA, Karani S, Bucknall CA, et al: Clinical outcome of coronary angioplasty for single-vessel disease. *Lancet* 1989; 2:546.
4. Essed CE, VandenBrand M, Becker AE: Transluminal coronary angioplasty and early restenosis: Fibrocellular occlusion after wall laceration. *Br Heart J* 1983; 49:393.
5. Austin GE, Ratliff NB, Hollman J, et al: Intimal proliferation of smooth muscle cells as an explanation for recurrent coronary artery stenosis after percutaneous transluminal coronary angioplasty. *J Am Coll Cardiol* 1985; 6:369.
6. Nobuyoshi M, Kimura T, Nosalea H, et al: Restenosis after successful percutaneous transluminal coronary angioplasty: Serial angiographic follow-up of 229 patients. *J Am Coll Cardiol* 1988; 12:616.
7. McBride W, Lange RA, Hills LD: Restenosis after successful coronary angioplasty. *N Engl J Med* 1988; 318:1735.

8. Fanelli C, Aronoff R: Restenosis following coronary angioplasty. *Am Heart J* 1990; 119:357.

9. Tobis J, Smolin M, Mallery J, et al: Laser-assisted thermal angioplasty in human peripheral artery occlusions: Mechanism of recanalization. *J Am Coll Cardiol* 1989; 13:1547.

10. Gerrity RG, Loop FD, Golding LAR, et al: Arterial response to laser operation for removal of atherosclerotic plaques. *J Thorac Cardiovasc Surg* 1983; 85:409–421.

11. Kjellstrom BT, Bylock AL, Bott-Silverman C, et al: Removal of surgically induced fibrous arterial plaques by argon ion laser angiosurgery using a multifiber delivery system. *J Thorac Cardiovasc Surg* 1988; 96:925.

12. Kramer JR, Feld MS, Cothren RM, et al: Laser angiosurgery: A biomedical system using photons to diagnose and treat atherosclerosis, in Vogel JHK, King SB (eds): *Future Directions in Interventional Cardiology*, ed 2. St Louis, Mosby–Year Book, 1990.

13. Partovi F, Izatt JA, Cothren RM, et al: A Model for Thermal Ablation of Biological Tissue Using Laser Radiation. *Lasers Surg Med* 1987; 7:141–154.

14. Cothren RM, Kittrell C, Hayes GB, et al: Controlled light delivery for laser angiosurgery. *IEEE J Quant Elect* 1986; 1:4–7.

15. Kittrell C, Tobin J, Rulnick J, et al: Plasma ablation of tissue (abstract). *Lasers Surg Med* 1986; 6:267.

16. Izatt JA, Albagli D, Britton M, et al: Wavelength dependence of pulsed laser ablation of calcified tissue. *Lasers Surg Med* 1991; 11:238.

17. Izatt JA, Albagli D, Itzkan I, et al: Pulsed laser ablation of calcified tissue: Physical mechanisms and fundamental parameters. Laser-tissue interaction. *Proc SPIE* 1990; 1202:133–140.

18. Grundfest WS, Litvack F, Forrester JS, et al: Laser ablation of human atherosclerotic plaque without adjacent tissue injury. *J Am Coll Cardiol* 1985; 6:929–933.

19. Srinivasan R, Dyer PE, Braren B: Ablation of polymers and biological tissue by ultraviolet lasers. *Science* 1986; 234:559–565.

20. Vanderleun JC: UV-carcinogenesis: Yearly review. *Photochem Photobiol* 1984; 39:861.

21. Friedman PS: Ultraviolet carcinogenesis in men and mice. *Br J Dermatol* 1983; 109:683.

22. Rasmussen RE, Hammer-Wilson M, Berns MW: Mutation and sister chromatid exchange induced in Chinese hamster ovary (CHO) cells by pulsed excimer laser radiation at 193 nm and 308 nm and continuous UV radiation at 254 nm. *Photochem Photobiol* 1989; 49:413.

23. Colella CM, Bogani P, Agati G, et al: Genetic effects of UV-B: Mutagenicity of 308 nm light in Chinese hamster V79 cells. *Photochem Photobiol* 1986; 43:437.

24. Tiphlova OA, Karu TI, Furzikov NP: Lethal and mutagenic action of XeCl laser radiation on *Escherichia coli*. *Lasers Life Sci* 1988; 2:155.

25. Freeman RG: Action spectrum for ultraviolet carcinogenesis. *Natl Cancer Inst Monogr* 1978; 50:27.

26. Hsu J, Forbes PD, Harber LC, et al: Induction of skin tumors in hairless mice by a single exposure to UV radiation. *Photochem Photobiol* 1975; 21:185.

27. Strickland PT, Burns FJ, Albert RE: Induction of skin tumors in the rat by single exposure to ultraviolet radiation. *Photochem Photobiol* 1979; 30:683.

28. Karsch KR, Haase KK, Voelker W, et al: Percutaneous coronary excimer laser angioplasty in patients with stable and unstable angina pectoris. *Circulation* 1990; 81:1849.

29. Litvak F, Grundfest WS, Goldberg T, et al: Percutaneous excimer laser angioplasty of aortocoronary saphenous vein grafts. *J Am Coll Cardiol* 1989; 14:803.

30. Smith WL, Bechtel JH, Bloembergen N: Picosecond laser-induced breakdown at 5321 and 3547 A: Observation of frequency-dependent behavior. *Phys Rev* 1977; 15:4039–4055.

31. Reif J: High power laser interaction with the surface of wide bandgap materials. *Optical Eng* 1989; 28:1122–1132.

32. Taylor RS, Leopold KE, Brimacombe RK, et al: Dependence of the damage and transmission properties of fused silica fibers on the excimer laser wavelength. *Appl Optics* 1988; 27:3124–3134.

33. Rainer F, Lowdermilk WH, Milam D: Bulk and surface damage thresholds of crystals and glasses at 248 nm. *Optical Eng* 1983; 22:431–434.

34. Albagli D, Izatt JA, Hayes GB, et al: Time dependence of laser-induced surface breakdown in fused silica at 355 nm in the nanosecond regime. *Proc SPIE* 1990; 1441:146–153.

35. Cothren RM, Hayes GB, Kramer JR, et al: A multifiber catheter with an optical shield for laser angiosurgery. *Lasers Life Sci* 1986; 1:1–12.

36. Haase KK, Mauser M, Baumbauch A, et al: Restenosis after excimer laser coronary atherectomy (abstract). *Circulation* 1990; 82(suppl 3):672.

37. Reeder GS, Bresnahan JF, Bresnahan DR, et al: ELCA Registry members: Excimer laser coronary angioplast (ELCA) in patients with restenosis after prior balloon angioplasty (BA) (abstract). *Circulation* 1990; 82(suppl 3):672.

38. Unterker W, Litvack F, Margolis J, et al: ELCA investigators: Excimer laser coronary angioplasty of saphenous vein grafts (abstract). *Circulation* 1990; 82(suppl 3):680.

39. Leon MB, Lu DY, Prevosti LG, et al: Human arterial surface fluorescence: Atherosclerotic plaque identification and effects of laser atheroma ablation. *J Am Coll Cardiol* 1988; 12:94–102.

40. Fitzmaurice M, Bordagaray G, Englemann G, et al: Argon ion laser induced autofluorescence in normal and atherosclerotic aorta and coronary artery: Morphologic studies. *Am Heart J* 1989; 118:1028.

41. Richards-Kortum R, Rava RP, Fitzmaurice M, et al: A one-layer model of laser-induced fluorescence for diagnosis of disease in human tissue: Applications to atherosclerosis. *IEEE Trans Biomed Eng* 1989; 36:122–132.

42. Richards-Kortum R, Rava RP, Cothren R, et al: A model for extraction of diagnostic information from laser induced fluorescence spectra of human artery wall (abstract). *Spectrochim Acta* 1988; 45:87.

43. Richards-Kortum R: *Fluorescence Spectroscopy as a Technique for Diagnosis of Pathologic Conditions in Human Arterial, Urinary Bladder, and Gastrointestinal Tissues* (thesis). Massachusetts Institute of Technology, Department of Health Science and Technology, June 1990.

44. Ball RY, Carpenter KLH, Mitchinson MJ: What is the significance of ceroid in human atherosclerosis? *Arch Pathol Lab Med* 1987; 111:1134–1140.

Pulsed Laser Ablation of Atherosclerotic Plaque in Blood Vessels

Alexander A. Oraevsky, Ph.D.

Vladilen S. Letokhov, Ph.D.

Laser angioplasty of blood vessels has been the subject of several investigations in many laboratories and clinics.[1-3] The main merit of this technique as compared with balloon angioplasty is that the vessels can be recanalized in the case of total occlusion as well as in the presence of highly calcified plaque. A number of medical and physical problems should be resolved for successful and wide application of this method clinically. The effects of lasers on vessel walls are among the medical questions that should be answered. The principal questions are how to avoid fast reocclusion and increase the rate of vessel healing, and whether ablation products are thrombogenic. The physical problems include the choice of optimal wavelengths and laser radiation regimen for effective removal of various plaques with minimal damage to their adjacent tissues as well as laser radiation dosimetry in tissue that is aimed at excluding vessel wall perforation.

This chapter considers the specific features of ablation of vessel tissue, particularly atherosclerotic plaque by pulsed laser radiation. This mode of ablation holds much promise for laser angioplasty. The practical recommendations given here on application of this method for laser destruction of plaque are based on the results of studies of the optical and thermal properties of tissue and the mechanism of the laser pulse interaction with the tissue of atherosclerotic vessels.

COMPARISON OF LASER ABLATION MODES: LONG AND SHORT PULSES

The fact that continuous-wave lasers are simple in design and convenient and reliable in operation can ex-plain why the so-called continuous mode of irradiation with "long" laser pulses has been applied in most experiments and clinical practice.[4,5] With the advent of pulsed and particularly excimer lasers in many laboratories, these lasers have found application in plaque ablation.[6,7] These two modes, however, for the sake of simplicity referred to as continuous (although the irradiation duration in the experiment is limited) and pulsed, have a qualitative difference. To understand this difference one should consider the penetration of laser radiation within absorbing and scattering tissue. The depth of this penetration is equal to the inverse value of the attenuation factor μ_{eff}:

$$l_{eff} = \mu_{eff}^{-1} = [3\mu_a(\mu_a + \mu'_s)]^{-1/2} \qquad (1)$$

where μ_a and μ'_s are the coefficients of absorption and effective scattering in inverse centimeters, respectively. Table 19–1 contains information on μ_a, μ'_s, and l_{eff} for the wavelengths of lasers frequently used. The value l_{eff} determines the depth of laser energy deposition. The absorbed energy is converted to heat at a very fast rate in a short time (usually faster than 10^{-8} sec) and heats the volume of irradiated plaque.

The heat from the irradiated volume of tissue can diffuse into the nonirradiated sides. The distance of heat propagation during the irradiation time is expressed as follows[16]:

$$l_{HD} = (M\chi\tau_p)^{1/2} \qquad (2)$$

where $\chi = 1.3 \times 10^{-3}$ cm^2/sec denotes the thermal diffusivity coefficient. M is a numerical coefficient dependent on the shape of the heated volume ($M = 8$ for a long cylinder, $M = 4$ for a disk, and $M = 27$ for a sphere). According to the results of Welch,[17] the thermal diffusivity varies from 1.4 cm^2/sec (calcified) to 1.1 cm^2/sec (fatty) for different types of plaques (calcified and fibrous or fatty) in the temperature range T from 20°C to 100°C. This value does not differ essentially from the values for water (1.4 to 1.5 cm^2/sec) and normal vessel wall (1.2 to 1.3 cm^2/sec). Table 19-1 gives values of l_{HD} for various lasers with different pulse durations, τ_p.

The most interesting case of tissue ablation is when the laser beam diameter (d_L) is considerably larger than the radiation attenuation depth, l_{eff}. In this case heat diffuses mainly through the bottom of an exposed volume into the biotissue as shown in Figure 19-1. The qualitative difference in ablation at continuous and pulsed irradiation is particularly vivid here.

In the case of continuous-wave action of laser radiation on vessel walls, heat due to diffusion propagates to all sides in the surrounding tissue at a distance $l_{HD} \gg l_{eff}$ (Fig 19-1,A). As a result of continuous-wave irradiation of atherosclerotic plaque, thermal damage to vessel wall tissue occurs.

In the case of pulsed action, the exposed tissue volume is only heated. Owing to ablation almost this entire volume of overheated tissue will be ejected outside[18] (Fig 19-1,B). For pulsed ablation the depth of thermal damage of the adjacent tissue is determined by the absorption and scattering coefficients as well as by the energy that did not escape with tissue during ablation. It is assumed here that the laser pulse duration (τ_p) is much shorter in comparison with the time of heat diffusion from the irradiated volume (V_{irr}):

$$V_{irr} \cong (\pi d_L^2/4)l_{eff} \qquad (3)$$

where d_L is the laser beam diameter (or the diameter of fiber tangent to the tissue surface) and l_{eff} is the effective depth of light penetration. For the case when the volume subjected to radiation is disk shaped, $l_{eff} \ll d_L$, Table 19-1 presents heat diffusion times for different types of lasers used in angioplasty. The restriction on τ_p arises from the condition that $\tau_p < \tau_{HD}$. The value of l_{HD} in this case is minimal. Besides the restriction on laser pulse duration, it is also necessary to restrict the pulse repetition rate in order to realize pulsed ablation. This condition dictates that the exposed tissue be cooled during the time gap (τ) between the two pulses. Hence, this interval (τ) should be much longer than the time of thermal diffusion from the irradiated volume (τ_{HD}). So the pulse repetition rate must be about ten times lower than $(\tau_{HD})^{-1}$.

A qualitative comparison between continuous and pulsed ablation shows that the latter not only minimizes overheating of the surrounding tissue but is also characterized by a higher efficiency relative to the energy deposited. Indeed, at pulsed irradiation the maximal part of deposited energy is spent to realize the process of ablation. With continuous irradiation a part of the deposited energy is lost to heat diffusion, and additional energy is needed to keep the acting fluence above the ablation threshold. The pulsed ablation efficiency at 465 nm (dye laser), for example, comes to 0.25 mg/J,[15] whereas the efficiency (η) of continuous ablation by an Ar^+ laser is just 2.5 times lower, $\eta \leq 0.1$ mg/J.[5] Histologic studies (Fig 19-2) confirm a qualitative difference between the pulsed and continuous modes of ablation. It can be seen from Figure 19-2 that the crater diameter with pulsed ablation corresponds to the laser beam diameter, the crater walls are even, and the tissue around the crater is not charred. On the other hand, the crater shape produced by continuous ablation is dis-

TABLE 19-1.

Optical Properties of Atherosclerotic (Fibrous) Plaque and Parameters of Ablation by Different Lasers*

Parameters	XeCl[9]	3ωNd:YAG[10]	Dye[11]	Argon[5]	2ωNd[10]	Nd:YAG[12]	Ho:YAG[13]	Er:YAG[14]	CO_2[15]
λ, nm	308	355	465	488/514	532	1064	2100	2940	10,600
τ_p	20–100 ns	10 ns	1 μs	10^{-3}–1 sec	15 ns	20 ns	200 μs	200 μs	2 μs
μ_a, cm^{-1}	25	15	7	6.0/4.0	3.5	0.1	22	10,000	500
μ'_s, cm^{-1}	85	62	33	32/29	26	10	—	—	—
l_{eff}, μm	110	170	345	380/500	570	5745	455	1	20
τ_{HD}, ms	23	55	228	280/490	700	31,735	400	0.002	0.8
f_{max}, Hz	4	2	0.5	0.4/0.2	0.1	0.003	0.25	50,000	130
η, mg/J	0.3	0.21	0.25	0.1/—	0.13	0.06	—	0.54	1.9
P_{thr}, W/cm^2	—	—	—	120/—	—	4800	—	—	—
ϕ_{thr}, J/cm^2	2.7	4.0	6.8	—/—	24	45	28	0.6	3.2

*Spectral properties of plaque for the ultraviolet and visible spectral range are from Oraevsky AA, Jacques SL: *Lasers Surg Med*, 1992, in press. The spectral properties for the infrared range are from Zolotarv VM, Morozov VN, Smirnov EV, et al: *IEEE J Quant Electr* 1987; 23:1751–1755.

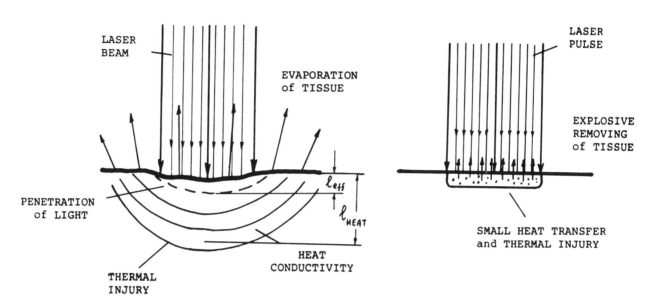

FIG 19–1.
Ablative destruction of biotissue under the action of a long **(A)** or short **(B)** laser pulse. *CW* = continuous wave.

torted due to heat diffusion, its diameter is larger than that of the laser beam, and the crater edges are charred and irregular. For angioplasty of coronary vessels the precision of plaque and occlusion removal without damaging the vessel wall is highly important.[19, 20]

The degree of thermal injury to tissue during ablation is vividly characterized by the coefficient Q_{inj}, that is, the ratio of the mass of adjacent tissue thermally damaged around the crater and not ejected by ablation (Δm_{inj}) to the mass of tissue removed on ablation (ΔM_{abl})[21]:

$$Q_{inj} = \Delta m_{inj}/\Delta M_{abl} \qquad (4)$$

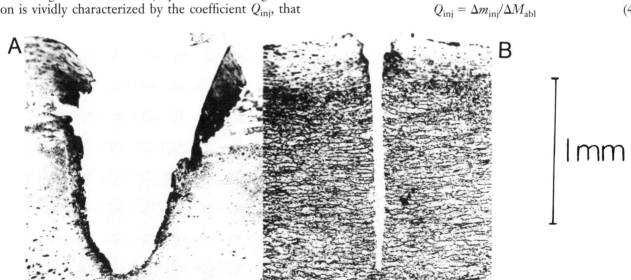

FIG 19–2.
Histologic sections of tissue ablated by continuous *(cw)* **(A)** and pulsed **(B)** laser radiation. (From Abil'siitov GA, Belgaev AA, Bragin EP: *Sov J Quant Electr* 1985; 12:1991–1992. Used by permission.)

As follows from the above, Q_{inj} depends on the laser energy deposited into the tissue and the heat diffusion rate. In the case of continuous ablation, Q_{inj} is determined by the ratio of the tissue removal rate to the rate of heat diffusion. The experimental value of Q_{inj} for stationary irradiation ranges from 1 (about threshold) to 0.1 (at a maximum rate of ablation). For pulsed irradiation Q_{inj} is determined by the ratio of the laser pulse duration plus the lifetime of the overheated tissue volume to the time of heat diffusion from the irradiated volume. The standard value of Q_{inj} in this case ranges from 0.1 for long pulses to 0.0001 for short ones.

It should be noted that the profile of the transverse intensity distribution in the laser beam affects the degree of thermal injury (see Fig 19–9).

PHOTOTHERMAL MODEL OF PULSED LASER ABLATION

The basic process in experimental and theoretical studies of the mechanism of pulsed laser ablation of atherosclerotic plaque at the present time is explosive boiling of the overheated tissue volume,[21, 22] analogous to the process of the metastable liquid boiling investigated previously.[23] The conditions for explosive boiling are fast transfer of tissue to a metastable state and production of the temperature of intense fluctuational formation of vapor bubbles.

Within this model the process of pulsed laser ablation can be divided into three stages: opticophysical, thermophysical, and gas-dynamic (Fig 19–3).

In the first stage, laser radiation is absorbed in the tissue. Depending on laser pulse wavelength, chromophores are either biomolecules (proteins of various types and lipids) or water. Only in the spectral range from 1.5 to 4 μm is laser radiation purely absorbed by water. In the rest of the optical spectrum the laser pulse energy excites biomolecules. In both cases water is a sort of reservoir for heat energy into which the light pulse energy is transferred. This transfer of laser energy to heat is very rapid when compared with laser pulse duration.[24] The first stage of ablation is over when the exposed tissue volume is heated and the temperature is higher than the threshold value.

The second, thermophysical, stage consists of the formation of gaseous bubbles in overheated tissue. This stage yields a sharp increase in pressure in the irradiated volume. Simultaneously, water is evaporated from the tissue surface. Because evaporation tissue surface is

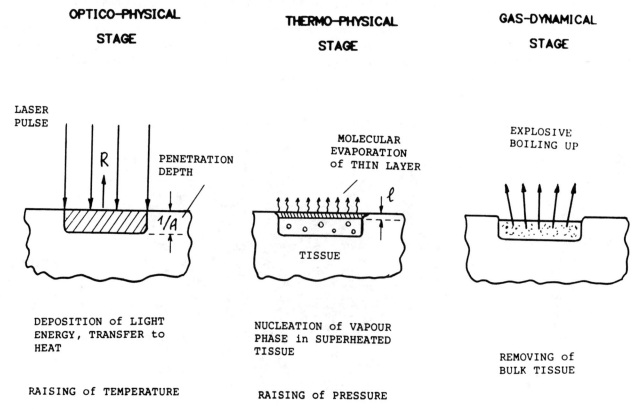

FIG 19–3.
Three stages of pulsed laser ablation of tissue.

cooled, the maximum temperature is achieved in the subsurface layer of the irradiated tissue volume.

Depending on laser pulse duration (the rate of heat deposition in the tissue volume), two versions of the thermophysical stage of ablation may be realized in principle. In the first case of short-pulse irradiation, explosive boiling of overheated water in the tissue, ejection of the vapor phase, and mechanical destruction of the "loose" matrix of biomolecules simultaneously occur due to very fast rate of superheating. The second version is realized at a comparatively slow rate of heat deposition into the plaque tissue by a long laser pulse (10^{-6} to 10^{-3} seconds). In this case water is totally evaporated from the exposed volume during a laser pulse. The tissue matrix is overheated by the pulse below the temperature of explosive boiling corresponding to the tissue composition and water content.

During the last, gas-dynamic, stage, removal of overheated tissue and gas-dynamic flow of the products take place. The initial velocity of ablation products essentially exceeds the speed of sound. The collisions of tissue microparticles, molecules, atoms, and radicals in a hot gas cloud with themselves and with the molecules of air are responsible for ablation product thermochemiluminescence.[12, 25] It is convenient to study the kinetics of the gas-dynamic stage of pulsed ablation by recording ablation product luminescence. Figure 19–4 shows typical oscillograms of luminescence pulses when a fibrous plaque is ablated by 20-ns laser pulses at $\lambda = 532$ nm.[12] The first pulse on the oscillogram is the laser pulse overlapping with the luminescence of excited electronic states of biomolecules and the second pulse, delayed with respect to the first one, is luminescence of ablation products. Thus, the oscillograms in Figure 19–4 present the three stages of the ablation process. The first pulse describes the kinetics of heat deposition. The interval between the pulses is a thermophysical stage of intense formation of gas bubbles. The second pulse describes the kinetics of ablation product blow-up and ejection. At the threshold laser fluence the duration of

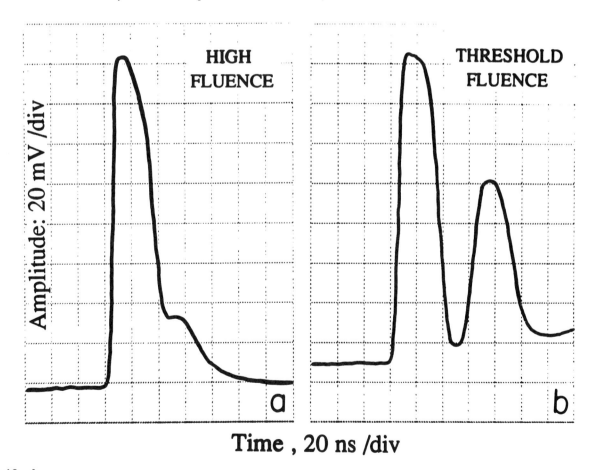

FIG 19–4.
Oscillograms of radiation pulses in tissue irradiated by a laser pulse with high **(a)** and threshold **(b)** energy fluence at $\lambda = 532$ nm. The first pulse is laser radiation and tissue fluorescence. The second pulse is luminescence of fibrous plaque ablation products. (From Oraevsky AA, Esenaliev RO, Letokhov VS: *Lasers Life Sci* 1991, 2; 5:75–93. Used by permission.)

the thermophysical stage is rather long, sometimes more than 100 ns (Fig 19–4,B). On the other hand, when incident laser fluence is high, the temperature of tissue overheating can be very significant. The duration of the thermophysical stage tends to zero. One can see an example of this in Figure 19–4,a, where both pulses are overlapping and fusing.

THRESHOLD CHARACTERISTICS OF ABLATION EFFICIENCY

The process of laser ablation has a laser pulse fluence threshold. The value of the threshold fluence is determined by the fact that the temperature in the volume of an atherosclerotic plaque must exceed the boiling temperature, so the time of formation of a critical-size vapor bubble is shorter than the time of heat diffusion from the overheated volume. Therefore, it is possible to determine the ablation threshold by measuring the lifetime of the superheated tissue volume before the onset of explosive boiling (the duration of the thermophysical metastable stage). At the ablation threshold the lifetime

of overheated tissue tends to the heat diffusion time. At high laser fluences the time before explosive boiling tends to the time of laser energy transformation to heat (the time of excited state relaxation), and ablation occurs even during a short nanosecond pulse. Figure 19–5 demonstrates the above-described processes on ablation of fibrous plaque by a third-harmonic pulse of an Nd: YAG laser ($\lambda = 355$ nm).[12] The threshold energy fluence measured by the method described accurately coincides with the threshold laser fluence measured by the standard technique. This standard technique consists of measuring the mass of the ablated tissue relative to the deposited energy as a function of the incident energy fluence. Similar curves are plotted in Figure 19–6 for different materials, including nonbiological ones.

Within the thermal model the threshold laser fluence (ϕ_{thr}) (in joules per square centimeter) is approximately determined[3] from the condition of heating of an irradiated volume (V_{irr}) (in cubic centimeters) to the critical temperature T^* of phase transition of biotissue to a metastable overheated state, i.e., from the condition of equality of the laser energy absorbed per unit volume

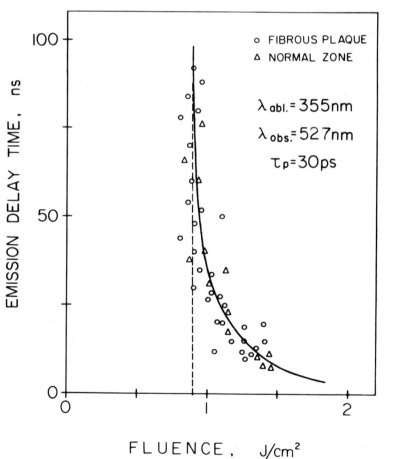

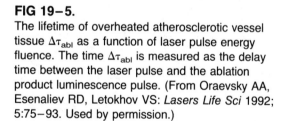

FIG 19–5.
The lifetime of overheated atherosclerotic vessel tissue $\Delta\tau_{abl}$ as a function of laser pulse energy fluence. The time $\Delta\tau_{abl}$ is measured as the delay time between the laser pulse and the ablation product luminescence pulse. (From Oraevsky AA, Esenaliev RD, Letokhov VS: *Lasers Life Sci* 1992; 5:75–93. Used by permission.)

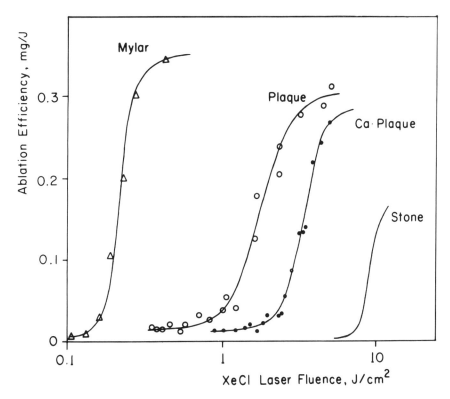

FIG 19–6.
Dependence of the ablation efficiency of various materials on the energy fluence of an exciter XeCl laser at $\lambda = 308$ nm.

$(\phi_{thr}) \cdot \mu_a$ and the required increase in thermal energy per unit volume $[c\rho (T^* - T_0)]$.

$$\phi_{thr} \cdot \mu_a = c\rho (T^* - T_0), \qquad (5)$$

where μ_a is the absorption coefficient, T_0 is the initial (usually room) temperature, and c and ρ are the heat capacity and the density of irradiated tissue. The density and the heat capacity of vessel tissue depend on the water percentage W and relate to it as follows[16, 26]:

$$\rho = (\rho_d - 0.3 \ W) \ (\text{g/cc}) \qquad (6)$$

$$c = (0.37 + 0.67 \ W/\rho) \ (\text{J/g/°C}) \qquad (7)$$

Assuming that the water content (W) in the tissue is 75% and the dry tissue density (ρ_d) is 1.3 g/cc, we have $\rho = 1.08$ g/cc and $c = 3.5$ J/g/°C. For different types of atherosclerotic plaque and normal vessel walls the value of $c\rho$ varies between 3.6 and 3.9 J/cm³/°C.

The larger the radiation absorption coefficient in tissues the smaller the volume of laser pulse energy and the higher the temperature of tissue heating. With the same absorption coefficient, the higher the threshold temperature of explosive boiling, the higher the thresh-

old laser fluence. For example, the coefficient of excimer XeCl laser radiation absorption in calcified plaque is higher than that in fibrous plaque. The threshold fluence for calcified plaque, however, is higher than that in fibrous plaque due to the higher boiling temperature of calcium salts.

Figure 19–7 presents absorption and scattering spectra for normal zones and fibrous plaques of an atherosclerotic aorta in the visible and near-ultraviolet (UV) ranges. One may see that both the absorption and scattering coefficients increase as the wavelength decreases from 800 to 300 nm.[9] In the infrared (IR) range the absorption coefficient increases again due to water absorption.[27] At the Er:YAG laser wavelength the absorption coefficient of water is at its maximum, $\mu_a = 13,000$ cm^{-1}. In this case the energy fluence threshold is lower than for all existing lasers (see Table 19–1). Figure 19–8 demonstrates the drop of the threshold energy fluence for various lasers as the coefficient of radiation attenuation by a plaque rises.

The existence of a threshold laser fluence for ablation explains the dependence of the thermal injury to adjacent tissue on the cross-sectional distribution of the laser beam intensity. It is obvious that the degree of thermal injury increases as the sharp intensity distribution at the edges of the laser spot becomes smooth. The afore-

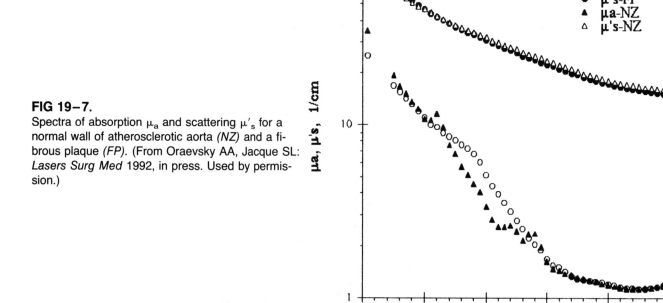

FIG 19–7.
Spectra of absorption μ_a and scattering μ'_s for a normal wall of atherosclerotic aorta *(NZ)* and a fibrous plaque *(FP)*. (From Oraevsky AA, Jacque SL: *Lasers Surg Med* 1992, in press. Used by permission.)

said is illustrated in Figure 19–9. The radiation on the periphery of the laser beam penetrates the tissue and causes thermal injury, but the energy fluence is not enough to realize tissue ablation at the edge of the irradiated volume.

SELECTIVE ABLATION OF PLAQUE VS. NORMAL VESSEL WALL

Selective ablation of atherosclerotic plaque at minimal action of a laser pulse on the normal zone of the

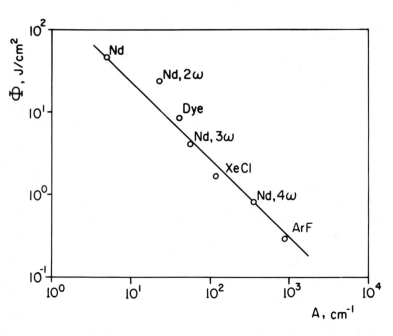

FIG 19–8.
Threshold energy fluence for atherosclerotic plaques ablated by pulses of various lasers as a function of the radiation attenuation coefficient of these lasers in plaque.

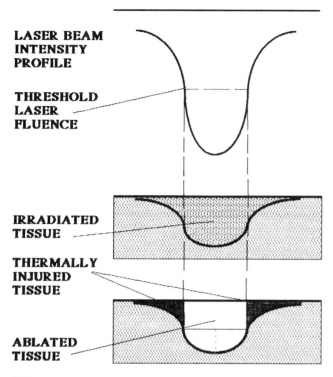

LASER BEAM
INTENSITY
PROFILE

THRESHOLD
LASER
FLUENCE

IRRADIATED
TISSUE

THERMALLY
INJURED
TISSUE

ABLATED
TISSUE

FIG 19–9.
Heat injury to tissues around the crater by a laser beam with smeared edges.

blood vessel wall decreases the risk of perforating the vessel wall and reduces the requirements for accurate dosimetry of the energy applied. There are two types of spectral selectivity: natural selectivity based on the difference in optical properties and selectivity based on sensitizers accumulated in the atherosclerotic plaque.

Natural selectivity of atherosclerotic plaque ablation is possible only in the green-blue range of wavelengths from 450 to 540 nm because plaque absorption is greater than that for normal vessel wall. As can be seen from Figure 19–7, the absorption coefficient μ_a^{FP} of fibrous plaque in this spectral range is somewhat higher than the absorption (μ_a^{NZ}) by a normal wall. The maximal ratio of the coefficients μ_a^{FP}/μ_a^{NZ} comes to about 1.5. The scattering coefficients in both types of tissue in this case are the same.

Since the effective depth of heat penetration into tissue is approximately proportional to the inverse of the attenuation coefficient, μ_{eff}, the difference in absorption coefficients between plaque and normal vessel tissue, according to Strikwerda et al.,[5] makes the ablation thresholds different. The maximal possible selectivity can be found from the following relationship:

$$\phi_{thr}^{NZ}/\phi_{thr}^{FR} \approx \mu_a^{FP}/\mu_a^{N2} = 1.5 \qquad (8)$$

This value is consistent with the selectivity of fibrous plaque ablation by the second harmonic of the Nd:YAG laser as demonstrated experimentally.[10]

Figure 19–10 shows the dependence of the ablation efficiency of the normal zone and a fibrous plaque of an atherosclerotic aorta as a function of the incident fluence of a laser pulse at $\lambda = 532$ nm. It can be seen that the energy fluence reaches its threshold for the normal wall, when the ablation efficiency of the fibrous plaque reaches its maximum.

Selective ablation of plaque was first demonstrated[11] by using a dye laser at $\lambda = 465$ nm. The natural spectral selectivity in this experiment was somewhat increased due to an accumulation of carotenoids in the plaque. The carotenoids, for example, can be given to patients as a special diet prior to treatment.

Introducing sensitizers into plaque is an alternative method of attaining selective ablation. The selectivity value in this case is determined by the product of the difference of sensitizer concentrations in the plaque and the normal wall and the sensitizer absorption coefficient at the laser radiation wavelength. This method is particularly attractive in combination with the technique of controllable substance transport that is now being developed. Sensitized selective ablation of fibrous plaques by Nd:YAG laser third-harmonic radiation was realized by Murphy-Chutorian et al.,[28] who treated atherosclerotic aorta with tetracycline having an intense absorption band at $\lambda = 355$ nm. The selectivity (the ratio of ablation efficiency of the plaque and the normal wall) obtained = 2.

ENERGY CONSUMPTION BY ABLATION. PLAQUE ABLATION EFFICIENCY

By knowing the optical properties of tissue and the ablation mechanism one can estimate the energy required to remove a certain volume of an atherosclerotic plaque by a laser pulse. Since the coefficients of radiation attenuation by tissue, μ_{eff}, for various types of lasers as well as the plaque ablation thresholds are known (see Table 19–1), the volume energy fluence required for ablation can be roughly estimated from the following expression:

$$E = \mu_{eff}(\phi_{thr} - \phi_R) - \phi_{fl} \ \text{(J/cc)}, \qquad (9)$$

where ϕ_{thr} is the fluence threshold of the incident energy, ϕ_R is the reflected energy fluence, and ϕ_{FL} is the escaped fluence of plaque fluorescence.

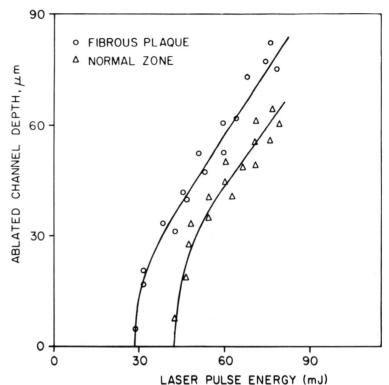

FIG 19–10.
Dependence of crater depth on laser pulse energy when the fibrous plaque and the normal wall of the aorta are ablated by nanosecond second-harmonic pulses of an Nd:YAG laser (λ = 532 nm). (From Esenaliev RO, Oraevsky AA, Letokhov VS: *IEEE Trans Biomed Eng* 1989; 36:1188–1194. Used by permission.)

The value of the total reflectance ranges from 75% to 5% when passing from the near-IR to the near-UV spectral range[26] (specular reflectance is included). The fluorescence quantum yield decreases from about 5% to 0% when passing back from UV to IR wavelengths.[26] Thus, from 25% to 90% of the incident pulse energy can be deposited into the volume under irradiation. In the case when the main ablation mechanism is explosive boiling of overheated tissue, one can assume that the energy is stored in the irradiated tissue volume as heat. With this assumption it is possible to estimate the thermal energy density deposited in the atherosclerotic plaque at the threshold. From the data in Table 19–1 for various types of lasers it is found that in the UV, visible, and near-IR wavelength ranges, the volume energy fluence required for ablation is similar (from 100 to 300 J/cm³). This conclusion qualitatively supports the validity of the thermal ablation mechanism. But there is also a quantitative paradox that has been observed earlier.[29, 30] The point is that the specific energy of water evaporation is equal to 2.6 kJ/g. Water is the basic component of "soft" atherosclerotic plaque and amounts to about 70% of the total mass. The structural proteins of tissue have a higher boiling temperature than water does, so, to ablate 1 cm³ of plaque one must apply an energy not less than that required to evaporate 1 cm³ of water. The solution to this paradox may be found from the following considerations.

First, vessel tissue and atherosclerotic plaque are optically inhomogeneous. The laser pulse radiation can be (in the wavelength range λ < 1.5 μm) absorbed by microchromophore centers of tissue whose volume is much less than the total irradiated volume. The explosive boiling of such overheated microcenters and mechanical removal of the whole irradiated volume of tissue lead to a sharp decrease in the volume energy fluence required to realize the ablation process. In the IR spectral range (λ > 1.5 μm) it is water that strongly absorbs laser radiation. The absorption is homogeneous within the irradiated volume. The threshold laser ablation fluence (ϕ_{thr}) relative to the attenuation coefficient (μ_{eff}) is much higher for this case in comparison with that in the visible range of the spectrum[13–15] (see Table 19–1). The ablation volume energy density required in the IR region is close to the specific heat of water evaporation.

The second essential point is that vessel tissue optics should be taken into account as well. The effect consists of increasing the energy fluence acting inside tissue as compared with the incident fluence. Due to strong diffuse reflection of laser radiation of the vessel wall or a plaque, the acting fluence is composed of the incident fluence and the fluence reflected back from internal tissue layers. As a result, the energy fluence maximum realized in the subsurface layer of a plaque may be 2 to 4 times higher than the incident fluence.[31]

Third, short laser pulses with duration less than the time of sound propagation from the overheated region to the tissue surface can cause huge pressure pulses within the irradiated sample.[32] This surplus pressure (up to hundreds of bars), arises and affects the explosion before the beginning of the gas-dynamic stage of ablation product expansion. This effect may change the depth of the ablation crater and the ablation efficiency, it may also decrease the threshold temperature of overheated tissue.

CONDITIONS OF EFFECTIVE LASER ABLATION

On the basis of the experiments performed and the thermal model of pulsed laser ablation of atherosclerotic plaque we can summarize the experimental characteristic features of the most efficient ablation.

1. The laser pulse wavelength should be such that the radiation absorption coefficient in a plaque is high. The lasers recommended for this purpose are XeCl (UV) and Ho:YAG (IR) (see Table 19–1). These lasers have comparatively low ablation thresholds and a high efficiency, and in addition, their radiation can be guided through a quartz fiber.

2. The laser pulse duration should be shorter than the time of heat diffusion from the irradiated volume, but not too short in order to avoid energy losses caused by nonlinear effects as the laser pulse is transported through an optical fiber. Pulses of 10^{-7} seconds are optimal in this case.

3. To exclude the effect of energy accumulation of several laser pulses, their repetition rate must be much less than the inverse time of thermal diffusion.

4. To decrease thermal injury to the adjacent tissue around the crater, the laser beam should have "sharp edges" and a rectangular intensity distribution in the spot.

5. The temperature of the plaque tissue heated by laser radiation must exceed the boiling temperature of both water and protein matrix. In this case effective and "fast" ablation can be realized with minimal overheating of the surrounding tissues. The term "fast" here means that the lifetime of the overheated tissue volume before the explosion is much shorter than the heat diffusion time from this volume.

REFERENCES

1. *IEEE J Quantum Electr* 1984; 20:12, 1987; 23:10, 1991; 27:20.
2. *IEEE Trans Biomed Eng* 1989; 36:12.
3. *Lasers in Life Science* 1992; 5:(entire issue).
4. Abela GS, Norman S, Cohen D, et al: Effects of carbon dioxide, Nd:YAG and argon laser radiation on coronary atheromatous plaques. *Am J Cardiol* 1982; 50:1199–1205.
5. Strikwerda S, Bott-Silverman C, Ratliff NB, et al: Dosimetry studies for argon ion laser light ablation of atheromatous plaque. *Lasers Surg Med* 1986; 6:270–276.
6. Grundfest WS, Litvack F, Forrester JS, et al: Laser ablation of human atherosclerotic plaque without adjacent tissue injury. *J Am Coll Cardiol* 1985; 5:929–933.
7. Sartori M, Henry PD, Sauerbrey R, et al: Tissue interactions and measurement of ablation rates with ultraviolet and visible lasers in canine and human arteries. *Lasers Surg Med* 1987; 7:300–306.
8. Wilson B, Park Y, Helez Y, et al: The potential of time-resolved reflectance measurement for the noninvasive determination of tissue optical properties, in *Thermal and Optical Interactions with Biological and Related Materials. SPIE* 1989; 1064:97–106.
9. Oraevsky AA, Jacques SL: XeCl ablation of atherosclerotic tissue. Optical properties and energy pathways. *Lasers Surg Med* 1992, in press.
10. Esenaliev RO, Oraevsky AA, Letokhov VS: Laser ablation of atherosclerotic blood tissue under various irradiation conditions. *IEEE Trans Biomed Eng* 1989; 36:1188–1194.
11. Prince MR, Deutch TF, Shapiro AH, et al: Selective ablation of atheromas using flashlamp-excited dye laser at 465 nm. *Proc Natl Acad Sci USA* 1986; 83:7064–7068.
12. Oraevsky AA, Esenaliev RO, Letokhov VS: Kinetics and mechanism of the pulsed laser ablation of atherosclerotic vessel tissue. *Lasers Life Sci* 1992; 5:75–93.
13. Kopchok GE, White RA, Tabbara M, et al: YAG laser ablation of vascular tissue. *Lasers Surg Med* 1990; 10:405–413.
14. Bonner RF, Smith PD, Leon MB, et al: Quantification of tissue effects due to a pulsed Er:YAG laser at 2.9 μm with beam delivery in a wet field via zirconium fluoride fibers, in Katzir A (ed): *Optical Fibers in Medicine II. SPIE* 1986; 713:2–8.
15. Walsh JT, Deutsch TF: Pulsed CO_2 laser tissue ablation: Measurement of ablation rate. *Lasers Surg Med* 1988; 8:264–275.
16. McKenzie AL: Physics of thermal processes in laser-tissue interaction. *Phys Med Biol* 1990; 35:1175–1209.
17. Welch AJ: The thermal response of laser irradiated tissue. *IEEE J Quant Electr* 1984; 20:1471–1481.
18. Isner JM, Clarke RH: The paradox of thermal laser ablation without thermal injury. *Lasers Med Sci* 1987; 2:165–173.
19. Choy DSJ, Stertzeer SH, Myler RK, et al: Human coronary laser recanalization. *Clin Cardiol* 1984; 7:37–38.
20. Abela G: laser recanalization: Peripheral and coronary application. *Cardiovasc Surg* 1988; 2: 131–135.
21. Dmitriev AK, Furzikov NP: Mechanism of laser ablation of biotissue. *Sov Phys Izvest* 1989; 53:1105–1110.
22. Furzikov NP, Letokhov VS, Oraevsky AA: Fundamentals of laser angioplasty. Photoablation and spectral diagnostics, in Chester AN et al (eds): *Laser Science and Technology*. New York, Plenum, 1988, pp 243–258.
23. Skripov VP: *Metastable Liquids*. Jerusalem, Wiley, Israel Program of Scientific Translations, 1974.

24. Baraga JJ, Taroni P, Park YD, et al: Ultraviolet laser induced fluorescence of human aorta. *Spectrochim Acta*, 1989; 45:95–99.

25. Oraevsky AA, Pettit GH: XeCl laser ablation of atherosclerotic tissue: Luminescence spectroscopy of ablation products. *Lasers Surg Med* 1992, in press.

26. Jacques SL, Prahl SA: Modeling optical and thermal distributions in tissue during laser irradiation. *Laser Surg Med* 1987; 6:494–503.

27. Hale GM, Querry MR: Optical constants of water in the 200 nm–200 μm wavelength region. *Appl Opt* 1973; 12:555–563.

28. Murphy-Chutorian D, Kosek J, Mok W, et al.: Selective absorption of ultraviolet laser energy by human atherosclerotic plaque with tetracycline. *Am J Cardiol* 1985; 55:1293–1297.

29. Furzikov NP: Different lasers for angioplasty: Thermooptical comparison. *IEEE J Quant Electr* 1987; 23:1751–1755.

30. Abil'siitov GA, Belyaev AA, Bragin EP, et al: A study into photoablation of atherosclerotic plaques by laser radiation. *Sov J Quant Electr* 1985; 12:1991–1992.

31. Jacques SL: Simple theory, measurements, and rules of thumb for dosimetry during photodynamic therapy. *SPIE* 1989; 1065:100–108.

32. Dingus RS, Scammon RJ: Grüneisen-stress induced ablation of biological tissue. *SPIE* 1992; 1427:45–54.

20

Infrared Laser Angioplasty: Clinical Experience With the Holmium:YAG Laser

Christopher J. White, M.D.
Stephen R. Ramee, M.D.

The development of a safe and effective coronary laser angioplasty system for percutaneous recanalization is an extremely complex task involving the selection of an optimal laser wavelength and coupling this energy source to a delivery catheter that can safely and effectively recanalize lesions in the coronary arteries. Laser angioplasty offers several potential advantages for percutaneous revascularization of coronary artery disease when compared with conventional balloon angioplasty, including (1) reducing the restenosis rate that occurs following balloon angioplasty in approximately one third of patients,[6, 10] (2) reducing the frequency of abrupt artery occlusion and emergency coronary bypass grafting following balloon angioplasty,[1] and (3) extending the indications for percutaneous recanalization to patients currently considered to be poor candidates for balloon angioplasty, such as those with unfavorable lesions or diffuse disease.[15, 18]

Two types of lasers are undergoing clinical trials for coronary laser angioplasty. One is an ultraviolet laser, also known as an excimer laser, and the other is the infrared holmium:YAG (yttrium-aluminum-garnet) laser. Both systems utilize multifiber catheter delivery systems composed of small-diameter silica fibers tightly packed together to minimize "dead space" between the fibers that transmit light from the laser source to the target tissue.

OPTIMAL LASER WAVELENGTH

There are several important criteria to be used when selecting a laser for intracoronary ablation of atherosclerotic tissue. First, the laser should be mechanically reliable and easy for the physician to operate. Lasers that require the presence of an on-site physicist for frequent adjustments to the laser or frequent alignment of the internal optics are not acceptable for general clinical use. The laser beam should be easily and efficiently coupled to optical delivery fibers ranging in diameter from 50 to 200 μm. Ideally, the laser should be pulsed to minimize thermal damage to surrounding tissues,[13] and the light should be highly absorbed by the target tissue to increase the efficiency and precision of tissue ablation.[2, 5, 13, 14, 17, 19–21]

LASER CATHETERS

The basic requirement for a laser delivery catheter is that the light from the laser source be efficiently transmitted through the optical fibers and that the catheter be able to reach the target lesion in tortuous and small (1.5 to 4.0 mm) coronary arteries. Infrared wavelengths less than 2.5 μm such as the holmium:YAG are easily and efficiently transmitted in commercially available silica glass fibers. The transmission of excimer laser energy presents a difficult problem because silica glass is relatively opaque to ultraviolet radiation. This inefficient energy transmission has required modification of the laser to "stretch" the normally very short pulses (~10 ns) to avoid destroying the fibers. The relatively narrow margin of safety between the energy required to ablate or vaporize tissue (threshold of ablation) and the fiber damage threshold limits the amount of excimer energy that can be used to ablate tissue.

The catheters must have the flexibility to reach coronary lesions, which requires that many small-diameter optical fibers (≤ 100 μm) be used rather than a single relatively stiff larger fiber. The smaller the fiber, the more important efficiency of energy transmission becomes, and in this regard infrared lasers have an advantage over ultraviolet lasers. The multifiber catheters currently available create channels in obstructed arteries approximately the same size as the catheter itself. To enhance the safety of laser angioplasty and limit coronary artery perforation, laser delivery catheters are kept very small (~2.0 mm in diameter). This results in the creation of relatively small channels and significantly limits the ability of the laser system to be used as a "stand-alone" device.

There are two general approaches to increasing the size of the lumen created by small laser catheters. The first method is to position the laser catheter in an eccentric position over a guidewire, and by rotating the catheter around the wire, the lumen size can be increased. The other approach is to place a diverging lens on the tip of the catheter so that the light leaving the catheter is spread out over a larger area.[22] As the area irradiated by the laser increases, the energy requirements increase dramatically. Current excimer lasers are unlikely to be able to transmit sufficient energy to ablate a larger area than the catheter itself without exceeding the fiber damage threshold of the optical fiber, whereas it is possible to ablate a larger-diameter hole than the catheter with holmium:YAG energy. Both of these solutions to enlarge the laser channel will require some mechanism of catheter guidance (i.e., angioscopy, ultrasound, or spectroscopy) during laser ablation to prevent laser perforation in eccentric stenoses.

LASER GUIDANCE

The ability to guide and control laser ablation of intravascular obstructions requires resolution far beyond what can be obtained with fluoroscopy. One approach to catheter guidance involves using spectroscopic analysis of the tissue to differentiate "plaque" from normal tissue. It has been shown that it is possible to differentiate normal tissue from atherosclerotic tissue by fluorescence spectroscopy.[8, 11] In theory, a nonablative light source would "interrogate" the target tissue prior to delivering the ablative energy. If plaque is detected, then the laser would fire; however, if normal tissue were detected, then the catheter could be repositioned to avoid damaging normal tissue or perforating the artery. In practice, however, this concept has not worked. The problem is that the obstructive atherosclerotic lesion does not exist on the intimal surface but deeply invades and replaces the medial layer of the vessel wall. Therefore, if the entire vessel wall is atherosclerotic, then the laser could easily perforate the artery.

Coronary angioscopy provides a three-dimensional view of the vascular lumen but does not visualize subsurface structures. In tortuous coronary arteries it may be very difficult to ensure a coaxial position of the angioscope, which would result in suboptimal guidance. Because the thickness of the vessel wall cannot be assessed with angioscopy, the luminal view provided by the scope would not prevent laser perforation of an eccentric lesion or a lesion on a bend in the artery.

Intravascular ultrasound imaging is the most promising candidate as a tool for guiding intravascular laser ablation. The cross-sectional ultrasound image provides an assessment of wall thickness and the ability to determine calcified vs. soft plaque and can determine the centric nature of the stenosis. The major limitation of intravascular ultrasound is that it is not "forward looking" and therefore cannot provide an image or view of the artery in front of the laser catheter.

Infrared Lasers

Vascular tissue and atherosclerotic plaque contain a large amount of water that has two strong absorption peaks for wavelengths at or near 1.9 and 2.8 μm (Fig. 20–1). The closer the laser wavelength to the absorption peak of water, the more efficient the energy absorption; this results in shallower penetration of the laser into the tissue, and less total energy will be needed to ablate the target tissue (Table 20-1).[4]

The holmium:YAG laser is an infrared laser with a primary wavelength at 2.1 μm and satisfies the above criteria for an ideal laser. It is a solid-state laser that greatly simplifies its daily use and minimizes the need for frequent adjustments and maintenance. The holmium:YAG laser beam is easily and efficiently transmitted by small-diameter glass (silica) fibers. It is a pulsed laser that can be operated in its normal, free-running mode with microsecond pulses or in the Q-switched mode with ultrashort, nanosecond pulses.[9]

HOLMIUM:YAG CLINICAL TRIAL

Patient Selection

Patients referred for elective percutaneous transluminal angioplasty (PTCA) were considered candidates for this experimental coronary laser angioplasty trial if they had evidence of coronary ischemia, including symptom-limiting stable angina pectoris, a positive exercise test,

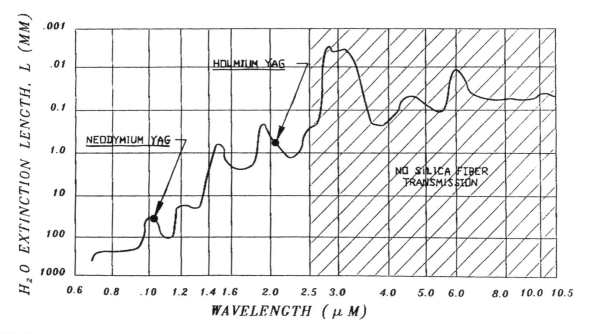

FIG 20–1.
Graph demonstrating water absorption over the infrared wavelengths. Note how close the peak at 1.9 μm is to the holmium:YAG wavelength. There is no fiberoptic transmission of infrared wavelengths greater than 2.5 μm.

or clinically unstable angina pectoris. The patients were required to have coronary artery lesion(s) suitable for elective PTCA and the ability to give informed consent. This protocol was approved by our hospital's institutional review board.

We enrolled 12 men and 2 women with an average age of 57.6 ± 10.8 years (range, 34 to 69 years) into the study. Unstable angina (angina at rest or accelerated angina pectoris) was present in 12 patients, and 2 had stable angina. Lesion types (American Heart Association/American College of Cardiologists [AHA/ACC] criteria modified by Ellis et al.)[3] treated included 1 type A lesion (6%), 8 type B2 lesions (47%), and 8 type C lesions (47%). Two patients had restenosis lesions treated. Fluoroscopic calcification was evident in 8 of 17 (47%) target lesions.

Laser Procedure

The holmium:YAG laser (SEO 1-2-3, Schwartz Electro-Optics, Orlando, Fla) delivered 240 to 450 mJ per pulse at a repetition rate of 4 Hz with a pulse duration of 250 μs in the free running mode. The 1.6- and 2.0-mm laser delivery catheter (Trimedyne, Santa Ana, Calif) contained 19 and 27 silica fibers (100 μm), respectively, arranged circumferentially around the central guidewire lumen and densely packed to minimize the dead space between fibers (Fig 20–2).

The target lesion was initially crossed with a 0.014-in. angioplasty guidewire, and the laser delivery catheter (1.6 or 2.0 mm) was advanced to be in contact with the target lesion. Laser energy was delivered in 2- to 5-second intervals with traction placed on the guidewire to

TABLE 20–1.
Comparison of Tissue Absorption Parameters for Near-Infrared Lasers*

Laser	Wavelength (μm)	a† (Tissue) (cm⁻¹)	Penetration Depth (μm)
Erbium:YAG	2.94	10,000	1
Holmium:YAG	2.06	35	286
Neodymium:YAG	1.06	4	2,500

*Adapted from Esterowitz L, Hoffman C, Storm M: A comparison of the erbium mid-IR laser and the short wavelength UV excimer lasers for medical applications. Presented at an international conference on lasers, 1986, pp 536–539.
†The absorption coefficients *(a)* assume a tissue water content of 60%.

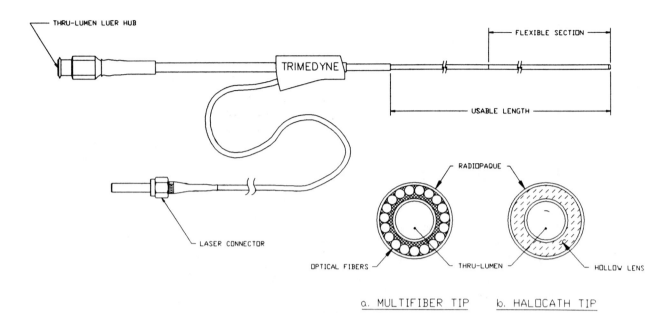

FIG 20–2.
Schematic repsentation of a multifiber catheter *(a)* and a lensed multifiber catheter *(b).*

"pull" the catheter across the stenosis. This passive method of advancing the catheter was used to avoid mechanical dilation of the stenosis.

If a significant stenosis remained (>30% diameter stenosis) following laser recanalization, adjunctive angioplasty with either a balloon or directional atherectomy (Devices for Vascular Intervention, Santa Clara, Calif) was performed. Following angioplasty, patients were observed in the catheterization laboratory for 15 minutes before the final angiogram was performed.

We defined a successful laser angioplasty as a reduction in the baseline stenosis by 20% or more, and procedural success was deemed to have been obtained when the final diameter stenosis was reduced to less than 50% diameter narrowing. An intraluminal thrombus was defined as a filling defect within the lumen of the vessel, and a dissection was defined as a linear contrast stain within the wall of the vessel. Perforation was defined as the extraluminal appearance of contrast material.

Results

Laser and procedural success were obtained in 13 of 14 (93%) patients and 16 of 17 (94%) lesions. The baseline diameter stenosis was reduced from 97.1% ± 4.9% to 38.8% ± 15.4% ($P < .001$) following laser angioplasty and further reduced to 8.4% ± 8.9% ($P < .01$) after balloon angioplasty or atherectomy. There was a statistically significant difference in the residual percent diameter stenosis (size of the neolumen) after the larger 2.0-mm catheter was used than with the smaller 1.6-mm catheter (Table 20–2). Stand-alone laser angioplasty was performed on only 1 stenosis, adjunctive balloon angioplasty was used in 8 lesions, and directional atherectomy was used in 7 lesions. The average laser energy required to successfully recanalize the 16 successful lesions was 300.9 ± 37.1 mJ per pulse (range, 240 to 350 mJ per pulse) with a mean fluence of 1,600 ± 344.5 mJ/mm² (range, 1,200 to 2,300 mJ/mm²). Because of its smaller surface area, the 1.6-mm catheter delivered a significantly higher fluence than did the 2.0-mm catheter (Table 20–3).

TABLE 20–2.
Angiographic Results in Successful Patients by Catheter Used

Catheter	Patients (n)	Lesions (n)	Baseline Stenosis (%)	Postlaser Stenosis (%)	Final Stenosis (%)
1.6 mm	7	8	98.5±1.4	47.5±13.9	10.6±8.6
2.0 mm	6	8	95.8±6.6	30.0±12.0	5.7±9.8
P value			.27	.017	.31

TABLE 20–3.

Lesion Parameters in Successful Patients by Laser Catheter Used

Catheter	Patients (n)	Lesions (n)	Vessel Diameter (mm)	Lesion Length (mm)	Energy (mJ/Pulse)	Fluence (mJ/mm²)
1.6 mm	7	8	3.0 ± 0.3	10.38 ± 7.2	286.3 ± 37.4	1,837 ± 329.2
2.0 mm	6	8	3.3 ± 0.5	13.38 ± 7.4	315.6 ± 32.6	1,362 ± 130.2
P value			.15	.42	.11	.002

Successful laser angioplasty was obtained in 11 native coronary arteries (left anterior descending, 4; left circumflex, 2; and right coronary, 5) and 2 saphenous vein coronary bypass grafts (Figs 20–3 and 20–4). Fluoroscopic calcification was present in 8 of 17 (47%) of the lesions, all of which were successfully treated. Eight lesions were treated with the 1.6-mm catheter and 8 with the 2.0-mm catheter. The average lesion length was 11.9 ± 7.2 mm (range, 1 to 25 mm) (Table 20–3).

Laser Failure

The single failure occurred in an ostial vein graft stenosis. We attempted to cross this noncalcified lesion with a 1.6-mm laser delivery catheter and were unsuccessful in delivering the maximum energy of 450 mJ per pulse (fluence, 2,600 mJ/mm²) permitted by our protocol. At this time angiography revealed contrast staining in the wall of the bypass graft consistent with a small perforation, and an occlusive dissection at the lesion site was present. Multiple attempts to open the graft with balloon angioplasty were unsuccessful and resulted in a non–Q-wave myocardial infarction.

Complications

As described above, there was one instance of an occlusive dissection and perforation following attempted laser recanalization of an ostial saphenous vein coronary bypass graft that resulted in a myocardial infarction. There were no instances of intraluminal thrombus formation. We did not observe any evidence of distal embolization following laser angioplasty, and the patients experienced no sensation other than occasional angina pectoris during laser energy delivery. One patient suffered reocclusion 6 hours following laser and directional atherectomy that was successfully redilated without infarction.

CONCLUSION

Our data suggest that holmium:YAG laser–assisted angioplasty in conjunction with multifiber catheters was effective in recanalizing lesions, the majority of which demonstrated morphology (type B2 or C) unfavorable for balloon angioplasty. Procedural success was obtained in 16 of 17 (94%) lesions overall, with 4 of 4 type C lesions and 8 of 9 type B2 lesions treated successfully, which compares favorably with the 61% and 72% success rates with balloon angioplasty reported for type C and B lesions, respectively.[3] All 8 lesions with fluoroscopic calcification were successfully recanalized with holmium energy, which is consistent with in vivo experiments demonstrating the holmium:YAG laser's ability to ablate calcified tissues.

In retrospect, the single failed lesion resulted from poor alignment of the guiding catheter with the ostium

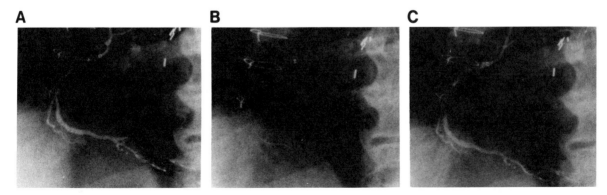

FIG 20–3.
Complex, calcified proximal right coronary lesion. **A**, baseline; **B**, 1.6-mm laser fiber; **C**, final result after laser and balloon angioplasty.

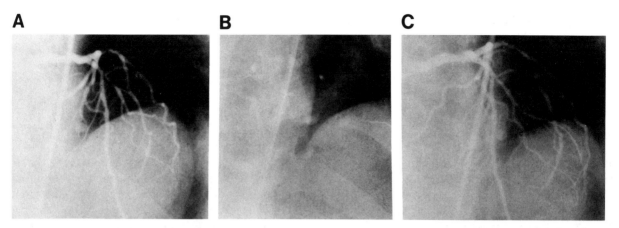

FIG 20–4.
Long lesion in a small diagonal branch. **A,** baseline; **B,** 1.6-mm laser fiber; **C,** final result after stand-alone lasing.

of the bypass graft. Attempts to cross this lesion were unsuccessful, and repeated attempts at higher energies resulted in perforation and an occlusive dissection that could not be redilated with balloon angioplasty. This complication may have been avoided by a more coaxial position of the guide catheter and the lumen of the graft and by not persisting in recanalization attempts after failing to cross with the highest energy allowed under the protocol.

The question of whether the predominant effect of the laser catheters is, in fact, tissue ablation or merely mechanical dilation of the lesion by crossing with the catheter remains. In one patient we used angioscopy to directly view the treated lesion and observed a qualitative improvement in the luminal diameter without evidence of thermal charring. We also obtained tissue samples with the atherectomy catheter following laser ablation, which confirmed a tissue effect of the laser without thermal charring. Further support for tissue ablation as the mechanism of improving the luminal diameter following holmium:YAG irradiation is that the minimum fluence delivered by the multifiber catheters (219 mJ/mm^2) is above the threshold required for ablation of noncalcified human atherosclerotic aorta tissue (160 mJ/mm^2).[9]

The multifiber laser catheters used in this study were prototype devices that will require improvement in the future. The distal tip of the catheter is relatively rigid and should be made more flexible to facilitate the catheter's ability to track over the angioplasty guidewire and remain in a concentric position with the lumen of the artery. Modifications are needed to decrease the "dead space" between the laser fibers and the catheter, as well as improvement in the catheter's performance, including both trackability and pushability.

For coronary laser angioplasty to succeed as a viable clinical technique it must stand alone as a percutaneous recanalization device and not rely on adjunctive balloon angioplasty to complete the procedure. One of the limitations of current laser angioplasty delivery systems is the small-diameter channels created with current multifiber laser angioplasty catheters.[7, 12, 16] The average diameter of coronary arteries currently approached with balloon angioplasty is much nearer to 3.0 mm; therefore, a stand-alone coronary laser system should be designed to create recanalized lumens 2.5 to 3.5 mm in diameter.

SUMMARY

Laser angioplasty, regardless of the wavelength selected for tissue ablation and Food and Drug Administration (FDA) approval, must still be considered an unproved approach for the treatment of atherosclerotic coronary artery disease. In evaluating the results of these initial trials one must maintain a perspective of the goals of these early procedures. It is unrealistic to expect these prototype devices to achieve results that are superior to conventional therapy. It must first be established that the procedure can be safely performed. Once this has been done, further catheter refinements can be made to increase the efficacy of the procedure.

The mystique of the laser must be divorced from the procedure. The laser is simply one of several tools available to recanalize an obstructed coronary artery. The laser recanalizes these arteries in a unique manner, with theoretical advantages over other methods of percutaneous revascularization. One advantage of laser energy over balloons or atherectomy devices is the potential for exceedingly precise tissue removal with minimal adverse effects on the adjacent arterial structures. It is hoped that this relatively atraumatic debulking procedure may have a favorable impact on the incidence of acute complications in complex lesions and possibly on restenosis following angioplasty.

Lasers are capable of delivering graded amounts of energy, which in theory allows a single catheter to achieve variable-sized lumens, depending on the tissue absorption and fiberoptic transmission characteristics of the laser wavelength. This phenomenon, the ability to create lumens larger in size than the catheter itself, is potentially a very important advantage of the laser. For this variable-diameter recanalization device to achieve clinical success, a guidance system such as angioscopy or ultrasound imaging will need to be developed to guard against arterial perforation.

The infrared laser wavelength used in this trial, holmium:YAG, 2.1 μm, has advantages over ultraviolet (excimer) wavelengths because the transmission of near-infrared energy through optical fibers is efficient and it has the potential to deliver adequate energy through a diverging lens to create a lumen larger than the catheter itself. Excimer lasers operate in a narrow range, which allows sufficient energy fluences to be transmitted through the optical fibers in order to ablate relatively small volumes of tissue but which limits the maximum energy transmitted as they quickly reach the energy levels that damage the optical fibers (fiber damage threshold). This fact makes it unlikely that excimer laser catheters will be able to deliver sufficient energy to ablate an area significantly larger than the catheter itself. If the goal of laser recanalization continues to be the ability to create neolumens of 2.5 to 3.5 mm in diameter or larger, the excimer wavelengths will require either the development of new fibers or the use of extremely large and potentially dangerous fiberoptic catheters.

With the increased need to reduce costs without compromising quality of care, the significant costs associated with laser angioplasty must be justified by enhanced clinical utility of these relatively expensive devices. In the final analysis, laser angioplasty systems will have to compete with less expensive technology. Prototype laser angioplasty systems with their small catheters are limited to an adjunctive role and as stand-alone devices are not currently capable of achieving comparable results to balloon catheters or atherectomy devices for routine angioplasty. A significant investment of both time and money is still required to develop laser angioplasty systems that will allow a fair comparison with alternative devices.

REFERENCES

1. Cowley MJ, et al: Emergency coronary bypass surgery after coronary angioplasty: The National Heart, Lung, and Blood Institute's percutaneous transluminal coronary angioplasty registry experience. *Am J Cardiol* 1984; 53:22.
2. Deckelbaum LI, et al: Elimination of pathologic injury associated with laser induced tissue ablation using pulsed energy delivery at low repetition rates (abstract). *J Am Coll Cardiol* 1985; 5:408.
3. Ellis SG, et al: Coronary morphologic and clinical determinants of procedural outcome with angioplasty for multivessel coronary disease: Implications for patient selection. *Circulation* 1990; 82:1193–1202.
4. Esterowitz L, Hoffman C, Storm M: A comparison of the erbium mid-IR laser and the short wavelength UV excimer lasers for medical applications. Proceedings of the International Conference on Lasers, 1986, pp 536–539.
5. Forrester JS, et al: The excimer laser: Current knowledge and future prospects. *J Intervent Cardiol* 1988; 1:75–80.
6. Holmes DR, et al: Restenosis after percutaneous transluminal coronary angioplasty (PTCA): A report from the PTCA registry of the National Heart, Lung, and Blood Institute. *Am J Cardiol* 1984; 53:77–81.
7. Karsch KR, et al: Percutaneous coronary excimer laser angioplasty in patients with stable and unstable angina pectoris. *Circulation* 1990; 81:1849–1859.
8. Kittrel C, et al: Diagnosis of fibrous arterial atherosclerosis using fluorescence. *Appl Optics* 1985; 24:2280–2281.
9. Kopchok GE, et al: Holmium:YAG laser ablation of vascular tissue. *Lasers Surg Med* 1990; 10:405–413.
10. Leimgruber PP, et al: Restenosis after successful coronary angioplasty in patients with single vessel disease. *Circulation* 1986; 73:710–717.
11. Leon MB, et al: Human arterial surface fluorescence: Atherosclerotic plaque identification and effects of laser atheroma ablation. *J Am Coll Cardiol* 1988; 12:94–102.
12. Litvack F, et al: Percutaneous excimer laser coronary angioplasty. *Am J Cardiol* 1990; 66:1027–1032.
13. Macruz R, et al: Laser surgery in enclosed spaces: A review. *Lasers Surg Med* 1985; 5:199–214.
14. Parrish JA, et al: Selective thermal effects with pulsed irradiation from lasers: From organ to organelle. *Dermatology* 1983; 80(suppl):75–80.
15. Ryan TJ, et al: Clinical competence in percutaneous transluminal coronary angioplasty. *Circulation* 1990; 81:2041–2046.
16. Sanborn TA, et al: Percutaneous excimer laser coronary angioplasty. *Lancet* 1989; 2:616.
17. Selzer PM, et al: Optimizing strategies for laser angioplasty. *Invest Radiol* 1985; 20:860–866.
18. Spies JB, et al: Guidelines for percutaneous transluminal angioplasty. *Radiology* 1990; 177:619–626.
19. Van Gemert MC, et al: Modeling of (coronary) laser-angioplasty. *Lasers Surg Med* 1985; 5:219–234.
20. Van Gemert MC, et al: Some physical concepts in laser angioplasty. *Semin Intervent Radiol* 1986; 3:27–38.
21. Welch AJ, et al: Effect of laser radiation on tissue during laser angioplasty. *Lasers Surg Med* 1985; 5:251–264.
22. White CJ, et al: Recanalization of totally occluded arteries using a holmium:YAG laser and lensed optical fiber (abstract). *Circulation* 1990; 82(suppl 3):667.

Excimer Laser Coronary Angioplasty

Arie Shefer, M.D.

Frank Litvack, M.D.

PHYSICAL CHARACTERISTICS OF THE EXCIMER LASERS

Excimer lasers are a relatively new entry to the medical field.[1] "Excimer" is a contraction of "excited dimer," which refers to the physical principle of laser energy production. The advantage of the excimer laser for medical applications is the strong absorption by tissue in the ultraviolet range, which minimizes heat penetration and provides for great precision. The argon fluoride laser at 193 nm has the strongest absorption but is not useful for coronary applications since this wavelength is difficult to transmit through current fiber optics. The xenon chloride and the xenon fluoride lasers are readily transmitted through high-purity silica–based fiber optics provided that the pulse width of the laser is long enough to keep the peak power in the fiber below its destruction threshold.

Laser energy is produced by a transverse pulsed high-voltage electric discharge across a mixture of a noble gas such as helium, neon, argon, krypton, or xenon and a highly diluted (0.1%) halogen compound such as hydrogen chloride or fluoride.[2] Excimer lasers are unique in that they operate in a two-level energy system. The gas mixture regenerates itself between pulses, which allows for a long sealed operation, in particular for the chloride lasers. The electric discharge causes electronic excitation of inert gas species such as xenon atoms and creates positively charged ions. Simultaneously, the electrons, freed after the discharge, produce negative halogen ions such as chloride anion. The positively charged xenon ion is strongly attracted to the negative halogen ion to produce an ionically bound molecule in the excited stage. This molecule is similar in electronic structure to a salt such as sodium chloride.

When this dimer molecule radiates, it goes to the lower ground level of xenon chloride, which is weakly covalently bound because the xenon cation has returned to its inert gas electronic state. This lower energy state of the xenon chloride molecule rapidly separates to the individual atoms. Therefore, the lower laser molecular level is lost as soon as it is formed, and there is only a very small population in this level to stop laser action.

XENON CHLORIDE EXCIMER LASER

As of now, the xenon chloride laser is the most appropriate excimer laser source for pulsed ultraviolet angioplasty since it is a relatively efficient laser device, with 1 to 4% of net laser energy output. Its gas mixture is the most benign and long-lived of all excimer lasers. The 308-nm ultraviolet energy is readily transmitted through fiber-optics without damaging the fibers when operated at pulse widths greater than 100 ns. Precise ablation of atherosclerotic plaque with insignificant thermal damage to the surrounding tissue has been demonstrated by using the 308-nm excimer laser with fiber-optic delivery.[3]. In vitro tissue studies have shown that this can be achieved with a pulse duration of 100 to 200 ns and with an energy density at the tip of the fiber between 35 and 100 mJ/mm^2 per pulse. If the same xenon chloride excimer laser were used with a fluence of less than 20 mJ/mm^2, the tissue would show signs of thermal damage with irregular rather than precisely cut edges. Furthermore, at any given pulse energy, a short pulse width (less than 10 ns) would result in direct damage to the fiber-optic delivery system because of a high peak power.

So far, more than 2,000 patients have been enrolled in a multicenter clinical trial using a 308-nm xenon chloride excimer laser for coronary interventions (Advanced Interventional Systems, Inc, Irvine, Calif). This laser unit emits up to 350 mJ per pulse with a pulse width of 200 to 300 ns. The pulse repetition rate can be varied from 2 to 30 Hz. The laser has a portable gas exchange system that blends the proper gas mixture and complies with the safety requirements of the Occupational Safety and Hazard Administration. The laser generator is shielded electrically and acoustically to suppress radio frequency interference and to dampen the acoustic effects of the high-voltage discharges.

LASER-TISSUE INTERACTION

Laser light is useful for surgical applications because of its ability to be concentrated in space and time and cause very high levels of local power deposition, which cannot be easily achieved with any other energy source. Light interacts with matter by the processes of absorption, transmission, reflection, refraction, diffraction, and several types of scattering. When an object appears colored under illumination by white light, it is due to selective absorption of light of the colors except that observed. The absorbed light of the other frequencies is most often converted into heat in the absorbing material. Most atoms and molecules have optical energy resonances only in the infrared and ultraviolet regions of the electromagnetic spectrum. Absorption of light by the irradiated material results directly in increasing the energy content of the material. This increased energy can be eliminated by reradiation of the absorbed photon. If the emitted photon has the same energy as the photon absorbed, there is no net increase in the energy of the material. If the absorbed photon is not reemitted or a photon with less energy than that absorbed is reemitted, as usually happens, some energy remains in the molecule. This absorbed energy is converted into mechanical resonance (heat) or electronic resonance (molecular excitation). Resonances in the visible region lie between 1.5 and 3 eV, too high a range for molecular rotation and vibration and too low in energy for most electronic excitations.

Energy that is not absorbed at the surface of the tissue can be scattered and absorbed in areas remote from the impact site of the radiation. The effect of the scattered energy depends on the depth of penetration of energy and the presence of absorbing molecules (chromophores). If the energy is delivered in short intense pulses, boiling, ejection of material, and acoustic transients can be set up within the tissue and cause caviation, which leads to loss of tissue architecture. When a very high peak power laser radiation is used, it produces a very intense local electric field causing the electric breakdown of atoms and production of local gaseous plasma. The sudden expansion of vaporized material produces a shock wave causing localized rupture of the tissue. This mechanism even works on materials that are normally transparent to the laser wavelength at low intensity and can also destroy optics and solid laser rods.[4]

There are four variables that should be optimized to control the tissue response to laser light irradiation: (1) the power or energy delivered per unit of time at the target, (2) the spot size of the target area irradiated, (3) the cumulated time of irradiation, and (4) if pulsed laser is used, the duration of the laser pulse. Average power is the energy delivered per unit of time, whereas peak power is the energy content of a single laser pulse divided by its pulse width. The energy fluence of a pulsed laser is the energy per pulse divided by the beam spot area and is expressed in millijoules per square millimeter.

THERMAL EFFECT

The tissue effect of continuous-wave and most pulsed lasers emitting in the visible and infrared ranges is caused by the conversion of the absorbed photons into heat. As heat is deposited into the irradiated target area, there is lateral thermal conduction to the surrounding tissue. Tissue welding by lasers occurs at relatively low temperatures. Heating the tissue to 43 to 50°C may allow for the uncoiling of collagen helices so that opposed tissue edges may be fused by reforming covalent bonds. As the tissue temperature increases to between 50° and 60°C, irreversible protein denaturation or coagulation and subsequent cell death occur. Beyond 60°C, cell death is inevitable. As temperatures reach 90 to 100°C, the underlying collagen and elastin structures begin to degrade.[5] At temperatures greater than 100°C, melting, boiling, and pyrolysis occur and result in tissue ablation.[6] Ablation temperatures for calcified tissue may exceed 500°C.

When laser energy is absorbed in the target area and partially or totally converted to heat, thermal diffusion begins. Diffusion of heat through the tissue is dependent on the thermal properties of the material. Vascular tissue usually has thermal diffusion constants between 1 and 10 μm/sec. Pulses longer than several microseconds will allow thermal energy to diffuse over a distance of 10 to 100 μm in a few milliseconds. Pulses in the millisecond range are sufficiently long to allow for the heat generated to diffuse 100 to 1,000 μm away from the irradiated target. The thermal relaxation or cooling phenomenon is influenced by the thermal coefficient of the surrounding tissue, the temperature gradient between the irradiated and nonirradiated tissue, and the cooling effect of the flowing blood (heat convection). To minimize the lateral thermal spread, either a pulsed laser with a pulse duration shorter than the characteristic thermal conduction time of the tissue should be used, or a very small target area should be irradiated.

PHOTOCHEMICAL ABLATION

The energy of an ultraviolet photon is greater than 3.0 eV, and it is sufficient to force transition of electron states in covalent bonds. When an ultraviolet photon is absorbed by a molecule, it can rupture the molecular bonds directly by thus breaking a large molecule to smaller fragmented molecules. This mechanism is called photochemical ablation, and it is operative only with a short pulse of ultraviolet wavelength.[7] The fragmented molecules, usually in gaseous form, leave the substrate in rapid expansion away from the tissue surface and carry with them much of the energy that was initially deposited within the target area. This layer-by-layer photochemical ablation mechanism produces clean incisions with minimal thermal heat retention in the nonirradiated tissue, provided that the pulse width is shorter than 1 μs.[8] During this photodisruption process, the rapidly expanding gaseous fragments can induce an acoustic shock wave after each laser pulse, which may rupture the adjacent plaque material. The combination of high repetition rates and short pulse width tends to produce a significant zone of blast injury. This phenomenon was described during laser fragmentation of urinary and biliary calculi.[9] The photochemical ablation is not 100% efficient, and some heat is also generated during this process. Thermal injury can occur with pulsed lasers either at high repetition rates, where there is insufficient time to allow for thermal relaxation of the tissue, or by prolonged irradiation with energy fluence lower than the ablation threshold.

Up to 50% to 60% of all coronary and 60% to 70% of all peripheral atheromas contain calcium. Very hard calcified lesions are not uncommon in either the peripheral or coronary arterial circulation. Thus, when choosing the appropriate laser for ablative processes, one must consider the tissue heterogeneity. None of the continuous-wave lasers, including the carbon dioxide, Nd:YAG, argon ion, and continuous-wave ultraviolet, are effective in ablating calcified tissue. In contrast, the 308-nm excimer laser and the Nd:YAG 266-nm harmonic laser can ablate calcified material.

FLUORESCENCE

Fluorescence occurs when photons are absorbed by tissue and reemitted at a longer visible wavelength. This rapid process, occurring in nanoseconds or less, is strongly affected by electronic bond structure and the chemical composition of the irradiated matter.[10] Fluorescence can be used to detect specific compounds that occur naturally or that have been added to the system. To date, this work has primarily focused on photodetection of hematoporphyrin derivatives, tetracycline, and carotenoids.[11, 12] Laser-induced fluorescence results when a portion of the laser light is absorbed and reradiated. Attempts to achieve ablation through chromophore enhancement are limited by the tissue variability or lack of chromophore uptake within many segments.[13]

EXCIMER LASER ABLATION IN THE VASCULAR SYSTEM

The 308-nm ultraviolet energy is totally absorbed within a short distance of blood, less than 100 μm. Thus, laser ablation of any tissue immersed in blood is possible only in direct contact with the tip of the fiber-optic catheter.[14] The short-wavelength energy is intensely absorbed at the atheroma surface and does not diffuse into adjacent, nontarget tissue.[3] The high power density of the excimer laser can instantly vaporize the atheromatous material with minimal thermal injury to the underlying tissue. The depth of a single-pulse ablation is about 100μ in noncalcified tissue. This phenomenon of layer-by-layer ablation is favorable for small vessels since it minimizes trauma to the deeper tissue of the vessel wall and may reduce the risk of subsequent acute thrombotic occlusion. The 308-nm ultraviolet energy is powerful enough to ablate calcified plaque without thermal injury to the surrounding tissue. While the ablation depth per pulse is smaller, it can be compensated with higher fluence and a higher pulse rate. Analysis of the fluorescent pattern is now under study for differentiating normal from arteriosclerotic and calcified tissue.[13, 15] This would allow target-specific laser angioplasty. However, laser-induced fluorescence is so sensitive to chemical changes that irradiated or ablated tissue may give different signals than normal or atherosclerotic tissue. Another source for concern is the enormous variability even within a few millimeters of the diseased arterial segment. Although laser-induced fluorescence spectroscopy may prove to be a valuable tool in the future for both diagnostic and therapeutic purposes, its current application is not sufficiently reliable for clinical use.

FIBER-OPTIC DELIVERY SYSTEM AND CATHETER DESIGN

To direct a beam of light from a laser source to the tissue site for a medical procedure, the process of reflection is used to steer the beam from the source through the target. Refraction or reflection from a curved surface is used to focus or defocus the spot size of the laser beam to either increase or decrease the power and the fluence delivered to the target. Fiber-optic transmission is another form of light beam propagation through an optical fiber guide by total internal reflection. The fiber-optic waveguide must be adequately housed within an appropriately designed catheter system.

Early evaluation of laser angioplasty clearly showed that bare-tipped and stiff fiber-optics are associated with a high incidence of vascular perforation and are difficult to steer to the target site.[16] The fiber-optic and catheter delivery system must be sufficiently flexible to enable navigation through the arterial tree to the segment being treated. For peripheral vascular application, this requirement is easily fulfilled. Coronary application by a percutaneous technique, however, requires catheters of significant flexibility. Fiber-optics, by virtue of their glass composition, are intrinsically inflexible, but the smaller the diameter, the greater the flexibility of the fiber. Therefore, smaller-diameter (50 through 300 μm) fiber-optics are required for coronary application. Unfortunately, small-diameter fiber creates an ablated channel of small diameter that matches the size of the fiber. Such channels are generally insufficient to provide meaningful augmentation of blood flow and are likely to occlude.[17]

In an attempt to balance the apparent opposed requirements of flexibility in large areas of ablation, investigators and engineers have been forced to modify designs. One such modification is the placement of a metallic cup at the fiber tip. Another modification is the use of multiple small fiber-optics grouped together in a bundle similar to what is used in a fiber-optic endoscope. With such a system, flexibility is maintained because of the individual characteristics of the thin fibers, yet a bundle can create a large and clinically relevant cross-sectional area of ablation. Multiple-fiber coupling enables a delivery system to have the same or larger cutting area as that of a large single fiber but with much greater flexibility. The cutting area is proportional to the square of the fiber diameter, whereas stiffness is proportional to the fourth power of the fiber diameter. Coupling a multiple-fiber delivery system to a laser requires stable and consistent performance from that laser.

Wasted space at the input of a multiple-fiber delivery system requires that the lasers have high energy output. Most multiple-fiber inputs would consist of a circular bundle. It is impossible, however, to group the fibers together without having air ducts between them. The portion of the laser beam that passes between the fiber input surfaces is not coupled to any fibers. Thus, a substantially greater input energy is required to achieve the same output density when a multiple-fiber delivery system is used. Furthermore, for a multiple-fiber system to operate safely, similar energy densities must be exiting from each fiber. If the energy delivered from the fiber tips is inhomogeneous, some fibers may be below the ablation threshold. It follows that since each input of a multiple-fiber bundle occupies a different portion of the laser beam, the beam must have uniform energy density.

Initial clinical experience in laser angioplasty, mainly with continuous-wave systems and single bare fibers, revealed two significant safety issues: laser perforation and mechanical trauma. A practical and improved technology uses the guidewire to maintain coaxiality in the vessel and provide a track over which the laser catheter may be advanced. The excimer laser catheter functions as a contact cutting device because blood is opaque to ultraviolet light.[14] The laser catheter cuts forward and remains coaxial within the vessel lumen, and the guidewire ensures that the laser energy is not directed at the vessel wall.

The second significant safety issue in laser angioplasty is mechanical trauma, which in the worst case results in vessel perforation. Mechanical trauma to the interior of the vessel wall can be avoided by blunting the distal tip of the fiber-optic delivery system. Coaxial orientation and flexibility are features of the delivery system that minimize the risk of mechanical perforation. Thus, design modifications made in the fiber-optic delivery systems were dedicated to these issues, toward more flexible atraumatic tips and coaxial orientation. We are currently evaluating a multifiber laser delivery system (Advanced International Systems, Inc.) in a multicenter clinical trial. The system for treatment of stenotic lesions incorporates from 12 to more than 300 flexible optical fibers concentrically arranged around the guidewire lumen within the catheter. Flexibility of the intracoronary segment and the tip is vital to this over-the-wire system to ensure good tracking over the guidewire tangential to the vessel wall.

CLINICAL PROTOCOL

An investigational protocol approved by the Food and Drug administration was initiated for percutaneous coronary 308-nm excimer laser angioplasty in late 1988.[18] The protocol has allowed for the use of the multiple-fiber over-the-wire system for the treatment of lesions in native coronary arteries and vein grafts. The trial was commenced with a 1.6-mm-diameter catheter constructed of twelve 200-μm fibers. This design was modified to the 50-μm fiber technology with more than 200 fibers in the same diameter. Recently, we have introduced 1.3- and 2-mm-diameter catheters (with about 350 individual 50-μm fibers) with the new design. A 2.2-mm-diameter catheter with "cobra head" design has been introduced recently, and a 2.4-mm-diameter catheter is available but requires a 10 F guiding catheter for its delivery. The procedure is performed by using an 8 or 9 F standard coronary guiding catheter and conventional over-the-wire percutaneous transluminal coronary angioplasty (PTCA) technique. The lesion is crossed with a 0.016- or 0.018-in. coronary guidewire under fluoroscopic guidance. The guidewire is custom-made and combines a floppy tip with a standard wire shaft for better axial support of the laser catheter (Advanced Cardiovascular Systems, Temecula, Calif). To maximize axial support the wire should be advanced as distal as possible so that the catheter tip rides the more rigid part of the wire. Major side branches of the treated artery are not protected. Laser energy emitted from the catheter tip can be calibrated at 35 to 60 mJ/mm^2, but the preferred fluence for noncalcified lesions is 45 to 50 mJ/mm^2. The laser catheter is then advanced over the guidewire until its tip is immediately proximal to the lesion. When treating total occlusion with stagnation of contrast medium in the proximal "stump," it is recommended that the contrast medium be flushed out with saline before the laser ablation to avoid interaction of ultraviolet energy with the contrast medium.

Under fluoroscopic control, the laser catheter is advanced slowly at a rate of 1 mm/sec across the lesion as laser pulses are delivered at 20 Hz. To prevent the accumulation of gaseous discharge and temperature rise in the treated plaque, it is strongly recommended that the train of pulses be limited to 3 seconds each, interposed with pauses of 3 seconds. After each passage through the lesion, the laser catheter is withdrawn, and selective contrast injection is done to demonstrate the morphology of the lesion after the ablation. It is recommended that repeated passes through the lesion be avoided except for aorto-ostial lesions, where it is possible to change the orientation of the tip of the guiding catheter and perform a few passes with different angulations to etch the ostial plaque.

In order to minimize the risk of perforation or dissection, the laser catheter diameter is undersized so as to be 30% smaller than the proximal normal segment of the treated artery. For example, a 1.3-mm laser catheter is used to treat arteries of up to 1.8 mm in diameter. A 1.6-mm laser catheter is used for treating arteries 2.3 mm in diameter, and a 2-mm laser catheter is used for arteries 3 mm in diameter. In cases of calcified plaque or tight lesions (luminal diameter less than 1 mm), it is recommended that one start with the lowest-profile catheter, 1.3 mm in diameter, and with high fluence, up to 60

mJ/mm^2. The 1.3-mm laser catheter can be exchanged with a larger catheter to complete the intervention.

Our recent experience has shown that a higher-than-usual fluence, 50 to 60 mJ/mm^2, is often required to ablate calcified plaque, and the pulse repetition rate may be increased to 30 Hz. Ablation speed, i.e., catheter advancement, is less than 1 mm/sec. For safety purposes, an autoperfusion balloon catheter should be readily available during all laser interventions. In case of perforation, insertion of an appropriate-sized autoperfusion balloon catheter and its inflation in the area of the perforation is recommended to minimize the extravascular leakage of blood into the pericardial sac while permitting distal myocardial perfusion.

INITIAL CLINICAL EXPERIENCE

In our initial group of 1,570 patients (1,917 lesions) treated in the multicenter trial of the excimer laser system, acute laser success was obtained in 79%, but only 34% were stand-alone laser procedures.[19] Overall procedural success (balloon and laser angioplasty combined) was obtained in 89% of the patients. Adjunctive balloon angioplasty was performed in 66% of all patients. Acute complications included acute occlusion, 7.2% (about half were transient); angiographically visible dissections, 14.0% (most of them without hemodynamic significance); perforation, 1.8%; in-hospital bypass surgery, 3.4%; acute myocardial infarction (including non–Q wave infarction), 2.9%; and death, 0.4%.

Excimer laser angioplasty was successful in 90% of the 114 ostial lesions attempted (96% overall procedural success (Fig 21–1) when adjunctive balloon angioplasty, which was performed in 64% of the procedures, was used. The complications were transient occlusion, 1.8%; non–Q wave myocardial infarction, 3.5%; distal embolization, 2.6%; dissection, 6.2%; perforation, 0.9%; and in-hospital aortocoronary bypass surgery, 2.6%. No transmural infarctions or death has occurred. The reported success rate with another type of atherectomy device in aorta-ostial lesions, however, has been less than 50%.

Excimer laser angioplasty was attempted in 152 patients with total occlusions; 70% had adjunct balloon angioplasty for an 86% laser success rate and a 93% procedural success rate (Fig 21–2). The acute complications were perforations, 1.3%; acute myocardial infarction, 2.6%; in-hospital aortocoronary bypass surgery, 0.7%; and death, 0.7%. After the introduction of the new 1.3-mm catheter, combined with higher fluence (55 to 65 mJ/mm^2), the procedural success reached 97%, and there were fewer complications.

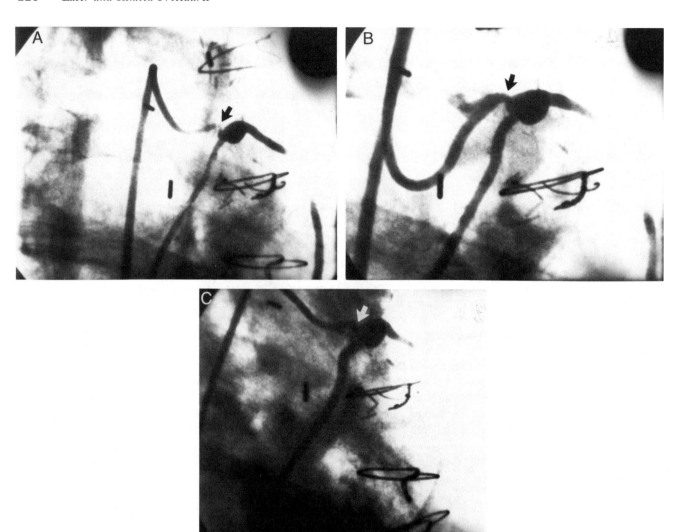

FIG 21–1.
A, aorto-ostial lesion in a sapheneous vein graft with end-to-side anastomosis of another vein graft in its proximal segment *(arrow).* **B,** the result after 1.3- and 2.0-mm-diameter stand-alone excimer laser angioplasty. **C,** angiographic follow-up (6 months) of the ostium.

In the 265 saphenous vein grafts that were attempted in 225 patients the procedural success rate was 97%; 69% required adjunctive balloon angioplasty. The complications were perforations, 1.1%; angiographically visible dissections, 5.3%; acute thrombosis, 3.0%; transient acute occlusion, 6.4%; and distal embolization, 3.7%. The clinical events were acute myocardial infarction, 3.7%; in-hospital aortocoronary bypass surgery, 0.7%; in-hospital repeat PTCA, 2.6%; and death, 0.4%.

Because of the referral bias, many of the lesions treated were unfavorable for balloon angioplasty due to morphologic attributes such as tubular shape, diffuseness, total occlusion, ostial location, or previous history of a failed attempt of balloon angioplasty or restenosis after PTCA. In the first 100 patients (105 lesions) treated with excimer laser coronary angioplasty in Cedars-Sinai Medical Center, 28% of the lesions were type A American College of Cardiology/American Heart Association (ACC/AHA) lesion: 5 (47%) were type B, and 25% were type C.[21] Despite the relatively high-risk morphology, the procedural success rate did not differ significantly between the subgroup with the low-risk morphology (discrete lesions shorter than 10 mm) and the highest-risk subgroup (lesions longer than 20 mm including total occlusions): 91% and 92%, respectively (Fig 21–3). Laser and procedural success rates were achieved in 83% and 97% of type A lesions, 88% and 96% in type B, and 85% and 88% in type C, respectively. These data contrast with the lower expected success rate for type C lesions, 50%, according to recent ACC/AHA Task Force classification.

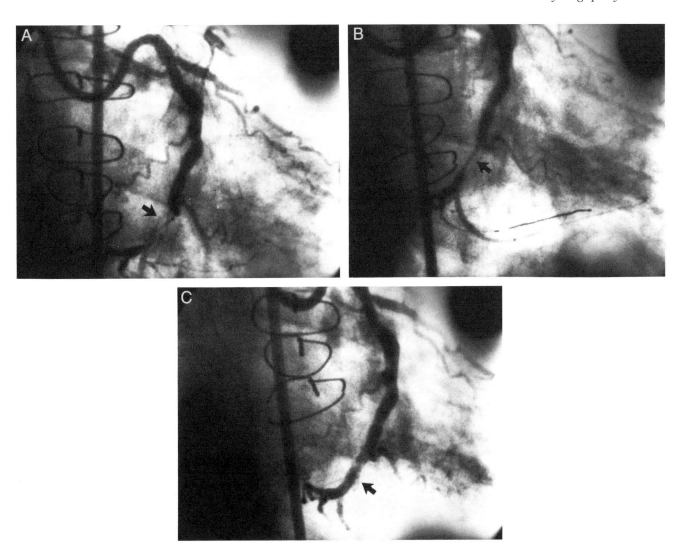

FIG 21–2.
A, total occlusion with bridging collaterals in the midsegment of a dominant left circumflex artery *(arrow).* **B,** recanalized artery after excimer laser angioplasty with a 1.3-mm catheter calibrated to 60 mJ/mm². **C,** final result after adjunct balloon angioplasty with a 3.0-mm balloon.

LATE RESTENOSIS AFTER EXCIMER LASER CORONARY ANGIOPLASTY

The overall restenosis rate in the first 812 lesions with completed 6-month follow-ups was 51% in the 468 cases with available angiographic follow-up. The clinical restenosis rate for the group was 29% (in 88% of the patients). The restenosis rate was 58% in total occlusions, 61% in saphenous vein grafts, and 47% in aorto-ostial lesions. Because of the relatively small proportion of patients who had 6-month angiographic follow-ups (58%), these "angiographic" follow-up rates are probably overestimated.

Only two procedural variables were significant predictors for late restenosis: percent residual stenosis immediately after angioplasty and laser fluence at the tip of the laser catheter. The higher the fluence, the lower was the rate of late restenosis. With low fluence in the range of 30 to 34 mJ/mm², the late restenosis rate was 69%, while for high fluence in the range of 50 to 54 mJ/mm², the late restenosis rate was only 26%. This trend suggests that there is a trade-off between pure ablation and mechanical dottering during the catheter passage through the lesion and that the higher the laser fluence, the less the mechanical trauma to the vessel wall. The current safety limit for the excimer laser system is a fluence of 60 mJ/mm² with a frequency of 30 Hz. The more liberal use of high fluence may result in lower restenosis rates in the future.

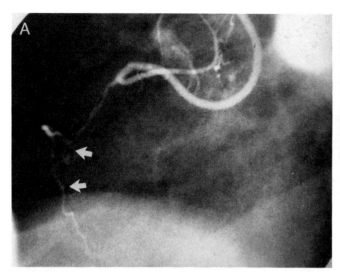 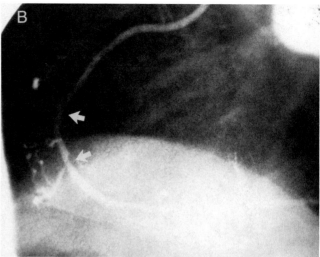

FIG 21–3.
A, total occlusion and proximal diffuse disease in a dominant right coronary artery *(arrow).* **B,** final result after 1.3 and 1.6-mm-diameter excimer laser angioplasty and adjunct balloon angioplasty of the proximal segment.

POTENTIAL INDICATIONS

Our initial experience suggests that excimer laser coronary angioplasty is an effective alternate treatment for lesions not favorable for balloon angioplasty, including long, tubular, and diffuse lesions; calcified plaques; ostial lesions; total occlusions; and lesions of saphenous vein grafts. Lesion length had been shown to increase acute closure and restenosis rates following balloon angioplasty, but only scarce data have been published about the effect of lesion length on acute procedural success rates. Our data suggest that in these lesions, excimer laser may be useful as either definitive therapy or to debulk a lesion prior to balloon angioplasty. For the time being, there is no obvious advantage of excimer laser angioplasty over balloon angioplasty for the treatment of discrete coronary stenosis without complicating features. In our study there was a selection bias toward more complex lesions, smaller-diameter arteries, and previously dilated lesions, which usually result in higher restenosis rates and higher complication rates.

CASE SELECTION

Analysis of the cumulative information acquired during the clinical multicenter trial resulted in tentative selection criteria to stratify lesions to risk subgroups. The following criteria are valid for the current catheter design and limitations and not necessarily inherent to excimer laser coronary angiography in principle.

A. Desirable lesions
   1. Diffuse disease (> 20 mm)
   2. Long lesions (> 10 mm)

   3. Aorto-ostial lesions
   4. Total occlusions crossable with a guidewire
   5. Saphenous vein graft lesions
   6. Nondilatable or noncrossable lesions by balloon angioplasty catheters
B. Acceptable lesions
   1. Ostial lesion of the left anterior descending (LAD) artery when the proximal LAD segment is in line with the left main trunk
   2. Restenotic lesions
   3. Diffusely atherosclerotic or thrombotic saphenous vein grafts
   4. Lesion involving a side branch
C. Contraindicated lesions
   1. Bifurcation lesion
   2. Highly eccentric lesions
   3. Lesions involving tight radius bends
   4. Mid-LAD lesions that terminate in a tight-radius intramyocardial bridge
   5. Any evidence of prior dissection (balloon or laser induced)

FUTURE DIRECTIONS

Over-the-wire multiple-fiber systems have a potential advantage for the treatment of coronary ostial stenoses and long coronary segments with diffuse disease and subtotal or short total occlusions. As opposed to balloon angioplasty, the excimer will not fracture the arterial wall. Removal of arteriosclerotic plaque with these systems has been demonstrated by angioscopy and ultrasound. A new 1.8-mm catheter with eccentric design has been developed and tested in an animal model, and the prototype is ready for pilot clinical trial. This catheter will enable excimer laser angioplasty in eccentric lesions in straight or even bent segments, and it has potential use in treating concentric lesions in vessels greater than 3.0 mm in diameter. Another new entry to the excimer laser arsenal is a deflectable and torquable multifiber laser catheter for recanalization of chronic total occlusions (provided that they are short and the distal segment can be opacified through collaterals). This device creates a pilot channel through the occlusion for an over-the-wire system to follow. Such a device is currently undergoing development and preclinical evaluation. A potential new indication for excimer laser coronary angioplasty is primary recanalization of acute thrombotic occlusion of the coronary arteries. This application has been studied in an animal model, and the preliminary results are encouraging.[22]

The excimer laser is a new entrant to interventional cardiology. It is likely that at least some types of lesions such as long, diffuse, or heavily calcified ones will do better with excimer than with balloon therapy alone. For recanalization of coronary occlusions, the excimer laser may have a role, especially in chronic or even calcified lesions unyielding to a conventional coronary guidewire. Since no angioplasty system is optimal for all possible lesion types and anatomic variations, the future angioplaster will have to match the lesion type with the device characteristics. Consequently, it will be necessary to combine two or more devices for the same lesion or for several lesions in the same patient to achieve optimal results with minimal risk.

The prospects for excimer laser angioplasty to become a clinically relevant procedure are encouraging, but only a larger clinical experience will determine its future role. New catheter designs will add more indications and be applicable to a greater number of patients. A unified registry for all the current interventional devices is being created, and it will enable us to determine the safety, efficacy, and long-term patency of the various angioplasty devices with respect to patients and lesion characteristics.

REFERENCES

1. Burham R, Harris NW, Djeu N: Xenon fluoride laser excitation by transverse electric discharge. *Appl Phys Lett* 1976; 28:86–87.
2. Laudenslager JB: Ion-molecule processes in lasers, in Ausloos P (ed): *Kinetics of Ion-Molecule Reactions.* New York, Plenum, 1978.
3. Grundfest S, Litvack F, Forrester JS, et al: Laser ablation of human atherosclerotic plaque without adjacent tissue injury. *J Am Coll Cardiol* 1985; 5:929–933.
4. Gorshkov BG, Epifanov AS, Manenkov AA, et al: Studies of laser-produced damage to transparent optical material in the UV region and in the crossed UV-IR beams. Proceedings of the Annual Symposium for Optical Materials for High Power Lasers, Boulder, Colo, 1981, pp 76–85.
5. Gorisch W, Boargen KP: Heat induced contraction of blood vessels. *Lasers Surg Med* 1982; 2:1–13.
6. Anderson RR, Parrish JA: Selective photothermolysis: Precise microsurgery by selective absorption of pulsed radiation. *Science* 1983; 220:524–527.
7. Srinivasan R: Ablation of polymers and biological tissue by ultraviolet lasers. *Science* 1986; 234:559–565.
8. Segalowitz J, Litvack F, Grundfest W, et al: Direct angioscopic observation of plaque ablation by excimer laser (abstracted). *Circulation* 1989; 80(suppl 2):1989.
9. Nishioka NS, Teng P, Deutsch TF, et al: Mechanisms of laser induced fragmentation of urinary and biliary calculi. *Lasers Life Sci* 1987; 1:231–245.
10. Prince MR, Deutsch TF, Mathews-Roth MM, et al: Preferential light absorption in atheromas in vitro: Implication for laser angioplasty. *J Clin Invest* 1986; 78:295–302.
11. Spears JR, Serur J, Shropshire D, et al: Fluorescence of experimental atheromatous plaques with hematoporphyrin derivative. *J Clin Invest* 1983; 71:395–399.
12. Abela GS, Barbieri E, Roxey T, et al: Laser enhanced plaque atherolysis with tetracycline (abstracted). *Circulation* 1986; 72(suppl 2):7.
13. Sartori MP, Weinbaecher D, Valderrama GL, et al: Laser induced autofluorescence of human arteries. *Circ Res* 1988; 63:1053–1059.
14. Chutorian DM, Selzer PM, Koshek J, et al: The interaction between excimer laser energy and vascular tissue. *Am Heart J* 1986; 112:739–745.
15. Leon MB, Almagor Y, Bartorelli AL, et al: Fluorescence-guided laser assisted balloon angioplasty in patients with femoropopliteal occlusions. *Circulation* 1990; 81:143–155.
16. Isner JM, Donaldson RF, Funai JT, et al: Factors contributing to perforations resulting from laser coronary angioplasty: Observations in an intact human postmortem preparation of intraoperative laser coronary angioplasty. *Coronary Artery Surg* 1985; 72(suppl 2):191–199.
17. Abela GS, Normann SJ, Cohen DM, et al: Laser recanalization of occluded atherosclerotic arteries in vivo and in vitro. *Circulation* 1985; 71:403–411.
18. Litvack F, Grunfest WS, Eigler N, et al: Percutaneous excimer laser coronary angioplasty. *Lancet* 1989; 2:102–103.
19. Holmes DR, Litvack FI, Goldenberg T, et al: Excimer laser coronary angioplasty (ELCA) registry; lesion length and outcome (abstracted). *Circulation* 1991; 84(suppl II):362.
20. Eigler NL, Douglas JS, Margolis JR, et al: Excimer laser angioplasty of aorto-ostial stenosis: Results of the ELCA registry (abstracted). Circulation 1991; 84(suppl II):251
21. Cook SL, Eigler NL, Shefer A, et al: Percutaneous excimer laser coronary angioplasty of lesion not ideal for balloon angioplasty. *Circulation* 1991; 84:632–643.
22. Shefer A, Forrester JS, Litvack F: Recanalization of acute thrombus: Comparison of acute success and short term patency after excimer laser coronary angioplasty, balloon angioplasty and intracoronary thrombolysis in pigs (abstracted). *J Am Coll Cardiol* 1991; 17:205.

22

Excimer Laser Coronary Angioplasty: Wire-Guided Techniques and Results From a Multicenter Trial

John A. Bittl, M.D.

The role of coronary eximer laser angioplasty is being investigated in large multicenter trials. After 3 years of clinical investigation, it is clear that excimer laser coronary angioplasty will not supplant balloon angioplasty. Instead, preliminary information from the large multicenter trials suggests that excimer laser coronary angioplasty has shown remarkable success with certain lesion types that are traditionally difficult for balloon angioplasty. Thus, further investigation of the efficacy of excimer laser angioplasty for these complex lesion types is warranted before absolute indications for the procedure can be established.

The purpose of this chapter is to review the current status of excimer laser coronary angioplasty and to focus on patient selection and special techniques for certain lesion types that are difficult for traditional balloon angioplasty. This chapter will not focus on the fundamental principles of excimer laser physics or laser-tissue interaction because it is understood that these topics will have already been covered by the interested reader.[1-4]

METHODS

The Excimer Laser System for Coronary Angioplasty

Percutaneous excimer laser coronary angioplasty is performed with the Spectranetics CVX-300 system (Spectranetics Corp., Colorado Springs), which is an XeCl excimer laser system that operates at 308 nm with an average output of 200 mJ per pulse at nominal voltage operation. The fluence at the laser catheter tip is set by the operator to a level of 40 to 60 mJ/mm^2 in this self-calibrating system. The minimum pulse width is 120 ns.

During angioplasty, a guiding catheter (e.g., Soft-tip, Schneider Corp., Minneapolis) intubates the coronary ostium. For laser catheters 1.4 or 1.7 mm in diameter, an 8 F guide catheter is used. For 2.0-mm laser catheters, a 9 F guide catheter is selected. An exchange-length 0.014-in. (0.36-mm) High-Torque Floppy guidewire (ACS, Advanced Cardiovascular Systems, Mountain View, Calif) or similar wire is advanced through the stenosis. The self-calibrating Spectranetics laser catheter is advanced over the guidewire to the stenosis. The Spectranetics laser catheter is a multifiber, over-the-wire, "end-firing" catheter with diameters that range from 1.4 to 2.0 mm and contains 20 to 85 100-μm optical fibers arranged coaxially around a 0.022-in. (0.56-mm) central lumen (Fig 22–1). The guidewire predominantly determines the course that the laser catheter will take in the coronary artery and is influenced to only a small degree by the operator. Thus, the term "wire-guided" excimer laser coronary angioplasty has been introduced to clarify the technique of performing excimer laser coronary angioplasty. The laser catheter is advanced through the guiding catheter over the guidewire to the origin of the stenosis. The position of the laser catheter is confirmed by injecting 3 cc of Hypaque-76 (diatrizoate meglumine and diatrizoate sodium) under cineangiography. Laser output from the generator is activated with a foot pedal as the catheter is advanced through the stenosis at a rate of 0.5 mm/sec, which is slower than the rate of tissue ablation.[2] Laser

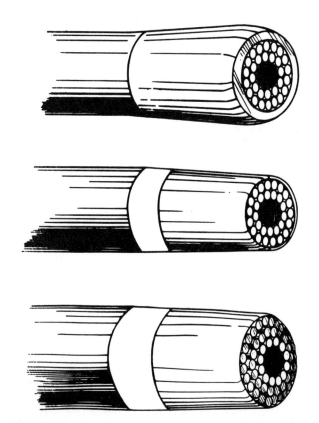

FIG 22–1.
Laser catheters. The figure illustrates the distal tip of three types of laser catheters that range in outer diameter from 1.8 mm *(top)* and 1.7 mm *(middle)* to 2.0 mm *(bottom).* Concentrically surrounding the 0.021-in. (0.53-mm) central lumen, which carries a guidewire that may range in size from 0.014 to 0.018 in. (0.36 to 0.46 mm), is an array of 100 μm-purified silica optical fibers that carry the laser radiation to the catheter tip.

energy is delivered in pulses of 120 ns, at a frequency of 25 sec, in trains of 0.04 to 5.0 seconds in duration, and at a fluence of 40 to 60 mJ/mm.[2] Each train of pulses is followed by a 15-second delay time, which minimizes energy loss to the optical fibers from absorption of ultraviolet light (e.g., band-gap phenomenon) and permits the operator to make a record of the laser catheter tip position on cineangiography. The laser catheter tip position remains unaltered during the 15-second delay period and need not be withdrawn proximally unless the catheter has been advanced completely along the length of the stenosis. After each passage of the laser catheter through the stenosis, the laser catheter is withdrawn into the proximal segment of the coronary artery, and contrast agent is injected to assess the residual stenosis. Typically, only one passage of the laser catheter is required. However, under conditions where an eccentric stenosis is involved, multiple passes may be used (see

TABLE 22–1
Clinical Sites

Mt. Sinai Medical Center, New York
Brigham & Women's Hospital, Boston
Arizona Heart Institute, Phoenix
St. Francis Hospital, Roslyn, NY
Duke University Medical Center, Durham, NC
Good Samaritan Hospital, Phoenix
Mills-Peninsula Hospital, Palo Alto, Calif
Northwestern Memorial Hospital, Chicago
Scott & White Clinic, Temple, Tex
St. Elizabeth's Hospital, Boston
Texas Heart Institute, Houston
University of Michigan, Ann Arbor
University of California, Irvine

below). Measuring laser output from the catheter before and after each procedure ensures that a known, constant fluence is delivered and allows comparisons to be made with other manufacturers' devices.

PATIENT ENROLLMENT

A multicenter trial of the Spectranetics CVX-300 excimer laser system commenced in May 1989 under Dr. Timothy A. Sanborn of Mt. Sinai Medical Center, New York. Twelve additional centers have participated in the trial (Table 22–1).

As of October 26, 1990, a total of 374 patients have undergone excimer laser coronary angioplasty with the Spectranetics system (Table 22–2). The average age of the patients was 59.9 years, and 79% of the patients were men. Seventy-five percent of the patients had Canadian Heart Association class III or IV angina before treatment.

A total of 408 stenoses were treated with excimer laser coronary angioplasty in the patients (Table 22–3). The distribution of lesions involved the three coronary arteries, the left main coronary artery, and saphenous vein bypass grafts. Fifty percent of the lesions were

TABLE 22–2
Patient Characteristics (374 Patients)

Average age, 60 ± 11 yr		
Gender		
M	296	(79%)
F	78	(21%)
Canadian Heart Association Classification:		
Asymptomatic	5	(1%)
Class I	15	(4%)
Class II	74	(20%)
Class III	148	(40%)
Class IV	132	(35%)

TABLE 22–3

Lesions Treated (*N* = 408)

Lesion	*n*	(%)
Left anterior descending artery	213	(52.2)
Right coronary artery	116	(28.4)
Left circumflex	53	(13.0)
Left main coronary artery	3	(0.7)
Saphenous vein graft/other	23	(5.6)

TABLE 22–4

Laser Catheters*

Diameter (mm)	*n*	(%)
1.4	137	(31)
1.7	284	(66)
2.0	11	(3)

*Note: Some lesions required more than one catheter. *N* = 432.

judged to be in the proximal segment of the coronary artery or graft, 42% were in the middle segment, and 6% were distally located. Sixty of the treated vessels (14.7%) were ≤2.0 mm in diameter, 30 (7.4%) were 2.1 to 2.5 mm, 198 (48.5%) were 2.6 to 3.0 mm, and 120 (29.4%) were >3.0 mm in diameter. Thus, more than 75% of the treated vessels were >2.5 mm in diameter.

Prospective recruitment of specific lesion types commenced after initial experience was gained at each participating site. Once proficiency was achieved (after 5 to 20 cases), each investigator then enrolled patients who were felt to be at increased risk for abrupt closure or restenosis with traditional balloon angioplasty. Twenty-seven percent of the lesions were "restenosis" lesions, having been dilated previously with balloon angioplasty. Forty-nine lesions (12.0%) were 11 to 19 mm in length, and 29 (7.1%) were ≥20 mm in length (≥50% stenosis along the entire length). One hundred seventy-six lesions (43.1%) were judged to be eccentric. Fifteen lesions (3.7%) were in old (>3 years) saphenous vein bypass grafts. Five lesions were documented chronic total occlusions.

All procedures were approved by the institutional review boards of the respective participating centers.

SUCCESS AND COMPLICATION RATES

Acute Success.—Of the 408 lesions treated with excimer laser angioplasty, successful passage of the laser catheter through the lesion was achieved in 332 (81.4%), with a reduction in the stenosis by 20% or greater. Procedural success was achieved in 379 lesions (92.8%), defined as 50% or less residual stenosis and avoidance of major complication such as death, myocardial infarction, or emergency bypass surgery.

Most patients were treated with the 1.4- and 1.7-mm laser catheters, which reflects their earlier introduction into use (Table 22–4).

Complications.—The risk of serious complications is low for excimer laser coronary angioplasty (Table 22–5). The risk of death was less than 1%, and the risk of acute myocardial infarction or need for bypass sur-

gery at any time during hospitalization was about 4%. Six patients experienced perforation of the coronary artery during laser angioplasty; two patients required surgery, and the others had uneventful courses with conservative management, such as prolonged inflation of the Stack perfusion catheter at the perforation site.[5]

We have evaluated the influence of clinical, angiographic, and procedural variables on the likelihood of success of excimer laser coronary angioplasty. Procedural success rates for lesions in the proximal segment of the coronary artery are equivalent to those in the mid and distal segments (92.3%, 90.8%, and 93.3%, respectively). Similarly, vessel diameter has no effect on laser success or procedural success (82.0% and 90.0% for vessels ≤2.0 mm, 82.6% and 87.0% for vessels 2.1 to 2.5 mm, 80.8% and 98.6% for vessels 2.6 to 3.0 mm, and 85.3% and 100% for vessels >3.0 mm, respectively). We observed no effect of lesion length on the likelihood of laser or procedural success (81.8% and 93.6% for lesions ≤10 mm and 80.2% and 91.6% for lesions >10 mm, respectively). These results compare favorably with current data on the efficacy of balloon angioplasty for long lesions: Ghazzal et al. recently reported that the clinical success rate for lesions >20 mm (entire segment contained a stenosis >30%) was 82% with a 9.7% incidence of major complications.[6]

Embolization.—Formation of debris during laser ablation has been reported for continuous-wave systems

TABLE 22–5

Complications in 374 Patients*

Complications	No.	(%)
Death	1	(0.3)
Bypass surgery during hospitalization	18	(4.8)
Q wave myocardial infarction	1	(0.3)
Non–Q wave myocardial infarction	17	(4.6)
Dissection	67	(17.9)
Minor	47	(12.6)
Clinically significant†	20	(5.4)
Perforation	6	(1.6)

*Includes death, myocardial infarction, or bypass surgery required at any time during hospitalization.

†Associated with major complication of death, myocardial infarction, bypass surgery, or dissection producing a flow of TIMI grade 2 or less.

such as the argon laser, which has been shown to produce particulate matter of diameter >50 μm during radiation of human cadaveric aorta.[7] The rate of ablation of tissue with excimer laser radiation is limited[2]; thus, the catheter should be advanced through the stenosis at a rate of 0.5 to 1.0 mm/sec. Advancement of the catheter at a rate faster than the rate of ablation may be associated with mechanical dilatation, tissue dissection, or embolization. Fortunately, the rate of embolization observed in large multicenter studies with excimer laser angioplasty has been low, ranging from 0.9% to 1.4%,[8, 9] with most of the events related to the use of adjunctive balloon angioplasty.

Thrombosis.—The risk of thrombosis from wire-guided excimer laser coronary angioplasty is theoretically less than that for thermal laser angioplasty.[10] However, the risk of thrombosis is not completely eliminated. Abrupt closure may occur in about 2% of patients undergoing excimer laser coronary angioplasty, and some of these cases are probably related to the presence of thrombosis.[8, 9]

Restenosis.—Of 94 consecutive patients who underwent excimer laser coronary angioplasty at either Mt. Sinai Hospital or the Brigham and Women's Hospital, 6-month clinical follow-up has been obtained in 91 (97%). Twenty-two of the 91 patients had a return of symptoms of angina, required repeat angioplasty, had myocardial infarction, or had a positive exercise test. Thus, the clinical restenosis rate was 24%. There were no deaths in this cohort. Angiographic follow-up at 6 months has been obtained in 71 of 94 (75%) patients, with a total of 79 lesions being evaluated. We observed 50% or greater stenosis at 51% of the treated sites. The risk of restenosis in this small cohort is not influenced by a history of restenosis after prior balloon angioplasty or location of the treated site.

TECHNICAL GUIDELINES LEARNED FROM THE MULTICENTER TRIAL

The use of relatively stiff prototype laser catheters places special demands on the adjunctive equipment used during angioplasty. In addition, the direction of the laser catheter in the vessel and through the stenosis is operator independent, being fixed by the course of the guidewire in the vessel. Thus, we have termed this type of intervention "wire-guided" excimer laser coronary angioplasty. We have identified the following set of guidelines from our experience with this intervention.

Guide Catheters.—The selection of the appropriate guide catheter is critical for the success of wire-guided

laser angioplasty. Laser catheters are stiffer than currently available balloon catheters and are thus more difficult to advance through the bends of a guide catheter and into the coronary artery. Certain features about the construction, size, and configuration of guide catheters have been identified to compensate for the limitations of the relatively stiff prototype laser catheters and to increase the likelihood of successful laser angioplasty.

For the left coronary artery, the Judkins shape is the configuration of first choice. The Amplatz shape can provide greater support, but this important characteristic of guide catheters for balloon angioplasty is ideally less important in wire-guided excimer laser angioplasty because advancement of the laser catheter through a stenosis depends on tissue ablation and not on forceful mechanical dilatation. In order to align the guide catheter tip with the left main coronary artery, the operator selects a Judkins catheter with a short tip configuration. Advancing the laser catheter into the coronary artery is simplified if the operator chooses a catheter with a Judkins curve size one-half size larger for laser angioplasty than for balloon angioplasty (e.g., JL4.5 short tip instead of JL4.0) in an effort to decrease the angle at the secondary bend in the catheter (Fig 22–2).

For the right coronary artery, the right Judkins 4.0 shape can be used successfully, but better guide catheter support for passage of the laser catheter through tortuous segments is provided by the left Amplatz shape (either AL1.0, 1.5, or 2.0).

Compliant guide catheters accommodate the relatively rigid prototype laser catheters better than stiff guide catheters do. In addition, a guide catheter should contain a central lumen lined with Teflon or other non-braided material for lubricity. One type of catheter that combines flexibility, shape, and construction for laser angioplasty is made by Schneider (Minneapolis).

For laser catheters of outer diameter <1.85 mm, an 8 F guide catheter with an internal diameter of 0.076 to 0.082 in. (1.93 to 2.08 mm) is used. For a laser catheter with an outer diameter ≥1.90 mm, a 9 F guide catheter with two-layer, thin-wall "superflow" construction and an inner diameter of 0.092 in. (2.34 mm) is required.

RECOMMENDATIONS FOR SPECIFIC LESIONS

Eccentric Lesions.—Some types of eccentric stenoses may be preferentially treated by wire-guided laser ablation than by balloon angioplasty. In comparison with directional atherectomy in which the operator rotates the cutting blade to face the lesion for ablation, the direction of ablation during laser angioplasty is operator in-

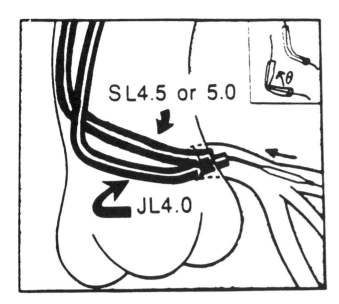

FIG 22–2.
Guide catheter selection. Judkins left guide catheters of small curve size such as the JL4.0 may be associated with an angle of less than 90 degrees at the secondary bend, which can lead to buckling of the central lumen around the guidewire *(inset)*. This can be prevented by selecting a guide catheter with a larger curve size, such as 4.5 or 5.0. The short tip design may minimize the likelihood of poor coaxial alignment of the guide with the left main coronary artery. Adapted from Clark DA: coronary angioplasty catheters and accessories, in Clark DA (ed): *Coronary Angioplasty.* New York, Alan R Liss, 1987, pp 9–27.

dependent and is determined instead by the course of the guidewire in the coronary artery. Certain types of eccentric stenoses have been consistently and successfully treated with wire-guided laser ablation.

If the guidewire abuts an eccentric lesion, laser ablation can be carried out easily. The lesion positions that are amenable to laser ablation include the proximal segment of the left anterior descending artery and the middle segments of the right coronary and left circumflex coronary arteries. Eccentric lesions that arise from the superior concave arc of the left anterior descending artery, which frequently is spanned by the guidewire, are disposed to wire-guided nondirectional laser atherectomy (Figs 22–3 and 22–4). Similarly, the outer concave arcs of the right coronary artery (Fig 22–5) and the left circumflex coronary artery also frequently carry the guidewire, thus allowing close apposition of eccentric stenosis with the ablating tip of the wire-guided laser catheter.

Bifurcation Lesions.—Although the risk of occluding a side branch that arises from a stenosis is theoretically less for an ablative procedure than for balloon angioplasty, any benefit of the laser technique is offset by the likelihood of wire-guided laser angioplasty to disrupt the delta-shaped tissue that lies between the two vessels. The resulting intimal flap, which is generated from dissection and not by the "snowplow" effect seen with balloon angioplasty,[11] can nevertheless occlude the side branch and produce ischemia. Thus, we recommend

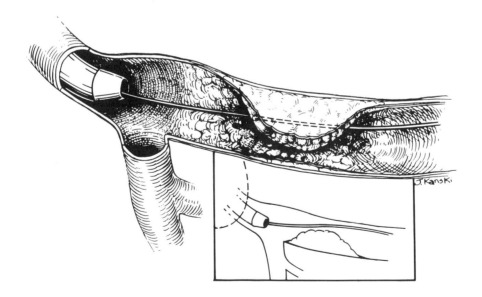

FIG 22–3.
Eccentric stenosis in the proximal segment of the left anterior descending artery. The eccentric stenosis that arises from the superior arc of the left anterior descending artery in the right anterior oblique view abuts the guidewire and is thus amenable to wire-guided laser angioplasty, whereas the lesion lying on the opposite wall remains in a position that cannot be reached by the guidewire *(inset)* and is difficult to ablate with laser angioplasty.

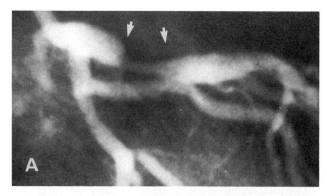

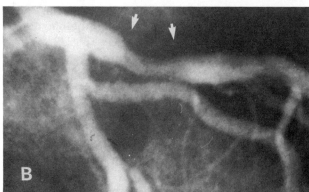

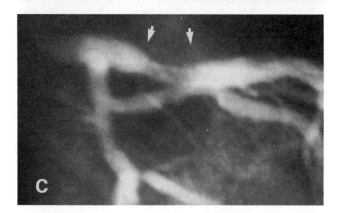

FIG 22–4.
Eccentric stenosis *(arrows).* **A,** the 80% stenosis in the proximal segment of the left anterior descending artery was treated with nine passages of the 1.7-mm laser catheter without the need for adjunctive balloon angioplasty. **B,** a residual 40% stenosis was left that remained unchanged at follow-up angiography **C.**

that the double-wire technique be used for large side branches that arise from the center of bifurcation lesions. This permits the laser catheter to be passed successively over the two wires, allows loose intimal flaps to be removed cleanly, and thus prevents side branch loss. On the other hand, it is extremely uncommon to observe side branch occlusion from treatment of a stenosis

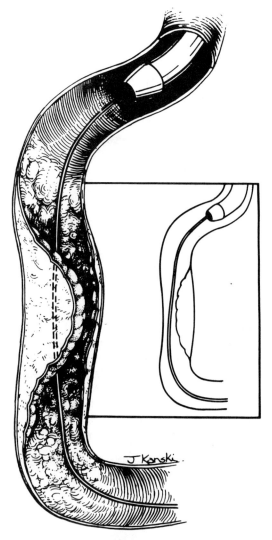

FIG 22–5.
Eccentric stenosis in the midportion of the right coronary artery. The stenosis that arises from the outer convex sweep of the midportion in the right coronary artery is spanned by the guidewire and is suitable for laser angioplasty. The stenosis positioned against the inner concave arc on the opposite wall is difficult to reach with the laser catheter *(inset).*

that terminates in a bifurcation because of the absence of the "snowplow" effect (Fig 22–6).

Total Occlusions.—Since passage of a guidewire through a stenosis must be achieved before wire-guided laser angioplasty can be performed, chronic total occlusions should be selected for treatment with laser angioplasty in the manner that they are chosen for balloon angioplasty. The ideal lesion consists of a tapered occlusion with no bridging collaterals[12] and one additional characteristic: the stenotic segment should be straight with no angles greater than 45 degrees (Fig 22–7). The

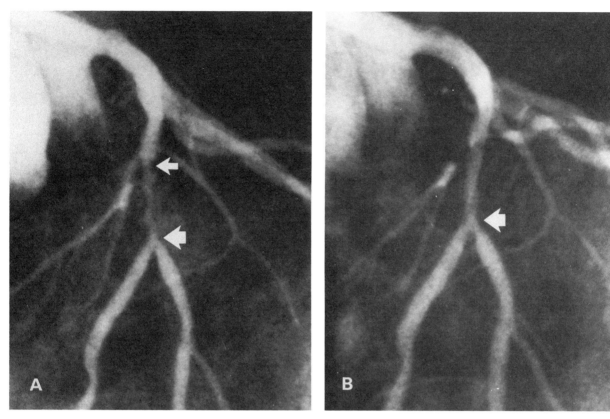

FIG 22–6.
Bifurcation lesion (single guidewire). A 10-mm stenosis of the proximal portion of the left anterior descending artery *(arrows)* terminates in the bifurcation with a large diagonal branch **(A)**. After treatment with a 2.0-mm laser catheter and no balloon, the origin of the side branch *(large arrow)* remains intact **(B)**.

total occlusion is then penetrated with the softest wire that will permit passage, but this often requires use of the high-torque standard (ACS) or steerable guidewire (USCI, Billerica, Mass.). The bare-wire technique can be used with an exchange or extendable system. On the other hand, a low-profile laser catheter can be used to direct the guidewire at the total occlusion in a manner similar to balloon angioplasty.

DISCUSSION

A perplexing variety of new coronary interventional devices is currently under evaluation. The interventional cardiologist must ferret out reliable information about each new device from reports that give no direct comparison with balloon angioplasty and yet conclude that the new procedure is "safe and effective." What useful information can be wrought from such studies whose only merits are that they are prospectively designed to gain broad clinical experience with the new technology? In the absence of a randomized trial, the results of such studies must be compared rigorously and fairly with known success and complication rates for percutaneous transluminal (balloon) coronary angioplasty. The refinements in balloon angioplasty catheters and in patient selection have produced superior success rates so that the results from the 1985–1986 National Heart, Lung, and Blood Institute (NHLBI) Registry are now obsolete. The common practice of comparing success rates for new interventional devices with those from the 1985–1986 NHLBI Registry is improper: the registry's angiographic success rate of 88%, overall clinical success rate of 78%, nonfatal infarction rate of 4.3%, and mortality rate of <1.0%[13] have been superseded at the current time. In an effort to control for variability in case mix, many investigators have compared results from new interventional devices with those for balloon angioplasty from the useful classification of lesion morphology generated by the American College of Cardiology/American Heart Association (ACC/AHA) Task Force for Angioplasty.[14] Such comparisons are problematic because the stated success rates in the task force report are estimates based on experienced opinion and

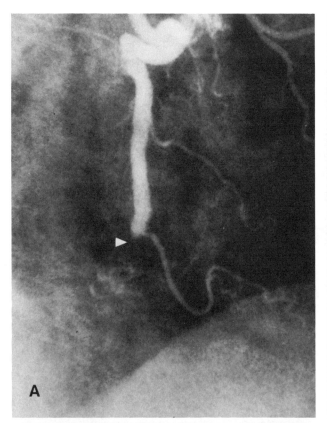

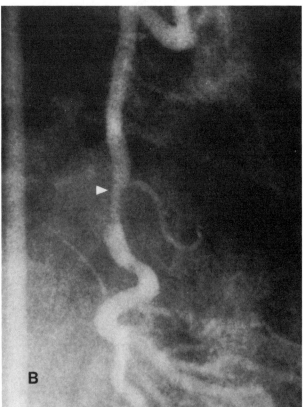

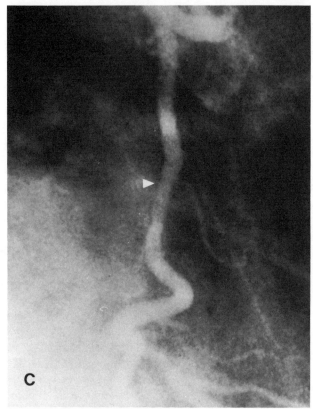

FIG 22–7.
Chronic total occlusion *(arrow).* The total occlusion in the midportion of the right coronary artery **(A),** documented to be totally occluded at coronary arteriography 4 months previously, was penetrated with a 0.014-in. (0.36-mm) steerable guidewire (USCI, Billerica, Mass) and treated with a 1.7-mm laser catheter; a residual 50% stenosis was left **(B).** This was dilated further with a 3.0-mm balloon **(C).**

TABLE 22–5

Potential Indications for the Use of Wire-Guided Excimer Laser Coronary Angioplasty

Long diffuse lesions
Eccentric lesions
Chronic total occlusions
Saphenous vein bypass grafts
Ostial lesions

not on original data. What, then, are the failings of balloon angioplasty that may be overcome by new interventional devices? Despite improvements in success rates and complication rates, balloon angioplasty has indisputable shortcomings: a 4% rate of abrupt closure[15, 16] and a 17% to 49% rate of angiographic restenosis.[17–19] The problems of abrupt closure[15] and restenosis[18] are more common for patients with long lesions (>4.8 to 9.0 mm) or >30% to 35% residual stenoses.

Excimer laser coronary angioplasty has been under investigation since 1989. The role of this expensive technology has not been defined. Based on little more than anecdotal experience, the procedure seems to be associated with a lower rate of abrupt closure for long lesions than in the case of balloon angioplasty. It is unclear whether the technique offers any advantage over balloon angioplasty for chronic total occlusions, certain types of eccentric lesions, ostial lesions, or lesions in old saphenous vein bypass grafts, but preliminary experience is promising. The overall restenosis rate of 50% after excimer laser angioplasty is disappointing and probably reflects no significant difference from balloon angioplasty if the same definition of restenosis is used and similarly complex lesions treated.

If excimer laser coronary angioplasty proves to be more effective than balloon angioplasty for these complex lesions (Table 22–5) the new procedure may then apply to about 15% to 20% of patients who undergo percutaneous angioplasty procedures. However, defining the indications for excimer laser coronary angioplasty awaits the results of focused investigation on complex lesions. In the absence of a randomized trial, the results of excimer laser angioplasty for complex lesions must be compared with the current success and restenosis rates for balloon angioplasty for matched lesions.

REFERENCES

1. Laudenslager JB: Ion-molecule processes in lasers, in Ausloos P (ed): *Kinetics of Ion-Molecule Reactions.* New York, Plenum, 1978, pp 405–436.
2. Litvack F, Forrester JS, Grundfest WS, et al: The excimer laser: From basic science to clinical application, in Vogel JHK, King SB III (eds): *Interventional cardiology: Future Directions.* St Louis, Mosby–Year Book, 1989, pp 170–181.
3. Isner JM, Clarke RH: *Cardiovascular Laser Therapy.* New York, Raven Press, 1989.
4. White RA, Grundfest WS: *Laser in Cardiovascular Disease: Clinical Applications, Alternative Angioplasty Devices, and Guidance Systems.* Chicago, Mosby–Year Book, 1989.
5. Parker JD, Ganz P, Selwyn AP, et al: Successful treatment of an excimer laser–associated coronary artery perforation with the Stack perfusion catheter. *Cathet Cardiovasc Diagn* 1991; 22:118–123.
6. Ghazzal ZMB, Weintraub WS, Ba'albaki HA, et al: PTCA of lesions longer than 20 mm: Initial outcome and restenosis (abstract). *Circulation* 1990; 82(suppl 3):509.
7. Grewe DD, Castañeda-Zuñiga WR, Nordstrom LA, et al: Debris analysis after laser photorecanalization of atherosclerotic plaque. *Semin Intervent Radiol* 1986; 3:53–60.
8. Bittl JA, Sanborn TA, Hershman RA, et al: Coronary excimer laser angioplasty: Results in 223 patients from a multicenter registry (abstract). *Circulation* 1990; 82(suppl):670.
9. Margolis JR, Litvack F, Krauthamer D, et al: Coronary angioplasty with laser and high frequency energy. *Herz* 1990; 15:223–232.
10. Sanborn TA, Alexopoulos D, Marmur JD, et al: Coronary excimer laser angioplasty: Reduced complications and indium-111 platelet accumulation compared with thermal laser angioplasty. *J Am Coll Cardiol* 1990; 16:502–506.
11. Meier B, Grüntzig AR, King SBI, et al: Risk of side branch occlusion during coronary angioplasty. *Am J Cardiol* 1984; 53:10–14.
12. Stone GW, Rutherford BD, McConahay DR, et al: Procedural outcome of angioplasty for total coronary artery occlusion: An analysis of 971 lesions in 905 patients. *J Am Coll Cardiol* 1990; 15:849–856.
13. Detre K, Holubkov R, Kelsey S, et al: Percutaneous transluminal coronary angioplasty in 1985–1986 and 1977–1981. The National Heart, Lung, and Blood Institute Registry. *N Engl J Med* 1988; 318:265–270.
14. Ryan TJ, Faxon DP, Gunnar RM, et al: Guidelines for percutaneous transluminal coronary angioplasty. A report of the American College of Cardiology/American Heart Association Task Force on Assessment of Diagnostic and Therapeutic Cardiovascular Procedures (Subcommittee on Percutaneous Transluminal Coronary Angioplasty). *Circulation* 1988; 78:486–502.
15. Ellis SG, Roubin GS, King SB I, et al: Angiographic and clinical predictors of acute closure after native vessel coronary angioplasty. *Circulation* 1988; 77:372–379.
16. Bredlau CE, Roubin G, Leimgruber P, et al: In-hospital morbidity and mortality in patients undergoing elective coronary angioplasty. *Circulation* 1985; 72:1044.
17. Fanelli C, Aronoff R: Restenosis following coronary angioplasty. *Am Heart J* 1990; 119:357–368.
18. Pepine CJ, Hirshfeld JW, Macdonald RG, et al: A controlled trial of corticosteroids to prevent restenosis after coronary angioplasty. *Circulation* 1990; 81:1753–1761.
19. Nobuyoshi M, Kimura T, Nosaka H, et al: Restenosis after successful percutaneous transluminal coronary angioplasty: Serial angiographic follow-up of 229 patients. *J Am Coll Cardiol* 1988; 12:616–623.

23

Experience in Peripheral Laser Angioplasty

Giancarlo Biamino, M.D.

Pia Skarabis, M.D.

Expansion of the simple Dotter[1] concept by transcutaneous balloon angioplasty[2, 3] has dramatically changed the management of obstructive arterial disease. The unique technological development of this method during the last few years has enabled worldwide primary success rates of 95% and more to be reported in attempts to recanalize stenotic peripheral or coronary arteries. However, the incapability of crossing occluded vessels in more than 50% of the cases remains an important limitation of arterial balloon angioplasty. This relevant limitation of the technique is magnified by the main disadvantage of balloon angioplasty: a high degree of restenosis or reocclusion of about 40%[4-15] in coronary and approximately 50% in peripheral arteries.[16-25]

Many new interventional techniques have been developed during the last 10 years.[26] In the early 1980s some groups picked up the innovative idea that laser energy might also be used to vaporize sclerotic material,[27-29] and laser angioplasty was introduced as a clinical modality very quickly.[24, 30-40]

Our group started a cardiovascular laser angioplasty program in November 1985. The main goal was the development of a technology for percutaneous application of laser energy that would be able to remove rather than mechanically reshape the lumen of the artery without causing relevant damage to adjacent tissue. Since January 1989 we have performed excimer laser–assisted angioplasty of peripheral vessels in more than 350 cases. In this article we will report our experiences in transcutaneous angioplasty of 260 patients with a follow-up longer than 6 months.

METHODS AND CLINICAL MATERIAL

Study inclusion criteria

Patients who had peripheral vascular disease for more than 6 months and were clinically symptomatic (gangrene, rest pain, or claudication at a walking distance of 200 m or less) were included in the study. In a few cases patients with claudication at a walking distance between 200 and 500 m were also included in the study if their quality of life was seriously affected because of their inability to walk longer distances.

All patients had single or multiple subtotal or total occlusions in the iliacal arteries or in the superficial femoral or popliteal artery with an infrapopliteal runoff of at least one vessel.

Patient Population

Since January 1989 recanalization with excimer laser–assisted angioplasty has been attempted in 260 peripheral vessels. A second laser angioplasty on the contralateral side was performed in approximately 21% of the patients, and these patients were included in the study twice. The ages of the 212 male and 48 female patients ranged from 40 to 81 years (mean, 65). The mean ankle-brachial index before the intervention was 0.58. Seventeen patients (6.5%) had rest pain or gangrene, 29 patients (11%) experienced claudication at a walking distance of less than 50 m, 188 patients (72%) experienced claudication at a walking distance between 50 and 200 m, and 26 patients (10%) could walk more than 200 m (Table 23–1).

TABLE 23–1.
Clinical Data of 260 Patients

Sex: 212 male, 48 female
Age: 40–81 yr (mean, 65)
Mean ankle-brachial index: 0.58
Symptoms:
  Rest pain: 17 pts* (6.5%)
  Claudication < 50 m: 29 pts (11.0%)
  Claudication at 50–200 m: 188 pts (72.5%)
  Claudication at 200–500 m: 26 pts (10.0%)
Previous PTCA* on angioplasty site: 31 pts (12.0%)

*pts = patients; PTCA = percutaneous transluminal coronary angioplasty.

Sixty patients (23%) had diabetes mellitus, 42 patients (16%) had systemic hypertension, 84 patients (32%) had additional coronary heart disease or a high-grade stenosis of the carotid arteries, and 25 patients (9.5%) had hypercholesterolemia (>250 mg/dL) at the time of intervention. Most patients had formerly been smokers, but only 27 patients (10%) admitted to still be heavy smokers at the time of the intervention.

Thirty-one patients (12%) had been previously treated by one and 3 patients by two previous balloon dilatations at the angioplasty site.

Angiographic Findings

Two hundred six lesions were located in the superficial femoral artery (SFA), 29 in the iliac arteries, and 25 lesions in the popliteal region. Forty percent of the lesions were subtotal (single or multiple) and 60% were total occlusions. Length of the lesion varied from 1 to 35 cm; 43 lesions (16.5%) were shorter than 3 cm, there were 81 lesions (31%) between 3 and 7 cm, and 73 lesions (28%) were between 7 and 12 cm. Sixty-three lesions (24%) were longer than 12 cm (43 even longer than 20 cm) (Table 23–2).

Follow-up

Before and 24 hours following the intervention all patients underwent color Doppler flow imaging analysis of the region of interest. Clinical follow-up included questionnaires, physical examination, treadmill exercise tests, brachial-ankle index determination, and color-flow

TABLE 23–2.
Lesion Length (1–35 cm) of 260 Peripheral Lesions

Lesion Length (cm)	n
<3	43 (16%)
3–7	81 (31%)
7–12	73 (28%)
>12	63 (24%)

Doppler 3, 6, 12, and 24 months after the intervention. Digital subtraction angiography was performed 6 months after the intervention in all patients who wanted to have an angiographic control and at variable times in all patients who experienced deterioration of their clinical situation.

Laser and Laser Catheters

A 308-nm pulsed ultraviolet xenon chloride excimer laser (MAX 10, Technolas, Germany) with a repetition rate of 20 Hz was used as an energy source. The pulse duration was 60 to 110 ns. When a xenon chloride 308-nm excimer laser is used, the ablation of the irradiated tissue is predominantly a local, very fast microexplosion provoked by an extremely high temperature rise of the irradiated volume with energy densities of about 3 to 6 J/cm^2.[41] Nevertheless, the thermal damage induced remains minimal even when high-energy densities (7.5 J/cm^2) are used.[42]

A 7 F multifiber catheter (containing 12 fibers with a core diameter of 260 μm incorporated around a central channel) was used in 35% of the cases to attempt recanalization, and a 9 F multifiber catheter (containing 18 fibers with a core diameter of 260 μm incorporated around a central channel) was used in 56% of the cases. In 8% of the lesions both catheter types were applied during the procedure. In a few cases a 5 F catheter (42 fibers with a core diameter of 100 μm) was used in the popliteal region.

The central channel of the 9 F catheter allowed the introduction of a guidewire with a maximum size of 0.035-in, and guidewires with a maximum size of 0.020 and 0.014 in. could be introduced into the central channel of the 7 and 5 French catheters, respectively.

Laser Angioplasty Treatment Protocol

After routine noninvasive arterial evaluation of the afflicted area via an antegrade puncture of the ipsilateral common femoral artery, a hemostatic introducer sheath (8 or 9 F) was introduced into the SFA. When the procedure was performed in the pelvic region, the sheath was placed into the common femoral artery/external iliacal artery by using standard coronary angiography techniques. Baseline angiography was obtained through the sheath with a digital road-mapping technique that permitted good fluoroscopic control of the coaxial guidance of the laser catheter's gold-marked tip.

Patients were not pretreated with acetylsalicylic acid and were not sedated. Intra-arterial heparin (5,000 units) was administered before the laser catheter was introduced.

In the case of subtotal stenoses in the femoropopliteal region the guidewire was first passed through the lesion under fluoroscopic control before the laser catheter was slowly advanced while firing. In the case of total occlusions, penetration of the blocking obstacle was not vigorously attempted to try to avoid subintimal laceration or a false lumina. After advancing the catheter, we tried to penetrate the most distal portion of the occlusion with the guidewire and avoid subintimal dissections or other mechanical injuries to the distal patent segment of the vessel. When the angiographic control through the proximal sheath clearly showed an intravascular position of the guidewire, the laser catheter would be advanced to the junction and the whole recanalized segment would be passed three to five times with the fibers firing while advancing and withdrawing the laser catheter. If the residual stenosis exceeded 50% of the lumen, an additional balloon dilatation was performed.

Before the sheath was removed, digital subtraction angiography was performed to document the results. The severity of the lesions before and after the intervention was visually estimated.

If there were no contraindications, patients with successful laser-assisted balloon angioplasty were treated with low-dose heparin and unlimited acetylsalicylic acid (100 to 300 mg/day). In a few cases continuous systemic heparin was infused for 24 to 36 hours after the intervention. Before patients were discharged 1 to 2 days after the intervention, a noninvasive evaluation of the peripheral arteries including physical examination, ankle-brachial index, and treadmill test was performed. In an attempt to validate a semiquantitative or approximate evaluation of primary success, our patients all underwent a color Doppler analysis of the region of interest before and after the intervention.

RESULTS

Recanalization of peripheral vessels was attempted in 260 cases. In our hands, the overall primary success rate was 73%. In the majority of cases complex lesions were present in the recanalized segment (Table 23–3). In the case of complete occlusion the angiographic criteria for successful recanalization were a restoration of blood flow and a residual luminal diameter 50% or less of the diameter of the cranial segment of the vessel. In the case of subtotal stenosis, the criterion was a residual stenosis 20% or less. The criteria for technically successful dilatation were the appearance of a normal groin Doppler pulse after the iliac procedure and the appearance of an adequate flow in color-coded Doppler combined with an increase of at least 0.15 in the ankle-brachial blood pressure index within 24 hours after femoropopliteal intervention.

TABLE 23–3.

Primary Success Rates in Different Peripheral Locations: Excimer Laser–Assisted Angioplasty (N = 260)

	Iliac Arteries	Superficial Femoral Artery	Popliteal Region Trifurcation
n	29	206	25
Primary success rate	80%	72%	76%

Superficial Femoral Artery

With regard to the size of the lesion, the 206 cases of obstructed SFAs were subdivided into four groups: (1) subtotal stenoses and occlusions up to 3 cm, (2) total occlusions between 3 and 7 cm in length (Figs 23–1 and 23–2), (3) occlusions between 3 and 12 cm in length, and (4) occlusions longer than 12 cm (Fig 23–3). The overall primary success rate in these four groups was 72% (Table 23–4).

Independent of the length and number, subtotal stenoses or occlusions up to 3 cm could successfully be recanalized in 31 of 34 cases, which corresponds to a primary success rate of 91%. In this group of patients a stand-alone laser procedure was performed in 11 cases with satisfactory angiographic results. All 3 unsuccessful cases of this group were short, heavily calcified occlusions. When the occlusion was located in the middle or distal part of the SFA and the length was between 3 and 7 cm (n = 46), the primary success rate remained high (81%)(Fig 23–4). In the third group with occlusions of the SFA longer than 7 cm (n = 61), the primary success rate decreased. This result might be due to the fact that the patients were not selected with regard to the duration of their ischemic symptoms, so patients who had clinical symptoms for more than 3 to 5 years were also accepted for laser angioplasty (Fig 23–5).

With regard to group 4 (12 to 25 cm, n = 65), in contrast to previous reports[43] there was a relevant increase in the primary success rate from below 50% for the first 100 patients to a 63.5% overall success rate. This very encouraging result may be due to the fact that during the last year each patient scheduled for laser angioplasty underwent not only the usual blood flow analysis by color-coded Doppler ultrasound but also a careful analysis of the structure of the occluded vessel segment by ultrasound. Only if the continuity of the

TABLE 23–4.

Acute Results of 206 Interventions in the Superficial Femoral Artery

Lesion Length (cm)	n	Primary Success
<3	34	31 (91%)
3–7	46	37 (81%)
7–12	61	41 (67%)
>12	65	41 (63%)

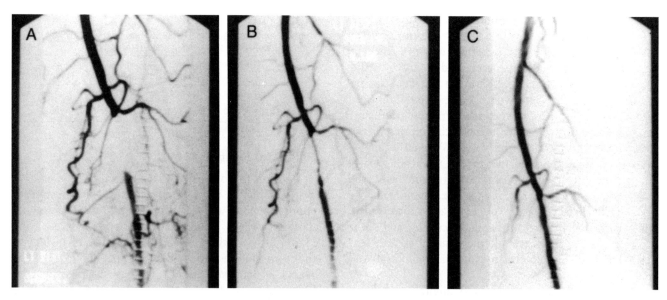

FIG 23–1.
Total occlusion of the superficial femoral artery (SFA), 3.5 cm in length **(A)**. After laser recanalization the size of the channel achieved is not satisfactory **(B)**. After dilatation with a 6-mm balloon, the angiographic result is optimal **(C)**.

blocked artery was detected by longitudinal ultrasound scan was the patient definitively selected for laser-assisted angioplasty.

Iliac Arteries

Iliac arteries are rarely straight, thus implying a theoretically higher risk of perforation with clinical sequelae than in the SFA, particularly when the obstructed section includes the aortoiliac junction. Therefore, the multifiber laser catheter was only advanced if it had been possible to traverse the lesion with a guidewire. With this precaution in mind when approaching the obstruction from the ipsilateral side, 23 of 29 iliac arteries selected for angioplasty could be recanalized.

When the obstruction was no longer than 3 cm, successful recanalization was achieved in 14 of 15 lesions (93%). In the group of longer occlusions the primary success rate decreased to 75% for lesions with a length between 3 and 7 cm. Only 3 of 6 occlusions longer than 7 cm could be successfully recanalized (Table 23–5).

It is obvious that when a 9 F laser catheter was used, the size of the new channel was approximately 3 mm in diameter which is not satisfactory, so in each case balloon dilatation terminated the intervention (Fig 23–6).

Popliteal Region

Recanalization was attempted in 25 patients with obstructions of the popliteal artery and also in obstructive lesions of the trifurcation area, where recanalization has always been regarded as a relatively high risk. Because the patients were carefully selected, a relatively low rate of primary failures was observed. The overall early success rate of crossing the popliteal lesion was 76%. Four of 6 failures in this group were due to final balloon dilatation. Our experience, which is limited to lesions in the third popliteal segment and the trifurcation area, seems to demonstrate that the stand-alone use of a 5 to 7 F multifiber catheter should be preferred instead of its use in combination with balloon dilatation. Nevertheless, more experiences with new types of catheters are necessary before a conclusive statement about the value of laser angioplasty in this area can be made.

Complications

Large dissections were observed in seven cases (2.7%) and sustained spasms without clinical implications in five patients (1.9%). The amount of serious local bleeding needing no surgical treatment is an acceptable risk at 1.15% (three patients). The rate of clinically

TABLE 23–5.
Acute Results of 29 Interventions in the Iliac Region of the Superficial Femoral Artery

Lesion Length (cm)	n	Primary Success
<3	15	14 (93%)
3–7	8	6 (75%)
>7	6	3 (50%)

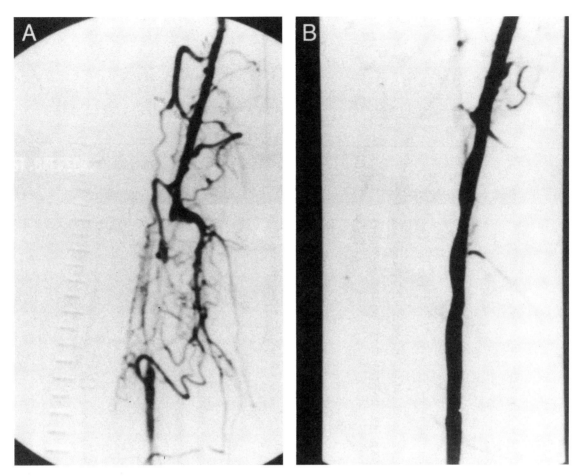

FIG 23–2.
Total occlusion (4.5 cm in length) of the midsegment of the SFA **(A).** After successful excimer laser recanalization (9 F multifiber catheter) without final percutaneous transluminal coronary angioplasty (PTCA) the angiographic result is excellent. Note the disappearance of collaterals after recanalization, which indicates high flow through the recanalized channel **(B).**

symptomatic peripheral macroembolizations is surprisingly low at 1.15% (three patients). Perforation or vessel rupture occurred in 7 patients (2.7%), but in only two cases was elective surgical treatment necessary. There were two acute reocclusions of the SFA a few hours after the intervention that both required acute surgical treatment because of deterioration of the clinical situation.

In summary, 11 complications were major (4.2%), 5 could be managed conservatively, and 6 needed surgical intervention. There was no death and no procedure-related amputation.

Follow-up

Since limitation of walking distance because of pain was a relatively objective and reproducible criterion, a patient was suspected of having developed restenosis when the improvement in exercise capability (defined by

the treadmill exercise test) after recanalization was relevantly reduced. When the suspicion of restenosis was confirmed by color-coded Doppler, an angiographic control was performed. This procedure clearly implies an uncontrolled selection of patients because in practice only the patients with clinical symptoms underwent further studies. On the other hand, it is hard to obtain consent from a symptom-free patient for a new angiogram when costs, risks, and the laboratory's capacity are considered.

Data collection after discharge was complicated by the fact that a large number of the patients treated in the first 18 months after clinical introduction of the excimer laser technique, reached our department from different, partially remote parts of the country. As a consequence, the collection of follow-up data could not be complete, particularly with regard to evaluable angiograms.

Nevertheless, we could collect the clinical and nonin-

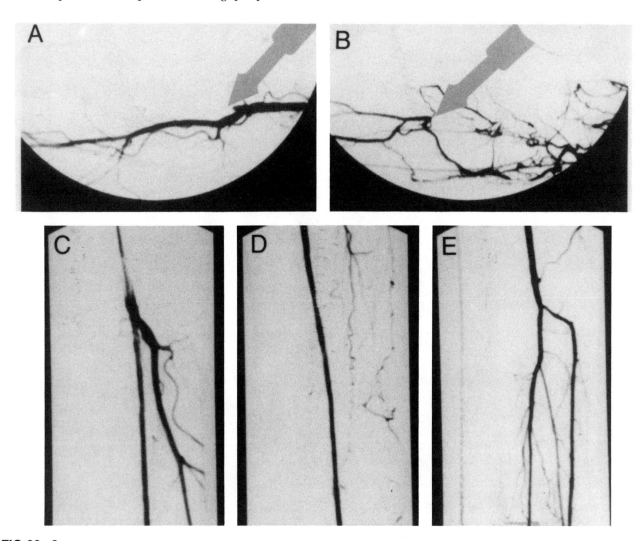

FIG 23–3.
Complete occlusion of the SFA from the origin **(A)** to the third part of the popliteal artery **(B)**, 32 cm long. After lasering with a 9 F catheter and partial dilatation a smooth, regular channel could be obtained with excellent runoff **(C–E)**.

vasive data of 170 successfully recanalized patients 3 months after discharge and the complete data of 130 patients including angiographic studies. The early reocclusion rate during the first 4 weeks after the intervention is surprisingly low at 4%. In contrast to the results of conventional percutaneous transluminal coronary angioplasty (PTCA), the patency rate after 3 months remains extremely high at 92.5%.

As expected, the majority of clinical and consequently angiographic deteriorations occurred between the third and sixth month after discharge. Nevertheless, the reocclusion rate after 6 months was only 26% (Table 23–6). The nonconclusive data of 90 patients of this group 1 year after intervention indicate that the patency rate remains nearly constant.

The follow-up results of recanalizations performed in the iliac region confirm the general trend that after a satisfactory initial result, the majority of the vessels will remain patent. Nevertheless, a patency rate of 95.5% in the iliac region 6 months after intervention is imposing, particularly if one considers the relatively large amount of initially totally occluded vessels in our series.

DISCUSSION

It has been shown during the last few years that the majority of laser wavelengths of the electromagnetic spectrum can debulk vessel material.[31, 34, 35, 42, 44–47] In vitro studies have shown that one of the main advantages of the excimer laser in comparison to other light sources was that even at higher energy densities (7.5

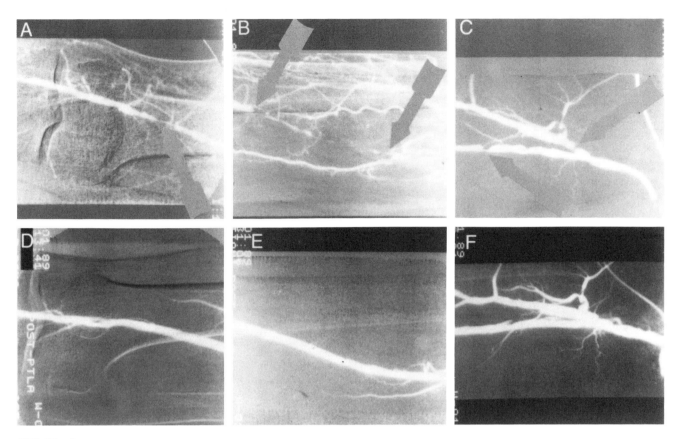

FIG 23-4.
A-C, multiple lesions of the SFA and the arteria femoralis profunda. After the occluded segment was lasered with a 7 F catheter, the distal and proximal stenoses were dilated **(D).** Finally the stenosis at the origin of the arteria femoralis profunda was cracked, **(E). F,** the optimal initial result was confirmed 1 year later by control angiography.

J/cm^2) the damage zone around the ablated channel remains minimal within a tolerable range of 50 μm.[42] Furthermore, the results obtained in human calcified coronary arteries demonstrate that ablation of calcified material is possible but there will be a reduced ablation rate for heavily calcified material.[43, 48, 49]

The main disadvantage associated with the excimer laser is that the size of the channel achieved is not significantly larger than the core diameter of the fiber used. Under certain circumstances larger recanalization channels could be achieved by utilizing an effect leading to local explosion of the target tissue.[43, 50] This may explain why when multifiber catheters incorporating 12 to

TABLE 23-6.
Patency Rates After Excimer Laser-Assisted Angioplasty

Follow-Up	Superficial Femoral Artery	Iliac Region
4 wk	96%	100%
3 mon	92.5%	95.5%
6 mon	74%	95.5%

18 fibers with a core diameter of 260 μm are used, a relatively smooth channel with a diameter up to 3 mm can be achieved, although the death zone of the catheter's tip is extremely large when compared with the sum of the fiber's ablating surfaces.[51] However, another phenomenon related to the explosion-like ablation effect at 308 nm seems to have clinical relevance: the induction of photoacoustic shock waves. This mechanism may partially explain the high incidence of dissections and spasms observed during coronary excimer laser angioplasty.[52] On the other hand, shock wave-related complications seem to be irrelevant for peripheral revascularization interventions. The following factors seem to have an influence on the amplitude of the shock waves: pulse length, configuration of the laser pulse, and the geometry of the tip of the multifiber laser catheter used.[51]

Successful obliteration of totally obstructed segments with a 7 or 9 F excimer laser catheter implies the formation of an angiographically estimated channel 2 to 3 mm in diameter. Consequently, appropriate balloon dilata-

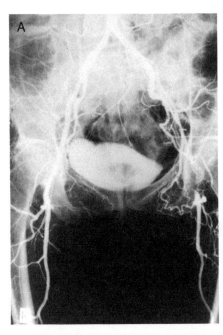 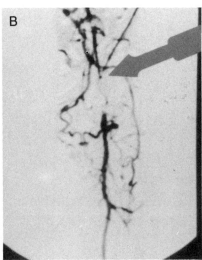 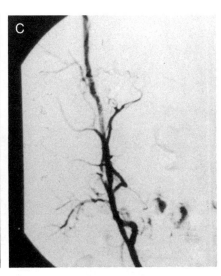

FIG 23–5.
Fifty-two-year-old woman with claudication symptoms for 7 years who in 1988 had bilateral femoropopliteal bypass surgery. After a pain-free period of 8 to 12 month, she experienced claudication again. Following a constant period of walking at a capacity of 300 to 500 m, a crescendo developed and left limited symptoms with a pain-free walking distance less than 50 m. The angiographic study showed total occlusion of the common femoral artery of about 5 cm in length **(A)**. In a crossover technique the tip of the 7 F laser catheter could be placed at the beginning of the occlusion **(B,** *arrow*). After laser recanalization and partial PTCA the result was satisfactory **(C)**. The patient recovered her walking capacity and stopped smoking. Eight months later after intensive vascular training she is practically free of symptoms.

tion is necessary. Only in a few cases (9%) was it possible to achieve a satisfactory channel with a narrowing less than 50% by passing the laser catheter through the lesion and back again three to five times. However, it is important to stress that in the majority of the cases final balloon dilatation was limited to one or two localized persistent narrowings to avoid stretching the total length of the primarily occluded segment and to consequently diminish the probability of dissection or other dilatation-related complications. The reduction in potential injury area could also have a positive influence on the long-term results of this technique.

In trying to validate the early clinical success of the excimer laser angioplasty method, it is important to stress that there is no uniform definition of clinical primary success of angioplasty in the peripheral arteries. Many groups mention a Doppler ankle-brachial index rise of at least 0.1[53] or 0.15,[19, 54, 55] a normalized index,[54, 56] or a Doppler pulsatility index increased by more than 20%[54, 57] as a criterion for early clinical success. An improvement of the patient's symptoms by at least one clinical category[57–59], diminution of symptoms,[55] or a doubling of the treadmill exercise distance[57] has also been required. Further criteria are the reappearance of missing relevant pulses, marked strengthening of weak pulses,[19, 21, 59] or a transformation of the monophasic Doppler waveforms to biphasic or triphasic waveforms.[57, 58] In our study clinical success was evident if there was a Doppler ankle-brachial index rise of at least 0.15 and a doubling of the treadmill exercise distance. Furthermore, all patients underwent color-flow Doppler analysis after the intervention. With this noninvasive technique it is possible to confirm and substantiate the visual assessment of the angiographic picture, but the determination of a reliable "quantitative" flow level is only possible when the runoff is not obstructed. Nevertheless, this noninvasive technique seems to be helpful in completing a total clinical evaluation of the primary success rate.

The results presented in this report clearly indicate that when the described technique is used, a high percentage of femoropopliteal stenoses and occlusions (94.5% to 63%) can be recanalized, thus confirming our data and the preliminary data of other groups.[43, 49, 60–65] Nevertheless, this young, continuously evolving technology with a primary success rate of nearly 70% in the case of total occlusions has demonstrated its superiority in comparison to conventional balloon angioplasty, which has initial failure rates greater than 50%.[3, 16, 21–25, 41]

Eximer laser–assisted angioplasty permits one to at-

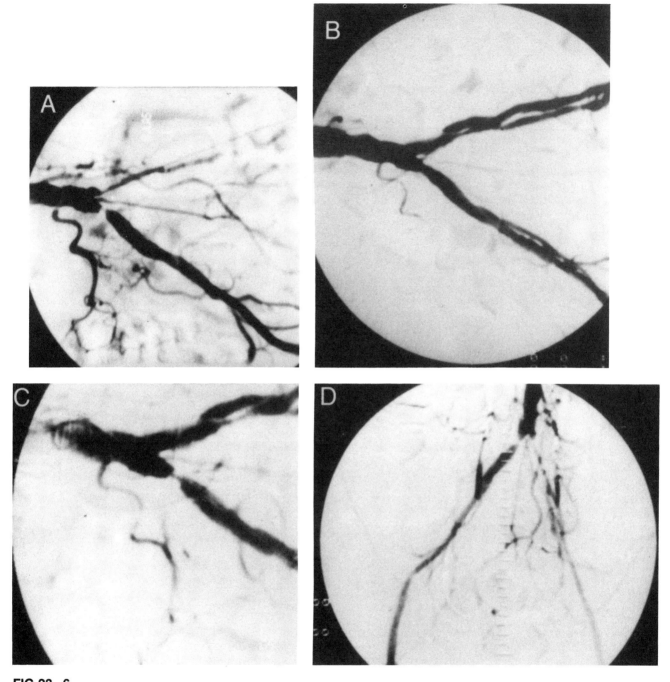

FIG 23–6.
Fifty-two-year-old man with an incomplete Leriche syndrome. Angiography showed a subtotal occlusion of the right and a long occlusion of the left common iliacal artery **(A)**. After the first pass with a 9 F multifiber laser catheter a small channel was achieved **(B)**. After multiple passes of the laser catheter and PTCA (7-mm balloon) a good angiographic result was achieved **(C)**. Three weeks later the subtotal stenosis on the right side was successfully recanalized **(D)**. The final angiogram shows an excellent result. The patient is completely pain free and plays tennis.

tempt recanalization of very long occlusions exceeding 15 cm, which are normally excluded from conventional PTCA. The longest femoropopliteal segment recanalized in our series was 35 cm.

The patency rate of our patient population after 3 months is very high, 92.5% in the femoral artery and 95.5% in the pelvic region. In contrast to the SFA where the patency rate drops to 74% after 6 months, no change in the patency rate of iliac arteries was observed between 3 and 6 months.

At the present stage it is nearly impossible to compare the different obliterating techniques in a realistic and neutral way because the patient populations treated in the different studies are too heterogenous and the number of patients in the single groups is often too small. We need more experience and intensive collaboration between the single groups with a generally accepted protocol that can be followed when different equipment or techniques are used.

In the near future laser technology will not solve problems related to transcutaneous interventions substantially. This young technology must continue to evolve to be able to leave the experimental state and become a standard interventional technique.

REFERENCES

1. Dotter CT, Judkins MP: Transluminal treatment of atherosclerotic obstructions: Description of a new technique and a preliminary report of its application. *Circulation* 1964; 30:654–670.
2. Grüntzig AR, Senning A, Siegenthaler WE: Nonoperative dilatation of coronary-artery stenosis: Percutaneous transluminal coronary angioplasty. *N Engl J Med* 1979; 301:61–68.
3. Zeitler E, Richter EI, Roth FL, et al: Results of percutaneous transluminal angioplasty. *Radiology* 1983; 146:57–60.
4. Bussman W, Kaltenbach M, Kober G, et al: The Frankfurt experience in restenosis after coronary angioplasty. *Am J Cardiol* 1987; 60:48–49.
5. Detre K, Holubkov R, Kelsey S, et al: Percutaneous transluminal coronary angioplasty in 1985–1986 and 1977–1981. *N Engl J Med* 1988; 318:265–270.
6. Ernst SMPG, van der Feltz TA, Bal ET, et al: Long-term angiographic follow-up, cardiac events, and survival in patients undergoing percutaneous transluminal coronary angioplasty. *Br Heart J* 1987; 57:220–225.
7. Holmes DR, Vlietstra RE, Smith HC, et al: Restenosis after percutaneous transluminal coronary angioplasty (PTCA): A report from the PTCA registry of the National Heart, Lung, and Blood Institute. *Am J Cardiol* 1984; 53:77–81.
8. King SB: Percutaneous transluminal coronary angioplasty: The second decade. *Am J Cardiol* 1988; 62:2–6.
9. Leimgruber PP, Roubin GS, Hollman J, et al: Restenosis after successful coronary angioplasty in patients with single-vessel disease. *Circulation* 1986; 73:710–717.
10. Levine S, Ewels CJ, Rosing DR, et al: Coronary angioplasty: Clinical and angiographic follow-up. *Am J Cardiol* 1985; 55:673–676.
11. Mata LA, Bosch X, David PR, et al: Clinical and angiographic assessment 6 months after double vessel percutaneous coronary angioplasty. *J Am Coll Cardiol* 1985; 6:1239–1244.
12. McBride W, Lange RA, Hillis LA: Restenosis after successful coronary angioplasty. *N Engl J Med* 1988; 318:1734–1737.
13. Roubin GS, King SB, Douglas JS: Restenosis after percutaneous transluminal coronary angioplasty: The Emory University Hospital experience. *Am J Cardiol* 1987; 60:39–43.
14. Val PG, Bourassa MG, David PR, et al: Restenosis after successful percutaneous transluminal coronary angioplasty: The Montreal Heart Institute experience. *Am J Cardiol* 1987; 60:50–55.
15. Vandormael MG, Deligonul U, Kern MJ, et al: Restenosis after multilesion percutaneous transluminal coronary angioplasty. *Am J Cardiol* 1987; 60:44–47.
16. Bergentz SV, Jonsson K: Percutaneous transluminal angioplasty. *Acta Chir Scand* 1983; 149:641–649.
17. Colapinto RF, Harries-Jones EP, Johnston KW: Percutaneous transluminal angioplasty of peripheral vascular disease: A two year experience. *Cardiovasc Intervent Radiol* 1980; 3:213–218.
18. Greenfield A: Femoral, popliteal, and tibial arteries: Percutaneous transluminal angioplasty. *AJR* 1980; 135:927–935.
19. Hewes RC, White RI, Murray RR, et al: Long-term results of superficial femoral artery angioplasty. *AJR* 1986; 146:1025–1029.
20. Johnston KW, Colapinto RF, Baird RJ: Transluminal dilation: An alternative? *Arch Surg* 1982; 117:1604–1610.
21. Krepel VM, van Andel GJ, van Erp WFM, et al: Percutaneous transluminal angioplasty of the femoropopliteal artery: Initial and long-term results. *Radiology* 1985; 156:325–328.
22. Kumpe DA, Jones DN: Percutaneous transluminal angioplasty. Radiologic viewpoint. *Appl Radiol* 1982; 11:29–40.
23. Lu CT, Zairns CK, Yang CF, et al: Long-segment arterial occlusion. Percutaneous transluminal angioplasty. *AJR* 1982; 138:119–122.
24. Probst P, Cerny P, Owens A, et al: Patency after femoral angioplasty: Correlation of angiographic appearance with clinical findings. *AJR* 1983; 140:1227–1232.
25. Spence RK, Freiman DB, Gatenby R, et al: Long-term results of transluminal angioplasty of the iliac and femoral arteries. *Arch Surg* 1981; 116:1377–1386.
26. Waller BF: Crackers, breakers, stretchers, drillers, scrapers, shavers, burners, welders and melters — The future treatment of atherosclerotic coronary artery disease: A clinical-morphologic assessment. *J Am Coll Cardiol* 1989; 13:969–987.
27. Choy DSJ: History of lasers in medicine. *Thorac Cardiovasc Surg* 1988; 36:114–117.
28. Choy DSJ, Stertzer SH, Myler RK, et al: Human coronary laser recanalization. *Clin Cardiol* 1984; 7:377–381.
29. Forrester JS, Litvack F, Grundfest WS: Laser angioplasty and cardiovascular disease. *Am J Cardiol* 1986; 57:990–992.
30. Abela GS: Laser arterial recanalization: A current perspective. *J Am Coll Cardiol* 1988; 12:103–105.
31. Abela GS, Normann S, Feldman RL, et al: Effects of carbon dioxide, Nd:YAG and argon laser radiation on coronary atheromatous plaques. *Am J Cardiol* 1982; 50:1199–1205.
32. Crea F, Davies G, McKenna W, et al: Percutaneous laser recanalisation of coronary arteries. *Lancet* 1986; 1:214–215.
33. Cumberland DC, Tayler DI, Welsh CL, et al: Percutaneous laser thermal angioplasty: Initial clinical results

with a laser probe in total peripheral artery occlusions. *Lancet* 1986; 1:1457–1459.

34. Geschwind HJ, Boussignac G, Teisseire B, et al: Conditions for effective Nd:YAG laser angioplasty. *Br Heart J* 1984; 52:484–489.

35. Ginsburg R, Kirr DS, Guthaner P, et al: Salvage of an ischemic limb by laser angioplasty: Description of a new technique. *Clin Cardiol* 7:54–58.

36. Ginsburg R, Wexler L, Mitchell RS, et al: Percutaneous transluminal laser angioplasty for treatment of peripheral vascular disease: Clinical experience with 16 patients. *Radiology* 1985; 156:619–624.

37. Ginsburg R: Percutaneous laser angioplasty in the treatment of peripheral vascular disease. *Thorac Cardiovasc Surg* 1988; 36:142–145.

38. Nordstrom LA, Castaneda-Zuniga WR, Lindeke CC, et al: Laser angioplasty: Controlled delivery of argon laser energy. *Radiology* 1988; 167:463–465.

39. Sanborn TA, Cumberland DC, Greenfield AJ, et al: Percutaneous laser thermal angioplasty: Initial results and 1-year follow-up in 129 femoropopliteal lesions. *Radiology* 1988; 168:121–125.

40. Welch AJ, Bradley AB, Torres JH, et al: Laser probe ablation of normal and atherosclerotic human aorta in vitro: A first thermographic and histologic analysis. *Circulation* 1987; 76:1353–1363.

41. Kar H: Anwendungen der Photoablation in der biomedizinischen Technik, in *Advances in Laser Medicine IV*. Ecomed Verlag, 1991, in press.

42. Biamino G, Dörschel K, Harnoss BM, et al: Experience in excimer laser photoablation of arteriosclerotic plaques, in Biamino G, Müller GJ (eds): *Advances in Laser Medicine I. First German Symposium on Laser Angioplasty*. Berlin, Ecomed Verlagsgesellschaft, 1988, pp 147–156.

43. Biamino G: Coronary and peripheral laser angioplasty, in *Interventional Cardiology*. Hogrefe & Huber, Göttingen, West Germany, 1990, pp 243–260.

44. Abela GS, Norman SJ, Cohen DM, et al: Laser recanalization of occluded atherosclerotic arteries: An in vivo and in vitro study. *Circulation* 1985; 71:403–411.

45. Deckelbaum LI, Isner JM, Donaldson RF, et al: Reduction of laser-induced pathologic tissue injury using pulsed energy delivery. *Am J Cardiol* 1985; 56:662–667.

46. Grundfest WS, Litvack F, Forrester JS, et al: Laser ablation of human atherosclerotic plaque without adjacent tissue injury. *J Am Coll Cardiol* 1985; 5:929–933.

47. Pacala TJ, McDermid IS, Laudenslager JB: Ultranarrow linewidth, magnetically switched, long pulse, xenon chloride laser. *Appl Phys Lett* 1984; 44:658–660.

48. Linsker R, Srinivasan R, Wynne JJ, et al: Far ultraviolet laser ablation of atherosclerotic lesions. *Lasers Surg Med* 1984; 4:201–206.

49. Litvack F, Grundfest W, Adler L, et al: Percutaneous excimer laser and excimer laser–assisted angioplasty of the lower extremities: Results of initial clinical trial. *Radiology* 1989; 172:331–335.

50. Berlien HPG, Müller GJ: Laser in medicine, in Biamino G, Müller GJ (eds): *Advances in Laser Medicine 1. First German Symposium on Laser Angioplasty*. Berlin, Ecomed Verlagsgesellschaft, 1988, pp 45–55.

51. Biamino G, Kar H, Fleck E, et al: Comparison of different excimer laser systems for coronary and peripheral angioplasty. Submitted for publication.

52. Karsch K, Haase K, Voelker W, et al: Percutaneous coronary excimer laser angioplasty in patients with stable and unstable angina pectoris. *Circulation* 1990; 00:1849–1859.

53. Nordstrom LA, Castaneda-Zuniga WR, Young EG, et al: Direct argon laser exposure for recanalization of peripheral arteries: Early results. *Radiology* 1988; 168:359–364.

54. Borozan PG, Schulter JJ, Spigos DG, et al: Long-term hemodynamic evaluation of lower extremity percutaneous transluminal angioplasty. *J Vasc Surg* 1985; 2:785–793.

55. Murray RR, Hewes RC, White RI, et al: Long-segment femoropopliteal stenoses: Is angioplasty a boon or a bust? *Radiology* 1987; 162:473–476.

56. Colapinto RF, Stronell RD, Johnston WK: Transluminal angioplasty of complete iliac obstructions. *AJR* 1986; 146:859–862.

57. Morin JF, Johnston W, Wasserman L, et al: Factors that determine the long-term results of percutaneous transluminal dilatation for peripheral arterial occlusion disease. *J Vasc Surg* 1986; 4:68–72.

58. Johnston KW, Rae M, Hogg-Johnston SA, et al: 5-year of a prospective study of percutaneous transluminal angioplasty. *Ann Surg* 1987; 10:403–413.

59. Walden R, Siegel Y, Rubinstein ZJ, et al: Percutaneous transluminal angioplasty: A suggested method for analysis of clinical, arteriographic, and hemodynamic factors affecting the results of treatment. *J Vasc Surg* 1986; 3:583–590.

60. Huppert PE, Duda SH, Seboldt H, et al: Periphere Excimer-Laserangioplastie. *Dtsch Med Wochenschr* 1991; 116:161–167.

61. Katzen B, Schwarten D, Kaplan J, et al: Initial experience with an excimer laser in peripheral lesions (abstract). *Circulation* 1988; 78(suppl 2): 47.

62. Litvack F, Grundfest W, Adler L, et al: Percutaneous excimer laser angioplasty in humans. *Circulation* 1988; 78(suppl 2):417.

63. Litvack F, Grundfest W, Segalowitz J, et al: Interventional cardiovascular therapy by laser and thermal angioplasty. *Circulation* 1990; 81(suppl 4):116.

64. McCarthy WJ, Vogelzang RL, Nemcek AA, et al: Eximer laser–assisted femoral angioplasty: Early results. *J Vasc Surg* 1991; 13:607–614.

65. Pokrovsky AV, Volynsky JD, Konov VI, et al: Recanalisation of occluded peripheral arteries by eximer laser. *Eur J Vasc Surg* 1990; 4:575–581.

66. Sanborn TA, Faxon DP, Haudenschild CC, et al: Experimental angioplasty circumferential distribution of laser thermal injury with a laser probe. *J Am Coll Cardiol* 1985; 5:934–938.

67. Zeitler E, Richter EI, Roth FL, et al: Results of percutaneous transluminal angioplasty. *Radiology* 1983; 146:57–60.

24

Direct Argon Laser Angioplasty for the Treatment of Peripheral and Coronary Vascular Lesions: A Progress Report

Leonard A. Nordstrom, M.D.

Nearly a decade has been devoted to conceptualizing, developing, and testing numerous laser delivery systems for use in treating atherosclerotic vascular disease. Yet today laser angioplasty remains experimental. The delivery of laser energy intravascularly to ablate lesions remote from a percutaneous access site, thought only feasible 10 years ago, is now a reality through progress in the technology. However, much work remains to be completed in determining the clinical utility of this treatment modality and to further improve the tissue ablation characteristics of laser delivery systems.

The following presents the experience at Park Nicollet Heart Center (Minneapolis) in performing 68 procedures in 63 patients with totally and subtotally occluded peripheral arteries with one such delivery system that utilizes direct argon laser energy (Lastac System, G.V. Medical, Inc., Minneapolis). Additionally, these results are compared with those of a larger multicenter trial. The early clinical experience in coronary arteries is also presented.

METHODS

The delivery system used in the series transmits argon laser energy to the vascular lesion by using a 200-nm quartz fiber inserted into the lumen of a "centering" balloon catheter (Fig 24–1A). This catheter is designed to lift the fiber from the arterial wall and align the fiber coaxially in the lumen. Beam direction is further controlled through an optical assembly mounted at

the fiber tip that diverges the light beam. Increasing beam divergence not only increases the diameter of the projected light spot and consequently the area of tissue removal but also dissipates the intensity of the beam such that tissue removal occurs only at distances close to the fiber tip (approximately 3 mm) where the beam direction can be controlled by the centering balloon catheter.

Arteries are recanalized by multiple laser exposures at 10-W power for 2 to 5 seconds. As laser exposures are delivered, heparinized saline is infused to clear blood and contrast media from the lasing field and to irrigate the irradiated tissue. As a pathway is created, the laser fiber and catheter are incrementally advanced until the lesion is traversed. Lasing is followed by balloon dilatation as the catheter system is removed. In the case of a long lesion, the lasing catheter is replaced with a 10-cm conventional balloon dilatation catheter and the lesion dilated further. This system has been described in detail previously.[1-3]

The first clinical use of this integrated system occurred on May 13, 1986. The Park Nicollet Heart Center series was part of a multicenter trial performed under the auspices of the U.S. Food and Drug Administration (FDA) to determine the safety and efficacy of the Lastac system as an adjunct to conventional balloon angioplasty in the peripheral vascular bed.

Success was evaluated by using two end points: primary success and clinical success. Primary success was defined as recanalization and reduction of the lesion to less than 50% stenosis accompanied by an increased an-

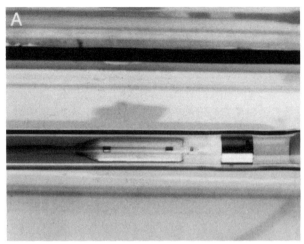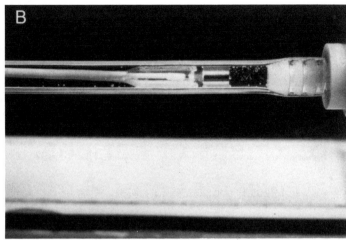

FIG 24–1.
A, inflation of the centering balloon in peripheral arteries lifts the fiber from the artery wall and centers the beam in the arterial lumen. (From Nordstrom LA, Castaneda-Zuniga WR, Young EG, et al: *Radiology* 1988; 168:359–364. Used by permission.) **B,** the balloon was further modified to provide even more precise control of the laser beam in coronary arteries by mounting the balloon at the catheter tip.

kle-brachial index (ABI) as well as improved distal pulses, measured immediately after the procedure was terminated and the catheters were removed. Clinical success, which considers both early (within 1 week) and late reclosures, was defined as the continued alleviation of symptoms at follow-up, again supported by improved distal pulses and ABI. Patients were followed over a period of 2 years after the laser procedure.

THE PARK NICOLLET HEART CENTER EXPERIENCE

Between May 1986 and October 1989, 63 patients underwent a total of 68 laser procedures for peripheral vascular disease.[4] Indications for treatment included life-style–limiting claudication in 82% of the patients, rest pain in 9%, nonhealing ulcers in 7%, and gangrene in 2%. The average age of the patients in this series was 66 years, and there were 34 women and 29 men. Diabetes was present in 16% of the patients, 77% had a positive smoking history, and 58% were undergoing treatment for hypertension. Patients with poor distal runoff composed 24% of the series.

Of the 68 lesions treated, 12 were femoropopliteal stenoses, the majority of which were selected early in the series. The remaining 56 lesions were total occlusions located in either the superficial femoral (42) or iliac (14) arteries and averaging 8 cm in length (range, 1 to 37 cm). Lesion characteristics are summarized in Table 24–1.

Although only 26% of the femoropopliteal total oc-

clusions in this series resulted in severe ischemia such that limb loss was a possibility, a disproportionate share of these lesions (73%) were short occlusions (less than or equal to 7 cm in length). In these patients, advanced disease was present at the level of the trifurcation and below in addition to the short total occlusions in the femoropopliteal segment, which contributed to the severity of the ischemic symptoms. Conversely, relatively few of the long lesions greater than 7 cm (27%) were involved in advanced disease. This observation had important ramifications in interpreting analyses of late patency.

Technical success was achieved in 87% (59/68) of the procedures. In successful procedures there was a significant increase in the mean ABI from 0.58 ± 0.16 to 0.82 ± 0.19 ($P < .0001$). There were 9 technical failures because of inadequate tissue removal, and thus it was not possible to negotiate the total occlusion.

The procedure was successful in all 12 femoropopliteal stenoses (100%). Criteria for selecting high-grade stenoses into the study was the inability to pass

TABLE 24–1.
Lesion Characteristics: Park Nicollet Medical Center

Lesion Location	Number of Lesions	Lesion Type		Lesion Length (Occlusions)	
		Occlusions	Stenoses	Mean (cm)	Range
Iliac	14	14	0	6	1–12
Femoropopliteal	54	42	12	9	1–37

the laser balloon catheter across the obstruction. The laser was then used to partially reopen the lesion, with residual occluding plaque dilated by using conventional balloon angioplasty. It is very likely that balloons with lower profiles could have negotiated these high-grade obstructions.

The primary success rate was 88% (37/42) in femoropopliteal occlusions (mean length, 9 cm). When stratified by lesion length, the primary success rate was 83% (15/18) in occlusions greater than 7 cm in length and 92% (22/24) for femoropopliteal occlusions less than or equal to 7 cm ($P = .63$). The design of the catheter system, which permits incrementally ablating plaque as it is advanced across the lesion, regardless of lesion length, could possibly explain the results in long total occlusions. This trend has been observed by others using this delivery system, further supporting this hypothesis.[5, 6]

A total of 10 of the 14 totally occluded iliac arteries (71%) was successfully reopened. The three of the 4 technical failures actually demonstrated angiographic evidence of recanalization. Yet when the sheath was removed, the ABI and distal pulses were not improved, which suggests the presence of soft thrombus that was not possible to dilate or possibly elastic recoil of the artery wall.[7, 8] The remaining failed iliac procedure involved a calcified fibrotic occlusion that could not be recanalized by the laser.

For the entire series, 5 arteries, or 7%, reclosed within the first 24 hours after the laser procedure due to acute thrombosis. The predominance of the thrombotic occlusions (4/5) occurred in the first 36 procedures.[2] At this point the data were reviewed, and it became apparent that long total occlusions in a setting of impaired runoff had a higher incidence of acute occlusion. In the later cohort of 32 procedures, those patients who demonstrated similar clinical characteristics were identified and were continued on a regimen of heparin after the procedure until the following morning. The heparin therapy was discontinued and the patients discharged. With this change in protocol only 1 thrombotic occlusion occurred in the subsequent 32 procedures.[4]

Complications included two intimal dissections resulting in technical failure of the procedures; three thermal arterial perforations, all of which were resolved without adverse sequelae; and three patients with groin hematomas that prolonged the hospital stay. In two of the three perforations the procedure was thought to be successful in terms of reopening the artery. Additionally, one superficial femoral artery (SFA) procedure and one femoropopliteal graft procedure resulted in distal embolization. The SFA occlusion was resolved with the use of streptokinase infused over a period of 24 hours, and the femoropopliteal graft involved embolectomy and revision of the graft and ultimately required amputation.

Long-term results were evaluated by using life table methods with a mean follow-up for the series of 1 year. A total of 39 patients demonstrated improved symptoms, distal pulses, and ABIs at the last follow-up. The overall 1-year patency rate for the series was 75%. Analysis by lesion location revealed 1-year patency rates as follows: total iliac occlusions, 79%; femoropopliteal stenoses, 91%; and femoropopliteal occlusions, 60%. Disease severity was the only variable that proved to be predictive of late patency: 85% of claudicants had a patent artery at 1 year vs. 23% of patients with procedures performed for limb salvage indications ($P = .0003$).

Although distal runoff correlated well with disease severity ($P = .07$), runoff was not predictive of patency, nor was lesion length. The 1-year patency rate was 72% for patients with good runoff as compared with 71% for those patients with poor runoff. In this series runoff was determined by the number of patent tibial arteries (0 to 1 indicates poor runoff, and 2 to 3 equates with good runoff). It has been proposed that the foot arch should be considered in determining runoff status, with patients with one patent tibial artery but an intact foot considered to have reasonable runoff as evidenced by improved long-term patency.[9] This type of patient, if present in this series, would have been misclassified as having poor runoff and thus would have diluted the results.

If only femoropopliteal occlusions are considered, both long (>7 cm) and short (≤ 7 cm) lesions had a 1-year patency rate of 60%. The patency rate for short femoropopliteal occlusions was lower than would be expected. Because of the large proportion of limb salvage procedures with short lesions, the data were further stratified by both lesion length and disease severity. Claudicants with short femoropopliteal occlusions had a 1-year patency rate of 84% as compared with 68% in long occlusions ($P = .36$). Patients with severe ischemia had a 1-year patency rate of 21% for short and 33% for long occlusions ($P = .38$). This disparity is probably a function of small numbers inasmuch as there were 11 short and 3 long occlusions treated for severe ischemia. Life table analyses are summarized in Table 24–2.

MULTICENTER EXPERIENCE

A larger data base for a collective of ten investigative centers was established to satisfy FDA requirements for market approval. Although FDA approval was granted in December 1988, many of the investigators continued

TABLE 24-2.
Results of Femoropopliteal Occlusion at the Park Nicollet Heart Center

Occlusions	Primary Success (%)	Cumulative Patency* (%)	1-yr (± SE)
Overall	87	75	(± 13)
Iliac total occlusions	71	79	(± 9)
Femoropopliteal stenoses	100	91	(± 9)
Femoropopliteal occlusions	88	60	(± 9)
≤7 cm	92	60	(± 12)
>7 cm	83	60	(± 15)
By indications			
Claudication	84	85	(± 6)
Severe ischemia	100	23	(± 13)
Claudication–femoropopliteal occlusions			
≤7 cm		84	(± 11)
>7 cm		68	(± 16)
Severe ischemia—femoropopliteal occlusions			
≤7 cm		21	(± 18)
>7 cm		33	(± 27)

*Patency rates were determined by Kaplin-Meyer life table methods.

to enter patients into this data base. A total of 536 procedures were documented between May 1986 and March 1990, which included the 68 procedures discussed above.[10] The patient selection criteria, treatment protocol, and measures of success were the same as those described earlier in the discussion.

For this group, indications for treatment were similar in that life-style–limiting claudication accounted for 78% of the patients; rest pain, 11%; nonhealing ulcers, 7%; and gangrene, 4%. Total occlusions represented 88% of the lesions treated and averaged 13 cm in length (range, 1 to 55 cm). Lesions were located predominantly in the SFA (81%), with iliac (11%) as well as popliteal and trifurcation vessels (8%) also treated.

The overall primary success rate for the multicenter trial was 82%. A total of 80% of all total occlusions and 98% of stenoses were successfully reopened. When stratified by location, primary success was achieved in 74% of iliac lesions, 82% of SFA lesions, and 91% of lesions in the popliteal and trifurcation vessels. Again, there was a slight trend toward improved primary success in shorter lesions less than or equal to 13 cm in length (83%) vs. longer lesions greater than 13 cm (77%), but this was not statistically significant ($P = .19$), nor was the severity of disease predictive of primary success, with success achieved in 82% of the procedures treated for claudication, 83% of those treated for rest pain, and 88% of those treated for nonhealing ulcers or gangrene.

A 3.5% incidence of mechanical perforation, either guidewire or catheter induced, and a 2.2% incidence of thermal perforation were documented for the multi-center trial. None required urgent treatment. Groin hematomas that prolonged the hospital stay occurred in 6.1% of the procedures. Distal embolization was reported in 2.7% of the cases.

With voluntary participation in this data base after FDA approval, the patency data available were limited to a smaller cohort of patients with more complete follow-up. The cumulative 1-year patency rate in 317 successful procedures was 64%. Stenoses had a higher patency rate (81%) than did total occlusions (60%) at the 1-year follow-up. Lesion location also influenced patency, with the patency rate for iliac arteries being 82% vs. 62% for femoropopliteal arteries. Patients with life-style–limiting claudication had a 1-year patency rate of 66% vs. 37% of those with limb-threatening ischemia ($P < .001$).

It is difficult to compare results with literature data for reasons exemplified in the Park Nicollet series. That is, differences in patient population characteristics can markedly influence the results, and unless literature studies clearly identify the patient population and stratify results, definitive comparisons are not possible. However, in the absence of randomized data, looking at the literature provides a general sense of how well a new treatment modality performs.

Primary success rates documented for angioplasty range from 86% to 95% for lesions less than 5 cm[11-14] in length and 59% to 86% for lesions greater than 5 cm.[13-15] The expected results are slightly lower for series composed predominantly of long total occlusions, 59%,[15] and/or limb salvage patients, 46% to 73%.[15, 16] As one would expect, disease severity greatly influences patency results, with patients with limb-threatening ischemia experiencing patency rates ranging from 39% to 77%, depending on the length of the lesion. For patients with life-style–limiting claudication as the indication for treatment, again, the expected patency varies by lesion length, with patency rates ranging from 74% to 93% for shorter lesions and 45% to 64% for longer obstructions.[11–13, 15] Although the results of the multicenter trial varied among centers, they do suggest that the Park Nicollet Heart Center experience is reproducible. Additionally, both the results of the Park Nicollet series and the multicenter trial compare favorably with the results documented in the literature for conventional percutaneous transluminal coronary angioplasty (PTCA).

EARLY CORONARY EXPERIENCE

Despite its short tip, the catheter that had been used in the peripheral arteries resulted in uniform thermal perforations when introduced into smaller, dynamic canine arteries. To remedy this problem the balloon was mounted directly on the end of the catheter to provide even more precise control in positioning the fiber (Fig 24–1,B). This in theory prevents the fiber tip from contacting the arterial wall. Experimental studies supported this concept.[17]

The following results are again a part of an investigational protocol approved by the FDA. This protocol called for laser angioplasty of high-grade stenoses and totally occluded coronary arteries. Early cases involved high-grade obstructions predominantly in the right coronary artery (seven procedures at Park Nicollet Heart Center). Although all arteries were successfully reopened with a combination of laser and balloon angioplasty (the energy delivered ranged between 10 and 360 J), the amount of tissue removed was small. It was felt in this setting that this particular system did not have much to offer for high-grade obstructions. Attention was then directed to totally occluded arteries, which could not be satisfactorily negotiated with a guidewire.

The trial in total occlusions is progressing at multiple centers as reported by Foschi et al.[18] From October 1988 to August 1989, 67 patients were treated with a combination of laser and balloon angioplasty – 57 were men, and 10 were women with an age range of 39 to 80 years. Included in this series were 48 patients with complete occlusions, 5 of whom had demonstrated high-grade stenoses in native coronary arteries. There were also 14 patients who presented with obstructive saphenous vein grafts – 7 were total occlusions, and 7 were high-grade stenoses. It was felt on the basis of clinical

symptoms that the duration of occlusion was approximately 2 months for most patients. Lesions were located in the native coronary vessels as follows: 33 in the right coronary artery, 16 in the left anterior descending coronary artery, and 4 in the circumflex artery. The mean length of the totally occluded arteries was 22 mm (± 2.1 SD).

Technical success was achieved in 51 of 67 patients, or 76%. Complications included 2 sudden occlusions, 1 of which was precipitated by an arterial dissection. Both patients required emergency coronary bypass surgery and had satisfactory outcomes. Distal embolization occurred in 1 patient. This person sustained a myocardial infarction and was treated medically. One mechanical perforation occurred that resolved spontaneously without requiring surgical intervention. Twenty-four hours later, angiography was performed and demonstrated a patent artery without adverse sequelae. One patient died post-treatment due to massive gastrointestinal bleeding. Limited follow-up data revealed that 42% of the patients had evidence of reclosure (patency rate, 58%).

Success in opening totally occluded arteries by using conventional balloon angioplasty ranges between 50% and 70% in most series (Table 24–3). The primary success rate in this series was 76%, and in that sense it is certainly comparable with other series in presenting better results. The authors made the point that there was an attempt to initially recanalize these arteries in a conventional manner. This might indicate that this was a cohort of patients where a lower success rate would have been expected had it not been for the use of this system. In the end this question will only be answered with a randomized study.

TABLE 24–3.

Literature Review: Angioplasty of Totally Occluded Coronary Arteries

First Author	Number in Series	Primary Success (%)	Patency at Follow-up (%)
Dervan,[19] 1983	13	54	57*
Holmes,[20] 1984	24	54	—
Kereiakes,[20] 1985	76	53	75†
Serruys,[22] 1985	49	57	64†
DiScascio,[23] 1986	46	64	52†
Melchior,[24] 1987	100	56	45*
Saffian,[25] 1988	271	68	—
LaVeau,[26] 1989	57	70	—
Meier,[27] 1989	50	60	—
Little,[28] 1990	64	73	—
Finici,[29] 1990	100	—	45*
Stone,[30] 1990	971	72	—

*Angiographic determination of patency.
†Patency determined by clinical symptoms.

Additional follow-up will be needed to determine the long-term effectiveness of this therapy. Preliminary long-term data suggest that reclosure can be expected in 40% to 45% of the patients. When PTCA is used for total occlusions, the long-term patency rate has remained approximately 45% to 75%, depending on the method of follow-up (symptoms vs. angiography, see Table 24–3). If this limited follow-up is compared with long-term success in conventional balloon angioplasty, it would appear that the results of laser angioplasty are going to be similar to conventional angioplasty. This would not be surprising in the sense that the final result is achieved with balloon angioplasty.

In summary, "progressing" best summarizes the status of laser angioplasty. We have learned that laser energy can be delivered intravascularly with a low risk of complications and that the laser may be a useful adjunct to angioplasty in reopening occluded arteries. However, the amount of material removed is small, and the final result must still be achieved with a balloon catheter. It seems unlikely that the current technology will alter the restenosis rate because of these limitations. Whether lasers play a critical role as an adjunct to reopening an occluded artery, be it peripheral or coronary, cannot be answered short of a randomized study.

Future developments will have to remove tissue more completely so that the final result will no longer be dependent on balloon angioplasty. This may be feasible through the use of different types of laser sources that more efficiently remove plaque tissue and with delivery systems that can control these energy sources. As with all technology, this will take time to develop, test, and redesign and retest. As elucidated by Isner and Clarke in 1986, "If laser angioplasty in its ultimate form proves more widely acceptable than balloon angioplasty, it is reasonable to expect that the price to be paid for this development both in terms of time and money, will be correspondingly greater."[31]

REFERENCES

1. Nordstrom LA, Castaneda-Zuniga WR, Lindeke CC, et al: Laser angioplasty: Controlled delivery of argon laser energy. *Radiology* 1988; 167:463–465.
2. Nordstrom LA: Early results of peripheral laser angioplasty and preliminary experimental work on coronary laser angioplasty, in Vogel JHK, King SB, (eds): *Interventional Cardiology: Future Directions.* St Louis, Mosby–Year Book, 1989, pp 134–144.
3. Nordstrom LA, Castaneda-Zuniga WR, Young EG, et al: Direct argon laser exposure for recanalization of peripheral arteries: Early results. *Radiology* 1988; 168:359–364.
4. Nordstrom LA, Castaneda-Zuniga WR, Von Seggern KB: An analysis of patency: One year after laser-assisted transluminal angioplasty for peripheral arterial obstructions. *Radiology* 1991; 181:515–520.
5. Cronin TG, Calandra JD, Sheridan PH, et al: Early clinical experience in treating long total occlusions of the peripheral arteries via direct laser angioplasty (abstract). *Radiology* 1988; 169(suppl):139.
6. Allen B, Loflin TG, Embry BM, et al: Occluded peripheral arteries: Clinical utility of argon laser recanalization. *Radiology* 1990; 176:543–547.
7. McNamara TO: Technique and results of "higher-dose" infusion. *Cardiovasc Intervent Radiol* 1982, suppl, pp 48–57.
8. Jenkins RD, Sinclair IN, Leonard BM, et al: Laser balloon angioplasty versus angioplasty in normal rabbit iliac arteries. *Lasers Surg Med* 1989; 9:237–247.
9. Karagacil S, Almgren B, Bergstrom R, et al: Postoperative predictive value of a new method of intraoperative angiographic assessment of runoff in femoropopliteal bypass grafting. *J Vasc Surg* 1989; 10:400–407.
10. GV Medical: LASTAC Clinical Results: Peripheral Arteries, March 1990. Available from G.V. Medical Inc, Minneapolis.
11. Gallino A, Mahler F, Probst P, et al: Percutaneous transluminal angioplasty of the arteries of the lower limbs: A 5 year follow-up. *Circulation* 1984; 70:619–623.
12. Krepel VM, van Andel GJ, van Erp WFM, et al: Percutaneous transluminal angioplasty of the femoropopliteal artery: Initial and long-term results. *Radiology* 1985; 156:325–328.
13. Henricksen LO, Jorgensen B, Holstein PE, et al: Percutaneous transluminal angioplasty of infrarenal arteries in intermittent claudication. *Acta Chir Scand* 1988; 154:573–576.
14. Morgenstern BR, Getrajdman GI, Laffey KJ, et al: Total occlusion of the femoropopliteal artery: High technical success rate of conventional balloon angioplasty. *Radiology* 1989; 172:937–940.
15. Zeitler E, Richter EI, Seyferth W: Primary results: Leg arteries, in Dotter CT, Grüntzig A, Schoop W, et al (eds): *Percutaneous Transluminal Angioplasty.* Berlin, Springer-Verlag, 1983.
16. Jorgenson B, Henriksen LO, Karle A, et al: Percutaneous transluminal angioplasty of iliac and femoral arteries in severe lower-limb ischemia. *Acta Chir Scand* 1988; 154:647–652.
17. Nordstrom LA: The experimental background preceding direct laser-assisted angioplasty in the human coronary anatomy. *Tex Heart Inst J* 1989; 16:158–162.
18. Foschi AE, Myers GD, Flamm MD, et al: Laser-enhanced coronary angioplasty: Combined early results of direct argon laser exposures in atherosclerotic native arteries and bypass grafts (abstract). *J Am Coll Cardiol* 1990; 15:272.
19. Dervan JP, Baim DS, Cherniles J, et al: Transluminal angioplasty of occluded coronary arteries: Use of a movable guide wire system. *Circulation* 1983; 68:776–784.
20. Holmes DR, Vlietstra RE, Reeder GS, et al: Angioplasty in total coronary artery occlusion. *J Am Coll Cardiol* 1984; 3:845–849.
21. Kereiakes DJ, Selmon MR, McAuley BJ, et al: Angioplasty in total coronary artery occlusion: Experience in 76 consecutive patients. *J Am Coll Cardiol* 1985; 6:526–533.
22. Serruys PW, Umans V, Heydrickx GR, et al: Elective

PTCA of totally occluded coronary arteries not associated with acute myocardial infarction: Short-term and long-term results. *Eur Heart J* 1985; 6:526–633.

23. DiSciascio G, Vetrovec GW, Cowley MJ, et al: Early and late outcome of percutaneous transluminal coronary angioplasty for subacute and chronic total coronary occlusion. *Am Heart J* 1986; 111:833–839.

24. Melchior JP, Meier B, Urban P, et al: Percutaneous transluminal coronary angioplasty for chronic total coronary occlusion. *Am J Cardiol* 1987; 59:535–538.

25. Saffian RD, McCabe CH, Sipperly ME, et al: Initial success and long-term follow-up of percutaneous transluminal coronary angioplasty in chronic total occlusions versus conventional stenoses. *Am J Cardiol* 1988; 61:23–28.

26. LaVeau PJ, Remetz MS, Cabin HS, et al: Predictors of success in percutaneous coronary angioplasty of chronic total occlusions. *Am J Cardiol* 1989; 64:1264–1269.

27. Meier B, Carlier M, Finci L, et al: Magnum wire for balloon recanalization of chronic total coronary occlusions. *Am J Cardiol* 1989; 64:148–154.

28. Little T, Rosenberg J, Seides S, et al: Probe angioplasty of total coronary occlusion using the Probing Catheter technique. *Cathet Cardiovasc Diagn* 1990; 21:124–127.

29. Finci L, Meier B, Favre J, et al: Long-term results of successful and failed angioplasty for chronic total coronary arterial occlusion. *Am J Cardiol* 1990; 66:660–662.

30. Stone GW, Rutherford BD, McConahay DR, et al: Procedure outcome of angioplasty for total coronary artery occlusion: An analysis of 971 lesions in 905 patients. *J Am Coll Cardiol* 1990; 15:849–56.

31. Isner JM, Clarke RH: Laser angioplasty: Unraveling the Gordian knot. *J Am Coll Cardiol* 1986; 7:705–708.

25

Laser Balloon Angioplasty: Therapeutic Mechanisms and Clinical Correlations

Ronald D. Jenkins, M.D.

J. Richard Spears, M.D.

Percutaneous transluminal coronary angioplasty (PTCA) continues to play an increasingly dominant role in coronary revascularization and is currently expected to be utilized in over 300,000 patients annually. While registry studies of PTCA since its early beginnings have demonstrated remarkably increasing success rates despite increasing complexity of procedures, a few clinical problems continue to limit the efficacy and safety of PTCA.[1, 2] Despite numerous clinical trials employing a variety of pharmacologic agents, balloon catheters, and PTCA techniques, there has been little convincing evidence that post-PTCA restenosis can be either prevented or when already present, treated successfully without risk of recurrence.[3-5] While the mortality associated with PTCA has improved substantially, there is still significant morbidity associated with the occurrence of acute closure, even when emergency coronary artery bypass surgery is avoided successfully with conventional measures, including long inflations, perfusion balloons, and thrombolytic therapy.[6-8]

Other clinical situations frequently not treated effectively with PTCA include total vessel occlusions, acute myocardial infarction, and coronary anatomy demonstrating diffuse disease, angulated lesions, eccentric or thrombotic lesions, and other similar lesions known to be at a higher risk for adverse outcome.[8-10]

Because of the obvious need to improve on current balloon technology there has been a remarkable proliferation of new devices that may address some of these clinical problems. This paper details the tissue effects of one of the new technologies, laser-balloon angioplasty (LBA) and, correlates these effects with clinical benefits or a lack thereof when applied to certain clinical situations.

LASER-BALLOON ANGIOPLASTY CONCEPT

The concept of LBA involves thermal remodeling of the atherosclerotic arterial wall by applying heat and pressure briefly to a diseased artery. This technique, outlined in Figure 25–1, consists of radial dispersion of 1.06-μm neodymium-YAG (Nd:YAG) laser energy along the midportion of a conventional-appearing angioplasty balloon during the process of coronary dilatation. The arterial wall is heated to sub-vaporization temperatures by direct absorption of laser radiation and is subsequently allowed to cool before balloon deflation.

LASER-BALLOON ANGIOPLASTY TECHNIQUE

For the performance of LBA, a 50-W continuous-wave, 1.06-μm Nd:YAG laser is utilized (Quantronix Corp., Smithtown, NY). The Spears LBA catheter (USCI, Division of C.R. Bard, Inc., Billerica, Mass) is a triple-lumen design with a central channel suitable for a conventional 0.014-in. guidewire for catheter advancement typical of most over-the-wire balloon catheter systems. Within the balloon of the LBA catheter (shown in Fig 25–2) and spiraling about the central channel is a

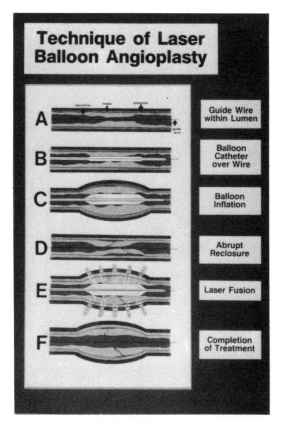

FIG 25–1.
Technique of laser balloon angioplasty following conventional angioplasty. During balloon inflation, laser energy is directed in a cylindrical pattern directly to tissues to a depth of about 3 mm surrounding the balloon *(E)*. Allowing the arterial wall temperature after laser exposure to normalize before balloon deflation facilitates thermal fusion of separated tissue layers and results in a reduction in viscoelastic recoil. Additional potentially useful effects include elimination of vasoconstriction, dehydration of thrombus, and destruction of smooth muscle cells.

helical diffusing tip that terminates the 100-μm fiberoptic coursing through the catheter from the laser interface. Balloon preparation is similar to that for conventional balloon catheters. Approximately 5 minutes of laser power calibration and safety checks are required before each procedure to be sure that both the laser and the selected catheter are functioning properly. Approximately 5 cc of flush solution is injected through the guiding catheter just as the LBA balloon is being inflated. This serves to hemodilute the small arterioles and vasa vasorum within the surrounding vessel, as well as "locking in" hemodiluted fluid distal to the inflated balloon. Animal studies previously performed suggested that this technique is helpful in reducing coagulation necrosis in small arterioles associated with microinfarction of perfused myocardium. While the balloon can be inflated up to 8 atm, laser energy is delivered generally

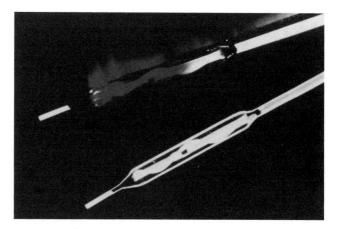

FIG 25–2.
This magnified photograph of the balloon assembly of the Spears USCI laser balloon angioplasty catheter demonstrates the helical diffusing tip within a 3-mm-diameter, 20-mm-long balloon, shown at the bottom with the HE:NE aiming laser activated. (From Jenkins, RD, Spears JR, LBA Study Group: *J Invasive Cardiol* 1990; 2:146–254. Used by permission.)

at balloon pressures of 4 atm to avoid collapse of the central lumen on the guidewire. The central lumen is flushed prior to, during, and subsequent to laser activation with 0.25 cc/sec of 37°C heparinized normal saline supplemented with 4 mEq/L of potassium chloride. Once the balloon is fully inflated, laser energy is delivered for 20 seconds by means of a hand-held triggering mechanism. The balloon is left inflated subsequently for an additional 20 to 30 seconds to allow the tissue to cool down to physiologic temperature. Premature balloon deflation may be associated with undesired tissue shrinkage. After the cool-down phase the balloon is deflated and the catheter pulled back into the guide catheter for subsequent angiography. Multiple doses can be given with a single catheter, although more than three doses at a single site is contraindicated because of excess tissue desiccation, which may excessively weaken the arterial wall structural integrity.

Occasional patients experience considerable burning chest discomfort during the latter half of laser energy delivery. It has been our experience that this is well managed with titrated doses of fentanyl administered in 50 to 100-μg doses intravenously, which allows for excellent sedation and tolerance of the laser doses.

TISSUE EFFECTS OF LASER-BALLOON ANGIOPLASTY

Thermal Fusion

Thermal fusion of soft tissues with laser energy has been demonstrated for a number of years. Jain and Gorisch in 1979 first demonstrated the ability of small vessels to be welded with an Nd:YAG laser.[11] The process involves mild coagulation necrosis while maintaining the structural integrity of connective tissue. Direct heating of vascular tissue to a specific depth by laser sources has been found to be more controllable than indirect tissue heating and thus able to avoid excess superficial heating and results in superior thermal fusion. Vascular anastomoses have been accomplished more recently with a variety of laser sources with evidence that tissue healing is associated with less scarring than in the case of sutured anastomoses.[12] The process of laser thermal fusion is suggested by Schober and colleagues to involve an interdigitation of collagen fibrillar elements secondary to thermal breakdown of noncovalent bonds and reformation of the bonds between adjacent collagen fibers upon tissue cooling.[13] Nd:YAG laser energy at 1.06 μm is not highly absorbed by tissue water and is therefore well suited to the task of thermal tissue fusion. At moderate doses, Nd:YAG laser energy penetrates into vascular tissue approximately 2 to 3 mm and imparts as thermal coagulation necrosis rather than tissue vaporization or carbonization, which may be seen at more highly absorbed wavelengths and/or at higher doses.

Previous in vitro investigations outlined the time and temperature profile of laser tissue fusion using the Nd:YAG laser,[14-16] as well as a number of clinical variables that may affect the strength of thermal tissue fusion.[17] Tissue temperatures between 80 and 130°C are associated with effective tissue thermal welds.[14] At least 10 seconds in this range is required for thermal fusion with little increment achieved from the application of laser energy for greater than 20 seconds.[15] A ramped format decreasing from higher to lower power is helpful in rapidly attaining an effective temperature range and limiting the required time and energy.[16] Variables such as the type of tissue, the degree of calcification, and the presence of blood between layers appear to have little effect on thermal tissue welding.[17]

Thermal sealing of arterial dissections was demonstrated in vivo in atherosclerotic rabbits with a prototype LBA system.[18] During clinical LBA studies, improvement in the grade of arterial dissection has been frequently noted.[19] An example of thermal sealing using LBA for dissection is demonstrated in Figure 25–3.

Thermal fusion can therefore be expected to result in an increased vascular lumen with fewer areas of flow separation common to the post-PTCA vessel. It is hypothesized that the improved rheology of the LBA-treated vessel may be associated with decreased deposition of microthrombi on exposed luminal surfaces.

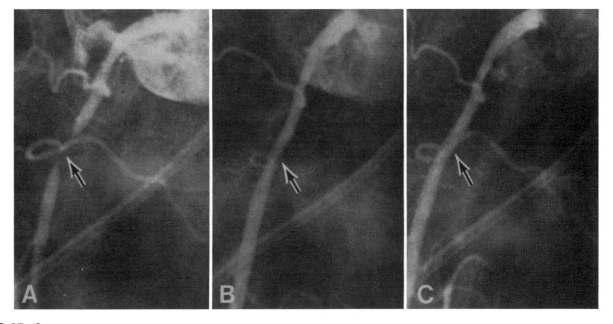

FIG 25–3.
Serial right coronary angiography of a 52-year-old man with postinfarction angina and severe right coronary artery stenosis *(arrows)* treated with PTCA and subsequent LBA. **A,** pretreatment baseline. **B,** post-PTCA result demonstrating arterial dissection and diminished flow in the acute marginal branch arising from the dissection flap. **C,** post-LBA result demonstrating sealing of the dissection, increased luminal diameter, and restoration of flow in the acute marginal branch. (From Jenkins RD, Spears JR, LBA Study Group: *J Invasive Cardiol* 1990; 2:146–254. Used by permission.)

LASER REDUCTION OF VISCOELASTIC RECOIL

Conventional balloon angioplasty, in the absence of arterial dissection, commonly results in at least some recoil of the elastic structural elements; which reduces the increase in luminal dimension. While stretching a vessel with oversized conventional balloons might result in decreased elastic recoil, an adverse outcome of severe dissection, thrombosis, and acute closure is more likely to occur, thus making this an impractical solution.[20, 21]

The application of laser energy to the arterial wall during balloon dilation very likely allows noncovalant bonds to break and reform, with realignment of the tertiary structure of connective tissue components, principally collagen and elastin. As long as the tissue is allowed to cool to physiologic temperatures so that these bonds are reformed while the balloon remains inflated, the vessel will remain dilated after balloon deflation nearly to the same degree as the stretch put upon it.

A reduction in elastic recoil following LBA as compared with balloon angioplasty was documented in 42 normal rabbit iliac arteries by using 3-mm-diameter prototype LBA balloons.[22] Although neointimal proliferation occurred after both balloon angioplasty and LBA, the arterial luminal dimensions of the LBA-treated vessels remained superior to those of balloon angioplasty–treated vessels acutely as well as chronically.

Coronary arteries of 17 dogs behaved similarly with reduced elastic recoil and no significant change in angiographic lumen diameter even after 1 month post-LBA.[17] Additionally, LBA appeared to inhibit vascular tone in these animals. Failure to vasoconstrict after ergonovine maleate administration curiously resulted in an unchangeable "cast" of the LBA balloon while the surrounding vasculature vasoconstricted. This phenomenon contrasts with the increased vasomotor tone observed following conventional PTCA, likely due to a loss of endothelial-derived relaxing factors and release of thromboxane A_2 from activated platelets.[23-25]

Clinically, an increment in the postprocedure luminal diameter is almost always evident after LBA as compared with the post-PTCA result (Fig 25–4). The major component of this luminal increase is thought to be a reduction in viscoelastic recoil. From the multicenter

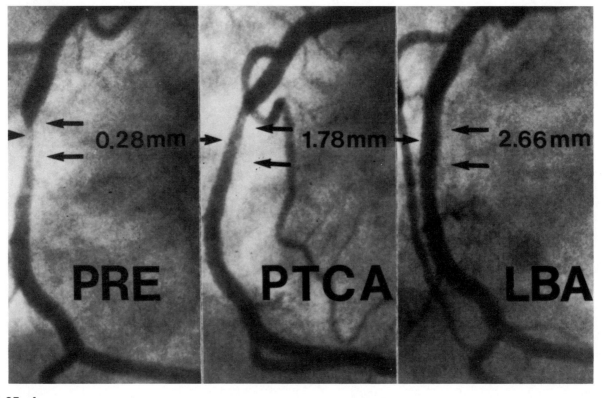

FIG 25–4.
Serial right coronary angiograms of a man undergoing elective PTCA and subsequent LBA for stable exertional angina. The Pretreatment angiogram at the *left* shows a severe concentric stenosis *(arrows)*. The post-PTCA angiogram in the *middle* shows a reasonable angiographic result *(arrows)*. The post-LBA result at the far *right* shows a further luminal increment *(arrows)* secondary to a laser effect on elastic recoil in the absence of dissection.

data comparing balloon angioplasty with LBA, in all patients excluding those with acute closure, the minimum luminal diameter increased from 0.62 ± 0.33 mm to 1.58 ± 0.61 mm after balloon angioplasty.[26] A further increment of approximately 0.5 mm in a 3.0 mm reference artery after LBA resulted in a minimal luminal diameter of 2.12 ± 0.40 mm that was maintained 1 month after angioplasty.

LASER TISSUE DESICCATION

During LBA tissue desiccation occurs secondary to tissue water evaporation. In vitro, a 15% to 20% weight reduction in postmortem atheromatous tissue was documented after repetitive 20-second Nd:YAG laser exposures. Significant rehydration does not appear to occur quickly, and therefore this effect may account for a portion of the luminal increment after LBA is used clinically. In situ thrombus appears to be desiccated to a greater proportion than surrounding vascular tissue. LBA performed in thrombus-containing vessels tends to dramatically improve the angiographic appearance of the artery.[19] Occasionally, thrombus has been observed to be adherent to the LBA balloon, adjacent to a "hot spot" on the diffusing tip, upon its withdrawal (Fig 25–5). Such adherence has not been noted since the more recent use of an LBA balloon with a more uniform diffusing tip.

Laser Effects on Thrombogenicity

Conflicting data have been obtained regarding the thrombogenic effect of LBA upon the arterial wall. Although Alexopoulos and colleagues noted increased

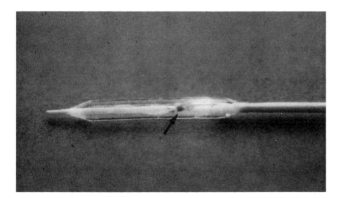

FIG 25–5.
Photograph of an LBA catheter after clinical use in a thrombotic lesion with desiccated thrombus firmly adherent to the LBA balloon *(arrow)*. The resultant angiogram showed interim restoration of flow in a previously occluded marginal vessel.

platelet deposition after LBA doses in rabbit iliac arteries,[27] in vivo LBA in both the dog coronary and rabbit iliac arteries failed to result in significant thrombus formation.[17, 22] In fact, in miniature swine there tended to be a high incidence of post procedure thrombosis in both sham LBA (PTCA only) and extremely low-dose LBA as compared with both moderate- and high-dose LBA-treated vessels.[28] In further studies (unpublished), LBA treatment of acutely thrombosed vessels in a dog model resulted in excellent short-and long-term angiographic patency rates and outcome. Therefore, there is reasonable support for the hypothesis that LBA would be useful in acute coronary syndromes.

CLINICAL CORRELATION OF TISSUE EFFECTS AND CLINICAL BENEFIT

Over 400 patients have been treated to date with LBA, most as part of a multicenter trial comparing both balloon angioplasty and LBA for both elective revascularization as well as for acute vessel closure involving dissection or thrombosis. Prior to study commencement it was hypothesized that LBA would be beneficial for the prevention of restenosis, reversal of acute closure, and management of higher-risk lesions such as those involving thrombus, severe eccentricity, greater length, significant angulation, or diffuse disease.

Prevention of PTCA Restenosis

When last reported over 200 patients were treated in a randomized unblinded trial of PTCA vs. LBA.[26] All patients were treated with appropriately sized PTCA balloons until the most satisfactory result could be obtained. Patients were then randomized to receive either a further PTCA inflation or one of three separate laser doses during LBA. The immediate and 6-month angiographic minimal luminal dimensions were collected and the clinical profile of each patient followed for at least 6 months.

While the safety profile of the LBA-treated patients was excellent, it became apparent that despite the initially improved luminal dimensions after LBA, the long-term angiographic luminal dimensions and restenosis rates were not significantly different between groups, with a mean percent stenosis at 6 months of 45% and 53% for the PTCA and three LBA groups, respectively.[29] Furthermore, there was no evidence that LBA was beneficial in treating a restenotic lesion as evidenced by the few patients in which LBA was used in this clinical setting. Therefore, although LBA-treated patients demonstrate improved luminal dimensions acutely, the arterial injury common to both balloon angioplasty and

LBA appears to outweigh this initial benefit chronically. While the procedure-related complication profile may be improved with LBA, the low frequency of such in elective PTCA patients does not warrant the routine clinical use of LBA for elective PTCA cases. In that light, further LBA use has been restricted to subgroups in which clinical benefit is more likely to be found.

Management of Acute Closure

Early in the clinical trials, LBA was rarely used in the setting of PTCA failure. This was initially done on a compassionate use basis inasmuch as the procedure was only to be used in the setting of acutely successful PTCA. After a number of successful reversals of acute closure, a formalized trial was instituted to study the potential clinical benefit of LBA in this setting. One hundred fifty-four patients with refractory acute closure after PTCA were treated with LBA.[30] Clinical inclusion criteria included the presence of abrupt vessel occlusion with Thrombolysis in Myocardial Infarction (TIMI) grade 0 or 1 flow or severe dissection with TIMI grade 2 or less flow and clinical signs of ischemia, as well as a failure to reestablish antegrade TIMI grade 3 flow by at least 3 minutes of balloon inflations with conventional or perfusion balloon catheters.

Eighty-three percent of patients experienced clinical success defined as a less than 50% diameter stenosis and avoidance of coronary artery bypass grafting or other major in-hospital complications following the performance of LBA.[30] There were no immediate device-related major complications in the clinically successful LBA group. Of 101 patients successfully treated with LBA for acute closure, 39% experienced a major clinical event within 6 months. This included death in 4 (3 of 4 occurred after bypass grafting surgery); myocardial infarction in 4 (2 non-Qwave); repeat PTCA, atherectomy, or stent placement in 17; and coronary artery bypass grafting in 14. In patients in whom angiographic follow-up was available, greater than 50% diameter stenosis was present in 65%, and 23% had developed interim total occlusions. Of note, 1 patient presented 1 week after successful LBA with acute myocardial infarction complicated by vessel perforation during emergency balloon angioplasty. It is yet unclear whether this perforation was a complication of prior LBA or due to mechanical misadventure during emergency PTCA. Two deaths occurred in the unsuccessful LBA group, 1 after bypass surgery. Of those patients who elected not to have angiographic follow-up, significantly more patients were asymptomatic (84%) than those with angiographic follow-up (29%), thus suggesting a bias to overestimate restenosis based on angiographic analysis alone.

Patients treated with LBA for acute closure appear to have a better outcome than otherwise expected. A review of the outcome of patients treated with prolonged balloon inflations for acute closure from Emory University shows a relatively high incidence of major complications even despite successful reversal of closure by using conventional means.[31] Inasmuch as the LBA protocol takes only the failures of this subset of patients, the clinical success rate and low incidence of major morbid events is remarkable.

Utilization Considerations

Factors to consider when choosing to utilize the LBA system for acute closure include the likelihood of success, adverse outcome, or restenosis; the time required to ready the device; and the cost. As shown above, success has been reasonably constant at approximately 80% in the avoidance of emergency surgery. It is well established that emergency bypass surgery carries greater morbidity and mortality than elective bypass surgery.[32] Even if all patients treated with LBA for acute closure required subsequent revascularization, the ability to perform further PTCA or bypass surgery electively under controlled circumstances is sufficient justification for LBA alone. The significant restenosis rate after reversal of acute closure is no surprise, given the amount of arterial injury, and does not necessarily imply that restenosis would occur following further PTCA of the restenotic lesion. The majority of patients who were successfully treated with LBA had no further major morbid events since the most frequent clinical events were restenosis requiring revascularization in approximately 31%. Fatal infarction was more likely to occur following bypass surgery than during the immediate period following LBA. The infarctions that were recognized periprocedure were almost exclusively related to the ischemic interval prior to gaining reperfusion, particularly in those patients who reoccluded after leaving the catheterization laboratory. A few infarctions did occur during the weeks and months following LBA. While some were due to nonstudy lesions, those few related to the study lesions are of concern. It is yet unclear whether these resulted from the mechanisms of LBA or whether the immediate post-LBA angiographic results were inadequate. Although not yet formally analyzed, this experience has been rare at centers electing to treat acute closures that appear thrombotic in origin with chronic oral anticoagulation.

The time required to warm up and ready the LBA system is approximately 15 to 20 minutes. In practice, the laser is warmed up at the first sign of possible adverse PTCA outcome. Initial power calibration and functional testing can be done by laboratory personnel often before a decision to proceed with LBA is even reached. The time delay is therefore generally not a hindrance since it usually takes a similar amount of time to redilate lesions further, particularly to attempt to use long inflations with perfusion balloons, before committing the patient to either LBA or emergency surgery. Although most patients who have a poor LBA result necessitating emergent or semi elective surgery nonetheless have adequate coronary flow, patients in whom dramatic improvement in flow after one to three LBA doses does not occur should have perfusion balloons replaced and emergency surgery performed. In general this can be done safely with little time lost due solely to the performance of LBA. In addition the safety of the surgery is not compromised with LBA as it may be following other alternative therapies such as the administration of additional thrombolytic or platelet-active agents.

The cost of the laser device required to be used with LBA catheters will likely exceed $100,000. When marketed, individual LBA catheters are likely to cost approximately $300 more than conventional balloon catheters. While the cost of such a system may be prohibitive for small laboratories, the LBA system has distinct clinical advantages for large-volume institutions seeking to deal with acute closure by nonsurgical means.

PTCA Failure Without Acute Closure or Ischemia

Subgroup analysis of patients with PTCA failure without acute closure or documented ischemia have also shown a very high LBA success rate and an intermediate restenosis rate.[33] These patients generally have clinical results deemed inadequate such that urgent coronary artery bypass grafting would still be necessary. It is our clinical impression that these patients are better served with immediate LBA with the realization that a 50% chance of restenosis may not be unreasonable. A more difficult dilemma occurs in dealing with patients with 40% to 70% residual stenosis post-PTCA. These patients, many of whom are clinically stable, have a high chance of restenosis, if left untreated. It is unclear whether LBA would have a positive or negative effect on their long-term outcome. At present, the clinical outcome of these patients with an inadequate PTCA result who are subsequently treated with LBA appears to be similar to the elective LBA group. The control group with these characteristics, however, is inadequately small to make reasonable correlations regarding the nat-

ural history of patients with these lesions left untreated after PTCA.

Total Coronary Occlusions

A small pilot study was attempted to determine whether LBA had any effect on the restenosis rate of total coronary occlusions, already known to be high following PTCA of these lesions.[34] At 6 months, the restenosis rate was nearly 90% in this group of patients, although the great majority of arteries remained patent. Because many presented with collaterals to the occluded artery initially, most of these procedures were accomplished without clinical morbid events. Given that LBA does not appear to change the proliferative response to injury, there is little reason to suspect any benefit from future application of LBA to total vessel occlusions out of the acute setting.

ACUTE CORONARY SYNDROMES

Subgroup analysis of LBA treatment electively for patients with class IV angina or recent myocardial infarction (within 2 weeks of the study procedure) demonstrated a high success rate with a low incidence of complications.[35] The excellent angiographic results likely stemmed from desiccation and remodeling of coronary thrombus in these patients. Furthermore, patients in the acute closure trial of LBA with intracoronary thrombus as the primary cause of vessel closure have been managed very effectively with LBA. Frequently, these are patients who otherwise continue to show unrelenting thrombosis despite repeated inflations, perfusion balloons, intracoronary thrombolysis, etc. An example of a patient treated successfully with LBA after failure of conventional measures is demonstrated in Figure 25-6.

High-Risk Lesions

Because the complication rate is elevated in lesions classified as type B or C according to the definitions of the American College of Cardiology/American Heart Association Task Force,[36] it has been hypothesized that patients exhibiting these lesions might have a lower incidence of procedure-related events if they were treated with LBA primarily rather than in the instance of failed PTCA. While the initial angiographic result after dilation and LBA in patients with type B and C lesions is similar to the overall cohort of patients (both with a minimal luminal diameter of 2.12 mm), the 6-month minimal luminal diameter is smaller for type B and C lesions treated with LBA[1, 22] vs. those treated electively with LBA, including all lesions. One might expect that

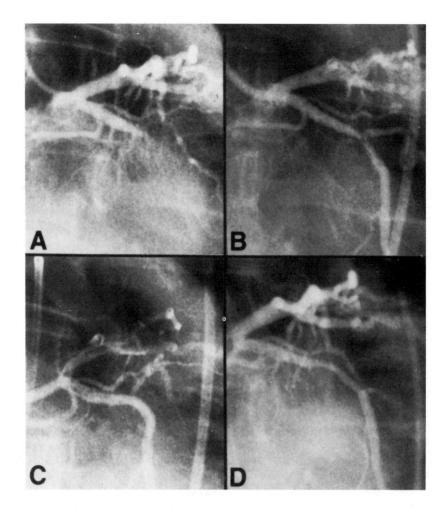

FIG 25–6.
Serial angiograms of the left coronary artery of a 62-year-old man presenting with unstable angina and subendocardial infarction. After initially successful PTCA, the patient developed clinical symptoms and electrocardiographic evidence of acute myocardial infarction occurring 4 hours after discontinuation of heparin infusion. **A,** initial angiogram upon return to the catheterization laboratory emergently. The left circumflex artery is totally occluded. **B,** the left circumflex artery remains severely compromised after multiple inflations of a perfusion balloon, effective anticoagulation, and local administration of a thrombolytic agent. **C,** 20 minutes following two LBA applications there is trivial residual stenosis, little evidence of further thrombus, and normalized flow. **D,** at the 6-month follow-up the patient is asymptomatic with mild residual stenosis and normal flow in the circumflex artery.

the restenosis rate for type B and C lesions treated with either PTCA or LBA will be increased. Clinical investigators are now struggling with the question of whether a clinical trial of LBA in high-risk lesions, primarily looking for a reduction in procedure-related events, is worthwhile given the restenosis data. An unknown potential effect is whether using LBA on the first balloon inflation will prevent severe dissection by facilitating plastic deformation of the artery, as opposed to attempting to repair a severely damaged artery after the fact. This potential effect might have implications regarding the amount and degree of tissue response to injury that would occur in either instance.

FUTURE OF LBA

Although data compiled for submission to the Food and Drug Administration (FDA) for premarket approval of the LBA system for the clinical indication of acute vessel closure following PTCA, the sponsor recently abandoned the study primarily because of financial considerations. The only alternative new technology at present is that of catheter placement of intracoronary stents.[37] While stent technology may be quite advantageous in settings of acute coronary dissection, difficult coronary architecture may prevent a significant number of devices from passing into such dissected lesions, and relatively small (<2.5 mm) vessels may not be suitable for stents. Stent placement for thrombotic closure also has theoretical limitations inasmuch as coronary thrombosis is still the leading concern regarding maintenance of stent patency. Therefore, it is likely that LBA may find a reasonable niche in clinical practice for the treatment of acute closure in the future (with an alternative sponsor). Once FDA approval for acute closure is accomplished, it is likely that clinical trials of this device for the treatment of acute myocardial infarction and high-risk lesions will very likely be pursued.

One interesting potential application of LBA is in the local delivery of medication to the arterial wall. Spears and colleagues have shown the ability to trap albumin microspheres at the luminal surface and in the arterial wall with LBA treatment.[38] Microspheres incorporated into the vessel wall by the coagulation necrosis that occurs with LBA are able to deliver encased medication over a protracted period of time. Heparin, for instance, may be delivered to potentially decrease the local thrombotic and proliferative responses to injury and may have a role in decreasing the restenotic response. Other antithrombin agents are also under consideration for local delivery to the lesion site.

CONCLUSIONS

LBA is a new technology that has been highly effective in reversing total vessel occlusions and may have a role in treating failed angioplasty without total vessel closure, as well as thrombotic and type B and C lesions. At present there is no clinical indication for LBA for the prevention or treatment of restenosis or the treatment of total vessel occlusions out of the acute setting. The mechanisms of laser thermal fusion, reduction of elastic recoil, and tissue desiccation appear to be responsible for these acute clinical effects.

REFERENCES

1. Detre K, Holubkov R, Kelsey S, et al: Percutaneous transluminal coronary angioplasty in 1985–1986 and 1977–1981: The National Heart, Lung, and Blood Institute registry. *N Engl J Med* 1988; 318:265–270.
2. Holmes DR, Vliestra RE, Smith HC, et al: Restenosis after percutaneious transluminal coronary angioplasty (PTCA): A report from the PTCA registry of the National Heart, Lung and Blood Institute. *Am J Cardiol* 1984; 53:77–81.
3. Roubin GS, King SB III, Douglas JS: Restenosis after percutaneous transluminal coronary angioplasty: The Emory University Hospital experience. *Am J Cardiol* 1987; 60:39–43.
4. Hermans WRM, Rensing BJ, Strauss BH, et al: Prevention of restenosis after percutaneous transluminal coronary angioplasty: The search for a "magic bullet." *Am Heart J* 1991; 122:171–187.
5. Popma JJ, Topol EJ: Factors influencing restenosis after coronary angioplasty. *Am J Med* 1990; 88:16–24.
6. Kaltenbach M, Beyer J, Walter S, et al: Prolonged application of pressure in transluminal coronary angioplasty. *Cathet Cardiovasc Diagn* 1984; 10:213–219.
7. Cowley MJ, Dorros G, Kelsey SF, et al: Acute coronary events associated with percutaneous transluminal coronary angioplasty. *Am J Cardiol* 1984; 53:12–16.
8. Ellis SG, Roubin GS, King SB III, et al: In-hospital cardiac mortality after acute closure from coronary angioplasty: Analysis of risk factors from 8,207 procedures. *J Am Coll Cardiol* 1988; 11:211–216.
9. Safian RD, McCabe CH, Sipperly ME, et al. Initial success and long-term follow-up of percutaneous transluminal coronary angioplasty in chronic total occlusions versus conventional stenoses. *Am J Cardiol* 1988; 61:23–28.
10. Ernst SMPG, van der Feltz TA, Bal ET, et al: Long-term angiographic follow-up, cardiac events, and survival in patients undergoing percutaneous transluminal coronary angioplasty. *Br Heart J* 1987; 57:220–225.
11. Jain KK, Gorisch W: Repair of small blood vessels with the neodymium-YAG laser: A preliminary report. *Surgery* 1979; 85:684.
12. White RA, Abergel RP, Lyons R, et al: Biological effects of laser welding on vascular heating. *Lasers Surg Med* 1988; 6:137.
13. Schober R, Ulrich F, Sander T, et al: Laser-induced alteration of collagen substructure allows microsurgical tissue welding. *Science* 1986; 232:1421.
14. Jenkins RD, Sinclair IN, Anand RK, et al: Laser balloon angioplasty: Effect of tissue temperature on weld strength of human postmortem intima-media separations. *Lasers Surg Med* 1988; 8:30–39.
15. Jenkins RD, Sinclair IN, Anand RK, et al: Laser balloon angioplasty: Effect of exposure duration on shear strength of welded layers of postmortem human aorta. *Lasers Surg Med* 1988; 8:392–396.
16. Anand RK, Sinclair IN, Jenkins RD, et al: Effect of constant temperature vs. constant power on tissue weld strength. *Lasers Surg Med* 1988; 8:40–44.
17. Spears JR, Sinclair IN, Jenkins RD: Laser balloon angioplasty: Experimental in vivo and in vitro studies, in Abela GS (ed): *Lasers in Cardiovascular Medicine and Surgery.* Norwell, Mass, Kluwer, 1989, pp 167–188.
18. Jenkins RD, Sinclair IN, McCall PE, et al: Laser balloon angioplasty: Thermal sealing of arterial dissections and perforations in atherosclerotic rabbits. *Lasers Life Sci* 1989; 3:13–30.
19. Reis GJ, Pomerantz RM, Jenkins RD, et al: Laser balloon angioplasty: Clinical, angiographic, and histologic results. *J Am Coll Cardiol* 1991; 18:193–202.
20. Steele PM, Chesebro JH, Stanson AW, et al: Balloon angioplasty: Natural history of the pathological response to injury in a pig model. *Circ Res* 1985; 57:105.
21. Sinclair IN, McCabe CH, Sipperly ME, et al: Predictors, therapeutic options, and long-term outcome of abrupt closure. *Am J Cardiol* 1988; 61:61–66.
22. Jenkins RD, Sinclair IN, Leonard BM, et al: Laser balloon angioplasty in normal rabbit iliac arteries. *Lasers Surg Med* 1989; 9:237–247.

23. Palmer RM, Ferrige AG, Moncada S: Nitric oxide release accounts for the biological activity of endothelium-derived relaxing factor. *Nature* 1987; 327:524.

24. Halushka PV, Dollery CT, MacDermot J: Thromboxane and prostacyline in disease: A review. *Q J Med* 1983; 52:461.

25. Chierchia S, Patrono C: Role of platelet and vascular eicosanoids in the pathophysiology of ischemic heart disease. *Fed Proc* 1987; 46:81.

26. Spears JR, Reyes VP, Wynne J, et al: Laser balloon angioplasty: Initial results of a multicenter experience. *J Am Coll Cardiol* 1990; 16:293–303.

27. Alexopoulos D, Sanborn TA, Marmur JD, et al: Biological response to laser balloon angioplasty in the atherosclerotic rabbit (abstract). *Circulation* 1989; 80(Suppl 2):476.

28. Jenkins RD, Spears JR, LBA Study Group: Laser balloon angioplasty: A review of the technique and clinical applications. *J Invasive Cardiol* 1990; 2:146–254.

29. Spears JR, Reyes VP, Plokker HWT, et al: Laser-balloon angioplasty: Coronary angiographic follow-up of a multicenter trial (abstract). *J Am Coll Cardiol* 1990; 15(suppl):26.

30. Ferguson JJ, Dear WE, Leatherman LL, et al: A multicenter trial of laser balloon angioplasty for abrupt closure following PTCA (abstract). *J Am Coll Cardiol* 1990; 15:25.

31. Ba'albaki HA, Weintraub WS, Tao X, et al: Restenosis after acute closure and successful reopening: Implications for new devices (abstract). *Circulation* 1990; 82(Suppl 3):314.

32. Cowley MJ, Dorros G, Kelsey SF, et al: Emergency coronary bypass surgery after coronary angioplasty: The National Heart, Lung, and Blood Institute's percutaneous transluminal coronary angioplasty registry experience. *Am J Cardiol* 1984; 53:22–26.

33. Safian RD, Reis GJ, Murice MC, et al: Failed PTCA: Salvage by laser balloon angioplasty. *Circulation* 1990; 82(Suppl 3):673.

34. Knudtson ML, Spindler BM, Traboulsi M, et al: Coronary laser balloon angioplasty in chronic total occlusion provides excellent short-term results (abstract). *Circulation* 1989; 80(Suppl 2):1894.

35. Jenkins RD, Safian RD, Dear WE, et al: Laser balloon angioplasty for unstable ischemic syndromes. *J Am Coll Cardiol* 1990; 15:245.

36. Ryan TJ, Faxon DP, Gunnar RM, et al: Guidelines for PTCA: A report of the American College of Cardiology/American Heart Association Task Force on Assessment of Diagnostic and Therapeutic Cardiovascular Procedures (Subcommittee on PTCA). *Circulation* 1988; 78:486–502.

37. Sigwart U, Urban P, Golf S, et al: Emergency stenting for acute occlusion after coronary balloon angioplasty. *Circulation* 1988; 78:1121–1127.

38. Spears JR, Kundu SK, McMath LP: Laser balloon angioplasty: Potential for reduction of the thrombogenicity of the injured arterial wall and for local application of bioprotective materials. *J Am Coll Cardiol* 1991; 17:179B–188B.

26

Laser Thrombolysis

Kenton W. Gregory, M.D.

Lasers have the potential to rapidly remove intravascular thrombi.[1-7] Laser energy is very reliably absorbed by all types of thrombi within a wide range of wavelengths and can result in rapid and efficient vaporization or ablation.[4,5] Thermal or other light-based effects may also have a favorable effect upon surface thrombogenicity.[8] Primary concerns limiting the deployment of lasers in this field include the risk of vessel wall perforation, the lack of a practical and safe means of laser energy delivery, and the lack of a reliable and reasonably priced laser system. The new technological developments described herein may eventually allow practical, safe, and efficient thrombolysis by utilizing advantages unique to lasers.

BACKGROUND

Arterial thrombosis can be treated with fibrinolytic drugs, balloon angioplasty or embolectomy, mechanical cutting or aspiration devices, lasers energy, as well as surgical techniques. A description of each of these entities is not within the scope of this chapter. Fibrinolytic drugs are the mainstay of many medical regimens and have revolutionized the treatment of a wide range of acute and chronic thrombotic disorders. A variety of success rates have been reported depending upon the agent, the means of administration, the site of thrombosis, and the indication; however, most results have been reported for trials of fibrinolysis for acute coronary thrombosis. While indications and regimens wax and wane, it appears that the majority of patients referred with acute coronary thrombosis for thrombolysis receive fibrinolytic drugs with reported success rates varying between 50% and 70%.[7-9] Since 30% to 50% of patients fail to benefit from these agents and another sig-

nificant group of patients has contraindications to their use, alternative, predominantly mechanical strategies have been developed. For coronary thrombosis, balloon angioplasty has been the strategy most commonly employed. In some centers with requisite facilities and manpower, balloon angioplasty has evolved to be the first line of therapy for acute coronary artery thrombosis.[12-14] Acute procedural success rates for percutaneous transluminal coronary angioplasty (PTCA) for acute myocardial infarction have been reported to be as high as 94%. In view of the acute success rate alone, the tactical problems and the high initial risk and cost aside, it would appear reasonable to proceed with acute PTCA as the first line of therapy in many instances. Drawbacks, however, appear in the immediate- and short-term follow-up phase, where a 15% acute closure rate and restenosis rates within 6 months ranging from 30% to 60% have been reported.[12-16]

The currently accepted etiology of most episodes of acute coronary thrombosis has been attributed to injury or disruption of the luminal surface, thereby exposing a subendothelial substrate rich in targets for platelet receptors. The most common precipitating event appears to be rupture or hemorrhage of atherosclerotic plaque.[17-19] A platelet nidus leading to aggregation of platelets and subsequent organization of a fibrin thrombus completes the initial maladaptive response to this breach of the integrity of the arterial lumen. Intuitively, therapies that entail compression of these platelet-rich thrombi saturated in procoagulation factors, vasoconstrictors, and subacute reactants such as mitogens and growth factors into the vessel wall while further injuring the site of initial injury might not be the ideal therapy. This may, in part, explain the acute thrombotic mischief and restenosis rates encountered following simple mechanical recanalization achieved by balloon dilation.[20,21]

OBJECTIVES OF THROMBOLYSIS

Objectives for optimal thrombolysis based upon the above-mentioned considerations are formidable. A safe and rapid removal of thrombus must result in a restoration of blood flow while maintaining vascular integrity. Removal of the platelet component of the thrombus as well as the fibrin component while minimizing any further injury to the vessel wall may lower the risk of acute thrombosis following the intervention as well as possibly decrease the effect of platelet- and injury-mediated subacute-phase reactants. Minimizing a systemic lytic state and the cost as well as the discomfort of the intervention would also be ideal.

SELECTIVE LASER THROMBOLYSIS

A unique potential of lasers in the treatment of vascular thrombosis is the opportunity to rapidly remove thrombi without incurring injury to the vessel wall or a systemic lytic state. Prior investigations utilizing laser energy to ablate thrombi have evaluated systems developed for catheter-based atherectomy whose propensity for perforation or other undesirable injury to the vessel wall during the process of removing the atheroma are well known and reported in animal and human trials.[1-3, 7] These nonselective laser systems are capable of ablating not only atheroma and thrombi but all other vascular wall constituents as well. The ultimate biological response to injury following deployment of these laser systems is not yet fully known but may be similar to other mechanical means of removing tissues.

In order to remove the thrombus with laser energy and reduce the possibility of inadvertent damage to nearby tissues that might magnify the acute and chronic responses to pre-existing tissue injury, our approach has been to exploit the difference in optical properties between thrombus and the arterial wall. The concept of selective photothermolysis was developed to allow laser treatment of vascular diseases of the skin such as port wine stains without damaging nearby normal structures.[22-24] Prince et al. reported that differential absorption of light at selected wavelengths between atheroma and normal constituents of arterial wall resulted in observations of modest differences in ablation thresholds between normal and pathologic tissues.[25, 26] Following this work, La Muraglia et al. reported a large difference in optical properties between various types of thrombus and vessel wall.[4] Acute coronary arterial thrombi were subsequently studied in an animal model of acute myocardial infarction; an increase of nearly two orders of magnitude in absorption of thrombus as compared with arterial wall was demonstrated in the wave band between 450 and 600 nm[5] as shown in Fig-

ure 26-1. These findings provided the foundation for the premise that a laser with a wavelength within the wave band of selective absorption may be used to remove highly absorptive thrombus with little risk of affecting vascular wall constituents because of their comparatively negligible absorption within this wave band.

LASER

From these tissue spectrophotometric studies, a laser emitting optical radiation within this wave band of selective absorption was developed (Dymed 3010 flashlamp-excited pulse dye laser, Dymed, Inc., Marlborough, Mass). This laser can emit selected wavelengths by exciting a variety of fluorescent dyes and is currently configured to emit 480-nm light. In order to minimize thermal injury to adjacent vascular structures during thrombus ablation, the light is emitted in 1- to 2-μs pulses, a time domain that is far below the 100-μs thermal relaxation time of vascular tissue, which is the time required for significant thermal diffusion beyond the zone of ablation. In vivo experiments with this laser system revealed an ablation threshold for thrombus at approximately 1.5 J/cm^{2,5} while the threshold for ablation of normal arterial tissues of animals and humans was nearly 150 J/cm^2.[5, 27]

FLUID-CORE LASER CATHETER

Delivery of laser energy for thrombolysis has been accomplished with a fluid-core light guide developed specifically for this task.[5, 6, 28] Rather than transmission of light through bundles of optical fibers, which can limit catheter flexibility and impose expensive technical problems, laser output can be launched into a low index of refraction tubing filled with an optically transparent fluid with the appropriate index of refraction to allow internal reflection. Furthermore, if the catheter is open ended and allows the optical fluid to flow, light can potentially be transmitted distally into the vessel as shown schematically in Figure 26-2. A flowing optical core has several potential advantages over quartz or fused silica fiber–based catheters, which are summarized in Table 26-1. The flowing optical fluid can flush away blood, which absorbs almost all laser wavelengths and could otherwise interfere with efficient delivery of light to the thrombus. Since light can be transmitted past the end of the catheter, catheter contact with the target is not necessary, as is the case for most other laser angioplasty catheters, and this feature may reduce mechanical injury to the vessel wall. If the fluid is radiopaque, real-time visualization of the catheter, the target, and the distal vas-

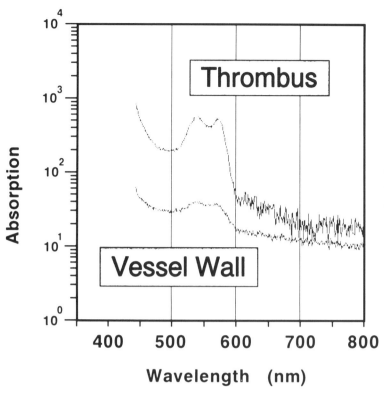

FIG 26–1.
The absorption curves derived from spectrophotometric studies of normal coronary wall and mixed acute coronary arterial thrombi demonstrate a marked difference in absorption between approximately 400 and 600 nm.

culature could be achieved so that the operator can continuously observe the effectiveness and consequences of laser energy delivery during fluoroscopy. Fortuitously, we discovered that conventional radiographic contrast material appears to be an excellent optical transmission medium. All types of contrast agents tested are transparent within the wave band of selective thrombus absorption and have the requisite high index of refraction necessary for total internal reflection.[6] Since it is filled with fluid, the optical channel adds no stiffness to the catheter, and there is no dead space in the optical channel such as exists between optical fibers in more conven-

tional laser catheters. From the consumer and manufacturing standpoint, these catheters can be simple and inexpensive since the optical channel presently consists of only a plastic or Teflon tube. A schematic drawing of a typical fluid-core optical catheter is shown in Figure 26–3. Light is delivered to the optical catheter via a conventional large-diameter fused-silica fiber that is placed into the laser catheter via an O-ring–Y adapter. The fiber is advanced to a point in the catheter where stiffness is advantageous for pushability, with the more distal aspect of the catheter with an open channel left where flexibility is needed for negotiating the angles of

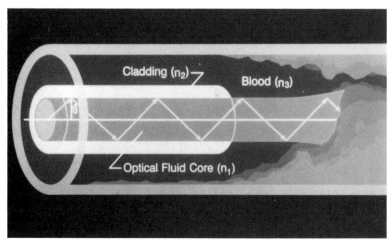

FIG 26–2.
A schematic drawing of a fluid-core catheter in a coronary artery where light is transmitted through the catheter and to a target in the vessel via total internal reflection when light is incident at an angle greater than a critical angle d given by $\sin d = n_2/n_1$ or n_3/n_1. (From Gregory KW, Anderson RR: *IEEE J Quant Electron* 1991; 26:2289–2296. Used by permission.)

TABLE 26–1.

Advantages of Fluid-Core Laser Catheters

Flexible and atraumatic
Optical and mechanical stability
Adequate laser spot size
Blood removal from the target area
Noncontact energy delivery
Real-time target and vessel imaging
Guidewire compatible
Simple, low-cost design

curvature encountered in coronary arteries. The internal diameter of the optical channel is 1.1 mm, which results in a laser spot diameter of similar dimensions. Iodinated contrast is delivered to the catheter at uniform flow rates by a conventional power injector set at a flow rate between 0.3 and 0.5 cc/sec, and this provides adequate flow for light transmission up to a centimeter from the tip of the catheter. During a typical 5- to 10-second round of laser pulses, 3 to 5 cc of the contrast agent is injected. The catheter is delivered to the target with conventional 8 F angioplasty guiding catheters and guidewires via a "monorail" lumen provided at the distal 15 cm of the laser catheter. A fluid-core laser catheter with a gold-tipped marker is shown in Figure 26–4; it delivers a 30-mJ (1 μs) laser pulse at 480 nm in a water bath.

TECHNIQUE OF LASER THROMBOLYSIS

Following a 5-minute warm-up and self-calibration, the laser is ready for use. The desired energy can be dialed in and increased at any time without retesting the output since pulse-to-pulse output is monitored continuously. The initial pulse energy setting is normally approximately 80 mJ (fiber output), which results in a fluence at the thrombus of approximately 8 J/cm.[2] Preparation of the laser catheter entails flushing the catheter with heparinized saline and connecting an injection hose to the power injector. Standard injector settings include a flow rate of 0.3 cc/sec with a maximum of 3 cc total volume at a pressure maximum of 300 psi. Angiovist 370 (Berlex Laboratories, Wayne, NJ) or Hexabrix (Malinkrodt, St Louis) preheated to 37°C were the contrast agents utilized during the animal and clinical trials. Any conventional power injector can be used with the fluid-core system as long as an electronic signal from the injector can be obtained and connected to a laser interlock. Most power injectors are equipped with such an output to gate exposures for film changers. This safety feature prevents the laser from firing when contrast is not flowing since optical transmission requires the presence of flowing contrast.

A sterile optical fiber is then removed from its package, and the proximal end is handed to an assistant who connects the fiber to the laser via a simple screw mount. Fiber output is measured with an external energy meter with a 5-second exposure. The fiber tip is then inserted through the O-ring of the laser catheter and placed approximately 20 cm from the distal endhole shown in Figure 26–3. The catheter is then filled with contrast dye and carefully inspected to exclude air bubbles. The catheter is now ready for insertion, with preparation generally requiring 2 to 4 minutes.

The fluid-core laser thrombolysis catheter can be deployed with conventional angioplasty equipment and techniques. Standard 8 F guiding catheters can be used to access the target vessel. Current laser catheters designed for intracoronary use are compatible with conventional 0.014- to 0.016-in. angioplasty guidewires via the "monorail" technique. A guidewire is passed through the O-ring of a Y adapter at the proximal end of the guiding catheter and passed to the distal end of the thrombosed vessel if possible. The laser catheter is then "backloaded" on the distal segment of the guidewire and passed over the guidewire to the area of thrombosis under fluoroscopy.

When the distal tip of the laser catheter is positioned approximately 2 to 3 mm from the proximal aspect of the thrombus, laser and injector activation is accom-

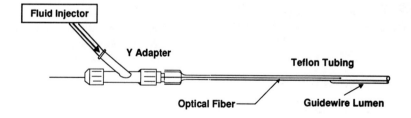

Fluid-core Laser Thrombolysis Catheter

FIG 26–3.
Schematic drawing of a coronary flowing, fluid-core laser thrombolysis catheter.

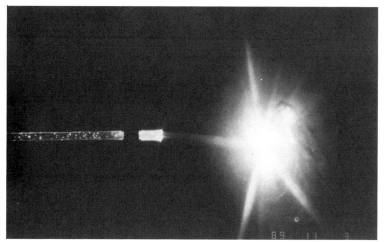

FIG 26–4.
A photograph of a flowing, fluid-core laser catheter transmitting a 480-nm, 1-μs pulse in a water bath to a target demonstrates the ability to conduct light in a fluid stream distal to the exit hole of the catheter. (From Gregory KW, Anderson RR: *IEEE J Quant Electron* 1991; 26:2289–2296. Used by permission.)

plished by stepping on a control foot pedal. A 1-second delay from injector initiation to laser activation is built into the system for the injector to achieve the desired fluid flow rate at the exit hole of the catheter. Five- to 10-second rounds of laser pulses at 3 Hz have been chosen empirically. Immediate cessation of laser output is possible by stepping off the foot pedal. Each round of laser firing produces an angiogram that allows the operator to follow thrombus removal. The catheter can be slowly advanced over the guidewire as the thrombus is removed. If inadequate thrombus removal occurs, the laser pulse energy can be increased to 100 mJ. Increasing the flow rate of the injector to 0.5 cc/sec can also potentially improve light transmission to recalcitrant thrombi. Generally, a fixed atherosclerotic obstruction is also present, and if this residual stenosis is significant, the laser catheter can be withdrawn, the guidewire left in place, and standard balloon PTCA accomplished. Patients generally receive aspirin and intravenous heparin infusions during the procedure and for 24 hours after the procedure. All personnel and the patient must wear safety glasses designed to block 480-nm light.

PRECLINICAL STUDIES

Fluid-core laser catheters delivering 1-μs laser pulses of 480-nm radiation from a pulsed dye laser were used to ablate coronary artery thrombi in a canine model of acute myocardial infarction. The model developed by Yasuda et al.[29] developed mixed platelet and fibrin thrombi in a traumatized circumflex or left anterior descending coronary artery with a superimposed distal 90% stenosis as shown in Figure 26–5. In an initial study, coronary artery thrombi were removed in 22 of 22 dogs without perforation, vasospasm, or other untoward events aside from reperfusion arrythmias.[5, 6] All thrombi were removed within 600 laser pulses (maxi-

mum, 120 seconds of laser activation). Thirteen of 13 animals that underwent attempted thrombolysis with the laser catheter and fluid injection without laser energy did not achieve a mechanical or hydraulic-mediated reperfusion. Four animals with thrombi that were not instrumented did not experience spontaneous reperfusion.

Interestingly, serial Doppler flow monitoring of the laser-treated vessel and follow-up angiography at mean of 1.5 hours after laser thrombolysis demonstrated an 80% patency rate vs. a 20% patency rate at 90 minutes when dogs were treated with recombinant tissue-type plasminogen activator (rt-PA) in this model in our laboratory. Coronary angiograms before and 2 hours after laser thrombolysis of a left circumflex coronary artery are shown in Figure 26–6,A and B. Light microscopy and scanning electron microscopy demonstrated remarkable removal of platelet-rich thrombi and a lack of readhesion and platelet aggregation up to 2 hours after laser thrombolysis[8] Control animals and animals treated with rt-PA were notable for large amounts of platelet-rich thrombi in the area of vascular injury proximal to the stenosis. Chronic animal studies subsequently demonstrated appropriate healing without evidence of rethrombosis or aneurysm formation in laser-treated vessels.

CLINICAL STUDIES

Based upon favorable animal studies of laser thrombolysis in acute myocardial infarction in terms of effective thrombus removal and lack of adverse complications, a Food and Drug Administration (FDA)-approved pilot study of laser thrombolysis for acute myocardial infarction in patients with contraindications for fibrinolytic drugs or for patients who fail to reperfuse with fibrinolytic drugs was begun. Initial results at St. Vincent

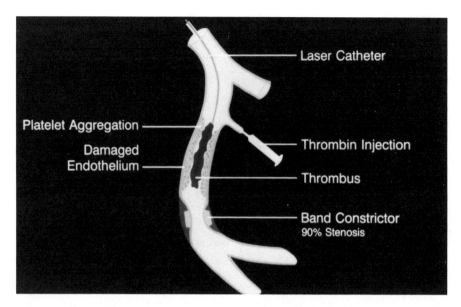

FIG 26-5.
The canine acute myocardial infarction model shown schematically with a mixed platelet and fibrin thrombus and superimposed high-grade stenosis. (From Gregory KW, Anderson RR: *IEEE J Quant Electron* 1991; 26:2289-2296. Used by permission.)

Hospital and Medical Center in Portland, Oregon, and the Academisch Ziekenhuis in Groningen, The Netherlands, have demonstrated the feasibility of this new means of thrombolysis. In the first 12 patients treated, no perforation or other adverse vascular consequence has occurred despite laser energy directed toward the arterial wall. Effective thrombus removal has been demonstrated with real-time visualization of the process and progress of thrombus removal under fluoroscopy. In Figure 26-7,A and B are photographs of angiograms before and after laser thrombolysis in a right coronary artery in a patient with acute inferior myocardial infarc-

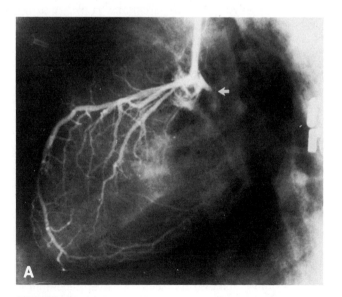
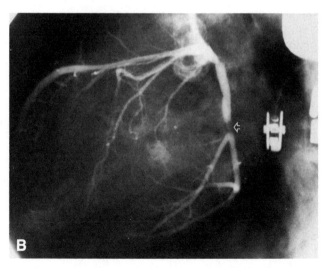

FIG 26-6.
Photographs of angiograms of a canine left coronary artery show complete thrombotic occlusion of the left circumflex branch *(filled arrow)* before **(A)** and after **(B)** laser thrombolysis, which completely removed the thrombus. The *open arrow* in **B** is the location of a 90% external hose clamp stenosis. (From Gregory KW, Anderson RR: *IEEE J Quant Electron* 1991; 26:2289-2296. Used by permission.)

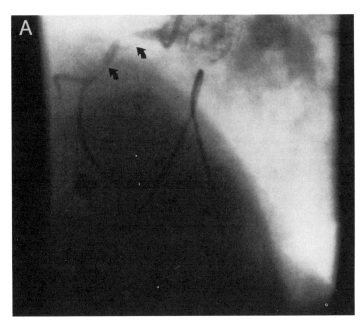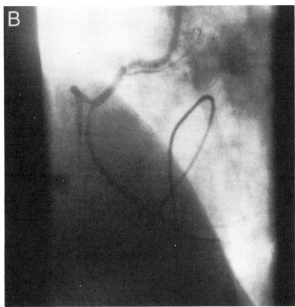

FIG 26–7.
Photographs of angiograms from a patient with acute inferior myocardial infarction after failed fibrinolysis with streptokinase show thrombosis of the proximal right coronary artery *(arrows)* before **(A)** and after **(B)** laser thrombolysis, which nearly completely removed the thrombus and established reperfusion to the distal part of the vessel. (Courtesy of Drs. Rene Van Dijk and Peter den Heijer, Groningen, The Netherlands.)

tion. Complications attributable to the laser thrombolysis procedure have been limited thus far to transient bradycardias probably secondary to the 5- to 10-second infusions of radiographic contrast agents and reperfusion arrythmias, both of which were reduced with placement of transvenous pacemaker wires in a demand mode in the right ventricle.

IMPLICATIONS

Selective laser thrombolysis with a flow-directed, fluid-core laser catheter may become a new means of treating vascular thrombosis in medium to large vessels. While the investigations thus far have centered around the treatment of acute coronary thrombosis, the treatment of other vascular sites of thrombosis such as peripheral artery or graft thrombosis, renal or pulmonary artery thrombosis, or venous thrombosis is well within the realm of possibilities for this technology. The treatment of less acute thrombosis for other cardiac disorders such as unstable angina, postangioplasty thrombosis, or coronary graft thrombosis is presently being planned.

CONCLUSIONS

Initial studies appear to indicate that laser thrombolysis is feasible and that thrombi can be removed rapidly

with a much lower potential risk of inflicting unwanted vascular injury than with other laser or mechanical angioplasty systems. While laser thrombolysis is unlikely to replace chemical fibrinolysis, it may become an important adjunct in the treatment of vascular thrombotic disorders.

REFERENCES

1. Lee G, et al: Effects of laser irradiation on human thrombus: Demonstration of a linear dissolution-dose relation between clot length and energy density. *Am J Cardiol* 1983; 52:876–877.
2. Crea F, Fenech A, Smith W, et al: Laser recanalization of acutely thrombosed coronary arteries in live dogs. *J Am Coll Cardiol* 1985; 6:1052–1056.
3. Marco J, et al: Complete patency in thrombus-occluded arteries two weeks after laser recanalization. *Lasers Surg Med* 1985; 5:291–296.
4. La Muraglia GM, Anderson RR, Parrish JA, et al: Selective laser ablation of venous thrombus: Implications for a new approach in the treatment of pulmonary embolus. *Lasers Surg Med* 1988; 8:486–493.
5. Gregory KW, Guerrero JL, Girsky M, et al: Coronary artery laser thrombolysis in acute canine myocardial infarction. *Circulation* 1989; 80:523.
6. Gregory KW, Anderson RR: Liquid core light guide for laser angioplasty. *IEEE J Quant Electron* 1990; 26:2289–2296.
7. Labs JD, Caslowitz PL Williams GM, et al: Experimen-

tal treatment of thrombotic vascular occlusion. *Lasers Surg Med* 1991; 11:363–371.

8. Gregory KW, Flotte T, Michaud N, et al: Laser-induced inhibition of platelet adhesion. *Circulation* 1989; 80(suppl 2):344.

9. Collen D, Topol EJ, Tiefenbrunn AJ, et al: Coronary thrombolysis with recombinant human tissue-type plasminogen activator: A prospective randomized placebo-controlled trial. *Circulation* 1984; 70:1012–1027.

10. The TIMI Study Group: The Thrombolysis in Myocardial Infarction (TIMI) trial: Phase I findings. *N Engl J Med* 1985; 312:932–936.

11. Gruppo Italiano per lo Studio della Streptochinasi Nell'Infarto Miocardio (GISSI): Effectiveness of intravenous thrombolytic treatment in acute myocardial infarction. *Lancet* 1986; 314:1465–1471.

12. Hartzler GO, Rutherford BD, McConahay DR: Percutaneous transluminal coronary angioplasty with and without thrombolytic therapy for acute myocardial infarction. *Am Heart J* 1983; 106:965–973.

13. O'Keefe JH, Rutherford BD, McConahay DR, et al: Early and late results of coronary angioplasty without antecedent thrombolytic therapy for acute myocardial infarction. *Am J Cardiol* 1989; 64:1221–1230.

14. Rothbaum DA, Linnemeier TJ, Landin RJ, et al: Emergency PTCA in acute myocardial infarction: A three year experience. *J Am Coll Cardiol* 1987; 10:264–272.

15. Ellis SG, O'Neill WW, Bates ER, et al: Implications for patient triage from survival and left ventricular functional recovery analysis in 500 patients treated with coronary angioplasty for acute myocardial infarction. *J Am Coll Cardiol* 1989; 13:1251–1259.

16. Hopkins J, Savage M, Zaluniski A: Recurrent Ischemia in the zone of prior myocardial infarction: Results of coronary angioplasty of the infarct related vessel. *Am Heart J* 1988; 115:14–19.

17. Davies MJ, Thomas A: Thrombosis and acute coronary artery lesions in sudden cardiac death. *N Engl J Med* 1984; 310:1137–1140.

18. Friedman M, Van Den Bovenkamp GJ: The pathogenesis of a coronary thrombus. *Am J Pathol* 1966; 48:19–44.

19. Fuster V, Badimon L, Cohen M, et al: Insights into the pathogenesis of acute ischemic syndromes. *Circulation* 1988; 77:1213–1220.

20. Harker LA: Role of platelets and thrombosis in mechanisms of acute occlusions and restenosis after angioplasty. *Am J Cardiol* 1987; 60:20–28.

21. Gulba DC, Daniel WG, Simon R, et al: Role of thrombolysis and thrombin in patients with acute coronary occlusion during PTCA. *J Am Cardiol* 1990; 16:563–568.

22. Anderson RR, Jaenke KF, Parrish JA: Mechanisms of selective vascular changes caused by dye lasers. *Lasers Surg Med* 1983; 3:211–215.

23. Anderson RR, Parrish JA: Microvasculature can be selectively damaged using dye lasers: A basic theory and experimental evidence in human skin. *Lasers Surg Med* 1981; 1:263–276.

24. Anderson RR, Parrish JA: Selective photothermolysis: Precise microsurgery by selective absorption of pulsed radiation. *Science* 1983; 220:524–527.

25. Prince MR, Deutsch TF, Mathews-Ross M, et al: Preferential light absorption in atheromas in vitro. *J Clin Invest* 1986; 78:295–302.

26. Prince MR, Deutsch TF, Shapiro AH, et al: Selective ablation of atheromas using a flashlamp-excited dye laser at 465 nm. *Proc Natl Acad Sci USA* 1986; 84:7064–7068.

27. Gregory KW, Prince MR, La Muraglia GM, et al: Effect of blood upon the selective ablation of atherosclerotic plaque with a pulsed dye laser. *Lasers Surg Med* 1990; 10:533–543.

28. Gregory KW, Anderson RR: Iodinated contrast fluid can replace quartz in laser catheters. *Circulation* 1989; 80(Suppl 2):107.

29. Yasuda T, Gold HK, Fallon JT, et al: A canine model of coronary artery thrombosis with superimposed high grade stenosis for the investigation of re-thrombosis after thrombolysis. *J Am Coll Cardiol* 1989; 13:1409–1414.

27

Microwave Balloon Angioplasty

Paul Walinsky, M.D.

Arye Rosen, M.S.

Antonio Martinez-Hernandez, M.D.

David L. Smith, M.D.

Donald T. Nardone, M.D.

Barry Bravette, M.D.

Although coronary angioplasty is a routine procedure for the treatment of coronary artery obstruction, two major problems remain unsolved. First, a less-than-optimal result or acute occlusion can be caused by dissection, thrombus, or elastic recoil of the vessel. Second, restenosis occurs in approximately 30% of patients. A variety of techniques have been proposed to overcome these current limitations. Thermal angioplasty is one of the approaches that have been studied in this regard.[1] Although laser is the thermal energy form that has been most extensively studied, alternative means of thermal energy delivery in conjunction with angioplasty are feasible. We have studied the potential application of microwave energy for thermal angioplasty.

We have been involved in the development of a prototype microwave balloon angioplasty system and have performed initial animal studies to evaluate the feasibility and efficacy of such a system. The system consists of a microwave generator that emits microwave energy at a frequency of 2,450 MHz. (Fig 27–1) The generator is coupled to a cable 0.023 to 0.035 in. in diameter. The cable terminates in an antenna that is inserted into the central lumen of a balloon catheter. When the cable is fully advanced, the antenna is in the center of the balloon. Energy radiates from the antenna, through the balloon, to the surrounding vessel wall. Different types of antennas can be designed that optimize radiating characteristics. An important feature of this energy form

is the fact that energy transmission occurs by radiation through the medium in the balloon to the surrounding tissue, and not primarily by conduction to the tissue by heating of the balloon contents. The balloon catheter has a thermocouple connected to the generator. Temperature rise is determined on-line, and generator output is controlled by sensing of temperature at the balloon surface.

Our initial studies using this technology were performed in the iliac arteries of normal rabbits. Following induction of anesthesia, the femoral arteries of the rabbits were isolated, and the catheter/cable system was positioned retrogradely in the external iliac artery. The interaction of three variables was evaluated in the study: the duration of heating and balloon inflation, the temperature attained, and peak balloon inflation pressure.

The period of balloon inflation was either 1 or 2 minutes, and the corresponding time of heating was either 30 or 60 seconds. The peak temperature varied from 50°C to 100°C, and the peak balloon inflation pressure was either 2 or 5 atm. Animals were sacrificed 1 week later. The arteries were perfusion fixed, sectioned, and stained with hemotoxylin and eosin, trichrome, and Verhoff–van Giesen stains.

The effect of microwave heating was analyzed by evaluating the presence and extent of injury to the media of the vessel and by the extent of intimal proliferation. An index relating the depth of medial injury, the

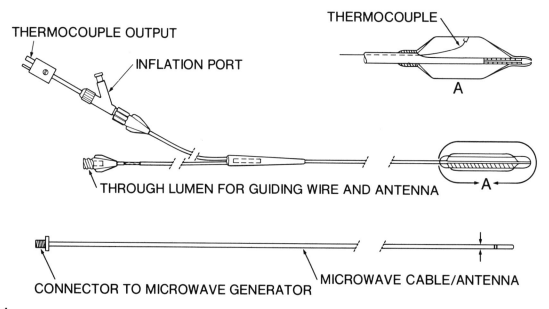

FIG 27–1.
The microwave balloon angioplasty system is illustrated. The microwave cable is inserted in the central lumen of the angioplasty catheter and is connected to a generator for energy delivery. The thermocouple in the balloon segment is indicated in enlargement *A*.

extent of intimal proliferation, and the percent circumferential involvement was used to express medial injury and intimal proliferation.

There was no correlation between medial injury or intimal proliferation and either the peak balloon inflation pressure or the time of heating or balloon inflation. We observed a direct correlation between the extent of medial injury and the peak temperature attained. We also noted an inverse relationship between the extent of medial injury and intimal proliferation. An example of the difference in response to low temperature vs. higher temperature is shown in Figure 27–2. Figure 27–2,A shows an artery that was heated to 50°C for 30 seconds. The media is intact, and prominent intimal proliferation is seen. In Figure 27–2,B an artery that was heated to 80°C is demonstrated. There is loss of cellularity in the media and replacement by fibrous elements. There is no evidence of intimal hyperplasia. Since ingrowth of smooth muscle cells from the media is thought to be one of the mechanisms responsible for restenosis, this information suggests the possibility that selective thermal injury to the media could modify this process.

Our next study was performed in an atherosclerotic rabbit model. After 2 weeks on a high-fat diet, endothelial denudation of the external iliac arteries was performed by positioning a balloon catheter in the external iliac artery and then withdrawing it to the distal segment of the aorta. This procedure predictably resulted in an atherosclerotic lesion at the site of denudation. Four to 6 weeks later these animals were brought back

to the laboratory, and bilateral femoral artery cutdowns were performed. The balloon catheter/cable system was then positioned in the atherosclerotic external iliac artery. Animals had microwave balloon angioplasty (MBA) performed on one external iliac artery and conventional balloon angioplasty (CBA) performed on the contralateral artery. Each animal thus served as its own control. Angioplasty was performed with a 3-mm balloon inflated to 5 atm for 1 minute. In the animals treated with MBA a similar procedure was performed with the addition of microwave energy for 30 seconds during the inflation. Energy was delivered to raise the temperature, as measured on the balloon surface, to 70°C or 85°C. After treatment of both vessels, angiography was performed and the femoral arteries ligated.

Four weeks after the initial angioplasty procedure, repeat angiography of the iliac arteries was performed, and the animals were sacrificed. Following perfusion fixation of the iliac arteries, the vessels were excised, fixed, sectioned, and stained in the same manner as described above. Histologic analysis and quantitative angiography of the vessels were performed.

Histologic analysis revealed that on the side treated with MBA there was a loss of lipid-laden cells and replacement in the intima, and in some cases in the media, with a hypocellular fibrotic matrix. Quantitative angiography of the iliac arteries revealed a significant improvement in the diameter of the arteries treated with MBA at 85°C both immediately and at 4 weeks. The increase in luminal diameter with microwave balloon angioplasty

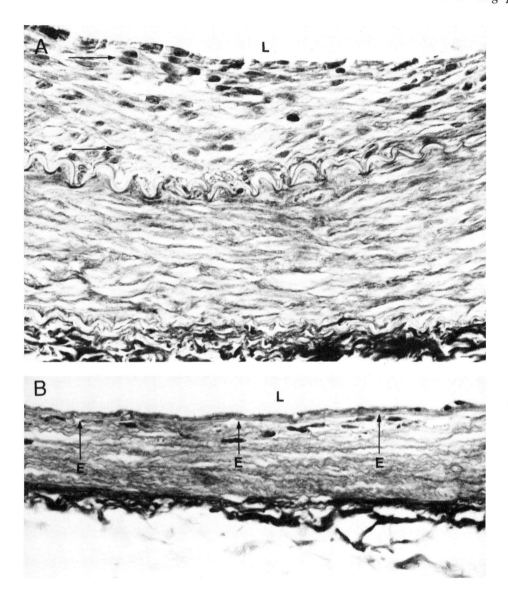

FIG 27–2.
A, artery exposed to 50°C for 30 seconds. There is prominent intimal proliferation *(arrows)*. The media is intact. *L* = lumen. Trichrome stain; original magnification × 200. **B,** artery exposed to 80°C for 30 seconds. There is extensive medial fibrosis. Smooth muscle cells are absent. The intima is composed of a single layer of endothelial cells. *E* = internal elastic lamella; *L* = lumen. Trichrome stain; original magnification × 200.

at 85°C was greater ($P < .05$) than that with conventional balloon angioplasty immediately postangioplasty. A trend toward enhanced benefit was also noted at 4 weeks. Although there was a trend for benefit immediately after the procedure in the animals treated with MBA at 70°C, this was not statistically significant. Furthermore, at 4 weeks there was a loss of the immediate benefit in the 70°C MBA vessels and no difference when compared with the control arteries treated with conventional angioplasty.

An example of the thermal effect is seen in Figure 27–3. In Figure 27–3,A angiography of the iliac arter-

ies in a rabbit is seen. Bilateral atherosclerotic lesions are noted. MBA was subsequently performed on the right and CBA on the left iliac artery. Immediately postangioplasty a dissection was noted on the left. A larger lumen without dissection is noted on the right (Fig 27–3,B). At 4 weeks postangioplasty there is sustained benefit on the right. Restenosis is noted on the left (Fig 27–3,C).

These studies demonstrated that MBA is technically feasible and that the initial results of angioplasty can be enhanced with MBA. The finding of sustained benefit at 4 weeks has encouraged us to further explore the poten-

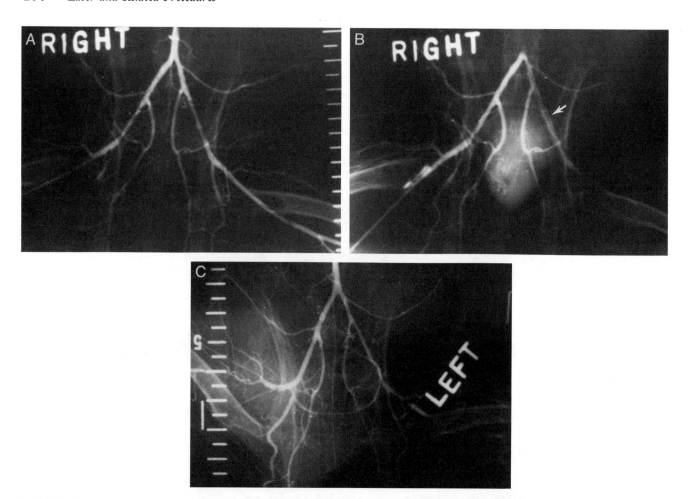

FIG 27–3.
A, Angiography of the iliac artery prior to angioplasty. Bilateral atherosclerotic lesions are seen. **B,** angiography of the iliac arteries following angioplasty. Microwave balloon angioplasty was performed on the right, and conventional balloon angioplasty was performed on the left. Note the dissection on the left *(arrow)*. **C,** angiography of the atherosclerotic iliac arteries 4 weeks following angioplasty. Restenosis is noted on the left.

tial of this modality in reducing the incidence of restenosis. At the current time, a target temperature of 85°C seems optimal for this effect.

Studies are also in progress to evaluate the potential of this technique to treat two additional mechanisms that may decrease coronary flow and lead to unsuccessful angioplasty. In the first study, the ability to seal dissections is being evaluated. Initial observations suggest that such tears in the vessel wall can be sealed by microwave thermal energy.[2]

A third problem that can complicate angioplasty is the presence or the development of thrombus at the site of angioplasty. We have performed studies in which thrombus was induced in the coronary artery of a dog. Following complete occlusion of the coronary artery with thrombus, the microwave balloon system was positioned across the thrombosed region. CBA was com-

pared with microwave angioplasty, with MBA balloon inflation for 60 seconds and microwave heating to 85°C for 30 seconds. This was compared with a 1-minute conventional angioplasty. Following a 30-minute period of observation, the animal was sacrificed and the artery excised and studied histologically. On angiography, five out of six animals that had received conventional angioplasty had evidence of thrombus, whereas two out of six that had received microwave angioplasty had evidence of thrombus. On examination of the histology, the vessels that had microwave angioplasty had less evidence of thrombus than those treated with conventional angioplasty did. Furthermore, following MBA, thermal coagulation of thrombus with peripheral lamination was seen. A satisfactory lumen was created in the center of this channel. This phenomenon was not seen following conventional angioplasty. Thus, it may be possible to coagulate and stabilize thrombi with MBA and subsequently achieve resolution of the thrombi without coronary occlusion.

Our understanding of the mechanisms and therapeutic applications of intravascular thermal energy, i.e., heat, whether by laser, microwave, or another energy form, is in an early stage. Complex changes occur in all layers of the vessel, and different thermal dosimetry profiles may be required to optimize therapeutic benefit. A high tissue temperature may be optimal for tissue welding in the therapy of dissection. Maintenance of vascular distension may be accomplished with a lower temperature. Modification of the injury response of the media may be best accomplished with yet another temperature profile. Coagulation and stabilization of thrombus is yet another therapeutic goal requiring its own thermal characterization. Clarification of the therapeutic potential of heating will be aided by further understanding of such thermal dosimetry.

Our studies thus far have led us to the conclusion that MBA is effective in enhancing the primary result of angioplasty. The addition of microwave energy is effective in increasing the diameter of the vessel postangioplasty and in sealing dissections and seems to be effective in aiding in the stabilization of thrombi. The role of microwave angioplasty in reducing the incidence of restenosis is a complex question. Although the restenosis rates following laser balloon angioplasty have been high, those results should not be transposed to MBA since the temperature reached and the energy form are different.

The MBA system is relatively easy to deploy, and the system is cost-effective when compared with alternative heating modalities.

REFERENCES

1. Spears JR, Reyes VP, Wynne J, et al: Percutaneous coronary laser balloon angioplasty: Initial results of a multicenter experience. *J Am Coll Cardiol* 1990; 16:292–303.
2. Landau C, Currier JW, Haudenschild CC, et al: Microwave balloon angioplasty to treat arterial dissections in an atherosclerotic rabbit model (abstract). *J Am Coll Cardiol* 1991; 17:234.

28

Ultrasound Angioplasty

Robert J. Siegel, M.D.

John R. Crew, M.D.

Russell Pflueger, B.S.

Anthony Don Michael, M.D.

Marilyn Dean, R.V.T.

Richard K. Myler, M.D.

David C. Cumberland, M.D.

The application of ultrasound for medical purposes is widely utilized for the removal of dental plaque,[1] emulsification of cataracts,[2] and destruction of renal and ureteral calculi.[3] It has also been shown to have a potential application for fragmentation of gallstones[4] and decalcification of cardiac valves.[1, 5] Because surgical ultrasound is relatively atraumatic to normal tissues and blood vessels, it is useful in facilitating the excision of intracranial and hepatic tumors.[6, 7] However the use of ultrasound as an endovascular therapeutic tool has been less widely used and studied.

In 1965 Anscheutz and Bernard suggested the potential of ultrasound for atherosclerotic plaque ablation.[8] In the 1970s the first experimental studies on the intravascular application of therapeutic ultrasound for clot lysis were initiated by Trubestein, Stumpff, and coworkers.[9, 10] They demonstrated the feasibility of clot lysis in vitro as well as in vivo in canine thrombotic occlusion models.

We began our studies of ultrasound for atherosclerotic plaque ablation and clot lysis in 1986. The following year, we reported on in vitro ablation of human atherosclerotic plaque by electrohydraulic and ultrasound energy.[11, 12] A number of studies have now shown the in vitro and in vivo potential of low-frequency, high-intensity ultrasound for clot dissolution and plaque ablation.[9–20] We performed in vivo studies in animals in which the feasibility of catheter-delivered ultrasound energy was demonstrated for clot dissolution, plaque ablation, and arterial recanalization.[12–14, 21, 22] On the basis of our in vitro studies, in vivo animal feasibility and safety studies, and extensive clinical data showing the safety of surgical ultrasound for nonvascular use, we initiated the first clinical application of percutaneous ultrasound angioplasty in patients with symptom-limiting peripheral vascular disease.[23]

IN VITRO STUDIES OF ULTRASOUND PLAQUE ABLATION AND ITS EFFECT ON THE ARTERIAL WALL

Our early feasibility studies evaluated the efficacy and potential safety of ultrasonic energy for the ablation of human atherosclerotic plaque in vitro.[11, 12] In the series of atherosclerotic segments studied ($n = 79$), there was a gross reduction in atheroma mass as well as microscopic disruption of fibrous and calcified plaque. All occlusions (length, 0.5 to 5.0 cm) were recanalized irrespective of the presence of calcium. As shown in Figure 28–1 light microscopy demonstrated that the ultrasound plaque ablation sites were smooth and conformed

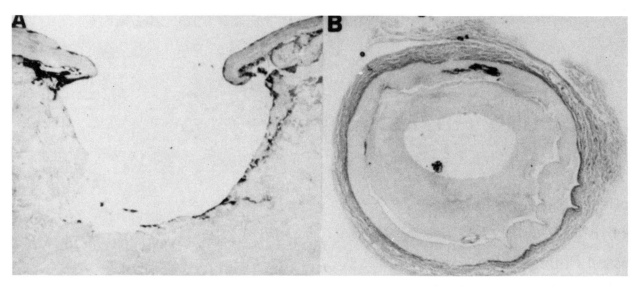

FIG 28–1.
Examples of in vitro results with the solid ball-tipped ultrasound wire probe in atherosclerotic human arteries. **A,** after application of the probe perpendicular to the intimal surface, a crater is created that is limited to the intimal plaque (hematoxylin-eosin stain; the black material in the crater is India ink used to identify sites of sonication). **B,** histologic cross section of an artery that had been totally occluded by atherosclerotic plaque before ultrasound recanalization. After recanalization, a smooth luminal surface conforming to the shape of the ball-tipped probe is present in both **A** and **B.** (From Siegel RJ, et al: *J Invasive Cardiol* 1991; 13: 135–143. Used by permission.)

to the shape of the rounded probe tip. The initial in vitro studies also showed that with continuous-wave ultrasound energy there was a potential for thermal damage and arterial perforation. However, with the use of pulsed-wave and lower-power energies, i.e., power outputs of less than 25 W, peak-to-peak probe tip amplitudes of 111 μm, and crystalloid flush of 20 mL/min, thermal damage and arterial perforation did not occur in vitro. After plaque ablation we analyzed the effluent generated by using a series of graded filters. We found that 90% to 98% of the particulate debris was less than 25 μm. Subsequently, Ernst et al. found the particulate debris to be primarily less than 10 μm.[20]

In vitro confirmation of ultrasonic plaque ablation has also been demonstrated by Rosenschein et al.[15] as well as by Drobinski and Kremer.[18] It has been suggested that there is an energy-dependent differential sparing effect of ultrasound on the normal arterial wall as compared with the plaque of fibrotic and calcified arteries.[20–22]

Demer and Siegel hypothesized that ultrasonic disruption may alter the mechanical properties of severely diseased vessels. In studies of postmortem human calcified arterial segments, they made pressure-volume measurements before and after the intra-arterial application of pulsed-wave ultrasound energy (20-kHz frequency, 25-W power output, and 111-μm peak-to-peak probe amplitude).[24] After exposure to ultrasound the pressure-volume curves shifted to the right, thus indicating a significant increase in arterial distensibility. These data suggest that ultrasonic alteration of calcific plaque by ultrasound enhancement of distensibility might make such lesions more amenable to balloon angioplasty.

IN VITRO STUDIES OF VASCULAR REACTIVITY

Application of ultrasound to arterial rings in vitro was shown by Chokshi and coworkers to result in vasodilation.[25] They proposed that this phenomenon was related to the release of endothelium-derived relaxant factor.[25] The effects of ultrasound on arterial vasomotion in whole-vessel rabbit aortas were studied in detail by Fischell et al.[26] They found that ultrasonic energy caused a dose-dependent relaxation that was independent of the presence or absence of endothelium. This occurred after precontraction with vasoconstrictor substances and was not related to thermal warming during sonication. These findings were corroborated in an in vivo canine model in which ultrasound induced vasodilation at a site of arterial spasm after arterial recanalization. Since it has been observed by cell biologists that ultrasound (20-kHz frequency) reversibly fragments actin filaments at lower energies than those necessary to disrupt cell membranes, Fischell et al. have suggested that the mechanism of ultrasound endothelium-independent vasodilation may be due to the reversible breaking of actin filaments in vascular smooth muscle.[26] This vasodilating effect occurring at energies and frequencies used to ablate plaque could improve the clinical outcome of recanalization procedures by decreasing the frequency and severity of vasospasm after arterial recanalization.

IN VIVO ANIMAL STUDIES

We have used canine models with implanted human atherosclerotic arterial xenografts to study the potential of intra-arterial ultrasound for in vivo recanalization of total occlusions.[21] The 13 atherosclerotic occlusions were 2 to 7 cm in length, 9 were calcified, and 12 were resistant to passage of a conventional guidewire or probe without ultrasound energy. Figure 28–2 demonstrates the in vivo results of ultrasound recanalization of atherosclerotic and calcific human arterial xenografts in a dog model. All 13 occluded atherosclerotic xenografts were recanalized in 15 seconds to 4 minutes (mean, 1.5 ± 1.3 minutes). In these arteries no evidence of vasospasm, thrombosis, dissection, or ultrasound-induced perforation was seen. After ultrasound recanalization

alone the residual stenosis was 62% ± 24%, and when combined with balloon angioplasty, it was 29% ± 13%. On high-resolution (nonscreen) angiograms there were nonocclusive emboli detected in 3 cases after balloon angioplasty that measured 500 to 2,000 μm. In addition, in these dogs 12 normal canine arteries were studied after an average of 3.6 minutes of exposure to ultrasound. Histologic assessment did not reveal evidence of thermal damage, cavitation injury, vacuolization, degeneration, or necrosis of smooth muscle cells in either the xenografts or normal arterial segments exposed to ultrasound. Histologic examination of recanalized segments treated only with ultrasound did not significantly differ from segments after balloon angioplasty: namely, there was focal cracking of plaque and mild separation of the plaque from the media. These studies suggested that it might be clinically feasible to use the ultrasound to create a lumen in an obstructed, guidewire-resistant lesion and that this method could be coupled with balloon angioplasty.

Studies of ultrasound ablation in porcine models of atherosclerosis have been more problematic and less successful. In collaborative studies with Drs. Jeffrey Brinker and Ray Plack, we have encountered complications of iliofemoral arterial dissection and perforation in a porcine atherosclerotic model. In this model it has

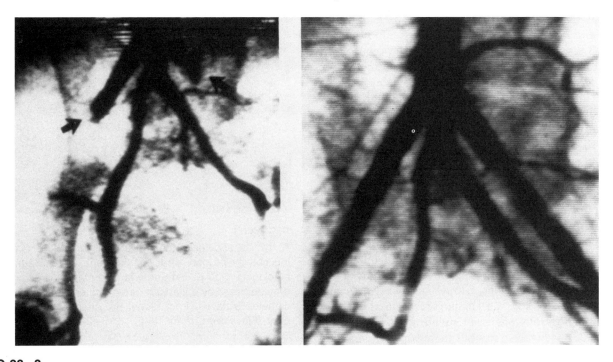

FIG 28–2.
The aortogram on the *left* from a dog shows bilateral external iliac xenograft occlusions *(arrow)*. The 4-cm xenograft occlusions on the *right* were each recanalized within 60 seconds with intermittent ultrasound. Each vessel was subjected to balloon angioplasty to enhance the arterial lumen area. (From Siegel RJ, Ariani M, Forrester JS, et al: *J Invasive Cardiol* 1989; 1:219–229. Used by permission.)

been unclear whether these complications were related to sonication or mechanical trauma from the stiff 0.030-in. titanium wire probe (personal communication). In similar studies by Freeman and coworkers using a 22-kHz system (Sonic Needle, Inc., Farmdale, NY) with 0.02- to 0.03-in. wires, they recanalized five arteries in four pigs. After 2 to 7 minutes of ultrasound the residual stenosis ranged from 20% to 30%. In three of their five cases, arteries were perforated during manipulation of the guide catheter, not during activation of the ultrasound probe.[19]

The chronic effects of ultrasound ablation have been assessed in the normal vasculature of rabbits, dogs, and pigs as well as in the atherosclerotic pig. The histologic findings have ranged from the type of sequelae expected from passage of a guidewire to that found after balloon angioplasty.

IN VITRO AND IN VIVO STUDIES OF THROMBUS DISSOLUTION

The initial studies of Trubestein and Stumpff documented the feasibility of thrombus dissolution in vitro as well as in vivo. They used a 26.8-kHz hollow metal probe 21 to 47 cm long. While this device allowed concomitant aspiration of the thrombus, inflexibility of the stiff metal tubular device limited catheter delivery. Nonetheless, they were able to perform thrombus dissolution in one human case with an acute femoral arterial occlusion. In our studies we have shown in vitro that continuous- or pulsed-wave ultrasound (20-kHz frequency) results in rapid (1 cc of thrombus in 15 seconds) dissolution.[13, 14] In vitro studies showed that the clot dissolution time was inversely related to the ultrasound power output and tip amplitude ($r = 0.95$). Residual particulate measurements with an electronic particle counter of the resistive pulse type revealed that 99% of the debris was less than 10 μm. We performed in vivo studies in 18 canine superficial femoral arteries. Thrombotic occlusions were induced by a combination of arterial crush injury and injection of 200 units of thrombin followed by 2 mL of a 72-hour-old autologous clot. After 4 to 6 hours baseline angiography was performed to document the presence and length of the femoral arterial occlusions. Ultrasound energy intermittently applied for less than 4 minutes recanalized all 18 arteries. Angiography was used for guidance in all 18 cases. Figure 28–3 demonstrates the angiographic findings at baseline and after ultrasound recanalization. In 9 cases angioscopy was also used to more precisely put the probe in direct contact with the intra-arterial thrombus. As shown in Plate 12, the probe can be seen directly against the clot. Angioscopy demonstrated that probe activation caused

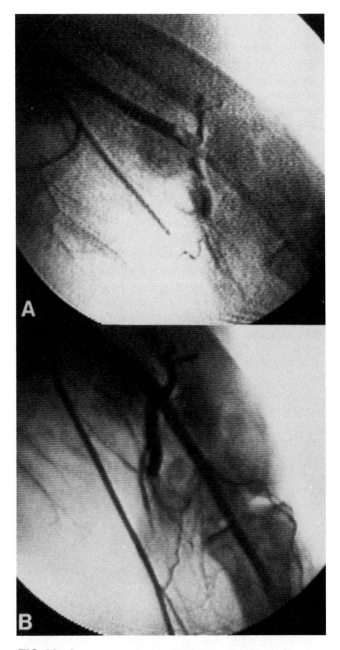

FIG 28–3.
A, canine superficial femoral arterial thrombotic occlusion induced by balloon abrasion, Gelfoam, and a 72-hour-old autologous clot. **B,** the artery is patent after ultrasound energy delivered by a titanium wire probe ensheathed in a 7 F catheter. (Adapted from Siegel RJ, Ariani M, Forrester JS, et al: *J Invasive Cardiol* 1989; 1:219–229.)

rapid clot dissolution without arterial disruption. In our experimental studies angioscopic guidance permitted more complete dissolution of intraluminal clots. Thus there was less residual fibrin deposition along the arterial luminal surface with angioscopically guided clot disruption than when angiography was used alone. Figure 28–4,A demonstrates the two-dimensional ultrasound cross-sectional image of an intraluminal thrombus imaged with a CVIS, Inc. 8 F, 20-mHz ultrasound imaging catheter. After exposure to high-intensity ultrasound, the thrombus has been disrupted and is no longer evident by intravascular ultrasound imaging (Fig 28–4,B). As seen in Figure 28–4,C, during activation of high-intensity, low-frequency ultrasound, cavitation and the resultant "bubbles" lead to a "contrast" effect that defines the arterial lumen.

We believe that our in vitro and in vivo results with high-intensity, low-frequency ultrasound as well as the findings of others[9, 10, 13–15] suggest that ultrasonic clot dissolution could be a potentially effective and safe alternative treatment for peripheral vascular arterial thromboses.

MECHANISM OF ULTRASOUND ABLATION

Ultrasound differs from other catheter-delivered higher-frequency forms of energy such as radiation and microwave in that it is a mechanical form of energy and is nonionizing. Therapeutic ultrasound differs significantly from diagnostic ultrasound in that lower frequencies and higher power intensities are used in therapeutic applications. Therapeutic frequencies of 20 to 100 kHz are used as opposed to 2 to 40 MHz for diagnostic imaging. These higher power intensities are translated in the form of higher amplitudes of probe

motion that give low-frequency ultrasound mechanical ablation characteristics not seen with its higher-frequency counterpart.

Most surgical ultrasound devices use frequencies ranging from 20 to 50 kHz with an amplitude of probe vibration from 10 to 300 μm. The effects of therapeutic ultrasound on tissue are thought to be (1) mechanical vibration, (2) sonic cavitation, (3) the formation of intracellular microcurrents, and (4) thermal warming. In calcified or densely fibrotic plaque the mechanism of action of the ultrasonic probe is primarily mechanical due to the rapid (approximately 20,000 cycles per second [cps] or greater) movement of the probe impacting on the rigid, noncompliant portions of the arterial wall. Normal blood vessels are not damaged due to the small amplitude (100 ± 50 μm) of motion of the ultrasound wire probe. This process is analogous to an orthopedic cast cutter, which saws through the rigid immobile plaster without affecting the normal (elastic) underlying skin, which moves away from the cutter's teeth. We believe that ultrasound dissolution of thrombi is primarily due to cavitation, which is the generation of vapor-filled cavities (bubbles) in tissues, fluids, or cells. There is a threshold intensity above which cavitation occurs. A plausible explanation for the formation of these cavitation nuclei is that they result from consolidation of gas dissolved in the medium or tissue. Several theoretical studies indicate that cavitation during pulsed- or continuous-wave ultrasound should be capable of producing effects in vivo when bubbles produced at the probe tip implode. Such implosions can generate up to and possibly in excess of 6 atm of pressure. Maximal cavitation

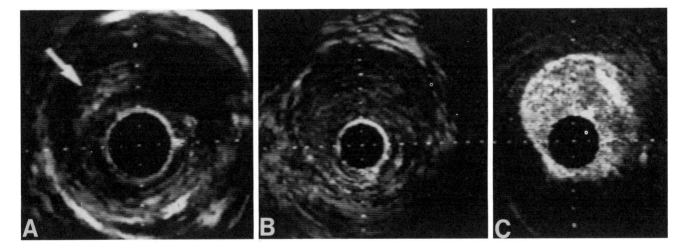

FIG 28–4.
A, intra-arterial two-dimensional ultrasound imaging identifies a thrombus *(arrow)* in vivo in a canine superficial femoral artery. **B,** after application of the ultrasound wire probe to the thrombus it is no longer evident by ultrasound imaging. **C,** intravascular ultrasound imaging during activation of the low-frequency, high-intensity ultrasound ablation probe demonstrates a contrast effect due to cavitation and the generation of microbubbles.

occurs at the interface of materials with differing acoustic impedance.

Heating of tissues may result from dissipation of the ultrasound probe's mechanical energy. When an irrigation solution is used to cool the ultrasound probe, thermal effects are minimal and generally below 40°C.[21] In the absence of irrigation, however, we have generated probe temperatures with continuous-wave energy in excess of 75°C.[22] Such thermal energy may either facilitate therapeutic tissue ablation or cause tissue damage.[12] For our ultrasound ablation studies in humans we have chosen to keep the probe cooled to avoid thermal effects.

ULTRASOUND PLAQUE ABLATION SYSTEM IN DEVELOPMENT

We utilize a low-frequency ultrasound system composed of an ultrasound generator, piezoelectric transducer, flexible metal waveguide, and catheter (Fig 28–5). The system features include a 19.5-kHz operational frequency with a 50% duty cycle operating at 30 ms on followed by 30 ms off. There is a variable power output control on the front panel of the generator that is capable of delivering 25 W maximum power measured calorimetrically at the transducer horn tip. A safety timer has been added to the system to limit the maximum activation of energy to the system to 15 seconds with a minimum of 5 seconds off. Power activation is controlled by a foot switch. Twenty to 25 cc/min of saline or a saline-contrast mixture is required for adequate cooling of the waveguide inside the catheter body. The ultrasound energy is devel-

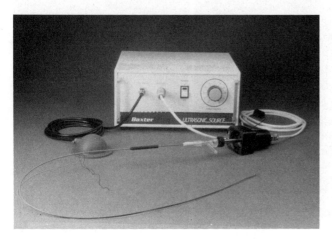

FIG 28–5.
Photograph of a Baxter-Edwards ultrasound generator, foot pedal *(left),* ultrasound transducer *(center),* and wire probe (waveguide) ensheathed in an angiographic catheter.

oped by alternately exciting the piezoelectric crystals inside the transducer with positive and negative sine wave voltage, thus inducing expansion and contraction of the crystals proportionate to the voltage applied across them. The mechanical amplitude generated from the crystals is amplified by a biased acoustic horn attached to the crystals. This action generates a longitudinal wave of energy, also known as a compressional wave, that is then imparted to the waveguide (ultrasound wire probe). Along the waveguide there are nodal points and antinodal points. The nodal points are areas within the metal where the molecules are stationary but are under maximum stress. The antinodal points are areas where the molecules show maximum displacement with minimal stress. The system is designed so that the antinodes occur at the transducer horn tip and the waveguide tip in order to produce maximum displacement. When applying ultrasound energy to a flexible system, waves of energy are also created perpendicular to the incident direction of the energy. These waves are known as transverse waves and cause the wire probe to whip back and forth. The true importance of this mode of energy is not yet fully understood, but it may play an important role in fatigue failure of the wire probe.

When selecting a specific alloy for a waveguide, there are several critical features that are important to its performance. The first is good acoustic transmission. This is a combination of many inherent qualities of a metal including density and hardness. The optimum metal will have high strength, a low modulus of elasticity, and a high proportional limit. These characteristics may be varied to suit the specific application and stresses expected.

Transducer

The transducer is hand-held during the procedure. It contains the piezoelectric elements and the acoustic horn, which is an amplifier that transmits the sound waves from the piezoceramic crystals to the wire probe. The range of power output at the acoustic horn are from 8 to 25 W depending on the setting used.

Wire Probe

To date in clinical trials we have used 0.020- and 0.030-in. wires 50 to 90 cm long with a distal 2-mm ball tip. Wires for clinical use have been made from titanium, while the early prototypes for experimental studies were fabricated out of Elgiloy (a cobalt-nickel alloy). Titanium has much greater durability and is less likely to fracture. With a power output of 8 to 25 W at the acoustic horn, the longitudinal amplitude of the wire probe is 63.5 to 111 μm. A 7 to 8 F guiding catheter ensheathes the ultrasound waveguide. Figure 28–5 shows an example of the generator, transducer, wire probe, and catheter system (Baxter-Edwards LIS, Irvine, Calif) used in our clinical trials.[28] Additional prototype catheters, including an over-the-wire system, are also in development.

METHOD OF PERCUTANEOUS ULTRASOUND ARTERIAL RECANALIZATION

We use an ipsilateral antegrade approach if the proximal segment of the superficial femoral artery is patent or use a retrograde ipsilateral percutaneous popliteal arterial puncture if the femoral artery is occluded at its origin. An introducer sheath is placed in the superficial femoral (7 to 9 F) or popliteal artery (7 F). Twenty to 25 mL of crystalloid per minute is infused through the guide catheter to facilitate cooling of the waveguide during ultrasound ablation. The ultrasound probe catheter system is guided by fluoroscopy. Contrast is intermittently injected through the introducer sheath to assess the progression of arterial recanalization. The ultrasound energy is applied in 15-second intervals for 1 to 5 minutes during passage of the probe through the occlusions and stenoses and during withdrawal of the probe. After crossing each lesion, an angiogram is performed to evaluate arterial patency, percent luminal diameter stenosis, the resultant arterial morphology produced by the probe, and the distal arterial bed for evidence of embolic debris. Medications during the procedure include local lidocaine (Xylocaine) at the catheter insertion site and 3,000 to 5,000 units of intra-arterial heparin. Because the application of ultrasound itself is painless, it does not require analgesia or sedation. Routinely patients have been discharged within 24 to 48 hours of the procedure on a regimen of aspirin (75 to 325 mg).

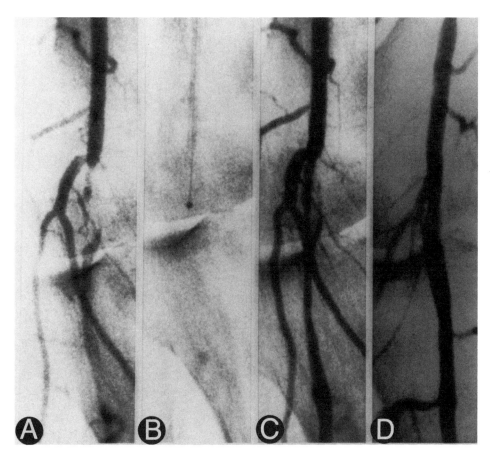

FIG 28–6.
A, total occlusion of the popliteal artery. **B,** ball-tipped ultrasound probe initiating arterial recanalization. **C,** the probe has traversed the lesion to produce an arterial lumen. **D,** definitive lumen produced after balloon angioplasty. (From Siegel RJ, Cumberland DC, Myler RK, et al: *Herz* 1990; 5:329–334. Used by permission.)

CLINICAL STUDIES

As of the end of 1990 we have treated a total of 30 atherosclerotic peripheral vascular obstructions in 27 patients[23, 27, 28] in the laboratories of Dr. David Cumberland (Sheffield, England) and Dr. John Crew (San Francisco). The patients' ages were between 41 and 79 years, and there were 8 women and 19 men. The indications for arterial recanalization were claudication or limb ischemia manifested by lower-extremity ulceration. There were 21 arterial occlusions 1 to 28 cm long. Arterial calcification was present in 10 cases. Of the 9 stenoses, 4 had greater than 85% diameter stenosis. There were 22 superficial femoral and 8 popliteal lesions.

Figure 28–6 demonstrates the angiographic results of ultrasound recanalization of an occluded popliteal artery. Figure 28–7 reveals the angiographic findings after ultrasound recanalization and subsequent balloon angioplasty of a subtotal occlusion of the superficial femoral artery. Figure 28–8 is a schematic showing the findings in the 21 occlusions at baseline, after ultrasound, and after follow-up percutaneous transluminal coronary angioplasty (PTCA). Of the 21 occlusions there were 3 unsuccessful cases. There were 2 cases in which distal access could not be achieved due to inadequate steerability of the probe and 1 case in which the ultrasound recanalization procedure was terminated due to mechanical arterial perforation. Figure 28–9 demonstrates the percent stenosis of the arterial stenoses at baseline, after ultrasound alone, and after follow-up balloon angioplasty. Note that in 6 of 9 stenoses there is a significant increase in lumen diameter whereas there is very little change in 3 cases. To summarize the findings for all cases the mean diameter stenosis fell from 94% ± 11% to 60% ± 20% after ultrasound alone, with the final residual stenosis after balloon angioplasty being 13% ± 7%.

Intraoperative treatment of seven occluded femoral arteries with a 1.6-mm-diameter wire ultrasound probe attached to an acoustic horn with a frequency of 20 kHz has been reported by Rosenschein et al.[29] They also studied six occluded control arteries that were crossed mechanically without activating the wire probe. They noted that the ultrasound-treated arteries, when compared with controls, had a greater recanalized lumen area (5.9 mm vs. 1.7 mm, $P < .05$), greater flow (49 vs. 12 mL/min, $P < .05$), and smaller plaque debris (19 vs. 87 μm, $P < .001$).

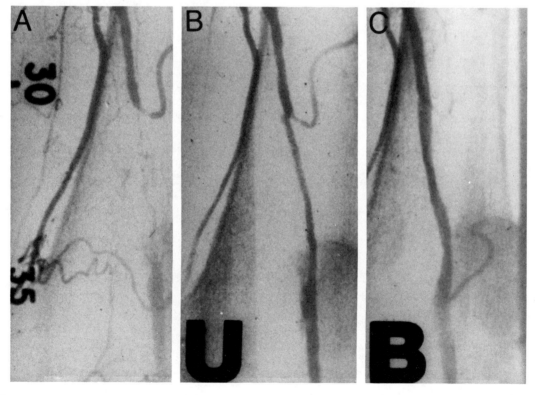

FIG 28–7.
Angiogram of a subtotal occlusion of the distal segment of the superficial femoral artery **(A).** The results of ultrasound recanalization alone are shown in **B.** The final result after further treatment with balloon angioplasty is shown in **C.** (From Siegel RJ, et al: *J Invasive Cardiol* 1991; 13:135–143. Used by permission.)

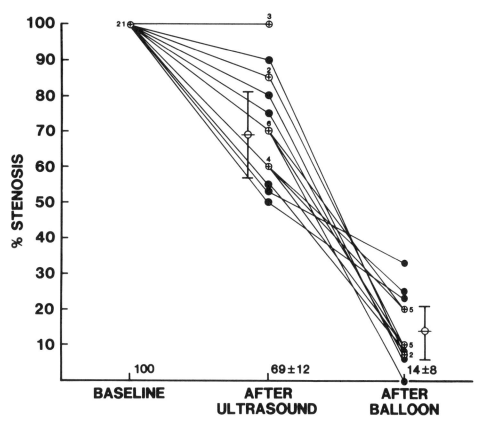

FIG 28–8.
This graph demonstrates the findings after ultrasound alone and subsequent balloon angioplasty in 21 total occlusions of the femoropopliteal arteries in human clinical trials.

Monteverde and coauthors have recently studied ten patients with claudication and peripheral vascular occlusions ($n = 6$) and stenoses ($n = 4$).[30] They used a prototype device with a frequency of 22 kHz and a titanium wire probe (Sonic Needle Inc., Farmdale, NY). All lesions were percutaneously recanalized in less than 80 seconds with a residual stenosis of 48% ± 6% that further fell to 11% ± 5% following balloon angioplasty. They reported no complications.

Restenosis data remain limited due to the relatively few numbers of patients studied. We have follow-up on 23 patients (24 lesions) over a mean of 11 months (range, 2 to 21 months).[27, 28] Patients have been followed symptomatically and with Doppler ankle-brachial indices. In those patients with 8 stenoses and 16 occlusions pretreatment, there have been 4 reocclusions after combined ultrasound and balloon angioplasty. These have been confirmed angiographically and occurred within 3 months of the procedure in 3 of 4 cases. In our limited series all cases in which restenosis has been detected occurred at a site of prior total occlusion. One of these patients underwent repeat balloon angioplasty and again reoccluded. Monteverde and coworkers have fol-

lowed their ten patients angiographically who underwent combined ultrasound and balloon angioplasty. None of their ten patients have had restenoses at 13 ± 2 weeks.[30]

SAFETY AND LIMITATIONS OF PERIPHERAL ULTRASONIC ANGIOPLASTY

With percutaneous application of a 0.020-in. wire ultrasound probe there were no perforations, dissections, emboli, or episodes of vasospasm detected in eight patients.[24, 25] However, the 0.030-in. probe is significantly stiffer and was consequently associated with mechanical trauma, i.e., three perforations and two dissections that were without clinical sequelae.[28] Thus a major and significant limitation of this technology remains the relatively poor flexibility and steerability of the titanium wire probes due to their stiffness. Unlike laser energy, which is readily transmitted via fiber optics around bends, ultrasound energy dissipates and poorly transmits around sharp angles or multiple bends. These factors limit the application of therapeutic intravascular ultra-

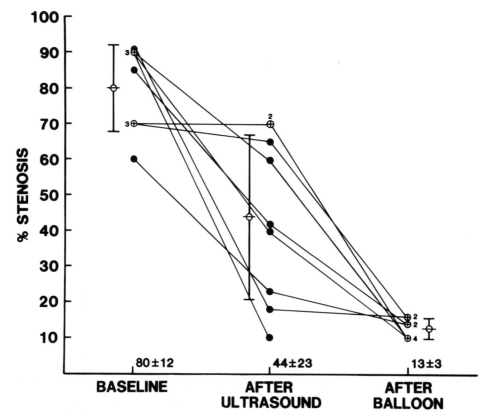

FIG 28–9.
This graph demonstrates the findings in nine stenoses after ultrasound alone and subsequent balloon angioplasty. Note that in five cases the residual stenosis was less than 50% and was 10% in one case after ultrasound alone.

sound to arterial sites that are directly accessible and do not require deployment of ultrasound energy around complex bends.

CONCLUSIONS

Experimental studies have shown that catheter-delivered therapeutic ultrasound recanalizes complete occlusions, reduces stenoses, dissolves thrombus, dilates vessels, and enhances arterial distensibility. The potential clinical applications of therapeutic ultrasound include recanalizing arterial occlusions, reducing arterial stenoses, dissolving thrombi, facilitating balloon angioplasty by increasing arterial compliance, and using it as a stand-alone angioplasty device.

At present, percutaneous peripheral ultrasound angioplasty should be considered in those patients with symptoms of claudication or resting limb ischemia. More specifically, the preferred lesions are those above the knee with a greater than 70% stenosis or an arterial occlusion that can be approached ipsilaterally. The current delivery system with the 0.030-in. wire probe (December 1990) is difficult to use and may result in me-

chanical trauma because of its relative stiffness and inflexibility. Improvements in wire flexibility through utilization of new titanium alloys as well as better wire probe and catheter designs should make this device more "user friendly." It is expected that newly designed over-the-wire ultrasound probes will allow the application of ultrasound angioplasty to lesions below the knee as well as to contralateral vascular occlusions. An intraoperative device for plaque ablation and arterial recanalization is in development for use in less accessible sites such as the coronary arteries.

Acknowledgment

The authors gratefully appreciate the technical skills of Theresa DeBell, R.N.

REFERENCES

1. Brown AH, Davies PG: Ultrasonic decalcification of calcified cardiac valves and annuli. *Br Med J* 1972; 3:274–277.
2. Davidson TA: No lift capsular bag phacoemulsification

and dialing technique for no-hole intraocular lens optic. *J Cataract Refract Surg* 1988; 14:346–349.

3. Brannen GE, Bush WH: Percutaneous ultrasonic versus surgical removal of kidney stones. *Surg Gynecol Obstet* 1985; 161:473–478.

4. Gacetta DJ, Cohen JM, Crummy AB, et al: Ultrasonic lithotripsy of gallstones after cholecystostomy. *Am J Radiol* 1984; 143:1088–1089.

5. Mindich BP, Guarino T, Krenz H, et al: Aortic valve salvage utilizing high frequency vibratory debridement (abstract). *J Am Coll Cardiol* 1987; 11:3.

6. Chan KK, Watmough DJ, Hope DT, et al: A new motor-driven surgical probe and its in vitro comparison with the cavitron ultrasonic surgical aspirator. *Ultrasound Med Biol* 1986; 12:279–283.

7. Hodgson WJB, Del Guercio LRM: Preliminary experience in liver surgery using the ultrasonic scalpel. *Surgery* 1984; 95:230–234.

8. Anscheutz R, Bernard HR: Ultrasonic irradiation and atherosclerosis. *Surgery* 1965; 57:549–553.

9. Trubestein G, Engel C, Etzel F, et al:Thrombolysis by ultrasound. *Clin Sci Mol Med* 1976; 51(suppl):697–698.

10. Stumpff U, Pohlman R, Trubestein G: A new method to cure thrombi by ultrasonic cavitation. *Ultrason Int Conf Proc* 1975; 273–275.

11. Siegel RJ, Fishbein MC, Don Michael TA: Ultrasonic and electrohydraulic atherosclerotic plaque dissolution. *Circulation* 1987; 76(suppl 4):46.

12. Siegel RJ, Fishbein MC, Forrester J, et al: Ultrasound plaque ablation: A new method for recanalization of partially or totally occluded arteries. *Circulation* 1988; 78:1443–1448.

13. Hong AS, Chae JS, Dubin SB, et al: Ultrasonic clot disruption: An in vitro study. *Am Heart J* 1990; 120:418–422.

14. Ariani M, Fishbein MC, Siegel RJ: Angioscopically guided dissolution of arterial thrombi by ultrasound (abstract). *J Am Coll Cardiol* 1991; 17:278.

15. Rosenschein U, Bernstein JJ, Di Segni E, et al: Experimental ultrasonic angioplasty: Disruption of atherosclerotic plaques and thrombi in vitro and arterial recanalization in vivo. *J Am Coll Cardiol* 1990; 15:711–717.

16. Marraccini P, Orsini E, Pelosi G, et al: Low frequency ultrasound energy for selective dissolution of atherosclerotic plaque (abstract). *Eur Heart J* 1988; 9:235.

17. Rosenschein U, Bernstein J, Bakst A, et al: Ultrasonic angioplasty device (abstract). *Circulation* 1988; 78(suppl 2):1077.

18. Drobinski G, Kremer D: Elaboration d'un systeme a ultrasons pour desobstruction des arteres coronaires. *Arch Mal coeur* 1989; 82:377–380.

19. Freeman I, Isner JM, Gal D, et al: Ultrasonic angioplasty using a new flexible wire system (abstract). *J Am Coll Cardiol* 1989; 13:4.

20. Ernst A, Schenk EA, Gracewski SM, et al: Can high-intensity ultrasound selectively destroy human atherosclerotic plaques and minimize residual debris size *Am J Cardiol* 1991; 68:242–246.

21. Siegel RJ, Don Michael TA, Fishbein MC, et al: In vivo ultrasound arterial recanalization of atherosclerotic total occlusion. *J Am Coll Cardiol* 1990; 15:345–351.

22. Siegel RJ, Ariani M, Forrester JS, et al: Cardiovascular applications of therapeutic ultrasound. *J Invasive Cardiol* 1989; 1:219–229.

23. Siegel RJ, Cumberland DC, Myler RK, et al: Percutaneous ultrasonic angioplasty: Initial clinical experience. *Lancet* 1989; 9:772–774.

24. Demer LL, Siegel RJ: Artery compliance improves after ultrasonic ablation of atherosclerotic lesions (abstract). *J Am Coll Cardiol* 1990; 15:104.

25. Chokshi SK, Rongione AJ, Freeman I, et al: Ultrasonic energy produces endothelium-dependent vasomotor relaxation in vitro (abstract). *Circulation* 1989; 80(suppl 2):565.

26. Fischell TA, Abbas M, Grant GW, et al: Ultrasonic energy causes dose-dependent, endothelium-independent arterial relaxation (abstract). *Circulation* 1990; 82(suppl 2):306.

27. Siegel RJ, Cumberland DC, Myler RK, et al: Percutaneous peripheral ultrasonic angioplasty. *Herz* 1990; 5:329–334.

28. Siegel RJ, Don Michael TA, Crew JR, et al: Percutaneous ultrasound angioplasty: Acute angiographic and angioscopic findings and long-term clinical results (abstract). *J Am Coll Cardiol* 1991; 17(suppl 3):236.

29. Rosenschein U, Kraus L, Marboe CC, et al: Ultrasonic angioplasty: Initial clinical results in peripheral vascular disease (abstract). *Circulation* 1990; 82(suppl 3):306.

30. Monteverde C, Velez M, Victorio R, et al: Percutaneous transluminal ultrasonic angioplasty in totally occluded peripheral arteries: Immediate and intermediate clinical results (abstract). *Circulation* 1990; 82(suppl 3):678.

PART V

Stents

29

Stents for Bailout and Restenosis

Spencer B. King III, M.D.

The mechanism of coronary angioplasty is expansion of the constricted arterial lumen to produce cracks in the intima, various degrees of splits into the media, and often separation of the plaque from the vessel wall. After the balloon is deflated and removed, the arterial pressure keeps the artery open, but some recoil of the tissues results in a lumen that is consistently smaller than the inflated balloon. On average that recoil amounts to about 30% of the diameter or 50% of the cross-sectional area. Closure of coronary arteries after angioplasty is obviously multifactorial, but the decreased lumen just after balloon deflation may play a role in both acute closure and late restenosis.

The concept of intracoronary stenting arises from a recognized need in some cases to counter this elastic recoil phenomenon and to reattach these separated plaque segments. If a prosthetic device is placed in the artery after balloon deflation, then the vessel may be held open to the same size as the balloon and the adjacent unobstructed artery. By leaving a larger lumen, the chance of early reclosure and late restenosis may be minimized. Some arteries are so severely dissected that acute occlusion immediately after angioplasty occurs. In those cases, dissected intimal flaps can be reapproximated to result in a restored functional lumen. Another mechanism by which stents are advantageous is by creating smoother walls of the dilated artery. The irregular geometry created by plaque fissuring and separation from the vessel wall is a perfect substrate for platelet deposition and thrombus formation.[1] Chesebro et al. have shown a direct correlation between the extent of injury and the amount of platelet deposition.[2] Stenting, by the mechanism of sealing flaps and cracks, creates a smoother inner surface of the lumen. Whether these beneficial effects of stenting, i.e., providing a wide and smoother lumen, will translate into a reduced risk of acute closure and late restenosis has been the subject of

ongoing stent investigations. In this chapter, I will describe some of the background experimental work on stenting, the various stent designs that are under investigation, the use of stents in the setting of acute closure, the potential for stents to reduce the rate of restenosis, and the future for stents as a local drug delivery system.

EXPERIMENTAL TESTING

Animal testing of stents has been instructive but has left more questions unanswered than answered. As early as the late 1960s, Dotter was placing wire coil grafts in dog femoral arteries and assessing long-term patency.[3] More recently the Palmaz-Schatz stent[4] and the Gianturco-Roubin stent[5] have been evaluated in dog coronary arteries. The healing phenomenon is very consistent and limited. Within a few days, cells resembling endothelial cells begin to cover the stent wires, and within 2 weeks there is a confluent covering. The neoendothelial lining thickens until about 8 weeks, reaches a maximal thickness of about 200 to 400 μm, and then begins to regress. Dog coronary arteries examined as late as 2 years show a thin covering over the stent.

Hypercholesterolemic rabbits with stents placed in the iliac arteries developed atherosclerosis internal and external to the stent.[6] At 1 month even though there was extensive atherosclerosis in the stented segment, the lumen of the stented iliac arteries retained greater patency than did the dilated but not stented control iliac arteries.

The pig coronary model has been used by the group at the Mayo Clinic and our group at Emory to test the balloon overstretch plus stent placement in an effort to duplicate the situation encountered in human angioplasty.[7, 8] These injured pig arteries sustained significant damage, and the healing process produces extensive proliferation within the stent. Thrombosis in the stented segment is a problem, and arteries harvested 4 hours after stent placement showed extensive thrombosis. It is felt that this normolipemic pig coronary model may be the best nonprimate model in which to test new strategies for successful stent placement.

TYPES OF STENTS UNDER INVESTIGATION

It is unclear whether the design of stents is of importance in achieving the results desired. Nonetheless, there are significant differences among stent designs. At the present time, more than 20 different stent designs have been proposed. The Medinvent stent is a self-expanding mesh that resembles a Chinese finger splint. In the relaxed state it is expanded. When pulled from the ends, it constricts in diameter and remains constrained by a covering membrane. When the membrane is removed, the stent is released and expands to the size of the artery in which it is deployed. The Palmaz-Schatz stent is composed of a cylindrical stainless steel tube with slots cut so that when it is expanded by a balloon it is deformed into a diamond-shaped matrix. The balloon expansion of the metal device overcomes any elastic component in the metal so that the stent remains deformed in the expanded state. Other balloon-expandable stents are made of stainless steel wire similar to suture material. The Cook (Gianturco-Roubin), Medtronic (Wiktor), and Cordis stents are examples of various coil configurations. Another stent by Boston Scientific (Strecker) is a wire mesh design. All these stents have the ability to perform a scaffolding function; however, there are differences. The Medinvent and Palmaz-Schatz stents provide the smoothest angiographic appearance of the dilated artery. The coil stents have wider interstices, and therefore some dimpling occurs in the vessel wall at the site of each wire loop. The coil stents have, on the other hand, excellent flexibility and can therefore be placed in arteries around moderate curves. Whether flexibility after placement, as is possible with the coil or mesh stents or a rigid artery segment as occurs with the Palmaz-Schatz stent, is important for long-term patency is unresolved.

STENTS AS BAILOUT DEVICES FOLLOWING FAILED ANGIOPLASTY

The most obvious use of stent technology is for the acutely dissected and obstructed coronary artery. The Medinvent, Palmaz-Schatz, and Cook stents have been used for this indication. Closure of coronary arteries following angioplasty occurred in 6.8% of patients treated in the National Heart, Lung and Blood Institute (NHLBI) registry in 1985 and 1986.[9] These patients who suffered acute closure had a five times greater mortality risk and a 27% risk of acute myocardial infarction. Most of these patients, of course, required urgent bypass surgery. Traditional therapy for acute closure has included repeat balloon inflations and prolonged balloon inflations, sometimes using perfusion balloons. If these measures fail, the usual approach to such patients, namely, emergency bypass surgery, has in the past been effective. The low mortality rate in such patients reported earlier by our group[10] has been difficult to maintain in more complex patients undergoing angioplasty. Placement of intracoronary stents in this setting is designed either as a bailout procedure to relieve the acute ischemia and move the patient to bypass surgery or for a more permanent restoration of flow.

The Medinvent stent was utilized for acute closure in 14 of 105 patients receiving the stent in the early experience.[11] In a separate report,[12] the results of stenting for acute closure were detailed; however, most of these patients (13) underwent subsequent early bypass surgery on a semielective basis.

Our major experience with stenting in the setting of acute closure is with the Gianturco-Roubin (Cook) stent. This balloon-expandable stainless steel coil stent had been tested extensively in our institution in animal models and seemed to be well tolerated. We began investigations in the fall of 1987 with a pilot study to assess the ability of the stent to open the artery. In this protocol, the patients were all taken to bypass surgery following stent placement.[13, 14] This experience showed that ischemia could be remarkably reversed by stent placement, that the angiographic lumen could be reestablished, and that normal angiographic flow could be reestablished predictably.

Subsequently a protocol was approved for stent placement in the setting of an acutely disrupted artery in which surgery was not mandated but was left to the discretion of the operator. By utilizing this protocol between September 1988 and December 1990, 100 stents were placed in 93 patients.[15] Patients included were those with complete occlusion at the time of or shortly following angioplasty that could not be resolved with repeat balloon inflations or evidence for imminent closure that consisted of severe dissections or intraluminal plaque that compromised greater than 50% of the lumen and could not be resolved with repeated balloon inflations. The decision to move to bypass surgery rested with the perceived consequence of recurrent arterial closure. Arteries supplying small areas of myocardium were suitable for continued observation of the stent without surgery, as were large arteries supplying critical areas of myocardium if good collateral systems feeding the distal segment existed. Relative exclusions to stenting were diffusely diseased arteries, multiple lesions in the same artery, the presence of triple-vessel disease, or significant impairment in left ventricular function, as well as akinetic contralateral ventricular wall motion. The smallest stent size available was 2.5 mm, and therefore segments smaller than this as well as segments involving severe bends or branch points that precluded stent placement were avoided. Contraindications to anticoagulation or antiplatelet therapy as well as obvious thrombus formation in the area to be stented were also exclusions.

Stent placement was accompanied by preprocedural therapies of aspirin, intravenous heparin, and calcium channel blocking agents plus dipyridamole, 75 mg, dextran 40 at a rate of 100 mL/hr, and intracoronary nitroglycerin. The dextran was continued at a rate of 100 mL/hr throughout stent placement and then reduced to 50 mL/hr until 500 mL had been administered. More recently, longer infusions of dextran have been advocated. Stents were selected to be slightly larger than the estimated diameter of the artery since this stent design exhibits slight elastic recoil. Additional heparin was given liberally at least every hour during the procedure, and following the procedure a continuous heparin infusion at approximately 1,000 units/hr was begun. Some sheaths were removed the same day after a temporary discontinuation of the heparin to allow the activated clotting time to decline to 150 seconds. Other patients received continuous heparin infusion without interruption until the next day that the sheaths were removed. Following sheath removal a bolus of heparin (2,000 to 5,000 units) and continued infusion were instituted and continued for 3 to 5 days. Further drug therapy included warfarin (Coumadin) adjusted to raise the prothrombin time to 1.5 to 2 times control; aspirin, 80 mg/day; dipyridamole, 75 mg three times a day; diltiazem (Cardizem), 60 mg 4 times a day; and a transdermal nitroglycerin patch. Creatine kinase concentrations and electrocardiograms were obtained serially, and the patients were typically discharged on the fifth day following stenting unless complications occurred.

One hundred two patients with acute closure or threatened acute closure underwent attempted stenting; 109 stents were used in 104 percutaneous transluminal coronary angioplasty (PTCA) procedures. In 9 patients, stents could not be deployed because of an inability to pass the stent through the guiding catheter or through the stenosis itself. All these were removed without losing any stents into the circulation. Ninety-three patients were therefore stented and their results evaluated. Ninety of the 93 stent placements were angiographically successful, that is, they reduced the diameter of the stenosis by greater than 50%. Three patients had successful stent placement, but angiographically the artery was not opened to this degree. Eighty-five of the placements were carried out in native arteries and 10 in saphenous vein grafts. Some characteristics of the stented patients included age, 57 ± 11 years; male, 79%; unstable angina, 79%; class III or IV angina, 73%; prior myocardial infarction, 33%; multivessel coronary disease, 43%; ejection fraction, $56 \pm 13\%$ and restenotic lesions, 44%. Some stent placements followed the use of other new technologies. Two patients had atherectomy, 6 had excimer laser therapy, and 7 had laser balloon angioplasty in attempts to solve their acute closure syndrome. The quantitative angiographic stenosis prior to stenting averaged 67%, and following stent placement it was 16%. Relief of ischemia was documented by the fact that of the 58 patients with angina just prior to stent placement, 51 had their angina relieved, and of the 57 patients with ST elevation prior to stenting, 46 patients had resolution of their ST segments to baseline.

Despite successful stent placement in these patients with acute occlusion, complications were relatively frequent. There were 5 deaths, 2 of which seemed unrelated to the stent placement. One had surgery and postoperative peptic ulcer disease with perforation and expired 2 months after the procedure without evidence of ischemia. Another patient suffering left main occlusion during diagnostic catheterization had a stent placed following a prolonged attempt at cardiopulmonary resuscitation; however myocardial function could not be reestablished. One patient with severe chronic obstructive pulmonary disease vomited and aspirated in the poststent follow-up period and sustained a cardiac arrest. The stent was found to be patent and thrombus free at the time of autopsy. Two patients, however, died either as a result of stent placement or because of complications of the antithrombotic therapy. One, who received two stents in the right coronary artery and went to bypass surgery because of severe hypotension documented when total occlusion was present, suffered sudden cardiogenic shock following postoperative protamine reversal. Although no autopsy was obtained, it was speculated that stent thrombosis occurred. Another patient suffered a fatal stroke several days following stenting while receiving heparin. This was assumed to be due to intracranial hemorrhage. In-hospital surgery was performed in 18.9%, Q wave myocardial infarction occurred in 5.2%, repeat PTCA in 5.2%, and subacute closure after the stenting procedure in 7.3%. Sixty-seven patients, or 74%, had none of these complications following stent placement. The other major problems were related to the femoral puncture site. Because of continued anticoagulation in a rather vigorous manner, femoral artery hematoma occurred in 33%, and pseudoaneurysm repair was required in 8%. During a 14-month follow-up period there have been 2 additional deaths, 1 from acute respiratory failure and 1 following bypass surgery. Bypass surgery was subsequently required in 11 patients, 2 patients suffered Q wave myocardial infarction, and 15 patients had repeat angioplasty.

Although restenosis was not the subject of this trial, angiographic follow-up postdischarge was obtained in 50 patients when they became eligible for a 6-month restudy. This represented 82% of the patients eligible for restudy (that is, those who did not have early bypass surgery). Of the 50 patients restudied, 25 had restenosis defined by 50% or greater diameter reduction. Restenosis was somewhat higher in the circumflex artery (79%) or in the saphenous vein grafts (100%) than in the left anterior descending (LAD) (42%) or right coronary artery (39%).

Restenosis occurring within the stents has been treated with redilatation in 16 patients. At the present time 8 of those patients have been restudied and 6 have developed a second restenosis. Repeat dilatation within the stent produces an excellent angiographic appearance with very little elastic recoil due to the rigid stent wires in the media. Although the numbers are small at the present time, the restenosis observed after such a procedure, however, remains disquieting.

In a small subset of the patients, a vigorous antiproliferative program was attempted. In addition to the previously mentioned antithrombotic and antiplatelet agents, hydrocortisone and colchicine were administered to a group of patients.[15] Among these patients, 16 have undergone late restudy to evaluate symptoms or to perform a 6-month routine restudy. The restenosis rate in this group is not different from the overall group; however, there were 6 patients who developed aneurysms within the stented segment, an indication of nonhealing. This is the first documentation of altered healing in angioplasty, and although it is not a desired result, it is of some interest in the future investigation of restenosis strategies.

Since the results presented here, we have continued to utilize this stent and the Palmaz-Schatz stent as bailout devices in acute closure situations and have modified the poststent anticoagulation program slightly. Experience from other stent programs teaches us that the long-term results in larger arteries are significantly superior to those in smaller arteries. It is important to note that in this series, approximately 25% of the patients received 2.5-mm stents. Whereas late restenosis is an undesired outcome in the setting of acute closure

with ischemic syndrome, the ability to bail out of that situation with a stent is quite desirable. The availability of stents for this purpose has become a major nonsurgical backup procedure for high-risk angioplasty. Virtually all patients undergoing angioplasty in our center are informed of the availability of stents and are asked to sign experimental protocols allowing the use of stents if necessary for the occurrence of a nonsolvable acute closure syndrome. However, because of the obvious added burden of prolonged anticoagulation and prolonged hospitalization, all efforts are aimed at solving the acute closure problems without stent placement.

STENTS USED FOR THE PREVENTION OF RESTENOSIS

The first large stent experience utilized for restenosis was with the self-expanding Wallstent in an investigation carried out entirely in Europe.[16] The first Wallstent was implanted in 1986. Between that time and March 1990, 265 patients were enrolled, with 308 lesions treated. One hundred seventy-three of those lesions were in native arteries and 135 in bypass grafts. Whereas the end point of the stent program was primarily to evaluate the effect on restenosis, some of the stents were placed for bailout purposes at the time of initial angioplasty. This occurred in 33% of the native stent implantations and in 4% of the vein graft implantations. Half of the native stent procedures were performed in restenotic lesions, and 21% of the bypass graft implantations were also for restenotic lesions. Anticoagulation was spottedly administered in the early portion of this experience, and there was a problem with thrombosis within 2 weeks of stent implantation in 15% of the patients. Of the patients who did not suffer early thrombotic closure, restenosis as defined by the 50% diameter definition occurred in 20% of the native coronary arteries and in 34% of the vein grafts. The restudy rate in this series was 82%, and it is important to emphasize that the studies were performed by automated edge detection quantitative angiographic measures in a core laboratory.

The conclusion that can be reasonably surmised from this data would suggest that whereas this particular stent, in the manner in which it was used, resulted in perhaps an unacceptable early thrombotic closure rate, the restenosis rate was respectable and perhaps reduced below what would have been expected for similar lesions not stented. This conclusion can only be speculative, of course, because a randomized trial has not been conducted.

The Palmaz-Schatz stent has undergone a carefully controlled trial to evaluate its effect on restenosis. An angiographic core laboratory has now been established to evaluate this stent.[17] Patients selected for this trial must have (1) objective evidence of ischemia, (2) critical stenoses greater than 70% by visual estimation, (3) preserved left ventricular function, and (4) suitability for coronary artery bypass surgery. Important exclusions were recent acute myocardial infarction, diffuse disease, ostial stenosis, large diseased side branches, pre-existent coronary thrombi, unprotected left main stenosis, and extreme vessel tortuosity. The protocol calls for aspirin therapy, 325 mg daily; dipyridamole, 75 mg three times a day; calcium channel antagonists; low–molecular-weight dextran; heparin, 1,000 units initially with continuous infusion or intermittent boluses to maintain activated clotting time greater than 300 seconds throughout the procedure; and following stent placement heparin administration continued for several days until warfarin therapy could increase the prothrombin time to greater than 16 seconds. Aspirin therapy is continued indefinitely, and dipyridamole and calcium antagonists are continued for 3 months. Coumadin anticoagulation is continued for 1 to 3 months. During the first phase of the trial of this stent, 226 patients underwent attempted placement, and 94%, or 213 patients, had successful stent placement. Subacute thrombosis, that is, thrombosis occurring within the first 2 weeks, occurred in 8 patients, or 3.8%. Excluding those patients, 205 patients were eligible for follow-up angiography, which was performed in 165 patients, or 80% of that group, 5.5 months following stent implantation. This study was limited to native coronary arteries; however, once again restenotic lesions were included and represent 65% of the total population.

Restenosis was determined by an automated edge detection computer-assisted quantitative methodology performed by a core angiographic laboratory. By utilizing the definition of a 50% stenosis at final follow-up, restenosis occurred in 34% of the patients. Subgroup analysis revealed some important differences. Placement of multiple stents resulted in a higher restenosis rate, with 21 of 40, or 53%, of the patients having restenosis. There was no difference in the restenosis rate relative to the artery stented. Previously observed higher restenosis rates with balloon angioplasty in the proximal anterior descending artery were not seen in this stent experience. Larger arteries had a better maintained patency, with arteries greater than 3.2 mm in diameter having a restenosis rate of 21% and arteries smaller than this having a restenosis rate of 37%. As mentioned, two thirds of these patients had restenotic lesions rather than de novo lesions. The restenosis rate for de novo lesions was 25% vs. 34% for restenotic lesions. In the subgroup that received a single stent for a de novo lesion, the restenosis rate was 13%. This study certainly achieved better early results, with perhaps more careful selection and vigorous anticoagulation playing a role. It is not clear whether the design of the stent, which as mentioned earlier differs significantly from the coil stents or the interdigitating mesh stents, is an important factor. There is clearly a broad range of restenosis rates depending on the type of lesion treated. This fact certainly calls for a randomized trial of stenting vs. balloon angioplasty in a wide array of lesions in which stenting shows promise. Such trials are currently in the planning stage.

FUTURE DIRECTIONS FOR CORONARY STENTING

Whereas coronary stenting seems to have proved to be an effective means of solving the abrupt closure of arteries, its effect on restenosis, although encouraging, needs significantly more study. The price of stenting remains high. The threat of thrombotic closure necessitates a vigorous anticoagulation program. The use of anticoagulants significantly increases the risk of bleeding complications, dramatically prolongs the patient's hospitalization, and increases costs. An effective anticoagulant and antiplatelet therapy that is administered systemically may reduce acute thrombotic closure but will not reduce the hemorrhagic complications unless some dramatic breakthroughs in antithrombotic therapy are achieved. Various agents including antithrombins and antiplatelet antibodies as well as polymers to inhibit platelet activity have been proposed and will soon undergo more extensive testing. Another approach is the application of such antithrombotic agents directly to stents, and many efforts are under way to incorporate these agents into the stent itself. This could be accomplished with the coating of existing metallic stents or the replacement of the metal stent with a totally polymer device. Such polymers could be biodegradeable or nondegradeable. In any case, the role for stenting in interventional cardiology will obviously be an important one for the future and, as with so many other breakthroughs, creates its own list of interesting problems for exploration by scientists in the future.

REFERENCES

1. Liu MW, Roubin GS, King SB III: Restenosis after coronary angioplasty: Potential biologic determinants and role of intimal hyperplasia. *Circulation* 1989; 79:1374–1387.
2. Chesebro JH, Lam JYT, Badimon L, et al: Restenosis after arterial angioplasty: A hemorrheologic response to injury. *Am J Cardiol* 1987; 60:10–16.
3. Dotter CT: Transluminally placed coil-spring endarterial

tube grafts, long-term patency in canine popliteal artery. *Invest Radiol* 1969; 4:329–332.

4. Schatz RA, Palmaz JC, Tio FO, et al: Balloon expandable intercoronary stents in the adult dog. *Circulation* 1987; 76:450–457.

5. Roubin GS, Robinson KA, King SB, et al: Early and late results of intracoronary arterial stenting after coronary angioplasty in dogs. *Circulation* 1987; 76:891–897.

6. Robinson KA, Roubin GS, Siegel RJ, et al: Intraarterial stenting in the atherosclerotic rabbit. *Circulation* 1988; 78:646–653.

7. Karas SP, Gravanis MB, Robinson KA, et al: Comparison of the response to coronary artery balloon injury and stenting in swine: An animal model of restenosis. *J Am Coll Cardiol*, in press.

8. Schwartz RS, Murphy JG, Edwards WD, et al: Restenosis after balloon angioplasty: Practical proliferative model in porcine coronary arteries. *Circulation* 1990; 82:2190–2200.

9. Detre KM, Holmes DR, Holubkov R, et al: Incidence and consequences of periprocedural occlusion. The 1985–1986 National Heart, Lung, and Blood Institute Percutaneous Transluminal Coronary Angioplasty Registry. *Circulation* 1990; 82:739–750.

10. Talley JD, Weintraub WS, Roubin GS, et al: Failed elective percutaneous transluminal coronary angioplasty requiring coronary artery bypass surgery: In-hospital and late clinical outcome at 5 years. *Circulation* 1990; 82:1203–1213.

11. Serruys PW, Strauss BH, Beatt KJ, et al: Angiographic follow-up after placement of a self-expanding coronary artery stent. *N Engl J Med* 1991; 324:13–17.

12. deFeyter PJ, DeScheerder I, van den Brand M, et al: Emergency stenting for refractory acute coronary artery occlusion during coronary angioplasty. *Am J Cardiol* 1990; 66:1147–1150.

13. Roubin GS, Douglas JS Jr, Lembo NJ, et al: Intracoronary stenting for acute closure following percutaneous transluminal coronary angioplasty (PTCA). *Circulation* 1988; 78(suppl 2):407.

14. Roubin GS, King SB III, Douglas JS Jr, et al: Intracoronary stenting during percutaneous transluminal coronary angioplasty. *Circulation* 1990; 81(suppl 4):92–100.

15. Hearn JA, King SB III: Restenosis after Gianturco-Roubin stent placement for acute closure, in Serruys, PW, Strauss B, Kings S (eds): *Restenosis*. Dodrecht, The Netherlands, Kluwer, in press.

16. Rab ST, King SB, Roubin GS, et al: Coronary aneurysms following stent placement: A suggestion of altered vessel healing in the presence of anti-inflammatory agents. *J Am Coll Cardiol*, in press.

17. Bertrand ME, Puel J, Meier B, et al: The Wallstent experience: 1986–1990, in Serruys PW, Strauss B, King S, (eds): *Restenosis*. Dodrecht, The Netherlands, Kluwer, in press.

18. Schatz RA, Baim DS, Leon M, et al: Clinical experience with the Palmaz-Schatz coronary stent. Initial results of a multicenter study. *Circulation* 1991; 83:148–161.

30

Nonsurgical Implantation of a Self-Expanding Intravascular Stent Prosthesis

George I. Frank, M.D.
Ulrich Sigwart, M.D.

CLINICAL BACKGROUND

Despite the considerable improvements that have been made in equipment and the developments made in clinical technique, percutaneous coronary angioplasty is still associated with a traumatic assault on the integrity of both arteriosclerotic and native vessel walls. The fluid dynamics of the acute postdilatation vessel and the long-term healing of the traumatized surfaces remain continuing problems. Acute occlusion occurs in 5% of cases, and restenosis rates may be as high as 35% within the first months of recovery.[1, 2] The fact that these statistics remained constant despite the experience and progress attained with angioplasty leads one to propose that a logical approach to preventing both acute occlusion and restenosis may be the use of an intraluminal scaffolding device, or stent, to support and smooth the traumatized lumen.

Early research work with various types of stent prostheses has shown that the metal surface is covered by cellular proliferation that encapsulates the device into the vessel wall and protects it from further contact with blood.[3, 4] None of the present design concepts, however, come reasonably close to the ideal intravascular stent, especially with respect to homogeneous force distribution, ease of access, conformability, and stability. Therefore, a new system was developed that combined a stainless steel, multifilament, self-expanding, macroporous prosthesis and an innovative delivery instrument (Medinvent, Lausanne, Switzerland). After successful animal trials, in 1986 this device became the first to be implanted into a human coronary artery.[5] Since then over 200 of these devices have been implanted in Lausanne and London. In this chapter we will summarize the results.

Methods

The stent is woven from a surgical-grade stainless steel alloy formulated to International Standards Organization prescriptions. Because of its design (Fig 30–1) and process of fabrication, the prosthesis can be made geometrically stable and self-expanding. The elastic and compliant properties of the prosthesis geometry allow for moderate longitudinal elongation to significantly decrease the diameter of the prosthesis. The prosthesis can therefore be constrained on a narrow delivery catheter, and as the constraining membrane is progressively removed, the device will return to its original, unconstrained diameter. When the device is implanted into a vessel whose caliber is smaller than the unconstrained prosthesis, there will be some residual elastic, radial force that will act against the vessel wall to prevent any elastic wall recoil and help to maintain the stent position.

The constrained wire mesh prosthesis is retained at the distal end of the delivery catheter by a double-layer membrane that can be progressively withdrawn by virtue of a fluid film between the layers. Low friction during the deployment process is maintained by filling of the intermediate space with contrast medium at approximately 3 bars of pressure. Two or three radiopaque metal markers on the delivery catheter permit identification of the extremities of the metal prosthesis at the time of deployment. The outer diameter of the loaded delivery system is 1.57 mm; a prosthesis up to 6.5 mm

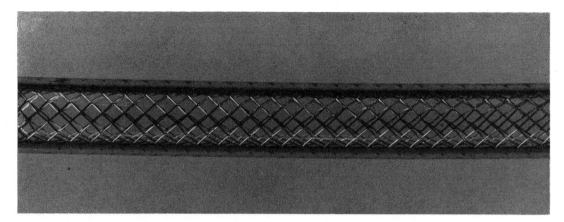

FIG 30–1.
Self-expanding, elastic, macroporous tubular prosthesis woven from stainless steel.

in nominal diameter can be mounted on such a delivery device. Large-diameter prostheses for peripheral use have a correspondingly larger delivery catheter.

Animal Experimentation

A prosthesis up to 6.5 mm in diameter mounted on the delivery catheter could be passed through conventional guiding catheters to the femoral, popliteal, and coronary arteries of animals without difficulty. Under pentobarbital anesthesia with fluoroscopic control, 15 stents were implanted into 25 to 35-kg mongrel dogs who received no anticoagulants or antiplatelet drugs before or after implantation. In general during catheterization the animals were given an intravenous heparin infusion of 25 units/kg body weight per hour. One dog received only 12.5 units of heparin per kilogram of body weight which led to an acute thrombosis of the prosthesis. This was spontaneously recanalized during the first 3 weeks of follow-up.

In three dogs, eight transluminal implants under adequate heparinazation were placed into branches of the femoral arteries at the level of the knee by way of the common femoral artery (Fig 30–2). The prostheses varied from 2 to 6.5 mm in diameter and between 20 to 70 mm in length. The prostheses were patent immediately after implantation and remained patent after successive angiographic controls at 3-month intervals up to 1 year. Weekly Doppler flow monitoring also indicated equally positive results. Two dogs were electively sacrificed after 6 and 9 months of survival. Three stents were perfectly patent, one of which demonstrated a mural thrombus. One stent demonstrated recanalization after retrograde perfusion in an artery that had been ligated proximally. The prostheses remained free from intimal hyperplasia, and moreover, all side branches leaving the

stented segments of the main vessel remained clearly patent (Figs 30–2 and 30–3).

In seven dogs, seven coronary stents were implanted by the femoral technique with 8 F coronary guiding catheters. Under fluoroscopy, one stent was placed in the right coronary artery, one stent was placed in the first marginal branch of the right coronary artery, and five prostheses were placed in the proximal segment of the left anterior descending coronary artery. Prosthesis dimensions varied between 2.5 and 3.5 mm in diameter and 15 and 20 mm in length. No anticoagulants were given after implantation, but heparin was infused intraoperatively. On control angiography at 3 and 6 months after implantation, no signs of obstruction either from thrombus or hyperplasia were seen. However, when the animals were sacrificed at 9 months, one case of nonobstructive mural thrombus was seen that was probably caused by diameter mismatch between the artery and stent.

Histologic Analysis

From previous trials with an early prosthesis design, histologic analyses at 24 hours, 4 weeks, 3 months, and 6 months, respectively, demonstrated the following four mechanisms of prosthesis–vessel wall interaction[6]:

1. There is an initial abrasion of the endothelial lining.
2. Within a period of 1 month the intima thickens, fills the spaces between the metal filaments of the prosthesis, and smoothly covers the entire prosthesis.
3. After 3 months the intimal covering is stabilized, and no further evolution occurs.
4. No perforation of the internal elastic lamina is seen, and no damage to the media is apparent as evidenced by a lack of vacuolization.

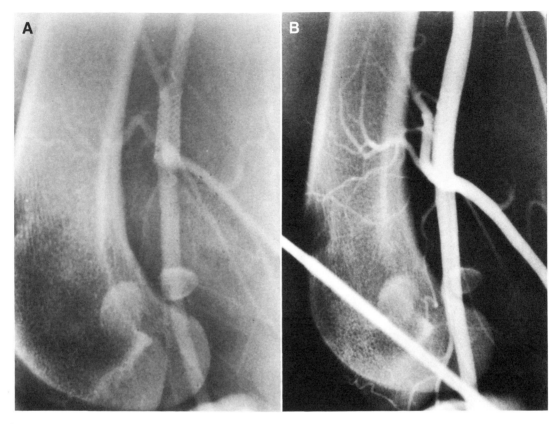

FIG 30–2.
The endoluminal stent prosthesis after implantation in a canine femoral artery. The faint contrast injection **(A)** allows for better identification of the stent and the side branch leaving the stented segment. **B**, artery with regular contrast injection.

Figure 30–3 gives an example of a prosthesis firmly embedded in the arterial wall. This specimen was recovered from a branch of the femoral artery at the level of the left knee 9 months after implantation. Scanning electron microscopy shows the intima filling the pores between the stent filaments in a rather smooth fashion. The thickness of the neointimal layer is about 450 μm, and no signs of necrosis due to continuous mural pressure from the stent are seen. The endothelial surface (Fig 30–4,A) is very similar to the original arterial endothelium (Fig 30–4,B). All side branches within the stented segments remained open. The stents were covered with smooth intimal lining when the arteries were removed for analysis after 9 months (Fig 30–5).

Initial Clinical Experience in Human Peripheral Vessels

Following the encouraging results from animal experiments, in early 1986 a proposal for human implantation was submitted to the hospital ethics committee. The protocol defined the indications, methods, and monitoring for stent implantation in peripheral and coronary arteries of patients.

For peripheral implants highly symptomatic patients were selected for the following:

1. Recanalization of the iliac or femoral artery with long and complex stenoses and in whom balloon angioplasty either failed or suggested a poor prognosis.
2. Iliac or femoral restenosis after previous angioplasty.

For coronary implants three conditions were considered to be indications for endoluminal stent implantation:

1. Restenosis of a major coronary artery after previous coronary angioplasty.
2. Stenosis of aortocoronary bypass grafts suggesting poor overall graft quality.
3. Acute occlusion secondary to intimal dissection following balloon angioplasty.

The protocol was accepted, and informed patient consent (in accordance with the Helsinki Declaration) was obtained from each patient before the intervention.

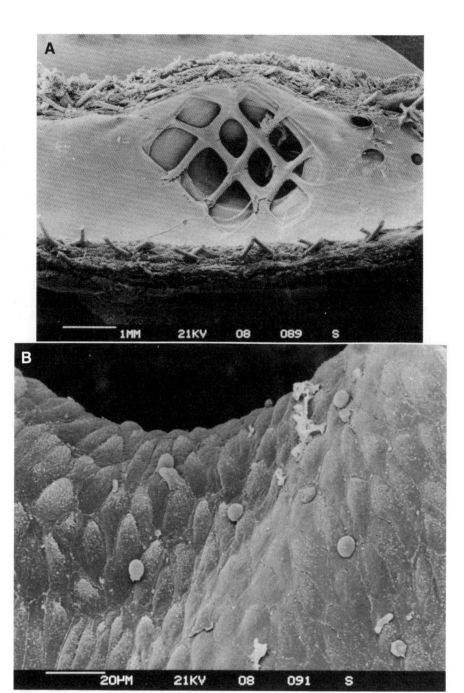

FIG 30–3.
A, scanning electron micrograph of a stent covering the orifice of a departing side branch of a canine femoral artery (see Fig 30–2). Nine months after implantation, the metal wires are totally coated with a smooth neointimal lining that does not interfere with blood flow to the branch artery. **B,** a high-magnification view of the neoendothelial surface of the junction between the stent and branch vessel.

Peripheral Implants

Implantation Technique

The early group of stent prostheses comprised 14 devices implanted in nine patients in femoral and iliac arteries. Stent diameters varied between 6 and 12 mm, and stent lengths were 30 to 80 mm. Prostheses up to 6.5-mm nominal diameter were delivered through an 8 F coronary guiding catheter. Larger stents were deployed by using an 8 F delivery system through an ordinary 9 F introducing sheath. Drug therapy consisted of 500 mg of aspirin the day before the intervention, a bo-

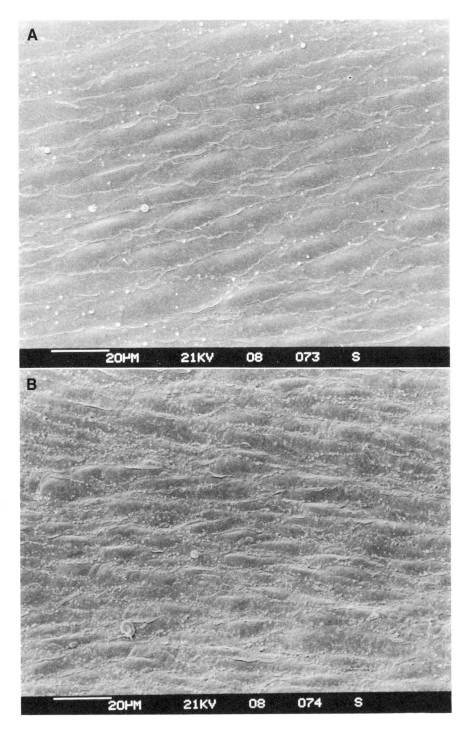

FIG 30–4.
A, scanning electron micrograph of the endothelial surface covering the prosthesis. (From Sigwart U, Puel J, Mirkovitch V, et al: *N Engl J Med* 1987; 316:701–706. Used with permission.) **B,** for comparison, the endothelium of the adjacent nonstented artery is shown. The specimen was recovered from a canine femoral artery 9 months after implantation.

lus injection of 15,000 units of heparin during the implantation, and a fixed combination of 330 mg of aspirin plus 75 mg of dipyridimole once daily in addition to oral anticoagulation with sodium warfarin (Coumadin) for the first 3 months of follow-up.

Results

In two patients totally occluded arteries were recanalized and stented. One patient had a left superficial femoral artery occlusion of 30 cm in length that failed to remain patent despite adequate balloon angioplasty fol-

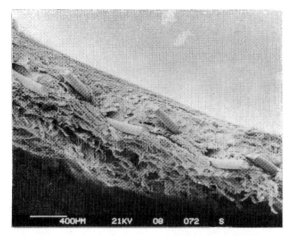

FIG 30–5.
Scanning electron micrograph of a prosthesis firmly embedded in the femoral artery of a dog at the level of the left knee 9 months after implantation (see the text for details).

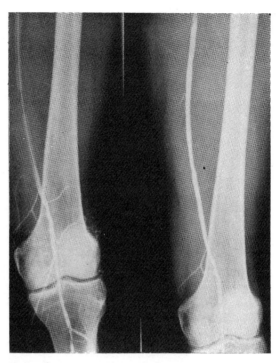

FIG 30–6.
Superficial femoral artery after mechanical recanalization of a 30-cm long total occlusion, followed by catheter implantation of two consecutive endoprostheses. For better visualization the right part of this figure shows injection of contrast medium distal to the two prostheses through a 4 F angiography catheter. Note the nonstented lesion 4 cm below the knee. Three more prostheses were implanted 3 months later, to treat severe lesions within nonstented segments.

lowed by local urokinase infusion. Two consecutive prostheses 6 mm in diameter and 8 cm in length (Fig 30–6) were implanted, and resulted in adequate blood flow and the disappearance of severe claudication. Symptoms reappeared after 3 months due to a high-grade stenosis of the nonstented segments of the previously occluded femoral artery both proximal to and between the stents. These stenoses were then dilated and supported by three additional stents, one bridging over the gap between the first two prostheses and two upstream to the first implant. Again symptoms were significantly ameliorated. The pressure gradient and peripheral flow were substantially improved when measured by peripheral Doppler. Some endothelial thickening was noted at the time of repeat angiography. However, this intimal hyperplasia was not enough to produce a significant modification of the Doppler flow signal. Unfortunately, local restenosis developed a year later. The most important lesions were removed with the help of an atherectomy device (Devices for Vascular Interventions, Redwood City, Calif), and no further restenosis has occurred since.

Another patient had a long-standing, 8-cm occlusion of the left external iliac artery that was mechanically recanalized and dilated. Since adequate flow was not obtained, the vessel was stented with a prosthesis 8 cm in length and 12 mm in diameter. No recurrence of symptoms occurred over a follow-up of 19 months.

All other prostheses were placed into suboccluded arteries that did not respond satisfactorily to conventional balloon angioplasty. There were no cases of recurrence as judged by the reappearance of symptoms, decrease of peripheral flow determined by Doppler measurements,

or control digital subtraction angiography. No side effects were reported.

Coronary Implants

Implantation Technique

All coronary stents were inserted by using the same basic pharmacologic protocol. Patients received a bolus of 15,000 units of heparin at the beginning of the procedure. After the sheath was removed, patients were maintained on a heparin drip until fully anticoagulated with warfarin. Low–molecular-weight dextran at 100 cc/1h was administered for 1 hour prior to the procedure and 1 hour after completion in the majority of cases. All patients received aspirin, 300 to 500 mg, before the procedure and were maintained on 75 to 100 mg, daily for 6 months afterward. Dipyridamole, 100 mg three times daily, was also continued for 6 months in most patients. A calcium antagonist, usually diltiazem, 60 mg three times daily, was administered for 6 months after the procedure. All patients received warfarin to maintain an INR of 2.5 to 3.5, which was continued until control angiography was performed, usually at 4 to 6 months. A small number of patients in the middle of the series also received sulfinpyrazone, 200 mg three times daily for 6 months.

When coronary stent implantation began, it was necessary to call the company each time a device was needed. Because of delays of 30 to 60 minutes, these early patients additionally received urokinase, 250,000 units, while the guidewire was across the lesion. Once the procedure became more routine, a supply of stents was kept in the catheterization laboratory and urokinase was no longer felt to be necessary.

All patients underwent standard balloon angioplasty before stent deployment, except those with bypass vein graft disease. Many of the latter group had friable-appearing lesions that were therefore stented prior to balloon dilatations in the hope of avoiding the potential for distal embolization. After successful balloon dilatations, the standard angioplasty balloon was exchanged over a 0.014 or 0.018-in guidewire for the stent delivery system. The delivery device was sufficiently supple to allow placement despite very tortuous vessels. High-resolution fluoroscopy was used to visualize stent positioning at the site of the previous balloon dilatation. Stents were chosen so that the unconstrained diameter of the device was 15% to 20% larger than the native vessel in order to maintain some residual radial force against the vessel wall and avoid the potential for vessel wall recoil and the possibility of stent migration (which has never occurred in our experience). The stents generally varied between 15 and 29 mm in length.

Over 200 stents have been deployed in 170 patients since the initial implantation in 1986. Nearly 10% of patients had more than one stent placed. Stent deployment was unsuccessful in only 1 early case when the delivery system failed and an alternative system was unavailable. Approximately 25% of the stents were inserted emergency for abrupt occlusion after standard angioplasty, 50% of the stents were deployed for re-

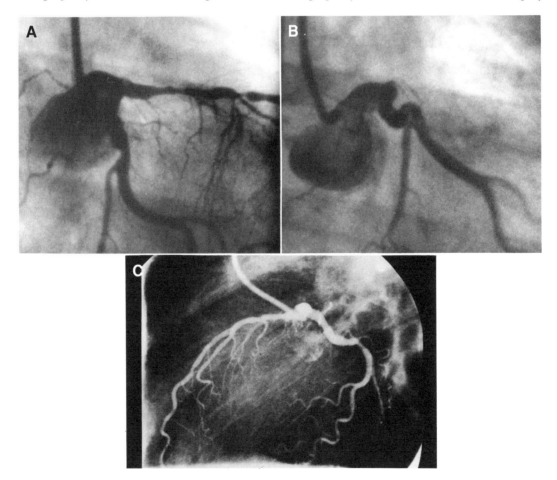

FIG 30–7.
Left coronary artery before angioplasty **(A)**, after angioplasty **(B)**, and 6 months after emergency recanalization and stent implantation of the left anterior descending (LAD) coronary artery **(C)**. The stent is invisible because of high contrast.

stenosis, and the remainder were placed because of bypass graft disease. Figure 30–7 shows the left coronary system in a patient who had abrupt occlusion of the left anterior descending artery after routine angioplasty and a 6-month follow-up angiogram of the stented vessel. In Figure 30–8 the same patient's right coronary artery is seen before and after stenting because of restenosis.

Patients were routinely followed weekly for the first month postprocedure and then monthly. They under-

went exercise tests at 2-month intervals, and control angiography was suggested between 4 and 6 months. If the stent was patent at the time of control angiography without evidence of significant restenosis, all drug therapy was stopped except for aspirin.

Results

In the group of patients stented for abrupt occlusion, 2% of the patients suffered thrombosis of the stent. Q

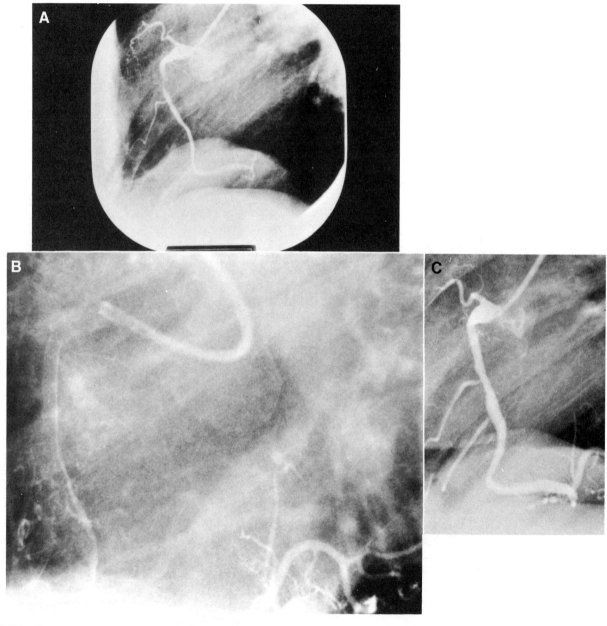

FIG 30–8.
Same patient as in Figure 30–7. **A,** restenosis 8 weeks after percutaneous transluminal coronary angioplasty (PTCA) of the right coronary artery. **B,** stenting of the redilated artery with an endoprosthesis 20 mm in length and 3.5 mm in nominal diameter. **C,** after 6 months follow-up.

wave infarctions occurred in 9% of this patient group. It is impossible to know whether this was related to the stent procedure or the period of time that the vessel was occluded prior to stenting. Patients for whom stents were placed because of documented restenosis experienced a 4% incidence of acute (Q wave) myocardial infarction. Early stent thrombosis occurred in 6% of this group, some of which were associated with a Q wave infarction. Half of the patients with acute stent thrombosis were successfully recanalized with a combination of thrombolytic therapy and repeat angioplasty. The other half required bypass surgery. One patient from the restenosis population died. This death deserves further comment.

The patient had a 90% narrowing of the proximal segment of the left anterior descending artery at angiography performed 1 week after a small anteroapical infarction. The patient underwent standard angioplasty and 2 months later developed symptomatic restenosis. The lesion was redilated and stented with an excellent result (see Fig 30–9,A and B). Two days later the patient underwent maximal exercise testing the results of which were normal. Shortly after the stress test, he developed a marked vagal reaction with electrocardiographic (ECG) evidence of anterolateral ischemia. Since angiographic facilities were not immediately available, the patient was sent for emergency surgery with implantation of a mammary artery to the left anterior descending artery. At the time of surgery there was no longer evidence of ischemia, and the stent was found to be patent. Postoperative recovery seemed uneventful except for minor problems of hemostasis and signs of mild cardiac tamponade. The following day the patient developed unexplained hypoxia and died. At the postmortem examination there were signs of cardiac tamponade, a patent mammary implant, and very recent thrombus (less than 1 hour old) on the stent.

Three late deaths occurred in the group of patients stented for restenosis. Two deaths were clearly stent related since these patients suffered a myocardial infarction in the distribution of the stented artery after discontinuing their anticoagulation program. One patient with far-advanced coronary artery disease died after surgical revascularization following the discovery of a new left mainstem stenosis.

Patients who were stented for bypass graft disease had a 2% incidence of stent thrombosis but an 11% incidence of Q wave myocardial infarction. Among this group of patients, 2% died either early or in late follow-up. The restenosis rate for all patients was calculated by using the number of those patients who returned for angiographic follow-up. In patients with bypass graft disease the rate is 25%. Long-term patient follow-up of stented patients from all three groups is over 95%, but

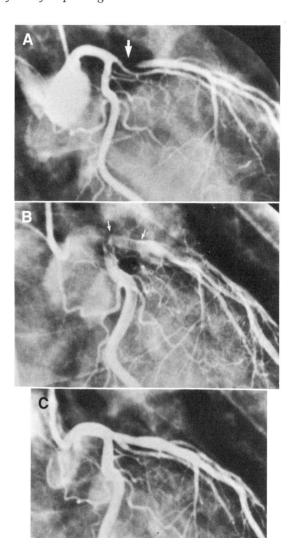

FIG 30–9.
Restenosis of the left anterior descending (LAD) coronary artery 6 weeks after the first angioplasty. **A,** there is a greater than 90% proximal LAD stenosis after implantation of the self-expanding endoprosthesis **(B).** A regular contrast injection reveals an almost perfect result.

only 75% have come to control angiography at 4 to 6 months either for clinical reasons or for stent research. Among those patients who have had control angiography, 16% have demonstrated stent restenosis. Overall in our patient population there was a 7.5% incidence of stent thrombosis, a 11% incidence of Q wave myocardial infarction, and a 3.8% incidence of death.

DISCUSSION

Restenosis and acute occlusion are the most vexing issues in interventional cardiology today. The applicability of PTCA for those patients with significant left ventricular dysfunction is limited by the risk of abrupt occlusion. the very high restenosis rates limit its role in multivessel disease.[7] Yet these subgroups of patients represent the majority who need interventional therapy. Moreover, the socioeconomic cost of restenosis is enormous and may outweigh the economic advantages of angioplasty when compared with bypass surgery.[8] Experience has demonstrated that the rates of abrupt occlusion and restenosis are not related to operator skill, the type of equipment, or the duration or magnitude of pressure used in balloon inflations. Attempts to modify the PTCA failure rate with drug therapy have proved unsuccessful to date. Research efforts are now directed at discovering the control mechanism for smooth muscle cell hyperplasia, which causes the majority of restenosis.

As we wait for basic research to unravel the biochemical and flow mechanisms that might effect smooth muscle cell proliferation, we need new devices to improve the success of coronary intervention today. Various new mechanical devices have entered clinical trials over the last few years, but none have overcome the combined problems of abrupt occlusion and restenosis. Shaving tools, lasers, and ablaters using high-speed rotational devices have all had their advocates early in their development. However, once clinical investigations have been reported, the enthusiasm for these new tools has waned.[9] Many investigators have concluded that an endoluminal support device for the diseased vessel is the best hope for immediately benefiting patients. Several different designs have been proposed, and some are under clinical investigation at this time. These designs include thermally expandable devices, balloon-deformable models, and biodegradable polymers with variable elastic properties.

The present generation of stent designs are based on earlier animal research. Endothelialization with uniform and consistent intimal thickening and collateral vessel patency as we described in dogs has also been found by other investigators evaluating different stent designs.[10] Research suggests that the rate of intimal thickening is related to the thickness of the metal wires of a stent. Wright et al. have reported only 30% covering of endothelium at 1 month for stents with wires 0.46 mm thick deployed in dogs while stent wires 0.09 mm thick were completely covered with endothelium within 3 weeks.[11] The relative porosity of the design also appears to alter results in animal models. Devices with less porosity are more likely to lead to higher levels of fibrin deposition with subsequent increased smooth muscle cell hyperplasia and luminal narrowing. Devices with too high a porosity can have insufficient structural support and suboptimal hemodynamics, which can cause

increased turbulence. These results have influenced the development of the present group of stents under clinical investigation.

The self-expanding mesh stent was designed with an 80% porosity factor. It is made from polished stainless steel 0.06 to 0.08 mm thick so that it is flexible enough to traverse serpinginous vessels with a profile low enough to allow placement under almost all circumstances encountered in coronary angioplasty. The initial results confirm that these design goals have been met. Only once in over 160 cases of stent deployment was placement unsuccessful, and that situation arose from a mechanically defective delivery catheter when a replacement device was unavailable. The results are in contrast to those reported by both Roubin using the Gianturco-Roubin stent and Schatz using the Palmaz-Schatz device.[12-14] Both of these designs have had some early problems with stent embollzation or premature dislodgement, as well as continuing difficulties in navigating tortuous vessels.

All three of these designs, however, have demonstrated common problems, the most significant being the rate of early or subacute stent thrombosis, which is reported to be between 3% and 10% for all three devices. Despite the animal research suggesting that thrombosis of these devices would not be an inherent risk, human trials have consistently demonstrated this to be the case. Several important points are raised by this issue. Clearly, no animal models of human arteriosclerosis exist that adequately mimic the conditions of a diseased human vessel. Human experimentation is necessary for an adequate assessment of any new mechanical device. It is also apparent that the present stent designs will need further modifications before they are ready for widespread clinical use.

Our results, however, confirm the early enthusiasm for an intraluminal scaffolding device despite some recent negative opinions.[9] Part of these issues may reflect misunderstanding of the data analyzed at the Thoraxcenter in Rotterdam. This group analyzes computerized measurements of coronary segments after stenting vs. follow-up angiography performed 4 to 6 months later. Their sensitivity for accurate measurements is 0.72 mm, and therefore the group has used this difference as one measure of restenosis.[15] Although there is little doubt that these differences can be assessed accurately, one can question what clinical significance such a measurement reflects. The average stent placed is 3.5 to 4.0 mm in coronary arteries. With a 3.5-mm stent, a 0.72-mm decrease in cross-sectional area at 6 months actually represents a 21% degree of narrowing. No one in clinical situations would consider this evidence of restenosis. The Rotterdam group has also analyzed the same group of angiograms by using a criterion of 50% narrowing representing restenosis. With this criterion, they found a restenosis rate of 14% in a very heterogeneous population, including the first 50 patients ever stented in the world.[16]

The restenosis rate of the self-expanding mesh stent is even more impressive when we examine the patients in which the devices were implanted. Most of our patients had either bypass vein graft disease or at least one prior episode of restenosis, which makes their likelihood of recurrent restenosis at least 50% according to most series.[17, 18] The risk of myocardial infarction and emergency surgery (2.3%) in our population is also quite low when compared with a similar patient population undergoing standard angioplasty. Finally, the acute and long-term follow-up mortality rate for our patient group, 3.8%, could be compared with the rate in those patients who have failed angioplasty and required emergency bypass surgery; in this group rates up to 15% have been reported.[19]

There is little question that results of stenting will improve as investigators gain experience with these new devices. We have analyzed our patient population by comparing the first 80 cases of stent deployment with the last 50 cases. In the latter group we had 4 cases of stent thrombosis (8%), only 1 of which was permanent (2%). One patient suffered a myocardial infarction, and 1 patient demonstrated new disease distal to the stent. None of the patients from this group has died. We have seen no cases of stent occlusion or restenosis among the 39 patients who have undergone control angiography. The significant improvement in these results primarily relates to improved patient selection.

We do not deploy stents in vessels in which the flow may be compromised, and we only insert stents 3.5 mm or greater in unconstrained luminal diameter. Proximal left anterior descending disease should be avoided if possible, and vessels that have demonstrated coronary spasm are not stented. If a clot is present in a diseased vessel, we believe that this represents a relative contraindication for stenting. In our experience the ideal situation for stent deployment involves a large right coronary vessel or a diseased vein bypass graft. When these circumstances exist, we feel that intracoronary stents may be considered primary therapy rather than a bailout device or a secondary attempt to prevent restenosis. Randomized trials based on these inclusion criteria are now being initiated.

CONCLUSION

Since the initial deployment of a self-expanding mesh stent in a human coronary artery in 1986, research has progressed to the point where the device may reasonably be considered as a primary form of therapy in certain situations. However, most disease that confronts the modern cardiologist still requires conventional balloon angioplasty or bypass surgery. This situation will change as new stent designs enter clinical investigation. The next generation of devices will be balloon expandable or radiopaque to ease insertion. They will be flexible and have low profiles allowing placement throughout the coronary tree. Almost certainly the stent designs will incorporate chemical or cellular bonding to provide a mechanism for the local and continuous instillation of therapy to the affected vessel site. This therapy may involve drugs like heparin or hirudin, a potent anticoagulant, or genetically engineered endothelial cells that release tissue-type plasminogen activator (t-PA), thus avoiding problems of early stent thrombosis. Both of these modalities are presently under clinical investigation. We feel that the primary mechanism for controlling restenosis is the maintenance of normal flow down a diseased vessel, which can be best achieved by an intraluminal supporting device. However, this device could well be temporary and made of biodegradable polymers that might dissolve over 3 to 9 months to provide sufficient time for the vessel to heal from the barotrauma inflicted by balloon angioplasty. If these goals are met, the socioeconomic impact of coronary artery disease will be substantially reduced, and interventional techniques will be applicable in many more clinical situations.

Acknowledgment

Dr. Frank was supported in part by a grant from Northwest Hospital Foundation, Seattle, Washington.

REFERENCES

1. Serruys PW, Luijten HE, Beat KJ, et al: Incidence of restenosis after successful coronary angioplasty: A time-related phenomenon. A quantitative angiographic study in 342 consecutive patients at 1, 2, 3, and 4 months. *Circulation* 1988; 77:361–371.
2. Detre K, Holubkov R, Kelsey S, et al: Percutaneous transluminal angioplasty in 1985–1986 and 1977–1981: The National Heart, Lung, and Blood Institute registry. *N Engl J Med* 1988; 318:265–270.
3. Palmaz JC, Sibbet RR, Reuter SR, et al: Expandable intraluminal graft: A preliminary study. *Radiology* 1985; 156:73–77.
4. Wright KC, Wallace S, Charnsangavi C, et al: Percutaneous endovascular stents: An experimental evaluation. *Radiology* 1985; 156:69–72.
5. Sigwart U, Puel J, Mirkovitch V, et al: Intravascular stents to prevent occlusion and restenosis after transluminal angioplasty. *N Engl J Med* 1987; 316:701–706.

6. Maass D, Kropf L, Egloff L, et al: Transluminal implantations of intravascular "double helix" spiral protheses: Technical and biological considerations. *Eur Soc Artificial Organs Proc* 1982; 9:252–256.
7. DiSciascio G, Cowley MJ, Vetrovec GW, et al: Triple vessel coronary angioplasty: Acute outcome and long-term results. *J Am Coll Cardiol* 1988; 12:42–47.
8. Black AJR, Roubin GS, Sutor C, et al: Comparative costs of percutaneous transluminal coronary angioplasty and coronary artery bypass grafting in multivessel coronary artery disease. *Am J Cardiol* 1988; 10:246–252.
9. Block P: Coronary artery stents and other endoluminal devices. *N Engl J Med* 1991; 324:52–53.
10. Schatz RA, Palmaz JC, Tio FO, et al: Balloon expandable intracoronary stents in the adult dog. *Circulation* 1987; 76:450–457.
11. Wright KC, Wallace S, Charnsangavej C, et al: Percutaneous endovascular stents: An experimental evaluation. *Radiology* 1985; 15:69–72.
12. Schatz RA, Leon MB, Baim DS, et al: Balloon expandable intracoronary stents: Initial results of a multicenter study. *Circulation* 1989; 80(suppl 2):174.
13. Baim DS, Schatz RA, Cleman M, et al: Predictors of unsuccessful placement of the Schatz-Palmaz coronary stent. *Circulation* 1989; 80(suppl 2):174.
14. Roubin GS, Douglas JS Jr, Lembo NJ, et al: Intracoronary stenting for acute closure following percutaneous transluminal coronary angioplasty (PTCA). *Circulation* 1988; 78(suppl 2):407.
15. Reiber JHC, Serruys PW, Kooijman CJ, et al: Assessment of short-, medium-, and long-term variations in arterial dimensions from computer-assisted quantification of coronary cineangiograms. *Circulation* 1985; 71:280–288.
16. Serruys PW, Bradley SH, Beatt KJ, et al: Angiographic follow-up after placement of a self-expanding coronary-artery stent. *N Engl J Med* 1991; 324:13–17.
17. Douglas JS Jr, King SB III, Roubin GS, et al: Percutaneous angioplasty of venous aortocoronary graft stenoses: Late angiographic and clinical outcome (abstract). *Circulation* 1986; 74(suppl 2):281.
18. Sugrue DD, Vlietstra RE, Hammes LN, et al: Repeat balloon angioplasty for symptomatic restenosis: A note of caution. *Eur Heart J* 1987; 8:697–701.
19. Satter P, Krause E, Skupin M: Mortality trends in cases of elective and emergency aorto-coronary bypass after percutaneous transluminal angioplasty. *Thorac Cardiovasc Surg* 1987; 35:2–5.

31

The Palmaz-Schatz Coronary Stent

Alexander Shaknovich, M.D.

Alexander A. Stratienko, M.D.

Paul S. Teirstein, M.D.

Richard A. Schatz, M.D.

This chapter is a clinically oriented review of the Palmaz-Schatz coronary stent. It will focus on (1) clinically relevant features of the stent design; (2) aspects of patient selection, preparation, and management; (3) strategies of stent delivery and deployment; and (4) analysis of the current international clinical experience with this device. For more information on the biology of vascular stents and other stents presently in clinical trials, several references are recommended.[1-3]

BACKGROUND

Since Grüntzig's first daring percutaneous transluminal coronary angioplasty (PTCA) in September 1977,[4] PTCA has become a widely accepted and generally safe treatment modality for coronary artery disease in appropriately selected patients. However, in spite of the rapid accumulation of clinical and operator experience and significant improvements in angioplasty and imaging equipment, PTCA remains associated with a significant incidence of restenosis and a measurable risk of procedure-related complications.

Restenosis remains the Achilles heel of conventional PTCA. Most series[5-8] report a 25% to 45% incidence of restenosis within the first 6 months following PTCA. The rate of restenosis may be higher for certain subsets of patients, such as diabetics[9, 10] and smokers who continue to smoke after the index PTCA,[9, 11] and certain lesion sites, such as the left anterior descending (LAD) coronary artery,[12-14] saphenous vein aorto-coronary bypass grafts,[15-17] coronary ostia,[18] and origins of major branches.[19] Restenosis rates of 26% to 45% have been reported in patients undergoing repeat PTCA for restenosis.[20-23] Newer treatment modalities such as ex-

cimer laser,[25, 26] laser balloon,[27] and various plaque-removing devices[28, 29] have failed to have any impact on the incidence of restenosis, with a possible exception of directional coronary atherectomy for de novo lesions in large proximal LAD coronary arteries.[29]

The 1979–1983 National Heart, Lung and Blood Institute (NHLBI) PTCA Registry reported the early experience with PTCA in the United States.[30] The primary success rate was 67%. Major coronary events occurred in 13.0% of patients, with myocardial infarctions in 5.5% urgent bypass surgery in 6.6%, and death in 0.9% of patients. The more current 1985–1986 NHLBI PTCA Registry reported[31] 4.3% of patients experiencing nonfatal myocardial infarctions, 3.4% requiring urgent bypass surgery, and a death rate of 1.0%. The primary success rate was 88%. Other representative high-volume institutions have reported similar success and major complication rates.[32, 33] In a comprehensive review of minor complications of 3,500 consecutive PTCAs at Emory University between 1980 and 1984, Bredlau et al.[34] reported a 0.9% incidence of vascular complications, with 0.6% of patients requiring surgical repair of the femoral artery and 0.3% of patients receiving transfusions.

The limitations and risks of conventional PTCA provide a context in which one can evaluate the accumulating clinical experience with the newer catheter-based percutaneous treatments of coronary artery disease, such as the Palmaz-Schatz coronary stent.

STENT DESIGN AND DELIVERY SYSTEM

The currently available Palmaz-Schatz coronary stent delivery system (SDS) was developed as a result of systematic and critical accumulation of clinical experience with the stent. This overview will reflect its evolution and improvements.

Initial implantation of the Palmaz-Schatz coronary stent, first in dogs by Schatz et al.[1] and then in clinical trials,[35, 36] beginning in December 1987, employed rigid stents identical in design to those originally used by Palmaz et al. in rabbit aortas.[37] Each coronary stent was a single tube of surgical-grade 316L stainless steel, 15 mm in length, 1.6 mm in diameter, and with a wall thickness of 0.003 in. (0.08 mm). The design of the stent is based on the concept of plastic deformation, whereby a metal will not change its shape after being stretched beyond a certain limit. The walls of the stent are etched into multiple rows of staggered rectangles that upon balloon inflation become diamond-shaped spaces and allow for stent expansion to a maximum diameter of 5 to 6 mm (expansion ratio of up to 4:1) and a minimal amount of metal composing the surface area when expanded (approximately 10%) (Fig 31–1). The original rigid coronary stent was slipped retrogradely over a collapsed delivery balloon and crimped down manually. The balloon/stent assembly was then passed through an 8 F or 9 F guiding catheter over a 0.014-in. PTCA guidewire down the target vessel into the predilated target lesion. The stent was deployed with a single 6- to 8-atm balloon inflation.[1] Because of the difficulty experienced in passing the rigid stent through the bends of most conventional guiding catheters, the guidewire and guiding catheter had to be removed after the initial predilatation and replaced with a preloaded guide/balloon/stent assembly. The predilated target lesion had to be recrossed with a guidewire before the balloon/stent assembly could be advanced into the target lesion.

The stent delivery strategy was simplified considerably with a modification of the stent design by Schatz,[2, 38] which introduced a 1-mm-long flexible strut between two 7-mm-long rigid segments (Fig 31–2). The assembly of a PTCA balloon and a monoconstructed articulated flexible stent could now be easily advanced through any standard 8 F or 9 F guiding catheter into the target vessel over a previously placed exchange-length 0.014-in. guidewire, thus eliminating the need for recrossing the lesion. The articulated stent is the stent used in the current SDS.

While the articulated stent design largely solved the problem of stent delivery to the origin of and into the proximal segment of the target vessel, it only partially addressed the difficulties encountered in advancing the balloon/stent assembly down relatively small-caliber and tortuous coronary arteries. Despite predilatation, attempts at deployment of an unprotected balloon/stent assembly were associated in a small percentage of pa-

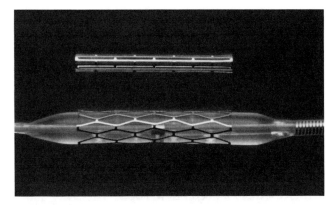

FIG 31–1.
Nonarticulated stent/balloon assembly.

tients with the stent snagging on diseased or dissected proximal vessel segments and resulted in failure of stent delivery in 5% of patients[39] and isolated cases of stent embolization.[35, 39] These problems were solved with the incorporation of 5 F and 6 F protective subselective delivery sheaths (Teleguide, Schneider, Minneapolis) into the SDS. Before introducing the device into the patient, the balloon/stent assembly is carefully inserted into the delivery sheath, with the tip of the balloon extending past the tip of the delivery sheath. This SDS prevents stent-wall contact until stent deployment and creates a gradual transition from the approximately 3 F tip of the balloon to the tip of the delivery sheath. The use of 6 F subselective sheaths was abandoned in favor of 5 F sheaths because of excessive stiffness. With the 5 F SDS, the stent delivery success rate is 99%, with no embolizations.[39]

A modified SDS (Johnson & Johnson Interventional Systems, Warren, NJ) is now available as a factory preassembled unit, with an articulated two-segment stent crimped on a specified-diameter balloon between two radiopaque balloon markers and preloaded into a transparent delivery sheath that also has a radiopaque

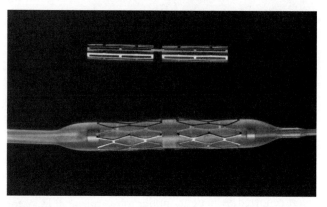

FIG 31–2.
Articulated stent/balloon assembly.

marker. The SDS is sized according to the diameter of the stent delivery balloon. Prior to deployment of the current SDS, the operator is required to flush the guidewire lumen of the balloon and the lumen of the delivery sheath.

In summary, the present SDS enjoys optimal component matching, requires minimal preparation prior to delivery, and allows easier manipulation of the protective sheath relative to the balloon/stent assembly and more optimal visualization of the relevant landmarks of the SDS.

PATIENT SELECTION, PREPARATION, AND MANAGEMENT

At the time of preparation of this chapter, the Palmaz-Schatz coronary stent remains an investigational device in the United States. Adult patients of any age are candidates for entry into the present nonrandomized multicenter clinical trial if they (1) have stable symptoms of angina pectoris despite medical therapy or abnormal thallium stress test results, (2) are able to give informed consent, (3) are candidates for coronary artery bypass surgery, (4) have no contraindications to anticoagulation or aspirin administration, and (5) have lesions less than 15 mm in length in native coronary arteries or saphenous vein aorto-coronary bypass grafts (between 2.5 and 5.0 mm in diameter). In the setting of abrupt closure after PTCA or after a recent myocardial infarction, coronary stents are not implanted if there is angiographic evidence of persistent thrombus in the target lesion despite intracoronary administration of an adequate amount of a thrombolytic agent.

Additional comments should be made regarding angiographic criteria for patient selection. Angiographic features of the target lesion and the target vessel proximal and distal to the target lesion must be carefully assessed. As indicated above, any discrete nonthrombotic lesion in a relatively large vessel (> 2.5 mm in diameter) is in principle suitable for stenting. Ostial lesions, restenoses after multiple previous conventional PTCAs,[40] suboptimal results of previous PTCAs, including dissections,[41] and totally occluded vessels can be stented with excellent angiographic results. Lesions in the left main coronary artery should not be stented unless protected by one or more bypass grafts. The clinical significance of branches of the target coronary artery in the immediate proximity of the target lesion must be carefully estimated; a loss of branches originating within a stented coronary segment is very uncommon (personal communication, David L. Fishman, M.D.), but an obstructing strut of the stent may preclude any subsequent attempts of catheter-based treatment of any current or future lesions in the branch. Clinical decision making has to be individualized to a given patient, but as a good rule of thumb, the operator should avoid obstructing a side branch if it is large enough to warrant a bypass graft if diseased.

While rare, acute and subacute stent closure appears to have occurred more frequently in those patients in whom there was impairment of inflow or outflow from the stented segment due to other untreated stenoses or dissections in the target vessel. Adequate inflow and in particular adequate runoff are thus two critical criteria for optimal selection of coronary lesions suitable for stenting. The operator must also carefully assess the location of the ostium of the target vessel and the tortuosity of the target vessel proximal to the lesion to be stented for guide selection and stent delivery, as described in greater detail elsewhere in this chapter.

At least 1 day prior to the procedure, patients selected for stenting are started on a regimen of one noncoated adult Bayer aspirin a day; dipyridamole, 75 mg three times a day; and a calcium channel blocker. Standard screening blood tests, electrocardiography, and if indicated, chest x-rays are performed prior to the procedure. On the day of stent implantation, low–molecular-weight dextran is administered intravenously beginning at least 2 hours prior to the procedure. Because isolated idiosyncratic reactions to dextran, including pulmonary edema, have been described,[42] a small initial intravenous test dose is advisable. Intravenous infusion of at least 200 cc of dextran prior to stent delivery is preferred; dextran administration is then continued at 50 cc/hr intravenously until 1 L has been infused. Ten thousand to 15,000 units of heparin is injected intravenously at the beginning of the procedure; continuous heparin infusion is not routinely started. The activated clotting time (ACT) is monitored periodically during the procedure, and additional heparin boluses are given intravenously as needed to keep the ACT greater than 300 seconds. An intracoronary thrombolytic agent is administered through the guiding catheter before attempting stent delivery if there is any angiographic suggestion of thrombus in the target lesion before or after stent deployment. After uncomplicated stent delivery, intravenous dextran is continued as noted above, but heparin is withheld until 4 hours after the sheaths have been removed. The ACT is followed immediately after the procedure so that removal of the sheaths is possible when it is less than 165 seconds. Hemostasis is achieved with direct manual compression or groin clamps. Meticulous technique is required in these patients while securing vascular access and when removing sheaths to minimize the risk of access-related complications such as bleeding requiring transfusions and pseudoaneurysms and hematomas requiring vascular surgery, the incidence of which remains high at 8% to 10%. Four to six hours after complete hemostasis at the vascular access sites has been ensured, the patient is re-heparinized to achieve a partial thromboplastin time (PTT) between 50 and 70 seconds. The PTT is followed closely during the next several days. Warfarin, 10 to 15 mg, is given the evening of the procedure and continued daily along with aspirin, dipyridamole, and intravenous heparin until the prothrombin time (PT) is greater than 16 seconds. At that point the heparin infusion is stopped, and another PT determination is performed 6 hours later. If the patient remains stable and free of access site complications, the patient can be gradually ambulated the day after the procedure and discharged when the PT remains greater than 16 seconds more than 6 hours after discontinuing heparin therapy. The PT is maintained between 16 and 18 seconds with warfarin for 1 month after stenting, at which point warfarin therapy is discontinued. Dipyridamole, 75 mg three times a day orally, is continued for 3 months, and one adult aspirin is prescribed daily indefinitely. Patient compliance with this regimen is crucial for the prevention of complications after coronary stenting and should be closely monitored, particularly during the first month after the implantation.

Even in properly selected patients compliant with the postprocedure medical regimen there is a small — 2% to 6%[41, 43–45] — risk of subacute closure, defined as stent thrombosis more than 24 hours after implantation. In a number of cases, this complication developed 7 to 12 days after the procedure, or after they had been discharged from the hospital. While it is imminently treatable,[43, 44] this complication of coronary stenting is potentially life-threatening and requires heightened awareness and recognition by both the patient and the physician for prompt and successful management. Any clinical suggestion of possible stent thrombosis, particularly when supported by electrocardiographic findings and especially during the first 2 weeks after the procedure, should lead to a very strong consideration of repeat coronary angiography. Subacute coronary stent thrombosis can be successfully treated with intracoronary thrombolytic agents, repeat PTCA, or emergency bypass surgery, but appears to be resistant to intravenous thrombolytic therapy.

Routine follow-up of patients receiving the coronary stent includes office visits necessary to maintain adequate anticoagulation, a submaximal stress test 4 weeks after the procedure, a thallium stress test 3 months after the procedure, and a repeat coronary angiogram 6 months after stenting as required by the current Food and Drug Administration (FDA)-approved protocol. Patients are given standard recommendations regarding antibiotic prophylaxis for intravascular prostheses for 3 months.[46] Patients may undergo nuclear magnetic resonance (NMR) imaging after receiving the coronary stent; because it is made from 316L steel, the stent should be expected to create a "black-hole" artifact on the NMR image.[47]

TECHNIQUE OF STENT DEPLOYMENT

The following discussion outlines a tested and successful[39] strategy for deployment of the Palmaz-Schatz coronary stent by utilizing the currently available SDS. It will, we hope, serve as a useful supplement to an operator's own skill, judgement, and accumulating experience with the stent.

It is most appropriate to begin a discussion of the techniques of deployment of the Palmaz-Schatz coronary stent by commenting on guiding catheter selection and use. In general, 8 F guiding catheters with an internal diameter of 0.079 in. or greater are used with the present SDS. Despite the improved SDS, successful delivery of the coronary stent often critically depends on the operator's ability to provide adequate guiding catheter support while advancing the SDS to its target. In most cases, much more guiding support is required with the coronary stent than with conventional PTCA. Consequently, careful assessment of the adequacy of guiding support is essential *before* proceeding even with the initial steps of preparation of the SDS. Several views of the origin and proximal segment of the target vessel may be necessary prior to selecting the first guiding catheter. Once the selected guiding catheter is engaged in the ostium of the target vessel, it should be subjected to the *push test*: as gentle firm pressure is applied to the guiding catheter, displacement of its tip relative to the target vessel is assessed. Forward intubation of the tip of the guiding catheter down the target vessel is sought. If the tip of the guiding catheter prolapses out of the target vessel, it is advisable to try a different guiding catheter before proceeding with stent delivery. On rare occasions, a 9 F guiding catheter may be required. A wide selection of available 8 F and 9 F guiding catheters is therefore recommended.

Angiograms of the target artery are performed with the appropriate guiding catheter, and the target lesion is visualized in multiple views that are available for review during stent delivery. It is advisable to work in a view that offers additional clues to help localize the target lesion, such as arterial branches or surgical clips, and to decide in advance on the desired position of the delivery balloon markers relative to the target lesion. While the stent slightly shortens during its expansion, the extent of stent shortening is minimal at 3.0 mm and thus can be discounted in smaller target vessels. However, at 5 to 6 mm of expanded diameter, foreshortening of as much as 1 mm can be expected. The diameter of the disease-free segments of the target artery immediately proximal and distal to the lesion is assessed by comparison to the guiding catheter, preferably with the help of electronic calipers, in order to select an appropriate-size SDS. Stent delivery systems are sized in 0.5-mm increments, beginning with 3.0 mm, according to the diameter of the stent delivery balloon in the SDS. Unlike with PTCA,[48] there appears to be a decrease in the rate of angiographic restenosis and no increase in the rate of acute complications when the stent delivery balloon is slightly oversized relative to the vessel adjacent to it.[49] The current recommendation is to select an SDS with an SDS–target vessel diameter ratio of greater than 1.0 (the *rule of over*). Excessive oversizing should be avoided to minimize the chance of disruption of the artery adjacent to the target lesion since the ends of the delivery balloon extend beyond the stent.

After the selected SDS is made ready, the lesion is crossed with a 0.014-in. exchange-length guidewire. At this point, the operator must decide whether the target lesion needs to be predilated prior to stenting, and if so, what size balloon should be used for predilatation. In general, target *vessels* too small for a 3.0-mm SDS (i.e., <2.5 mm in diameter) should not be stented. All *lesions* should be *under*dilated with a 2.5-mm balloon regardless of the size of the target vessel (the *rule of under*). The aim is to prevent excessive disruption of the lesion prior to stent deployment, which may be associated with a somewhat higher incidence of complications after stenting.[44] During predilatation, placement of the balloon should be precise to avoid trauma to the adjacent normal vessel not intended to be covered with the stent in order to minimize platelet activation[50] and stimulation of smooth muscle cell turnover.[51] With heavily calcified lesions or lesions known to be resistant to balloon dilatation at usual inflation pressures, one may consider predilating with a balloon matched to vessel size to ensure the ability to fully expand the stent once it is delivered into the lesion. Finally, if the SDS cannot be advanced into the lesion despite optimal guiding catheter support, it may be necessary to redilate the lesion with a larger balloon.

Once an adequate channel through the target lesion is available, the SDS is advanced over the guidewire into the lesion, with the assistant gently pulling on the guidewire and the operator applying firm pressure on the guiding catheter. After the SDS has been advanced

out of the guiding catheter, test injections through the guiding catheter may require the use of a smaller-diameter, 2-cc glass syringe for adequate visualization of the target artery. The SDS is advanced as a unit until the balloon markers come to bracket the target lesion. It is absolutely essential to confirm that the lesion is well encompassed by the stent before proceeding any further. Once that is so, the delivery sheath is pulled as far back as the SDS will allow to expose the entire length of the balloon/stent assembly. Great care is taken to keep the balloon/stent assembly stationary within the target vessel during the delivery sheath pullback. The location of the balloon/stent assembly within the target vessel is again assessed with contrast injections through the guiding catheter (or delivery sheath), and gentle minor adjustments in the position of the now unprotected balloon/stent assembly are made, painstakingly avoiding forceful or abrupt displacements. After the balloon/stent assembly has been exposed, the operator must never attempt to pull it back into the delivery sheath because it may cause stent dislodgement and embolization. Only after the optimal position of the balloon/stent assembly is established is the delivery balloon prepared by applying negative pressure; accidental balloon expansion must be avoided during its preparation. The stent is deployed with a single balloon inflation to a desired pressure sufficient to ensure full and uniform balloon expansion (usually 10 to 15 seconds), after which the balloon is deflated and withdrawn and the guidewire left across the stented lesion.

Repeat angiograms of the target vessel are performed in multiple projections at this time to assess the diameter of the stented segment relative to the diameter of the vessel immediately proximal and distal to it. The optimal angiographic appearance of the stented segment of the target artery will have a slight "step-up" from the target vessel proximal to the stent, a slight indentation in the middle of the stented segment that corresponds to the articulation of the stent, and a "step-down" to the target vessel distal to the stent. If necessary, the stented segment of target artery may be dilated with another, larger-sized, preferably short balloon or with another balloon of the same size as the delivery balloon, but inflated to higher pressures. Final angiograms, with the wire still across the stented segment, should be examined for any evidence of haziness or filling defects within the stented segment (which may indicate thrombus formation requiring intracoronary administration of a thrombolytic agent) or the presence of balloon-induced dissection of the vessel proximal or distal to the stent.

Although elective use of multiple stents may result in significantly higher rates of restenosis when compared

TABLE 31–1.

Strategy for Palmaz-Schatz Coronary Stent Deployment

Step 1—Guiding catheter selection
  Views of the *origin* of and the *proximal* target artery
  Choose an *8 F guide* with the best anticipated fit
  The *"push test"* (see the text)
  If this fails, try other 8 F guides
Step 2—Target lesion imaging
  Multiple projections, available for review during the procedure
  Assess proximal vessel tortuosity, location of branches, other lesions in the vessel, presence of
    calcification
  If possible, identify *additional markers* that may be helpful in localizing the lesion: branches of the
    target or other arteries, surgical clips, etc.
  If possible, confirm lesion length and artery diameter with electronic calipers.
Step 3—SDS selection and preparation
  Select an SDS with a balloon size slightly larger than the diameter of the normal artery (the *"rule
    of over,"* see the text)
  Flush the wire lumen of the balloon and the lumen of the delivery sheath
  Do not prepare the balloon until the balloon/stent assembly is in the target lesion
Step 4—Crossing the lesion with a guidewire
  Use 0.014-in. *exchange-length* guidewires
  Advance the tip of the guidewire as far down the target artery as safely possible
Step 5—Target lesion predilatation
  Avoid stenting *vessels* too small for a 3.0-mm SDS
  Predilate *lesions* with a *2.5-mm balloon* irrespective of the actual size of the normal artery (the
    "under" rule, see the text)
  Consider predilating heavily calcified lesions or lesions known to be resistant to balloon dilatation
    with the balloon matched to the vessel size
  Consider repeat predilatation of the lesion with a larger balloon if unable to advance the SDS past
    the lesion after the initial predilatation
  Consider stenting *all* dilated segments in the target artery
Step 6—Stent deployment
  Change the control syringe to a smaller-diameter (e.g., 2-cc glass) syringe
  Measure the *ACT* and keep it *>300* seconds
  With gentle pulling on the guidewire by the assistant and firm pressure on the guiding catheter by
    the operator, *advance the SDS*
  Bracket the lesion with the balloon markers
  Gently *pull the delivery sheath back* while keeping the balloon markers stationary
  Confirm the position of the balloon/stent assembly and carefully adjust it if necessary
  Prepare the balloon and again confirm the position of the balloon/stent assembly in the lesion
  Deploy the stent by fully inflating the balloon for 10–15 sec
  Withdraw the balloon and leave the guidewire in place
  Repeat angiograms; if necessary, dilate the stent further with larger-size balloon(s)

with single stents,[36, 40] their use may be required if the operator elects to stent a lesion longer than 15 mm or stent more than one lesion in the same artery. The distal end of the lesion or the more distal of the multiple lesions should always be stented first. If multiple stents are used in the same lesion, no gaps should be left between the stents, and excessive overlap should be avoided to minimize the area of increased density of metal, which may serve as a nidus for increased neointimal proliferation in the future. If lesions in more than one vessel are to be stented, procedures should be staged, ideally 4 weeks apart or more.

As long as the balloon/stent assembly has not been exposed and remains within the subselective delivery sheath, the attempted stent delivery may be aborted, as when the SDS cannot be advanced into the lesion, sim-

ply by withdrawing the entire SDS as a unit out of the target artery into the guiding catheter and leaving the exchange-length guidewire across the lesion. The strategy for delivering Palmaz-Schatz coronary stents that is outlined above is summarized in Table 31–1. Figures 31–3 through 31–5 show angiograms of various native coronary lesions treated with the Palmaz-Schatz coronary stent.

CURRENT CLINICAL EXPERIENCE

Complications of Coronary Stenting

Implantation of the Palmaz-Schatz coronary stent has been performed since early 1988 at ten hospitals in the United States in a multicenter trial and by several

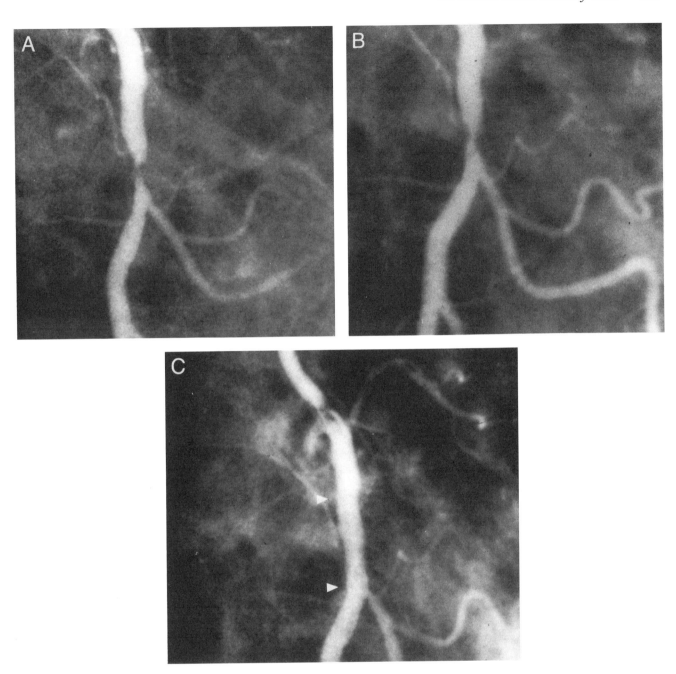

FIG 31–3.
A, right coronary artery stenosis before predilation. **B,** right coronary artery stenosis after predilation. **C,** right coronary artery stenosis after Palmaz-Schatz stent deployment; *arrowheads* indicate the stent.

European groups. Schatz et al. reviewed the United States multicenter experience with this stent in the first 263 patients.[52] Stent delivery was successful in 94% of the patients. As also noted by Baim et al.,[39] the delivery success rate improved to greater than 99%, with no stent embolizations, after the introduction of a 5 F subselective protective sheath into the SDS. Acute closure, or stent thrombosis within 24 hours of implantation, did

not occur. Subacute thrombosis, defined as total stent thrombosis between 24 hours and 2 weeks after implantation, occurred in 7 (2.8%) patients. Of these 7 patients, 3 (1.2%) developed myocardial infarctions, 1 of which was a Q wave infarction. Emergency bypass surgery was performed in 1 patient with subacute closure and 3 other patients because of guiding catheter or wire dissection. No patients died because of stent thrombo-

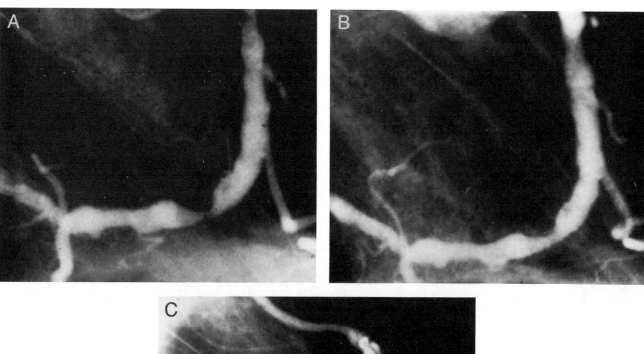

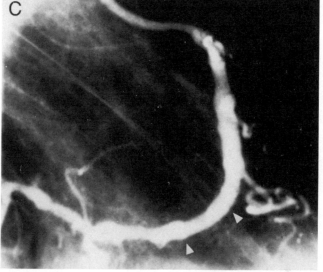

FIG 31–4.
A, right coronary artery stenosis before predilation. **B,** right coronary artery stenosis after predilation. **C,** right coronary artery stenosis after Palmaz-Schatz stent deployment; *arrowheads* indicate the stent.

sis. One patient died after a cerebrovascular accident 2 months after receiving a coronary stent, 1 patient with normal recent stress test findings and no recurrence of angina died suddenly 4 months after stenting, and 1 patient died of a malignancy 2 years after stent implantation. Therefore, major complications such as death, myocardial infarction, or urgent bypass surgery occurred in 10 (4.0%) patients. Vascular access–related complications requiring transfusions or, in a small minority of these patients, vascular surgery occurred in 24 (9.7%) patients.

In the review of their initial single-institution experience within the multicenter trial, Levine et al.[36] re-

ported procedural success in 35 (94%) of the 37 patients with attempted right coronary artery (RCA) implantations of the Palmaz-Schatz stent at the Beth Israel Hospital in Boston. In 2 patients, failure resulted from an inability to pass the stent across the target lesion; in 1 of these patients, a rigid stent was used. The rigid stent embolized into the pelvic vasculature without sequelae during attempted removal of the delivery system from the body. There were no acute closures, no myocardial infarctions, and no deaths; no patient required emergency bypass surgery. One out of 35 patients (2.9%) with successfully delivered stents developed subacute closure after mistaken discontinuation of warfarin ther-

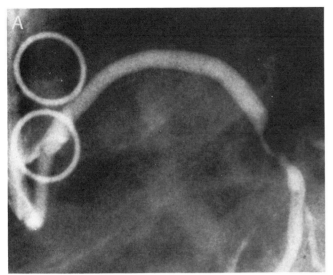

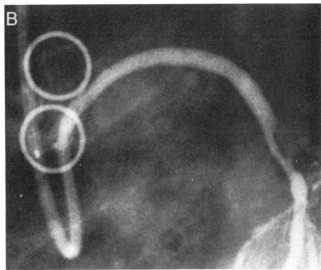

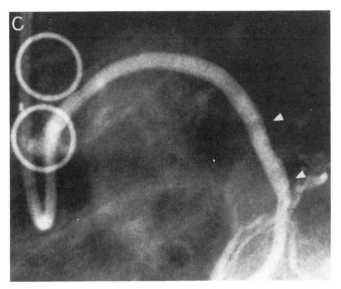

FIG 31–5.
A, saphenous vein bypass graft before predilation. **B,** saphenous vein bypass graft after predilation. **C,** saphenous vein bypass graft after Palmaz-Schatz stent deployment; *arrowheads* indicate the stent.

apy; the vessel was reopened with thrombolytic therapy and repeat dilatation. Six of these 35 patients (17.1%) developed vascular access–related complications: 4 had false aneurysms requiring surgical repair under local anesthesia, 1 developed a large groin hematoma, and 1 had a retroperitoneal hemorrhage.

Fajadet et al. reviewed complications related to Palmaz-Schatz stent implantation in a consecutive series of the first 160 patients at Clinique Pasteur in Toulouse, France.[43] Stent delivery was successful in 149 (93%) patients. Five of 11 patients with unsuccessful stent delivery subsequently underwent successful PTCA. Major complications were reported in 6 (3.8%) patients. Abrupt closure was seen in 5 (3.4%) cases, 4 of which

were successfully recanalized. One patient died 5 days after receiving a single stent in the LAD artery, and 1 patient underwent emergency bypass surgery for a dissection of the ostium of the RCA. There was a 5-fold decrease in the rate of complications, from 6.5% to 1.3%, between the first and second 80 patients who received stents. Stent undersizing and inadequate runoff were among the strongest predictors of stent closure.

Patients with suboptimal angiographic results after PTCA such as significant intimal dissections and residual stenosis greater that 35% to 50% have a particularly high — 10% to 20% — incidence of major complications.[34, 53, 54] Two groups have reported their experience with the Palmaz-Schatz stent in such patients.

Haude et al. reported their series of 15 patients receiving bailout Palmaz-Schatz coronary stents for persistent dissection with objective evidence of ongoing ischemia after PTCA at University of Mainz in West Germany.[41] A total of 22 stents were implanted without any procedure-related problems. Acute stent thrombosis was successfully treated with thrombolysis in 1 patient, and 1 patient was sent for bypass surgery 24 hours after stent implantation for persistent angina. All other patients had patent stents at 24-hour angiograms.

Schatz et al. reviewed complications of coronary stenting in a subset of 116 patients in the United States multicenter trial following suboptimal PTCA of a native coronary artery.[44] All patients had one or more of the following: persistent filling defects, >50% residual narrowing, and persistent dissection. In this subset of patients, there were no cases of acute closure or deaths. Subacute closure was reported in 4 (3.4%) patients, myocardial infarction occurred in 2 (1.7%) patients, and 2 (1.7%) patients underwent urgent bypass surgery. Dissection prior to stenting predicted almost a twofold increase (3.4% vs. 1.8%) in subacute thrombosis when compared with patients without dissection who received stents. This would suggest that avoidance of dissection may be the appropriate treatment strategy for PTCA prior to stenting in order to reduce the risk of subacute thrombosis.

Restenosis in Native Coronary Arteries

Schatz et al. reviewed clinical outcomes in the first 213 patients with successfully implanted Palmaz-Schatz stents in native coronary artery.[52] Seventy-seven percent of patients were male. Patients ranged in age from 26 to 86 years; the mean age for the group was 56 years. The distribution of vessels stented was as follows: RCA in 134 patients, LAD coronary artery in 74 patients, circumflex coronary artery and obtuse marginal branches in 17 patients, and protected left main coronary artery in 1 patient. Seventy percent of the patients had previous PTCAs; 188 patients received single stents, and 42 were stented with multiple (two to six) contiguous stents. At follow-up angiography 4 to 6 months after coronary stent implantation, restenosis, defined as narrowing of 50% or more within the stent, was seen in 20% of patients with single stents and 50% of patients with multiple stents. Clinical restenosis, or recurrent symptoms of angina pectoris or positive stress test results requiring repeat PTCA or bypass surgery, occurred in approximately half of the patients with greater than 50% angiographic restenosis in single stents. When the definition for restenosis of Serruys et al.[56]—greater than 0.72-mm thickness of intimal growth within the stent—was applied, 50% of patients with single stents had restenosis. From these observations, further corroborated by Ellis et al.,[49] the authors concluded that the Palmaz-Schatz coronary stent does not inhibit smooth muscle cell growth but results in a low incidence of clinical and angiographic (>50% lumen narrowing) restenosis because it provides an optimal initial vessel lumen diameter so that the expected intimal hyperplasia does not compromise the vessel lumen.

Among the 37 patients with attempted RCA implantation of the Palmaz-Schatz stent who were reported by Levine et al.,[36] 21 (57%) had restenosis after conventional PTCA (of which 10 had two or more previous PTCAs), 17 (46%) had markedly eccentric lesions, 5 (14%) had flaplike or ulcerated lesions, and 2 (5%) had total occlusions. There was, for the group of 35 patients with successful stent delivery, a change in mean diameter stenosis from 83% ± 14% at baseline study to 42% ± 14% after conventional angioplasty and to −3% ± 12% after stent placement. Eighteen (54%) patients had a suboptimal angiographic result after conventional PTCA. Twenty-seven (77.1%) of the 35 patients received single stents, 7 patients received two stents, and 1 patient had four stents placed for an extensive dissection following conventional PTCA. At clinical follow-up after stenting, only 2 out of the 35 patients developed recurrent angina or had evidence of reversible ischemia on thallium exercise testing. Routine follow-up angiography 4 to 6 months after stent implantation in 25 patients showed 7 (28.0%) with restenosis, defined in this study as narrowing of 60% or greater anywhere within or immediately adjacent to the stented segment. Restenosis was present in 3 of 18 patients with single stents (16.7%) and 4 of 7 patients with multiple stents (57.1%). Of the 7 patients with restenosis, 1 with an asymptomatic total occlusion of the four stents placed for an extensive post-PTCA dissection was managed medically, and the remaining 6 underwent successful redilatation of the within-stent stenosis, with the mean within-stent narrowing reduced from 80% ± 12% to 13% ± 21%.

Fajadet et al. presented their findings in 79 patients who underwent successful implantations of a single Palmaz-Schatz coronary stent in a native coronary artery.[45] Approximately one third of these patients had restenosis after previous PTCAs. Thirty-seven (46.8%) patients received a stent in the LAD coronary artery, 16 (20.3%) patients had stents implanted in the circumflex coronary artery, and 26 (32.9%) patients received stents in the RCA. At follow-up coronary angiography 3 to 6 months (mean, 4.4 months) after stenting, restenosis, defined as >50% narrowing, was observed in 12 (15.2%) patients. Restenosis rates were 21.6% for LAD artery stents, 12.5% for stents in the circumflex coronary artery, and 7.7% for RCA stents.

Because of the above evidence strongly suggesting lower rates of restenosis after native coronary artery implantation of the single Palmaz-Schatz stent than after conventional PTCA, several multicenter randomized trials have been initiated to compare these two treatments.

Restenosis in Aortocoronary Bypass Grafts

Leon et al.[55] reviewed the early multicenter experience with the Palmaz-Schatz stent in saphenous vein aortocoronary bypass grafts (SVBGs) in 90 consecutive patients. The mean age of the patients was 64 ($\pm$ 10) years. The mean age of the SVBG stented was 8.5 ($\pm$ 3.8) years. Fifty-nine percent of the patients had had prior PTCA of the lesion stented. One hundred seventeen stents were deployed in 109 lesions. The mean present narrowing was 81% ($\pm$ 15%). The mean lesion length was 5.5 ($\pm$4.0) mm. The mean poststenting residual stenosis was 7% ($\pm$ 9%), and the mean expanded stent diameter ws 3.4 ($\pm$ 0.6) mm. Early angiographic follow-up on the average 2.7 ($\pm$ 18) months after stenting demonstrated angiographic restenosis in 17% of patients.

Included in the series of 83 patients with follow-up angiograms 3 to 6 months after the implantation of a single Palmaz-Schatz stent of Fajadet et al.[45] there were 6 patients with the SVBG stents. Two of these six patients, or 33.3%, had greater than 50% within-stent stenosis at follow-up.

While the rate of restenosis after implantation of the Palmaz-Schatz stent appears to be higher in the SVBGs than in the native coronary arteries, this rate of restenosis compares favorably to the rates of restenosis reported after SVBG PTCA.[15–17]

Management of Restenosis

While the incidence of restenosis appears to be lower after coronary stenting with the single Palmaz-Schatz stent than following PTCA,[36, 40, 45, 52, 57] within-stent restenosis does occur. Current management of restenosis after coronary stenting has been recently analyzed by several authors. Levine et al. reviewed the experience of the ongoing United States multicenter trial.[57] In the cohort of 186 patients with follow-up angiograms 4 to 6 months after stent placement, 50 patients, or 27%, had restenosis, defined as angiographic narrowing of greater than 60% within or immediately adjacent to a coronary stent. Fifty-six percent of the 50 patients with restenosis had anginal symptoms, and 44% were asymptomatic. Thirteen of 50 patients with restenosis, most of whom had mild restenoses or collateralized total occlusions, were managed medically. Fifteen patients underwent

elective coronary artery bypass surgery, and 22 patients had PTCA of the restenosis. In all 22 patients, PTCA was successful, with reduction in luminal stenosis from 81% $\pm$ 12% to 9% $\pm$ 13%. Post-PTCA vessel contour was smooth in 21 patients, with a small dissection noted in only 1 patient, which suggests that with the stent firmly incorporated into the arterial wall 4 to 6 months after implantation, the artery exhibits plastic rather than elastic behavior, a fact that may contribute to the safety and effectiveness of PTCA within the stented segment.

Fajadet et al. reported on their management of restenosis following successful implantation of a single Palmaz-Schatz stent.[45] In their cohort of 83 patients, the mean interval from stent implantation to follow-up angiography was 4.4 months. Fourteen patients, or 16.9% of the total group, had restenosis, defined as >50% narrowing, at follow-up angiography. One late closure was found. Five patients, or 35.7% of those with restenosis, were asymptomatic, had moderate restenosis of 50% to 70% and normal thallium scintigraphy findings, and were treated medically. Of the 8 patients with symptoms and angiographic restenosis of >70%, 1 patient had elective bypass surgery, 1 was treated with atherectomy, and 6 patients had successful PTCA.

CONCLUSION

In summary, results of the ongoing clinical trials with the Palmaz-Schatz coronary stent attest to its safety and efficacy. When compared with the published series of patients undergoing PTCA of a native coronary artery, coronary implantation of single Palmaz-Schatz stents appears to be associated with a lower incidence of restenosis despite a higher proportion of patients with recurrent restenosis in the initial stent trials and a determination of rates of restenosis based on angiographic rather than clinical criteria. Restenosis rates are especially favorable in de novo lesions in the native coronary arteries treated with single stents. Several multicenter randomized trials comparing rates of angiographic restenosis after PTCA and after coronary stenting with the single Palmaz-Schatz stent are in progress. Restenosis within the stent can be managed with any of the clinically appropriate currently available strategies, with most patients being safely and successfully treated with repeat PTCA. Long-term outcomes of stent restenoses treated with PTCA remain to be determined. The incidence of clinical restenosis remains approximately half that of angiographic restenosis.

The rate of major complications after implantation of the Palmaz-Schatz stent compares favorably with that reported after PTCA. The rates of acute and subacute thrombosis range from 0% to 6% and may be increased in patients receiving the Palmaz-Schatz stent for suboptimal outcomes of PTCA (but still substantially below those reported with PTCA alone).[34, 53, 54] The incidence of complications decreases with operator experience.[43] Vascular access–related complications are higher in patients receiving stents than after PTCA and are related to the more rigorous anticoagulation regimen.

Even while the current Palmaz-Schatz coronary stent and the SDS are in clinical trials, concerted research efforts are being made to make coronary stenting more effective. Krupski et al. found that infusion of a new synthetic antithrombin, D-phenylalanyl-L-prolyl-L-arginyl-chloromethylketone (D-FPRCH2C1), but not infusion of heparin prevents thrombus formation on stents implanted in baboons.[58] Bailey et al. reported less local platelet deposition and less vascular spasm with polymer-coated stents when compared with uncoated stents in rabbits.[59] In their elegant study, Dichek et al. demonstrated the feasibility of seeding Palmaz-Schatz stents with endothelial cells genetically engineered to secrete tissue-type plasminogen activator (t-PA) and showed persistent stent adherence of such cells after balloon expansion of the stent.[60] There is every reason to hope that in the near future improved understanding of thrombosis and atherosclerosis will ultimately result in the availability of antithrombotic and possibly antimitotic stent coatings.

The Palmaz-Schatz balloon-expandable coronary stent is an exciting, safe, and effective new nonsurgical treatment modality for coronary stenoses in properly selected patients.

REFERENCES

1. Schatz RA, Palmaz JC, Tio FO, et al: Balloon-expandable intracoronary stents in the adult dog. *Circulation* 1987; 76:450.
2. Schatz RA: A view of vascular stents. *Circulation* 1989; 79:445–457.
3. Topol EJ (ed): *Textbook of Interventional Cardiology.* Philadelphia, WB Saunders, 1990.
4. Grüntzig AR: Transluminal dilatation of coronary artery stenosis (letter). *Lancet* 1978; 1:263.
5. Grüntzig AR, King SB, Schlumpf M, et al: Long-term follow-up after percutaneous coronary angioplasty. *N Engl J Med* 1987; 316:1127–1132.
6. Holmes DR, Vliestra RE, Smith HC, et al: Restenosis after percutaneous transluminal coronary angioplasty (PTCA): A report from the Coronary Angioplasty Registry of the National Heart, Lung, and Blood Institute. *Am J Cardiol* 1984; 53:77–81.
7. Nobuyoshi M, Kimura T, Nosaka H, et al: Restenosis after successful percutaneous coronary angioplasty: Serial angiographic follow-up of 229 patients. *J Am Coll Cardiol* 1988; 12:616–623.
8. Serruys PW, Luijten HE, Beatt KJ, et al: Incidence of restenosis after successful coronary angioplasty: A time-related phenomenon. A quantitative angiographic study in 342 consecutive patients at 1, 2, 3, and 4 months. *Circulation* 1988; 77:361–371.
9. Myler RK, Topol EJ, Shaw RE, et al: Multiple vessel coronary angioplasty: Classification, results, and patterns of restenosis in 494 consecutive patients. *Cathet Cardiovasc Diagn* 1987; 13:1–15.
10. Fleck E, Regitz V, Lehnert A, et al: Restenosis after balloon dilatation of coronary stenosis: Multivariant analysis of potential risk factors. *Eur Heart J* 1988; 9:15–18.
11. Galan KM, Deligonul U, Kern MJ, et al: Increased frequency of restenosis in patients continuing to smoke cigarettes after percutaneous transluminal coronary angioplasty. *Am J Cardiol* 1988; 61:260–263.
12. Mata LA, Bosch X, David PR, et al: Clinical and angiographic assessment 6 months after double vessel percutaneous coronary angioplasty. *J Am Coll Cardiol* 1985; 6:1239–1244.
13. Leimgruber PP, Roubin GS, Hollman J, et al: Restenosis after successful coronary angioplasty in patients with single-vessel disease. *Circulation* 1986; 73:710–717.
14. Vandormael MG, Deligonul U, Kern MJ, et al: Multilesion coronary angioplasty: Clinical and angiographic follow-up. *J Am Coll Cardiol* 1987; 10:246–252.
15. Cote G, Myler RK, Stertzer SH, et al: Percutaneous transluminal angioplasty of stenotic coronary artery bypass grafts: 5 years' experience. *J Am Coll Cardiol* 1987; 9:8–17.
16. Douglas JS, King SB, Roubin GS, et al: Percutaneous angioplasty of venous aortocoronary graft stenoses: Late angiographic and clinical outcome. *Circulation* 1986; 74(suppl 2):281.
17. Webb JG, Myler RK, Shaw RE, et al: Coronary angioplasty after coronary bypass surgery: Initial results and late outcome in 422 patients. *J Am Coll Cardiol* 1990; 16:812–820.
18. Topol EJ, Ellis SG, Fishman J, et al: Multicenter study of percutaneous transluminal angioplasty for right coronary artery ostial stenosis. *J Am Coll Cardiol* 1987; 9:1214–1218.
19. Whitworth HB, Pilcher GS, Roubin GS, et al: Do proximal lesions involving the origin of the proximal left anterior descending artery (LAD) have a higher restenosis rate after coronary angioplasty (PTCA) (abstract)? *Circulation* 1985; 72(suppl 3):398.
20. Meier B, King SB, Grüntzig AR, et al: Repeat coronary angioplasty. *J Am Coll Cardiol* 1984; 4:463–466.
21. Quigley PJ, Hlatky MA, Hinohara T, et al: Repeat percutaneous transluminal coronary angioplasty and predictors of recurrent stenosis. *Am J Cardiol* 1989; 63:409–413.
22. Williams DO, Grüntzig AR, Kent KM, et al: Efficacy of repeat percutaneous transluminal coronary angioplasty for coronary restenosis. *Am J Cardiol* 1984; 53:32–35.
23. Teirstein PS, Hoover CA, Ligon RW, et al: Repeat restenosis: Efficacy of a third angioplasty for a second restenosis. *J Am Coll Cardiol* 1989; 13:291–296.
24. Haase KK, Mauser M, Baumbach A, et al: Restenosis after excimer laser coronary atherectomy (abstract). *Circulation* 1990; 82(suppl 3):672.
25. Reeder GS, Bresnahan JF, Bresnahan DR, et al: Excimer

laser coronary angioplasty (ELCA) in patients with restenosis after prior balloon angioplasty (BA) (abstract). *Circulation* 1990; 82(suppl 3):672.

26. Reis GJ, Pomerantz RM, Jenkins RD, et al: Laser balloon angioplasty: Clinical, angiographic, and histologic results (abstract). *Circulation* 1990; 82(suppl 3):672.

27. Sketch MH, O'Neill WW, Tcheng JE, et al: Early and late outcome following coronary transluminal extraction-endarterectomy: A multicenter experience (abstract). *Circulation* 1990; 82(suppl 3):310.

28. U.S. Directional Coronary Atherectomy Investigator Group: Restenosis following directional coronary atherectomy in a multicenter experience. *Circulation* 1990; 82(suppl 3):679.

29. Simpson JB, Rowe MH, Selmon MR, et al: Restenosis following directional coronary atherectomy in de novo lesions in native coronary arteries (abstract). *Circulation* 1990; 82(suppl 3):313.

30. Cowley MJ, Dorros G, Kelsey SF, et al: Acute coronary events associated with percutaneous transluminal coronary angioplasty. *Am J Cardiol* 1984; 53:12–16.

31. Detre KM, Holubkov R, Kelsey SF, et al: Percutaneous transluminal coronary angioplasty in 1985–1986 and 1977–1981. *N Engl J Med* 1988; 318:265–270.

32. Tuzcu EM, Simpfendorfer C, Badhwar K, et al: Determinants of primary success in elective percutaneous transluminal coronary angioplasty for significant narrowing of a major single coronary artery. *Am J Cardiol* 1988; 62:873–875.

33. Park DD, Laramee LA, Tierstein PS, et al: Major complications during PTCA: An analysis of 5413 cases (abstract). *J Am Coll Cardiol* 1988; 11:237.

34. Bredlau CE, Roubin GS, Leimgruber PP, et al: In-hospital morbidity and mortality in patients undergoing elective coronary angioplasty. *Circulation* 1985; 72:1044–1052.

35. Schatz RA, Palmaz JC: Balloon expandable intravascular stents (BEIS) in human coronary arteries: Report of initial experience (abstract). *Circulation* 1988; 78 (suppl 3):1625.

36. Levine MJ, Leonard BM, Burke JA, et al: Clinical and angiographic results of balloon-expandable intracoronary stents in right coronary artery stenoses. *J Am Coll Cardiol* 1990; 16:332–339.

37. Palmaz JC, Windelar SA, Garcia F, et al: Balloon expandable intraluminal grafting of atherosclerotic rabbit aortas. *Radiology* 1986; 160:723–726.

38. Schatz RA, Palmaz JC, Tio F, et al: Report of a new articulated balloon expandable intravascular stent (ABEIS). *Circulation* 1988; 78(suppl 3):1789.

39. Baim DS, Bailey S, Curry C, et al: Improved success and safety of Palmaz-Schatz coronary stenting with a new delivery system (abstract). *Circulation* 1990; 82(suppl 3):657.

40. Teirstein PS, Cleman MW, Hirshfield JW, et al: Influence of prior restenosis on subsequent restenosis after intracoronary stenting (abstract). *Circulation* 1990; 82(suppl 3):675.

41. Haude M, Erbel R, Straub U, et al: Intracoronary stent implantation in patients with symptomatic dissections after balloon angioplasty — short- and long-term results (abstract). *Circulation* 1990; 82(suppl 3):655.

42. Kaplan AI, Sabin S: Dextran 40: Another cause of drug-induced noncardiogenic pulmonary edema. *Chest* 1975; 68:376–377.

43. Fajadet JC, Marco J, Cassagneau BG, et al: Balloon expandable intracoronary stent: Analysis of complications in a consecutive series of 160 patients (abstract). *Circulation* 1990; 82(suppl 3):539.

44. Schatz RA, Goldberg S, Leon MB, et al: Coronary stenting following "suboptimal" coronary angioplasty results (abstract). *Circulation* 1990; 82(suppl 3):540.

45. Fajadet JC, Marco J, Cassagneau BG, et al: Restenosis following successful single Palmaz-Schatz stent implantation (abstract). *Circulation* 1990; 82(suppl(supp 3):314.

46. Dajani AS, Bisno AL, Chung KJ, et al: Prevention of bacterial endocarditis. Recommendations by the American Heart Association. *JAMA* 1990; 264:2919–2922.

47. Teitelbaum GP, Bradley WG, Klein BD: MR imaging artifacts, ferromagnetism, and magnetic torque of intravascular filters, stents, and coils. *Radiology* 1988; 166:657–664.

48. Nichols AB, Smith R, Berke AD, et al: Importance of balloon size in coronary angioplasty. *J Am Coll Cardiol* 1990; 13:1094–1100.

49. Ellis SG, Fishman DL, Hirshfeld JW, et al: Mechanism of stent benefit to limit restenosis following coronary angioplasty: Regrowth vs. larger initial lumen (abstract) *Circulation* 1990; 82(suppl 3):540.

50. Steele PM, Chesebro JH, Stanson AW, et al: Balloon angioplasty: Natural history of the pathophysiological response to injury in a pig model. *Circ Res* 1985; 57:105–112.

51. Leung DY, Glagov S, Mathews MB: Cyclic stretching stimulates synthesis of matrix components by arterial smooth muscle cells in vitro. *Science* 1976; 191:475–477.

52. Schatz RA, Baim DS, Leon M, et al: Clinical experience with the Palmaz-Schatz coronary stent: Initial results of a multicenter study. *Circulation*, 1991; 83:148–161.

53. Ellis SG, Roubin GS, King SB, et al: Angiographic and clinical predictors of acute closure after native vessel coronary angioplasty. *Circulation* 1988; 77:372–379.

54. Detre KM, Holmes DR, Holubkov R, et al: The 1985–1986 NHLBI PTCA Registry: Incidence and consequences of periprocedural occlusion. *Circulation* 1990; 82:739–750.

55. Leon MB, Pichard AD, Baim DS, et al: Early results of stent implantation in aortocoronary saphenous vein grafts. *Circulation* 1990; 82(suppl 3):679.

56. Serruys PW, Beatt KJ, Van Der Giessen WJ: Stenting of coronary arteries. Are we the sorcerer's apprentice? *Eur Heart J* 1989; 10:774–782.

57. Levine MJ, Cleman MW, Schatz RA, et al: Management of restenosis following stenting: Multicenter results (abstract). *Circulation* 1990; 82(suppl 3):657.

58. Krupski WC, Bass A, Kelly AB, et al: Heparin-resistant thrombus formation by endovascular stents in baboons. Interruption by a synthetic antithrombin. *Circulation* 1990; 82:570–577.

59. Bailey SR, Guy DM, Garcia OJ, et al: Polymer coating of Palmaz-Schatz stent attenuates vascular spasm after stent placement (abstract). *Circulation* 1990; 82(suppl 3):541.

60. Dichek DA, Neville RF, Zwiebel JA, et al: Seeding of intravascular stents with genetically engineered endothelial cells. *Circulation* 1989; 80:1347–1353.

32

The Wallstent Experience: 1986–1990*

Patrick W. Serruys, M.D., Ph.D.
Bradley Strauss, M.D., Ph.D.

In 1986, the first coronary Wallstent implantation ushered in a new era in interventional cardiology with the purpose of circumventing the two major limitations of coronary angioplasty, early acute occlusion and late restenosis.[1] As with all new procedures, operators of the device had to struggle with their own learning curves at the same time that anticoagulation regimens and clinical indications and contraindications evolved from their clinical experience.

Since March 1986, the coronary Wallstent has been the most intensively studied endovascular prosthesis in Europe. As a result of cooperation among the six participating European centers, a central core laboratory was set up in Rotterdam to objectively assess the follow-up of stents with quantitative coronary angiography.

A previous publication from our group reported the late angiographic and clinical follow-up of the initial 105 patients who received implants between 1986 and 1988.[2] In the period from January 1989 until March 1990, a further 160 patients underwent stent implantation in the coronary circulation.

In this chapter, we compare the late quantitative angiographic and clinical follow-up of this second group of patients with the initial group, and to further characterize the factors associated with angiographic restenosis within the stented segment, we retrospectively studied the predictive ability of several angiographic variables.

*This study was supported in part by grants from the Dutch Ministry of Science and Education, Den Haag, The Netherlands (87159) and the Swiss National Fund (3.835.083).

METHODS

Study Patients

Two hundred sixty-five patients (308 lesions) were enrolled after obtaining informed consent between March 1986 and March 1990 at the participating centers. The study patients were grouped according to the date of implantation (prior to or after January 1, 1988; groups 1 and 2, respectively) and the vessel type stented (native vessel vs. bypass graft) (Tables 32–1 and 32–2).

In group 1, 117 stents were implanted in 114 lesions, 82% of which were in native vessels (and in particular the left anterior descending artery). In group 2, 266 stents were implanted in 194 lesions, predominantly in bypass grafts (60% of cases). In this group, the right coronary artery was the most common vessel stented in the native circulation.

The indications for stenting also differed between the two vessel types (Fig 32–1). Native vessels were primarily stented to prevent a second restenosis or as a bailout procedure for angioplasties complicated by abrupt closure or large dissections that interrupted anterograde flow and were associated with clinical and electrocardiographic signs of ischemia. However, in bypass grafts, the principle indication was for primary lesions in bypass grafts that had not been previously treated with angioplasty.

In the overall group, angiographic follow-up was obtained in 218 patients (82%). However, in-hospital occlusions occurred in 40 patients (41 lesions). Follow-up angiograms were quantitatively analyzed in 176 patients (78%) of the 225 patients who were discharged from the

TABLE 32–1

Stent Implantations According to Date of Implantation

	Group 1 (March 1986–Dec 1988)	Group 2 (Jan 1989–March 1990)
Vessels	107	175
Bypass	18%	60%
Native*	82%	40%
LAD	54%	15%
Cx	7%	5%
RCA	21%	20%
Stent lesions	117/114	266/194

*LAD = left anterior descending; Cx = circumflex; RCA = right coronary artery.

TABLE 32–2

Stent Implantations According to Vessel Type

	Group 1 (March 1986–Dec 1988) Native	Group 2 (Jan 1989–March 1990) Bypass Grafts
Patients	166	101
Vessels	171	110
Stent/lesion*	193/173	192/135
LAD	55%	
Cx	10%	
RCA	35%	

*LAD = left anterior descending; Cx = circumflex; RCA = right coronary artery.

hospital without known occlusion (Figs 32–2 and 32–3). They had a total of 259 stents implanted in 214 lesions. The mean length of angiographic follow-up in the study group was 6.6 ± 4.8 months.

The anticoagulation for the first period of implantation has previously been described.[2] Based on this initial clinical experience, a uniform anticoagulation schedule was followed at the centers. Acetylsalicylic acid, 1 g orally, was started 1 day before the procedure. At the beginning of the procedure, patients received heparin, 10,000 IU intravenously, and in some cases, dextran infusions (500 mg/4 hr) were also given. Additional heparin (10,000 IU) and intracoronary urokinase, 100,000 units, were administered during the procedure. Following the procedure, the heparin infusion was adjusted according to the activated partial thromboplastin time

(APTT; 80 to 120 seconds) in addition to initiating oral vitamin K antagonist therapy. Heparin therapy was discontinued after the therapeutic oral anticoagulation level was stabilized (international normalized ratio of 2.3 or more). Acetylsalicylic acid, 100 mg daily, dipyridamole, 300 to 450 mg/day, and in some patients sulfinpyrazone, 400 mg daily, were also administered.

In this trial, the endovascular prosthesis Wallstent was provided by Medinvent SA, Lausanne, Switzerland. The method of implantation and description of this stent has previously been reported.[1, 2] This stent is a self-expandable stainless steel woven mesh prosthesis that can be positioned in the coronary artery by using standard over-the-wire technique through a 8 F or 9 F guiding catheter. The device is constructed of 16 wire filaments, each 0.08 mm wide. It is constrained in an

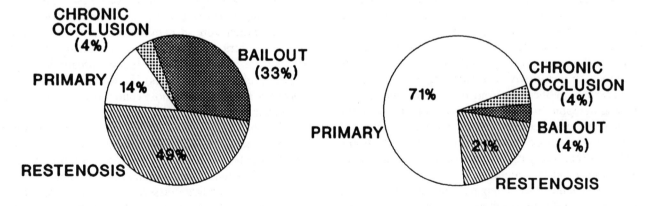

NATIVE   BYPASS

FIG 32–1.

The indications for stenting in native arteries and bypass grafts. *Primary* = primary atherosclerotic lesion that has not been previously treated by percutaneous transluminal coronary angioplasty [PTCA] or stenting.

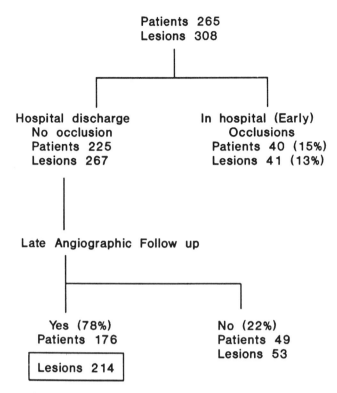

Patients 265
Lesions 308

Hospital discharge
No occlusion
Patients 225
Lesions 267

In hospital (Early)
Occlusions
Patients 40 (15%)
Lesions 41 (13%)

Late Angiographic Follow up

Yes (78%)
Patients 176

Lesions 214

No (22%)
Patients 49
Lesions 53

FIG 32–2.
Flow diagram showing the angiographic follow-up in 265 stented lesions. In-hospital (early) occlusions occurred in 40 patients (15%). In the remaining 225 patients who were discharged from the hospital without known stent occlusion, 176 patients (78%) with 214 stented lesions had quantitative angiographic follow-up.

elongated configuration on a 1.57-mm-diameter delivery catheter with the distal end covered by a removable plastic sleeve. As the sleeve is withdrawn, the constrained device returns to its original unconstrained larger diameter and becomes anchored against the vessel wall. The unconstrained stent diameter ranged from 2.5 to 6 mm and was selected to be 0.50 mm larger than the stented vessel based on a visual estimate of the prestent angiogram by the investigator. In an effort to alleviate the problem of acute thrombosis, the stent design was changed in April 1989 with the introduction of a polymer-coated stent (Biogold) for certain stent sizes. By August 1989, all manufactured stents contained this particular polymer coating.

Quantitative Coronary Arteriography

All cineangiograms were analyzed at the core laboratory in Rotterdam by using a computer-assisted cardiovascular angiography analysis system (CAAS) that has previously been discussed in detail.[3, 4] The important

steps will be briefly described. Selected areas of the cineframe encompassing the desire arterial segment (from side branch to side branch) are optically magnified, displayed in a video format, and then digitally converted. Vessel contour is determined automatically from the weighted sum of the first and second derivative functions applied to the digitized brightness information. A computer-derived estimation of the original arterial dimension at the site of the obstruction is used to define interpolated reference diameter and area. The absolute diameter of the stenosis as well as the reference diameter is measured by the computer, which uses the known guiding catheter diameter as a calibration factor after correction for pincushion distortion. The percent diameter of the narrowed segment is derived by comparing the observed stenosis dimensions to the reference values. *The length* of the lesion (millimeters) is determined from the diameter function on the basis of a curvature analysis. By using the reconstructed borders of the vessel, the computer can calculate a symmetry coefficient for the stenosis. Differences in distance between the actual and reconstructed vessel contours on both sides of the lesion are measured. *Symmetry* is determined by the ratio of these two differences, with the largest distance between actual and reconstructed contours becoming the denominator. Values for symmetry range from 0 for extreme eccentricity to 1 for maximal symmetry (that is, equal distance on both sides between reconstructed and actual contours). The angiographic analysis was done before and after angioplasty, immediately after stent implantation, and at long-term follow-up in all patients by using the average of multiple matched views with orthogonal projections wherever possible.

Restenosis

Two different set of criteria were applied to determine the restenosis rate. We have found a change in minimal luminal diameter (MLD) of 0.72 mm or more to be a reliable indicator of angiographic progression of vessel narrowing, but this by no means implies functional or clinical significance.[3, 4] This value takes into account the limitations of coronary angiographic measurements and represents two times the long-term variability (i.e., the 95% confidence intervals) for repeat measurements of a coronary obstruction with CAAS. The other criterion for restenosis chosen was an increase in the diameter of stenosis from less than 50% after stent implantation to greater than or equal to 50% at follow-up. This criterion was selected since common clinical practice continues to assess lesion severity by

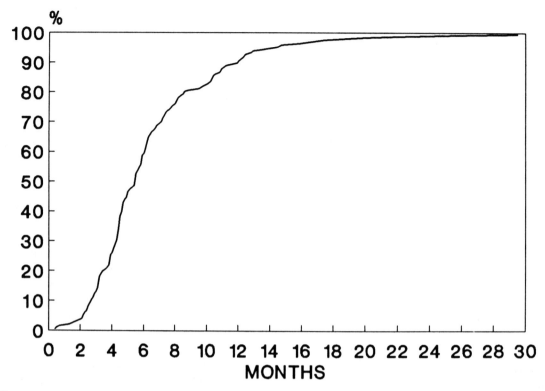

FIG 32–3.
Timing of late angiographic follow-up after stent implantation. In this cumulative curve, the interval (in months) between the date of implantation and final angiographic follow-up is shown for the study group.

percent stenosis. The two criteria were assessed within the stent and in the segment immediately adjacent (proximal and distal) to the stent.

Late (i.e., documented after initial discharge from the hospital) occlusions ($n = 10$ patients, 16 lesions) were regarded as restenoses.

Angiographic Variables

Based on the quantitative angiographic data, multiple variables were identified and recorded for each lesion. These variables, either discrete (two or three distinct responses) or continuous (a range of responses), were grouped according to lesion, stent, or procedural factors (Tables 32–3 and 32–4). These particular variables were of a priori clinical interest on the basis of previously published PTCA and stent reports.[5–11]

Statistical Methods

The data obtained by quantitative angiographic analysis are given as means ± SD. The mean of each angiographic variable pre-PTCA, poststent, and at follow-up were compared by using analysis of variance. If significance differences were found, two-tailed *t*-tests were ap-

plied to pairs of data. The occlusion and restenosis rates were compared by using a chi-squared test. A statistical probability of less than .05 was considered significant.

A relative-risk analysis was performed for the aforementioned discrete and continuous variables.[12] The continuous variables were dichotomized for the risk ratio analysis. To avoid arbitrary subdivision of data in continuous variables, cut points were derived by dividing the data into two groups, each containing roughly

TABLE 32–3
Angiographic Follow-up

Implantations (lesions/patients)	308/265
Early occlusions	41/40
Late follow-up	214/176
Total	255/216 (82%)
No angiographic follow-up	53/49 (18%)
Death	10 (4%)
Early CABG*	11 (4%)
Refusal	25 (9%)
Technical	3 (1%)
Time to angiographic follow-up	
Excluding early occlusions	6.6 ± 4.8
Including early occlusions	5.7 ± 5.0
*CABG = coronary artery bypass grafting.	

TABLE 32–4

Angiographic Results: Early Occlusions

	Total	Group 1	Group 2	Native Vessels	Bypass Grafts
Lesions	308/265	114/105	194/160	173/166	135/101
Early occlusions	40 (13%)/39 (15%)	21 (18%)/21 (20%)	20 (10%)/19 (12%)	32 (18%)/32 (19%)	9 (7%)/8 (8%)

50% of the total population. This method of subdivision has the advantage of being consistent for all variables and thus avoids any bias in selection of subgroups that might be undertaken to emphasize a particular point. The incidence of restenosis in the two groups was compared by using a relative-risk analysis. A relative risk of 1 for a particular variable implies that the presence of that variable poses no additional risk for restenosis; relative risks greater than 1 or less than 1 imply additional or reduced risk, respectively. For example, a relative risk

of 2 for a particular parameter implies that the presence of that factor increases the likelihood of restenosis by a factor of 2. The 95% confidence intervals were calculated to describe the statistical certainty. Statistical significance was defined as $P < .05$ and was determined by using the Pearson chi-squared test (BMDP) statistical software, University of California, Berkeley, 1990). Late clinical follow-up was determined according to a life table format by using the Kaplan-Meier method.[13]

The following events were considered clinical end

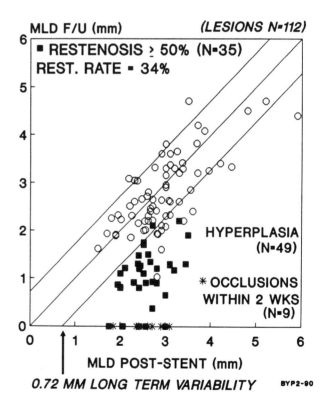

FIG 32–4.
Change is the minimal luminal diameter *(MLD)* for individual lesions in native vessels **(A)** and in bypass grafts **(B)** between stent implantation and angiographic follow-up *(F/U)*. The diameter of each segment immediately after implantation is plotted against the diameter at follow-up. The lines on each side of the identity line *(diagonal)* represent the limits of long-term variability of repeat measurements (a change of $\geq$ 0.72 mm *[arrow]*). All symbols below the *right-hand* line represent stents with involvement of angiographically detectable hyperplasia. The *filled squares* represents lesions with a follow-up diameter stenosis of 50% or greater. Occlusions are located along the x-axis, and those lesions that occurred within the first 2 weeks are marked with an *asterisk.*

points: death, myocardial infarction, and bypass surgery or nonsurgical revascularization (PTCA or atherectomy). The life table was constructed according to the initial clinical event.

RESULTS

Occlusion and Restenosis Rate

The angiographic follow-up for the entire study population was 82% (see Table 32–3). This includes patients with documented early occlusions during hospital admission ($n = 40$) in addition to patients who had late (after the initial hospital discharge) angiographically confirmed occlusions. The reasons why follow-up angiography could not be performed are listed in Table 32–3). The time to angiographic follow-up was 6.6 ± 4.8 months if early occlusions are excluded and 5.7 ± 5.0 months with the early occlusions.

The angiographic data for individual lesions in bypass grafts and native vessels are presented in Figure 32–4,A and B. In native vessels, there was a mean increase in MLD from 1.17 ± .52 mm to 2.53 ± .53 mm immediately poststenting but a late deterioration to 1.99 ± .81 mm if early occlusions are excluded and 1.59 ±

1.08 mm with the inclusion of the early occlusions ($P <$ .0001) (Fig 32–5). Similarly, the MLD increased in bypass lesions from 1.39 ± 0.64 mm to 2.81 ± 0.69 mm poststenting with a late reduction to 2.21 ± 1.16 mm and 2.03 ± 1.27 mm with the exclusion and inclusion of early occlusions, respectively ($P <$ .0001). Diameter stenosis was reduced immediately poststenting in bypass grafts from 60% ± 14% to 23% ± 10% but increased at late follow-up to 43% ± 31% and to 38% ± 27% with and without the early occlusions, respectively ($P <$ .0001). Similar changes were observed in native vessels (data not shown).

In the overall group, the incidence of early in-hospital occlusion was 15% by patient and 13% by lesion (Table 32–4). In bypass grafts, early occlusions were documented in 7% of lesions (8% of patients) vs. 18% of lesions (19% of patients) in native vessels (by lesion, $P = .005$; by patient, $P = .016$). Three of these native vessel occlusions occurred during the procedure and could not be recanalized. The remaining occlusions presented clinically as acute ischemic syndromes following a successful stenting procedure. Early occlusions were less frequent in group 2 patients (12%) than in group 1 (20%) but not statistically significant. Detectable angiographic narrowing (0.72 mm loss in MLD) in the over-

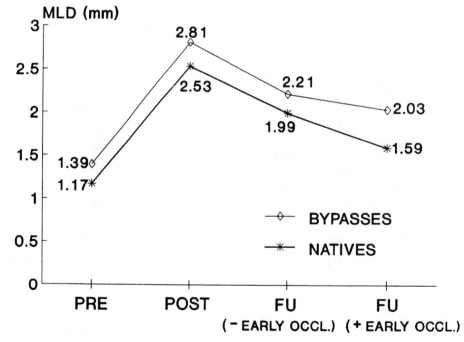

CHANGE IN MINIMAL LUMINAL DIAMETER

FIG 32–5.
Minimal luminal diameter *(MLD)* of native vessels and bypass grafts preprocedure, poststenting, and at follow-up. The mean values at follow-up have been calculated with and without the inclusion of the early in-hospital occlusions.

TABLE 32–5

Late Angiographic Follow-Up: Restenosis Within and Immediately Adjacent to the Stent

	Total	Group 1	Group 2	Native Vessel	Bypass Grafts
Lesions/patients	214/176	85/75	129/101	111/104	103/74
0.72-mm criterion					
Within stent	75/61	25/21	50/40	34/30	40/31
Adjacent to stent	14/14	5/5	9/9	5/5	9/9
Total	89/75	30/26	59/49	40/35	49/40
	(42%/43%)	(37%/35%)	(46%/49%)	(36%/34%)	(48%/54%)
50% DS* criterion					
Within stent	51/42	17/15	34/27	21/18	30/24
Adjacent to stent	6/6	1/1	5/5	1/1	5/5
Total	57/48	18/16	39/32	22/19	35/29
	(27%/27%)	(22%/21%)	(30%/32%)	(20%/18%)	(34%/39%)

*DS = diameter stenosis.

all group was 42% by lesion and 43 % by patient (Table 32–5). With the 50% diameter stenosis criterion, restenosis occurred in 27% of lesions (27% of patients).

Restenosis according to either definition was significantly higher in bypass grafts (MLD criterion, 54% by patient; diameter stent [DS] criterion, 39% by patient) than in native vessels (34% and 18%, respectively) (MLD, $P = .016$; DS, $P = .001$). Group 2 patients (MLD criterion, 49% by patient; DS criterion, 32% by patient) did not have significantly greater restenosis than group 1 patients (MLD criterion, 35%; DS criterion, 21%).

Relative-Risk Analysis

The relative risk and 95% confidence intervals for each variable with either of the two criteria for restenosis are shown in Figure 32–6. The variables with statistically significant associations with restenosis when the 0.72-mm criterion was applied were multiple stents and oversizing the stent (unconstrained diameter) with respect to the reference diameter by more than 0.70 mm, which had relative-risk ratios (RR) (and 95% confidence intervals [Cl] of 1.56 (1.08 to 2.25) and 1.64 (1.10 to 2.45), respectively. The second criterion, ≥ 50% diameter stenosis at follow-up, was associated with oversizing

by > 0.70 mm (RR, 1.93; 95% Cl, 1.13 to 3.31), bypass grafts (RR, 1.62; 95% Cl, 0.98 to 2.66), multiple stents per lesion (RR, 1.61; 95% Cl, 0.97 to 2.67), and residual diameter stenosis > 20% poststenting (RR, 1.51; 95% Cl, 0.91 to 2.50). The actual restenosis rates for these variables are included in Tables 32–6 and 32–7.

Long-Term Follow-Up

The overall mortality rate during the study period was 8.9% for bypass grafts and 6.6% for native vessels (7.9% and 6% at 1 year, respectively). In the bypass group, four of the nine deaths occurred during the initial hospitalization. Two of these deaths resulted from intracerebral hematomas related to the anticoagulation, and two were from myocardial infarctions due to stent occlusion. Two of the five late deaths were sudden (at 2 and 18 months), two were clearly unrelated to the stent (chronic congestive heart failure, chronic renal failure), and the other death occurred after bypass surgery. In the group with native vessels, 7 of the 11 deaths were in-hospital. These were all due to myocardial infarctions

TABLE 32–6

Restenosis Rates According to Criterion 1 (≥ 0.72-mm Loss in Minimal Luminal Diameter)

Stent	n	Restenosis Rate
Number		
Multiple	22/44	50%
Single	53/165	32%
Oversize		
> 0.7mm	40/90	44%
≤ 0.7 mm	26/96	27%

TABLE 32–7

Restenosis Rates According to Criterion 2 (> 50% Diameter Stenosis at Follow-up)

Parameter	n	Restenosis Rate
Vessel type		
Bypass	30/103	30%
Native	20/111	19%
Stent oversize		
> 0.7 mm	29/90	32%
≤ 0.7 mm	16/96	17%
Diameter stenosis		
Poststent		
> 20%	30/107	28%
≤ 20%	19/102	19%

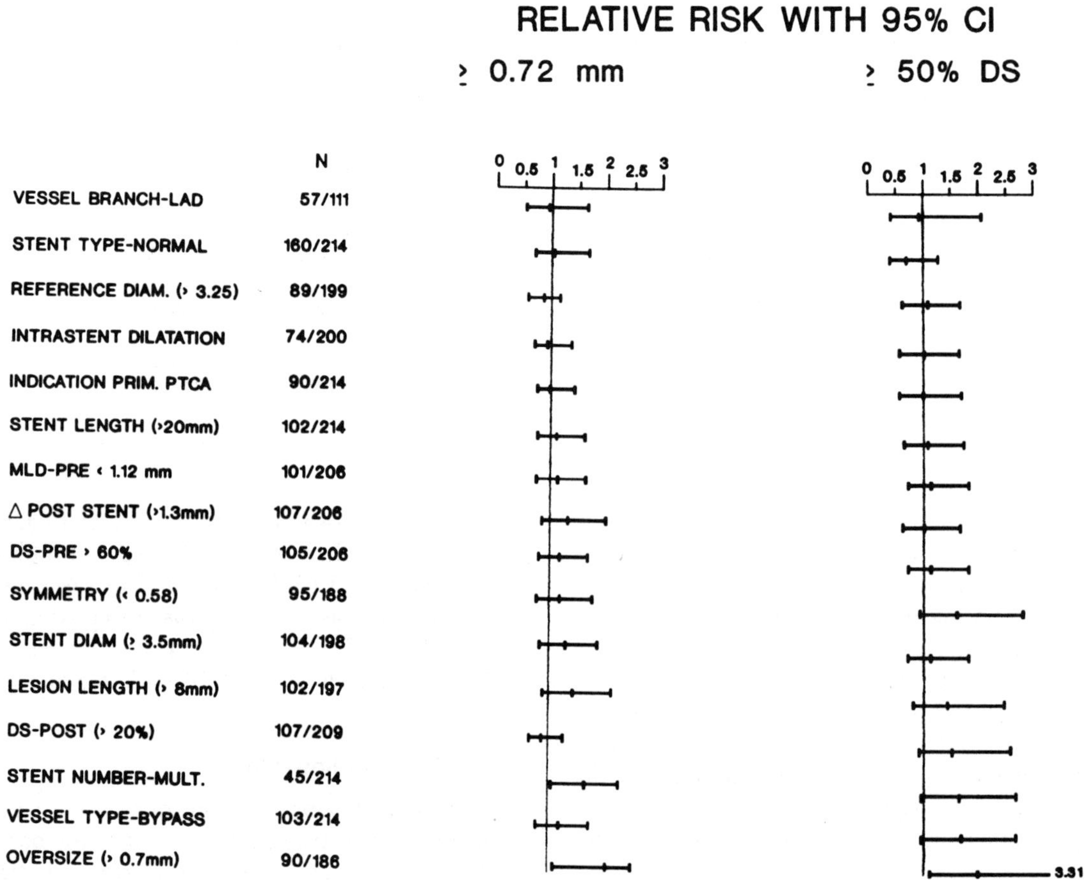

RELATIVE RISK WITH 95% CI

≥ 0.72 mm   ≥ 50% DS

	N
VESSEL BRANCH-LAD	57/111
STENT TYPE-NORMAL	160/214
REFERENCE DIAM. (› 3.25)	89/199
INTRASTENT DILATATION	74/200
INDICATION PRIM. PTCA	90/214
STENT LENGTH (›20mm)	102/214
MLD-PRE ‹ 1.12 mm	101/206
Δ POST STENT (›1.3mm)	107/206
DS-PRE › 60%	105/206
SYMMETRY (‹ 0.58)	95/188
STENT DIAM (≥ 3.5mm)	104/198
LESION LENGTH (› 8mm)	102/197
DS-POST (› 20%)	107/209
STENT NUMBER-MULT.	45/214
VESSEL TYPE-BYPASS	103/214
OVERSIZE (› 0.7mm)	90/186

FIG 32–6.
Relative risk ratios (with 95% confidence intervals) for the angiographic variables by using the two restenosis criteria (≥0.72-mm loss in minimal luminal diameter from immediately poststenting to follow-up and a diameter stenosis of 50% or greater at follow-up). The relative risk is indicated by the *thick vertical line* in the center, and the outside vertical line represent the 95% confidence limits. The *hatched vertical line* signifies a relative risk of 1 (no additional risk for restenosis). Variables with values greater than or less than 1 imply additional or a reduction in risk, respectively (see the text for details). The variables are listed in the *left-hand* column. *N* represents the number of lesions analyzed for each particular variable. Although 214 lesions were analyzed in total, some lesions could not be analyzed for certain variables. The denominator for vessel branch (111) represents the total number of lesions that were stented in native vessels. *CI* = confidence interval; *DS* = diameter stenosis; *LAD* = left anterior descending artery; *DIAM* = diameter; *PRIM* = primary; *PTCA* = percutaneous transluminal coronary angioplasty; *MLD* = minimal luminal diameter; / = absolute change; *MULT.* = multiple.

resulting from stent occlusion with the exception of 1 intracerebral bleed and 1 patient who was stented 24 hours after an extensive myocardial infarction with cardiogenic shock. Two of the 4 late deaths were sudden (at 1.5 and 19 months), 1 was noncardiac (pneumonia), and the other resulted from complications after bypass surgery.

The actuarial event-free survival rate (freedom from death, myocardial infarction, bypass surgery, or PTCA) for patients with native arteries was 46% at 40 months, and for patients with bypass grafts it was 37% at 20 months (Fig 32–7).

DISCUSSION

Despite progress in techniques and equipment, the rate of late angiographic narrowing following PTCA, a process popularly termed "restenosis," has not been altered since its clinical introduction 13 years ago. This failure has provided the impetus for the development of newer alternative forms of coronary revascularization such as stenting, atherectomy, and laser treatment. However the effectiveness of all forms of nonoperative coronary interventions remains limited by the restenosis process(es).

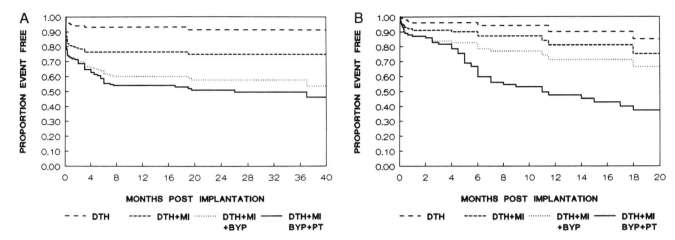

FIG 32–7.
Clinical follow-up in native vessels up to 40 months **(A)** and bypass grafts up to 20 months **(B)**. Death *(DTH)*, myocardial infarction *(MI)*, bypass surgery *(BYP)*, and PTCA *(PT)*, or atherectomy were considered clinical end points.

Early Occlusion, Late Restenosis

The coronary Wallstent was initially introduced as an endovascular device to prevent the late restenosis process that limits PTCA. The indications for and management of patients who had this particular prosthesis implanted have evolved as experience and knowledge have increased. In this study, an attempt has been made to separate two important factors in the late outcome of patients with stent implantations. The first division, according to the date of implantation, provides the clearest picture of the changes in stent applications based on the early experience. Investigators originally believed that the stent could be safely implanted in native vessels and that the benefit of stents would be most apparent in lesions that had already become restenosed on at least one occasion. However, a high in-hospital occlusion rate was noted, particularly in patients with unstable syndromes, evolving myocardial infarction, or angiographic evidence of thrombus. These occlusions, often with disastrous clinical sequelae, convinced most of the investigators that native vessels in general and particularly the left anterior descending artery (due to the large territory at risk) should only be stented in bailout situations. Group 2 mainly consisted of patients with bypass grafts that were stented for primary lesions and native vessels that were stented as part of a bailout strategy following complicated balloon angioplasty. Bypass grafts in particular were selected for stent implantations due to an extremely high rate of restenosis after PTCA alone and because the larger diameter of these grafts seemed less likely to become thrombosed than smaller-caliber native arterial vessels.[14–17] Bypass lesions, which were the majority of lesions stented in group 2, were more

complex in general than group 1 lesions due to the advanced age and diffuse nature of the disease in the bypass grafts. As a result, more stents per lesion (1.4 vs. 1.1 in native vessels) were required to cover these lesions. Therefore, the significantly lower rate of in-hospital occlusion in patients with bypass grafts vs. patients with native vessels (8% vs. 19%) and the trend in group 2 vs. group 1 (12% vs. 20%) are indicative of several possible factors, including improvements in anticoagulation regimens, operator experience, and/or larger-caliber vessels despite more complex case selection.

The initial clinical experience with the Palmaz-Schatz stent has recently been reported.[18] With a similar anticoagulation schedule in 174 patients, a 0.6% in-hospital occlusion rate was demonstrated. The discrepancy between a substantially higher occlusion rate in our series with the Wallstent and the Schatz study cannot be entirely explained. The stent itself does not appear to be more thrombogenic. In a model of stents placed inside a polytetrafluoroethylene graft in exteriorized arteriovenous shunts in baboons, no difference in acute platelet deposition and thrombus formation was noted between the two types of stents.[19] Differences in study design such as patient selection (collateralized vessels, predominantly right coronary arteries, and exclusion of patients with recent myocardial infarction and abrupt closure following PTCA in the Schatz study) may account for some of the differences.

Higher restenosis rates by both criteria were demonstrated in bypass grafts than in native vessels and in group 2 than in group 1. There are two possible explanations for this increase. First, bypass grafts, which are overrepresented in group 2, are known to have higher restenosis rates than native vessels.[14–16] Second, higher restenosis rates may be the "price" for lower occlusion rates. Organization of a thrombus at the site of intimal damage may be an important cause of late restenosis after stenting. Although it is often difficult to histologically differentiate thrombus organization from intimal hyperplasia, we have observed an extremely disorganized pattern of intimal thickening in the stented segments of several bypass grafts that have been surgically retrieved or obtained by atherectomy 1 to 5 months following stent implantation.[20] By diminishing the formation of early occlusive thrombus with more effective anticoagulation, the residual nonoccluding thrombus could form the substrate for late restenosis. Although the second group had a higher proportion of bailout cases, we did not identify increased relative risk for restenosis from bailout cases in comparison to stent implantations performed in primary or restenosed lesions.[21]

Relative-Risk Analysis

Restenosis is a complex process that is only partially understood. Pathologic studies of patients who have died more than 1 month following angioplasty have demonstrated the presence of intimal hyperplasia, presumably due to proliferation and migration of medial smooth muscle cells into the intima, and associated production of extracellular matrix collagen and proteoaminoglycans.[22, 23] It has been suggested by Liu et al. that the two major factors that determine the absolute amount of intimal hyperplasia are (1) the depth of injury and (2) the regional flow characteristics (which are determined by the geometry of the dilated lumen of the lesion and blood flow velocity patterns across that lumen).[24] Two separate PTCA follow-up reports support the concept that the greater the diameter change post-PTCA (implying a greater degree of disruption to the vessel wall), the more extensive is the absolute amount of reactive hyperplasia.[25, 26] On the basis of several angiographic studies from the Thoraxcenter, immediate results following stent implantation are superior to angioplasty alone (mean MLD of 2.5 mm vs. 2.0 to 2.1 mm) and thus favor a more aggressive proliferative response postprocedure.[2, 4, 27] The second factor is illustrated by the inverse relationship between the level of wall shear stress and subsequent intimal thickening. In the presence of a significant residual stenosis, the poststenotic region is a site of flow separation and low wall shear stress. This may retard endothelial recovery and prolong the period of smooth muscle cell proliferation, which is partially dependent on restoration of a regenerated endothelial barrier.[28] Stenting appears to diminish

the effect of poststenotic wall shear stress by significantly improving the hemodynamic effects of the stenosis (based on the calculated reductions in Poisseuille flow and turbulent contributions to flow resistance).[29]

It is extremely difficult if not impossible to predict restenosis in the individual patient following PTCA.[30] This problem can be partially understood when one considers that the two factors (i.e., depth of injury and regional flow characteristics) affecting the extent of intimal proliferation act in opposition to the other and thus make it hazardous to predict the outcome of this interaction in a particular patient. In a large population of patients, relative-risk analyses following PTCA have identified several patient, lesion, and procedural variables that predict late restenosis. However, the situation following stenting may be different where the mean loss of MLD at late follow-up is twice that of PTCA alone (0.62 mm vs. 0.31 mm).[2, 27] Therefore, this study was designed to identify factors that were associated with an increased risk of restenosis following stenting.

Lesion Factors

Stented bypass grafts had a greater risk of restenosis than native vessels did (30% vs. 19%), but this finding was restricted to the diameter stenosis criterion. The increased susceptibility of bypass grafts to the restenosis process has previously been documented following PTCA.[9, 31-35] Although left anterior descending coronary artery lesions have been shown to be a risk factor in several PTCA studies,[5] this was not evident in our study. The reference diameter of the vessel also had no relationship to restenosis. Forty-three percent of the vessels had reference diameters between 3 and 4 mm, and 43% were 3 mm or less. Lesion length and the severity of the lesion, in absolute MLD or diameter stenosis, prior to the procedure have been cited by several authors as important risk factors for restenosis following angioplasty, although our data did not show this association.[5-7] Lesion length is probably not an important factor for restenosis if the lesion can be covered by a single stent (see below). We believe that this is due to a more uniform and optimal dilatation with stenting. Long lesions treated with angioplasty are frequently less successfully dilated along the entire length of the lesion, and the ragged irregular surface of the vessel may predispose to rheologic factors critically involved in restenosis. Total occlusions have been reported as an important predictor of restenosis in angioplasty studies. However, this accounted for only 4.5% of the lesions in our study, which was too few for this analysis. Although there was a trend for higher restenosis in more eccentric lesions, this was not statistically significant.

Stent Factors

Multiple stents (RR: MLD, 1.56 [1.08 to 2.25]); DS, 1.61 [0.97 to 2.67]) and unconstrained stent diameter exceeding the reference diameter by greater than 0.7 mm (RR: MLD, 1.64 [1.10 to 2.45]; DS, 1.93 [1.13 to 3.31]) significantly predicted restenosis with both criteria. Preliminary reports from four separate groups working with the Palmaz-Schatz stent have shown a similar relationship between multiple stents per lesion and restenosis.[36–39] In our study, multiple stents placed in tandem were overlapped at the extremities (so-called telescoping), which may be the reason for the observed increase in restenosis rates. The segment of the vessel that was covered by the overlapping stents was subjected to the dilating force of two separate stents as well as an increased density of metal. We have observed that restenosis commonly occurred at these sites of overlapping between stents. Since the length of the lesion and the absolute length of the stent required to cover a lesion were not significant predictors, it seems prudent to implant longer stents rather than two or more shorter stents in tandem.

Selecting an oversized stent (unconstrained diameter >0.7 mm larger than the reference diameter) was a particularly important stimulus for hyperplasia with the self-expanding Wallstent. Schwartz et al. have described an aggressive proliferative response in a porcine model as a result of severe stent oversizing (0.5 to 1.5 mm).[40] This effect, which they attributed to penetration of the internal elastic lamina by the stent wires and subsequent deep medial injury, was much less pronounced when the stent diameter was matched more closely to the vessel diameter. Furthermore, due to its self-expanding property, the Wallstent (and particularly when it is oversized) continues to expand the vessel wall for at least 24 hours postimplantation.[41] The vessel is subjected to increasingly higher wall stress than after implantation of a balloon-expandable stent (which is maximally expanded at the time of implantation), a factor that may adversely stimulate the proliferative process. It may seem paradoxical that oversizing the stent by >0.7 mm would result in a higher restenosis rate with the 50% diameter stenosis criterion. However, the diameter stenosis poststent was not different in the two groups despite the oversizing. The main effect of oversizing then was not particularly a superior immediate result but rather a more aggressive "hyperplastic" reaction and a smaller MLD at follow-up than if less-oversized stents were implanted. The absolute value of the unconstrained stent diameter and the addition of the polymer coating (Biogold) had no significant relationship to late restenosis.

Procedural Factors

No significant relative risk could be attributed to a particular indication for the procedure. Restenosis rates for primary cases were not significantly different than for bailout or restenosis cases (MLD criterion: 37%, 42%, 33%; DS criterion: 24%, 27%, 24%), although an increased rate of restenosis has been described with the Palmaz-Schatz stent in patients with previous restenosis.[39] The absolute change in diameter from the prestent to the poststent result and dilatation within the stent after implantation (the so-called Swiss kiss) did not appear to affect the late restenosis. This poststent dilatation was performed to dissipate clot within the stent and to accelerate early expansion of the stent. A poststent diameter stenosis greater than 20% tended to be predictive of a follow-up diameter stenosis greater than 50% (RR, 1.51; 95% Cl, 0.91 to 2.50), although not for the MLD criteria. The larger the residual stenosis following stenting (i.e., less optimal result), the less hyperplasia required to reach a particular diameter stenosis at follow-up such as the 50% diameter stenosis criterion.

Limitations of the Study

Several important limitations of this study must be mentioned. Although this study suggests several factors that may be predictive of restenosis following stenting, it does not address the actual mechanisms of restenosis in the stented vessel. By comparing the predictors of restenosis following stenting with angioplasty, we have assumed that the underlying mechanism(s) responsible for late angiographic narrowing are similar (i.e., primarily intimal hyperplasia). Although almost every stenting procedure was accompanied by balloon dilatation at some particular time during the procedure, several other mechanisms may be important. Elastic recoil, which in the first few days following the procedure may be a significant factor in causing renarrowing, may be less important in stented vessels than angioplasty alone due to the scaffolding function of the stent. Although organization of thrombus at the site of intimal damage following PTCA has been recognized as a cause for late restenosis, it has not been particularly regarded as an important factor based on late pathologic studies following PTCA. However, this may be an extremely important cause of late restenosis after stenting. Although it is difficult to histologically discriminate thrombus organization from intimal hyperplasia, we have observed a disorganized layer of intimal thickening directly above the stent wire that is associated with remnants of thrombus in segments of several bypass grafts surgically retrieved up to 10 months following stent implanta-

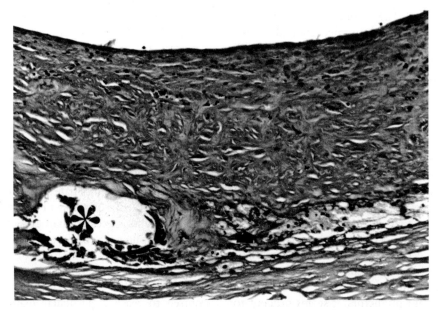

FIG 32–8.
Light micrograph of stented bypass graft removed 10 months after stent implantation. The void (*) represents a 70-μm-diameter stent wire. Immediately adjacent to the stent wire are cellular debris and foam cells *(arrowhead)*. Directly above the stent wire is a layer of disorganized fibrointimal hyperplasia. (Courtesy of H.M.M. van Beusekom.)

tion[20, 42] (Fig 32–8). Therefore we consider organization of residual thrombus to be a potentially important cause of late angiographic narrowing in addition to the major occlusion problems early after stenting. This may partially explain why commonly regarded determinants of restenosis following PTCA (e.g., lesion length, left anterior descending artery) do not appear to be significant in this analysis since different pathologic processes may predominate. This also has important clinical implications since therapy to limit smooth muscle proliferation may be quite different from therapy to minimize thrombus formation. There are two statistical limitations to this study. Due to the relatively small sample size, we cannot rule out a significant beta error. Second, in performing multiple statistical comparisons, there is a risk that some of them may be significant by chance alone. Therefore, these data require confirmation by other studies.

In conclusion, the European coronary Wallstent experience has demonstrated that restenosis following stenting is increased in bypass grafts and in the presence of multiple stents and excessive oversizing of the stent (>0.7 mm) and has shown less optimal results immediately poststenting (>20% diameter stenosis). Since some of these factors can be modified, we recommend against the use of multiple stents and excessive oversizing to reduce the probability of late restenosis.

Short- and Long-Term Follow-Up: Clinical Events

The problems of prolonged anticoagulation are an additional consideration. Increased morbidity (increased femoral hematomas, gastrointestinal and genitourinary tract bleeding) and mortality (three patients died of intracerebral hemorrhage) are directly attributable to the intensive anticoagulation regimen. The duration of hospitalization is also lengthened to ensure therapeutic levels of anticoagulation.

The high incidence of late adverse clinical events in stented patients is a cause for concern. A mortality rate of 8.9% in bypass grafts and 6.6% in native vessels is higher than in reported PTCA studies.[43–45] However, it must be stressed that a large number of stents in native vessels were implanted for abrupt closure following PTCA, which dramatically increases the risk of the procedure.[45] The actuarial event-free survival (freedom from death, myocardial infarction, bypass surgery, or repeat PTCA or atherectomy) rates were 37% at 20 months in bypass patients and 46% at 40 months in native vessels. In the bypass group, about 30% of the adverse events were unrelated to the stented lesion and were due to worsening of a different lesion or to the development of new lesions. In the native vessel group, 12% of the adverse events were unrelated to the stented lesion. In addition, 9 of the 30 bypass operations in patients with stented native vessels were performed as part of a protocol for patients stented for the bailout indication.[46] Although there are no comparable series of native vessel stents in the literature because of the unique set of indications in our study, three recent reports have been published of late clinical follow-up (Kaplan-Meier analysis) after PTCA in bypass grafts. The Thoraxcenter reported that only 41% of patients were alive and event free (myocardial infarction, repeat coronary artery bypass grafting [CABG], repeat PTCA) at a median follow-up of 2.1 years.[47] A review of the overall Dutch experience also showed limited late beneficial results, with 2-year and 5-year event-free survival rates of 52% and 26% respectively in 454 bypass patients.[48] Webb et al. have described a 71% rate of freedom from death, infarction, and surgery at 5 years in bypass patients who underwent PTCA at their institution, but they did not include the 27% incidence of second angioplasty procedures also required in their patient group.[14] However, it must be stressed that our study was not a randomized trial designed to compare stenting with PTCA but rather an observational study with a first-generation coronary stent. Nevertheless, all of these late follow-up studies of nonoperative coronary revascularization clearly show that these are palliative procedures and not long-term solutions to the underlying problems of progression of underlying coronary disease and iatrogenically induced restenosis. Several important points emerge from this study. First, although in-hospital occlusion rates improved in the later experience, Wallstent coronary thrombosis continues to limit its use. Restenosis rates with the 50% diameter stenosis criterion do not seem to be significantly improved when compared with historical postangioplasty results, although definitive statements must await randomized trials. Bypass grafts in particular have a high incidence of late restenosis, although early occlusion occurred less significantly than in patients with native vessels. Based on our experience, there is insufficient evidence at this time to suggest implantation of this particular stent outside of a randomized trial with the following exceptions: (1) bailout for abrupt occlusion, (2) suboptimal (inadequate dilatation) results following PTCA, and (3) bypass grafts at high risk for distal embolization with PTCA (friable lesions that may benefit from the scaffolding property of the Wallstent). If the low occlusion rate with the Palmaz-Schatz stent is confirmed in other studies, that particular stent would appear to be a more suitable candidate for randomized trials of presently available stents.

Acknowledgment

We gratefully acknowledge the assistance of Hanneke Roerade in preparation of the manuscript and Dr. Edward Murphy (Portland, Oregon) for critical comments. We appreciated the technical assistance of Marie-Angèle Morel and Eline Montauban van Swijndregt. Participating centers and collaborators: Catheterization Laboratory for Clinical and Experimental Image Processing, Thoraxcenter, Rotterdam, The Netherlands: B.H. Strauss, M.D., K.J. Beatt, M.B., B.S., M. van den Brand, M.D., P.J. de Feyter, M.D., H. Suryapranata, M.D., I.K. de Scheerder, M.D., J.R.T.C. Roelandt, M.D., P.W. Serruys, M.D.; Department of Cardiology, Hôpital Cardiologique, Lille, France: M.E. Bertrand; Department of Invasive Cardiology, The Royal Bromptom and National Heart Institute, London: A.F. Rickards, M.D., U Sigwart, M.D.; Department of Clinical and Experimental Cardiology, CHRU Rangeuil, Toulouse, France: J.P. Bounhoure, M.D., A Courtault, M.D., F. Joffre, M.D., J. Puel, M.D., H. Rousseau, M.D.; Division of Cardiology, Department of Medicine, CHUV, Lausanne, Switzerland: J.-J. Goy, M.D., J-C Stauffer, M.D., U Kaufmann, M.D., L. Kappenberger, M.D., P. Urban, M.D.; Cardiology Center, University Hospital, Geneva, Switzerland: B. Meier, P. Urban.

REFERENCES

1. Sigwart U, Puel J, Mirkovitch V, et al: Intravascular stents to prevent occlusion and restenosis after transluminal angioplasty. *N Engl J Med* 1987; 316:701–706.
2. Serruys PW, Strauss BH, Beatt KJ, et al: Quantitative follow-up after placement of a self-expanding coronary stent. *N Engl J Med* 1991; 324:13–17.
3. Reiber JHC, Serruys PW, Kooijman CJ, et al: Assessment of short-, medium-, and long-term variations in arterial dimensions from computer-assisted quantitation of coronary cineangiograms. *Circulation* 1985; 72:280–288.
4. Serruys PW, Luijten HE, Beatt KJ, et al: Incidence of restenosis after successful angioplasty: A time related phenomenon. *Circulation* 1988; 77:361–371.
5. Leimgruber PP, Roubin GS, Hollman J, et al: Restenosis after succesful coronary angioplasty in patients with single-vessel disease. *Circulation* 1986; 73:710–717.
6. Myler RK, Topol EJ, Shaw RE, et al: Multiple vessel coronary angioplasty: Classification, results, and patterns of restenosis in 494 consecutive patients. *Cathet Cardiovasc Diagn* 1987; 13:1–15.
7. Vandormael MG, Deligonul U, Kern MJ, et al: Multilesion coronary angioplasty: Clinical and angiographic follow-up. *J Am Coll Cardiol* 1987; 10:246–252.
8. Mata LA, Bosch X, David PR, et al: Clinical and angiographic assessment 6 months after double vessel percutaneous coronary angioplasty. *J Am Coll Cardiol* 1985; 6:1239–1244.
9. Holmes DR Jr, Vliestra RE, Smith HC, et al: Restenosis after percutaneous transluminal coronary angioplasty (PTCA): A report from the PTCA registry of the Na-

tional Heart, Lung, and Blood Institute. *Am J Cardiol* 1984; 53:77–81.

10. Levine S, Ewels CJ, Rosing DR, et al: Coronary angioplasty: Clinical and angiographic follow-up. *Am J Cardiol* 1985; 55:673–676.

11. Disciascio G, Cowley MJ, Vetrovec GW: Angiographic patterns of restenosis after angioplasty of multiple coronary arteries. *Am J Cardiol* 1986; 58:922–925.

12. Gardner MJ, Altman DG: *Statistics With Confidence.* Belfast, The Universities Press, 1989.

13. Kaplan EL, Meier P: Nonparametric estimation from incomplete observations. *J Am Stat Assoc* 1958; 53:457–481.

14. Webb JG, Myler RK, Shaw RE, et al: Coronary angioplasty after coronary bypass surgery: Initial results and late outcome in 422 patients. *J Am Coll Cardiol* 1990; 16:812–820.

15. Douglas JS, Grüntzig AR, King SB III, et al: Percutaneous transluminal coronary angioplasty in patients with prior coronary bypass surgery. *J Am Coll Cardiol* 1983; 2:745–754.

16. Block PC, Cowley MJ, Kaltenbach M, et al: Percutaneous angioplasty of stenoses of bypass grafts or of bypass graft anastomosis sites. *Am J Cardiol* 1984; 53:666–668.

17. Bucz JJJ, de Scheerder I, Beatt K, et al: The importance of adequate anticoagulation to prevent early thrombosis following stenting of stenosed venous bypass grafts. *Am Heart J* 1991; 121:1309–1396.

18. Schatz RA, Baim DS, Leon M, et al: Clinical experience with the Palmaz-Schatz coronary stent. Initial results of a multicenter study. *Circulation* 1991; 83:148–161.

19. Krupski WC, Bass A, Kelly AB, et al: Heparin-resistant thrombus formation by endovascular stents in baboons: Interruption by a synthetic antithrombin. *Circulation* 1990; 82:570–577.

20. Serruys PW, Strauss BH, van Beusekom HM, et al: Stenting of coronary arteries. Has a modern Pandora's box been opened? *J Am Coll Cardiol* 1991; 17:143–154.

21. Strauss BH, Serruys PW, de Scheerder IK, et al: A relative risk analysis of the angiographic predictors of restenosis in the coronary Wallstent (abstract). *Circulation* 1990; 82(suppl 3):540.

22. Austin GE, Ratliff NB, Hollman J, et al: Intimal proliferation of smooth muscle cells as an explanation for recurrent coronary artery stenosis after percutaneous transluminal coronary angioplasty. *J Am Coll Cardiol* 1985; 6:369–375.

23. Waller BF, Gorfinkel HJ, Rogers FJ, et al: Early and late morphologic changes in major epicardial coronary arteries after percutaneous transluminal coronary angioplasty. *Am J Cardiol* 1984; 53:42–47.

24. Liu MW, Roubin GS, King SB III: Restenosis after coronary angioplasty: Potential biologic determinants and role of intimal hyperplasia. *Circulation* 1989; 79:1374–1387.

25. Beatt KJ, Luijten HE, Suryapranata H, et al: Suboptimal post angioplasty result, the principle risk factor for "restenosis" (abstract). *Circulation* 1989; 80(suppl 2):257.

26. Liu MW, Roubin GS, King SB III: Does an optimal luminal result after PTCA reduce restenosis (abstract)? *Circulation* 1989; 80(suppl):63.

27. Serruys PW, Rutsch W, Heyndrickx G, et al: Effect of long term thromboxane A^2 receptor blockade on angio-

graphic restenosis and clinical events after coronary angioplasty. The CARPORT study (abstract). *J Am Coll Cardiol* 1991; 17:2:283.

28. Haudenschild CC, Schwartz SM: Endothelial regeneration. Restitution of endothelial continuity. *Lab Invest* 1979; 41:407–418.

29. Serruys PW, Juilliere Y, Bertrand ME, et al: Additional improvement of stenosis geometry in human coronary arteries by stenting after balloon dilatation. *Am J Cardiol* 1988; 61:71–76.

30. Renkin J, Melin J, Robert A, et al: Detection of restenosis after successful coronary angioplasty: improved clinical decision making with the use of a logistic model combining procedural and follow-up variables. *J Am Coll Cardiol* 1990; 6:1333–1340.

31. Douglas JS, Grüntzig AR, King SB III, et al: Percutaneous transluminal coronary angioplasty in patients with prior coronary bypass surgery. *J Am Coll Cardiol* 1983; 2:745–754.

32. Block PC, Cowley MJ, Kaltenbach M, et al: Percutaneous angioplasty of stenoses of bypass grafts or of bypass graft anastomosis sites. *Am J Cardiol* 1984; 53:666–668.

33. Corbell J, Franco I, Hollman J, et al: Percutaneous transluminal coronary angioplasty after previous coronary artery bypass surgery. *Am J Cardiol* 1985; 56:398–403.

34. Pinkerton CA, Slack JD, Orr CM: Percutaneous transluminal angioplasty in patients with prior myocardial revascularization surgery. *Am J Cardiol* 1988; 61:15–22.

35. Webb JG, Myler RK, Shaw RE, et al: Coronary angioplasty after coronary bypass surgery: Initial results and late outcome in 422 patients. *J Am Coll Cardiol* 1990; 16:812–820.

36. Ellis SG, Savage M, Baim D, et al: Intracoronary stenting to prevent restenosis. Preliminary results of a multicenter study using the Palmaz-Schatz stent suggest benefit in selected high risk patients (abstract). *J Am Coll Cardiol* 1990; 15:18.

37. Levine MJ, Leonard BM, Burke JA, et al: Clinical and angiographic results of balloon-expandable intracoronary stents in right coronary artery stenoses. *J Am Coll Cardiol* 1990; 16:332–339.

38. Schatz RA, Goldberg S, Leon MB, et al: Coronary stenting following "suboptimal" coronary angioplasty results (abstract). *Circulation* 1990; 82(suppl 3):540.

39. Teirstein PS, Cleman MW, Hirshfeld JW, et al: Influence of prior restenosis on subsequent restenosis after intracoronary stenting (abstract). *Circulation* 1990; 82(suppl 3):657.

40. Schwartz RS, Murphy JG, Edwards WD, et al: Restenosis after balloon angioplasty. A practical proliferative model in porcine coronary arteries. *Circulation* 1990; 82:2190–2200.

41. Beatt KJ, Bertrand M, Puel J, et al: Additional improvement in vessel lumen in the first 24 hours after stent implantation due to radial dilating force (abstract). *J Am Coll Cardiol* 1989; 13:244.

42. van Beusekom HMM, Serruys PW, van der Giessen WJ, et al: Histological features 3 to 320 days after stenting of human saphenous vein bypass grafts (abstract). *J Am Coll Cardiol* 1991; 17:53.

43. Kent KM, Bentivoglio LG, Block PC, et al: Long-term efficacy of percutaneous transluminal coronary angioplasty (PTCA): Report from the National Heart, Lung,

and Blood Institute PTCA Registry. *Am J Cardiol* 1984; 53:27–31.

44. Grüntzig AR, King SB III, Schlumpf M, et al: Long-term follow-up after percutaneous transluminal coronary angioplasty. The early Zurich experience. *N Engl J Med* 1987; 316:1127–1132.

45. Detre K, Holubkov R, Kelsey S, et al: One-year follow-up results of the 1985–1986 National Heart, Lung, and Blood Institute's percutaneous transluminal coronary angioplasty registry. *Circulation* 1989; 80:421–428.

46. de Feyter PJ, de Scheerder I, van den Brand M, et al: Emergency stenting for refractory acute coronary artery occlusion during coronary angioplasty. *Am J Cardiol* 1990; 66:1147–1150.

47. Meester BJ, Samson M, Suryapranata H, et al: Long-term follow-up after attempted angioplasty of saphenous vein grafts: The Thoraxcenter experience 1981–1988. *Eur Heart J* 1991; 12:640–653.

48. Plokker HWT, Meester BH, Serruys PW: The Dutch experience in percutaneous transluminal angioplasty of narrowed saphenous veins used for aortocoronary arterial bypass. *Am J Cardiol* 1991; 67:361–366.

33

Temporary Coronary Stenting: Preliminary Experience With a Heat-Activated Recoverable Temporary Stent

Neal L. Eigler, M.D.

Mehran J. Khorsandi, M.D.

Although metallic stents have been successfully deployed in several thousand human coronary arteries, both for primary treatment of stenosis and for lumen-compromising intimal dissection following angioplasty, these devices currently suffer three major limitations: (1) subacute thrombosis, (2) bleeding, and (3) continuous vascular injury inciting intimal proliferation and restenosis.[1-6] Many investigators are attempting to solve these problems through a host of means including (1) nonthrombogenic coatings, (2) new stent geometries, (3) new alloys such as tantalum, (4) local drug delivery to prevent restenosis, and (5) biodegradable polymer stents. An alternative approach is the development of a temporary metallic stent that is removable hours to days following implantation.[7] In this chapter, we describe the results of early feasibility testing for implanting and retrieving a heat-activated recoverable temporary stent (HARTS) and the effects of temporary stenting on the angiographic, gross, and histologic appearance of a normal canine coronary artery wall.[8] Our long-range objective is to determine whether temporary stenting will confer the benefits of permanently implanted stents and potentially minimize their limitations.

HARTS DEVICE

The prototype HARTS device (Advanced Coronary Technologies, Menlo Park, Calif) is constructed from multiple segments of nickel-titanium alloy (nitinol) wire 0.009 in. in diameter. The wire segments are connected by stainless steel tubing crimp joints to form a tubular, meshed stent (Fig 33–1,A). The undeployed stent is 15 mm in length and has an outer diameter of 1.5 mm. The HARTS device is balloon expandable to a diameter of 4.0 mm. Nitinol stands for Nickel-Titanium Naval Ordnance Laboratory. This unique alloy has been used in engineering for many years to provide mechanical motion where circumstances do not allow the use of conventional mechanical devices.[9] Nitinol exists in either a martensite or austenite crystal phase. At body temperature, the alloy contains a higher martensitic fraction, which gives it a deformable structure. The HARTS device is inserted in the collapsed configuration mounted on a balloon. It is deployed by balloon expansion (Fig 33–1,B). Such deformation further increases the martensitic fraction, which further improves the axial flexibility of the device. The shape memory properties of nitinol were selected so that upon heating the expanded stent to 55° C it undergoes a thermoelastic transition with return to the austenitic phase; this results in recovery and collapse of the stent to its original unexpanded configuration (Fig 33–1,C). This phase change occurs at the speed of sound and with considerable force such that the stent grips the recovery catheter tightly, thereby providing a mechanism for recovery and removing an expanded, deployed stent. Thus, our stent differs significantly from the nitinol stents developed by Dotter et al. Their stents and other iterations of the nit-

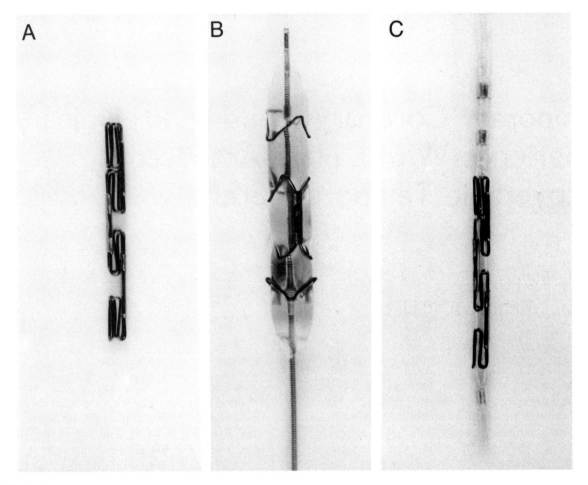

FIG 33–1.
Prototype HARTS device. **A,** unexpanded stent. **B,** expanded stent on a delivery balloon. **C,** collapsed stent on a recovery catheter.

inol stents use the shape memory properties of the nickel-titanium alloy as a mechanism for deployment only. To our knowledge, this is the first stent to exploit the austenitic phase transition of nitinol to achieve stent collapse and removal.

STENT DEPLOYMENT

We tested this device in 13 adult mongrel dogs that were pretreated with aspirin (325 mg) and dipyridamole (75 mg) 1 day prior to the procedure. The activated clotting time (ACT) was maintained at greater than 300 seconds by bolus heparin infusions until the stent was implanted. Low–molecular-weight dextran (Rheomacrodex, Pharmacia, Inc., Piscataway, NJ) was administered at a rate of 50 cc/hr for the duration of the procedure. A 8 F percutaneous transluminal coronary angioplasty (PTCA) guide catheter (Schneider, Minneapolis) with a JR5 or hockey stick curve was positioned selectively into the left coronary artery. A custom-made 3- to 4-mm-diameter over-the-wire balloon catheter (Advanced Coronary Technologies, Meadow Park, Calif) approximately 20% larger in diameter than the target vessel was chosen. The HARTS device was crimped over the collapsed balloon to complete the stent delivery system. This was advanced into the selected coronary segment by using standard angioplasty techniques and a 0.014-in. high-torque floppy guidewire (Advanced Cardiovascular Systems, Inc., Temecula, Calif). Two dilatations of 6 to 8 atm for 15 seconds were performed to expand the stent. The deflated balloon and guidewire were then removed with the expanded stent left embedded in the vessel wall. Patency was confirmed by repeat angiography. A total of 47 HARTS devices were placed in the mid to distal regions of the left circumflex (LCx), left anterior descending (LAD), and diagonal branches of the LAD artery of 13 dogs. A different segment of the same vessel was chosen on many occasions to place a second stent after removal of the first (Table 33–1).

TABLE 33–1.
Summary of the Number of Stented Segments and Duration of Implantation in Each Animal

| Dog No. | Stents Implanted* | | Duration (hr) | | |
	LAD	LCx	0.5	1.5–5	24
1	2	2	4	—	—
2	2	1	3	—	—
3	3	2	4	1	—
4	1	2	2	1	—
5	2	2	2	2	—
6	2	1	1	2	—
7	1	3	2	2	—
8	3	2	3	2	—
9	0	4	3	1	—
10	2	2	2	2	—
11	2	2	2	2	—
12	1	1	—	—	2
13	1	1	—	—	2

*LAD = left anterior descending; LCx = left circumflex.

There were 22 LAD and 25 LCx stent placements. An additional experiment was performed in which an animal was not pretreated with aspirin and dipyridamole. Because this was not per protocol, the results are not included in the summarized data. One of the two stents implanted in this animal thrombosed after 30 minutes. Microscopic inspection revealed a white, platelet-rich thrombus.

STENT RECOVERY

Stents were recovered 30 minutes to 24 hours after deployment (Table 33–1). After angiographic confirmation of vessel patency, a 0.014-in. PTCA guidewire was placed through the device and advanced into the distal segment of the artery. A stent recovery catheter (Advanced Coronary Technologies, Menlo Park, Calif) was advanced coaxially through the implanted stent until the two platinum markers that delineate the 20-mm landing zone straddled the stent (Fig 33–2,C). To collapse the stent, 3 to 5 mL of lactated Ringer's solution preheated to 75 to 80° C was hand-injected proximal to the stent through multiple sideholes in the stent recovery catheter. In bench simulation, this technique delivers a pulse of 65 to 70° C liquid at the distal delivery site. The stent-catheter recovery system was then withdrawn from the coronary artery and either removed through the guide catheter or by pull back through the introducer sheath.

RESULTS OF TEMPORARY STENTING

The stents were easily visible under fluoroscopy. All stents were successfully delivered to the target vessels without embolization, migration, dissection, or spasm visualized on the postdelivery angiogram (Fig 33–2,E). All stented vessels remained patent without angiographic evidence of thrombus or side branch occlusion. The stent had sufficient structural strength to maintain an arterial luminal diameter larger than baseline for the duration of the implantation. The stented segments of the vessels were 12% ± 6% larger in diameter than the adjacent unstented segments (Fig 33–3).

The transcatheter/sheath recovery procedure was successful in all 47 stent implantations. Each stent was observed to collapse on the recovery catheter between the angiographic markers without embolization. Stented arterial segments maintained a diameter equal or greater than the adjacent proximal segments after removal of the stent (Fig 33–3). The mean diameter of these segments was 6% ± 3% larger than the adjacent unstented segment. There were no arrhythmias or hemodynamic changes associated with intracoronary injection of the thermal bolus. The ease of stent recovery was the most notable characteristic of the device. The dynamic recovery process (stent collapse) was always well visualized by fluoroscopy. The vessel and the device cooled within seconds to body temperature as coronary blood flow dispersed the thermal bolus. This cooling did not affect the collapsed stent dimensions. In every case the stent tightly gripped the recovery catheter.

PATHOLOGIC STUDIES

Under a dissecting microscope, the stents appeared free of thrombus or vascular tissue. Gross examination of the hearts revealed limited periadventitial hemorrhage at the site of stent deployment in 6 of 47 stented

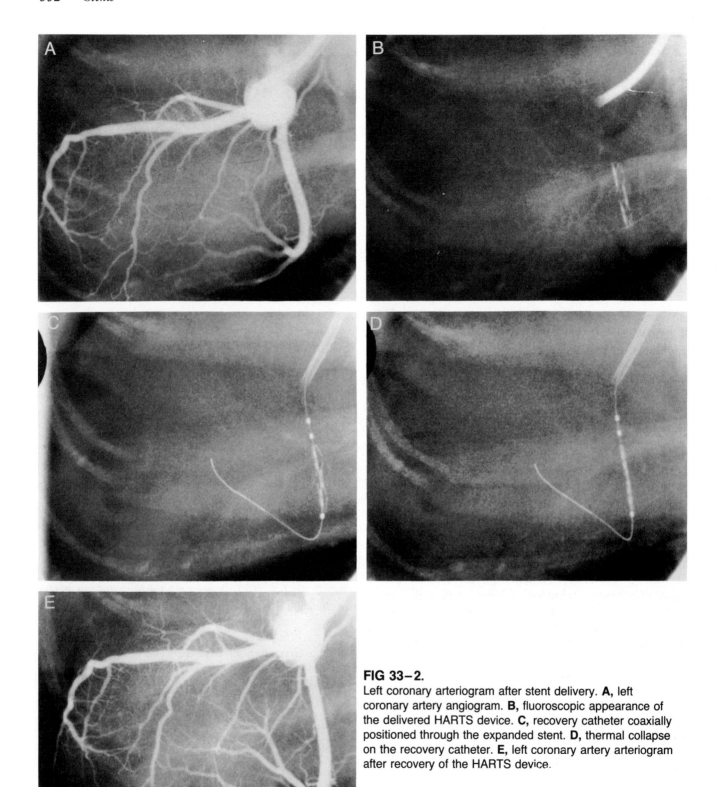

FIG 33–2.
Left coronary arteriogram after stent delivery. **A,** left
coronary artery angiogram. **B,** fluoroscopic appearance of
the delivered HARTS device. **C,** recovery catheter coaxially
positioned through the expanded stent. **D,** thermal collapse
on the recovery catheter. **E,** left coronary artery arteriogram
after recovery of the HARTS device.

Normalized Vessel Diameter(Baseline = 1)

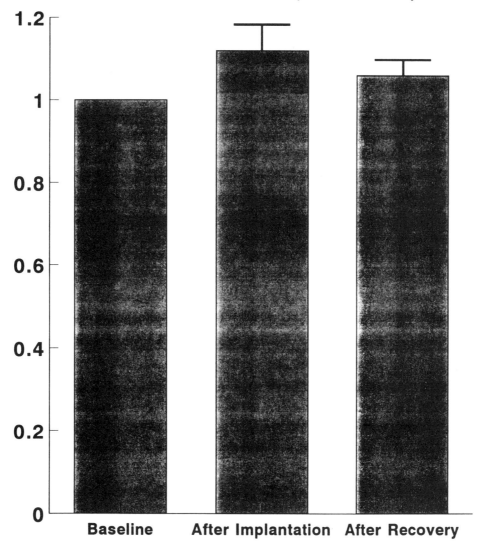

FIG 33–3.
Vessel diameter after implantation and recovery. The y-axis values are normalized for baseline (the adjacent unstented segment = 1). The mean vessel diameter after implantation was 12% ± 6% larger than the adjacent segment. The mean vessel diameter after recovery was 6% ± 3% larger than the adjacent segment.

segments. This appeared as myocardial staining in the area immediately next to the arterial segment. In all such cases the ratio of balloon-to-vessel diameter exceeded 1.4:1. Histologic evaluation revealed evidence of minor intimal injury in 31 stented segments (66%, Fig 33–4,A and Table 33–2). This consisted of focal endothelial damage and disturbance of the internal elastic lamina in the stented segments. There were microscopic platelet-fibrin thrombi in 10 stented segments (21%, Fig 33–4,B). The 6 arterial segments with gross periadventitial hemorrhage showed medial disruption on microscopic examination (13%, Fig 33–4,C). There was

no evidence of distal embolization on serial cuts through the myocardium. The extent of vascular injury appeared to be related to the degree of vessel overexpansion and not to the duration of implantation. Minimal changes were noted in the 24-hour stent exposures (Fig 33–5).

POTENTIAL CLINICAL APPLICATIONS

The clinical value of a removable stent is yet to be demonstrated. All metallic coronary stents are capable

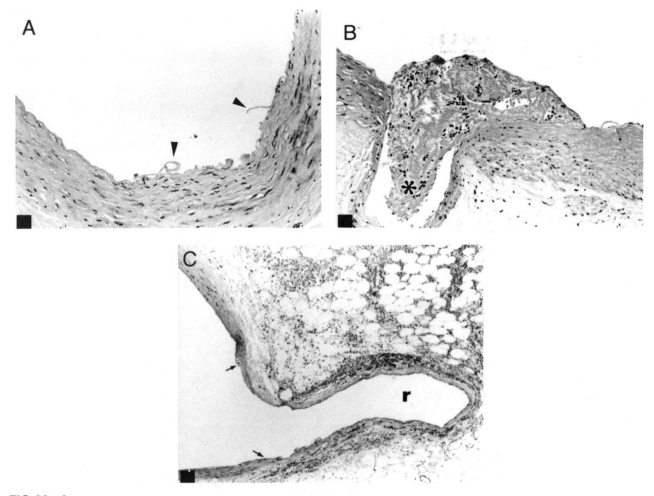

FIG 33–4.
Histologic changes following stenting. **A,** stented segment of the LAD artery in dog no. 12 after removal of a HARTS device that had been implanted for 24 hours. Mild intimal injury is present. Note the fragmentation of internal elastic lamina *(arrowheads)*. The media and adventitia are intact. **B,** section of a stented segment of the LCx coronary artery in dog no. 13. The HARTS device was removed 24 hours after implantation. A focus of platelet fibrin thrombus is seen attached to the vessel wall at a small branch site *(asterisk)*. **C,** section of a segment of the LAD artery in dog no. 2 where perivascular hemorrhage was seen on gross inspection. The HARTS device was removed 30 minutes after implantation. Note the site of transmural rupture of the vessel wall *(arrows)* with hemorrhage into the adventitia adjacent to the rupture *(r)* site (hematoxylin-eosin stain; original magnification: A = 50×; B = 50×; C = 25×).

of restoring flow in acute intimal dissection or suboptimal balloon dilatation. There is preliminary evidence that one of the stents may lower the restenosis rate when implanted in previously undilated vessels of suitable size.[10] Permanent stents, however, are associated with a significantly increased incidence of subacute thrombosis (3% to 27%) that occurs from several days to 4 weeks after implantation. Consequently, extensive antiplatelet and anticoagulant therapy is required, which in turn necessitates prolonged hospitalization.[11] The antithrombotic measures are associated with a 7% to 10% incidence of major bleeding or vascular complications requiring transfusion and/or surgery. A temporary stent may have a role in the treatment of flow-compromising

intimal dissection since prolonged balloon inflation for minutes or several hours has been reported to stabilize many lumen-compromising dissections. Potentially, intimal "tacking" for several hours to a few days could stabilize the dissection and yet allow the stent to be removed prior to the peak incidence of subacute thrombosis (days 4 to 10).[12] Conceivably, anticoagulation would not be required following device removal, which would reduce hospital costs and complications related to prolonged anticoagulation. Further study will be needed to determine whether removing the stent days to hours following implantation confers any of these potential advantages.

A second application for stenting is to enlarge the lu-

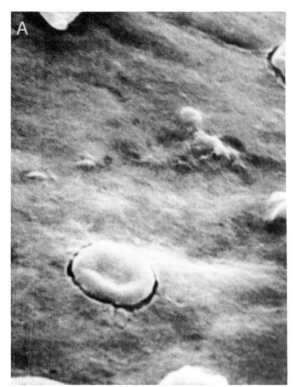
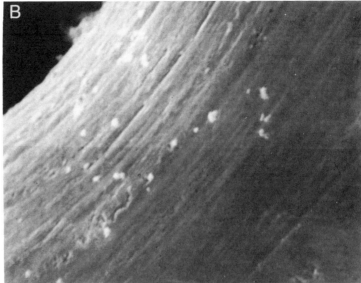
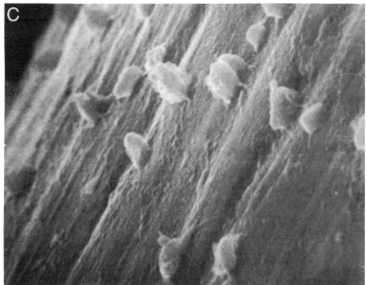

FIG 33–5.
Scanning electron microscopic specimens of a HARTS device removed 24 hours after implantation. **A,** stent covered with an amorphous layer of protein with a red cell on it. **B,** paucity of platelets *(arrow)* on the collapsed stent. **C,** on higher magnification occasional fibrin strands are seen attached to the surface of the stent and platelets.

minal diameter when balloon angioplasty results are suboptimal. It is possible that temporary stenting for hours to days could achieve a similar effect. Finally, permanent stents may reduce restenosis by eliminating elastic recoil. Schwartz et al. have shown, however, that permanently implanted stents can also be a potent stimulus to smooth muscle cell proliferation and restenosis.[13] It therefore appears that a reduction in restenosis

TABLE 33–2.
Arterial Histology After Implantation and Recovery

Minimal intimal injury only	31 (66%)
Microscopic platelet-fibrin thrombus	10 (21%)
Transmural tear	6 (13%)
Total	47 (100%)

involves a trade-off between maximal luminal expansion and induced intimal hyperplasia. It is conceivable that temporary stenting could inhibit elastic recoil, thereby maintaining luminal expansion without inducing the degree of intimal proliferation associated with the permanent implant. As with the other hypothetical advantages of temporary stenting, these speculations will require extensive preclinical and clinical study.

Other means of temporary flow support are now being evaluated. Whitlow et al. are developing removable flow support stent-catheters that have been deployed in humans up to 60 minutes for abrupt closure following PTCA.[14] This was successful in preventing bypass surgery in a minority of patients. Another group has developed a temporary stent very similar to a wire snare that is kept open across an intimal flap.[15] These devices may be limited by a radial expansive force inadequate to support vessel patency (<0.5 atm) as well as continuous attachment to an external catheter, thus limiting the duration of the implantation. These bulky devices may also limit flow when compared with a free stent, and thus we believe that they will have limited applicability.

Despite our encouraging early results, they should be considered preliminary and subject to several significant limitations. First, the normal canine coronary artery is not necessarily comparable to a diseased human coronary artery. It may be more forgiving to mechanical intervention. On the other hand, it is probably more prone to rupture under the study circumstances because the stent has to be expanded to a size greater than the vessel to ensure implantation in these normal vessels. Second, our study did not deal with the capability of this device to "tack" intimal dissections or to produce sustained vascular dilatation after removal. Third, we did not determine the effects of longer periods of temporary stenting, which might be expected to induce greater trauma on removal, because tissue grows over the device surface.

In summary we have demonstrated the feasibility of a new method of temporary stenting of the coronary arteries that uses the special thermoelastic properties of nitinol to permit satisfactory deployment, balloon expansion, and recovery of the device in normal canine coronary arteries. Extensive further research will be required to determine whether temporary stent placement has useful clinical applications.

REFERENCES

1. Schatz RA, Baim DS, Leon M, et al: Clinical experience with the Palmaz-Schatz coronary stent: Initial results of a multicenter study. *Circulation* 1991; 83:148–161.

2. Surreys PW, Strauss BH, Beatt KJ, et al: Angiographic follow-up after placement of a self expanding coronary artery stent. *N Engl J Med* 1991; 324:13–17.

3. Urban P, Sigwart U, Golf S, et al: Intravascular stenting for aortocoronary venous bypass grafts. *J Am Coll Cardiol* 1989; 13:1085–1091.

4. Roubin GS, King SB, Douglas JS, et al: Intracoronary stenting during percutaneous transluminal coronary angioplasty. *Circulation* 1990; 81(suppl 4):92–100.

5. Haude M, Erbel R, Straub U, et al: Results of intracoronary stents for management of coronary dissection after balloon angioplasty. *Am J Cardiol* 1991; 67:691–696.

6. Topol EJ: Promises and pitfalls of new devices for coronary artery disease. *Circulation* 1991; 83:689–694.

7. Litvack F: Intravascular stenting for prevention of restenosis: In search of the magic bullet. *J Am Coll Cardiol* 1989; 13:1092–1093.

8. Khorsandi MJ, Eigler NL, Hess RL, et al: Implantation and recovery of balloon delivered metallic stents (abstract). *J Am Coll Cardiol* 1992; 19:218.

9. Shetky LM: Shape-memory alloys. *Sci Am* 1979; 241:74–83.

10. Leon MB, Ellis SG, Pichard AD, et al: Stents may be the preferred treatment for focal aortocoronary vein graft disease (abstract). *Circulation* 1991; 84(suppl 2):249.

11. Haude M, Erbel R, Straub U, et al: Results of intracoronary stents for management of coronary dissection after balloon angioplasty. *Am J Cardiol* 1991; 67:691–696.

12. Brenner AS, Brown KF: Five hour balloon inflation to resolve recurrent reocclusion during coronary angioplasty. *Cathet Cardiovasc Diagn* 1991; 22:107–111.

13. Schwartz RS, Murphy JG, Edwards WD, et al: Restenosis after balloon angioplasty: A practical proliferative model in porcine coronary arteries (abstract). *Circulation* 1990; 82:2190–2300.

14. Whitlow P, Gaspard P, Kent K, et al: Improvement of coronary dissection with a removable flow support catheter: Acute results (abstract). *J Am Coll Cardiol* 1992; 19:218.

15. Simari RD, Schwartz RS, Higano ST, et al: A new temporary intracoronary stent: In vitro pressure-flow characteristics (abstract). *Circulation* 1991; 84(suppl 2):266.

PART VI

Interventional Procedures for Acute Myocardial Infarction

Angioplasty Therapy for Acute Myocardial Infarction: Current Status and Future Directions

William W. O'Neill, M.D.

HISTORICAL PERSPECTIVE

The invasive therapy for acute myocardial infarction (MI) has its origins in the early 1970s. At that time, centers in the United States and Europe were exploring the role of emergency coronary artery bypass in the management of MI.[1, 2] Initially a surgical approach was considered feasible only for patients who were already hospitalized.[3] Berg and his group at Spokane, however, tested emergency surgery for patients presenting to the emergency room.[4] Similarly, Rentrop et al.[5] tested emergency surgery in Europe. In order to perform emergency surgery, emergency cardiac catheterization was required to delineate the coronary anatomy. The Spokane group determined that thrombotic coronary occlusion was present in the large majority of patients undergoing catheterization prior to bypass. In fact, Rentrop et al.[6] pioneered mechanical recanalization during this era by attempting guidewire recanalization of an occluded left anterior descending artery. Once it was apparent that total coronary occlusion was frequently present, a natural extension was application of intracoronary thrombolytic therapy.[7, 8] Although thrombolytic therapy had been actively tested in Europe in the 1970s, this therapy was not widely accepted. Conflicting data concerning efficacy existed. More importantly, conceptually most investigators had not accepted the crucial role of thrombotic occlusion as the nidus for myocardial infarction.[9] The interventional studies of the 1970s provided crucial evidence that thrombotic occlusion frequently caused acute MI. These studies provided the impetus for studying both intracoronary and intravenous thrombolytic therapy. Soon after Rentrop's pioneering studies with intracoronary streptokinase, Kennedy et al.[10] and Hugenholtz[11] demonstrated that this therapy lowered mortality when compared with conventional therapy. In 1985, the modern era of thrombolytic therapy began with Tognoni's report of the Gruppo Italiano per lo Studio della Streptochinasi nell' Infarcto Miocardio (GISSI) study[12] of intravenous streptokinase therapy. Although intravenous thrombolytic therapy was widely applicable, an intense interest in interventional therapy remained in the United States and Europe.

The interest in invasive therapy existed because of early reports suggesting that percutaneous transluminal coronary angioplasty (PTCA) therapy resulted in impressive improvements in global ventricular function.[13, 14] The greater improvement in ventricular function when compared with thrombolytic therapy was felt to be due to relief of the underlying residual stenosis. Because of the concern about the detrimental impact of the persistent residual stenosis, PTCA therapy was further tested. In addition, early experience with intravenous streptokinase[15] suggested that early recanalization occurred in only 50% to 60% of patients. Fung et al.[16] demonstrated that PTCA therapy was highly effective in opening occluded vessels and successfully dilating stenotic vessels after pretreatment with intravenous streptokinase. In the mid-1980s intravenous streptokinase was felt to be effective but had major limitations.

For this reason a dual approach to the management of MI was evolving. Investigators were testing new thrombolytic agents[17] that might be more effective than streptokinase in recanalizing vessels. At the same time, the timing and role of angioplasty therapy after intravenous thrombolytic therapy were tested. Three large prospective studies were performed in the United States and Europe. The Thrombolysis and Angioplasty in Myocardial Infarction (TAMI) study tested whether immediate PTCA was required after successful thrombolytic therapy.[18] The European Co-operative Study[19] tested whether PTCA therapy was better than a noninvasive approach in presenting ventricular function. Finally, the Thrombolysis in Myocardial Infarction (TIMI) II-B study[20] tested the impact of PTCA and cardiac catheterization on survival. After these studies were completed, a consensus emerged concerning invasive therapy *after* intravenous thrombolytic therapy with recombinant tissue-type plasminogen activator (rt-PA). First, no additive preservation of ventricular function is achieved by PTCA performed after rt-PA therapy. Second, no improvement in survival probability occurs with immediate or delayed aggressive intervention. In fact, a disturbing trend toward a *higher* mortality rate was present in the aggressively treated patients. Finally, aggressive therapy is associated with greater morbidity. Thus, as the 1980s drew to a close, interventional therapy for MI appeared headed to the museum of antiquated therapies. Interestingly, however, PTCA therapy still has appeal to a number of investigators and clinicians. This chapter will discuss why an interventional approach may in fact still have merit.

DEFICIENCIES OF THROMBOLYTIC THERAPY

Thrombolytic therapy is now the standard of care for management of patients with electrocardiographic transmural injury pattern. Major deficiencies of this therapy exist, however. In spite of aggressive dosing regimens including front-loaded rt-PA,[21] combination therapy,[22] and the addition of intravenous heparin and oral aspirin,[23] a ceiling of early reperfusion exists. In other words, regardless of the intravenous therapy chosen, 20% to 36% of patients will have failed therapy. Califf et al. have demonstrated that patients who initially fail thrombolytic therapy have a much worse prognosis.[24] It is now apparent that delayed recanalization does occur for some patients not achieving early reperfusion. Angiographic studies[25] demonstrated that 80% to 85% of patients have patent infarct-related arteries 24 hours after therapy. Although delayed recanalization may provide an improved survival probability,[26] Califf et al.[27] have demonstrated that an aggressive interventional strategy is more likely to result in greater myocardial salvage and fewer complications (Table 34–1).

TABLE 34–1.

Clinical Events: TAMI-V Trial

Cumulative Adverse Events*	t-PA† (%)	UK† (%)	Combination (%)	Catheterization Strategy (%)
Aggressive catheterization	37	36	28	33‡
Deferred catheterization	44	54	37	45
Drug strategy	40	45	32§	

*P = .009 for all events.
††t-PA = tissue-type plasminogen activator; UK = urokinase.
‡P = .005 for a comparison of catheterization strategy.
§P = .04 for a comparison of drug strategy.

In the TAMI-V Study, Califf demonstrated that a strategy of early catheterization and mechanical recanalization for patients failing early thrombolytic therapy resulted in a 30% reduction of adverse events during hospitalization. This occurred in spite of the fact that both aggressively treated patients and patients treated with "watchful" waiting had greater than 90% arterial patency at the time of hospital discharge. Thus, benefit is derived from achieving maximal rates of early arterial recanalization. At present, this requires mechanical intervention.

After thrombolytic recanalization is achieved, a substantial risk of recurrent ischemia and reocclusion exists. Reocclusion may be clinically silent or evident only by reelevation of cardiac enzymes. It also may be catastrophic with pulmonary edema or cardiogenic shock resulting. Since a purely thrombolytic strategy does not employ early catheterization, there is no way to risk-stratify those patients at greatest risk. For instance, patients with severe left main or severe three-vessel disease cannot be identified noninvasively. Irrespective of the use of intervention, early catheterization allows a delineation of coronary anatomy and ventricular function. These data are extraordinarily useful in triage decisions and risk stratification of patients.

The fact that the TIMI II-B study could not substantiate a value for early catheterization is not related to the failure of this strategy as much as the fact that a very low-risk cohort of patients was enrolled in the TIMI-II study. The low-risk features of a thrombolytic-eligible population has been clearly stated by Cragg et al.[28] He reviewed the overall impact of thrombolytic therapy at our institution during the recruitment phases of the TIMI-IIB, Third International Study of Infarct Survival (ISIS-III) and Trial of Eminase for Acute Myocardial Infarction (TEAM)-III studies. Only 15% of the 1,409 patients with proven MI treated at our hospital were eligible for thrombolytic therapy. More important than the low proportion of patients eligible, were the baseline characteristics analyzed (Table 34–2). Multiple clinical characteristics that have previously been shown

TABLE 34-2.
Clinical Characteristics for Patients Excluded From Thrombolytic Therapy

Characteristic	Thrombolysis Treated	Thrombolysis Excluded	P Value
n	235	1,235	
Mean age (yr)	58	69	<.00001
Male (%)	79	60	<.00001
History of hypertension (%)	37	48	<.002
Prior MI* (%)	10	35	<.00001
Chronic angina (%)	16	36	<.0001
In-hospital mortality (%)	3.9	18.6	<.00001

*MI = myocardial infarction.

to denote increased risk after MI were analyzed. All were more severe or more frequent in the thrombolytic-ineligible patients. Thrombolytic-treated patients were younger and more often male and had fewer previous MIs, less chronic angina, and less incidence of hypertension. Given these low-risk features, it is not surprising that an early strategy of catheterization did not improve outcome. The TIMI-IIB study did identify a high-risk group of thrombolytic-eligible patients. Garrahy et al.[29] reviewed the TIMI-IIB experience with patients in cardiogenic shock after t-PA therapy. They found that patients treated strictly noninvasively had a 22% survival rate vs. a 78% survival rate for patients in shock after rt-PA therapy who had aggressive intervention including PTCA or bypass.

Because of the shortcomings of thrombolytic therapy, alternative recanalization strategies are important to study. We wished to determine whether thrombolytic therapy was required at all when angioplasty therapy was employed. Previous randomized trials all pretreated patients with thrombolytic therapy prior to PTCA. These studies (Table 34-3) found that the combined

approach was detrimental when compared with thrombolytic therapy alone. Angioplasty therapy alone had never been tested.

To this end, the Streptokinase Angioplasty Myocardial Infarction (SAMI) trial was organized.[30] Patients with entry criteria identical to the TIMI-II study were enrolled. Patients were treated immediately with 10,000 units of heparin intravenously and aspirin, 325 mg. They were then randomized to therapy with placebo or streptokinase, 1.5 million units. Both subgroups were taken immediately to the cardiac catheterization laboratory and had immediate coronary angiography. Those patients with suitable coronary anatomy underwent immediate PTCA. At the time of catheterization, contrast ventriculography was performed. Follow-up included radionuclide ventriculography at 24 hours and 6 weeks with repeat coronary angiography at 6 months.

The purpose of this study was to determine whether concomitant treatment with intravenous streptokinase augmented improvement in ventricular function or altered the clinical course after PTCA therapy (Table 34-4). We found that angioplasty was highly successful in both subgroups. The addition of streptokinase increased the likelihood of emergency or urgent bypass. No decrease in reocclusion rates was achieved. Streptokinase in fact prolonged hospital stays, markedly increased the need for blood transfusions, and significantly increased hospitalization costs. In addition to the deleterious effect on clinical course, no additional improvement in ventricular function occurred. Serial radionuclide ventriculograms were performed, and no improvement in global ventricular function was noted. At 6 months, there was ventricular function improvement for the whole group, but no differences were detected whether streptokinase had been used or not.

The SAMI study must be taken in context with the other randomized PTCA thrombolytic trials. This study

TABLE 34-3.
Adverse Outcomes of Immediate PTCA After Thrombolytic Therapy

Therapy/Outcome	Clinical Trial*			
	TAMI	TIMI II-A	SWIFT	SAMI
Thrombolytic agent†	t-PA	t-PA	APSAC	SK
Emergency bypass (%)	7	4	15	10
Transfusions (%)	20	20	19	39
Mortality (early PTCA) (%)	4	7	3.3	5

*TAMI = Thrombolysis and Angioplasty in Myocardial Infarction; TIMI = Thrombolysis in Myocardial Infarction; SWIFT = Should We Intervene Following Thrombolysis; SAMI = Streptokinase Angioplasty Myocardial Infarction.
†t-PA = tissue-type plasminogen activator; APSAC = anisoylated plasminogen streptokinase activator complex; SK = streptokinase.

TABLE 34-4.
Clinical Outcome of Angioplasty Alone vs. Combined Angioplasty/Streptokinase Therapy

Outcome	Combined Therapy	PTCA Alone	P Value
n	58	63	.20
Successful PTCA	98%	92%	.40
Need for bypass*	10.3%	1.6%	.03
Transfusions	39%	8%	.0001
Vascular complications	29%	5%	.004
Systemic bleeding	10%	0%	.01
Recurrent ischemia	12%	16%	.42
Hospital stay (days)	9.3 ± 5	7.7 ± 4.0	.046
Total cost ($1000s)	25.2 ± 15.4	19.6 ± 7.2	.02

*Bypass occurring within 5 days of admission.

corroborates the morbidity of combined angioplasty and thrombolytic therapy. Importantly, it also corroborates the disturbing increase in need for urgent surgery in these patients. The fact that patients treated with angioplasty therapy alone had a more benign course is intriguing. This fact suggests that the previous conclusions about the efficacy of PTCA and thrombolytic therapy cannot be extrapolated to PTCA therapy alone. This study also demonstrates that PTCA therapy can be optimally performed without adjunctive intravenous thrombolytic therapy.

The lack of need for thrombolytic therapy has major ramifications. First, interventional therapy may have much less morbidity than previously thought. More importantly, patients at increased risk for hemorrhage with thrombolytic therapy may be optimally treated with PTCA therapy alone. Cragg et al.[28] have shown that patients with previous stroke or bleeding risk are a high-risk subset and have a 24% hospital mortality with conventional care. In addition, some patients with relative contraindications such as those with uncontrolled hypertension or a remote history of gastrointestinal bleeding may be more safely treated with PTCA therapy alone. Finally, patients in whom the diagnosis of evolving MI is in doubt (i.e., complete left bundle-branch block) might be more optimally treated by emergency catheterization and infarct angioplasty. Whether patients who are good candidates for thrombolytic therapy do better or worse with infarct angioplasty alone remains to be answered by prospective randomized clinical trials. Such a trial is in progress in the United States (and in France) in 11 centers. This study, the Primary Angioplasty Myocardial Infarction (PAMI) trial randomized patients to therapy with PTCA alone or rt-PA therapy alone.[31a]

REVIEW OF MAJOR CLINICAL SERIES

Although there is a paucity of randomized data concerning infarct angioplasty alone, three large clinical series have been reported. These reports provide useful insight into the technical aspects and patient selection for lone PTCA therapy. Tables 34–5 and 34–6 summarize the clinical characteristics and outcome of the large reported series.

The earliest clinical study of infarct angioplasty occurred at the Mid-American Heart Institute. Hartzler initially reported[14] a dramatic 16% increase in global ejection fraction for patients treated with infarct angioplasty. This seminal study was a major impetus for evaluation of infarct angioplasty in the United States and

TABLE 34–5.

Clinical Characteristics of Angioplasty Therapy in Large Series

Characteristic	Ellis[33]	O'Keefe[32]	Brodie[34]	PAR*[35]
n	500	500	383	206
Eligible for PTCA (%)	NR*	NR	94	92
Mean age (yr)	56 ± 11	59 ± 11	57 ± 10	58 ± 12
Male (%)	78	73	72	74
Time to treatment (hr)	4.7	5.2	4.7	4.3
Shock (%)	12	8	5.7	0
Anterior MI (%)	46	43	45	40
Multivessel CAD* (%)	55	57	53	56
Successful PTCA (%)	78	94	91	95

*PAR = Primary Angioplasty Recanalization; NR = not recorded; CAD = coronary artery disease.

Europe. The overall updated clinical experience from this center has recently been reported by O'Keefe, et al.[32] A consecutive series of 500 patients were treated. Importantly, many elderly patients, those with previous bypass, those in cardiogenic shock, and those with contraindications to thrombolytic therapy were treated. Overall, PTCA was successful in 94% of cases. Subgroup analysis identified three important subgroups with an extremely favorable outcome when compared with historical controls. First, patients who were eligible for thrombolytic therapy but were treated by PTCA alone had a 1.8% hospital mortality rate. Second, patients with single-vessel disease had a 1.4% mortality rate. This subgroup is important because it represents 40% to 50% of all thrombolytic-eligible patients. Finally, patients in cardiogenic shock had a 59% survival rate. This is in keeping with other reports of PTCA in cardiogenic shock and a significant improvement in survival vs. historical controls. Alternatively, subgroups with less favorable outcome were identified. Patients with multivessel disease had an 11.5% mortality rate. Patients with failed angioplasty had a 34% mortality rate. Finally, patients older than 70 years of age had a 17% mortality rate.

The next major report relates to the University of Michigan experience.[33] Unlike the Kansas City experience, a heterogeneous treatment strategy existed for the 500 patients consecutively treated in Ann Arbor. In this series, 229 patients were pretreated with rt-PA, had combination rt-PA and urokinase pretreatment, or received intravenous streptokinase as part of prospective clinical trials. Infarct angioplasty alone was performed on 271 patients. This series included elderly patients, patients in shock (12%), and patients with contraindications to thrombolytic therapy. An overall 10% mortality rate occurred. The procedural success rate was 78%. Multivariate analysis identified subgroups that benefited

TABLE 34–6.

Outcome of Angioplasty Therapy in Large Series

Outcome	Survival (%)			
	Ellis[33]	O'Keefe[32]	Brodie[34]	PAR*[35]
Overall survival	90	93	91	96
Shock	68	59	50	0
Thrombolytic eligibility	NR*	98.2	96.1	NA*
Anterior MI	87	89	NR	NR
Inferior MI	93	96	NR	NR
Single-vessel disease	NR	99	97	98
Multivessel disease	NR	88	86	95
Elderly	84 (>70)	82 (>70)	70 (>75)	NR
Young	95 (<70)	95 (<70)	93 (<75)	NR

*PAR = Primary Angioplasty Recanalization; NR = not reported; NA = not applicable.

from angioplasty. These included those patients not pretreated with thrombolytic therapy, those with occluded infarct arteries, patients older than 65 years of age, patients in cardiogenic shock, and patients with anterior MI. Like the Kansas City experience, multivessel disease lessened the probability of successful PTCA. This was especially true for patients with triple-vessel disease who presented in cardiogenic shock. Here survival was disappointingly low.

A third large clinical series was reported by Brodie et al.[34] in 1991. These investigators treated 383 MI patients with angioplasty therapy alone. The authors report that 63% of all MI patients presenting to their institution were eligible and treated with PTCA therapy. This is in dramatic contrast to the 14% of MI patients eligible for thrombolytic therapy that was reported by Cragg et al.[28] (Table 34–7). Brodie further subdivided outcomes of patients for thrombolytic therapy. On the basis of clinical eligibility, Cragg has demonstrated that thrombolytic-ineligible patients have high-risk clinical features. Brodie found that they also have high-risk anatomic features. Thrombolytic-ineligible patients were more likely to have left anterior descending artery involvement, were more likely to have multivessel disease, and had lower left ventricular ejection fraction values.

In keeping with these findings, the mortality rate was 3.9% for thrombolytic-eligible and 24% for thrombolytic-ineligible patients who were treated with PTCA therapy. The greatest proportion of deaths in the ineligible patients occurred for those patients presenting in cardiogenic shock. The mortality rate was 50% for the 22 patients who were treated. When the patients with cardiogenic shock are excluded, a 16% mortality rate for thrombolytic-ineligible patients occurred. In addition to cardiogenic shock, Brodie found that age over 75 years, unsuccessful PTCA, multivessel disease, and delayed treatment were all independently associated with increased mortality. In addition to hospital outcomes, Brodie reported on the long-term angiographic follow-up of 63% of the surviving patients. An angiographic patency of 85% existed for the infarct-related artery. Thrombolytic-eligible patients had a mean 4.4% increase in ejection fraction, and thrombolytic-ineligible patients had a 10.5% increase ($P = .002$).

In addition to these large series, a new prospective registry of angioplasty therapy alone is being conducted in six major centers in the United States. This registry is known as the Primary Angioplasty Recanalization (PAR) Registry.[35] The purpose of this registry is to collect prospective, quality-controlled data concerning infarct angioplasty. Duke University is serving as the data monitoring center and angiographic core laboratory. To date, 157 patients have had completed data forms submitted to the monitoring center for analysis. This prospective registry has documented the extremely high success rate of infarct angioplasty performed at experienced, high-volume centers. In association with this a very low mortality and very favorable hospital course appear to occur. Further detailed analysis of predictors of procedural success and complications as well as 6-month patency rates and restenosis rates will be forthcoming.

TABLE 34–7.

Therapeutic Eligibility

Eligibility	Series	
	Brodie[34]	Cragg[28]
Therapy	PTCA	Thrombolytic therapy
n	609	1,470
Clinically eligible	383 (63%)	209 (14%)
Clinically ineligible	201 (33%)	1,283 (86%)
Angiographically ineligible	25 (4%)	

PATIENT SELECTION FOR ANGIOPLASTY THERAPY

The clinical series just reviewed provide insight into clinical and angiographic selection criteria for angioplasty therapy. It must be emphasized that the major limitation of angioplasty therapy is a logistic one. If there are no catheterization facilities and operators in an institution, then this form of therapy is impractical. In locations where angioplasty is logistically possible, identification of patients most likely to benefit is imperative. The strongest data exist for aggressive interventional management of patients in cardiogenic shock. Survival rates of greater than 50% are consistently reported[36] after angioplasty therapy. Survival is most likely for shock patients with one- or two-vessel disease. Both Ellis et al. and Lee et al. have found that angioplasty is less successful and the outcome worse for patients with triple-vessel disease who present in shock. This is related to the inferior technical outcome of angioplasty, the greater chance for procedural mortality, and the less complete revascularization with infarct vessel angioplasty alone. In addition, survival for patients with cardiogenic shock who are older than 75 years is extremely unlikely. We do not recommend aggressive therapy for these patients. In any event, patients in cardiogenic shock and younger than 75 years are most likely to survive if they have a catheterization-based treatment strategy that subsequently involves angioplasty or emergency coronary bypass. The other major subgroup at great clinical risk involves those patients with a risk of intracerebral or systemic hemorrhage. Currently, these patients are primarily receiving conservative care. Mortality rates of over 20% are to be expected with conservative treatment. Almany et al.[37] have demonstrated that elderly patients and patients presenting late after symptom onset have a major survival advantage when angioplasty therapy is employed. Other high-risk clinical subgroups that may benefit from angioplasty therapy are patients with anterior MI or a second MI.

Angiographic studies have demonstrated subgroups where angioplasty therapy is less likely to be effective. Ellis et al. carefully analyzed 300 patients treated with angioplasty therapy. Worsened results were achieved with triple-vessel disease, with poor ventricular function, and with bend points greater than 45 degrees. The Mid-American Heart Institute experience and the Greensboro experience also corroborate the worsened procedural and clinical outcome of patients with triple-vessel disease. Conversely, those patients with single-vessel disease have a superb clinical outcome with less than a 2% hospital mortality rate. It appears from these

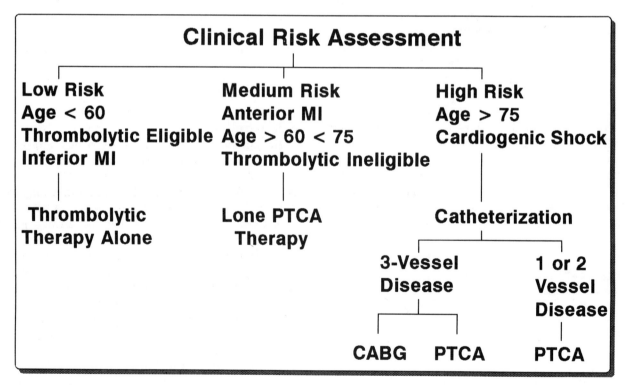

FIG 34–1.
Treatment algorithm. *CABG* = coronary artery bypass graft.

studies that angioplasty therapy is most likely to be successful in patients with high clinical risk (shock, elderly, anterior MI, second MI) who have low-risk angiographic findings (single- or double-vessel disease, ejection fraction greater than 25%). Based on this information, a treatment algorithm can be constructed (Fig 34–1).

FUTURE DIRECTIONS FOR RESEARCH

Of paramount importance, prospective comparative clinical trials of PTCA therapy alone and thrombolytic therapy alone are required. Such trials are currently under way in Spokane, at the Mayo Clinic, and by the PAMI investigation. These studies will demonstrate whether angioplasty therapy will have a role in the treatment of thrombolytic-eligible patients. Presently, no data exist that demonstrate the superiority of *either* thrombolytic or angioplasty therapy. Irrespective of these studies, further work on mechanical revascularization techniques are required. As has been discussed, mechanical revascularization has a role for high-risk patients and thrombolytic-ineligible patients. Ideally, a mechanical approach that provides greater than a 95% success rate and negligible reocclusion rates is required. Adjunctive pharmacologic therapy such as hirudin or antiplatelet antibody is promising. Alternative mechanical devices including the transluminal extraction catheter, thermal balloon angioplasty, and excimer coronary laser are all undergoing early clinical trials. In the interim, there is optimism that mechanical revascularization will become an increasingly important method of therapy for high-risk MI patients.

REFERENCES

1. Pifarre R, Spinazzola A, Memickas R, et al: Emergency aorto-coronary bypass for acute myocardial infarction. *Arch Surg* 1971; 103:525.
2. Reul GJ, Morris GC, Howell JF, et al: Emergency coronary artery bypass grafting in the treatment of myocardial infarction. *Circulation* 1973; 47(suppl 3):177.
3. Cheanvechai C, Effler DB, Loop FD, et al: Aortocoronary artery graft during early and late phases of acute myocardial infarction. *Ann Thorac Surg* 1973; 16:249.
4. Berg R, Kendall RW, Duvoisin GE, et al: Acute myocardial infarction: A surgical emergency. *J Thorac Cardiovasc Surg* 1975; 70:432.
5. Rentrop P, Blanke H, Karsch KR, et al: Initial experience with transluminal recanalization of the recently occluded infarct-related coronary artery in acute myocardial infarction — comparison with conventionally treated patients. *Clin Cardiol* 1979; 2:92.
6. Rentrop P, DeVivie ER, Karsch KR, et al: Acute coronary occlusion with impending infarction as an angiographic complication relieved by guidewire recanalization. *Clin Cardiol* 1978; 1:101.
7. Rentrop KP: Thrombolytic therapy in patients with acute myocardial infarction. *Circulation* 1985; 71:626.
8. Chazov EI, Matveeva LS, Mazaev AV, et al: Intracoronary administration of fibrinolysin in acute myocardial infarction. *Ter Arkh* 1976; 48:8–19.
9. O'Neill W, Topol E, Pitt B: Reperfusion therapy of acute myocardial infarction. *Cardiovasc Dis* 1988; 30:235–266.
10. Kennedy JW, Ritchie JL, Davis KB, et al: Western Washington randomized trial of intracoronary streptokinase in acute myocardial infarction. *N Engl J Med* 1983; 309:1477–1482.
11. Hugenholtz PG: Acute coronary artery obstruction in myocardial infarction: Overview of thrombolytic therapy. *J Am Coll Cardiol* 1987; 9:1375–1384.
12. Gruppo Italiano per lo Studio della Streptochinasi nell'Infarto Miocardio (GISSI): Effectiveness of intravenous thrombolytic treatment in acute myocardial infarction. *Lancet* 1986; 1:397–402.
13. O'Neill W, Timmis G, Bourdillon P, et al: A prospective randomized clinical trial of intracoronary streptokinase versus coronary angioplasty for acute myocardial infarction. *N Engl J Med* 1986; 314:812–818.
14. Hartzler GO, Rutherford BD, McConahay DR, et al: Percutaneous transluminal coronary angioplasty with and without thrombolytic therapy of acute myocardial infarction. *Am Heart J* 1983; 106:965–973.
15. Schroder R, Biamino G, Leitner E, et al: Intravenous short-term infusion of streptokinase in acute myocardial infarction. *Circulation* 1983; 67:536–548.
16. Fung A, Lai P, Topol E, et al: Value of percutaneous transluminal coronary angioplasty after unsuccessful intravenous streptokinase therapy in acute myocardial infarction. *Am J Cardiol* 1986; 58:686–691.
17. TIMI Study Group: The thrombolysis in myocardial infarction (TIMI) trial. *N Engl J Med* 1985; 312:932–936.
18. Topol EJ, Califf RM, George BS, et al: A randomized trial of immediate versus delayed elective angioplasty after intravenous tissue plasminogen activator in acute myocardial infarction. *N Engl J Med* 1987; 317:581–588.
19. Anderson J, McIlvaine P, Marshall H, et al: Long-term follow-up after intracoronary streptokinase for myocardial infarction: A randomized, controlled study. *Am Heart J* 1984; 108:1402–1408.
20. Guerci A, Ross R: TIMI-II and the role of angioplasty in acute myocardial infarction. *N Engl J Med* 1989; 320:663–665.
21. Neuhaus K-L, Feuerer W, Jeep-Tebbe S, et al: Improved thrombolysis with a modified dose regimen of recombinant tissue-type plasminogen activator. *J Am Coll Cardiol* 1989; 14:1566–1569.
22. Grines C, Nissen S, Booth D, et al: A new thrombolytic regimen for acute myocardial infarction using combination half dose tissue-type plasminogen activator with full dose streptokinase: A pilot study. *J Am Coll Cardiol* 1989; 14:573–580.
23. White H: GISSI-2 and the heparin controversy. *Lancet* 1990; 336:297–298.
24. Califf RM, Topol EJ, George BS, et al: Characteristics and outcome of patients in whom reperfusion with intravenous tissue-type plasminogen activator fails: results of

the Thrombolysis and Angioplasty in Myocardial Infarction (TAMI) Trial. *Circulation* 1988; 77:1090–1099.

25. PRIMI Trial study group: Randomized double-blind trial of recombinant provrokinase against streptokinase in acute myocardial infarction. *Lancet* 1989; 1:863–868.

26. Califf R, Topol E, Gersh B: From myocardial salvage to patient salvage in acute myocardial infarction: The role of reperfusion therapy. *J Am Coll Cardiol* 1989; 14:1382–1388.

27. Califf R, Topol E, Stack R, et al: Evaluation of combination thrombolytic therapy and timing of cardiac catheterization in acute myocardial infarction – Results of thrombolysis and angioplasty in myocardial infarction – Phase 5 randomized trial. *Circulation* 1991; 83:1543–1556.

28. Cragg DR, Friedman HZ, Bonema JD, et al: Outcome of patients with acute myocardial infarction who are ineligible for thrombolytic therapy. *Ann Intern Med* 1991; 115:173–177.

29. Garrahy PJ, Henzlova MJ, Forman S, et al: Has thrombolytic therapy improved survival from cardiogenic shock? Thrombolysis in Myocardial Infarction (TIMI II) results. *Circulation* 1989; 80(suppl 2):623.

30. O'Neill WW, Weintraub R, Grines CL, et al: A prospective placebo-controlled randomized trial of intravenous streptokinase and angioplasty vs. lone angioplasty therapy of acute myocardial infarction. *Circulation* (in press).

31. Grines CL, Browne K, Rothbaum D, et al: The Primary Angioplasty in Myocardial Infarction (PAMI) Trial: Pre-liminary report (abstract) *Circulation* 1991; 84(suppl II):II–537.

31a. Grines CL, Browne KF, Vandormaal M, et al: Primary Angioplasty in Myocardial Infarction (PAMI) Trial. *Circulation* 1992; 86(suppl II).

32. O'Keefe JH, Rutherford BD, McConahay DR, et al: Early and late results of coronary angioplasty without antecedent thrombolytic therapy for acute myocardial infarction. *Am J Cardiol* 1989; 64:1221–1230.

33. Ellis SG, O'Neill WW, Bates ER, et al: Implications for patient triage from survival and left ventricular functional recovery analyses in 500 patients treated with coronary angioplasty for acute myocardial infarction. *J Am Coll Cardiol* 1989; 13:1251–1259.

34. Brodie B, Weintraub R, Stuckey T, et al: Outcomes of direct coronary angioplasty for acute myocardial infarction in candidates and non-candidates for thrombolytic therapy. *Am J Cardiol* 1991; 67:7–12.

35. O'Neill WW, Brodie B, Knopf W, et al: Initial report of the Primary Angioplasty Revascularization (PAR) multicenter registry (abstract). *Circulation* 1991; 84(suppl II):II–536.

36. Lee L, Bates E, Pitt B, et al: Percutaneous transluminal coronary angioplasty improves survival in acute myocardial infarction complicated by cardiogenic shock. *Circulation* 1988; 78:1345–1351.

37. Almany SL, Meany TB, Cragg DR, et al: Long term patency incidence of restenosis after primary angioplasty therapy of acute myocardial infarction (abstract). *J Am Coll Cardiol* 1991; 17:336.

35

The Role of Angioplasty in the Treatment of Acute Myocardial Infarction

Allan M. Ross, M.D.

The application of percutaneous transluminal coronary angioplasty (PTCA) within the broad scheme of the treatment of acute myocardial infarction (MI) falls into three categories based predominantly on the timing of the intervention. In this discussion, "primary PTCA" is emergency recanalization by interventional techniques, "sequential PTCA" refers to the combination of early administration of intravenous (IV) lytic agents followed very closely by angioplasty, and "adjunctive PTCA" implies angiography and angioplasty delayed by at least several days and possibly reserved for selected patients (as opposed to the nonselective approach implicit in the first two strategies) (Table 35–1).

PTCA as a primary intervention refers to the immediate use of guidewire, balloon catheter, and/or other intracoronary devices to effect disruption of the infarct causing occlusive thrombus. In addition to providing direct and immediate reperfusion, these techniques also allow for a reduction in the severe atherosclerotic obstruction that commonly exists at the site of a total interruption of antegrade coronary flow. The successful use of PTCA as primary therapy in acute MI has been reported from numerous centers, Hartzler et al. being among the earliest operators to demonstrate the feasibility of this approach.[1]

In highly experienced hands, primary PTCA without the use of lytic drugs can effect reperfusion with a frequency comparable if not superior to that obtained with the most efficient plasminogen activators, that is, in the range of 75% to 95% of attempts. It has the additional advantages of early definition of the total coronary circulation, which identifies candidates such as those with an obstructed left main artery who would presumably benefit from very early operative intervention, and on the other end of the spectrum, identifies those patients with single-vessel disease, who are potential candidates for very early discharge.[2] The main conceptual benefit, however, of primary PTCA is the rapid conversion of a total occlusion to a widely patent infarct artery very early in the course of disease. Data from O'Neill and colleagues[3] and other workers have demonstrated that immediately after reperfusion is accomplished by primary PTCA the infarct-related artery demonstrates a mean residual stenosis of less than 50%, whereas after chemical thrombolysis the former site of occlusion is left initially with a far more severe residual obstruction (83% in the series of O'Neill et al.). See the comparison of residual stenosis with lytic therapy and PTCA in Table 35–2. While it is now recognized that over time (that is, days to a week) continued clot dissolution after lytic therapy results in an increasingly patent infarct artery (shown with careful quantitative methodology by Serruys and coworkers[4] and other researchers), there has been suspicion and some supportive data for the concept that greater early reperfusion flow may effect greater myocardial salvage. Data from Sheehan and colleagues[7] have reported that an infarct-related coronary artery cross-sectional area of 4 mm^2 or greater is associated with improving left ventricular (LV) regional wall motion during follow-up, whereas smaller lumen areas have not been associated with such benefits. Analogous experimental data exist that utilize postocclusion coronary flow control to demonstrate greater salvage with increased blood flow.[8]

Early clinical substantiation of this principle was shown by the Michigan group,[3] who demonstrated considerably augmented improvement in LV function among infarct patients reperfused by PTCA as compared with those in whom reflow was accomplished pharmacologically. Furthermore, the augmented benefit

TABLE 35–1.

Angioplasty in Acute Myocardial Infarction

Application	Definition	Advantages	Disadvantages
Primary	Immediate transport to catheterization laboratory for clot perforation and lesion dilatation without lytic drugs	High rate of reperfusion; minimizes residual stenosis	Often prolonged time from infarct to treatment Requires emergency transport. Therapeutic scheme not available to majority of population
Sequential	IV lytic therapy is given first, then patient is transported for angiography-PTCA within hours	Avoids initial time-to-treatment delay Reduces residual stenosis severity Identifies lytic failures relatively early	Emergency transport still required Not available to significant percentage of population Randomized trials not encouraging
Adjunctive	Angiography and angioplasty performed later (1 or 2 days to a week) after lytic therapy Can be applied routinely or by some selection process	Avoids initial time-to-treatment delay Dilatation performed remote from thrombosis and in patients selected by severity of stenosis and/or other criteria Transport nonemergent	Early recurrent ischemia and reocclusion not interdicted Lytic failure not identified until presumably too late Severe residual stenosis not relieved until presumably beyond the salvage window

correlated directly with the considerably improved infarct artery diameter achieved by PTCA.

Thus there is theoretical, experimental, and clinical support for primary PTCA in acute MI. The limitations of this approach, however, are also clearly evident and are based on the complexity of the required logistics. From a variety of lines of evidence it has become established that for most infarct victims, meaningful myocardial salvage attends reperfusion accomplished within the very first few hours of onset of the clinical syndrome, with a benefit curve steeply declining from 1 or 2 hours after infarction and becoming almost immeasurable for treatment beyond 4 to 6 hours after an MI. The delays inherent in patient response, triage, and transportation render prompt PTCA within a short time frame (prob-

ably) unaccomplishable for most patients with acute MI given the currently constituted public awareness and response systems. Furthermore, extremely skilled interventionalists in the emergency setting, with laboratories and staffs instantly available on an around-the-clock basis, are required commodities for primary PTCA to work and are simply not available in most communities. Thus at the present time this mode of therapy can be favored in only very selected environments as a routine approach and more widely for the occasional patient whose infarction begins fortuitously when and where all the resources are locally available.

An interesting and somewhat unexpected observation regarding direct or primary angioplasty for acute MI has been the failure to confirm a lower reocclusion rate for PTCA as compared with plasminogen activator therapy. It had been generally expected that rapid reduction of the percent stenosis in the infarct-related artery would lessen the likelihood of reocclusion. Table 35–3 displays the angiographically proven reocclusion incidence after primary PTCA and after lytic therapy alone from several of the largest published reports on the subject.

Current logistic limitations regarding primary PTCA notwithstanding, clinicians and investigators, have been interested in the assessment of the comparative clinical value of PTCA vs. thrombolytic therapy when compared head to head in resource-rich institutions capable of rapidly performing either therapy. Several small series in which candidates for either therapy have been

TABLE 35–2.

Percent Residual Stenosis in the Infarct-Related Artery (Patent Vessels)

	Lytic Therapy Alone	
Serruys[4] (median stenosis)	IV rt-PA	80%
O'Neill[3] (mean stenosis)	IC streptokinase	83%
Erbel[5] (mean stenosis)	IV streptokinase	73%
	PTCA	
Erbel[5]	After IV streptokinase	47%
Rothbaum[6]	No lytic therapy	29%
O'Neill[3]	No lytic therapy	43%

*rt-PA = recombinant tissue-type plasminogen activator; IC = intracoronary.

TABLE 35–3.
Reocclusion After Various Reperfusion Strategies

First Author	Lytic Therapy Only	Lytic Therapy and PTCA	PTCA Only
Uebis[9]	4% (5/130)	9% (13/147)	
Erbel[5]	20% (14/71)	14% (10/69)	
Topol[10]	13% (13/98)	11% (11/99)	
O'Keefe[11]			15% (47/307)
Lee[12]			10% (10/105)
Rothbaum[6]			9% (8/85)
Ohman[13]	12% (91/714)		

randomized to one or the other approach are under way, and preliminary observations from two such studies have been disseminated.

A comparison is being performed of IV lytic therapy with a tissue-type plasminogen activator vs. random assignment to primary PTCA in the Spokane, Washington area. DeWood and colleagues[14] have presented very preliminary findings. Surprisingly, the time to treatment favored PTCA (owing to a substantial delay in starting thrombolytic infusions in the medically treated cohort). Seventy-two percent of those assigned to each group had angiographically proven patency 90 minutes after the start of therapy. No clinical outcome differences have thus far been seen in this trial, although as expected, the early residual infarct artery percent stenosis was less after PTCA than following lytic therapy alone.

Another small trial from Brazil randomized 100 infarct patients to either PTCA or intravenous streptokinase.[15] Time to treatment significantly favored pharmacologic therapy (180 minutes from pain vs. 240 minutes). Patency measured at 48 hours was 80% for those administered streptokinase and 74% in those who had angioplasty. Outcome left ventricular ejection fractions (LVEF) (hospital discharge) were equivalent. At least two other direct comparisons of PTCA and lytic therapy are under way with as yet no results reported.

Although it can probably be stated with near certainty that direct PTCA is an effective therapy for acute MI, this approach has some unique disadvantages beyond the obvious logistic ones. There are anatomic contradictions to angioplasty, for example, significant left main coronary plaque in a patient with more distal left anterior descending (LAD) artery occlusion, which may result in the operator declining to proceed with the attempt. In this cited example it would be due to a reluctance to seat a large guide catheter in the left main artery. In a reported series of direct or adjunctive PTCA in MI, anatomic considerations have accounted for the fact that at least 10% of patients taken to the catheter-

ization laboratory for PTCA do not get the procedure. For those who were to have PTCA as the sole reperfusion method, this problem adds considerable time to when a lytic agent is finally infused.

The second potential problem is distal embolization of a thrombus. When carefully sought, the fragments of the dilated clot can be found angiographically in distal branches as often as 15% of the time. Although the course is often benign, such events can produce paradoxically increased ischemia. This in fact forms one of the arguments for combining a plasminogen activator with an angioplasty attempt.

The overall impression at the present time appears to be that direct PTCA for acute infarction is an effective method of reperfusion so long as it can be accomplished in the same time frame as can pharmacologic reperfusion. Since plasminogen activators result in arterial patency in approximately 45 minutes, the challenge to interventionalists is to transport the patient, assemble the team, and complete the PTCA within about an hour of making the diagnosis. Greater delays are likely to render this therapy less efficacious than immediate intravenous thrombolysis. The Kansas group[11] has shown striking differences in outcome mortality rates based upon elapsed time from infarct onset to successful PTCA. When angioplasty was accomplished within 2 hours of pain onset, the hospital fatality rate was 4%; but when the delay was 6 or more hours, the mortality rate was 11%. This urgency in speed to treatment (to salvage myocardium) precisely parallels the experience gained in large thrombolytic treatment trials.

DIRECT PTCA WHEN THROMBOLYSIS IS CONTRAINDICATED

For many patients, PTCA is the reperfusion method of choice because of a relative or absolute contraindication to the use of a plasminogen activator. Whereas this approach is highly logical, it has been shown that some of the contraindications to lytic therapy (advanced age, recent major surgery, bleeding diathesis, etc.) represent a population in whom PTCA also carries a greater-than-usual risk and constitutes a group in whom the clinical outcome is somewhat compromised.

Brodie et al.[16] contrasted the outcome after direct PTCA in good thrombolytic therapy candidates (success rate, 95%; hospital mortality rate, 2%) with those who had contraindications to lytic agents (success rate, 88%; mortality rate, 15%). Other reports on primary angioplasty have demonstrated that the elderly suffer a high post-PTCA mortality rate quite analogous to that seen after lytic therapy.[12]

ANGIOPLASTY AFTER LYTIC THERAPY

Because rapidity of reperfusion has been recognized as the most important single variable in producing clinical benefits and since transportation and procedure time preclude the possibility of most infarct victims' receiving early PTCA as effective primary therapy, a larger experience exists in adding angioplasty to the management strategy of patients who first are treated with an intravenous thrombolytic agent. From a theoretical basis, this sequence of lysis followed promptly by angiography and angioplasty is highly attractive. It combines the rapidity afforded by initial IV pharmacologic lysis with the additional benefits of angiography and PTCA discussed above. Conceptually it is an ideal algorithm for solving the problems of reocclusion, reinfarction, and recurrent ischemia. Furthermore, from a logistic point of view it affords more orderly transfer of patients after initial therapy to laboratories equipped to receive such patients under slightly less urgent conditions.

"Sequential" angioplasty (IV thrombolysis quickly followed by PTCA) is motivated by the dual goals of reperfusing patients who are not perfused adequately on IV lytic drug therapy (20% to 25% with recombinant tissue-type plasminogen activator [rt-PA] and higher with IV streptokinase) and having a favorable impact on the reocclusion and recurrent ischemia rates seen after thrombolytic therapy. The frequency of recurrent coronary occlusion after thrombolysis has shown considerable variability from study to study, but now with very large numbers of pooled data available it can be reasonably estimated to be between 10% and 15%. Actual reinfarction at the time of reocclusion occurs at a somewhat lower frequency owing to several probable factors, including the reality that not all reperfusion leads to clinically important salvage (thus little myocardium is at risk to reinfarct) and perhaps the development of substantial collateral flow between the first episode of occlusion and the second one.

The setting for reocclusion is the persistence of a severe coronary narrowing and some thrombus at the previously occluded site. Logic, therefore, would dictate that conversion of a tight to a mild obstruction by sequential PTCA ought to very favorably influence the rate of reclosure.

Recurrent ischemic events ascribable to the zone of salvaged myocardium and the severe postlysis stenosis in the infarct-related artery have also been well documented and are even more frequent than the problem of reocclusion. Again, the occurrence of this phenomenon is dependent on initial salvage of substantial muscle, which in turn is dependent on the efficiency of the lytic

agent selected and the time of delay from symptom onset to reperfusion. The range of reported recurrent ischemia is therefore even wider than the reported rates of reocclusion, but with effective early lysis, recurrent ischemia may be estimated to occur in up to 20% of patients during early and intermediate-term follow-up (and in some small series with an even higher incidence). Here too the concept that sequential PTCA would reduce the likelihood of recurrent ischemia has been highly attractive.

The careful evaluation of this strategy, that is, IV lytic therapy and then sequential PTCA, has followed the usual progression from clinical observations to more structured randomized trials. Early observations have been published by Uebis and associates[9] who, somewhat surprisingly, found a slightly higher early reocclusion rate (3 days after initial therapy) of 8.8% among 147 patients offered sequential PTCA than the 3.8% reocclusion rate seen in 130 patients with no PTCA (not significant). By late follow-up in this series (26 weeks) both groups had equivalent total reocclusion rates (14.2% and 16.1% respectively). It is to be noted, however, that this was not a randomized trial. The first formally randomized series on lytic therapy with or without sequential PTCA was published by Erbel and colleagues.[5] PTCA patients in whom the procedure was successful did display a reduced reocclusion rate. However, owing to a significant fraction of procedural failures in comparing the total group randomized to PTCA with the total group managed conservatively, the sequential PTCA strategy did not lead to a final reocclusion benefit.

The three most prominent studies of the role of PTCA after lytic therapy to date have been the Transluminal Angioplasty in Myocardial Infarction (TAMI) trial,[10] the Thrombolysis in Myocardial Infarction (TIMI-II) trial,[17, 18] and the European Cooperative Group trial.[19] All three study groups selected rt-PA as the intravenous lytic agent because of its higher coronary reperfusion rate than streptokinase.

In TAMI 197 patients were randomized with stenotic and dilatable infarct-related arteries to either immediate PTCA or conservative therapy for a week. The major trial end points included reocclusion rate and ventricular function after a week's follow-up. Perhaps surprisingly, the reocclusion rates of 11% for PTCA vs. 13% for conservative therapy (see Table 35–3) and the final LV function (global and regional) were not different based on treatment assignment. More patients in the immediate PTCA group suffered bleeding problems and had emergency coronary artery bypass graft (CABG), whereas more of those in the conservatively treated group needed urgent nonprotocol PTCA or CABG between the first and seventh days. Thus at the end of the hospitalization period, early PTCA had shown no particular benefit in terms of pre-established end points.

Additional important observations by the TAMI investigators concerned the prognosis of nonrandomized patients in whom lytic therapy failed to produce reperfusion. Finding and mechanically reperfusing this subgroup of approximately 20% of infarct patients administered rt-PA has been one of the important motivators of the strategy to perform very early angiography and angioplasty. In 95 such patients reported in the TAMI trial, PTCA failed in 15% and resulted in luminal opening but then early or delayed reclosure in more than a third of the remaining patients. Thus about half of the patients in this group had a closed artery at 1 week despite the procedure, and the group's early mortality rate (15%) was twice that of those in whom rt-PA had proved effective. No group benefit in outcome LV function was observed.

TIMI-II was a complex two-part trial.[17, 18] TIMI-IIA studied 600 patients randomized into three groups: (1) IV rt-PA and heparin with immediate angiography and PTCA if the infarct-related artery was occluded or highly stenotic; (2) IV rt-PA and heparin plus delayed angiography and PTCA (performed 18 to 48 hours after the start of therapy), with PTCA mandated for stenotic but not persistently totally occluded arteries; and (3) rt-PA and heparin plus a conservative course (i.e., no angiography until 7 to 10 days post-MI unless clinically mandated by recurrent ischemia).

The principal end point was predischarge LVEF, which was equivalent in all three groups. Moreover, infarct artery patency at hospital discharge was equivalent (84%). Patients who had PTCA had less residual stenosis (51%) than did those who were treated conservatively (67%). In the opposite direction, all complications were more common for the strategy of thrombolysis followed by immediate angioplasty.

The TIMI-IIB trial was much larger (3,262 patients) and randomized to lytic therapy alone (the "conservative strategy") or lysis, angiography, and PTCA, if appropriate, 18 to 48 hours later (the "invasive strategy"). The primary end point in this comparison was combined reinfarction and death, seen in 10.9% of those in the invasive group and 9.7% in the conservative arm. The outcome LV function was equivalent.

It should be noted that the "conservative management strategy" was intended to include catheterization laboratory interventions if recurrent ischemia was encountered, which occurred in 13% within 14 days. What the trial documents is that a treatment algorithm in which *only* selected patients are offered catheterization laboratory–directed therapy produces a clinical outcome that is comparable if not superior to a strategy that assigns "all comers" to a post–lytic therapy interventional approach.

Very similar conclusions were reached by the European Cooperative Study Group,[19] i.e., more bleeding complications, no advantage in LV function, and a somewhat higher mortality rate in patients subjected to postlytic PTCA routinely when compared with a more conservative and selected approach.

DOES PLASMINOGEN ACTIVATOR HAVE AN IMPACT ON THE OUTCOME OF POST-THROMBOLYTIC PTCA?

There are often discussed notions that infarct PTCA is disadvantaged by the presence of fibrin-specific lytic agents (such as rt-Pa) and/or that systemic plasminogen activators (like streptokinase, APSAC [anisoylated plasminogen streptokinase activator complex] or urokinase) provide a better "milieu" in which to perform angioplasty than does a fibrin-specific agent like rt-PA. On these related issues there are numerous small reports allowing no firm conclusion.

SWIFT (*Should We Intervene Following Thrombolysis?*)[20] was a trial quite similar to TIMI-II but performed with APSAC as the lytic therapy, followed by an invasive, catheterization laboratory based follow-up strategy within 48 hours, or a "conservative," sign and symptom–driven use of interventional techniques. No statistically significant differences in the stated end points (mortality, reinfarction, recurrent ischemia, or LV function) were found when the two strategies were compared.

Recently the notion has been suggested that a combination of both kinds of plasminogen activators, fibrin specific (i.e., rt-PA) and systemic (i.e., streptokinase or urokinase), provide a better environment for subsequent angioplasty.[21] This approach is being investigated in several ongoing larger trials.

THE SPECIFIC ISSUE OF RESCUE ANGIOPLASTY

"Rescue" or "salvage" angioplasty is the name applied to angioplasty attempts at mechanically reopening an infarct vessel that failed to respond to plasminogen activator therapy. It has been mentioned previously in connection with the formerly popular strategy of "sequential" PTCA.

Although rescue angioplasty is often performed, firm conclusions regarding this treatment are difficult to reach. Abbotsmith et al.[22] reported on the clinical outcome of 192 patients, within the large series of TAMI trials, in whom rescue was attempted. Outcome in these 192 was compared with 607 patients within the studies who had achieved infarct artery patency subsequent to plasminogen activator therapy alone. The results in these rescue attempts were PTCA success in 78%, reocclusion in 21% within the first week, and a 1-week mortality rate of 5.9%. The rescue group did not demonstrate infarct zone ventricular functional recovery to the degree that pharmacologically reperfused patients did.

The precise value of rescue angioplasty would only be established by a substantially sized clinical trial in which patients with failed thrombolysis were randomized to a rescue attempt or medical therapy. Such trials are being attempted but suffer from two major recruitment-suppressing limitations. At present, no bedside marker of lysis or failed lysis has been persuasively shown to be fast and highly accurate; hence to do a rescue trial, early angiography in most lytic-treated MI patients is required and, as has been discussed above, is a strategy falling out of favor. Second, once in the catheterization laboratory with a patient whose infarct vessel has been shown to be occluded, most interventionalists find it difficult to randomize, with a 50% chance that the patient will be assigned to the group in which no PTCA is to be attempted. It would seem that clarification of this entire rather important issue may have to await rapid strategies for noninvasive identification of failed thrombolysis, such as fast enzyme or myoglobin analysis or one of the computerized continuous multi-channeled ST segment monitoring systems.

PTCA FOR CARDIOGENIC SHOCK AFTER MYOCARDIAL INFARCTION

Perhaps least controversial among the applications of angioplasty after infarction is its use in the setting of severe hemodynamic compromise. When seen in the early post-MI hours, such a picture generally indicates a totally occluded infarct-related artery even if a plasminogen activator has been administered. Urgent angioplasty reperfusion in this setting has been associated with a gratifying salvage rate of an otherwise usually fatal outcome. Lee et al.[23] reported a 54% 2-year survival rate for patients in cardiogenic shock consequent to a successful emergency PTCA.

CONCLUSION

The role of PTCA in the management of acute MI is an evolving one. Primary PTCA is proving to be an increasingly useful approach when the logistic problems can be overcome and has a quite important role when lytic therapy is contraindicated. Sequential angioplasty after lytic therapy is presently out of favor due to trial results incorporating thousands of patients. Adjunctive use of angioplasty is a very common choice among physicians caring for MI patients and is probably applied in up to a third of patients first treated with a plasminogen activator.

The issue of the best pharmacologic milieu for doing PTCA in the presence of a clot remains unsettled, but there are exiting new agents that may come to play an important supportive role (second-generation antiplatelet and antithrombolytic drugs).

"Rescue" angioplasty is an ideal concept that has unfortunately been hard to validate. Finally, PTCA for early post-MI cardiogenic shock has become the standard of practice.

REFERENCES

1. Hartzler GO, Rutherford BD, McConahay DR, et al: Percutaneous transluminal coronary angioplasty with and without thrombolytic therapy for treatment of acute myocardial infarction. *Am Heart J* 1983; 106:965–973.
2. Topol EJ, Califf RM, Kereiakes DJ, et al: Thrombolysis and Angioplasty in Myocardial Infarction (TAMI) trial. *J Am Coll Cardiol* 1987; 10:65–74.
3. O'Neill WO, Timis GC, Bourdillon PD, et al: A prospective randomized clinical trial of intracoronary streptokinase versus coronary angioplasty for acute myocardial infarction. *N Engl J Med* 1986; 314:812–818.
4. Serruys PW, Arnold AER, Brower RW, et al: European Co-operative Study Group for Recombinant Tissue Type Plasminogen Activator. *Eur Heart J* 1987; 8:1172–1181.
5. Erbel R, Pop T, Henrirhs KJ, et al: Percutaneous transluminal coronary angioplasty after thrombolytic therapy: A prospective controlled randomized trial. *J Am Coll Cardiol* 1987; 8:485–495.
6. Rothbaum DA, Linnemeier TJ, Landin RJ, et al: Emergency percutaneous transluminary coronary angioplasty in acute myocardial infarction: A 3 year experience. *J Am Coll Cardiol* 1987; 10:264–272.
7. Sheehan FH, Mathey DG, Schofer J, et al: Factors that determine recovery of the left ventricular function after thrombolysis in patients with acute myocardial infarction. *Circulation* 1985; 71:1121–1128.
8. Schmidt SB, Varghese PJ, Bloom S, et al: The influence of residual coronary stenosis on size of infarction after reperfusion in a canine preparation. *Circulation* 1986; 73:1354–1359.
9. Uebis R, Reynen K, Dorr R, et al: Frequency of coronary reocclusion after successful intracoronary thrombolysis in acute myocardial infarction: Comparison of immediate PTCA with subsequent medical treatment (abstract). *J Am Coll Cardiol* 1987; 9:232.
10. Topol EJ, Califf RM, George BS, et al: A randomized trial of immediate versus delayed elective angioplasty after intravenous tissue plasminogen activator in acute myocardial infarction. *N Engl J Med* 1987; 317:581–588.

11. O'Keefe JH Jr, Rutherford BD, McConahay DR, et al: Early and late results of coronary angioplasty without antecedent thrombolytic therapy for acute myocardial infarction. *Am J Cardiol* 1989; 64:1221–1230.
12. Lee TC, Laramee LA, Rutherford BD, et al: Emergency percutaneous transluminal coronary angioplasty for acute myocardial infarction in patients 70 years of age and older. *Am J Cardiol* 1990; 66:663–667.
13. Ohman EM, Califf RM, Topol EJ, et al: Consequences of reocclusion after successful reperfusion therapy in acute myocardial infarction. *Circulation* 1990; 82:781–791.
14. DeWood MA, Fisher MJ, et al: Direct PTCA versus intravenous r-tPA in acute myocardial infarction: Preliminary results from a prospective randomized trial. *Circulation* 1989; 80:1663.
15. Ribeiro EE, Silva LA, Carneiro R, et al: A randomized trial of direct PTCA vs. intravenous streptokinase in acute myocardial infarction (abstract). *J Am Coll Cardiol* 1991; 17:152.
16. Brodie BR, Weintraub RA, Stuckey TD, et al: Outcomes of direct coronary angioplasty for acute myocardial infarction in candidates and non-candidates for thrombolytic therapy. *Am J Cardiol* 1991; 67:7–12.
17. Immediate vs delayed catheterization and angioplasty following thrombolytic therapy for acute myocardial infarction. *JAMA* 1988; 260:2849–2858.
18. Comparison of invasive and conservative strategies after treatment with intravenous tissue plasminogen activator in acute myocardial infarction. *N Engl J Med* 1989; 320:618–627.
19. Simoons ML, Arnold AER, Betriu A, et al: Thrombolysis with tissue plasminogen activator in acute myocardial infarction: No additional benefit from immediate percutaneous coronary angioplasty. *Lancet* 1988; 1:197–203.
20. SWIFT trial of delayed elective intervention v conservative treatment after thrombolysis with anistreplase in acute myocardial infarction. *Br J Med* 1991; 302:555–600.
21. Topol EJ, Califf RM, George BS, et al: Coronary arterial thrombolysis with combined infusion of recombinant tissue-type plasminogen activator and urokinase in patients with acute myocardial infarction. *Circulation* 1988; 77:1100–1107.
22. Abbottsmith CW, Topol EJ, George BS, et al: Fate of patients with acute myocardial infarction with patency of the infarct-related vessel achieved with successful thrombolysis versus rescue angioplasty. *J Am Coll Cardiol* 1990; 16:770–778.
23. Lee L, Erbel R, Brown TM, et al: Multicenter registry of angioplasty therapy of cardiogenic shock: Initial and long-term survival. *J Am Coll Cardiol* 1991; 17:599–603.

Thrombolytic Therapy for Acute Myocardial Infarction: Implications of the Randomized Trials

Cindy L. Grines, M.D.

Over the past decade it has become increasingly clear that timely administration of thrombolytic therapy decreases infarction size, lessens the incidence of congestive heart failure, and improves ventricular function as well as short- and long-term survival.[1-6] Because of overwhelming evidence of clinical benefit provided by reperfusion therapy, several placebo-controlled trials were terminated prior to their planned end point. It was the opinion of these investigators that there were ethical implications in withholding reperfusion therapy during the early hours of myocardial infarction (MI). However, since thrombolytic drugs also have the potential for serious and even life-threatening bleeding complications, appropriate patient, drug, and dose selection is critical.

CONTROVERSIES REGARDING PATIENT SELECTION FOR THROMBOLYTIC THERAPY

Placebo-controlled thrombolytic studies conducted in the 1970s and 1980s were performed primarily to determine whether lytic therapy was efficacious and which patient subgroups might benefit.[1-8] On the basis of the early trials, it was readily accepted that patients who presented within 6 hours of symptom onset with anterior ST segment elevation would benefit from lytic therapy. Patient subgroups in whom the risk-benefit ratio of thrombolytic therapy has been controversial have

included inferior MI, absence of ST segment elevation, patients who present more than 6 hours from symptom onset, and patients considered to be at high risk of bleeding such as elderly or hypertensive patients.

Inferior Myocardial Infarction

Given the low mortality rate in patients with inferior infarction, it has been difficult to achieve a significant improvement in survival with thrombolytic therapy. However, these trials demonstrate that although the mortality benefit may be less for patients with inferior infarction, thrombolytic treatment is worthwhile in most cases. Three large international studies demonstrated a reduction in mortality after thrombolysis that was entirely independent of infarct location.[6-8] Furthermore, as demonstrated in Figure 36–1, pooled data involving more than 12,000 inferior infarction patients indicate a reduced mortality rate in the thrombolytic group (6.8%) as compared with the control group (8.7%, $P <.0001$).[9] In no large mortality trial did inferior MI patients have a worsened outcome from complications of thrombolysis. Several additional trials have demonstrated a significant improvement in left ventricular ejection fraction as well as infarct zone function after reperfusion therapy for inferior MI.[10] Therefore, in the absence of contraindications, patients with acute inferior MI should undergo treatment with thrombolytic drugs.

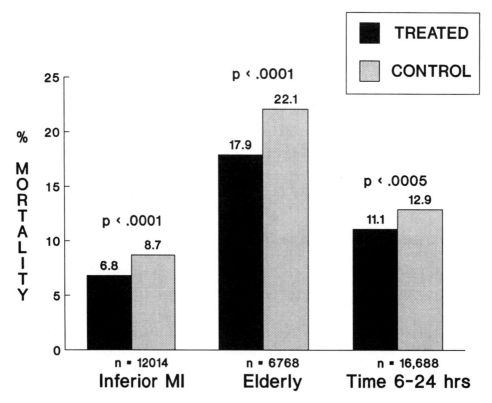

FIG 36–1.
Pooled mortality data in patient subsets in which the risk-benefit ration has been controversial. (Adapted from Grines CL, De-Mario AN: *J Am Coll Cardiol* 1990; 16:223–231.

Electrocardiographic Criteria

Currently, physicians generally require the presence of ST segment elevation on electrocardiograms (ECG) prior to initiating thrombolytic therapy. Patients who present with chest pain and a normal ECG have a very low mortality in both treated and control groups.[6, 8] Conversely, patients manifesting chest pain with isolated ST segment depression appear to have a very high mortality with minimal benefit from thrombolytic therapy.[5, 8] It has been reported that the high mortality in this subgroup may be due to unfavorable baseline characteristics such as advanced age, female sex, prior infarction, and multivessel coronary artery disease.[11] Therefore, these patients may benefit from a more aggressive approach with early catheterization to define the need for angioplasty or bypass grafting. Patients who present with good clinical evidence for infarction but whose ECGs manifest left bundle-branch block should be considered for thrombolytic therapy since the Second International Study of Infarct Survival (ISIS-2) trial found a 50% reduction in mortality rate in this subgroup after treatment with streptokinase and aspirin.[8]

Delayed Presentation

Primarily as a result of animal experiments and the Gruppo Italiana per lo Studio della Streptochinasi nell'Infarcto Miocardico (GISSI)-I trial's results with streptokinase,[5] it has been thought that the benefit from thrombolytic therapy may be chiefly confined to patients treated early after the onset of symptoms. However, pooled data analyzed by Yusuf et al. and the randomized ISIS-2 data suggests improved survival in patients treated between 6 and 24 hours after symptom onset.[8, 12] The preliminary report of the Estudio Multicentrico Estreptoquinasa Republicas de America del Sur (EMERAS) trial were recently presented.[13] In this study, 4,474 patients with suspected MI who presented between 6 and 24 hours from symptom onset were treated with aspirin and randomized to streptokinase or placebo. Patients treated between 6 and 12 hours from chest pain onset had a 13% reduction in mortality rate; however, this difference did not achieve statistical significance. Pooling all available data, the ISIS investigators concluded that there was a "definite" mortality advantage for the application of thrombolytic therapy within the first 6 hours, a "probable" advantage between hours 7 and 12, and a "possible" advantage between 13 and 24 hours.[14] It is interesting that these results were achieved with streptokinase, an agent that has been found to be relatively ineffective at achieving infarct vessel patency when administered in the late hours of infarction. Until the results of the ongoing Late Assessment of Thrombolytic Efficacy (LATE) trial, which is comparing tissue-type plasminogen activator (t-PA) to placebo, and complete data from the EMERAS and ISIS-3 trials are available, the routine administration of thrombolytic drugs cannot be advocated for patients who present late. However, serious consideration should be given to patients with a stuttering onset of chest pain, continued pain beyond the 6-hour window, large infarctions, or hemodynamic instability.

Elderly

Elderly patients traditionally have been excluded from thrombolytic trials due to the perceived increased risk of intracranial hemorrhage. As is apparent from many investigations, the mortality rate in older age groups is much greater than that of the overall infarct population.[1-8] If one calculates the difference in mortality rate between placebo and treatment groups to determine the number of lives saved per 100 patients treated, it becomes apparent that the greatest benefit of thrombolytic therapy may be in the elderly population. In fact, the lifesaving potential for the elderly appears to be two to three times that of the overall study population. As demonstrated in Figure 36–1, pooled data from five large trials demonstrated significant reduction in mortality rates after thrombolytic therapy in the elderly (17.9% vs. 21.1% in control patients, $P <.0001$).[9] Therefore, these data suggest that age in and of itself should not be considered an absolute contraindication to thrombolytic therapy.

Other Controversial Patient Selection Areas

Although hypertension is a risk factor for intracranial bleeding, a reduction in mortality produced by thrombolytic therapy may offset this risk in the hypertensive patient. Although "severe persistent hypertension" was a relative contraindication in the ISIS-2 trial, among the 1,141 patients who presented with a systolic blood pressure greater than 175 mm Hg, streptokinase resulted in improved mortality rates when compared with placebo control.[8] Therefore, although hypertensive patients may be at increased risk of intracranial bleeding, mortality in the group with moderate hypertension remains lower after treatment when compared with the control group.

However, it must be noted that the benefits of thrombolytic therapy in the severely hypertensive patient, i.e., diastolic blood pressure greater than 120 mm Hg, have yet to be determined.

In the past, cardiopulmonary resuscitation (CPR) has been considered a contraindication for thrombolytics. Califf et al. reported a series of patients who had undergone CPR without any increased risk of bleeding as assessed by transfusion requirement and change in hematocrit, and no cases of hemothorax or tamponade were identified.[15] Likewise, the ISIS-3 investigators reported that patients with a prior history of stroke or gastrointestinal bleeding had no increase in bleeding complications after lytic therapy and should not be routinely excluded.[14]

Table 36–1 outlines a practical and updated approach to select patients for thrombolytic therapy. Patients who present with chest pain of greater than 30 minutes' duration with ST segment elevation (regardless of location) will probably benefit from thrombolytic therapy. Furthermore, special consideration should be given to patients with good clinical evidence for MI whose ECGs manifest left bundle-branch block or anterior ST depression, which may represent a true posterior MI. Although the time window for treatment re-

TABLE 36–1.

Patient Selection for Thrombolytic Therapy

Indications
  Chest pain >30 min
  ECG:
    ST elevation >1 mm in 2 contiguous leads
    Anterior ST depression consistent with true posterior MI
    Left bundle-branch block
  Time window:
    <6 hr: routine treatment
    6–24 hr: high risk, continued chest pain
  Special subsets (treat in absence of other contraindications):
    Remote (>6 mo) history of nonhemorrhagic stroke or gastrointestinal bleeding
    Past history (>2 mo) of gastrointestinal bleeding
    Elderly
    Hypotension or moderate hypertension
    Cardiopulmonary resuscitation
Contraindications
  Absolute:
    Active internal bleeding
    Prior intracranial bleeding or cerebral neoplasm
    Cerebrovascular events or head trauma (within 6 mo)
    Known allergy to a drug considered for use
  Relative:
    Recent (<2 mo) surgery, gastrointestinal bleeding
    Pregnancy or within 1 mo postpartum
    Severe, persistent hypertension (diastolic BP >110 mm Hg)
    Recent (<2 wk) trauma including CPR with rib fractures

mains controversial, it is clear that thrombolytic drugs should be routinely administered if the patient presents within 6 hours of symptom onset. Since there is evidence to suggest that patients may continue to benefit beyond 6 hours, thrombolytic therapy should be considered in this group, particularly if the patient is in a high-risk subgroup or has a stuttering onset of chest pain or evidence of continued ischemia. In the absence of other contraindications, there are special subsets traditionally excluded from thrombolytic therapy in whom the benefit may outweigh the risk. These include patients with a remote history of nonhemorrhagic stroke or gastrointestinal bleeding, the elderly, patients who present with moderate hypertension or in shock, and those who have undergone CPR.

THROMBOLYTIC AGENTS

It is well established that complete thrombotic coronary occlusion occurs in the majority of patients presenting with acute MI. This is due to ruptured vascular endothelium at the site of an atherosclerotic plaque. In response to vessel injury, platelets adhere to the damaged endothelium and activate coagulation factors, and this results in fibrin formation and thrombotic coronary occlusion. Although their precise mechanisms of action differ, all thrombolytic drugs act by activation of plasminogen to the active enzyme plasmin, which digests the clot's fibrin component. As demonstrated in Table 36–2, differences between the drugs relate to the degree of fibrin specificity, duration of action, potential to cause allergic reactions, and cost.

Streptokinase

Streptokinase works by joining to plasminogen in a complex that converts neighboring plasminogen to plasmin.[16] Streptokinase activates fibrin-bound and circulating plasminogen equally and thus lacks significant fibrin specificity. The breakdown of circulating fibrinogen into fibrin degradation products results in antiplatelet and anticoagulant effects as well as a reduction in serum viscosity.[17,20] Since streptokinase is a product of β-hemolytic streptococci, it is antigenic and may produce allergic reactions in patients with recent streptococcal infections. Allergic reactions consisting of pruritus, rash, or fevers occur in 5% of patients, are usually quite mild, and are easily treated with antihistamines or antipyretics. The incidence of anaphylaxis is approximately 0.1%.[16] The recommended dose of streptokinase (1.5 million units) is usually sufficient to overcome the neutralizing effect of antibodies; therefore most patients will develop systemic fibrinolysis. Although the pharmacologic half-life of streptokinase is 30 minutes, depletion of fibrinogen usually lasts for 24 hours.[21] Antibodies develop approximately 5 days after streptokinase therapy and persist for 6 months to 1 year; therefore, it is recommended that patients not be retreated with streptokinase (or its derivative, APSAC) during that time interval. Hypotension due to vasodilatation occurs in approximately 10% to 15% of patients administered streptokinase. Patients who exhibit hypotension can be easily treated by temporarily stopping or decreasing the infusion rate of streptokinase and administering intravenous fluids. The advantages of streptokinase, with the proven additive effect of aspirin,[8] include its proven

TABLE 36–2.

Characteristics of Currently Available Thrombolytic Agents

Characteristics	Streptokinase	t-PA*	APSAC*	Urokinase†
IV dose	1.5 million units	100 mg	30 units	3 million units
Administration	1-hr infusion	60 mg/20 mg/20mg over hours 1, 2, & 3	bolus 2–5 min	1.5 MU bolus; 1.5 MU infusion/1 hr
Systemic lysis/bleeding risk	High/high	Low/high	High/high	High/high
Antigenicity	Yes	No	Yes	No
Allergic reactions/ hypotension	Yes	No	Yes	No
Acute coronary patency rates	40%–60%	60%–85%	60%–70%	50%–70%
Pharmacy cost‡	$87–$300	$2,300	$1,700	$2000–$3000
Mortality reduction	Yes	Yes	Yes	NA*

*t-PA = tissue-type plasminogen activator (Activase); APSAC = anisoylated plasminogen streptokinase activator complex (Eminase); NA = not available.
†Not Food and Drug Administration (FDA) approved for intravenous use.
‡Range in pharmacy costs at hospitals in the midwest.

track record in tens of thousands of patients, its ability to improve left ventricular function and save lives, and its cost saving (only $87 to $300 per dose). Disadvantages of streptokinase include the potential for allergic reactions and hypotension (although some believe that afterload reduction is beneficial after an MI). Although coronary reperfusion occurs more slowly with streptokinase than with other available agents, this has not translated into worsened clinical outcome.

Tissue Plasminogen Activator (Activase)

t-PA is a naturally occurring human protein that is nonantigenic and may be readministered immediately in the event of reinfarction.[16] Derived by recombinant DNA technology, t-PA is "fibrin specific." Therefore, t-PA selectively binds to the fibrin of clots, and the resulting complex converts neighboring plasminogen to plasmin, thereby producing more localized thrombolysis. Although this has resulted in lesser depletion of circulating fibrinogen, fibrin specificity has not resulted in a reduced incidence of bleeding complications.[21] Furthermore, the short half-life of t-PA (5 minutes) may result in a higher rate of infract vessel reocclusion and has resulted in the widespread use of concomitant intravenous heparin. The recommended dose of t-PA is 100 mg over a 3-hour period (60 mg, 20 mg, and 20 mg over hours 1, 2, and 3, respectively). Patients with a small body size have been shown to have an increased risk of bleeding complications with t-PA therapy. Therefore, in patients who weigh less than 65 kg, a total dose of 1.25 mg/kg is administered over a period of 3 hours, with 10% as a bolus, 50% over the first hour, and 40% over the last 2 hours. Advantages of t-PA include its lack of antigenicity and allergic reactions and no hypotension during infusion. Acute reperfusion rates have been demonstrated to be higher than that of streptokinase therapy.[22-26] However, reocclusion may also be higher, and clinical end points of left ventricular function, long-term patency, and mortality have been quite similar between the two agents. Disadvantages of t-PA include the complicated dosing regimen, the need for concomitant heparin administration, the higher rate of stroke, and its cost, which is $2,300.00 for a single dose.

Anisoylated Plasminogen Streptokinase Activator Complex (Eminase)

Anisoylated plasminogen streptokinase activator complex (APSAC) is a new second-generation thrombolytic agent that has been recently approved for intravenous use.[16] This drug was developed to overcome some of the limitations of intravenous streptokinase therapy. Temporary protection of the active enzymatic site of the plasminogen streptokinase complex by acylation allows APSAC to be given by rapid injection, thus improving bioavailability at the site of the clot and prolonging fibrinolytic action. This acylated derivative of streptokinase has several properties that differ from the parent compound, including greater fibrin binding and a longer duration of action (pharmacologic half-life of 90 minutes). These properties simplify intravenous administration and potentially improve coronary reperfusion and reduce reocclusion rates. The currently approved 30-unit dose has been demonstrated to result in acute infarct vessel patency rates of approximately 60% to 70%, improved ventricular function, and reduced mortality.[7, 27] As with streptokinase, its effectiveness at acutely opening coronary arteries is reduced in the later hours of MI (more than 4 hours from chest pain onset), but 24-hour patency rates are similar to other available agents. Advantages of APSAC include the ability to administer the entire dose as a bolus over a period of 2 to 5 minutes, moderate expense, and the ability to acutely open more arteries than with streptokinase therapy. However, the potential for allergic and hypotensive reactions remain, and this agent has not been demonstrated to be superior to streptokinase or t-PA with regard to improvement in ventricular function or reduction in mortality.

Urokinase

Urokinase is a proteolytic enzyme produced from human fetal kidney tissue cultures.[16] Although urokinase is approved for intracoronary use, the intravenous route of administration has yet to achieve Food and Drug Administration (FDA) approval. This naturally occurring enzyme has several advantages over streptokinase; however its use has been limited by the cost of this agent, which is approximately $2000 to $3000 per dose. Clinical trials demonstrated that after intravenous urokinase, the rate of coronary patency is approximately 50% to 70% and that of reocclusion, 5% to 10%.[28-30] At the usual dose of 3 million units of urokinase, depletion of fibrinogen commonly occurs. However, when compared with streptokinase, little or no hypotension, allergic reactions, or resistance to therapy has been noted. Urokinase is commonly given as a 3-million-unit dose consisting of 1.5 million units as a bolus and an additional 1.5 million units over a 1-hour period. Advantages of this therapy include the lack of antigenicity, allergic reactions, or hypotension, with disadvantages being the relative expense and lack of experience with this agent.

CLINICAL END POINTS AFTER THROMBOLYTIC THERAPY

In order to select a particular thrombolytic agent, it is important to compare the clinical benefits derived from various thrombolytic drugs. Clinical end points after thrombolytic therapy have included infarct vessel patency, left ventricular function, mortality, and complications, i.e., bleeding, reocclusion, or allergic reactions.

Patency of the Infarct-Related Artery

Since it is known that patients with acute MI have thrombotic coronary occlusion and that thrombi could be lysed by fibrinolytic agents, coronary patency has been used to judge the efficacy of different thrombolytic drugs. As demonstrated in Table 36–2, acute patency rates may be highest with intravenous t-PA,[22–26] intermediate with APSAC[27] or urokinase,[28–30] and lowest with streptokinase.[22, 23] A major rationale for the use of t-PA was its ability to achieve reperfusion within the first few hours of administration. Although patency of the infarct-related artery is associated with a lower mortality, fewer arrhythmias, and a reduction in size of the left ventricle, the optimal timing at which to determine patency has not been determined.[31] Studies employing acute angiography have used the time point of 90 minutes after initiation of thrombolytic therapy to determine patency. However, coronary artery patency is a dynamic process with continued thrombolysis as well as intermittent reocclusion.[32, 33] Perhaps, due to the differences in half-lives and fibrin specificity, t-PA appears to have a higher early reocclusion rate and streptokinase a greater frequency of late reperfusion, which has been referred to as the "catch-up phenomenon" (Fig 36–2). This may account for the fact that 24-hour patency rates were similar between t-PA– and streptokinase-treated groups. Likewise, infarct vessel patency rates at 1 to 3 weeks were identical for all of the available agents[34–38] (Table 36–3). Whether early patency or sustained patency is a more important prognostic factor has yet to be determined.

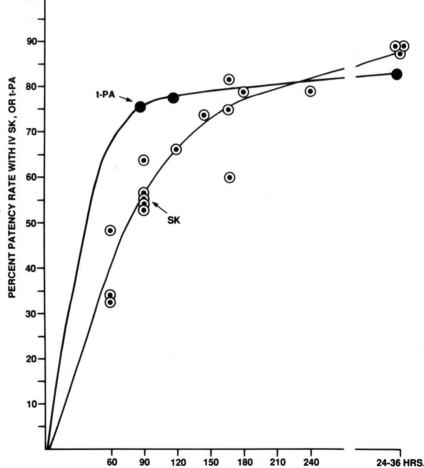

FIG 36–2.
Coronary patency rates after initiation of streptokinase *(SK)* or tissue-type plasminogen activator *(t-PA)* from angiographic studies in which thrombolytic therapy was initiated approximatedly 3 hours after symptom onset. (From Sherry S, Marder VJ: *Ann Intern Med* 1991; 114:417–423. Used by permission.)

TABLE 36–3.

Infarct Vessel Patency Rates 1–3 Weeks After Thrombolysis

Therapy	Patency (%)
t-PA	
TIMI-I[34]	72
White[35]	75
PAIMS[36]	81
Bassand[37]	75
Streptokinase	
TIMI-I[34]	72
White[35]	76
PAIMS[36]	74
APSAC	
Bassand[37]	72
APSIM[38]	77

Left Ventricular Function

Before the thrombolytic era, it was well established that left ventricular function was an important predictor of prognosis after acute MI.[39] All thrombolytic drugs have been demonstrated to improve regional and global ventricular function when compared with placebo.[40] Trials that directly compared streptokinase with t-PA showed that the two agents were similar in preserving left ventricular function. In phase I of the TIMI trial, the predischarge ejection fraction averaged 49.1% with streptokinase and 49.9% with t-PA.[41] In the Plasminogen Activator Italian Multicenter Study (PAIMS) trial, the mean ejection fraction as measured by contrast ventriculography 4 days after therapy demonstrated no significant difference between t-PA– and streptokinase-treated groups.[36] Similarly, in the study by White et al. the ejection fraction 3 weeks after infarction was identical in t-PA– and streptokinase-treated groups.[35] The GISSI-2 study group randomized 12,490 patients to either t-PA or streptokinase and performed predischarge two-dimensional echocardiograms.[42] They found no difference in left ventricular function or the incidence of congestive heart failure between the two groups. Trials directly comparing APSAC to t-PA with regard to ventricular function have shown similar findings.[37] It is not entirely clear why the high acute patency rates observed after t-PA administration have not resulted in greater preservation of ventricular function. Some have suggested that most patients are treated too late to have substantial limitation in infarct size, which may occur only if perfusion occurs in the first 1 or 2 hours.[31] Later application of thrombolytic drugs may improve survival by a reduction in infarct expansion, aneurysm formation, and malignant arrhythmias.[43] Unfortunately, due to patient and institutional delays, the majority of patients are being treated more than 3 hours from symptom onset, when minimal recovery in ventricular function can be expected.

Mortality

The most obvious clinical benefit of thrombolytic therapy is its lifesaving potential. The placebo-controlled trials have demonstrated that the use of streptokinase,[1–5, 8] t-PA,[6] or APSAC[7] will save lives. Prior to the availability of direct mortality comparisons, it was suggested that t-PA–treated patients had a lower mortality rate.[44] It is important to realize, however, that the t-PA studies enrolled a low-risk population by exclusion of elderly patients and those with cardiogenic shock, patients who were included in many of the streptokinase trials. Although it is difficult to compare trials that have different entry criteria and different patient populations and ancillary treatments, these data were all that were available until recently. Furthermore, since the time of eligibility varied from 4 hours to 24 hours among the early trials, analysis of mortality differences within the first 6 hours of infarction would provide a more useful comparison. In light of the differences in control group mortality rate between the various studies, ranging from 4% to 13%, it is also important to consider both the number of lives saved as well as the percent reduction in mortality. For example, the Anglo-Scandinavian Study of Early Thrombolysis (ASSET) demonstrated a reduction in mortality rate from 3% to 1.6% (a 50% reduction) in patients treated with t-PA in the setting of a normal ECG. In the APSAC Interventional Mortality Study (AIMS) trial, the 30-day mortality rate was 12.2% in the placebo group but only 6.4% in the APSAC group, a 47% reduction. In either case, the reduction in mortality rate was 50%. However, only 1 life was saved in the first example as compared with six lives being saved per 100 patients treated in the second example.

As demonstrated in Table 36–4, three thrombolytic agents (streptokinase, t-PA, and APSAC) have been shown to reduce mortality when compared with placebo. All agents appear to reduce the mortality rate by 30% (or save 3 lives per 100 patients treated) when administered within the first 3 hours of chest pain onset. When administered to 100 patients who present between 3 and 6 hours of chest pain onset, approximately 2 lives will be saved (a 20% reduction in mortality rate). At first glance, APSAC appears to be far superior at

TABLE 36–4.

Mortality Reduction Based on Thrombolytic Drug and Time to Treatment

| Time to Treatment | Mortality (%) | | %Reduction | No. of Lives Saved |
	Treated	Control		
0–3 hr				
Streptokinase[5, 8]	526/6,350 (8.3)	741/6,371 (11.6)	28	3.3
t-PA*[6, 45]	87/1,171 (7.4)	124/1,186 (10.5)	30	3.1
APSAC*[7]	18/334 (5.4)	30/326 (9.2)	41	3.8
3–6 hr				
Streptokinase[5, 8]	524/5,268 (9.9)	639/5,161 (12.4)	20	2.5
t-PA (3–5 hr)[6, 45]	111/1,680 (6.6)	141/1,647 (8.6)	23	2.0
APSAC[7]	14/168 (8.3)	31/176 (17.6)	53	9.3

*t-PA = tissue-type plasminogen activator (Activase); APSAC = anisoylated plasminogen streptokinase activator complex (Eminase).

achieving a mortality reduction (41% and 53% during hours 0 to 3 and 3 to 6, respectively). It must be kept in mind, however, that the AIMS trial was prematurely terminated in light of the large difference in survival at the interim analysis.[7] Therefore, the estimate of reduction in mortality may be exaggerated. Furthermore, the small patient numbers in the AIMS trial make the 95% confidence intervals quite wide, and one must conclude that the reduction in mortality is quite similar among all three thrombolytic agents. Most recently, direct comparisons incorporating nearly 70,000 patients demonstrated mortality to be virtually identical in patients treated with the available thrombolytic agent.[42, 46, 47]

The GISSI-2[42] plus its international extension[46] was a multicenter, randomized 2 × 2 factorial design that randomized 20,891 patients to t-PA vs. streptokinase, with a second randomization to subcutaneous heparin, 12,500 units twice daily started at hour 12, vs. no heparin (Table 36–5). As demonstrated in Table 36–6, there was no difference in mortality rates between t-PA– and streptokinase-treated patients (8.9% vs. 8.5%, respectively; not significant). Major cardiac events including reinfarction, congestive heart failure, and progression to cardiogenic shock were similar between t-PA– and streptokinase-treated groups. As expected,

hypotension and allergic reactions occurred more frequently after streptokinase therapy. Although t-PA was associated with a significantly higher incidence of stroke as compared with streptokinase (1.3% vs 1.0%), some attributed this to an "inadequate" heparin regimen that may have resulted in more embolic strokes.

These results, however, were confirmed in the ISIS-3 trial.[47] This was a multicenter randomized double-blind trial in which 46,092 patients with "clear" indications for thrombolytics were randomized to t-PA, streptokinase, or APSAC, with a second randomization to subcutaneous heparin, 12,500 units twice daily started at hour 4, or no heparin. Patients with uncertain indication were randomized to fibrinolytic vs. placebo therapy. There was no evidence of any difference in mortality between streptokinase, t-PA, and APSAC, either overall or in the subgroup with ST segment elevation randomized less than 6 hours from symptom onset. Disturbingly, t-PA was again associated with a higher incidence of stroke when compared with streptokinase (1.5% vs. 1.1%, $P = .001$), which appeared to be due to an increased rate of probable cerebral hemorrhage (0.7% vs. 0.3%; $P = 0001$).

Therefore, despite randomization of nearly 70,000 patients, there is no good evidence of any difference in

TABLE 36–5.

Mortality Trials Directly Comparing Thrombolytics: Protocols

Study	N	Time	Lytics*	Heparin	Adjunctive Therapy
International Study[42, 46]	20,891 (12,490 from GISSI-2)	0–6 hr	SK vs. t-PA	12,500 units SC b.i.d. started at 12 hr vs. no heparin	Aspirin, 325 mg; IV atenolol
ISIS-3[47]	46,000	0–24 hr	SK vs. t-PA vs. APSAC	12,500 units SC b.i.d. started at 4 hr vs no heparin	Aspirin, 160 mg; β-blockade

*SK = streptokinase; t-PA = tissue-type plasminogen activator; APSAC = anisoylated plasminogen streptokinase activator complex.

TABLE 36–6.
Mortality Trails Directly Comparing Thrombolytics: Results

| Result | International (GISSI-2[46]) | | ISIS-3[4] | | |
	SK*	t-PA*	SK	t-PA	APSAC*
Mortality	8.5	8.9	10.5	10.3	10.6
Reinfarction	3.0	2.6	3.6	3.1†	3.8
Stroke	1.0	1.3†	1.1†	1.5	1.4
All bleeds	3.9	5.0	4.6	5.3	5.6
Transfusions	0.9	0.6†	0.9	0.9	1.0
Hypotension	4.4	2.0†	6.8	4.3†	7.2
Allergy	1.7	0.2†			

*SK = streptokinase; t-PA = tissue-type plasminogen activator; APSAC = anisoylated plasminogen streptokinase
  activator complex.
†$P < .05$.

early mortality between streptokinase, t-PA, and AP-SAC. In addition, streptokinase appears to be safer than t-PA or APSAC since the rates of stroke and cerebral hemorrhage are significantly lower. The ISIS -3 investigators concluded that U.S. physicians began to use streptokinase routinely instead of t-PA, this might avoid hundreds of strokes a year and save more than $100 million a year.[48]

WHAT IS THE BEST DRUG, DOSE, AND HEPARIN REGIMEN

The major criticism of the GISSI-2 and ISIS-3 trials has been the use of high-dose subcutaneous heparin rather than intravenous heparin. Intravenous heparin appears to be superior to placebo at maintaining infarct vessel patency after t-PA[49–51] but whether it is superior to subcutaneous heparin is unknown. It is clear that subcutaneous heparin increases the risk of serious bleeding complications, including intracranial hemorrhage.[42, 46, 47] Furthermore, 10% of patients enrolled in the ISIS-3 trial received intravenous heparin per physician discretion, and heparin was associated with a doubling of the stroke rate.[47] Therefore, since t-PA is associated with a greater rate of cerebral hemorrhage than streptokinase is, a more aggressive heparin regimen may further aggravate serious bleeding complications.

Additionally, Genentech, Inc., the producer of Activase, has stated that the ISIS-3 results may not be valid due to the use of Burroughs Wellcome's version of t-PA (Duteplase) rather than Activase. However, since Genentech won the patent suit by claiming that the two drugs were "equivalent," this argument does not seem plausible.

To address these issues and determine whether new lytic regimens designed to maximize patency will fur-ther reduce mortality, a large international thrombolytic mortality trial entitled Global Utilization of Streptokinase and Tissue Plasminogen Activator (t-PA) for Occluded Coronary Arteries (GUSTO) was recently initiated. The GUSTO trial will enroll patients of any age who present within 6 hours of chest pain onset with ST segment elevation in two or more ECG leads. Aspirin, 160 mg, will be administered to all patients, as will intravenous β-blockers if no contraindications exist. Patients will be randomized to one of four thrombolytic strategies: intravenous herparin plus "front-loaded" t-PA, intravenous heparin plus combination t-PA/streptokinase, intravenous heparin plus streptokinase, or subcutaneous heparin plus streptokinase. To determine rates of infarct vessel patency and reocclusion an angiographic substudy involving 2,400 patients will be conducted. Patients will be randomly assigned to four groups: no early catheterization, catheterization at 90 minutes, catheterization at 3 hours, or catheterization at 24 hours. All patients in this substudy will undergo catheterization at 7 days. The target enrollment for the overall study will be 40,000 patients to determine an absolute mortality rate difference of 1% between treatment groups. It is anticipated that 1.5 to 2 years will be required for completion of the trial.

Choice of a Thrombolytic Drug

There appears to be few scientific data to advocate one thrombolytic drug over another when considering sustained patency, left ventricular function, or mortality. Furthermore, both the GISSI-2 and ISIS-3 trials have documented that streptokinase produces comparable survival with fewer strokes and less expense than t-PA. Although the appropriate dose and route of administration of heparin remains controversial, it is difficult to justify the use of agents that are 10 to 20 times more costly than streptokinase on the speculation that they *may* be better. Therefore, until proved otherwise, strep-tokinase has to be considered the "gold standard" in the management of acute MI.

Acknowledgment

The author extends appreciation to Phyllis McKinney for manuscript preparation.

REFERENCES

1. European Cooperative Study Group: Streptokinase in acute myocardial infarction. *N Engl J Med* 1979; 301:797–802.
2. Kennedy JW, Ritchie JL, Davis KB, et al: Western Washington randomized trial of intracoronary streptokinase in acute myocardial infarction. *N Engl J Med* 1983; 309:1477–1482.
3. Simoons ML, Serryts PW, van den Brand M, et al: Early thrombolysis in acute myocardial infarction: Limitation of infarct size and improved survival. *J Am Coll Cardiol* 1986; 7:717–728.
4. Schroder R, Neuhaus K-L, Leizorovica A, et al: A prospective placebo-controlled double-blind multicenter trial of intravenous streptokinase in acute myocardial infarction (ISAM): Long-term mortality and morbidity. *J Am Coll Cardiol* 1987; 9:197–203.
5. Gruppo Italiana per lo Studio della Streptochinasi nell'Infarcto Miocardico (GISSI): Effectiveness of intravenous thrombolytic treatment in acute myocardial infarction. *Lancet* 1986; 1:349–360.
6. Wilcox RB, Olsson CG, Skene AM, et al: Trial of tissue plasminogen activator for mortality reduction in acute myocardial infarction. *Lancet* 1988; 1:525–530.
7. AIMS Trial Study Group: Effect of intravenous APSAC on mortality after acute myocardial infarction: Preliminary report of a placebo-controlled clinical trial. *Lancet* 1988; 1:545–549.
8. ISIS-2 (Second International Study of Infarct Survival) Collaborative Group: Randomised trial of intravenous streptokinase, oral aspirin, both, or neither among 17,187 cases of suspected acute myocardial infarction: ISIS-2. *Lancet* 1988; 2:349–360.
9. Grines CL, DeMaria AN: Optimal utilization of thrombolytic therapy for acute myocardial infarction: Concepts and controversies. *J Am Coll Cardiol* 1990; 16:223–231.
'10. Bates ER: Reperfusion therapy in inferior myocardial infarction. *J Am Coll Cardiol* 1988; 12(suppl A):44–51.
11. MacDonnel AH, Grines CL: Absence of ST elevation during myocardial infarction identifies a patient population with advanced age and increased need for revascularization (abstract). *J Am Coll Cardiol* 1991; 17:45.
12. Yusuf S, Collins R, Peto R, et al: Intravenous and intracoronary fibrinolytic therapy in acute myocardial infarction: Overview of results on mortality, reinfarction and side-effects from 33 randomized controlled trials. *Eur Heart J* 1985; 6:556–585.
13. Paolasso E: EMERAS Trial: Results and discussion. Presented at the American College of Cardiology 40th Annual Scientific Session, March 1991.
14. Peto R: Which patients to treat with fibrinolysis: Overview of ISIS-3, EMERAS, et al. Presented at the American College of Cardiology 40th Annual Scientific Session, March 1991.
15. Califf RM, Topol EJ, Kereiakes DJ, et al: Cardiac resuscitation should not be a contraindication to thrombolytic therapy for myocardial infarction (abstract). *Circulation* 1988; 78(suppl H2):–127.
16. Sherry S: Appraisal of various thrombolytic agents in the treatment of acute myocardial infarction. *Am J Med* 1987; 83(suppl 2A):31–46.
17. Larrieu MJ: Comparative effects of fibrinogen degradation products D and E on coagulation. *Br J Haematol* 1973; 72:719.
18. Thorsen LI, Brossad F, Gogstad G, et al: Competitions between fibrinogen with its degradation products for interactions with the platelet-fibrinogen receptor. *Thromb Res* 1986; 44:611–623.
19. Wilson PA, McNicol GP, Douglas AS: Effect of fibrinogen degradation products on platelet aggregation. *J Clin Pathol* 1968; 21:141–153.
20. Neuhof H, Hey E, Glaser E, et al: Hemodynamic reactions induced by streptokinase therapy in patients with acute myocardial infarction. *Eur J Intensive Care Med* 1975; 1:27–30.
21. Rao AK, Pratt C, Berke A, et al: Thrombolysis in Myocardial Infarction (TIMI) trial — phase I: Hemorrhagic manifestations and changes in plasma fibrinogen and the fibrinolytic system in patients treated with recombinant tissue plasminogen activator and streptokinase. *J Am Coll Cardiol* 1988; 11:1–11.
22. Verstraete M, Bory M, Collen D, et al: Randomized trial of intravenous recombinant tissue-type plasminogen activator versus intravenous streptokinase in acute myocardial infarction. *Lancet* 1985; 1:842–847.
23. The TIMI Study Group: The Thrombolysis in Myocardial Infarction (TIMI) trial. *N Engl J Med* 1985; 312:932–936.
24. Topol E, Califf R, George B, et al: A randomized trial of immediate versus delayed elective angioplasty after intravenous tissue plasminogen activator in acute myocardial infarction. *N Engl J Med* 1987; 317:581–588.
25. Topol E, Moois D, Smalling R, et al: A multicenter, randomized, placebo-controlled trial of a new form of intravenous recombinant tissue-type plasminogen activator (Activase) in acute myocardial infarction. *J Am Coll Cardiol* 1987; 9:1205–1213.
26. Verstraete M, Arnold A, Brower R, et al: Acute coronary thrombolysis with recombinant human tissue type plasminogen activator: Initial patency and influence of maintained infusion on reocclusion rate. *Am J Cardiol* 1987; 60:231–237.
27. Anderson JL: Reperfusion patency and reocclusion with anistreplase (APSAC) in acute myocardial infarction. *Am J Cardiol* 1990; 64:12–17.
28. Wall T, Phillips H, Stack R, et al: Results of high dose intravenous urokinase for acute myocardial infarction. *Am J Cardiol* 1990; 65:124–131.
29. Neuhaus KL, Tebbe U, Gottwik M, et al: Intravenous rt-PA and urokinase in acute myocardial infarction: Results of the German Activator Urokinase Study (GAUS). *J Am Coll Cardiol* 1988; 12:581–587.
30. Califf R, Topol E, Stack R, et al: Evaluation of combination thrombolytic therapy and timing of cardiac catheter-

ization in acute myocardial infarction – results of Thrombolysis and Angioplasty in Myocardial Infarction – Phase 5 (TAMI-5) randomized trial. *Circulation* 1991; 83:1543–1556.

31. Sherry S, Marder VJ: Streptokinase and recombinant tissue plasminogen activator (rt-PA) are equally effective in treating acute myocardial infarction. *Ann Intern Med* 1991; 114:417–423.

32. PRIMI Trial Study Group: Randomized double blind trial of recombinant prourokinase against streptokinase in acute myocardial infarction. *Lancet* 1989; 1:863–867.

33. Grines CL, Topol EJ, Bates ER, et al: Infarct vessel status after intravenous tissue plasminogen activator and acute coronary angioplasty: Prediction of clinical outcome. *Am Heart J* 1988; 115:1–7.

34. Chesebro HK, Knatterud G, Roberts R, et al: Thrombolysis in myocardial infarction (TIMI) trial, phase 1: Comparison between intravenous tissue plasminogen activator and intravenous streptokinase: Clinical findings through hospital discharge. *Circulation* 1987; 76:142–154.

35. White HD, Rivers JT, Maslowski AH, et al: Effects of intravenous streptokinase as compared with that of tissue plasminogen activator on left ventricular function after first myocardial infarction. *N Engl J Med* 1989; 320:817–821.

36. Magnani B, for the PAIMS Investigators: Plasminogen Activators Italian Multicenter Study (PAIMS): Comparison of intravenous recombinant single-chain human tissue-type plasminogen activator (rt-PA) with intravenous streptokinase in acute myocardial infarction. *J Am Coll Cardiol* 1989; 13:19–26.

37. Bassand JP, Cassagnes J, Machecourt J, et al: A multicenter, double-blind trial aimed at comparing the efficacy and safety of alteplase and anistreplase in acute myocardial infarction (abstract). *Circulation* 1990; 82(suppl 3):665.

38. Bassand JP et al, for the APSIM Study Investigators: Multicenter trial of intravenous anisoylated plasminogen streptokinase activator complex (APSAC) in acute myocardial infarction: Effect on infarct size and left ventricular function. *J Am Coll Cardiol* 1989; 13:988–997.

39. The Multicenter Postinfarction Research Group: Risk stratification and survival after myocardial infarction. *N Engl J Med* 1983; 309:331–336.

40. Sheehan FH: Measurement of left ventricular function as an end point in trials of thrombolytic therapy. *Coronary Artery Dis* 1990; 1:13–22.

41. Sheehan FH, Braunwald E, Canner P, et al: The effect of intravenous thrombolytic therapy on left ventricular function: A report on tissue-type plasminogen activator and streptokinase from the Thrombolysis in Myocardial Infarction (TIMI, phase 1) Trial. *Circulation* 1987; 75:817–829.

42. Gruppo Italiano per lo Studio della Streptochinasi nell'Infarto Miocardico: GISSI-2: A factorial randomised trial of alteplase versus streptokinase and heparin versus no heparin among 12,490 patients with acute myocardial infarction. *Lancet* 1990; 336:65–71.

43. Califf RM, Topol EJ, Gersh BJ: From myocardial salvage to patient salvage in acute myocardial infarction: The role of reperfusion therapy. *J Am Coll Cardiol* 1989; 14:1382–1388.

44. Tiefenbrunn AJ, Sobel BE: The impact of coronary thrombolysis on myocardial infarction. *Fibrinolysis* 1989; 3:1–15.

45. Van de Werf F, Arnold AER, European Cooperative Study Group for Recombinant Tissue Type Plasminogen Activator (rt-PA): Intravenous tissue plasminogen activator and size of infarct, left ventricular function and survival in acute myocardial infarction. *Br Med J* 1988; 297:1374–1379.

46. The International Study Group: In-hospital mortality and clinical course of 20,891 patients with suspected acute myocardial infarction randomized between alteplase and streptokinase with or without heparin. *Lancet* 1990; 336:71–75.

47. Third International Study of Infarct Survival Collaborative Group: ISIS-3: A randomised comparison of streptokinase vs tissue plasminogen activator vs antistreplase and of aspirin plus heparin vs aspirin alone among 41,299 cases of suspected acute myocardial infarction. *Lancet* 1992; 339:1815–1823.

48. ISIS press release: ISIS-3 results. March 2, 1991.

49. Hsia J, Hamilton WP, Kleiman N, et al: The Heparin-Aspirin Reperfusion Trial (HART): A randomized trial of heparin versus aspirin adjunctive to tissue plasminogen activator–induced thrombolysis in acute myocardial infarction. *N Engl J Med* 1990; 323:1433–1437.

50. Bleich SD, Nichols TC, Schumacher RR, et al: Effect of heparin on coronary arterial patency after thrombolysis with tissue plasminogen activator in acute myocardial infarction. *Am J Cardiol* 1990; 66:1412–1417.

51. DeBono DP, on behalf of the European Cooperative Study Group: The need for anticoagulation with heparin after rt-PA, an angiographic study of 650 patients treated with rt-PA with or without intravenous heparin. Presented at the European Congress of Cardiology, September 20, 1990, Stockholm.

Thrombolysis in Acute Myocardial Infarction in the Community Hospital

John H.K. Vogel, M.D.

Barry J. Coughlin, M.D.

Ramachandra K. Setty, M.D.

Rosa M. Avolio, R.N.

R. Bruce McFadden, M.D.

The major determinate of morbidity and mortality in coronary artery disease is the status of myocardial function.[1] Thus the thrust of our therapy has been directed toward maintenance of normal ventricular function and prevention of loss of heart muscle.[1] In acute myocardial infarction (MI), coronary thrombolysis occurs spontaneously in approximately 20% of patients[2, 3] in the early hours after the event, and studies have shown that lytic agents may produce lysis in an additional 40% to 70% of patients. In 1976 Chazov and associates[4] reported successful thrombolysis and in 1978 Rentrop and associates[5] reported their encouraging experience with intracoronary streptokinase. The combination of thrombolytic therapy and spontaneous thrombolysis has achieved an early reperfusion rate of 70% to 90%.[6] However, it is clear that "time means muscle," and strategies that have evolved relate to reducing the time from acute occlusion to thrombolysis. If thrombolysis occurs within 30 minutes of the acute event, there is a high salvage rate of cardiac muscle; if it occurs within 90 minutes of the event, substantial benefits have been demonstrated, but after 3 hours the advantage diminishes.[7-9]

In 1981 and 1983 Schroder and associates[10, 11] reported on the use of early, short-time intravenous streptokinase for thrombolysis in acute MI. It was their thesis that if the majority of people with acute MI were to benefit by thrombolysis it would have to be early, by the intravenous route. They reported patency of the infarct-related artery in more than 80% of their patients and emphasized the importance of an early peaking of the MB fraction of creatine kinase (CK-MB) as an indicator of early reperfusion. In view of the promising nature of their results, in 1981 we initiated an intravenous streptokinase protocol in Goleta Valley Community Hospital in Santa Barbara, California, Marion Hospital in Santa Maria, California, and Lompoc Hospital in Lompoc, California. Our experience now extends beyond 10 years' time. With the release of tissue-type plasminogen activator (t-PA) in 1987, a protocol was developed for its use also.

INDICATIONS FOR THROMBOLYSIS

All patients with acute MI are candidates for intravenous thrombolytic therapy if seen less than 6 hours after the onset of the episode (longer than 6 hours if severe, continuing pain and/or ischemia is evident; unless you see the development of acute ECG changes, you cannot be certain what the time delay has been) and they have no known potential bleeding problems. We have administered intravenous streptokinase in patients over 75 years of age since it is evident that these people are at great risk and may benefit the most[12] (see also Chapter

36). If the patient is going *immediately* to the catheterization laboratory, 10,000 units of intravenous heparin and 0.3 g of oral acetysalicylic acid (ASA) are administered. We have utilized intravenous thrombolysis for preinfarction angina and acute, delayed rethrombosis following angioplasty, as well as intracoronary lytic agents for coronary artery thrombosis during cardiac catheterization and in patients with occlusion during angioplasty. *Consider all myocardial infarctions to be dangerous!*

Potential bleeding problems that would serve as a contraindication include active internal bleeding, recent surgery or major trauma, active ulcer disease, recent puncture of noncompressible vessels, *severe* uncontrolled systemic hypertension, known bleeding diathesis, history of recent cerebrovascular accident (CVA) (2 months), and recent intracranial surgery or known tumor. In our institutions if cardiopulmonary resuscitation has been of short duration with no obvious trauma, it is not considered a contraindication.[13]

PROCEDURE

Upon entering the emergency room the patient is seen immediately by the emergency room physician, and if the electrocardiogram (ECG) indicates the presence of acute MI the question is asked whether the patient is a candidate for thrombolytic therapy. Consultation is obtained immediately with the cardiologist. Time to treatment is shortened by developing a protocol allowing the emergency room physician to begin therapy, within 30 minutes if possible. Therapy should *not* be delayed waiting for a cardiologist. A FAX machine is *invaluable* for receiving the ECG! If the answer is yes, intravenous streptokinase, t-PA, or both are started. If the catheterization laboratory is immediately available, we (Goleta Valley Community Hospital) may consider the possibility of immediate study with percutaneous transluminal coronary angioplasty (PTCA) in the patient with a major MI and/or shock or in those ineligible for lytic therapy; 10,000 units of heparin, IV, and .3 g of ASA, PO, are given on the way to the lab. Laser thrombolysis, now under clinical evaluation, may prove useful[15] (see Chapter 26). Catheterization should be performed by an experienced angiographer expert in entering and caring for arteries. When the patient is seen in a hospital without a laboratory (Marion Hospital, Lompoc Hospital), thrombolytic therapy is initiated immediately and transport considered if there is evidence of early arterial opening or the patient remains unstable. Our hospital heliport facilitates immediate transport by helicopter. If the patient is in a stable condition, we prefer to wait 24 to 48 hours before study or transport. This has been the protocol followed in our

TABLE 37–1.

Protocol for Intravenous Streptokinase Therapy for Acute Myocardial Infarctions

1. *Handle the patient gently!*
2. Start two IV lines—one with an 18-gauge catheter with a 3-way stopcock to draw blood.
3. Obtain the following as soon as possible (preferably from the stopcock of the 18-gauge IV catheter) PTT, CBC, PT, cardiac enzymes, chemistry panel, platelet count, fibrinogen.
4. Premedication:
    Methylprednisolone, 250 mg IV
    Heparin, 5000 units IV
    ASA 0.3 g po
    Individualize β-blockers, calcium channel blockers, IV nitroglycerine, sedation, diuretics, digoxin, antiarrythmics, afterload reduction, H_2 blockers, warfarin (Coumadin)
5. Nitroglycerine, 1/150g subliqually as required for chest pain.
6. Check the patient for venous or arterial puncture sites. All puncture sites should have pressure dressings applied to them.
7. Begin infusion via an 18-gauge IV catheter, 1.5 million units SK in 50–100 cc normal saline to infuse over 30 min via IMED pump. Follow this infusion with 500 cc D_5W with 10,000 units heparin at 1,000 units/hr (50 cc/hr via IMED).
8. ECG before infusion of SK is begun, then 1 hr after infusion, or if sudden change in pain; monitor ST segment changes.
9. Chest x-ray.
10. Foley catheter as required; *handle gently!*
11. PTT q 2–4 h to start 2 hr after completion of SK infusion (attempt to draw these and any other laboratory work from the stopcock of the IV catheter). Call results to M.D. each time.
12. CPK and CPK-MB q2hr × 24 to start from completion of SK infusion.
13. Monitor patient's vital signs and quality of hemostasis, and document every 15 min until SK infusion completed or longer if clinically indicated.
14. Avoid excessive venipunctures and arterial punctures before start of SK and at least 24 hr after completion of infusion. *No IM injections.*
15. Two-dimensional echocardiogram whenever feasible (not to interfere with the infusion of SK).

institutions over the past 10 years (see Table 37–1). Streptokinase, 1.5 million units, is administered over a 30-minute period. If hypotension occurs, the rate is slowed, feet are elevated, and volume given. As noted, .3 g ASA, PO, is given and 5000 units of heparin is administered intravenously at the beginning and a drip started at a rate of 1,000 units/hr after streptokinase has been administered. Steroids are administered and depending on the clinical situation, other adjunctive therapy may be utilized. There is evidence to suggest that the use of calcium channel blockers and perhaps β-blockers widen the window of opportunity to preserve muscle with early reopening and reduce mortality.[14, 15, 15a] However, calcium channel blockers may be detrimental in patients with significant left ventricular dysfunction. Initially we establish two intravenous lines. Most important is to be extremely gentle with the patient, both in moving the patient and with any subsequent interventions. Intramuscular medicines are contraindicated, and if intravenous punctures are performed, pressure bandages should be applied. Arterial sticks are to be avoided. Carelessness in this regard leads to the highest number of complications with thrombolytic therapy. Thus the *nurse* assumes an extremely important role in management of the patient. We do not delay therapy to obtain an echocardiogram. The CK-MB fractions are determined at 2-hour intervals for 24 hours. The partial thromboplastin time (PTT) is followed closely after 2 to 4 hours. We attempt to maintain the PTT at 80 seconds. Time is of the essence, and none of the tests should delay the immediate commencement of thrombolytic therapy. The t-PA protocol utilized since November 1987 is similar to that used for streptokinase and is outlined in Table 37–2. If there is no evidence of reperfusion within 30 minutes of completion of the streptokinase infusion or there is evidence of reocclusion, 20 mg of t-PA may be given by intravenous push

(IVP). Also, in the patient with a large MI this may be done initially.

RESULTS

From November 1981 to January 1990, 174 patients were treated with streptokinase, including 140 men with an average age of 57 (range, 31 to 79 years) and 34 women with an average age of 64 (range, 43 to 77 years). There were 95 inferior wall MIs and 79 anterior wall MIs. The regional distribution of patients is seen in Figure 37–1.

The clinical criteria for luminal opening included an early peaking of the CK-MB fraction within 12 hours, sudden relief of pain in the early minutes (on the average 30 to 60 minutes after starting thrombolytic therapy), sudden emergence of arrhythmias or a change in the arrhythmia background accompanied by resolution of ST segment changes, advanced atrioventricular (AV) block, or cardiogenic shock. Serial echocardiograms are useful, but since these changes occur over a period of several days, they are of little help in indicating early reperfusion. A most useful sign of early reperfusion is sudden relief of pain followed by ventricular arrhythmias. This is not an uncommon event. *Determining reperfusion is best done by staying at or near the bedside and following the patient's signs and symptoms closely.* Automated analysis of ST segments and rapid sequential enzyme analysis may be useful. Representative CK-MB curves are shown in Figure 37–2. The flat curve has been seen in approximately 3% of patients and is associated with early reperfusion and a small or no infarction. The delayed peaking at approximately 20 hours is associated with a failure to reperfuse. Two types of early peaking curves are shown, one with a fairly rapid washout indicating excellent blood flow and early reperfusion

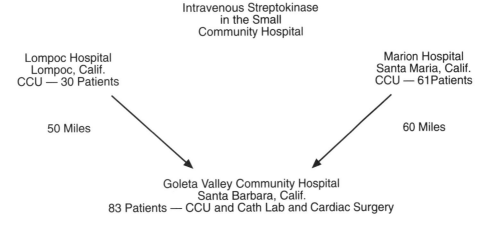

FIG 37–1.
Regional distribution of patients referred to Goleta Valley Community Hospital, including the hospitals involved, the number of patients referred, and the distance. *CCU* = coronary care unit.

TABLE 37–2.

Protocol for Intravenous t-PA Therapy for Acute Myocardial Infarction

1. *Handle the patient gently!*
2. Start two IV lines, one with an 18-gauge catheter with a 3-way stopcock to draw blood.
3. Obtain the following as soon as possible (preferably from the stopcock of the 18-gauge IV catheter): PTT, CBC, PT, cardiac enzymes, chemistry panel, platelet count, fibrinogen.
4. Premedication:
    Heparin, 5000 units by IV push
    ASA, 0.3 g po
    Individualize β-blockers, calcium channel blockers, IV nitroglycerin, sedation, diuretics, digoxin, antiarrhythmics, afterload reduction, H_2 blockers, and warfarin (Coumadin).
5. Check the patient for venous or arterial puncture sites. All puncture sites should have pressure dressings.
6. Begin t-PA.
    10 mg t-PA by IV push.
    Follow with 1 mg/kg (minus the 10 mg for IV push) to infuse over 60 min. Maximum dose, 90 mg first hour.[16, 17]
    Then begin t-PA infusion, 0.5 mg/kg over period of 1 hr.
    Maximum dose, 100 mg t-PA.
7. After the first hour of t-PA begin infusion of 500 cc D_5W with 10,000 units heparin at 1000 units/hr (50 cc/hr via IMED).
8. ECG before infusion of t-PA and 1 hr after infusion or if sudden change in pain, and monitor ST segment changes.
9. Foley catheter as needed—Handle gently!
10. PTT q 2–4 hr to start 2 hr after completion of t-PA infusion (attempt to draw these and any other laboratory work from the stopcock of the IV catheter). Call results to M.D. each time.
11. Chest x-ray.
12. CPK and CPK-MB q2h × 24 hr to start after first hour of t-PA infusion.
13. Nitroglycerine, 1/150 g sublingually as needed for chest pain.
14. Check vital signs every 15 min until infusion completed.
15. Avoid venous punctures and arterial punctures; no IM injections!
16. Two-dimensional echocardiogram whenever feasible. (Not to interfere with the infusion of TPA.)

and a somewhat flat curve generally associated with a very tight residual lesion and slow blood flow. In the protocol 157 patients demonstrated clinical signs of early reperfusion. The average time from initiation of streptokinase therapy to their peak CK-MB concentration was 7¾ ± 3¾ hours, with a range of 2 to 15 hours. Seventeen patients did not have clinical luminal opening and their average streptokinase peak CK-MB time was 20 ± 2 hours with a range of 12 to 24 hours. This correlated nicely with the report of Schroder and associates[11] wherein the time to peak CK-MB levels after the start of streptokinase infusion was less than 14 hours in all cases with early reperfusion and more than 16 hours in those patients who remained occluded.

The average time from the onset of pain to arriving in the emergency room in our experience was 83 minutes, and the time from arrival to the emergency room to beginning streptokinase therapy averaged 65 minutes. Thirty-five percent of the patients were treated within 30 minutes or less after arrival in the emergency room. The average time from the onset of pain to receiving streptokinase in those patients who had early reperfusion averaged 115 ± 90 minutes with a range of 15 to

300 minutes, whereas in those patients who remained occluded the average time to treatment was 228 ± 47 minutes with a range of 75 to 420 minutes. All patients treated within 60 minutes of the onset of their pain were open clinically. The dosage of streptokinase was increased from 250,000 units in 1 patient to 1.5 million units in the last 162 patients.

Documented arrhythmias of ventricular origin were common after streptokinase therapy (Table 37–3).

TABLE 37–3.

Arrhythmias After Streptokinase Therapy

Event	Pre-SK	Post-SK
Premature ventricular contraction	23*	55
Ventricular fibrillation	15	11
Complete heart block	10	5
Sinus bradycardia	6	4
Junctional rhythm	0	2
Wenckebach phenomenon	0	3
Ventricular tachycardia	1	7

*No. of patients.

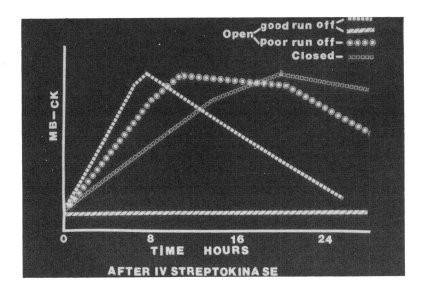

FIG 37–2.
A family of curves illustrating typical disease courses are shown. The flat curve represents a typical curve for those patients undergoing early reperfusion with no significant infarction. The late-peaking curve is typical of those patients who did not have early reperfusion. Two curves are shown with early peaking, one showing a rapid runoff that is typical of those patients who have early luminal opening and good runoff and a slow curve typical of those who have luminal opening but poor runoff.

Complete heart block resolved in nine patients after streptokinase therapy. The occurrence of ventricular fibrillation after streptokinase was an excellent indicator of early reperfusion since all those patients had luminal opening at catheterization. It is our thought that ventricular tachycardia and ventricular fibrillation, occurring before treatment, may represent intermittent reperfusion. Spontaneous reperfusion may account for late-onset ventricular fibrillation since it has been shown that there is continued spontaneous luminal opening several hours after the acute event.[2] Again, if one remains at the patient's bedside during thrombolytic therapy, the changes in pain, arrhythmias, ST segments, and hemodynamic status are generally obvious with reperfu-

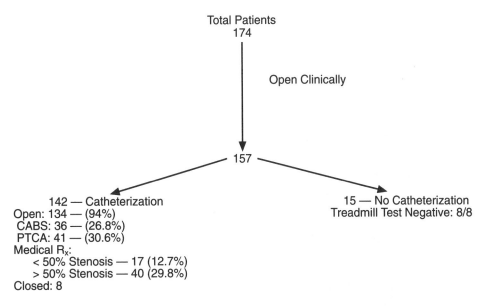

FIG 37–3.
Illustration of the number of patients who had luminal opening and underwent catheterization and the subsequent results. *CABS* = coronary artery bypass surgery; *PTCA* = percutaneous transluminal coronary angioplasty.

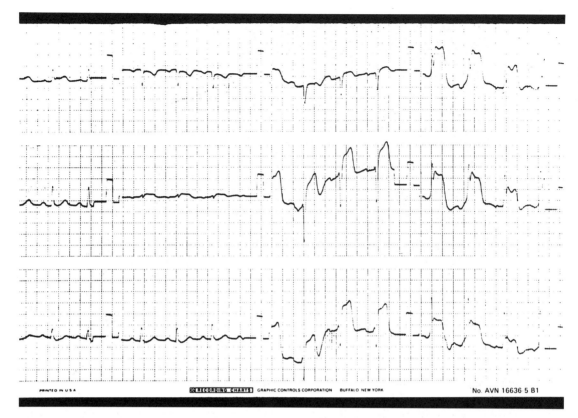

FIG 37–4.
Control ECG immediately preceding intravenous streptokinase administration shows acute anterior wall MI.

sion. Transient hypotension is not uncommon and usually responds to positioning the legs up and increased fluids.

As shown in Figure 37–3, of the 157 patients open clinically, 142 underwent cardiac catheterization. The relationship of time to treatment with streptokinase and time to study and the percentage of patients studied are shown in Table 37–4. During the first 2 years of our experience not all patients underwent catheterization. If they were stable following early reperfusion, they were treated conservatively. However, it became apparent that it was not clear what the potential dangers were after early reperfusion. Thus in order to effectively indi-

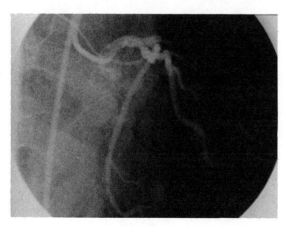

FIG 37–5.
Selective RAO coronary artery cineangiogram showing occlusion of the LAD coronary artery.

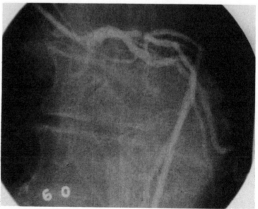

FIG 37–6.
RAO cineangiogram showing perfusion of the LAD coronary artery with residual proximal obstruction 60 minutes after intracoronary streptokinase infusion.

TABLE 37–4.
Time to Treatment With Intravenous Streptokinase and Percentage of Patients Studied

Time to Treatment	Patients Open Clinically (%)	Percentage of Total Patients
0–2 hr	96	63
2–3 hr	86	20
3–4 hr	83	6
4 hr	50	11

Patients	Patients Studied (%)	Patients Studied 1–48 hr After Therapy (%)
0–40	55	50
41–80	90	47
81–120	100	58
121–174	92	74

vidualize our treatment of the patient, we though it important to assess the coronary anatomy. Since 1983 virtually all patients with evidence of early reperfusion have undergone catheterization prior to discharge. As noted, 134 of the 142 patients (94%) studied had luminal opening. Subsequently, 36 of these patients under-

went coronary artery bypass surgery, and 41 patients were treated by PTCA. The remainder of the patients have been treated medically. Of note is that 17 (12%) of the patients had less than 50% stenosis. These patients have remained stable. Of the 15 patients who did not undergo catheterization, the majority had negative treadmill stress tests. In those that were open clinically but closed at catheterization (8 patients), heparin had not been administered to 3 patients and was inadequate or discontinued early in the remainder. Late reclosure was generally evident clinically. The early reclosure rate in our experience was approximately 5%.

Of the 17 patients who were closed clinically, 11 underwent catheterization. All were closed. One patient had luminal opening with intracoronary streptokinase, and another patient had luminal opening after PTCA.

CASE EXAMPLES

In Figure 37–4 is shown the ECG from our first patient, a 65-year-old man who received intravenous streptokinase, 500,000 units, at 2 hours. The control

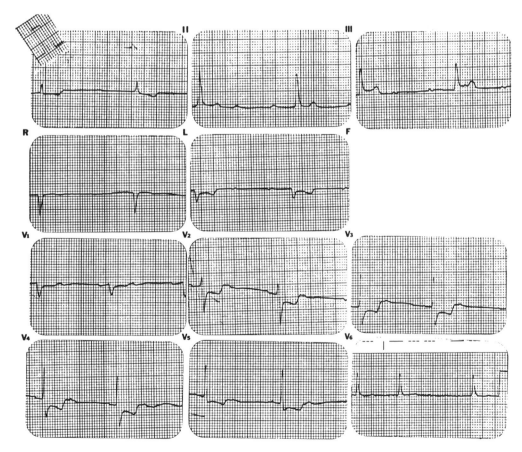

FIG 37–7.
Control ECG obtained immediately before streptokinase therapy shows acute inferior wall MI and complete heart block.

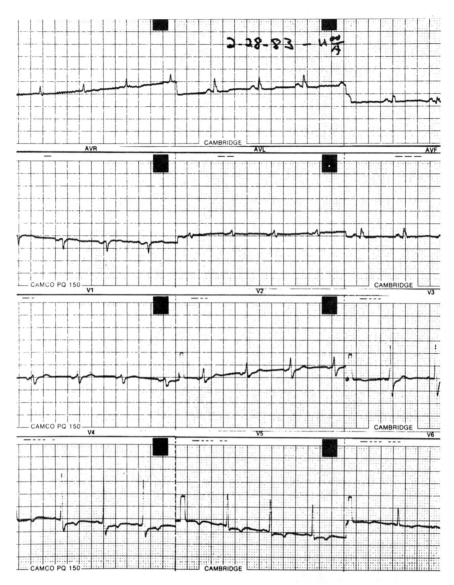

FIG 37–8.
ECG obtained immediately following intravenous streptokinase administration shows significant normalization and return of sinus rhythm.

tracing shows acute anterior wall MI. When luminal opening had not occurred within 20 minutes, he was taken to the catheterization laboratory (streptokinase running) where the right anterior oblique (RAO) angiogram showed an occluded left anterior descending (LAD) coronary artery (Fig 37–5), that spontaneously opened within minutes with no further therapy. This was associated with spontaneous ventricular fibrillation, readily converted with shock treatment. The vessel then reoccluded, and intracoronary streptokinase was administered with subsequent luminal reopening in 15 minutes. In Figure 37–6 is shown the cineangiogram at 60 minutes, which demonstrates the open LAD coronary

artery. An 80% diameter stenosis appears to be present. No collaterals were present. No further intervention was performed. This patient remained asymptomatic with a negative maximal treadmill stress test 8 years later. Sudden death occurred in the ninth year.

In Figure 37–7 is shown the ECG from a 59-year-old man with an acute inferior wall MI complicated by hypotension and advanced AV block. One hour after the onset of pain he received 1.5 million units of intravenous streptokinase. Thirty minutes later there was spontaneous relief of pain, resolution of the AV block, and normalization of the blood pressure. The CK-MB fraction peaked at 8 hours. The ECG showed considerable resolution (Fig 37–8). Because of the patient's instability before early reperfusion, it was deemed reasonable to study him, and he was transferred from Lompoc Hospital to Goleta Valley Community Hospital for study the following morning. In Figure 37–9 can be seen a significant lesion in a large circumflex artery with a crater and clot, disease in the main left coronary artery, and involvement of the LAD coronary artery system. He subsequently underwent internal mammary artery (IMA) bypass into the LAD coronary artery and saphenous vein bypass into the circumflex artery. Figure 37–10 shows the inferior wall akinesis. ECG on discharge showed minor residual ST-T wave changes in the inferior and lateral leads (Fig 37–11). He remains asymptomatic with normal treadmill test results 8 years later.

In Figure 37–12 is shown the ECG from a 50-year-old man with acute anterior wall MI changes. He received 1.5 million units of intravenous streptokinase within 30 minutes of the onset of pain, with relief of pain within 30 minutes. His subsequent ECG showed normalization (Fig 37–13). Because he normalized but had an acute anterior wall MI in progress and no enzyme rise, it was deemed reasonable to study him. The study done the following morning revealed 80% diameter stenosis of the LAD coronary artery (Fig 37–14). Figure 37–15 represents diastolic and systolic frames from the left ventricular cineangiogram showing normal function. Because of continued rest angina and ventricular arrhythmias, revascularization was performed (IMA to LAD). The treadmill results remain negative after 7 years.

Another 46-year-old man with acute inferior wall MI received 1.5 million units of intravenous streptokinase within 90 minutes of the onset of pain. Resolution of chest pain and ventricular arrhythmias occurred at 30 minutes. A subsequent ECG showed near normalization of the ECG. Sixty-eight hours later he underwent study, and in Figure 37–16, biplane views show a 45% diame-

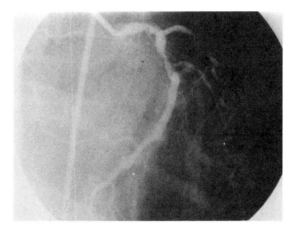
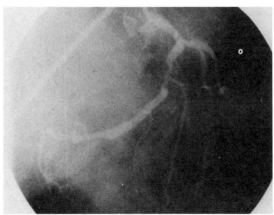

FIG 37–9.
Selective coronary cineangiograms show a significant lesion in the circumflex artery with involvement of the main left and LAD coronary arteries.

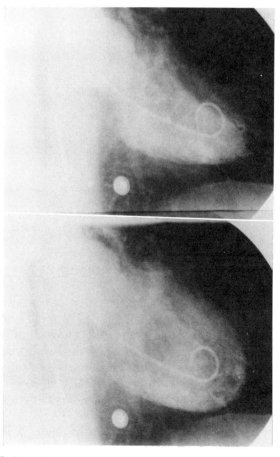

FIG 37–10.
Systolic and diastolic views of the left ventricular cineangiogram reveal inferior wall akinesis.

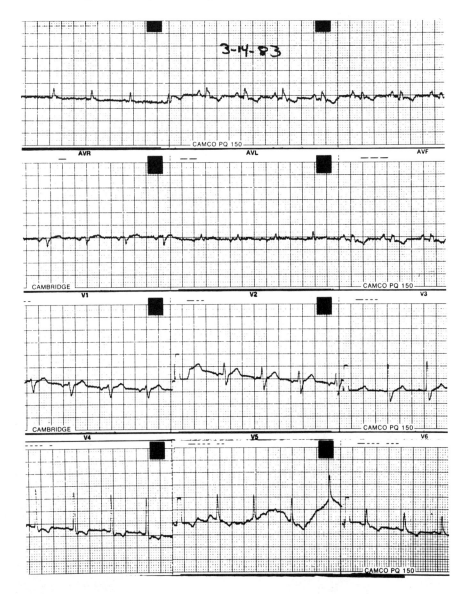

FIG 37–11.
ECG at discharge shows nonspecific residual ST-T wave changes and sinus rhythm.

ter stenosis of the right coronary artery. No collaterals were seen. The ventriculogram (Fig 37–17) shows slight akinesis of the inferior wall. The patient was treated medically and recently had a negative maximal exercise treadmill stress test. This case serves to emphasize how a vessel may have noncritical stenosis over a short period of time. Indeed, in the Thrombolysis and Angioplasty in Myocardial Infarction (TAMI) trial,[18] those patients directed to the elective "late" PTCA group had a 14% incidence of less than 50% stenosis on follow-up.

In Figure 37–18,A and B are shown serial strips from a 78-year-old man with marked ischemic lability. Because the patient was alternating between ST segment depression and elevation, as shown in the top two strips, he was given streptokinase. Approximately 15 minutes into the infusion, his pain intensified with recurrent ST segment elevation as shown on the fourth strip. At this point, intravenous nitroglycerin was administered, and the patient received 10 mg of nifedipine (Procardia) sublingually. Atropine was administered intravenously. The remainder of the streptokinase was infused within a few minutes. As the ST segments rose, blood pressure became unobtainable, and the patient was unresponsive. Within 2 minutes the ST segments began to come down, slightly oscillating as shown in the second and third panels and then tending to become negative at 5 minutes. At this point, the blood pressure returned to

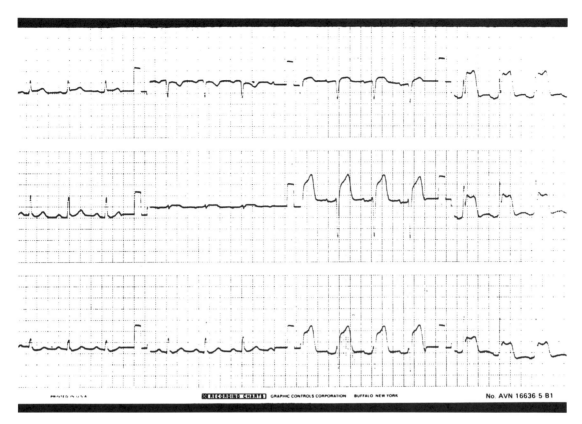

FIG 37–12.
Control ECG immediately before intravenous streptokinase infusion shows extensive anterior wall changes.

normal, the patient became alert, and his pain resolved. Figure 37–19 shows the ECG associated with severe pain and loss of blood pressure, and Figure 37–20 shows the subsequent tracing after the pain had resolved. This sequence suggests vasospasm plus clot as reported by Hackett and associates.[19] It was apparent that when occluded the patient could not survive and that a severe underlying lesion(s) was present. The CK-MB fraction peaked at 6 hours. Therefore the following morning he underwent study. As shown in Figure 37–21, there was near-total occlusion of a giant right coronary artery and 90% narrowing of the LAD coronary artery. Thus he underwent IMA-to-LAD coronary artery bypass and saphenous vein-to-right coronary artery bypass without complication. He was discharged 6 days later from the hospital. Treadmill stress test findings were negative 4 years postoperatively.

In Figure 37–22 is shown the ECG of a 66-year-old man with an acute anterior wall MI. He received intravenous streptokinase within 60 minutes of the onset of acute chest pain. Within 30 minutes of beginning the infusion there was resolution of pain and a burst of ventricular tachycardia. The subsequent ECG showed considerable normalization (Fig 37–23). The patient continued to have recurrent rest pain and ventricular arrhythmias and thus underwent study the following day after having been transported to Goleta Valley Community Hospital. The CK-MB fraction peaked at 8 hours. In Figure 37–24 is shown a high-grade lesion in the proximal segment of the LAD coronary artery. The gradient was 60 mm Hg. In Figure 37–25 is shown the result after PTCA: a widely patent vessel with no gradient. This patient remained asymptomatic for 1 year and then developed preinfarction syndrome. Studies showed a 90% stenosis of the circumflex artery and an old anterior wall infarction. The LAD coronary artery was widely patent. The ejection fraction was 20%. The circumflex artery supplied the only moving wall. Percutaneous cardiopulmonary-supported angioplasty was performed with an excellent result. Three months later restenosis developed in the circumflex artery, and he had successful bypass surgery with the left IMA to the circumflex.

Our overall results are summarized in Table 37–5. All patients have been followed at least 1 month and up to 96 months. At the time of the last follow-up, 164 of the 174 patients were known to be living, with a range of 1 month to 96 months. There were 5 hospital deaths.

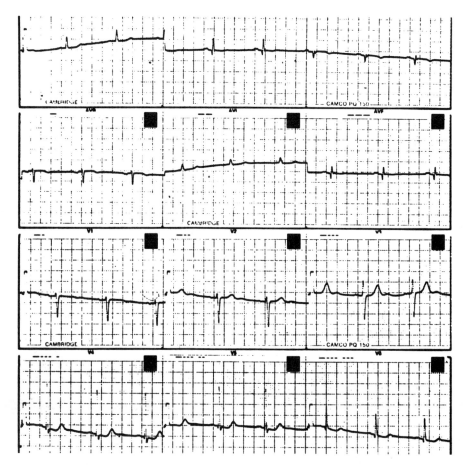

FIG 37–13.
ECG obtained immediately after the infusion of intravenous streptokinase shows normalization of the ECG.

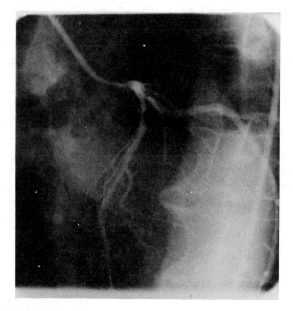

FIG 37–14.
Selective left anterior oblique (LAO) cineangiography reveals 80% diameter stenosis of the proximal segment of the LAD coronary artery.

Four major morbidity problems have resulted from arterial and venous intravenous lines. There were no cerebral bleeds. Nausea has been a common complaint, occurring in about 50% of patients, and transient hypotension is not uncommon. Clinically 157 out 174 patients (90%) had luminal opening, and at catheterization 134 of 142 patients (94%) had luminal opening.

MANAGEMENT AFTER THROMBOLYTIC THERAPY

Who should be catheterized after thrombolytic therapy? In our institutions nearly all patients receiving lytic therapy who have luminal opening clinically undergo study before discharge. Also, patients who remain unstable without early luminal opening undergo catheterization. Patients who remain stable but who do not have luminal opening are studied, depending on their clinical course, for example, recurrent angina and results of stress testing. *When to catheterize* depends on the clinical situation. Early study is considered within hours if the initial presentation was critical, for example, the patient

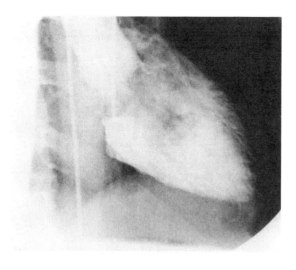

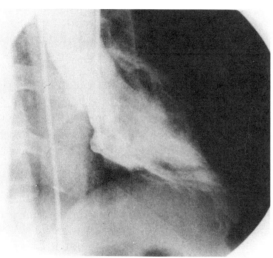

FIG 37–15.
Systolic and diastolic frames from the left ventricular cineangiogram show normal function.

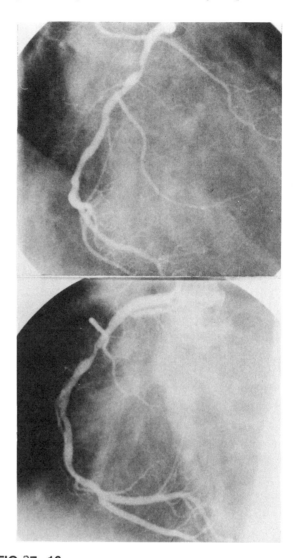

FIG 37–16.
Selective biplane coronary artery cineangiograms show 45% diameter stenosis of the proximal segment of the right coronary artery.

was in shock or had a complete heart block whose symptoms were then reversed with lytic therapy; early study is also feasible in the patient who has early reperfusion and no significant infarction, truly representing an opportunity to protect muscle, and in those patients with threatened extension. Study is delayed for a few days in those patients who had no complications or remain without complications but then have late recurrence of pain. This allows further "cleanup" to occur. This is the strategy that we have evolved over the past 10 years.

It is important to consider *all MIs to be dangerous.* When early reperfusion has been achieved, one does not know what might have happened, and we believe that it is important to ascertain what the coronary anatomy is for proper individualization of treatment (Figs 37–26 and 37–27).

DISCUSSION

The 10-year experience involving our three community hospitals has illustrated the effectiveness of intravenous thrombolytic therapy and the feasibility of initiating such therapy in the community hospital without a catheterization laboratory. The morbidity, mortality, and subsequent results in our patients are consistent with this approach. Our results show the importance of *early treatment* since all patients treated within 60 minutes of onset of their acute MI had clinical evidence of early reperfusion (see Table 37–4). Recently Topol and associates[20] have reported on their experience with the community hospital relationship and have noted excellent results. Although ours was not a randomized study, the occurrence of but five hospital deaths in our patients

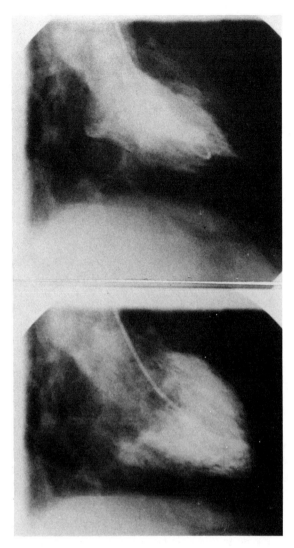

FIG 37–17.
Systolic and diastolic views of the left ventricular cineangiogram reveal minor akinesis of the inferior wall.

TABLE 37–5.
Results of Intravenous Streptokinase Therapy in 174 Patients With Myocardial Infarction

Living	164/174 at 1–96 mos
Mortality rate	
5 Hospital	2.8%
5 Late	2.8%
Morbidity	
1 Arm: compartment syndrome— hematoma	
1 Severe nosebleed	
1 Hematoma in arm (arterial stick)	
1 Hemoptysis	
Luminal opening clinically	157/174 (90%)
Luminal opening clinically and by catheterization	134/142 (94%)

indicates the usefulness of intravenous thrombolytic therapy. Similar results have been obtained by Hartman and associates (Table 37–6).[21] Table 37–7 presents the results from past trials. It is clear that with thrombolytic therapy, whether it consists of streptokinase, anisoylated plasminogen streptokinase activation complex (APSAC), or t-PA, mortality has decreased. In the Gruppo Italiano per lo Studio della Sopravivenza nell Infarto Miocardio (GISSI-2)[34] trial, results have been published that show no difference in mortality when t-PA was compared with streptokinase. This was a multicenter randomized trial involving 20,891 patients treated with t-PA vs. streptokinase with a second randomization to subcutaneous heparin, 12,500 units twice daily started at 12 hours vs. no heparin. There was no difference in mortality between t-PA– and streptokinase-treated patients,

8.9 % vs. 8.5%, respectively, nor in major cardiac events including cardiogenic shock, reinfarction, or congestive heart failure. Interestingly, in the original Thrombolysis in Myocardial Infarction (TIMI-1) trial in which the average time to treatment was nearly 4.8 hours,[35] although there was a higher recanalization rate at 90 minutes with t-PA vs. streptokinase, 62% vs. 31%, there was no significant difference in mortality, reinfarction, change in ventricular function, or major bleeding events. Of note is that patency rates several hours later were *similar.* When this happened is not clear. Although there was no difference in morbidity, mortality, or function, the difference in 90-minute patency *created the image* that t-PA was superior with a marked impact on practice habits.[36] Perhaps the trial design for GUSTO (Global Utilization of Streptokinase and Tissue Plasminogen Activation For Occluded Coronary Arteries) will serve as a model to avoid such scenarios in the future.[37] The results of the GISSI-2 trial were substantiated by the Third International Study of Infarct Survival (ISIS-3) trial in which 41,299 patients were randomized in a double-blind trial either to t-PA, streptokinase, or APSAC with a second randomization to either subcutaneous heparin, 12,500 units twice daily started at hour 4, or no heparin. There was *no* differ-

TABLE 37–6.
Intravenous Streptokinase in Acute Myocardial Infarction*

Event	Total	Percentage
Clinical reperfusion	98/110	89.0
Angiographic reperfusion	94/106	89.0
Mortality		
In-hospital	2	1.8
Late	1	0.9
Total	3	2.7

*From Hartmann J, McKeever L, Bufalino V, et al: *Clin Cardiol* 1988; 11:813. Used by permission.

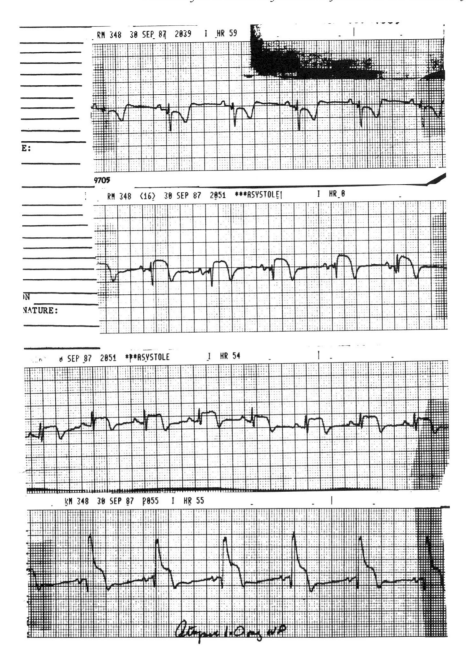

FIG 37–18.

A, serial rhythm strips reveal variable ST segment displacement. The top strip shows ST-T wave depression with slight elevation of the ST segments in strip 2 and then marked ST segment elevation in strip 4. **B,** further rhythm strips illustrating subsequent reduction in ST segment elevation in the second strip, then recurrent elevation in the third strip, and finally in the fourth strip normalization of the ST segment with T wave inversion.

(Continued.)

ence in mortality (SK 10.6% vs. t-PA 10.3%) or morbity (except that CVAs were slightly *less* with streptokinase) between streptokinase, t-PA, or APSAC.[38]

These studies have been criticized as flawed because heparin was administered several hours after thrombolytic therapy and was given subcutaneously. Investigators reported that nearly 3,000 of the 40,000 patients in the ISIS-3 trial were in fact treated with intravenous heparin before t-PA or streptokinase. Although this was not controlled or randomized, the numbers in both groups were similar, and there was no difference in mortality rates between streptokinase and t-PA.

In the GISSI II randomized trial, there was a total stroke rate of .94% with streptokinase and 1.33% with t-PA. The hemorrhage stroke rate was .29% with SK and .42% with t-PA.[38a]

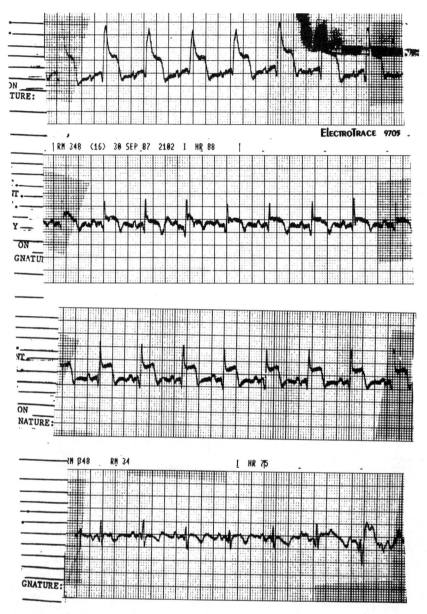

FIG 37–18. (cont'd.).

In another trial by Hogg and associates,[39] there was no evidence to suggest any benefits of APSAC over streptokinase. In fact, their studies showed strikingly similar 90-minute rates of reperfusion with no difference in end points.

In view of recent trials such as the Heparin Aspirin Reperfusion Trial (HART),[40] which have showed the importance of intravenous heparin in maintaining patency after t-PA, it is indeed possible that the initial benefit of t-PA was not realized in these trials.

To clarify these issues, the GUSTO trial[37] has been started. This trial, which administers aspirin to all patients, will evaluate the effectiveness of intravenous hep-

arin in patients treated with either t-PA, streptokinase, or a combination thereof. In addition, intravenous β-blockade will be assessed, and the primary end point will be 30-day mortality. However, at this time there appears to be few scientific data to advocate one thrombolytic drug over another in terms of sustained patency, left ventricular function, or mortality. Our excellent results are more likely related to the *early* treatment, 63% having been treated in two hours, and the high patency rate.[40a]

At Goleta Valley Community Hospital, all three agents are available. As shown in Table 37–8, the current cost to the hospital of 1.5 million units of strep-

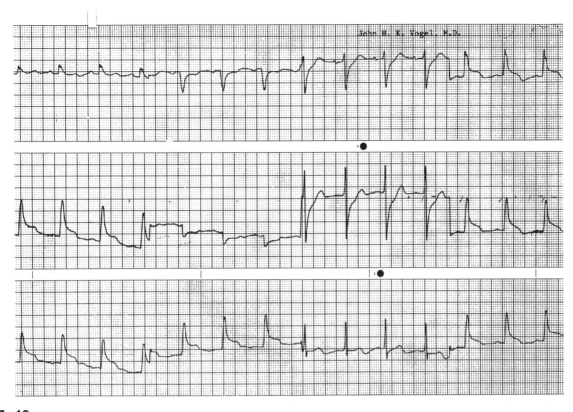

FIG 37–19.
Twelve-lead ECG obtained from a patient during maximal ST segment change. The rhythm strips reveal an acute inferior lateral wall current of injury.

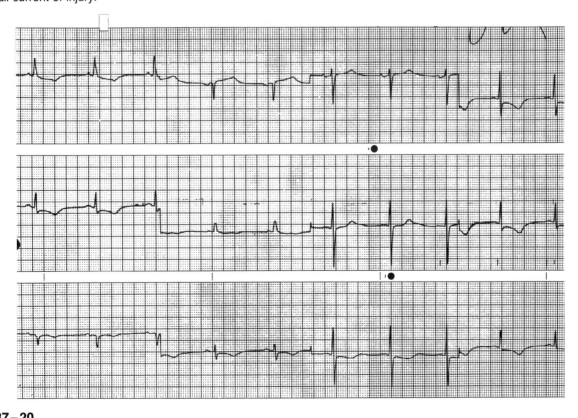

FIG 37–20.
ECG obtained immediately following intravenous streptokinase infusion shows reversion from the current of injury to marked ST segment depression, somewhat generalized.

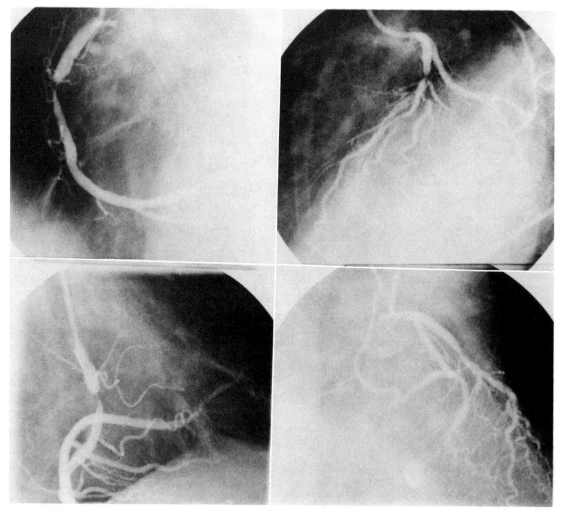

FIG 37–21.
A, a selective biplane right coronary artery cineangiogram shows near-total occlusion of a giant right coronary artery. **B,** a selective biplane coronary artery angiogram of the left coronary artery shows 90% diameter stenosis of the LAD coronary artery.

tokinase is $183.00; for 100 mg of t-PA, $2300.00; and for 30 mg of APSAC, $1695.00. Also shown is the charge to the patient which varies considerably from institution to institution. The diagnosis-related group (DRG) for uncomplicated MI reimbursement is $4300.00. Thus, the cost of the thrombolytic agent is exceedingly important in these times of limited funding. However, a recent survey indicated that many physicians were not aware of these specific costs and that 75% used t-PA.[41] Clearly, as physicians we need to be extremely conscious of costs so that we may allocate our ever-decreasing resources in the best possible way. Consequently, based on current studies, we find it difficult to justify the use of an expensive thrombolytic agent when a cheaper one or a combination does the job just

as well, unless specific contraindications exist.[42, 43, 44] An indication for t-PA is prior use of streptokinase.

Grines (Chapter 36) has pointed out the importance of expanding our indications for lytic therapy. Thus, in patients with inferior wall MI, pooled date combined from over 12,000 patients showed a reduction in the mortality rate from 8.7% to 6.8% with thrombolytic therapy (see Chapter 36). In addition, patients with left bundle-branch block who were treated with aspirin and streptokinase in the ISIS-2 trial experienced a 50% reduction in mortality rate.

Also, some data have suggested that treatment beyond 6 hours and up to 24 hours may be beneficial[33], although it has not been conclusive in all studies (see Chapter 36). The LATE trial may resolve some of these

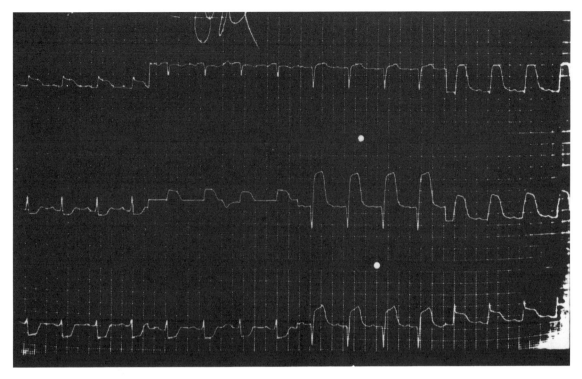

FIG 37–22.
ECG obtained immediately before intravenous streptokinase infusion shows acute anterior wall MI.

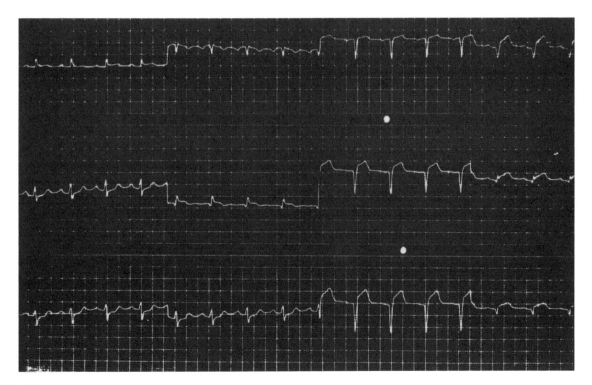

FIG 37–23.
ECG obtained immediately after streptokinase infusion shows normalization of the ST segments with a pattern suggestive of "old" anteroseptal wall MI.

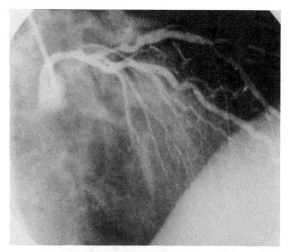

FIG 37–24.
Selective angiography of the left coronary artery shows a high-grade lesion in the proximal segment of the LAD coronary artery.

issues. At the present time, it is recommended that therapy be restricted to patients with under 6 hours of symptoms (perhaps 12 hours) unless there is evidence of a stuttering infarct, i.e., instability. Most important is extending therapy to the elderly, i.e., more than 75 years of age. Recently, Weaver and associates have shown the importance of age as a determining factor of mortality in those patients arriving at the hospital with acute MI.[12] Thus, in patients under 55 years of age, 39% of whom received thrombolytic therapy, the mortality rate was 2.5% in those treated vs. 1.5% in those

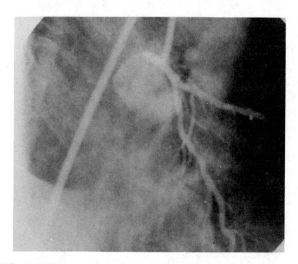

FIG 37–25.
Selective cineangiography of the left coronary artery following PTCA demonstrates the vessel to be widely patent. The predilatation gradient was 60 mm Hg, and the postdilatation gradient was 0 mm Hg.

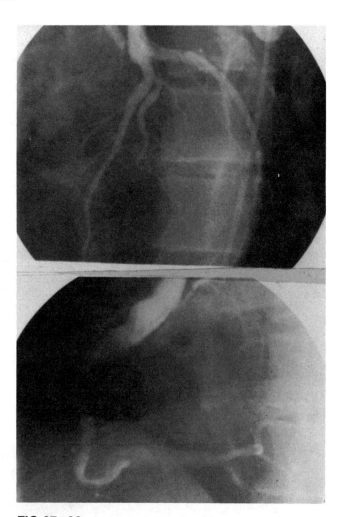

FIG 37–26.
Top panel, left coronary artery LAO projection. *Bottom panel,* LAO projection, right coronary artery. Note the aneurysmal dilatation.

not receiving lytic therapy. In contrast, the elderly demonstrated a significant reduction in mortality with treatment; thus, in those patients over 75 years of age, only 5% of whom were treated with thrombolytic therapy, the mortality rate was reduced from 18.4% in those not receiving lytic therapy to 11.5% in those receiving lytic therapy. These observations show the importance of age, not only in terms of the efficacy of treatment but also in terms of how age distribution may influence the results of trials. In five trials reviewed by Grines, mortality in the elderly treated with lytic therapy was reduced from 22.1% to 17.9% (see Chapter 36). Hypertension remains a controversial factor in terms of whether to give lytic therapy. In the ISIS-2 trial, those with systolic pressure over 175 mm Hg had a reduction in mortality, although there was concern about treating those patients with a diastolic pressure over 120 mm

TABLE 37–7.

Results of Recent Trials Using Intravenous Thrombolytic Therapy

Early Results	Type of Therapy*	Mortality (%)	
		Control	IV Therapy
Western Washington[22]	IVSK	9.7	6.3
<3 hr		11.3	5.2
>3 hr		7.5	7.5
New Zealand[23]	IVSK	12.9	2.5
ISAM[24, 25]	IVSK	7.1	6.3
GISSI[26]	IVSK		
<1 hr		15.4	8.2
>3 hr		12.2	9.2
AIMS (1 mon)[27]	IV APSAC	12.2	6.4
TICO (100)[28]	IV rt-PA	5.5	5.5
Hopkins (80)[29]	IV rt-PA	7.6	5.6
TIMI-IIA (100)[30]	IV rt-PA		
PTCA, 2 hr			7.2
PTCA, 33 hr			5.7
European (100) (patency at 90 min—89%) (100)[31]	IV rt-PA		3.0
Plus PTCA—at 1 hr (at 3 mon)			7.0
European Coop. Trial (100)[32]	rt-PA		
At discharge		6.8	3.7
At 3 mon		7.9	5.1
ISIS-2[33]	IVSK	12.3	8.2
<4 hr	IVSK and ASA	13.1	6.4

*IVSK = intravenous streptokinase; rt-PA = recombinant tissue-type plasminogen activator; ASA = acetylsalicylic acid. Numbers in parentheses are milligrams of t-PA.

Hg. A recent report showed no increased hazard in treating those patients who had received short-term cardiopulmonary resuscitation (CPR).[13]

In any event, whatever agent is used or patient treated, it is beneficial to delay catheterization a few days if possible since there is considerable "cleanup" after lysis, with some patients ending up with noncritical lesions as compared with their appearance immediately after lysis. Thus, unnecessary procedures and risks may be avoided since it appears clear that there is increased hazard with PTCA done urgently in association with lytic therapy as compared with late (elective PTCA) (see Table 37–7).

Revascularization procedures, i.e., salvage angioplasty, should be considered if there is continued ischemic instability with recurrent angina, arrhythmias, cardiogenic shock, or reocclusion (see Chapter 34). Recent studies have shown the feasibility, and at least the equivalence, of direct angioplasty to lytic therapy in acute MI, as well as in patients with cardiogenic shock.[48,51] If direct angioplasty is a consideration, we usually give 10,000 units of heparin intravenously and aspirin orally. However, if there is going to be a delay of over 30 minutes in going to the catheterization laboratory, one should consider the possibility of lytic therapy. In addition, under certain conditions direct angioplasty may be

TABLE 37–8.

Acute Myocardial Infarction Costs at Goleta Valley Community Hospital

Treatment*	Cost	
	Hospital	Patient
SK, 1.5 million units	$183.00	$290.00
t-PA, 100 mg	$2,300.00	$2,900.00
t-PA, 20 mg	$460.00	$550.00
Urokinase, 250,000 units	$270.00	$350.00
APSAC, 30 mg	$1,695.00	$1,995.00

*SK = streptokinase; t-PA = tissue-type plasminogen activator; APSAC = anisoylated plasminogen streptokinase activator complex.

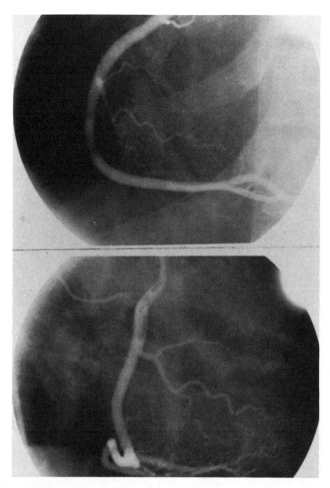

FIG 37–27.
Top panel, LAO projection. *Bottom panel,* RAO projection, right coronary artery. Note the absence of any significant obstructive lesion.

a consideration in the hospital without on-site surgical back-up (see Chapter 38).[49] This is so particularly in view of the preliminary PAMI results showing a 0% emergency CABS rate and a 97% procedural success with primary angioplasty; a significant reduction in re-cuttent ischemia and total stroke as compared to t-PA lytic therapy, and a lower death rate of 3.2% vs. 6.6%.[49a] If these results can be substantiated, infarct angioplasty centers may become a common reality in this country. Although PTCA is less effective in three-vessel disease, poor ventricular function, and severe bend points; open vessels result in less mortality and time from onset of pain to relief of pain; and, PTCA is most likely to be effective in high-risk patients with shock, anterior infarcts, second infarcts, low-risk angiographic findings (i.e., one- and two-vessel disease, ejection fraction over 25%), and in the elderly.

It is realized that it may be difficult to determine who has not reperfused and who may benefit by early study.

In our experience, clinical observation at the bedside has been quite effective, particularly when we have treated the patient very early. Perhaps new approaches to enzyme analysis and quantitation of ST wave changes will enhance this ability. However, observation of the level of pain in association with changing ST segments, changes in arrhythmia background, and clinical status are generally all powerful indicators when observed continuously at the bedside in determining the state of perfusion. Also, it is apparent that combinations of drugs may be useful in the individual patient,[44] and this may best be determined by careful clinical observation. We have found a 20 mg bolus of t-PA to be helpful with reocclusion or delayed opening following SK. Neuhaus and associates[50] have shown enhanced benefit of front loading with t-PA.

CONCLUSION

A 10-year experience with intravenous streptokinase as well as other lytic agents for the treatment of acute MI in the community hospital, with and without a catheterization laboratory facility, is presented. We have shown that intravenous streptokinase may be utilized very effectively in the community hospital without a catheterization laboratory when a close relationship exists with another hospital possessing full catheterization and surgical backup. In this study, two hospitals located approximately 1 hour's driving time from a third hospital that has a catheterization laboratory engaged in a highly satisfactory protocol of short-term, high-dose intravenous streptokinase. No problems were encountered in transportation of patients from the two hospitals without a catheterization laboratory and surgical backup to the facility with the laboratory. Results indicate that it is feasible to initiate intravenous streptokinase in a community hospital without a catheterization laboratory. The patient is followed closely, and if there is evidence of luminal opening clinically, observation is continued. If there is evidence of a potentially very large infarct or unstable situation or there is normalization with no evidence of infarction, transfer is initiated soon for catheterization. In the stable patient with early luminal opening, transfer may be delayed 2 to 4 days, with studies being done, however, before discharge. In the patient who remains unstable or has questionable luminal opening, transport is initiated as soon as possible after administering lytic therapy. In view of the tendency for many vessels to clean up over a matter of hours, an effort is made to wait a few days before study to obtain a better picture of what the final appearance may be.

In view of the benefit of *salvage angioplasty* (see Chapter 34) and the demonstrated effectiveness of PTCA in hospitals without on-site surgical backup[49] (see Chapter 38), perhaps consideration should be given to performance of *emergency* PTCA by *qualified* angioplasters in hospitals without surgical backup. The risk-benefit value of such an approach needs to be addressed.

The patient seen in the facility with a catheterization laboratory is managed in much the same way. However, if a large infarct is present and the laboratory is open, study may be performed immediately. With the administration of lytic therapy, if there is no evidence of opening within 30 to 60 minutes, supplemental t-PA may be administered, and if there is no effect, the patient may undergo study. If the patient is in shock, the patient goes to the laboratory immediately. Of note is that a number of patients seen in the outlying hospitals with hypotension and heart block responded dramatically to intravenous thrombolytic therapy. At the time of catheterization, if there is less than 50% stenosis and the patient is asymptomatic, medical therapy is given. Some patients have suffered restenosis and then have had PTCA. In those patients with over 70% residual stenosis who are symptomatic with positive stress testing results, revascularization is considered, the form and type depending on the extent of disease. If the patient is symptomatic but stable, PTCA may be delayed. In the patient with total occlusion who is unstable, early study and emergent PTCA should be attempted. Approximately 25% of our patients ultimately underwent PTCA, and approximately 25% had coronary artery bypass surgery. Fifty percent have been treated medically.

These results are consistent with the experience of other investigators in community hospitals and reflect the excellent results that are possible in such a setting with individualized evaluation and therapy. We believe that all patients with acute MI are candidates for intravenous thrombolysis unless specific potential bleeding problems are present.[45] The importance of time to treatment is clearly shown by the MITI trial results with a mortality rate of <1% and infarct size <5% in those treated less than 70 minutes from onset of pain, as compared to a mortality rate >10% and infarct size 11% in those treated after 70 minutes.[49]

Finally, we believe that almost all patients who demonstrate luminal opening clinically should undergo study before discharge, earlier study being performed in those patients who were critically unstable before thrombolytic therapy was administered and in those patients who had total resolution without infarction. Although controversy exists regarding the role of catheterization after lytic therapy,[46] we believe that it is the most powerful tool for individualization of subsequent treatment (Table 37-9).

It is important not to let uncertainty about which antithrombotic or fibrinolytic regimen to use routinely en-

TABLE 37-9.

Reasons for Catheterization After Lytic Therapy

Is vessel open?
Second-chance therapy!
Identify "clotters"
No major obstruction
Aneurysm vessels
Multivessel coronary disease—main left
Establish work, exercise status
Young patient
Individualized therapy!

gender uncertainty about whether to use antithrombotic and fibrinolytic therapies routinely.[38] It is clear that newer adjuvant agents may be helpful such as those that remodel the heart,[52] better antithrombin drugs, and new antiplatelet drugs. *However, the most important factor is still time to treatment and the necessity to educate our patients, emergency room teams, and doctors on the importance of prompt evaluation and treatment of chest pain.*

REFERENCES

1. Vogel, JHK: Coronary thrombolysis: Second chance therapy – Maximizing the advantage. *J Am Coll Cardiol* 1986; 8:1218–1219.
2. DeWood MA, Spores J, Notske R, et al: Prevalence of total coronary occlusion during the early hours of transmural MI. *N Engl J Med* 303:987, 1980.
3. Chesebro JH, et al: Thrombolysis in myocardial infarction (TIMI) trial, phase I: A comparison between intravenous tissue plasminogen activator and intravenous streptokinase. *Circulation* 1987; 76:142–154.
4. Chazov EL, Mateeva LS, Mazaev AV, et al: Intracoronary administration of fibrinolysis in acute myocardial infarction. *Ter Arkh* 1976; 48:8.
5. Rentrop KP, De Vivie ER, Karsch KR, et al: Acute coronary occlusion with impending infarction as an angiographic complication relieved by a guidewire recanalization. *Clin Cardiol* 1978; 1:101.
6. Rentrop KP: Thrombolytic therapy in patients with acute myocardial infarction. *Circulation* 1985; 71:627.
7. Italian Group for the Study of Streptokinase in Myocardial Infarction (GISSI): Effectiveness of intravenous thrombolytic treatment in acute myocardial infarction. *Lancet* 1986; 1:397–402.
8. Koren G, Weiss AT, Hasin Y, et al: Prevention of myocardial damage in acute myocardial ischemia by early treatment with intravenous streptokinase. *N Engl J Med* 1985; 313:1384–1389.
9. Sheehan FH: Determinants of improved left ventricular function after thrombolytic therapy in acute myocardial infarction. *J Am Coll Cardiol* 1987; 9:937–944.
10. Schroder R, Biamino G, Leitner ER: Intravenous short-term thrombolysis in acute myocardial infarction. *Circulation* 1981; 64(suppl 4):10.
11. Schroder R, Biamino G, Leitner ER, et al: Intravenous short-term infusion of streptokinase in acute myocardial infarction. *Circulation* 1983; 67:536.

12. Weaver WD, Litwin PE, Martin JS, et al: Effect of age on use of thrombolytic therapy and mortality in acute myocardial infarction. *J Am Coll Cardiol* 1991; 18:657–662.

13. Tenaglia AN, Califf RM, Candela RJ, et al: Thrombolytic therapy in patients requiring cardiopulmonary resuscitation. *Am J Cardiol* 1991; 68:1015–1019.

14. Sobel BE: Coronary thrombolysis with tissue-type plasminogen activator: Emerging strategies. *J Am Coll Cardiol* 1986; 8:1220–1225.

15. TIMI Study Group: Comparison of invasive and conservative strategies after treatment with intravenous tissue plasminogen activator in acute myocardial infarction. Results of Thrombolysis in Myocardial Infarction (TIMI) phase II trial. *N Engl J Med* 1989; 320:618–627.

15a. Olsson G, et al: Metoprolol-induced reduction in postinfarction mortality: Pooled results from five double-blind randomized trials. *Eur Heart J* 1992; 13:28–32.

16. Neuhaus KL, Feuerer W, Jeep-Tebbe S, et al: Improved thrombolysis with a modified dose regimen of recombinant tissue-type plasminogen activator. *J Am Coll Cardiol* 1989; 14:1566–1569.

17. Carney R, Brandt T, Daley P, et al: Increased efficacy of rt-PA by more rapid administration: The RAAMI trial. *Circulation* 1990; 82(suppl 3):538.

18. Topol EJ, Califf RM, George BS, et al: A randomized trial of immediate versus delayed elective PTCA after intravenous tissue plasminogen activator in acute myocardial infarction. *N Engl J Med* 1987; 317:581–588.

19. Hackett D, Davies G, Chierchia S, et al: Intermittent coronary occlusion in acute myocardial infarction: Value of combined thrombolytic and vasodilator therapy. *N Engl J Med* 1987; 317:1055–1059.

20. Topol EJ, Bates ER, Walton JA Jr, et al: Community hospital administration of intravenous tissue plasminogen activator in acute myocardial infarction: Improved timing, thrombolytic efficacy and ventricular function. *J Am Coll Cardiol* 1987; 10:1173–1177.

21. Hartman J, McKeever L, Bufalino V, et al: Intravenous streptokinase in acute myocardial infarction in community hospitals served by paramedics: A three year experience. *Clin Cardiol* 1988; 11:813.

22. Kennedy JW, Martin GV, David KB, et al: The Western Washington Intravenous Streptokinase in Acute Myocardial Infarction Randomized Trial. *Circulation* 1988; 77:345–352.

23. White HD, et al: Effect of intravenous streptokinase on left ventricular function and early survival after acute myocardial infarction. *N Engl J Med* 1987; 317:850–855.

24. The ISAM Study Group: A prospective trial of intravenous streptokinase in acute myocardial infarction (ISAM): Mortality, morbidity, and infarct size at 21 days. *N Engl J Med* 1988; 314:1465.

25. Schroder R, Neuhaus KL, Leizorovicz A, et al: A prospective placebo-controlled double-blind multicenter trial of intravenous streptokinase in acute myocardial infarction (ISAM): Long-term mortality and morbidity. *J Am Coll Cardiol* 1987; 9:197.

26. Italian Group for the Study of Streptokinase in Myocardial Infarction (GISSI): Long-term effects of intravenous thrombolysis in acute myocardial infarction: Final report the GISSI study. *Lancet* 1987; 2:871.

27. Aims Trial Study Group: Effect of intravenous ASPAC on mortality after acute myocardial infarction: Preliminary report of a placebo-controlled clinical trial. *Lancet* 1988; 1:545–549.

28. O'Rourke M, Baron D, Keogh A, et al: Limitation of myocardial infarction by early infusion of recombinant tissue-type plasminogen activation. *Circulation* 1988; 77:1311–1315.

29. Guerci AU, et al: A randomized trial of intravenous tissue plasminogen activation for acute myocardial infarction with subsequent randomization to elective coronary angioplasty. *N Engl J Med* 1987; 317:1613–1618.

30. TIMI Research Group: Immediate vs delayed catheterization and angioplasty following thrombolytic therapy for acute myocardial infarction. TIMI A results. *JAMA* 1988; 260:2849–2858.

31. Simoons ML, European Cooperative Study Group: Thrombolysis with tissue plasminogen activation in acute myocardial infarction: No additional benefit from immediate percutaneous coronary angioplasty. *Lancet* 1988; 1:197–202.

32. Van de Werf F, Arnold AER, European Cooperative Study Group: Effect of intravenous tissue plasminogen activation on infarct size, left ventricular function, and survival in patients with acute MI. Presented at an American College of Cardiology Meeting, 1988.

33. Collaborative Group: Second internal study of infarct survival (ISIS-2). Lancet 1988; 2:349–360.

34. Gruppo Italiano Per Lo Studio della Sopravivenza Nell Infarto Miocardico: GISSI-2. A factorial randomized trial of alteplase versus streptokinase and heparin versus no heparin among 12,490 patients with acute myocardial infarction. *Lancet* 1990; 336:65–71.

35. The TIMI Study Group: The Thrombolysis in Myocardial Infarction (TIMI) trials. *N Engl J Med* 1985; 312:932–936.

36. Sherry S, Marder JV: Creation of the recombinant tissue plasminogen activator (rt-PA) image and its influence on practice habits. *J Am Coll Cardiol* 1991; 18:1579–1582.

37. Topol EJ, Armstrong P, Van de Werf F, et al: Confronting the issues of patient safety and investigator conflict of interest in an international clinical trial of myocardial reperfusion. *J Am Coll Cardiol* 1992, in press.

38. ISIS-3 Collaborative Group: A randomized comparison of streptokinase vs tissue plasminogen activator vs anistreplase and of aspirin plus heparin vs heparin alone among 41,299 cases of suspected acute myocardial infarction. *Lancet* 1992; 339:753–770.

38a. Maggioni AP, Franzosi MG, Santoro E, et al: The risk of stroke in patients with acute myocardial infarction after thrombolytic and antithrombotic treatment. *N Engl J Med* 1992; 327:1–6.

39. Hogg KJ, Gemmill JD, Burns JMA, et al: Angiographic patency study of anistreplase versus streptokinase in acute myocardial infarction. *Lancet* 1990; 335:254–258.

40. Chsia J, Hamilton WP, Kleinman N, et al: A comparison between heparin and low-dose aspirin as adjunctive therapy with tissue plasminogen activator for acute myocardial infarction. *N Engl J Med* 1990; 323:1433–1437.

40a. Ohman EM, Califf RM, Topol EJ, et al: Consequences of reocclusion after successful reperfusion therapy in acute myocardial infarction. *Circulation* 1990; 82:781–791.

41. Vogel JHK: Management of acute myocardial infarction 1990: A prospective. *Clin Cardiol* 1991; 14:5–9.

42. Vogel JHK: Thrombolytic therapy of myocardial

infarction – It's time for science, not marketing. The perspective of a practicing cardiologist. *Clin Cardiol* 1991; 14:348.

43. Sherry S, Marder VJ: Streptokinase and recombinant tissue plasminogen activator (rt-PA) are equally effective in treating acute myocardial infarctions. *Ann Intern Med* 1991; 114:417–423.

44. Grines CL, Nissen SE, Booth, DC, et al: A new thrombolytic regimen for acute myocardial infarction using combination half dose tissue-type plasminogen activator with full dose streptokinase: A pilot study. *J Am Coll Cardiol* 1989; 14:573–580.

45. Vogel JHK, Setty, Ram K, et al: Intravenous streptokinase in acute myocardial infarction at the community hospital: A six-year experience. *J Am Coll Cardiol* 1988; 62:25–27.

46. Butman SM: What would I want to know if my dad had a heart attack? Good sense, versus dollars and cents. *J Am Coll Cardiol* 1991; 18:1220–1222.

47. Kahn JK, Rutherford BD, McConahay DR, et al: Catheterization laboratory events and hospital outcome with direct angioplasty for acute myocardial infarction. *Circulation* 1990; 82:1910–1915.

48. Grines CL, on behalf of the PAMI investigators. Primary Angioplasty in Myocardial Infarction (PAMI) Trial: Second European Workshop on Future Directions in Interventional Cardiology. Monaco, June 5–7, 1992.

49. Weaver WP, Lifwin PE, Maynard C, for the MITI Project. Primary angioplasty for AMI performed in hospitals with and without on-site surgical back-up. *Circulation* 1991; 84 (suppl 2):536.

49a. Grines CL, Browne KF, Vandormaal M, et al: Primary Angioplasty in Myocardial Infarction (PAMI) trial. *Circulation* 1992; 86(suppl II).

50. Neuhaus KL, Von Essen R, Tebbe A, et al: Improved thrombolysis in acute myocardial infarction with front-loaded administration of alteplase: Results of the rt-PA-APSAC patency study (TAPS). *JACC* 1992; 19:885–891.

51. Hibbard MD, Holmes DR, Bailey KR, et al: Percutaneous transluminal coronary angioplasty in patients with cardiogenic shock. *JACC* 1992; 19:639–646.

52. Mitchell GF, Lamas GA, Vaughan DE, et al: Left ventricular remodeling in the year after first anterior myocardial infarction: A quantitative analysis of contractile segment lengths and ventricular shape. *JACC* 1992; 19:1136–1144.

PART VII

Circulatory Support During Balloon Angioplasty

Guidelines for Surgical Standby in Patients Undergoing Percutaneous Transluminal Coronary Angioplasty

John H.K. Vogel, M.D.

In 1990, over 280,000 patients underwent percutaneous transluminal coronary angioplasty (PTCA) in the United States. The first PTCA was performed by Dr. Andreas Grünzig on September 16, 1977. In order to provide maximum safety to the patient, he insisted on immediate surgical backup should the angioplasty fail. In view of the not infrequent failure in the early experience with PTCA and the lack of methods for dealing with failure other than immediate surgery, the American College of Cardiology/American Heart Association Task Force Subcommittee in 1988 published guidelines for PTCA.[1] This report stated that

> An experienced cardiovascular surgical team should be available within the institution for emergency surgery for *all* angioplasty procedures. Transportation of patients to off-site facilities for emergency CABG fails to meet the standards of care exercised by prudent physicians and *cannot* be condoned.

However, with increasing experience, the development of new technology, and characterization of a number of preprocedural and intraprocedural factors, failure rates have declined.[2-4]

PREPROCEDURAL FACTORS

Patient selection plays a major role in outcome as evidenced by an increased failure rate in diabetics, elderly patients, and females. In addition, many have been concerned with the increased risk of PTCA and unstable angina in the presence of clot and unstable plaque.[5,6] The anatomy is also of importance, with lesion morphology and left ventricular (LV) function influencing results. The importance of lesion morphology has been shown by Ellis and associates[4] (Table 38–1). Although there is controversy regarding classification of lesions, their studies suggest that characterization of the lesions is helpful. Type A, B_1, B_2, and C lesions have been described and characterized and are summarized in Table 38–2. Generally, "simpler" lesions, easily approached, have been associated with less complication and higher success rates. From their results and others, one can anticipate a higher failure rate and increased complication rate with increasing lesion complexity.

INTRAPROCEDURAL FACTORS

The technology explosion has had a great impact on improving the success of PTCA as well as its safety. Advances in guiders, balloons, and wires have all had an impact on the success of these procedures. In addition, the advent of the laser balloon (see Chapter 25), directional rotational atherectomy (Chapter 15), and stents (Chapters 29, 31, and 34) has played a pivotal role in dealing with dissection and acute closure. Perfusion

TABLE 38–1.

Procedural Outcome After Multivessel PTCA (1.9 per Patient)*

Lesion Type	Success (%)	Complication (%)
A	92	2
B_1	84	4
B_2	76	10
C	61	21

*From Ellis SG, Vandormael MG, Cowley MJ, et al: *Circulation* 1990; 82:1193–1202. Used by permission.

TABLE 38–3.

Graded Inflation to Achieve Full Balloon Expansion*

Study Group (100 Patients)	Control (200 Patients)
0 Emergency CABG†	2% Emergency CABG
0 Deaths	1 Death
2% MI†	2.5% MI
≤8 atm (92%)	≤8 atm (86%)
98% success	97% success

*From Kahn JK, Rutherford BD, McConahay DR, et al: *Cathet Cardiovasc Diagn* 1990; 21:144–147. Used by permission.)
†CABG = coronary artery bypass graft; MI = myocardial infarction.

techniques, both active using various pump systems with blood (see Chapters 39 to 41) or Fluosol as well as passive perfusion catheters (Chapter 42), have enhanced safety. Technique may also play a significant role in terms of balloon inflation. Kahn and associates suggest that graded inflation to achieve full balloon expansion may be associated with a lower complication rate (Table 38–3).[7] Roubin and associates demonstrated that proper balloon sizing with avoidance of oversizing resulted in a lower complication rate (Table 38–4),[8] and Spielberg and associates[9] have noted the importance of completely coated guidewires used in association with the monorail technique (Table 38–5). Directional atherectomy has been associated with a reduced incidence of acute closure and has been effective in dealing with flaps and some forms of dissection. Perhaps most impressive has been the results with stents in dealing with acute closure. Although stents have essentially eliminated acute closure problems, there remains the problem of subacute closure and problems with anticoagulation (Table 38–6) (see Chapters 29 and 31).

O'Keefe and associates have noted a reduction in the need for urgent coronary artery bypass grafting (CABG) to only 1% in multivessel angioplasty as compared with 2.1% with single-vessel angioplasty, as well as reduced complications with complete revascularization with an urgent CABG rate of 0.1% vs. 2.4% with incomplete revascularization.[10] Of note has been the excellent results and low complication rates in direct infarct angioplasty as reported by Kahn and associates.[11] Urgent CABG was only required in 1 of 200 infarcts involving the left anterior descending (LAD) and right coronary artery (RCA) systems (Table 38–7). Webb and associates have reported an extremely low emergency CABG rate in patients under 40 years of age, only 0.7% (Table 38–8)[12]

TABLE 38–2.

Characteristics of Type A, B, and C Lesions*

Type A Lesions	Type B Lesions	Type C Lesions
High Success, 85%; low risk	Moderate success, 60%–70%; moderate risk	Low success, 60%; high risk
Discrete (<10 mm in length)	Tubular (10–20 mm in length)	Diffuse (>2 cm in length)
Concentric	Eccentric	
Readily accessible	Moderate tortuosity of the proximal segment	Excessive tortuosity of the proximal segment
Nonangulated segment, <45 degrees	Moderately angulated, >45 but <90 degrees	Extremely angulated, >90 degrees
Smooth contour, little or no calcification	Moderate to heavy calcification	
Less than totally occlusive	Total occlusion <3 mo old	Total occlusion >3 mo old
Not ostial in location	Ostial in location	Inability to protect major side branches
No major branch involvement	Bifurcation lesions requiring double guidewires	Degenerated vein grafts with friable lesions
Absence of thrombus	Some thrombus present	

*Adapted from Ellis SG, Vandormael MG, Cowley MJ, et al: *Circulation* 1990; 82:1193–1202.

TABLE 38-4.

Acute Complications*

	Total (n = 336)	Larger Balloon (n = 169)	Smaller Balloon (n = 167)	P
Total MI†	18 (5.4%)	13 (7.7%)	5 (3%)	.056
Q wave MI	4 (1.2%)	3 (1.8%)	1 (0.6%)	
NonQ wave MI	14 (4.2%)	10 (5.9%)	4 (2.4%)	
CABG†				
Total	19 (5.7%)	13 (7.7%)	6 (3.6%)	
Emergency	18 (5.4%)	12 (7.1%)	6 (3.6%)	.15
Elective	1 (0.3%)	1 (0.6%)	0	
Death	0	0	0	

*From Roubin GS, et al: *Circulation* 1988; 78:562. Used by permission.
†MI = myocardial infarction; CABG = coronary artery bypass graft surgery.

TABLE 38-5.

Acute Complications of PTCA of 725 Lesions in 660 Patients*

Complication	Group 1	Group 2	Group 3	Group 4
No. of lesions	192	91	232	210
Intermittent occlusions	3 (1.6)†	7 (7.7)	19 (8.2)	7 (3.3)
Recurrent occlusions	2 (1.0)	0	5 (2.2)	1 (0.5)
Permanent occlusions	7 (3.6)	8 (8.8)	24 (10.3)	4 (1.9)
Occlusion of the side branch	4 (2.1)	5 (5.5)	8 (3.4)	6 (2.9)
Coronary thrombus	5 (2.6)	5 (5.5)	15 (6.5)	2 (1.0)
Emergency CABG‡	1 (0.5)	2 (2.2)	5 (2.1)	1 (0.5)
PTCA‡-related death	1 (0.5)	1 (1.1)	5 (2.1)	1 (0.5)
No. of patients with ≥1 of these complications	17 (9.6)	16 (20)	49 (23)	19 (9.8)

*From Spielberg C, Schnitzer L, Linderer T: *Cathet Cardiovasc Diagn* 1990; 21:72–76. Used by permission.
†In Parentheses are the percentages of complications relative to all lesions treated within each group.
‡CABG = coronary artery bypass graft; PTCA = percutaneous transluminal coronary angioplasty.

TABLE 38-6.

Palmaz-Shatz Stent

For closure—acute
If wire across and
Vessel ≥ 2.5 mm
Guider ≥ .079 in
99% success
No closure—24 hr

TABLE 38-7.

Catheterization Events During Direct Infarct Angioplasty in 250 Patients*

Event	LAD† Infarct (n = 100)	RCA† Infarct (n = 100)	LCx† Infarct (n = 50)
Death	1	0	0
Urgent surgery	1	0	2
IABP†	10	4	4

*From Kahn JK, Rutherford BD, McConahay DR, et al: *Circulation* 1990; 82:19101915. Used by permission.)
†LAD = left anterior descending; RCA = right coronary artery; LCx = left circumflex; IABP = inta-aortic balloon pumping.

TABLE 38-8.

PTCA Demographics*

PTCA patients < 40 yr Old
148 patients
Success, 90.5%
SV†-PTCA, 70%; MV†-PTCA, 30%
Complications, 2%

Emergency CABG†	0.7% (1)
Nonfatal MI†	0.7% (1)
Fatal MI	0.7% (1)

*From Webb JG, Myler RK, Shaw RE, et al: *J Am Coll Cardiol* 1990; 16:15691574. Used by permission.)
†SV = single vessel; MV = multivessel; CABG = coronary artery bypass grafting; MI = myocardial infarction.

TABLE 38–9.

Goleta Valley Community Hospital—1990

Standby (operating room open—surgeon available)	65%
No standby	35%
Emergency CABG*	0
Deaths	0
AMI*	2%
Dissection 7	7%
Acute closure	2%

*CABG = coronary artery bypass graft; AMI = acute myocardial infarction.

TABLE 38–11.

Emory Survey of University Physician Fees

Physician Fees	Fee	Insurance Payment Yes
Surgeon (STBY)*	$443 ($50–$800)	68%
Anesthesiologist (STBY)	$422 ($200–$600)	67%
Cardiologist (PTCA)	$1946 ($1,000–$4,000)	NA

*STBY = Surgical standby.

With increasing experience, it became apparent that not all patients had to go to surgery following failed angioplasty and that individualization of standby might be a consideration. Thus, as shown in Table 38–9, in our facility during 1990, one third of our patients had no standby. Perhaps not representative, but during this time no emergency CABG was required, and no deaths were encountered. In fact, some 386 consecutive patients underwent PTCA without emergency CABG or death. Not unexpectedly, since then there has been 1 death in a patient requiring emergency coronary artery bypass surgery (CABS) secondary to pump failure after CABG.

In view of the infrequent necessity for surgical assistance and the enormous cost in terms of dollars and manpower being expended to provide this infrequently used service, a survey was conducted among our colleagues to ascertain practice patterns throughout the country. Thus, surveys of practice patterns of interventional cardiologists attending the Emory PTCA Conference, April 1990, the Geneva PTCA Conference, June 1990, and the ACC Santa Barbara Interventional Conference, September 1990, were conducted. Table 38–10 summarizes the demographics of the groups surveyed. A wide representation was obtained, with physicians from 31 states participating in the Emory and Santa Barbara conferences and physicians from 13 countries taking part in the Geneva study.

A remarkably consistent 86% of PTCAs were elective, and 14% were emergent. For elective PTCA, routine standby was requested or planned in 89% of the patients in the Emory group vs. 65% in the Geneva group, with lower percentages for emergency PTCA, Emory being 73% and Geneva 46%. Interestingly, over a third of physicians said that they would consider elective PTCA without surgical standby.

Cost was considered important by the majority of physicians in the Emory/Santa Barbara groups and less important in the European group. Not surprisingly, in spite of a concern about cost, only a small percentage actually knew the cost involved for the surgeon, the anesthesiologist, or the operating room. Physician fees reported are shown in Table 38–11.

COST ANALYSIS

Based on an estimated 282,000 PTCAs performed in the United States in 1990, in Table 38–12 are shown possible costs involved. By utilizing the percentages of standby reported in the Emory survey, an operating room cost of $990.00 for the first hour, but not including physician fees, packs, or pump setup and assuming a 2% emergency CABG rate, the estimated cost per patient was approximately $50,000 for those going to sur-

TABLE 38–10.

Surveys of PTCA Experience

	Geneva (Europe, Canada, Mexico)	Emory (USA)	Santa Barbara (USA)
No. countries/states	13	31	19
Average no. PTCA/yr	391	80	183
% doing < 100/yr	8%	64%	39%
Average experience, yr	5.2	4.7	6.6
No. responses	24	75	31
Average no. operating rooms	3.0	2.3	3.6

TABLE 38–12.

Estimated Cost for Standby 1990—United States

270,595	Patients
$990.00	(1 hr)
$267,889,050.00	Patient cost

- $156,945,100.00—Estimates actual hospital cost
- Does not include surgeon, anesthesiologist fees
- Packs not opened
- Pump not set up

Assume 2.0% emergency CABG*

Cost per patient proceeding to CABG, $49,499.00

*CABG = coronary artery bypass grafting.

gery. Obviously, these costs are substantially higher if one includes the fees. Wilson and associates have reported a cost for standby of $1,700.00 per patient which approximates our results.[13]

STRATEGIES FOR STANDBY

Intra-aortic balloon pumps and auto perfusion catheters such as the Stack device are present in virtually all laboratories in the United States. The newer technologies, not approved in the United States, are more prevalent in Europe. Obviously, the percentage of directional atherectomy devices will increase in the United States with the release of the Simpson directional atherectomy device. Interestingly, in regard to stents, although they are quite common in Europe, a low percentage actually had used them in this regard, whereas in the United States, wherein few centers have stents, they have been used enthusiastically, thus indicating confidence in the stent as a standby device. Similarly, with cardiopulmonary support (CPS), a system that has become fairly prevalent, it appears to have been used less in Europe, whereas in the United States confidence has been exhibited in using this device for standby. In contrast, directional atherectomy has not been perceived as a strong standby device.

PTCA IN HOSPITALS WITHOUT SURGICAL BACKUP

In Table 38–13 are shown the summary of responses to the question of whether participants performed or knew of other physicians who performed PTCA in hospitals without surgical backup. The percentage is high in the European contingent at 41%, whereas in the Emory response it was only 6% and somewhat higher at 22% in the Santa Barbara group. Clearly, PTCA is being done in hospitals without surgical backup in the United States.

At Victoria Hospital in London, Ontario (personal

TABLE 38–13.

PTCA in Hospitals Without Surgical Backup

Study	Percent	Distance to Backup
Geneva	41%	8–60 km 10–60 min Ambulance, helicopter
Emory	6%	60–150 miles 30 min Helicopter
Santa Barbara	22%	2–30 miles 15–20 min

TABLE 38–14.

Placement of Patients in Standby or No-Standby Groups on the Basis of Risk at Victoria Hospital, London, Ontario, Canada (Director of Cardiac Catheterization Laboratory: Robert Brown, M.D.)

400 Cases/yr
  50% Standby–operating room and surgeons ready
    Large area of risk
    Proximal segment of LAD* etc.
  50% Without standby
    Emergency—AMI*
    Salvage, shock
    Good collaterals
    Total occlusion with collaterals
    Small vessels
    Nonsurgical
Emergency CABG,* 3%
Mortality, <1%

*LAD = left anterior descending; AMI = acute myocardial infarction; CABG = coronary artery bypass grafting.

communication, Dr. Robert Brown), patients have been actively placed in standby or no-standby groups (Table 38–14). As noted, with patients selected on the basis of risk, the mortality rate has been less than 1%. For the past several months, they have utilized the Johnson & Johnson stent, with which they have been able to control all cases of acute closure with none going to the operating room.

There are three well-established PTCA programs in Canada without in-house surgical backup (Table 38–15). The oldest program at the Royal Alexandra Hospital, under the direction of Dr. W. Peter Klinke, has performed over 800 PTCAs during the past 10 years. Emergency bypass was required in 1.6% with an average time to surgery of 164 minutes and no deaths.[14] (personal communication). Also, at the Sir Mortimer B. Davis Jewish General Hospital in Montreal, Quebec, excellent results have been obtained by utilizing a defensive program (personal communication, Dr. L. N. Dragatakis) (Table 38–16). Their strategy includes working only during daytime hours with the backup of intra-aortic balloon pumping, reperfusion

TABLE 38–15.

Canadian System: Three PTCA Programs Without In-house Surgery

Royal Alexandra Hospital
  (1981) Edmonton, Alberta
St. Luc Hospital
  (1985) Montreal, Quebec
Sir Mortimer B. Davis Jewish General Hospital
  (1986) Montreal, Quebec

*Date program started.

TABLE 38–16.
PTCA Program at Sir Mortimer B. Davis Jewish General
Hospital, Montreal, Quebec (Director, L.N. Dragatakis, M.D.)

500 cases
3 emergency CABG—times to surgery: 45 min, 45 min, 120 min
3 deaths—none related to unavailability of surgery
AMI,* 2%–5%
Distance to hospital and surgical backup
2 km (10–20 min by ambulance)

*AMI = acute myocardial infarction.

catheters, perfusion balloons and atherectomy. They avoid left main artery disease and lesions over 5 mm in length, and they stage multi vessel LAD and RCA angioplasty.

An extensive experience in PTCA without on-site surgical backup has been reported by Richardson and associates from Belfast City Hospital.[15] Their report on 444 cases with an in-depth analysis concluded that the absence of immediate surgical help did not influence the outcome in any patient. In fact, the time to bypass was somewhat faster than for patients in the hospital that they referred to. Ninety percent of their cases were single-vessel disease. They concluded that with careful selection of patients, coronary angioplasty may be safely performed in a hospital without on-site cardiac surgical facilities, provided that these are available at a nearby center. At the Red Cross Hospital Center in Frankfurt, over 10,000 cases of PTCA have been performed without in-hospital surgery backup, with an emergency CABS rate of .2% and mortality rate of .2%, their time to the backup hospital is 12 minutes. (Dr. W. Reifart, personal communication). It is stated that 50% of cases in Germany are performed without in-house surgical backup.

Recently, Dr. Bernie Meier of Geneva reported on an in-depth prospective analysis of standby vs. no standby. The standby group was characterized by a PTCA site proximal to the largest vessel of the patient unless it was totally occluded, known to have been previously occluded (preinfarcted), or visible through collaterals or a bypass graft. All others were allocated to no standby. There were 189 patients in the standby group and 811 patients in the no-standby group. It was concluded that the absence of in-town surgical facilities would not have increased the risk of the no-standby patients and that among the 189 patients deemed to need surgical standby, only 1 potentially benefited from it, but even this patient would have been transportable for out-of-town surgery. He concluded that PTCA by an

experienced team without surgical backup proved ethically feasible when staying away from the patient's most important vessel, unless it was or had been totally occluded or was well collateralized or unless the patient was inoperable. Even for higher-risk indications, no clear benefit of surgical standby was documented in his analysis of 1,000 consecutive patients.[16] However, current recommendations of the Swiss Cardiology Society are for on-site surgical standby with individualized consultation on high-risk patients.

In the United Kingdom, it is the view of the working party of the British Cardiac Society that in carefully selected patients, it is ethical to attempt PTCA in the absence of immediate surgical standby.[17] Such cases might include previous CABS, poor LV function, and severe concomitant illness.

Recommendations in France suggest that PTCA is acceptable with or without standby on site, provided that the pump time is within 60 minutes, the operating room is open, and the ambulance has a console for IABP.[18]

Similarly, in Germany, organization is the important issue, such that operating room standby must be available in "short time" in an organized sequence with IABP available with or without on-site standby.[19]

Also, in Scotland, a large experience without on-site standby has suggested a "decision to pump" time of 120 minutes. They report a 1.7% emergency CABS rate, .25% mortality rate, and 5% acute closure with 97% successful management in the laboratory. They are 3 miles from the standby operating room.[20]

ISSUES AND CANDIDATES FOR NO STANDBY

The challenge is identifying those patients who can be treated medically after failed PTCA and identifying those patients in whom we can control the ischemia with failed PTCA and to what extent this is possible. Characterization of these factors is a pressing problem needing continual evaluation. The major challenge of failed PTCA is reducing myocardial ischemia and the incidence of myocardial infarction. Clearly, stabilization and elimination of myocardial ischemia prior to CABS improves the immediate- and long-term outlook. This may be especially true in elderly women and in patients with multivessel disease and diminished LV function. An evaluation of the results of CABG after failed elective PTCA in patients with prior CABG by Weintraub and associates illustrates the importance of controlling ischemia (Table 38–17).[21] In those patients without

TABLE 38–17.

In-Hospital Complications in the 46 Study Patients*

Hospital Stay and Complication	Coronary Bypass Surgery With Ischemia (n = 33)	Coronary Bypass Surgery Without Ischemia (n = 13)	Total (n = 46)
Mean length of hospital stay (days)	10.4 ± 7.8	6.8 ± 3.7	9.4 ± 7.0†
>9 Days	15 (45.5)‡	1 (7.7)	16 (34.8)§
Neurologic event	2 (6.1)	0 (0)	2 (4.3)
Wound infection	1 (3.0)	0 (0)	1 (2.2)
Nonfatal Q wave MI	11 (33.3)	0 (0)	11 (23.9)§
Death	3 (9.1)	0(0)	3(6.5)
Death or Q Wave MI	14 (42.2)	0(0)	14 (30.4)¶

*From Weintraub WS, Cohen CL, Curling PE, et al: *J Am Coll Cardiol* 1990; 16:1344. Used by permission.
†*P* = .04.
‡Values in parentheses are percentages.
§*P* = .02.
¶*P* = .005.

ischemia, there was no mortality, whereas in those with ischemia the mortality rate was 9.1%. In fact, those with ischemia were patients who were taken almost immediately to surgery, whereas in those without ischemia, the situation had been stabilized and surgery was performed later. This involved an analysis of 46 patients going to surgery out of a cohort of 1,263 patients undergoing PTCA. Talley and associates noted an increased incidence of nonfatal myocardial infarction in those going to CABG with ongoing ischemia as compared with those without ischemia, 25% vs. 3.5%, and a diminished 5-year survival rate of 65.6% in those with ischemia and 93.8% in those without ischemia.[2] However, the immediate mortality rate was not significantly different, being 1.4% with ischemia and 1.2% without ischemia.

THERAPY FOR FAILED PTCA

Clearly, factors involved in failed PTCA include operator experience, available technology, patient selection, lesion morphology, and ventricular function. In Table 38–18, the defensive armamentarium enabling individualization of standby is summarized. In terms of direct coronary support, stents, although investigational, have shown great promise for dealing with acute occlusion (see Chapter 29). Active perfusion using blood and/or Fluosol has been effective in controlling ischemia, and autoperfusion utilizing a Stack balloon has also been effective. Directional atherectomy appears to have a lower incidence of acute closure (see Chapter 15) when compared with balloon angioplasty and may be useful in salvaging some local occlusive dissection problems. Perforation remains a risk. The risks of stents continue to be subacute closure and problems of anticoagulation. Laser balloon angioplasty has shown promise in salvaging acute closure problems and dissection (see Chapter 25). Intra-aortic balloon pumping is a necessity for backup, and cardiopulmonary support has proved extremely powerful in controlling acute collapse in the short term (see Chapter 40).

In Table 38–19 practical factors are outlined for *avoiding trouble.* The degree to which one approaches lesions of different morphology is an individual matter that is influenced by experience and judgment. Certainly, having the available technology on site and

TABLE 38–18.

Therapy for Failed PTCA: Defensive Technology to Decrease Myocardial Ischemia

Coronary*	Systemic*
Stents	CPS
Auto-perfusion	IABP
Active perfusion	
DA	
LBA	

*DA = directional atherectomy; LBA = laser balloon angioplasty; CPS = cardiopulmonary support; IABP = intraaortic pump balloon.

TABLE 38–19.

Avoiding Trouble

Quit While Ahead (PTCA)
    Target vessel only
    Stage procedures
    Avoid B$_2$, C lesions
    Avoid ischemia
Have available technology and know how to use it
Consider other revascularization i.e., internal mammary
    artery-CABG
Continue medical therapy—Delay PTCA i.e. unstable angina
    Allow healing of plaque

knowing how to use it are important factors. With the increasing array of technology available, it is clear that fewer and fewer individual operators will have the necessary expertise to utilize all of the technology in a highly proficient way. Thus, with increasing complexity of the patient, many patients will probably be treated in tertiary centers with vast experience in utilizing all available technology in a given patient as indicated. Certainly, other revascularization methods such as the internal mammary artery should always be entertained.[22] The results with an internal mammary artery-to-LAD bypass are superb and may be superior to PTCA in proximal LAD lesions. Numerous studies suggest that somewhat delayed PTCA may be advantageous over immediate PTCA in acute ischemic syndromes. Balancing the results of various trials with careful judgment and personal experience should provide the best individualization of treatment.

SUGGESTED GUIDELINES FOR SURGICAL STANDBY FOR PTCA

In Table 38–20 an outline is proposed for standby:

1. *Active surgical standby* is defined as the prearranged, immediate availability of open heart surgery on site, that is, the cardiac surgeon, operating team, and operating suite are immediately available. In Table 38–21 are listed high-priority lesions for which active standby would be reasonable.

2. *Passive surgical backup* means that the next available operating room would be utilized following a failed angioplasty. The cardiac surgeon, his team, and the operating room are aware that PTCA is in progress but are not necessarily immediately available. In Table 38–22 are listed situations in which this strategy might be employed.

It is appreciated that in the very large centers wherein four or five operating rooms are being utilized there already exists a mix of active and passive standby with considerable overlap of these strategies. In some cases, with large-volume centers specific consultation is

TABLE 38–20.

Suggested Standby Classifications

I. OR* open—surgeon ready: *Active*
II. Next OR open—surgeon available *Passive*
III. No standby
Off-site PTCA
    (?)AMI*—Salvage—not lytic eligible
    (?) No standby patients
      i.e., failed PTCA—medical treatment

*OR = operating room; AMI = acute myocardial infarction

TABLE 38–21.

Active Standby, Operating Room Open—Surgeon Available

Proximal LAD*
LV Dys. EF* < 40%
Vessel → Major blood supply
    Closure → Shock
Dominant RCA,* circumflex
"Last" vessel
Multivessel angioplasty
Non-MI* vessel in AMI,* saphenous vein graft with occluded native vessel
Left main equivalent or unprotected left main
Anyone would operate if failed PTCA
B₂, C lesions

*LAD = left anterior descending; LVEF = left ventricular ejection fraction; RCA = right coronary artery; MI = myocardial infarction; AMI = acute myocardial infarction.

not obtained other than knowledge by the cardiac surgeons and the operating room personnel that PTCA is being conducted throughout the day and their next available room may be needed at any time during the day. However, in the vast majority of hospitals in the United States, only one to two operating rooms are being utilized, and thus a more specific strategy has to be developed for each individual patient regarding standby classification.

3. *No standby — no CABG.* This category includes the patient, who for various reasons, under no condition will undergo emergency bypass and for whom no standby is necessary. Table 38–23 lists potential situations in which this would apply.

4. *Off-site PTCA.* The possibility of performing PTCA without on-site surgical backup is highly controversial. In the United States, there is little justification for elective PTCA without on-site surgical backup because there is a plethora of surgical programs available

TABLE 38–22.

Passive Standby Operating Room Not Open—Surgeon Available

Small vessels or Midvessel disease
Total occlusion
Infarct vessel, AMI,* salvage
Small area at risk, vessel serves scar
Good LV*
Branch vessels
Grüntzig vessel
Mid-LAD*
Small grafts (not host vessel)
Elderly
Saphenous grafts with stent
Collateral protection

*AMI = acute myocardial infarction; LV = left ventricle; LAD = left anterior descending.

TABLE 38-23.
No Standby-No CABG

Patient absolutely refuses—agrees to accept consequences (death)
Surgeon refuses case
Nonsurgical—cancer, COPD*
Non-dominant RCA*
Closure less dangerous than CABG*
Total Occlusion (RCA) with collateral
Small area at risk—graft protected RCA

*COPD = chronic obstructive pulmonary disease; RCA = right coronary artery; CABG = coronary artery bypass grafting.

to patients throughout this country who are undergoing elective PTCA. However, many centers outside the United States have established safe, well-organized programs for PTCA without on-site facilities. One situation wherein PTCA might be justified in the United States, without on-site surgical backup, would be in the patient with acute myocardial infarction. With the increasing interest in the role of direct angioplasty in acute myocardial infarction, the low risk of PTCA,[11] and the value of revascularization for cardiogenic shock,[25, 26] this bears consideration. Clearly, many patients are not candidates for thrombolytic therapy and have unstable situations that may benefit from immediate direct angioplasty. The Primary Angioplasty Trial in Acute Myocardial Infarction (PAMI) has already shown fewer strokes with direct angioplsty than with lytic therapy (see Chapter 34). Experienced angioplasters might be effectively utilized in hospitals without on-site surgical backup for managing such patients. Similarly, in such a setting, perhaps a limited number of patients who are absolutely not candidates for CABG might be considered.

The feasibility of PTCA for AMI without on-site backup is supported by the MITI study reported by Weaver et al.,[23] wherein 238 consecutive AMI patients underwent PTCA in hospitals without on-site backup and were compared to 208 patients who had direct PTCA for AMI in hospitals with surgical backup. There were 3 deaths in the first group and 7 in the second, a nonsignificant difference. Only 1 patient in the nonsurgical group required emergency CABS, which was started within 45 minutes, as compared to 6 patients in group 2, in which surgery was begun in an average of 48 minutes.

Similar results have been obtained by others.[24] However, despite these excellent results, Professional Review stated on June 11, 1991, that HCFA has informed all PROS that the practice of performing PTCAs in settings where immediate in-house surgical intervention is not available is considered to be an unacceptable practice and

should be pursued as a quality problem; this judgement based on the old guidelines! The resultant effect has been consideration of a proliferation of low-volume surgical centers. Clearly, if PAMI and related trials show substantial benefits of direct angioplasty, then consideration has to be given to the development of "infarct angioplasty centers" without on-site surgical backup, particularly in view of the large number of patients who are "ineligible" for lytic therapy.

CONCLUSION

Since the first PTCA by Dr. Andreas Grünzig, September 16, 1977, several hundred thousand patients have now undergone PTCA with increasing success and low complication rates. Improved operator technique, increased awareness of patient risks, improved characterization of morphologic and anatomic factors, and the development of new technological tools such as lasers, atherectomy devices, stents, and perfusion pumps and balloons have extended this procedure to the more seriously ill patients. It is suggested that with the new technologies and the increased awareness of risk factors, active surgical standby can be markedly reduced, thereby resulting in enormous cost reductions and more appropriate patient care.

REFERENCES

1. Ryan TJ, Faxon DP, Gunnar RM, et al: Guidelines for percutaneous transluminal coronary angioplasty. *J Am Coll Cardiol* 1988; 82:529–545.
2. Tally JD, Weintraub WS, Roubin GS, et al: Failed elective percutaneous transluminal coronary angioplasty requiring coronary artery bypass surgery. In-hospital and late clinical outcome at 5 years. *Circulation* 1990; 82:1203–1213.
3. Tuzcu EM, Simpfendorfer C, Dorosti K, et al: Changing patterns in percutaneous transluminal coronary angioplasty. *Am Heart J* 1989; 117:1374–1377.
4. Ellis SG, Vandormael MG, Cowley MJ, et al: Coronary morphologic and clinical determinants of procedural outcome with angioplasty for multivessel coronary disease. Implications for patient selection. *Circulation* 1990; 82:1193–1202.
5. Laskey MAL, Deutsch E, Barnathan E, et al: Influence of heparin therapy on percutaneous transluminal coronary angioplasty outcome in unstable angina pectoris. *Am J Cardiol* 1990; 65:1425–1429.
6. Myler RK, Bell W: Thrombogenesis and thrombolysis in acute ischemic syndromes. Pathophysiological and pharmacological rationales for and limitations of thrombolytic, antithrombin, antiplatelet therapy and angioplasty. *J Invasive Cardiol* 1991; 3:95–114.
7. Kahn JK, Rutherford BD, McConahay DR, et al: Inflation pressure requirements during coronary angioplasty. *Cathet Cardiovasc Diagn* 1990; 21:144–147.

8. Roubin GS, et al: *Circulation* 1988; 78:562.

9. Spielberg C, Schnitzer L, Linderer T, et al: Influence of catheter technology and adjuvant medication on acute complications in percutaneous coronary angioplasty. *Cathet Cardiovasc Diagn* 1990; 21:72–76.

10. O'Keefe JH, Rutherford BD, McConahay DR, et al: Multivessel coronary angioplasty from 1980 to 1989: Procedural results and long-term outcome. *J Am Coll Cardiol* 1990; 16:1097–1102.

11. Kahn JK, Rutherford BD, McConahay DR, et al: Catheterization laboratory events and hospital outcome with direct angioplasty for acute myocardial infarction. *Circulation* 1990; 82:1910–1915.

12. Webb JG, Myler RK, Shaw RE, et al: Coronary angioplasty in young adults: Initial results and late outcome. *J Am Coll Cardiol* 1990; 16:1569–1574.

13. Wilson JM, Dunn EJ, Wright BD, et al: The cost of simultaneous surgical standby for PTCA. *J Thorac Cardiovasc Surg* 1986; 91:362–370.

14. Klinke WP, Hui WK, Hendriks R: Complications of percutaneous transluminal coronary angioplasty performed in a hospital without on-site cardiac surgery. *Catheterization Cardiovasc Diagn*, 1992, vol 23.

15. Richardson SG, Morton P, Murtagh JG, et al: Management of acute coronary occlusion during percutaneous transluminal coronary angioplasty: Experience of complications in a hospital without on site facilities for cardiac surgery. *Br Med J* 1990; 300:355–358.

16. Meier B, Urban P, Dorsaz PA, et al: Surgical standby for coronary balloon angioplasty. *JAMA* (in press).

17. Report of a working party of the British Cardiac Scoienty: Coronary Angioplasty in the United Kingdom. *Br Heart J* 1991; 66:325–331.

18. Monassier JP, Bertrand M, Cherrier F, et al: Recommendations concernant la formation des medicins coronarographistes et d'angioplastie coronaire transluminale. *Arch Mal Coeur* 1991; 84:1783–1787.

19. Herau gegenben von der Deutschen Gesellschaft fur Herz-und Kreislaufforschung: Empfehlungen fur die durchfuhrang der perkatanen transluminal en Koronarangioplastie (PTCA). *Z Kardiol* 1987; 76:382–385.

20. Shaw TRD, Starkey IR, Essop AR, et al: Emergency coronary bypass surgery after vessel occlusion at angioplasty in centres without on-site cardiac surgery. *Br Heart J* 1989; 61:438.

21. Weintraub WS, Cohen CL, Curling PE, et al: Results of coronary surgery after failed elective coronary angioplasty in patients with prior coronary surgery. *J Am Coll Cardiol* 1990; 16:1341–1347.

22. Vogel JHK, McFadden RB, Spence R, et al: Quantitative assessment of myocardial performance and graft patency following coronary bypass with the internal mammary artery. *J Thorac Cardiovasc Surg* 1978; 75:487–498.

23. Weaver WD, Litwin PE, Maynard C, for the MITI Project: Primary angioplasty for AMI performed in hospitals with and without on-site surgical backup. *Circulation* 1991; 4(suppl II):536.

24. Weatherly GK: Personal communication. 1992.

25. Goldberg RJ, Gore JM, Alpert JS, et al: Cardiogenic shock after acute myocardial infarction. *N Engl J Med* 1991; 325:1117–1127.

26. Lee L, Bates EK, Pitt B, et al: Percutaneous transluminal coronary angioplasty improves survival in acute myocardial infarction complicated by cardiogenic shock. *Circulation* 1988; 78:1345–1351.

Use of Prophylactic and Standby Circulatory Support During High-Risk Coronary Angioplasty

Robert A. Vogel, M.D.

Although first envisioned as an intervention for patients with single-vessel coronary artery disease and good left ventricular function,[1] coronary angioplasty has been increasingly utilized in those with more extensive coronary disease, severe and acute chest pain syndromes, and poor ventricular function. This progress has been facilitated by the technical advances in guidewires and dilatation catheters that have taken place during the 1980s and more recently by the introduction of laser and atherectomy catheters and intracoronary stents. Three other factors fostering the expanding applications of coronary angioplasty are increasing operator experience, improving radiographic and intravascular imaging equipment, and prophylactic use of myocardial and systemic circulatory support devices in high-risk patients. This chapter describes the use of cardiopulmonary bypass to support the systemic circulation in patients at the highest risk for circulatory collapse during coronary artery intervention, a technique termed *supported angioplasty*.

FACTORS DEFINING PATIENT RISK

The factors determining the risk of coronary angioplasty can be divided into two groups: technical/anatomic risks and clinical parameters.[2] Technical/anatomic risks refer to the location and morphology of the target stenosis. These factors determine the feasibility of dilatation and include stenosis severity, length, and calcification; vessel tortuosity; and branching and guiding catheter access.[3] Although these factors were crucial for the early angioplasty success of operators utilizing primitive equipment, more recent data from the National Heart, Lung, and Blood Institute Percutaneous Transluminal Coronary Angioplasty (PTCA) Registry suggests that these factors are of decreasing importance for operators with high skill levels.[4, 5]

Whereas technical success is more related to anatomic factors, patient procedural mortality is determined by more general clinical features. Hartzler et al.[6] have described the clinical parameters defining low-and high-risk patients (Table 39–1). Patients without clinical risk factors should undergo coronary angioplasty with a procedure-related mortality rate of about 0.25%. The performance of multivessel angioplasty and patient age greater than 70 years significantly increases the risk. The two most important factors determining procedural mortality, however, are the amount of left ventricular myocardium perfused by any single target vessel and overall left ventricular function.[7] In addition to procedural mortality, dilatation of vessels perfusing large amounts of myocardium exposes patients to higher subsequent mortality due to vessel restenosis or occlusion. This problem appears to be greatest for left main stenosis dilatations. Three-year survivorship in patients with protected left main stenosis is 87%, but only 40% for patients with unprotected left main stenosis.[6]

Unlike the situation of left main coronary stenosis, fewer data exist on the risk of coronary angioplasty in patients undergoing dilatation of other vessels perfusing substantial amounts of myocardium. An example of the latter would be dilatation of a proximal stenosis in a vessel providing extensive collateralization to another ma-

TABLE 39–1.

Coronary Angioplasty Procedural Mortality*

Factor	Mortality (%)
Total group	0.7
Low risk	0.25
PTCA of 3 vessels	1.3
Age > 70 yr	1.4
Left main equivalent	2.6
Ejection fraction < 40%	2.9
Left main stenosis	3.4

*Adapted from Hartzler GO, Rutherford BD, McConahay DR, et al: *Am J Cardiol* 1988; 61: 33–37.

jor distribution. Recent experience with dilatation of patients' only patent coronary vessel, which has been made possible through the use of systemic circulatory support, suggests that only about 40% of such individuals can tolerate even transient vessel occlusion. We have also found that although dilatation of less critical stenoses and patients with poor ventricular function has been better tolerated than originally predicted, individual patient response cannot always be predicted by clinical criteria. Some patients have developed irreversible hemodynamic collapse following even brief and successful dilatations. Thus, there appears to be an important role for myocardial and systemic circulatory support for many high-risk patients.

MYOCARDIAL PERFUSION

During experiments in canine preparations, Grüntzig found that ventricular dysfunction and arrhythmias were common and promptly followed balloon occlusion. Before the first clinical interventions were performed, Grüntzig developed a pump system that would maintain blood flow distal to the balloon occlusion.[8] The early, low-risk patients undergoing angioplasty tolerated balloon occlusion better than expected, however, and this precluded the early need for coronary perfusion. As more high-risk cases were undertaken, several approaches to distal coronary perfusion during angioplasty have been developed. These include use of the autoperfusion catheter and pump perfusion of blood and Fluosol-DA, 20%. Characteristics of these three approaches are summarized in Table 39–2.[9] Preservation of ventricular function and metabolism has been demonstrated by using autologous blood pumped through a balloon catheter in both experimental and clinical studies. Meier et al.[10] infused blood through the lumen of an angioplasty catheter during prolonged balloon occlusion in 11 dogs and noted preservation of ventricular function in 8 of 9 surviving animals. These authors, however, noted the development of thrombosis around the catheter and hemolysis. Most approaches to antegrade coronary perfusion through the dilatation catheter require removal of the guidewire. Failure to remove the guidewire results in hemolysis and potassium release at flow rates as low as 60 mL/min,[11] the minimum rate thought to be fully protective for perfusion of the left anterior descending coronary artery. In addition to the problems of hemolysis and thrombosis, antegrade perfusion of autologous blood requires an arterial source. This has most commonly been achieved through the use of an oversized femoral sheath or contralateral arterial puncture.

Despite these limitations, antegrade autologous blood perfusion at 60 mL/min has been shown to reduce anginal pain and ST segment depression during clinical coronary angioplasty.[11–13] Although not widely employed, antegrade perfusion has been used in unstable patients and in those undergoing dilatation of vessels supplying substantial amounts of myocardium. Guidewire removal and use of at least moderate-profile catheters to preclude hemolysis and thrombosis are necessary. In general, protracted antegrade pump perfusion is not advised, and fixed wire systems cannot be employed.

In an attempt to reduce hemolysis and thrombosis, antegrade oxygen-carrying fluorocarbon perfusion has

TABLE 39–2.

Antegrade Perfusion During Angioplasty*

Feature	Autoperfusion Catheter	Pump Blood Perfusion	Pump Fluosol Perfusion
O$_2$ capacity	Normal	Normal	Decreased
Viscosity	High	High	Moderate
Vascular access	No	Yes	No
Pump	No	Yes	Yes
Disadvantages	High profile Lower flow rate Less effective in hypotension	Possible hemolysis thrombosis	Reduced O$_2$ delivery

*Adapted from Rossen JD: *Cardiology* 1986; 6:103–106.

been tried. The most commonly used oxygen carrier is Fluosol-DA, 20%, which is a moderate-viscosity emulsion of perfluorodecaline and perfluorotripropylamine. It has a lower oxygen affinity than blood and requires hyperoxygenation at a pO_2 of 600 mm Hg to carry approximately one third of the oxygen-saturated blood concentration. In experimental studies, Fluosol infusion has improved regional left ventricular dysfunction during balloon occlusion but was less effective than autologous blood perfusion.[14] Variable results have been found in clinical studies. Anderson et al. found only a modest increment in time to the onset of angina associated with oxygenated Fluosol infusion.[15] In contrast, Cleman et al.[16] using echocardiography, demonstrated a marked reduction in ischemic myocardial dysfunction when distal Fluosol perfusion was used during 45- to 60-second occlusions. Prolonged Fluosol perfusion appears to be well tolerated but cannot be expected to preclude ischemia in all patients.

Due to its linear oxygen uptake, Fluosol is saturated with 95% oxygen and 5% carbon dioxide by bubbling the gas mixture through the body-temperature emulsion. A new cartridge system permitting rapid oxygenation has reduced the saturation time from 30 minutes to about 60 seconds. Fluosol, however, requires about 20 minutes to thaw, a process that should not be done more than 3 hours before use.[17] An additional benefit of Fluosol is that it reduces polymorphonuclear leukocyte function, which may have benefit in reducing free radical injury during acute myocardial infarction.[18, 19]

In an attempt to eliminate the need for additional arterial access and pump technology, several autoperfusion balloon catheter systems have been evaluated in experimental and clinical studies.[20–24] Autoperfusion balloon catheters have in common the presence of multiple shaft side holes proximal and distal to the balloon and a central lumen that allows blood to flow passively. Distal coronary perfusion is directly related to perfusion pressure, and flows of 40 to 60 mL/min are provided with only near-normal systemic blood pressure. Under these conditions, autoperfusion appears adequate during prolonged balloon inflations to maintain near-normal ventricular function. Under hypotensive conditions, however, inadequate perfusion may result, and vasopressors have been found helpful to maintain flow through the catheter.

A 4.5 F polyethylene catheter with 14 side holes over its distal 10 cm has recently been clinically introduced (Stack Perfusion Catheter, Advanced Cardiovascular Systems, Inc.). The device can be passed over a 0.018-in. guidewire, but because of its larger profile, it is generally limited to proximal major coronary artery loca-

tions. At times, predilatation using a 2.0-mm low-profile catheter has been found necessary to allow passage of the perfusion balloon catheter. The guidewire is withdrawn prior to balloon inflation, which is gradually augmented up to a maximum of 8 atm. The central lumen is periodically flushed with heparinized saline under clinical conditions. During balloon inflation, it is also helpful to disengage the guiding catheter from the coronary ostium to maximize coronary blood flow. The perfusion balloon catheter appears to be a helpful system for dilatations of large proximal coronary vessels in patients with initially adequate blood pressures. Unfortunately, early evidence does not suggest that prolonged balloon inflations reduce arterial restenosis, although they appear to be helpful in situations of inadequate dilatation, in the presence of intraluminal thrombus, and following acute vessel closure.[25] The utility of the perfusion balloon catheter in enabling high-risk angioplasty to be performed has yet to be determined.

Another approach to providing myocardial nutrition is through coronary sinus retroperfusion. This approach consists of electrocardiographically (ECG) synchronized diastolic retroperfusion at flow rates up to 150 mL/min. This approach appears to be of value for preventing coronary ischemia during dilatation of the left anterior descending system, but its efficacy for other distributions is as yet unproved. Two advantages of this technique are that myocardial perfusion can be provided without direct coronary artery access and that pharmacologic agents can be delivered to ischemic areas in high concentrations.[26–28]

SYSTEMIC CIRCULATORY SUPPORT

Systemic circulatory support has been accomplished with the intra-aortic balloon pump and by percutaneous femorofemoral cardiopulmonary bypass in the most high-risk patients. A comparison of these two techniques is summarized in Table 39–3. Intra-aortic balloon pumping increases cardiac output 20% to 30% in patients without significant rhythm disturbances. Several studies have reported that patients with ejection fractions as low as 20% and those undergoing dilatation of critical coronary vessels appear to do well when intra-aortic balloon pumping is initiated prior to angioplasty.[29–32] The role of the intra-aortic balloon appears best suited to moderate-risk patients who begin with or develop moderate systemic hypotension but retain stable rhythms (see below).

Attempting to undertake elective angioplasty in patients with the most severe ventricular dysfunction and/or target vessels supplying the majority of viable

TABLE 39–3.

Comparison of Intra-aortic Balloon Pump With Percutaneous Femorofemoral Cardiopulmonary Bypass

Feature	Intra-aortic Balloon Pump	Cardiopulmonary Bypass
Arterial assess	12–14 F	17–20 F
Venous access	No	18–20 F
Augmentation of cardiac output	20%–30%	4–6 L/min
Rhythm dependent	Yes	No
Duration of support	Days	Hours

myocardium, we began to place patients prophylactically on cardiopulmonary bypass in 1987, a technique we termed "supporting angioplasty."[33–38] The procedure is designed to be performed in the cardiac catheterization laboratory under local anesthesia, but intraoperative angioplasty on cardiopulmonary bypass has also been reported.[39] In the catheterization laboratory, cardiopulmonary support has been accomplished by using a portable, Food and Drug Administration (FDA) approved, centrifugal pump oxygenator system (CPS, C.R. Bard, Inc.) previously employed in emergency situations. This device differs from traditional heart-lung systems by placement of a centrifugal pump directly in line with the venous cannula. This allows active aspiration of blood from the right atrium and enables the use of 16 to 20 F cannulas. Up to 5-L/min flow can be provided with a combination of 19 F venous and 17 F arterial cannulas, and up to 3.5 L/min can be provided with a combination of 18 F venous and 16 F arterial cannulas. In contrast to the intra-aortic balloon, systemic flow is provided independent of intrinsic cardiac output or rhythm. Although the systemic circulation is fully supported by this approach, even during periods of cardiac arrest, myocardial perfusion is not augmented during balloon inflation, and segmental ventricular dysfunction has been shown to develop. For as yet unclear reasons, however, chest pain and ECG changes suggesting ischemia develop infrequently during coronary dilatation with patients on cardiopulmonary bypass.

SUPPORTED ANGIOPLASTY TECHNIQUE

We employ prophylactic cardiopulmonary bypass for patients at very high risk of hemodynamic collapse, i.e., severe ventricular dysfunction and/or target vessels supplying a large majority of viable myocardium. It is not entirely possible, however, to precisely predict those patients who will become hemodynamically unstable during interventions. We have also utilized standby femorofemoral support for patients at somewhat lesser risk.

Procedures are performed in the catheterization laboratory by a team composed of two interventional cardiologists, a perfusionist, an anesthesiologist, and two laboratory technicians. Local anesthesia and mild sedation are employed. Although femoral artery cannula insertion was initially performed by using surgical cutdown and vessel puncture under direct visualization, we have more recently utilized the percutaneous insertion technique developed by Shawl and coworkers.[37] Due to the large diameter of the cannulas employed, the size, level of bifurcation, and presence of vessel stenosis of the left femoral artery are determined prior to insertion by iliac angiography. Once vessel adequacy is established, guidewires are placed in the artery and vein by using the Seldinger technique. A long sheath is passed over the guidewires to facilitate subsequent passage of stiffer (0.038-in) guidewires. Progressively large dilators (12, 14 F) are then introduced into the artery, followed by passage of the cannula, which is sutured in place. Under fluoroscopic guidance, the longer venous cannula is positioned at the right atrial–inferior vena caval junction. Heparin is administered in a 300-unit kg dose prior to cannula insertion, and premedication with aspirin, nitroglycerin, and a calcium channel blocking agent is routinely given. The activated clotting time (ACT) is maintained at greater than 400 seconds during circulatory support. Heparin-bonded oxygenators requiring only clinically indicated anticoagulation have recently been developed. Heparin action is not reversed with protamine following support. Heparin treatment is reinstituted following cannula removal for a few days to prevent subacute vessel closure.

Standby support has been increasingly employed for high-risk, but not critical individuals.[40, 41] Our laboratory performs iliac angiography, sheath placement, and pump priming in such cases. If hemodynamic instability or vessel closure occurs, cannulation and initiation of cardiopulmonary bypass can be instituted in less than 2 to 3 minutes. Laboratories performing standby supported angioplasty have found that only 5% to 10% of patients require circulatory support, although it may be difficult to select those who will require it in advance.

Coronary angioplasty is performed once adequate circulatory support is established. Support allows prolonged balloon inflations of up to 5 to 7 minutes, and signs and symptoms of myocardial ischemia have been observed in only 20% to 25% of patients. The circulatory stability allows a greater number of balloon inflations and sequential use of different guiding and/or balloon catheters, thereby increasing the likelihood of optimal vessel opening.

Following successful angioplasty, pump flow is gradually decreased over a period of 3 to 5 minutes. Two methods are commonly employed for cannula removal. Most centers performing supported angioplasty remove the cannulas 4 to 6 hours following the procedure, when the ACT is about 240 seconds. A mechanical groin clamp is used to achieve hemostasis following cannula removal. Progressively lessening clamp pressure requires an additional 2 to 6 hours. If hemostasis cannot be obtained, surgical closure is performed. Other centers prefer to perform direct surgical closure immediately following the procedure, even if cannulas were placed percutaneously.

Patients sustaining vessel closure during supported angioplasty or unsupported angioplasty can be taken to the operating room on femorofemoral bypass with assurance of hemodynamic stability. The more time-consuming procedure of internal mammary grafting can be employed in these instances, although conversion to thoracic bypass is usually accomplished. Ventricular unloading has proved satisfactory on cardiopulmonary support as long as sinus rhythm is maintained. Autoperfusion ("bailout") catheters have been found additionally helpful following sustained vessel closure.

NATIONAL REGISTRY OF SUPPORTED ANGIOPLASTY

Data on more than 455 patients undergoing elective supported angioplasty in 21 centers have been collated in a national registry. Data included the entire experience of each center. Participating principal investigators and centers are listed in Table 39–4. Patients were considered supported angioplasty candidates if they had severe or unstable angina, a dilatable lesion, and a target vessel supply more than half the residual viable left ventricular myocardium or a left ventricular ejection fraction less than 25%.[36, 38] Trends in the registry's experience are listed in Table 39–5. Standby use of cardiopulmonary bypass increased from 1988 to 1989, the registry's first 2 years. During that time, percutaneous cannulation became widespread, with that technique being associated with lower mortality and morbidity than with the use of cutdown insertion. Initial vascular morbidity was high with percutaneous cannulation but declined significantly with procedural refinement.

Total hospital mortality fell slightly during the registry's first 2 years, with a majority being due to subacute vessel closure following initially successful procedures. Due to this experience, longer periods of heparin anti-

TABLE 39–4.
Elective Supported Angioplasty Registry

Robert Vogel, M.D.	Coordinator, University of Maryland
Gerald Dorros, M.D.	St. Lukes Hospital, Milwaukee
James Fergurson, III, M.D.	St. Lukes Hospital, Houston
Robert Freedman, Jr., M.D.	St. Francis Cabrini Hospital, Alexandria, Va
Barry George, M.D.	Riverside Hospital, Columbus, Ohio
Kenneth Kent, M.D.	Georgetown University Hospital, Washington, DC
Jeffrey Moses, M.D.	Lenox Hill Hospital, New York
Michael Mooney, M.D.	Minneapolis Heart Institute
William O'Neill, M.D.	Wm. Beaumont Hospital, Royal Oak, Mich
James O'Toole, M.D.	Shadyside Hospital, Pittsburgh
Paul Overlie, M.D.	Methodist Hospital, Lubbock, Tex
Fayaz Shawl, M.D.	Washington Adventist Hospital, Takoma Park, Md
Edward Simon, M.D.	Baptist Hospital, Miami
Sidney Smith Jr., M.D.	Sharp Memorial Hospital, San Diego
Simon Stertzer, M.D.	Seton Medical Center, San Francisco
Carl Tommaso, M.D.	University of Maryland Hospital
K. Kam Tabari, M.D.	San Jose Hospital
Paul Tierstein, M.D.	Scripps Clinic, La Jolla, Calif
Eric Topol, M.D.	University of Michigan Hospital, Ann Arbo
Michael Vandormael, M.D.	St. Louis University Hospital
John Vogel, M.D.	Goleta Valley Community Hospital
Christopher White, M.D.	Oschner Foundation Hospital, New Orleans

TABLE 39–5.

National Registry of Elective Supported Angioplasty

Results	1988	1989
Total patients	105	350
Institutions	14	20
Standby use	3.0%	26%
Percutaneous cannulation	55%	77%
Total morbidity	39%	18%
Hospital mortality	7.6%	5.8%
Mortality due to late vessel closure	3.8%	3.1%

TABLE 39–6.

Hospital Mortality of Elective Supported Angioplasty: Subgroup Analysis

Subgroups	Mortality (%)	Patients
CABG* inoperable	2.8	108
LVEF* <20%	3.9	76
PTCA only patent vessel	12	86
Left main coronary disease	20	55
Total	6.4	455

*CABG = Coronary artery bypass graft; LVEF = left ventricular ejection fraction.

coagulation are currently recommended. As is seen in Table 39–6, specific subgroups had very different outcomes. Patients who were deemed coronary bypass surgically inoperable and those with very low ejection fractions (<20%) did well, with a total hospital mortality rate of 3% to 4%. Those undergoing dilatation of their only patent coronary vessel and those with left main stenosis did less well. Patients with left main disease who were undergoing dilatation of any vessel did especially poorly.[42] The registry's experience was not randomized, and other reports on high-risk angioplasty may include different patient characteristics. With this caution in mind, intra-aortic balloon supported angioplasty has also been reported to have low hospital mortality.[32] Bypass surgery, however, in patients with left ventricular ejection fractions less than 20% appears to be high risk by comparison (26%).[43]

The outcome of the first 100 patients undergoing standby supported angioplasty is summarized in Figure 39–1. Only 8 patients required emergency initiation of cardiopulmonary bypass, although patient characteristics were similar to those undergoing prophylactic support, except for slightly better ventricular function (no ejection fractions <14%). Late vessel closure was the cause of death in all fatalities in those not requiring bypass and in 1 of the 2 who required bypass and surgery.

In all 8 instances, emergency cardiopulmonary bypass was initiated successfully. Five patients were stabilized without a need for surgery. This experience suggests that the use of standby or prophylactic circulatory support reduces the mortality of high-risk angioplasty about 50%. No differences in mortality were evident between standby and prophylactic bypass use, although the standby patients had lower vascular morbidity and transfusion requirements since cannulation was undertaken in a minority of cases.

Overall, the group underwent a mean of 1.8 dilatations per patient with a primary success rate of 95%. Ninety percent of patients were New York Heart Association (NYHA) anginal class III or IV prior to supported angioplasty. At a mean follow-up of 11 months, gratifyingly, 90% were anginal class I or II. This group's mean ejection fraction increased from 29% to 38%. Long-term survival also appears to be especially good for patients with such severe disease, with the 2-year survival rate being 80% (Fig 39–2).

CLINICAL PRACTICE

At present, there are no clear guidelines regarding utilization of any of the above myocardial and periph-

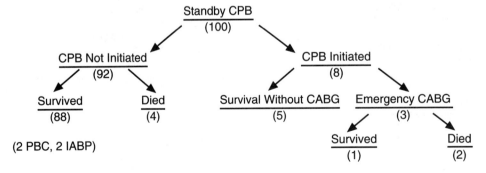

FIG 39–1.
Outcome of the first 100 patients undergoing standby supported angioplasty. Only eight patients required circulatory support, of whom five survived without bypass surgery.

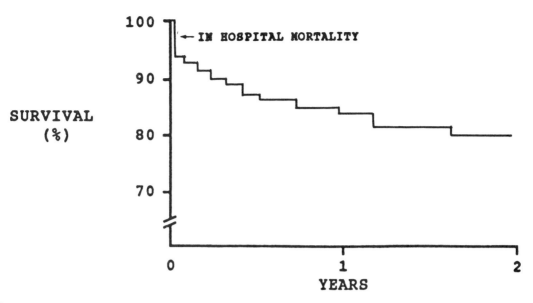

FIG 39–2.
Two-year survival curve for patients undergoing standby and prophylactic cardiopulmonary bypass supported angioplasty. Approximately one third of the total mortality occurred during the initial hospitalization.

eral circulatory support systems in specific clinical situations. Table 39–7 summarizes the two high-risk classes of angioplasty patients as judged at our institution. Clearly, patients with normal ventricular function and a limited extent of coronary disease require no circulatory support. The same is generally true of patients with moderate left ventricular dysfunction and/or triple-vessel disease. Many of these individuals are best treated with "staged" angioplasty to preclude the situation of multiple acute vessel closure. It is not reasonable to perform multiple-vessel angioplasty on these individuals even with circulatory support because they will be subject to acute vessel closure following the procedure.

Patients with more advanced disease, defined by ejection fractions between 21% and 30% and/or target vessels supplying the majority of viable myocardium, will

probably benefit from prophylactic or standby circulatory assistance. Standby cardiopulmonary bypass or intra-aortic balloon pumping are close alternatives. If technically feasible, perfusion balloon angioplasty appears useful for managing patients at this level of risk, as long as systemic pressure can be maintained. Unfortunately, it appears difficult to predict which patients in this category will undergo circulatory collapse. Patients at the highest risk include those with ejection fractions less than 21%, those undergoing dilatation of their only patent coronary vessel, and those who develop extreme hemodynamic instability during balloon inflation. We believe that such individuals are best handled with prophylactic femorofemoral cardiopulmonary bypass. As a group, circulatory support has clearly extended the use of coronary angioplasty to patients who were previously

TABLE 39–7.
Recommended Use of Circulatory Support During High-Risk Coronary Angioplasty

Risk	Patient Characteristics	Circulatory Support Options
High	PTCA vessel supplying >½ viable myocardium and/or LVEF* 15%–25%	Standby CPB* Perfusion balloon IABP* CS retroperfusion
Very high	Only patent vessel LVEF < 15% or Hemodynamic collapse during PTCA	Prophylactic CPB Hemopump LV assist

*CPB = cardiopulmonary bypass; IABP = intra-aortic balloon pumping; LVEF = left ventricular ejection fraction; CS = coronary sinus.

not considered appropriate candidates. Fortunately, many of these patients appear to benefit substantially from this option.

REFERENCES

1. Grüntzig AR, Senning A, Seigenthaler WE: Non-operative dilatation of coronary artery site: Percutaneous transluminal coronary angioplasty. *N Engl J Med* 1979; 301:61–68.
2. Tommaso CL: Management of high-risk coronary angioplasty. *Am J Cardiol* 1989; 64:33–37.
3. Ryan TJ, Faxon DP, Gunner RM, et al: Guidelines for percutaneous transluminal coronary angioplasty. *J Am Coll Cardiol* 1988; 12:529–545.
4. Bentivoglio LG, VanRaden MJ, Kelsey SF, et al: Percutaneous transluminal coronary angioplasty (PTCA) in patients with relative counterindications: Results of the National Heart, Lung, and Blood Institute PTCA Registry. *Am J Cardiol* 1984; 53:82–88.
5. Ellis SG, Topol EJ: Results of percutaneous transluminal coronary angioplasty of high-risk angulated stenosis. *Am J Cardiol* 1990; 66:932–937.
6. Hartzler GO, Rutherford BD, McConahay DR et al: "High-risk" percutaneous transluminal coronary angioplasty. *Am J Cardiol* 1988; 61:33–37.
7. Kohli RS, DiSciascio G, Cowley MJ et al: Coronary angioplasty in patients with severe ventricular dysfunction. *J Am Coll Cardiol* 1990; 16:807–811.
8. Hurst JW: The first coronary angioplasty as described by Andreas Grüntzig. *Am J Cardiol* 1986; 57:185–186.
9. Rossen JD: Perfusion during coronary angioplasty. *Cardiology* 1989; 6:103–106.
10. Meier B, Grüntzig AR, Dekmezian RH, et al: Percutaneous perfusion of occluded coronary arteries with blood from the femoral artery: A dog study. *Cathet Cardiovasc Diagn* 1985; 11:81–87.
11. Lehmann KG, Atwood E, Snyder EL, et al: Autologous blood perfusion for myocardial protection during coronary angioplasty: A feasibility study. *Circulation* 1987; 76:312–323.
12. Angelini P, Heibig J, Leachman R: Distal hemoperfusion during percutaneous transluminal coronary angioplasty. *Am J Cardiol* 1986; 58:252–255.
13. Heibig J, Angelini P, Leachman DR, et al: Use of mechanical devices for distal hemoperfusion during balloon catheter coronary angioplasty. *Cathet Cardiovasc Diagn* 1988; 15:143–149.
14. Tokioka H, Miyazoki A, Fung P, et al: Effects of intracoronary perfusion of arterial blood or Fluosol-DA 20% on regional myacardial metabolism and function during brief coronary artery occlusions. *Circulation* 1987; 75:473–481.
15. Anderson HV, Leimgruber PP, Roubin GS, et al: Distal coronary artery perfusion during percutaneous transluminal coronary angioplasty. *Am Heart J* 1985; 110:720–726.
16. Cleman M, Jaffee CC, Wohlgelernter D: Prevention of ischemia during percutaneous transluminal coronary angioplasty by transcatheter infusion of oxygenated Fluosol DA 20%. *Circulation* 1986; 74:555–562.
17. Cleman MW, LaSala JM: Protected PTCA, in Topol EJ (ed): *Textbook of Interventional Cardiology*, Philadelphia, WB Saunders, 1990, pp 496–514.
18. Lane TA, Lamkin GE: Paralysis of phagocyte migration due to an artificial blood substitute. *Blood* 1984; 64:400–405.
19. Schaer GL, Karas SP, Santoian EC, et al: Reduction in reperfusion injury by blood-free reperfusion after experimental myocardial infarction. *J Am Coll Cardiol* 1990; 15:1385–1393.
20. Quigley PJ, Hinohora T, Phillips HR, et al: Myocardial protection during coronary angioplasty with an autoperfusion balloon catheter in humans. *Circulation* 1988; 78:1128–1134.
21. Turi ZG, Campbell CA, Gottimukkala MV, et al: Preservation of distal coronary perfusion during prolonged balloon inflation with an autoperfusion angioplasty catheter. *Circulation* 1987; 75:1273–1280.
22. Turi ZG, Pezkalla S, Campbell CA, et al: Amelioration of ischemia during angioplasty of the left anterior descending coronary artery with an autoperfusion catheter. *Am J Cardiol* 1988; 62:513–517.
23. Erbel R, Clas W, Bursch U, et al: New balloon catheter for prolonged percutaneous transluminal coronary angioplasty and bypass flow in occluded vessels. *Cathet Cardiovasc Diagn* 1986; 12:116–123.
24. Stack RS, Quigley PJ, Collins G, et al: Perfusion balloon catheter. *Am J Cardiol* 1988; 61:77–80.
25. Kereiakes DJ, Stack RS: Perfusion angioplasty, in Topol EJ (ed): *Textbook of Interventional Cardiology*. Philadelphia, WB Saunders, 1990, pp 452–466.
26. Yamazaki S, Drury K, Meerbaum S, et al: Synchronized coronary venous retroperfusion: Prompt improvement of the left ventricular function in experimental myocardial ischemia. *J Am Coll Cardiol* 1985; 5:655–663.
27. Drury JK, Yamazaki S, Fishbein MC, et al: Synchronized diastolic coronary venous retroperfusion; results of a preclinical safety and efficacy study. *J Am Coll Cardiol* 1985; 6:328–335.
28. Gore JM, Weiner BH, Benotti JR, et al: Preliminary experience with synchronized coronary sinus retroperfusion in humans. *Circulation* 1986; 74:381–388.
29. Margolis JR: The role of the percutaneous intra-aortic balloon in emergency situations following percutaneous transluminal coronary angioplasty, in Kaltenbach M, Grüntzig A, Rentrop P, et al (eds): *Transluminal Coronary Angioplasty and Intracoronary Thrombolysis*. Berlin, Springer-Verlag, 1982, pp 145–150.
30. Alcan KE, Stertzer SH, Walsh JE, et al: The role of intra-aortic balloon counterpulsation in patients undergoing percutaneous transluminal coronary angioplasty. *Am Heart J* 1983; 105:527–530.
31. Szatmary LJ, Marco J, Fajadet J, et al: The combined use of diastolic counterpulsation and coronary dilatation in unstable angina due to multivessel disease under unstable hemodynamic conditions. *Int J Cardiol* 1988; 19:59–66.
32. Kahn JK, Rutherford BD, McConahay DR, et al: Supported "high-risk" coronary angioplasty using intraaortic balloon pump counterpulsation. *J Am Coll Cardiol* 1990; 15:1151–1155.
33. Vogel R, Tommaso C, Gundry S: Initial experience with angioplasty and aortic valvuloplasty using elective semi-

percutaneous cardiopulmonary support. *Am J Cardiol* 1988; 62:811–813.

34. Vogel RA: The Maryland experience: Angioplasty and valvuloplasty using percutaneous cardiopulmonary support. *Am J Cardiol* 1988; 62:11–14.

35. Vogel JHK, Ruiz CE, Janke EJ, et al: Percutaneous (non-surgical) supported angioplasty in unprotected left main disease and severe left ventricular dysfunction. *Clin Cardiol* 1989; 12:297–300.

36. Vogel RA, Shawl F, Tommaso C, et al: Initial report of the National Registry of elective cardiopulmonary bypass supported coronary angioplasty. *J Am Coll Cardiol* 1990; 15:23–29.

37. Shawl FA, Domanski MJ, Punja S, et al: Percutaneous cardiopulmonary bypass support in high-risk patients undergoing percutaneous transluminal coronary angioplasty. *Am Heart J* 1989; 64:1258–1263.

38. Vogel RA, Tommaso CL: Elective supported angioplasty: Initial report of the National Registry. *Cathet Cardiovasc Diagn* 1990; 20:22–26.

39. Jones EL, King SB: Intraoperative balloon catheter dilatation in the treatment of coronary artery disease. *Am Heart J* 1984; 107:836–837.

40. Tommaso CL, Vogel RA: Supported vs standby supported angioplasty (abstract) *Circulation* 1989; 80(suppl 2):272.

41. Teirstein PS, Vogel RA, Dorros G, et al: Prophylactic vs standby cardiopulmonary support for high-risk PTCA (abstract) *Circulation* 1990; 82(suppl 3):680.

42. Tommaso CL, Deligonul U, Vogel JHK et al: Angioplasty of the left main coronary artery: Results of the supported angioplasty registry (abstract). *Circulation* 1990; 82(suppl 3):654.

43. Hannan EL, Kilburn H Jr, O'Donnell JF et al: Adult open heart surgery in New York State: An analysis of risk factors and hospital mortality rates. *JAMA* 1990; 264:2768–2774.

Percutaneous Cardiopulmonary Bypass Support: Current Technique and Future Directions

Fayaz A. Shawl, M.D.

Coronary artery disease remains the most common cause of death in the industrialized countries. The first major advance in the treatment of atherosclerosis was coronary artery bypass graft surgery. The subsequent introduction of percutaneous transluminal coronary angioplasty (PTCA) began a new era of treatment of cardiovascular disease.

The growth of PTCA has continued, and the complexity of approachable lesions has increased since its introduction by Dr. Grüntzig in 1977.[1] PTCA was initially limited to patients with single-vessel coronary artery disease and normal left ventricular function.[2] However, with advances in catheter technology, including guiding catheter development and increased operator experience, the application of PTCA has been extended to patients with multivessel coronary disease, unstable angina, and acute myocardial infarction and to symptomatic patients with prior coronary bypass graft surgery.[3–5]

Despite the dramatic increase in the number of PTCAs, there remain certain limitations such as abrupt closure, which occurs in approximately 5% of cases.[6,7] While most patients tolerate abrupt closure, it is nonetheless associated with a mortality rate between 2% and 12%, as well as a Q wave myocardial infarction rate of more than 25% when such patients are sent for emergency coronary bypass graft surgery.[8,9] Some patients, particularly those with poor left ventricular function or those in whom the target vessel supplies a large amount of viable myocardium, may experience hemodynamic collapse following abrupt closure, and these patients may not even tolerate transient ischemia during balloon dilatation.

The cardiac catheterization laboratory has been transformed from a purely diagnostic to an interventional setting. Coronary intervention is being undertaken in increasingly high-risk patients, and therefore, there is a clear need to provide effective, temporary circulatory support.

Recently femorofemoral cardiopulmonary bypass support has been introduced to provide hemodynamic support to certain high-risk patients undergoing PTCA,[10] but the necessity for surgical cutdown has limited its use in the catheterization laboratory, particularly in emergencies.

The author has recently developed a percutaneous technique for establishing femorofemoral cardiopulmonary bypass support in awake, conscious patients in the catheterization laboratory.[11, 12] This chapter describes the technique, physiology of cardiopulmonary bypass, suggested indications, patient management while on cardiopulmonary bypass support, and complications encountered during percutaneously established cardiopulmonary support.

SUGGESTED INDICATIONS

In the past, cardiopulmonary bypass support using the femoral approach has been used predominantly in emergency situations outside the cardiac catheterization laboratory. Lande et al.[13] instituted cardiopulmonary bypass support in the emergency room in 18 patients with either cardiogenic shock, cardiac arrest, or pulmonary insufficiency. The time of cardiopulmonary bypass support varied from 45 minutes to 2 hours. Sixteen patients showed marked improvement, and these were 3 long-term survivors. Subsequently, Baird and his colleagues[14] treated 25 patients in cardiac arrest with cardiopulmonary bypass support. Twenty-eight of these otherwise terminally ill patients survived when the femoral approach was used. Also, Mattox and Beall[15] describe the application of portable cardiopulmonary bypass support in 43 patients who were at the point of death. There were 17 long-term survivors (up to 10 years). However, it was not until 1982 that Phillips and his coworkers[16] described the percutaneous initiation of cardiopulmonary bypass support in 5 patients with refractory cardiac arrest. They used 12 F cannulas and achieved a flow rate of 2 to 2.5 L/min.

The application of a portable cardiopulmonary bypass support system in the setting of coronary angioplasty was first reported by Kanter and his coworkers,[17] who used it to revive six patients with cardiac arrest or cardiogenic shock as a result of complications due to coronary angioplasty. These patients were unresponsive to conventional resuscitation, including intra-aortic balloon pumping. Subsequently, Vogel et al.[10] described three patients in whom coronary angioplasty was performed with prophylactic cardiopulmonary bypass support. In these three patients and in Kanter's group,[17] cardiopulmonary bypass support was instituted by using 18 or 20 F bypass cannulas placed by surgical cutdown.

In 1988 the author introduced the technique of percutaneous cardiopulmonary bypass support (PCPS) using 18 F or 20 F cannulas in the catheterization labora-

tory for patients undergoing emergency as well as elective high-risk interventions.[11]

The indications for the institution of PCPS can be categorized as either elective or emergent.[18-24] PCPS may be instituted electively as a prophylactic measure during high-risk coronary angioplasty (supported angioplasty). Patients considered for emergent PCPS include those in cardiogenic shock from acute myocardial infarction as well as patients who sustain cardiac arrest in the catheterization laboratory. Other suggested indications for the institution of PCPS are shown in Table 40-1.

CONTRAINDICATIONS

PCPS requires the use of intense anticoagulation, which makes the procedure inappropriate in patients with contraindications to anticoagulation. The other important contraindication is severe peripheral vascular disease. In selected patients, iliofemoral angioplasty has been performed prior to insertion of the bypass cannula. The contraindications are summarized in Table 40-2.

TECHNIQUE OF ELECTIVE PERCUTANEOUS CARDIOPULMONARY BYPASS SUPPORT

Patients are prepared and draped in the catheterization laboratory in the usual sterile manner, with both groin creases exposed. All items necessary for percutaneous cannula insertion (Fig 40-1) are available in a compact kit (Percutaneous Insertion Kit, Shawl Technique, C.R. Bard, Inc., Billerica, Mass).

TABLE 40-1.
Suggested Indications for Percutaneous Cardiopulmonary Bypass Support

Abrupt vessel closure associated with hemodynamic collapse
Cardiac arrest in the catheterization laboratory
High-risk coronary angioplasty
High-risk valvuloplasty
Cardiogenic shock due to acute myocardial infarction
Massive pulmonary embolism prior to pulmonary embolectomy
Prevention of reperfusion injury with the use of cardioplegic solution
During electrophysiologic testing, compromising ventricular tachycardia
Hypothermia
Thoracic aneurysm
Prior to repeat coronary bypass surgery
Near-drowning
Drug overdose
Bridge to other mechanical assist devices or cardiac transplantation

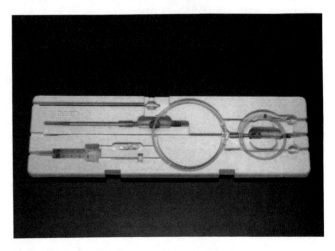

FIG 40-1.
Equipment necessary for percutaneous cannula insertion (commercially available percutaneous kit), including 18 arterial and venous cannulas, dilators, guidewires, syringe, needle, and scalpel blade.

TABLE 40-2.
Contraindication to the Institution of Percutaneous
Cardiopulmonary Bypass Support

Severe peripheral atherosclerotic disease
History of recent cerebro vascular accident
Pre-existing coagulopathy
Active bleeding
Untreatable or terminal disease
Suspected traumatic closed head injury
Unwitnessed normothermic cardiac arrest
Refracted cardiac arrest of long duration (normothermic)
Severe aortic regurgitation

ILIOFEMORAL ANGIOGRAPHY

By using the Seldinger technique, a 7 F pigtail catheter is introduced into the right femoral artery in order to perform iliofemoral angiography, initially visualizing the left (Fig 40–2) and then, if necessary, the right side. The tip of the pigtail is positioned just above the bifurcation of the aorta, and 16 cc of a contrast agent is power-injected at a rate of 8 cc/sec. Prior to angiography, a needle (the same as that used for percutaneous vascular access) is placed along the groin crease as a marker to establish the relationship of the skin crease to the bifurcation of the femoral system and as a guide for arterial entry (Fig 40–2,B). If the left iliofemoral system (Fig

40–3 and 40–4) has suitable anatomy, a Swan-Ganz catheter is placed in the right femoral vein and advanced to the pulmonary artery for monitoring hemodynamic parameters prior to, during, and after the procedure. If the anatomy of the left iliofemoral system is unsuitable (small caliber or critically diseased) for bypass cannulas, angiography is performed on the right side by using the same technique. If the left iliofemoral system reveals acceptable anatomy for the institution of bypass cannulas, the pigtail catheter is exchanged over a standard 0.038-in. guidewire for a standard 8 F long angioplasty sheath (USCI Division, C.R. Bard, Billerica, Mass), which is introduced into the right femoral artery.

CANNULATION

Access to the left femoral artery and vein is obtained by using a standard single-wall needle, and 7 or 8 F sheaths are left in place. With knowledge of the iliofemoral anatomy together with its relationship to the skin crease (needle marker), the common femoral artery (Fig 40–4) or femoral artery below the bifurcation (if of adequate caliber) is entered (Fig 40–2 and 40–3). Care is taken to ensure that the actual arterial puncture site is below the inguinal ligament (the line joining the iliac crest and symphysis pubis) in order to facilitate subse-

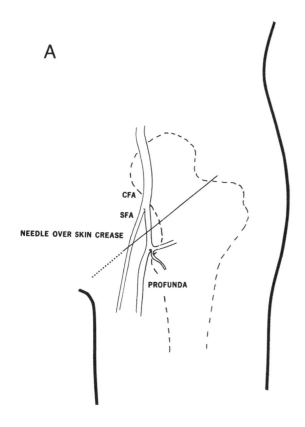

A

CFA

SFA

NEEDLE OVER SKIN CREASE

PROFUNDA

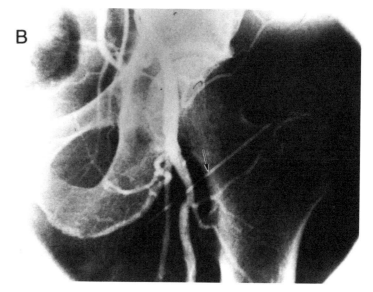

B

FIG 40-2.
A, left iliofemoral cineangiogram performed prior to cannulation to assess the adequacy for cannula placement. The skin crease is marked with a radiopaque needle *(arrow)* placed on the surface of the skin before angiography. **B,** Schematic representation of the iliofemoral system with the needle marker in place. Note that the angiogram allows selection of the appropriate vessel for cannulation (profunda rather than superficial femoral artery *[SFA]* or common femoral artery *[CFA]* in this case).

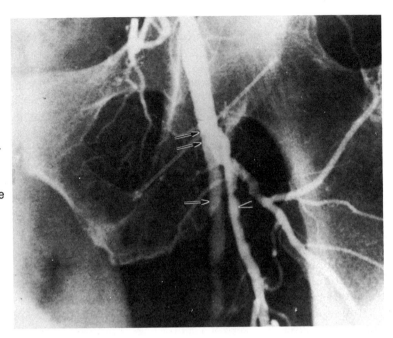

FIG 40–3.
Left iliofemoral cineangiogram with a needle maker left in place. Note that the appropriate vessel for cannulation is the superficial femoral artery *(arrow)* or common femoral *(double arrows)* rather than the profunda *(arrowhead).*

quent external clamp placement for hemostasis. Patients are then heparinized with 225 units of heparin (as a single bolus) per kilogram of body weight to obtain an activated clotting time of ≥400 seconds, which is checked after 10 or 15 minutes. The percutaneous insertion kit that contains the 18 F cannulas is opened next. Then, the 0.038-in. flexible guidewire is introduced through the arterial sheath (the arterial bypass cannula is introduced before the venous cannula). With this 0.038-in. flexible guidewire kept in place, the arterial sheath is re-

moved, and a long 8 F dilator is introduced. The tip of this long dilator usually lies above the bifurcation of the descending aorta. The 0.038-in. flexible guidewire is removed and replaced with the stiff 0.038-in. guidewire with a flexible tip. With the stiff guidewire held in place (its soft tip should remain above the level of the diaphram), the long 8 F dilator is removed, and the vessel is then dilated with a 12 F and then a 14 F dilator. Before the 14 F dilator is removed, a 1- to 2-mm skin incision is made at the entry site by using a no. 11 blade

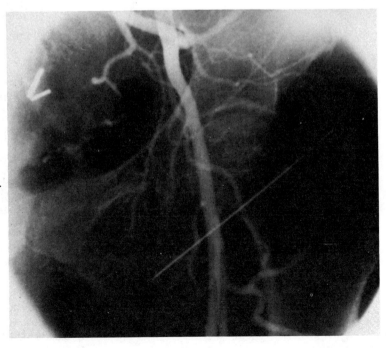

FIG 40–4.
Left iliofemoral cineangiogram showing a low bifurcation of the common femoral artery. Here, the appropriate vessel for cannulation is the common femoral *(arrow).*

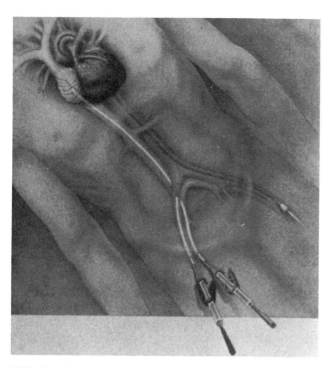

FIG 40–5.
Schematic representation of the appropriate position of the arterial and venous cannulas. Note placement of the tip of the venous cannula just above the junction of the inferior vena cava and right atrium. The aterial cannula is advanced until the hub is flush with the skin. Also note that a right femoral approach is shown in the diagram whereas the left femoral approach is more commonly used in elective cases, with PTCA performed from the contralateral side. (From Shawl FA, Domanski MJ, Wish MH: *Am Heart J* 1990; 120:195—203. Used with permission.)

to accommodate the bypass cannulas. The 14 F dilator is removed, and an 18 F arterial cannula (C.R. Bard, Inc.) is advanced over the stiff guidewire in a rotary motion, care being taken to advance both dilator and cannula assembly as a single unit so that the cannula does not buckle. This is best accomplished by having an assistant hold the proximal end of the cannula and dilator firmly together. After introduction of the 18 F arterial cannula (in our initial series 20 F cannulas were used), the guidewire and the dilator are removed, and the tubing is quickly closed by using the available Robert's clamp (see Fig 40–6). In a similar approach, an 18 F multihole venous cannula (C.R. Bard, Inc.) is advanced until the tip is positioned just above the junction of the inferior vena cava and the right atrium (Fig 40–5). During advancement of the venous cannula, the soft tip of the stiff guidewire is positioned in the superior vena cava.

Iliofemoral angiography is not performed in patients who present with cardiac arrest. Bypass cannulas are

placed in these patients by using previous arterial and venous access sites or obtaining bypass cannula access from the right femoral approach. After the patient has been placed on cardiopulmonary bypass support, the contralateral femoral vessel is used for angiography or intervention if indicated. In patients with cardiogenic shock, diagnostic angiography is performed after bypass support is initiated.

It takes less than 4 minutes to cannulate a patient for PCPS using the author's technique after venous and arterial access is obtained. While cannulation is being performed, a perfusionist primes the disposable perfusion circuit (C.R. Bard, Inc.).

ADDITIONAL TECHNICAL CONSIDERATIONS

1. *Tortuous iliofemoral arterial system.* A tortuous but patent iliofemoral system does not preclude cannula placement if the vessels are of adequate size (Fig 40–6). In approaching a tortuous system it is important to first pass a very flexible guidewire into the descending aorta. A long dilator (see Fig 40–1) is then advanced over the flexible guidewire, and the flexible guidewire is exchanged for a stiff guidewire via the long dilator. The long dilator is then removed over the stiff guidewire and the tip of the stiff guidewire left above the level of the diaphram. The stiff guidewire straightens the artery (Fig 40–6,D) and allows safe placement of the arterial cannula (Fig 40–6,E). If the contralateral vessel is of adequate size and is less tortuous, it may be used instead.

2. *Critical iliofemoral stenoses.* Severe iliofemoral disease should prompt arteriography of the contralateral system. If both systems are severely diseased, angioplasty of the iliofemoral system may be performed if feasible, followed by immediate cannula placement (Fig 40–7). Iliofemoral disease sufficiently severe to require angioplasty prior to cannula placement has been infrequent because patients with symptoms suggestive of peripheral vascular disease are usually excluded.

3. *Abdominal aortic aneurysm.* Although our experience has been limited (four cases), the presence of an abdominal aortic aneurysm does not appear to preclude cannula placement because the tip of the arterial cannula is generally at or below the aortic bifurcation.

PORTABLE CARDIOPULMONARY SUPPORT SYSTEM

The cardiopulmonary bypass support system (CPS, C.R. Bard, Inc.) is a battery-operated portable system on a hospital cart (Fig 40–8) with a disposable CPS cir-

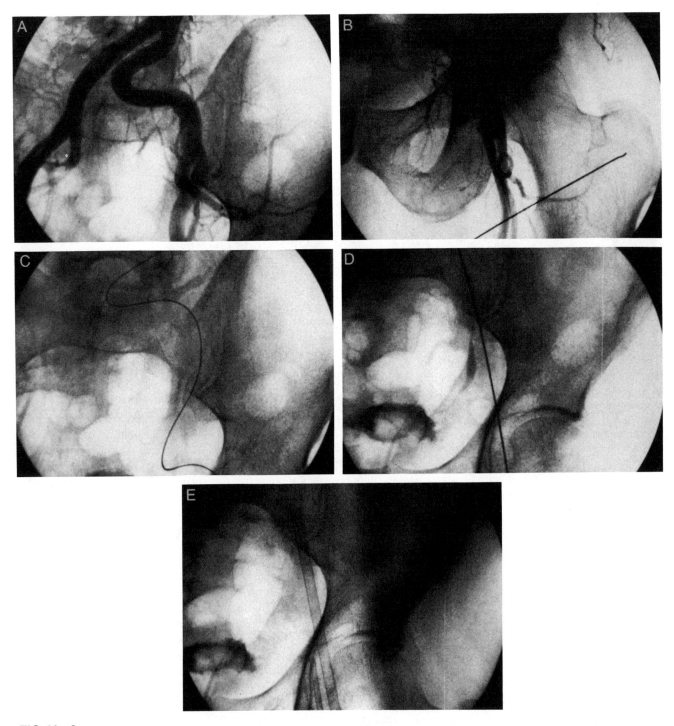

FIG 40–6.
A and **B,** cineangiograms prior to cannula placement show severe tortuosity of the left iliofemoral system. **C,** flexible guidewire in place in the left iliofemoral system. The J tip should be positioned above the level of the diaphram (not shown here). Passage of the wire is facilitated by advancing the long dilator. **D,** the stiff guidewire in place (note straightening of the tortuous artery by the stiff guidewire). **E,** arterial bypass cannula in place (note the continued straightening of the initially tortuous vessel).

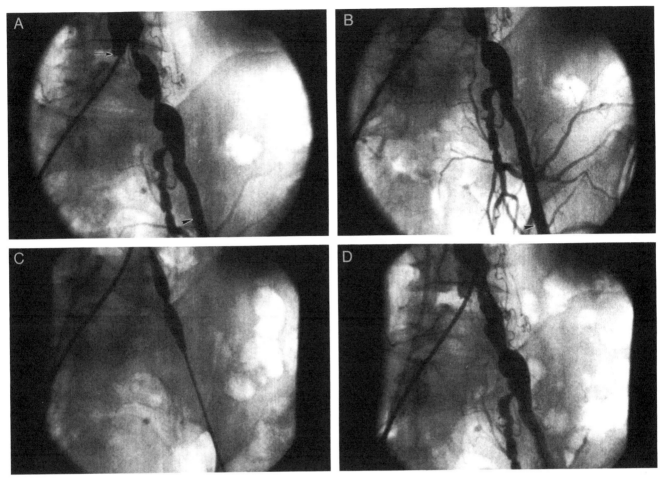

FIG 40–7.
A and **B,** cineangiograms prior to cannula placement show a totally occluded right common iliac *(arrow)* and critical stenoses involving the left iliac system but disease-free common femoral *(arrowheads).* **C,** peripheral angioplasty of the left iliac stenosis prior to cannulation. **D,** postangioplasty result in the left iliac.

cuit that includes a centrifugal, nonocclusive pump (Bio-Pump), a polypropylene hollow-fiber membrane oxygenator, clamps, connectors, and a heat exchanger. The perfusion circuit is primed by a perfusionist with 1,300 cc of Normosol. It takes less than 10 minutes to set up and prime this system.

With a vortex pump, blood is aspirated directly from the right atrium and vena cava; this has two advantages over the standard gravity drainage used in the standard heart-lung bypass machine. With this system, greater blood flow can be achieved with smaller cannulas, and the nonocclusive nature of the centrifugal pump does not allow excessive pressure to develop if an outlet of the pump is occluded.[25] These both are major problems with conventional roller pumps. After the blood is aspirated into the venous cannula (Fig 40–9), it is directed into the water-based heat exchanger. Blood then leaves the heat exchanger and is pumped into the central core

of the hollow-fiber membrane oxygenator. There are many potential advantages to this type of membrane. Gas exchange may be relatively atraumatic when compared with other membrane oxygenators.[26–28] The use of this design also results in a very low pressure drop across the membrane (40 mm Hg, with a 6-L/min blood flow), which allows for higher flows at lower pressures.[25] Again, a low-pressure system is safe from cavitation or explosion. Another advantage of CPS is that it is relatively safe from the hazard of introduction of air. The vortex nature of the centrifugal pump will lock any massive amount of air in the pump and prevent delivery of the air into the patient. Small amounts of air are trapped in the membrane system and diffuse out the gas path. Because of the ease of setup, priming, and operation, combined with the inherent safety features of the system, the technical perfusion skills are simplified.[25] These features make this system ideal in the cardiac

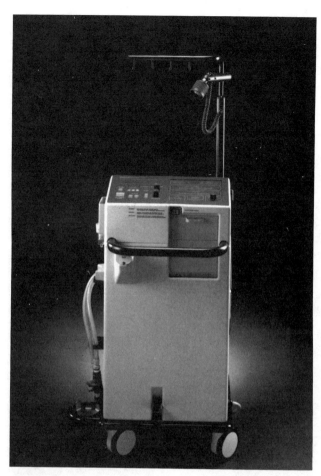

FIG 40–8.
Portable cardiopulmonary bypass support system.

catheterization laboratory in conjunction with a well-coordinated team approach.

BASIC PHYSIOLOGY OF CARDIOPULMONARY BYPASS

During operation of the PCPS in the cardiac catheterization laboratory, there is a reduction in pulmonary capillary wedge pressure (or pulmonary artery diastolic pressure) to approximately 0 to 5 mm Hg in approximately 90% of cases. There is also a reduction in systolic arterial pressure, with a slight increase in diastolic pressure, the latter feature known to be present with nonpulsatile flow.

During the initiation of cardiopulmonary bypass a drop in mean arterial pressure often occurs. This drop may be due in part to the sudden decrease in viscosity upon introduction of the crystalloid priming volume. As bypass progresses, the mean arterial pressure will gradually increase partly due to the increased viscosity as the circulating blood volume and the prime become homogeneous and increasingly extravascular fluid shift occurs.

If significant hypotension (mean pressure < 60 mm Hg) occurs, the goal is to add volume to the intravascular space without significantly altering the blood chemistry. When the type of volume solution available during cardiopulmonary bypass is selected, four options are available. Crystalloid solutions, which are the major priming and volume replacement agent during bypass, should contain normal electrolyte values and have a pH adjusted to 7.4 to prevent an inadvertent buffer base effect. In addition, some type of hyperosmotic and hyperoncotic solution should be available for control of the

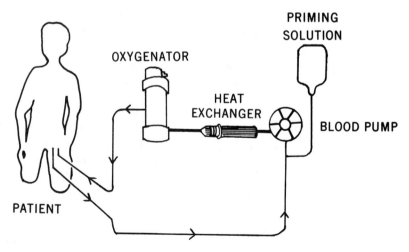

FIG 40–9.
Schematic of the cardiopulmonary bypass support system show active aspiration of venous blood by a vortex pump with subsequent passage of blood through the heat exchanger to the membrane oxygenator and return to the patient.

blood osmolarity and oncotic pressure when excessive crystalloid administration is required. Control of the colloid oncotic pressure and blood osmolarity is critical in controlling the degree of extravascular fluid shift commonly associated with bypass. This is especially evident in the application of cardiopulmonary bypass in resuscitation of the cardiac arrest patient who is unresponsive to conventional volume addition resuscitation. Several common solutions utilized are hetastarch solutions and varying concentrations of serum albumin solutions. The fourth product that should be made available is either autologus or homologous red cell products for their oncotic and hemoglobin benefit.

In the author's experience, the administration of 50 to 100 cc of 25% albumin to the priming volume has significantly reduced the additional volume requirement during PCPS supported interventions.

With 20 F cannulas, a flow of 4 to 6 L/min can be achieved; with 18 F cannulas, a flow of up to 5 L/min can be achieved, provided that the patient is well hydrated prior to the institution of cardiopulmonary bypass support. In most patients, angina or ischemic electrocardiographic changes are absent despite prolonged balloon inflation. Echocardiography of patients on bypass prior to balloon inflation has revealed a reduction in left atrial and left ventricular dimensions. These observations, together with reduction in the preload and afterload, suggest that cardiopulmonary bypass support reduces myocardial oxygen demand. These facts may be partially responsible for the lessening or absence of angina or electrocardiographic changes during balloon inflation. However, segmental wall motion abnormalities are worsened during balloon inflation, thus indicating ischemia distal to the occlusion.

INITIATION OF CARDIOPULMONARY BYPASS SUPPORT

Baseline hemodynamic measurements, which include systemic arterial, pulmonary artery, and pulmonary capillary wedge pressures, are obtained prior to the insertion of bypass cannulas. The arterial cannula is backbled by opening the Robert's clamp prior to its connection to the primed perfusion circuit. Next, venous and arterial cannulas are attached to the PCPS perfusion circuit while making sure that there are no air bubbles, particularly on the arterial side. Before the initiation of any flow, it is important to keep venous lines closed to the atmosphere. Elective patients are kept well hydrated before the initiation of cardiopulmonary bypass support. If the pulmonary artery diastolic (or pulmonary capillary wedge) pressure is less than 8 mm Hg, rapid volume infusion through the pump is given prior to full institution of bypass flow.

During elective supported angioplasty, cardiopulmonary bypass support is started by using 2 L of flow per minute (Fig 40–10), with increments of 0.5 L/min if the pulmonary artery diastolic (or pulmonary capillary wedge) pressure is greater than 5 mm Hg (Fig 40–10,B) or greater than 50% of the baseline (Fig 40–11) or if chest pain or electrocardiographic changes occur with an increase in the filling pressure after less than 2 minutes of balloon inflation (Fig 40–10,C–E).

At times, a "chattering" (vibration) of the venous line occurs during an attempt to increase the flow rate with a reduction in blood flow, as reflected on the blood flowmeter. This is an indication of intermittent collapse of the vena cava around the venous cannula, which can be resolved by reducing the speed of the blood pump, adding volume, and then increasing pump speed until a corresponding increase in blood flow cannot be demonstrated.

Significant hypotension, defined as a mean pressure of less than 60 mm Hg (a lower blood pressure can be tolerated if the patient is awake and responding to verbal commands), can be corrected in most patients by volume infusion through the pump (Fig 40–12). In certain circumstances, particularly if the systemic vascular resistance is low, phenylephrine (Neo-Synephrine) infusion may be necessary.

In patients in cardiogenic shock or cardiac arrest, an estimate of the blood flow requirement can be calculated from the patient's body surface area or body weight (2.2 to 2.4 L/m^2 or 50 to 60 mL/kg of body weight).

The activated clotting time is measured every 15 minutes and is maintained at or above 400 seconds. Arterial blood gas and mixed venous oxygen saturation, are determined periodically in all patients. All patients who have sustained cardiac arrest are intubated.

PTCA TECHNIQUE IN THE ELECTIVE GROUP

Patients who undergo elective supported angioplasty are premedicated with aspirin, 325 mg daily, prior to the procedure when this is feasible. An infusion of low–molecular-weight dextran is started 3 to 4 hours prior to the procedure at a rate of 50 mL/min unless the patient is in congestive cardiac failure. PTCA is then performed from the contralateral femoral artery in the standard fashion after the establishment of cardiopulmonary bypass support. PTCA of the culprit vessel (based upon vessel size and amount of myocardium in

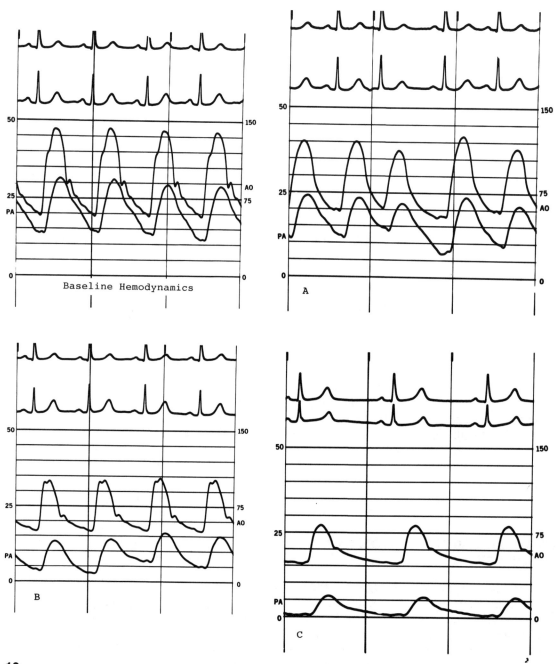

FIG 40–10.

Case example of a patient undergoing elective supported PTCA with a baseline blood pressure (BP) of 140/60 mm Hg and a pulmonary artery *(PA)* pressure of 40/22 mm Hg (pulmonary capillary wedge pressure of 22 mm Hg) *(upper left).* Aortic *(AO)* and PA pressures at **A,** 2 L/min of bypass flow. **B,** 2.5 L/min of bypass flow. **C,** further reduction in AO and PA pressure present 5 minutes after increasing the flow to 2.5 L/min. (Note the minimal change in the diastolic BP.) **D,** during balloon inflation there is no increase in the PA diastolic pressure. Note the reduced pulse pressure in the AO pressure tracing secondary to a reduced left ventricular ejection. **E,** return of left ventricular ejection as demonstrated by an increase in AO pulse pressure.

(Continued.)

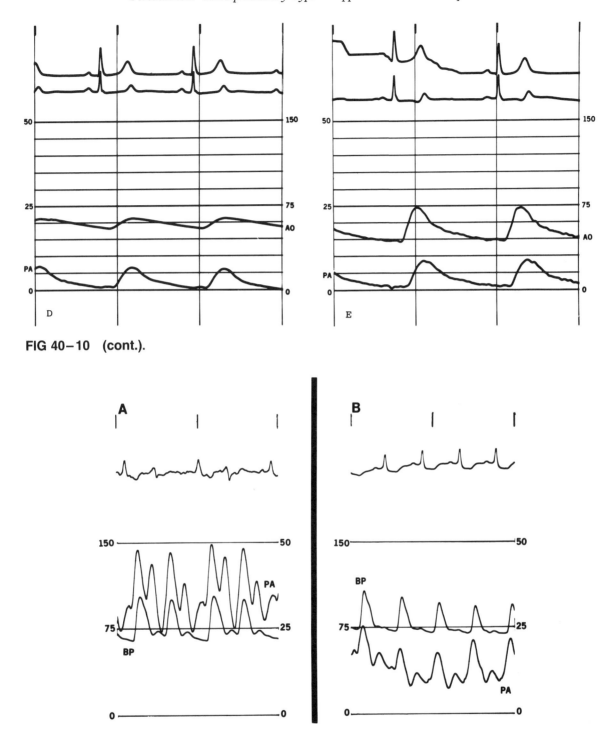

FIG 40–10 (cont.).

FIG 40–11.
Example of a patient undergoing elective, supported PTCA requiring 3.5-L/min flow to reduce the pulmonary artery *(PA)* diastolic pressure to less than 50% **(B)** of baseline **(A).** *BP* = blood pressure.

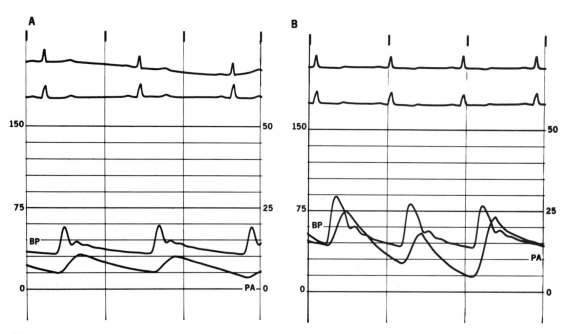

FIG 40–12.
Elevation of systemic blood pressure *(BP)* on bypass in response to volume infusion **(B)**. This is the expected response when the filling pressure is low **(A)**.

jeopardy) is initially performed, and if successful, additional vessels are also attempted. If patients are receiving intravenous nitroglycerin or heparin prior to PTCA (e.g., in unstable angina), both are continued. The heparin infusion is discontinued after the standard bolus of heparin at the time of cannulation for PCPS.

SUBSEQUENT THERAPY IN CARDIOGENIC SHOCK AND CARDIAC ARREST

In patients in cardiogenic shock, left ventriculography and coronary angiography are performed after hemodynamic stability is achieved. If feasible, the infarct-related vessel is dilated. Other critically narrowed vessels are also dilated if a good result is obtained in the infarct vessel and lesion characteristics (low risk) in the noninfarct vessel(s) appear amenable to PTCA. If the patient's coronary anatomy is not favorable for PTCA, emergency coronary bypass surgery is undertaken.

Patients in cardiac arrest with ventricular fibrillation are defibrillated (Fig 40–13). Patients who are initially asystolic usually return to sinus or junctional rhythm within a few minutes following institution of bypass, and pacemaker insertion is rarely necessary.

Patients who are not candidates for revascularization are gradually weaned from bypass over the next few hours.

Patients who undergo emergency bypass graft surgery are transported to the operating room on PCPS, which is terminated after standard cardiopulmonary bypass support (right atrium to aorta) is established. In order to avoid air embolism, care should be taken to be certain that PCPS is terminated before atrial cannulation for standard cardiopulmonary bypass. Also, no venous entry should be attempted while the patient is still on PCPS to avoid air embolus.

TERMINATION OF CARDIOPULMONARY BYPASS SUPPORT (ELECTIVE GROUP)

Following the completion of successful PTCA in the elective group, cardiopulmonary bypass support is gradually weaned over a period of 3 to 5 minutes by gradually reducing the bypass flow rate. Generally, bypass flow is reduced by about 0.5 L every minute. Volume is infused as necessary to increase the left ventricular filling pressure (estimated by the pulmonary capillary wedge/pulmonary artery diastolic pressure) to at least 8 to 10 mm Hg or to the prebypass level (whichever is less).

In some patients, particularly those with severe left ventricular dysfunction or recent myocardial infarction, inotropic agents (dopamine or dobutamine infusions) may be necessary in order to wean the patient from bypass. Rarely is an intra-aortic balloon pump necessary,

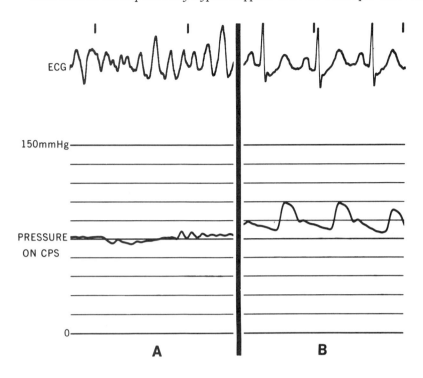

FIG 40–13.

A 72-year-old male who developed refractory cardiac arrest following abrupt closure (dissection) of the left circumflex after coronary angioplasty. **A,** mean blood pressure of 75 mm Hg on percutaneous cardiopulmonary support *(CPS)* at a flow rate of 5 L/min. The electrocardiogram (ECG) demonstrates ventricular fibrillation with the patient awake and responsive to verbal commands. **B,** after defibrillation and prior to emergency coronary artery bypass graft surgery. (From Shawl FA, Domanski MJ, Wish MH, et al: *Cathet Cardiovasc Diagn* 1990; 19:8–12. Used by permission.)

but if needed, it is placed via the contralateral femoral artery.

The patient is then transferred to the coronary care unit on a stretcher. Weaning and subsequent termination of PCPS can be done in the coronary care unit if the patient is not weaned in the catheterization laboratory within about 30 minutes, which happens very rarely. The stretcher commonly used (Haustead, Medina, Ohio) consists of a flat metal surface with an adjustable head support. A mattress with an egg crate supplement and a pillow with the head elevated approximately 15 degrees is used for patient comfort.

A cell saver is used to autotransfuse the blood remaining in the bypass perfusion circuit. After autotransfusion is completed, the activated clotting time is checked in the coronary care unit.

REMOVAL OF BYPASS CANNULAS (ELECTIVE GROUP)

Bypass cannulas are removed when the activated clotting time falls below 240 seconds. It takes 5 to 8 hours after the last dose of heparin to achieve this level of ac-

tivated clotting time. After the cannulas are removed, manual compression for hemostasis is performed for 15 to 20 minutes (Table 40–3). During this period of manual compression, an assessment of the appropriate point for clamp compression is made. Also, after 15 or 20 minutes of local compression, the pressure is slightly relaxed (without allowing bleeding) in order to assess the status of the pedal pulse. This allows an estimation of the degree of clamp pressure necessary for subsequent clamp compression.

Then a new, modified disk (Comfort Disc, Instromedix, Hillsboro, Ore) along with a locked compression clamp (Compressar, Instromedix) system is applied (Fig 40–14 and 40–15). Clamp compression is adjusted so

TABLE 40–3.

Percutaneous Cardiopulmonary Bypass Support Cannula Removal Protocol

Remove cannulas once ACT* is <240 sec
Manual compression for 15–20 min
Full clamp compression for 90 min
Gradual release of clamp: 2 mm every 15–20 min

*ACT = activated clotting time.

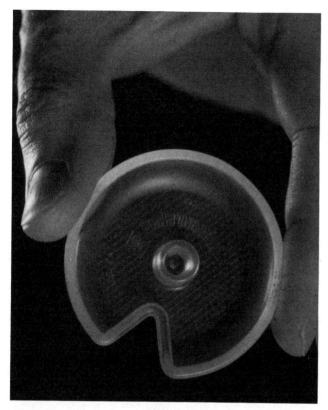

FIG 40–14.
Compression disk used for hemostasis.

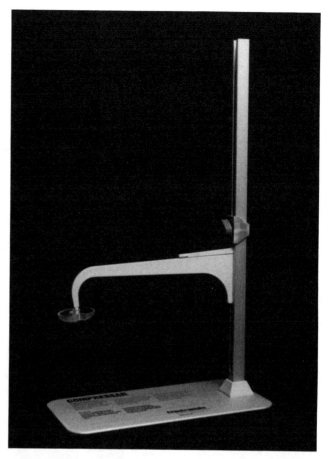

FIG 40–15.
Compression clamp with the lock and comfort disk in place.

that the pedal pulse remains palpable (or present on Doppler examinations if it was not palpable prior to the procedure). Gradual clamp release (2 to 3 mm every 20 minutes) is started after 90 minutes of compression if no bleeding is encountered.

A low-dose heparin (600 to 800 units/hr) infusion is started after the partial thromboplastin time declines to less than 70 seconds or the activated clotting time declines to less than 180 seconds and is continued until the patient is fully ambulatory. Other post-PCPS orders are found in Table 40–4. The angioplasty sheath and the Swan-Ganz catheter are removed the following day. Most patients are discharged no sooner than 72 hours after the procedure.

TERMINATION OF CARDIOPULMONARY BYPASS SUPPORT (EMERGENT GROUP)

In patients with cardiogenic shock who have undergone PTCA, termination of bypass support is similar to the elective group. However, in this group of patients weaning may take longer than in the elective group. Bypass cannulas can be left in place for up to 24 hours or longer (with full heparinization) if late instability appears likely.

In the cardiac arrest group, cannulas are left in place until definitive therapy is performed (PTCA or surgery). If patients are sent to emergency coronary bypass or other surgical procedures, PCPS is terminated after conventional bypass (right atrium to aorta) is instituted. In these patients, the femoral bypass cannulas are removed by the surgeon after completion of the surgical procedure, and the femoral artery and vein are sutured under direct vision. Patients in whom neither PTCA nor coronary bypass is possible are transferred to the coronary care unit on bypass. In this group, every effort is made to wean the patient from bypass in less than 6 to 7 hours. Other circulatory support (e.g., intra-aortic balloon pump) may be necessary to help wean the patient from PCPS.

OBSERVATION ON CARDIOPULMONARY BYPASS SUPPORT DURING ELECTIVE INTERVENTION

Once cardiopulmonary bypass support is instituted and the flow is increased, the patients usually complain

TABLE 40–4.

Orders After Supported Angioplasty Orders

Laboratory and Computer:
1. ACT* qh after completion of autotransfusion until ≤240 sec
2. PTT* q2h after completion of autotransfusion until <70, then qm* while taking heparin.
3. SMA* 7 with first PTT, then qm × 1
4. CBC* in A.M.
5. H&H* q8h × 3 upon completion of autotransfusion
6. Cardiac isoenzymes q6h × 4 (start with first PTT)
7. 0₂, 2 L by nasal cannula or _____
8. ABGs* upon arrival to CCU* and in A.M.
9. 12-Lead ECG* upon arrival to CCU and in A.M.
10. Clear liquids 1st 8 hr, then advance to previous diet as tolerated

IVs:
1. Maintenance IV D₅NS* (or NS if diabetic) at _____ cc/hr
2. Increase maintenance IV to 999 cc/hr for BP* ≤90 mm Hg systolic until 100 mm Hg systolic as long as PAD* < 16
3. Dextran at 50 cc/hr until _____
4. Restart heparin at 600 units/hr when PTT 70 or below.

Medications:
1. Resume pre-PTCA* medications
2. Prochlorperazine (Companize), 3–5 mg slow IV push q6h prn* for nausea
3. Morphine, 3–5 mg IV q3–4h prn for pain
4. Diazepam (Valium), 2–5 mg IV q6h prn for anxiety/restlessness
5. Flurazepam, (Dalmane), 30 mg po qhs* prn for sleep.
6. KCl, 20 mEq/100 cc D₅W* over 2-hr period prn K⁺ < 3.7 via central line
7. Transfuse 1 unit RBCs for Hb 8.0 g or less, followed by posttransfusion H & H
8. Cefazolin (Kefzol), 1 g IV q8h × 2 days

Monitoring and Misc.:
1. VS* every 15 min × 1 hr, every 30 min × 2 hr, then q1–2h
2. CO* every shift × 3
3. Measure thigh distal to CPS* site on admission, then q4h × 3
4. When ACT < 240 sec, after cannulas out, place C clamp after 15 min of manual compression
5. Release C clamp, after 90 min 2–3 mm every 20 min as long as no oozing or bleeding is noted
6. Soft restraints to R&L ankle and knee strap on the bypass side
7. Check _____ pulse (RT)/(LT)* by palpation or Doppler
8. Accept capillary return (+)– if no pedal pulse prior to procedure
9. Silvadene, 1% local cream with dressing on bypass site

Heparin standing orders:
Routine PCPS*
   1. Accept PTT of 55–70. Increase heparin drip by *200* units/hr if PTT < 55. If PTT is 71–100, reduce by *100* units/hr. If PTT≥101 hold heparin 1 hr, then resume by *200* units less
Emergent or acute PCPS only
   2. Accept PTT of 70–100. If PTT < 70, give *2,000* units heparin bolus and increase heparin drip by 200 units/hr. If PTT ≥ 101, reduce by 200 units less
   3. Hold heparin drip only if bleeding, and call MD.

Recheck PTT 1 hr after any heparin change both routine and acute pre-PTCA Medications:
1. _____
2. _____
3. _____

*ACT = activated clotting time; PTT = partial thromboplastin time; qm = every morning; SMA = Sequential Multiple Analyzer; CBC = complete blood count; H&H = hematocrit and hemoglobin; ABG= arterial blood gases; CCU = Critical case unit; ECG = electrocardiogram; D₅NS = 5% dextrose in normal saline; BP = blood pressure; PAD = pulmonary artery diastolic; prn = as needed; qhs = every hour of sleep; D₅W = 5% dextrose in water; VS = vital signs; CO = cardiac output; CPS = cardiopulmonary support; RT/LT = right thigh/left thigh; PCPS = percutaneous cardiopulmonary bypass support.

of generalized warmth and, in some cases, feelings of nausea. The administration of 5 mg of prochlorperazine (Compazine) intravenously prior to the initiation of cardiopulmonary bypass has substantially reduced the incidence of nausea. Nausea has also been substantially reduced by starting the flow at 0.5 L/min and increasing by 0.5 L/min every 30 seconds until a flow rate of 2 L/min is achieved. With the current use of 18 F cannulas, a flow up to 5 L/min can be achieved if the patients are well hydrated prior to the procedure.

With the initiation of cardiopulmonary bypass support, there is a rapid fall (over a few minutes) in the filling pressures as manifested by a reduction in the pulmonary capillary wedge pressure (or pulmonary diastolic pressure). There is also a reduction in systolic arterial blood pressure with a slight increase in diastolic pressure, the latter feature known to be present with a nonpulsatile flow (see Fig 40–10 and 40–13). Echocardiography performed during cardiopulmonary bypass support demonstrates a reduction in the left atrial and left ventricular dimensions. These observations, together with reduction of the preload (see Fig 40–10,D) and afterload, suggest that PCPS reduces myocardial oxygen demand, which may be partially responsible for the absence of angina during balloon inflation in most patients undergoing supported angioplasty. Nonetheless, segmental wall motion abnormalities and reduced pulse pressure (Figure 40–10,D) are present during balloon inflation and thus indicate ischemia distal to the occlusion.

The patient may experience numbness and tingling in the leg when PCPS cannulas are inserted. In such cases, sedation in the form of intravenous diazepam or morphine may be necessary. In some cases, intravenous nitroglycerin or sublingual nifedipine (as a vasodilator) may be helpful to counteract any spasm, particularly when iliofemoral angiography has revealed a good-caliber vessel prior to cannulation. Also, in patients with good-caliber iliofemoral vessels, such complaints may disappear spontaneously.

The flow rate that is necessary depends upon

whether the patient is on complete or partial bypass (left ventricle still ejecting while on bypass). During partial bypass in elective patients undergoing high-risk PTCA, the average flow rate necessary is about 3.0 L/min.[18] In cardiogenic shock the average flow requirement has been 4.0 L/min,[19] while in cardiac arrest (full bypass support) it is 4.8 L/min.[20] The average bypass time for elective high-risk angioplasty has been 37 minutes, 1.8 hours for cardiogenic shock, and 2.7 hours for cardiac arrest.[20]

With the initiation of cardiopulmonary bypass support, pulmonary artery and systolic blood pressures decline (see Fig 40–13 and 40–14). In the elective group as well as in cardiogenic shock patients, pulmonary capillary wedge (or pulmonary artery diastolic) pressure declines to 0 to 5 mm Hg in 90% of patients.

Patients with very poor left ventricular function and severe pulmonary hypertension and patients with prolonged cardiac arrest are among those in whom complete unloading is not possible. These patients may benefit from left ventricular venting. Also, when cardiopulmonary bypass flow is commenced, it may take a few minutes before a decline in the left ventricular filling pressure occurs (Fig 40–13,A).

In some patients, significant hypotension (defined as a mean blood pressure of 60 mm Hg or even lower as long as the patient is awake) may occur during bypass or when the flow rate is increased. This is more common and pronounced in patients who are volume depleted or have low filling pressures in the setting of a dilated, poorly functioning left ventricle. Therefore, it is imperative to have adequate filling pressures prior to institution of bypass flow. If the patient's pulmonary artery diastolic (or pulmonary capillary wedge) pressure is less than 8 to 10 mm Hg, volume can be given rapidly through the bypass perfusion circuit when the flow rate is inadequate. Urinary output increases after the institution of PCPS. Therefore, inserting a Foley catheter prior to the procedure is necessary.

In most patients in whom PCPS is terminated in the catheterization laboratory, volume infusion of 150 to 1,000 cc (through the bypass system) is necessary prior to termination of PCPS. Recently, 25% albumin (50 to 100 cc) has been given at the start of the procedure through the pump and has resulted in a dramatic decrease in volume requirement during the procedure.

OBSERVATION AFTER THE TERMINATION OF BYPASS SUPPORT

Some patients may complain of numbness and a tingling sensation in the leg when cannulas are still in place while waiting for the activated clotting time to fall below 240 seconds in the coronary care unit. Such patients may require sedation, as well as vasodilators (intravenous nitroglycerin or sublingual nifedipine). Interestingly, these complaints are usually transient and disappear in an hour or so. Observation is safe as long as there is good capillary filling.

The total clamp compression time necessary for hemostasis when the current method is used is less than 3 hours, with maximum compression for 90 minutes followed by subsequent gradual release over the next 90 minutes.

COMPLICATIONS

The complications due to PCPS are listed in Tables 40–5 and 40–6. Only 1 complication (repair of a femoral artery in a patient in the emergent group) was encountered in the last 33 patients in this series when the current cannula removal technique was used (Fig 40–16). Also, the requirement for blood transfusion has been significantly reduced with the current method, as well as with the use of a cell saver (Fig 40–17).

TABLE 40–5.
Percutaneous Cardiopulmonary Bypass Supported Interventions: Complication in 129 Procedures (Elective and Emergent) Requiring Local Surgery

Complication	No.
Pseudoaneurysm	6*
Enlarging hematoma	3
Infection	1
Embolus to popliteal artery	1
Arteriovenous fistula	1
Total	13(11%)†

*Noted on follow-up.
†Complication rate of less than 1.5% when the current cannula removal protocol is used.

TABLE 40–6.
Percutaneous Cardiopulmonary Bypass Supported Interventions: Complications in 129 Procedures (Elective and Emergent), Nonsurgical

Complication	No.
Minor superficial skin infection	6
Femoral nerve weakness	5*
Superficial skin necrosis	5*
Minor gastrointestinal bleeding	2
Deep venous thrombosis	1
TIA† (48 hr post procedure)	1
Air embolus	1
Diabetic ketoacidosis	1
Total	22 (18%)

*Due to clamping (early experience); none in the current series using the new cannula removal protocol.
†TIA = transient ischemic attack.

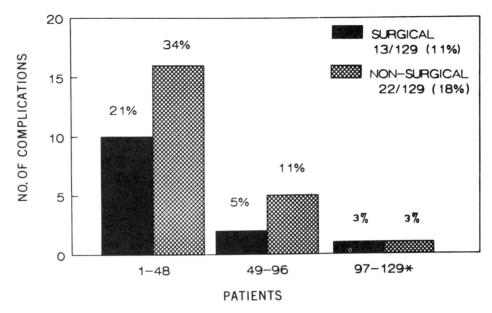

FIG 40–16.
Complication rate for elective and emergent procedures (129 procedures). A marked reduction in complications is noted in the last 33 cases when the current cannula removal technique was used *(asterisk)*.

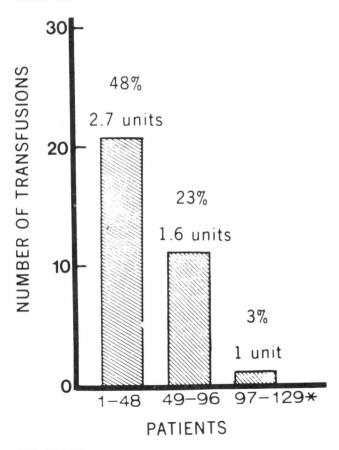

FIG 40–17.
Significant reduction in transfusion requirement in the last 33 procedures when the current cannula removal technique was used *(asterisk)*.

There is no evidence of significant hemolysis or thrombocytopenia, even when bypass support is extended to 6 hours.

COMMENTS

In the author's experience, PCPS is feasible and has an acceptable morbidity. In spite of the high-risk patient population, there has been no mortality directly due to PCPS.

The most common complications due to PCPS occur at the cannula site. The local complications usually occur after removal of the bypass cannulas. In our initial series (the first 78 elective cases), bypass cannulas were removed in the catheterization laboratory once the patient was considered clinically as well as hemodynamically stable. Since patients had received a large bolus of heparin before the initiation of cardiopulmonary bypass, a large amount of circulating heparin remained at the time of cannula removal. With the technique of early cannula removal, it took a longer time for hemostasis when external clamp compression was used. Because of this prolonged clamping (Fig 40–18), there were significant local complications as well as a need for blood transfusion. None of the complications that occurred in the entire series were life-threatening.

Local complications in the elective series have been reduced with the current removal technique (Fig 40–19) because there is a lesser amount of circulating heparin at the time of removal, thus allowing rapid he-

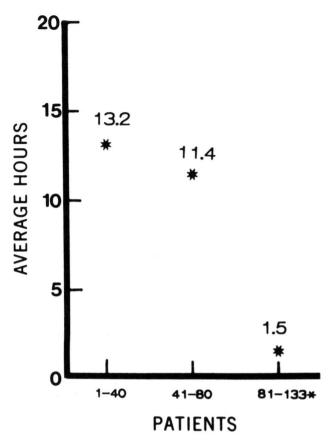

FIG 40–18.
Duration of clamp compression in the entire series of 133 procedures. Note the dramatic decrease in the necessary clamp time in the last 53 procedures when the current cannula removal technique was used *(asterisk).*

mostasis (<2 hours). Also, less external clamp compression time (full compression requirement of ≤90 minutes) is needed. The current cannula removal technique allows reinstitution of cardiopulmonary bypass in the coronary care unit in the event of hemodynamic compromise due to abrupt closure. This would not be possible if the vessels were sutured surgically after the completion of the procedure (an important advantage of the percutaneous approach).

Femorofemoral cardiopulmonary bypass support instituted percutaneously in the catheterization laboratory makes interventional procedures feasible in patients who were not previously candidates. Also, PCPS reduces operator anxiety and allows the achievement of an optimal result. If necessary, PCPS may be used if abrupt closure occurs during supported PTCA. Otherwise, these high-risk patients may not survive long enough to reach the operating room.

Currently, PCPS is the only practical circulatory support system for the catheterization laboratory that

provides complete hemodynamic support even in the absence of an intrinsic cardiac rhythm. Also, PCPS permits prolonged balloon inflation, which may reduce restenosis and improve immediate results.[29]

However, PCPS does not eliminate ischemia distal to an occlusion. Therefore, should abrupt closure occur that is not amenable to repeat PTCA, patients should undergo immediate coronary bypass surgery. Coronary perfusion in such patients with a separate roller pump is under investigation and may eliminate ischemia distal to the occlusion. If adequate coronary perfusion distal to an occluded vessel proves effective, then this form of support may be the most ideal, "total cardiopulmonary bypass support."

Because PCPS provides adequate systemic perfusion even in the absence of an intrinsic cardiac rhythm, it is superior to the intra-aortic balloon pump.[30] The ability of PCPS to provide hemodynamic support in patients with cardiogenic shock or cardiac arrest has been impressive.[19, 21] The hemodynamic stability achieved with PCPS allowed these patients to undergo complex PTCA or coronary bypass surgery and has resulted in improved survival that was greatest when PCPS was instituted early, followed by definitive therapy.[20]

There are two major advantages to instituting cardiopulmonary bypass support with the percutaneous femoral approach described here. First, the technique of cannula placement is simple and requires no extraordinary skill from an interventionalist. Definition of iliofemoral anatomy by angiography, which is obtained routinely prior to elective supported interventions, also enhances safety by reducing the likelihood of vascular injury. Also, in patients who have sustained cardiac arrest, cannulas can be placed while cardiopulmonary resuscitation is in progress. The second advantage of this approach is that by leaving the cannulas in for 5 to 7 hours (while waiting for the activated clotting time to drop below 240 seconds), any hemodynamic compromise during this period can be immediately reversed by restarting PCPS.

There are, however, three limitations (Table 40–7) of PCPS, including incomplete left ventricular unloading, particularly after a prolonged cardiac arrest; ischemia distal to an occluded vessel; and an inability to use the system for more than 6 hours. Also, the use of 18 F cannulas requires exclusion of patients with significant iliofemoral disease.

TABLE 40–7.
Limitations of Cardiopulmonary Bypass Support

Incomplete left ventricular unloading
Lack of coronary perfusion distal to the coronary occlusion
Inability to use for prolonged periods

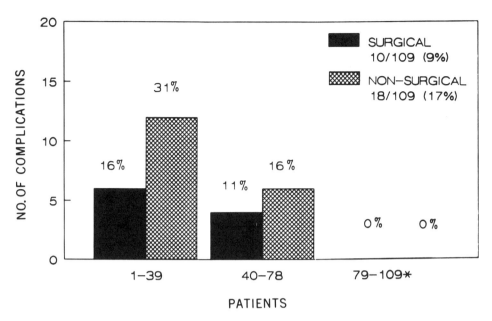

FIG 40–19.
Elimination of local complications in the last 31 elective procedures when the current cannula removal technique was used *(asterisk).*

Other modalities, however, may be useful in the support of high-risk angioplasty. The intra-aortic balloon pump has been used but is ineffective in patients in cardiac arrest or those in whom left ventricular function is sufficiently compromised.[30] The Hemopump may provide adequate support even in patients with profound dysfunction.[31] At present, however, the device requires surgical insertion. Also, the necessity of placing the device across the aortic valve may make it difficult to use in the setting of cardiac arrest.

Antegrade or retrograde perfusion catheters that provide blood flow to myocardium served by an occluded vessel may maintain adequate blood flow following abrupt closure or during balloon inflation.[32–35] These devices may prove useful when used alone or may be an effective adjunct to PCPS. However, because of a rather large profile, coronary perfusion catheters may not be feasible in tortuous vessels or in distal lesions. Also, such catheters require a mean pressure of at least 70 mm Hg for adequate perfusion. All of the current support modalities, including PCPS, are in a state of evolution, and the ultimate role of each remains to be defined.[36]

FUTURE DIRECTIONS

It appears that there are two major limitations to PCPS. The first is incomplete left ventricular unloading, which is present following prolonged cardiac arrest, with severe global ischemia and severe pulmonary hypertension, and in patients with severe left ventricular failure. One of the approaches to this limitation could be left ventricular venting, which can be accomplished by pump aspiration through a specially designed pigtail catheter placed in the left ventricle (Fig 40–20) or by retrograde[37] venting of the pulmonary artery (by making the pulmonic valve incompetent). In our experience, it appears that defibrillation of patients with prolonged cardiac arrest is facilitated by left ventricular venting. Left ventricular venting may also prove useful in reducing left ventricular myocardial oxygen consumption during acute myocardial infarction. Recent evidence suggests that myocardial reperfusion in an unloaded state,[38] as well as after the institution of cardioplegia,[39] may prevent reperfusion injury. Whether similar results can be achieved during PTCA for acute myocardial infarction requires further study.

The second limitation is the absence of perfusion distal to an occlusion. This may be remedied by using a separate roller pump to provide continuous antegrade perfusion (Fig 40–21) or by using currently available autoperfusion catheters. The lack of distal perfusion is of concern only if a vessel closes acutely during PTCA and flow is not reestablished quickly.

The combination of venting and antegrade coronary perfusion in conjunction with PCPS may provide an improved degree of circulatory support.[40]

The role of PCPS as a bridge to other left ventricular assist devices or cardiac transplantation requires evaluation.

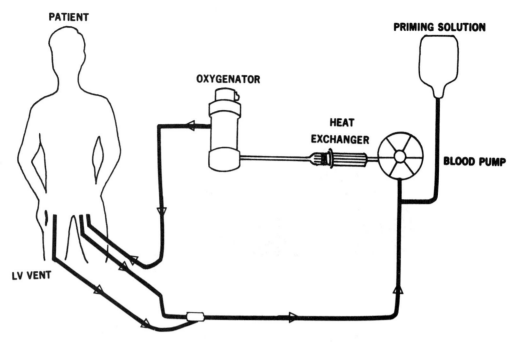

FIG 40–20.
Schematic of the cardiopulmonary bypass support system showing the technique of the left ventricular venting.

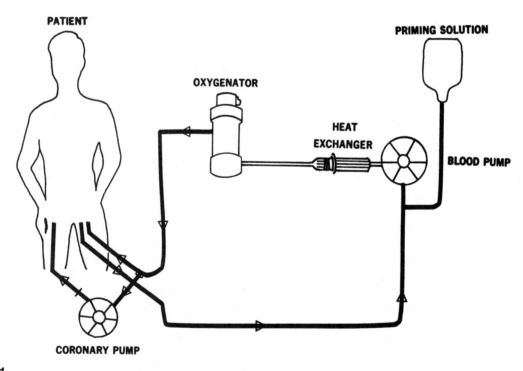

FIG 40–21.
Schematic of the cardiopulmonary bypass support system showing the technique of coronary perfusion (distal to coronary occlusion) with a separate roller pump.

CONCLUSION

A safe and easily applied technique of PCPS has been developed for use in the cardiac catheterization laboratory. The importance of this technique lies in its ability to maintain hemodynamic stability during high-risk interventional procedures regardless of intrinsic cardiac function. Eighteen French venous and arterial cannulas are inserted percutaneously over a stiff guidewire after sequential dilatation with 12 F and 14 F dilators. Bypass flow rates up to 5 L/min can be achieved.

This technique can be applied to support patients with cardiac arrest, with hemodynamic collapse following abrupt closure during coronary angioplasty, and with cardiogenic shock, as well as those undergoing high-risk elective angioplasty. This form of support also permits transport of patients to the operating room in a stable condition following a failed angioplasty. The complications are mostly related to cannula removal and can be minimized or eliminated by the use of proper technique. Although the ultimate role of this new technique remains to be completely defined, it appears that it will expand the patient population to whom coronary interventions can be applied.

Acknowledgment

The excellent contributions of my colleague, Dr. Michael J. Domanski, in the preparation of this manuscript are gratefully recognized. The contributions of the Interventional Cardiology Team of Washington Adventist Hospital are greatly appreciated. The secretarial assistance of Grace Murtagh is also very much appreciated.

REFERENCES

1. Grüntzig AR: Transluminal dilatation of coronary artery stenosis. *Lancet* 1978; 1:263–266.
2. Grüntzig AR, Senning A, Seigenthaler WE: Nonoperative dilatation of coronary artery stenosis: Percutaneous transluminal coronary angioplasty. *N Engl J Med* 1979; 301:61–68.
3. Cowley MJ, Vetrovec GM, DiSciascio G, et al: Coronary angioplasty of multiple vessels: Short term outcome and long term results. *Circulation* 1985; 72:1314–1320.
4. Quigley RJ, Erwin J, Maurer BJ, et al: Percutaneous transluminal coronary angioplasty in unstable angina: Comparison with stable angina. *Br Heart J* 1986; 55:227–230.
5. Holmes DR, Vliestra RE: Percutaneous transluminal coronary angioplasty: Current status of future trends. *Mayo Clin Proc* 1986; 61:865.
6. Dorros G, Cowley MJ, Janke L, et al: In-hospital mortality rate in the National Heart, Lung and Blood Institute Percutaneous Transluminal Coronary Angioplasty Registry. *Am J Cardiol* 1984; 53:17–21.
7. Cowley MJ, Dorros G, Kelsey SF, et al: Acute coronary events associated with percutaneous transluminal coronary angioplasty. *Am J Cardiol* 1984; 53:12–16.
8. Bredlau CE, Roubin GS, Leimgruber PP, et al: In-hospital morbidity and mortality in patients undergoing elective coronary angioplasty. *Circulation* 1985; 72:1044–1052.
9. Cowley MJ, Dorros G, Kelsey SF, et al: Emergency coronary bypass surgery after coronary angioplasty: The National Heart, Lung, and Blood Institute's Percutaneous Transluminal Coronary Angioplasty Registry Experience. *Am J Cardiol* 1984; 53:22–26.
10. Vogel RA, Tommaso CL, Gundry SR: Initial experience with coronary angioplasty and aortic valvuloplasty using elective semipercutaneous cardiopulmonary support. *Am J Cardiol* 1988: 62:811–813.
11. Shawl FA, Domanski MJ, Punja S, et al: Percutaneous institution of cardiopulmonary (bypass) support: Technique and complications (abstract). *J Am Coll Cardiol* 1989; 13:159.
12. Shawl FA, Domanski MJ, Wish MH, et al: Percutaneous cardiopulmonary bypass support in the catheterization laboratory: Technique and complications. *Am Heart J* 1990; 120:195–203.
13. Lande HA, Edwards L, Bloch JH, et al: Clinical experience with emergency use of prolonged cardiopulmonary bypass with membrane pump oxygenator. *J Thorac Surg* 1970; 10:409–423.
14. Baird RJ, Rocha AJ, Miyagishimart, et al: Assisted circulation following myocardial infarction: A review of 25 patients treated before 1971. *Can Med Assoc J* 1972; 107:287–291.
15. Mattox KL, Beall AC: Application of portable cardiopulmonary bypass to emergency intrumentation. *Med Instrum* 1977; 11:347–349.
16. Phillips SJ, Ballentine B, Slonine D, et al: Percutaneous initiation of cardiopulmonary bypass. *J Thorac Surg* 1983; 36:223–225.
17. Kanter KR, Binington DG, Vandormael M, et al: Emergency rescusitation with extracorporeal membrane oxygenation for failed angioplasty (abstract). *J Am Coll Cardiol* 1988; 11:149.
18. Shawl FA, Domanski MJ, Punja S: Percutaneous cardiopulmonary bypass support in high risk patients undergoing percutaneous transluminal coronary angioplasty. *Am J Cardiol* 1989; 64:1258–1263.
19. Shawl FA, Domanski MJ, Hernandez TJ, et al: Emergency percutaneous cardiopulmonary bypass with cardiogenic shock from acute myocardial infarction. *Am J Cardiol* 1989; 64:967–970.
20. Shawl FA, Domanski MJ, Wish MH, et al: Emergency cardiopulmonary bypass support in patients with cardiac arrest in the catheterization laboratory. *Cathet Cardiovasc Diagn* 1990; 19:8–12.
21. Shawl FA, Domanski MJ, Yackee JM, et al: Left ventricular rupture complicating percutaneous mitral commissurotomy: Salvage using percutaneous cardiopulmonary bypass support. *Cathet Cardiovasc Diagn* 1990; 21:26–27.
22. Shawl FA: Percutaneous cardiopulmonary bypass support in high risk coronary angioplasty. *Cardiol Clin* 1989; 87:865–875.

23. Shawl FA: Percutaneous cardiopulmonary bypass support in high risk interventions. *J Invasive Cardiol* 1989; 5:287–293.

24. Vogel RA, Shawl FA, Tammasco C. et al: Initial report of the National Registry of Elective Cardiopulmonary Bypass Supported Angioplasty. *J Am Coll Cardiol* 1990; 15:23–29.

25. Roberts C, Litziek F: *Cardiopulmonary Bypass Support System: Technical Specification Reference Manual.* Billerica, Mass, Bard Cardiosurgery, 1986.

26. Boers M, van den Dungen JJ, Karliczek GF, et al: Two membrane oxygenators and a bubbler: A clinical comparison. *Ann Thorac Surg* 1983; 35:455–462.

27. Clark RE, Beauchamp RA, Magrath RA, et al: Comparison of bubble and membrane oxygenators in short and long perfusions. *J Thorac Cardiovasc Surg* 1979; 78:655–666.

28. Volkmer I, Nienhaus KH, Meyers F, et al: Blood trauma during extracorporeal circulation: A comparison between two bubble and two membrane oxygenators in a standardized dog model. *Thorac Cardiovasc Surg* 1981; 29:323–327.

29. Kaltenbach M, Beyer J, Walter S, et al: Prolonged application of pressure in transluminal coronary angioplasty. *Cathet Cardiovasc Diagn* 1984; 10:213–219.

30. Alcan KE, Stertzer SH, Walsh JE, et al: The role of intra-aortic balloon counterpulsation in patients undergoing percutaneous transluminal coronary angioplasty. *Am Heart J* 1983; 105:527–530.

31. Smalling RW, Cassidy DB, Merhige M, et al: Improved hemodynamic and left ventricular unloading during acute ischemia using the left ventricular assist device compared to intra-aortic balloon counterpulsation (abstract). *J Am Coll Cardiol* 1989; 13:160.

32. Corday E, Meerbaum S, Dorey JK: The coronary sinus: Alternative channel for administration of arterial blood and pharmalogical agents for protection and treatment of cardiac ischemia. *J Am Coll Cardiol* 1986: 7:711–714.

33. Drury JK, Yamazaki S, Fishbein MC, et al: Synchronized diastolic coronary sinus venous retroperfusion: Results of preclinical safety and efficacy study. *J Am Coll Cardiol* 1985; 6:328–335.

34. Lehman KG, Atwood JE, Snyder EL, et al: Autologous blood perfusion for myocardial protection during coronary angioplasty: A feasibility study. *Circulation* 1987; 76:312–323.

35. Hinohara T, Simpson JB, Philips HR, et al: Transluminal intracoronary perfusion catheter. A device to maintain coronary reperfusion between failed angioplasty and emergency coronary bypass surgery. *J Am Coll Cardiol* 1988; 11:977–982.

36. Topol EJ: Emergency strategies for failed transluminal coronary angioplasty. *Am J Cardiol* 1989; 63:249–250.

37. Kolobow T, Rossi F, Borelli M, et al: Long term closed chest partial and total cardiopulmonary bypass by peripheral cannulation for severe right and/or left ventricular failure. The use of a percutaneous spring in pulmonary artery position to decompress the left heart. *Trans Am Soc Artif Intern Organs* 1988; 345:485–489.

38. Laschinger JC, Grossi, EA, Cunningham JN, et al: Adjunctive left ventricular unloading during myocardial reperfusion plays a major role in minimizing myocardial infarct size. *J Thorac Cardiovasc Surg* 1985; 90:80–85.

39. Allen BS, Okamoto F, Buckberg GD, et al: Studies of controlled reperfusion after ischemia. Improved functional recovery after 6 hours of regional ischemia by careful control of conditions of reperfusion and composition of reperfusate. *J Thorac Cardiovasc Surg* 1986; 92(suppl):621.

40. Shawl FA: Percutaneous cardiopulmonary bypass support: Technique, indications and complications, in Shawl FA (ed): *Supported Complex and High Risk Coronary Angioplasty.* Boston, Kluwer Academic Publishers, 1991, pp 65–100.

41

Myocardial Protection During Coronary Angioplasty

Paolo Angelini, M.D.

D. Richard Leachman, M.D.

Germano DiSciascio, M.D.

Michael J. Cowley, M.D.

Jeffrey A. Brinker, M.D.

Balloon coronary angioplasty, by its nature, requires temporary occlusion of the arterial segment being treated. Even when coronary angioplasty was first undertaken, Dr. Andreas Grüntzig explored the possibility of preserving coronary flow through the double-lumen balloon catheter.[1] While facing unresolved technical problems[2,3] with the available pumps, Grüntzig soon realized that balloon angioplasty could be safely and effectively done in selected cases[1] in the absence of myocardial protection. Interestingly, extracorporeal circulation was used during the first clinical coronary angioplasty[4] but was soon considered nonessential and thus abandoned. The technological improvements that occurred in coronary balloon angioplasty after 1977 were focused on the capacity of the balloon to cross a lesion, and as a result, more maneuverable, trackable, pushable, lower-profile balloon systems were introduced.

At this time, it seems that the role of balloon angioplasty has been well established but still has substantial limitations, in particular, (1) the significant incidence of abrupt closure (about 5%),[5] (2) a restenosis rate of 25 to 40% (within 4 to 6 months after a successful procedure),[6] and (3) the exclusion of some patients who have passable coronary lesions but might poorly tolerate balloon inflation (sudden occlusion)[7,8] or those for whom surgical backup is not immediately available.

At this time, our knowledge of the efficacy of balloon angioplasty is based on procedures done within the time constraints (or limiting the duration of inflation) imposed by the patient's tolerance to ischemia. Substantial, although preliminary evidence[6,9-13] has suggested that early and late success rates could be improved if the balloon could be inflated without limiting the duration of inflation (prolonged, single, or gradual onset).

The primary focus of this chapter is to review the results of a prospective multicenter study in which a new balloon catheter/coronary pump system was used in angioplasty procedures. Our goal was to make hemoperfusion through the balloon catheter routinely available during clinical angioplasty. In addition, alternative methods of myocardial protection are discussed.

MYOCARDIAL OXYGEN REQUIREMENTS

Coronary blood flow represents about 5% of the cardiac output, or 3 cc/kg of body weight.[14,15] Whereas only 20% of the coronary flow is required to preserve the viability of the myocardial cell, 80% is required for the myocardial contractile activity.[15] The time for circulatory flow through the coronary vessels averages 4 seconds.

The coronary bed is highly reactive and normally capable of increasing four to six times above baseline (coronary reserve).[14, 15] Myocardial oxygen consumption, which is mainly influenced by the left ventricular pressure and heart rate, is the major determinant of instantaneous coronary flow, within the limits of the effective coronary reserve.[14]

Coronary flow is obviously phasic within the left ventricular mass where intramural systolic pressure tends to exceed aortic pressure,[16] especially in the subendocardium, and can lead to total arrest or even backward flow in the epicardial coronary arteries during systole. Conversely, in the right ventricular myocardium, the coronary circulation is basically continuous, only phasically changing with aortic and right ventricular pressures. Whereas normal resting coronary flow and coronary reserve are relatively well-defined concepts, the minimal flow required to match the metabolic needs of the dependent myocardium during sudden coronary occlusion is not well defined but is clinically very useful to the angioplasty operation. During our experience with active hemoperfusion during balloon inflation, our group has come to identify minimal adequate coronary (MAC) flow as that required to prevent ischemic manifestations during balloon inflation. We knew from the literature[17] that regional segmental wall motion tends to deteriorate when blood flow is decreased to less than 50% of the normal (Fig 41–1). Empirically, we could determine how much blood flow was required in order to prevent angina or ST elevation, systemic blood pressure drop, and ventricular arrhythmias — the basic parameters monitored during balloon angioplasty — when we started selective hemoperfusion through the catheter with known and adaptable flow rates during balloon inflation. Great variations in MAC flows were observed in different anatomic segments, myocardial states, and clinical conditions. The usage of arterial blood (mean O_2 saturation, 98%) did not result in significant decreases in MAC flows with respect to the usage of renal vein blood during O_2 supplementation by nasal cannula (mean renal vein O_2 saturation, 89%).

The major conceptual error in our method was related to the fact that we could artificially supply blood during balloon inflation only to the vessel distal to the balloon, but not to any side branches that should have originated at the level of the balloon. With this limitation in mind, we have made the following observations:[18, 19]

1. Coronary branches that are totally and chronically occluded have a MAC flow of zero and do not require any distal blood supply during balloon inflation unless the inflated balloon compromises collateral flow.

2. Coronary branches that are subtotally occluded

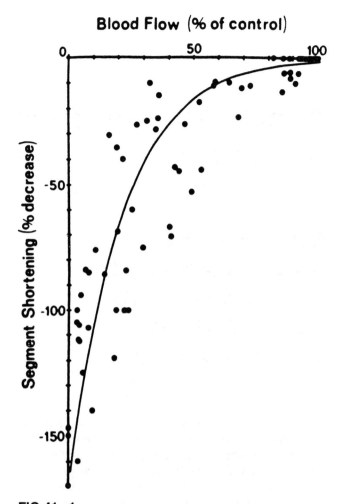

FIG 41–1.
Segmental wall motion in a dog's heart during a progressive decrease in coronary blood flow. Myocardial contractile performance is not affected by a <50% decrease in blood flow with respect to baseline. (From Vatner SF: *Circ Res* 1980; 47:201–207. Used by permission.)

with obvious collateral flow behave like total, chronic occlusions.

3. Coronary branches serving scarred or stunned myocardium from old, completed, or advanced infarctions have zero MAC flow.

4. Critical lesions related to resting angina frequently have baseline ischemia ("hibernating" myocardium, with segmental wall hypokinesia and T inversion). This condition is usually associated with a shorter tolerance time to sudden occlusion (by balloon) but lower blood flow requirements to suppress the onset of a more advanced state of ischemia. Actually, in this latter setting we have observed that baseline hypokinesia of the involved segment could improve quickly (within 2 to 5 minutes) after the initiation of active hemoperfusion.

5. The typical lesion targeted for coronary angioplasty is moderately severe with no collateral flow. In this case, the blood flow required to suppress ischemic manifestations is close to 50% of the normal baseline flow for that vessel. Usually, less blood flow is required to eliminate ischemic manifestations in smaller branches. Maintenance of segmental wall motion, as assessed by two-dimensional echocardiography, frequently requires slightly higher blood flows (10 to 20%) than those required to prevent angina or ST changes. In the absence of hemoperfusion during balloon angioplasty, hypotension only occurs in cases of critical compromise of the functional myocardial mass (Fig 41–2). Mitral insufficiency could also occur or become worse in some cases because of papillary muscle dysfunction (Fig 41–3). Arrhythmias, as a manifestation of ischemia, usually follow the onset of ST elevation (Fig 41–4).

Initial experience has shown that MAC flows range from 30 to 60 cc/min for most clinically indicated coronary angioplasty procedures. Only when a left main lesion or equivalent is considered would MAC flow exceed 70 to 80 cc, which is the maximum flow rate of the Corflo system (Leocor, Inc., Houston). The potential usage of two pumps, in parallel, with two balloon catheters positioned in a "kissing" fashion (one in the left anterior descending artery and one in the circumflex) could solve the technical problem of left main artery di-

latation. We have observed that when ischemic side branches compromised during balloon inflation are the cause of residual ischemic manifestations during hemoperfusion, increasing the blood flow rate will not result in an appreciable clinical effect.

Mechanical support during balloon angioplasty may be directed toward global cardiac function (cardiopulmonary bypass machine and intra-aortic balloon counterpulsation) or the affected area of myocardium (autoperfusion/active prograde perfusion or retroperfusion catheters). Pharmacologic support may be directed toward suppressing the perception of ischemia (general sedation/anesthesia) or decreasing myocardial oxygen requirements (calcium antagonists, β-blockers). In the following sections, we will comment on the technical and clinical aspects of these primary methods of support.

METHODS OF MYOCARDIAL PROTECTION

Passive Hemoperfusion/Autoperfusion

In this hemoperfusion technique of preserving coronary blood flow during balloon angioplasty, the aortic pressure serves as the driving force, and a special lumen inside the balloon is used as the channel for hemoperfusion.[20–22] Side holes in the inner shaft of the bal-

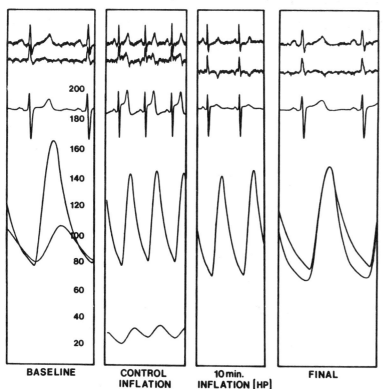

FIG 41–2.
Typical behavior of the electrocardiogram (L₁, aVL, V₃) and systemic blood pressure during balloon angioplasty of the left anterior descending coronary artery. During controlled balloon inflation *(second panel),* the ST segment is elevated in aVL and V₃, and there are systemic blood pressure decreases of 20 mm Hg after 30 seconds. During hemoperfusion (50 cc/min), balloon inflation does not result in any blood pressure change. The ST changes normalize even after 10 minutes of balloon inflation *(third panel).* The T wave is inverted in aVL, probably as a result of local hypothermia. The translesional pressure gradient is totally eliminated at the end of the procedure *(last panel).*

FIG 41–3.
Electrocardiographic tracings from a patient with mitral valve prolapse and severe obstruction of a dominant circumflex artery. There was no significant increase in the "v" wave in the wedge pressure *(first panel, middle pressure tracing)*. The controlled balloon inflation caused dyspnea, ST elevation (L$_2$, L$_3$), and clear elevation of the "v" wave to 42 mm Hg. Inflation supported by hemoperfusion of 40 cc/min resulted in effective protection at 10 minutes *(last panel)*.

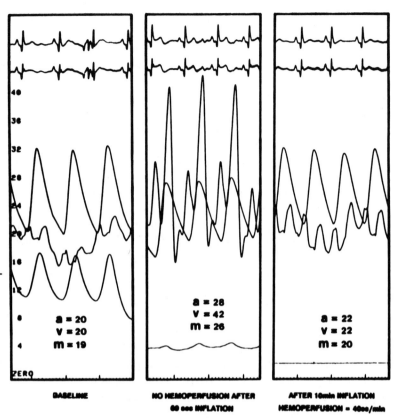

FIG 41–4.
Balloon inflation without protection resulted in the sudden onset of a burst of ventricular tachycardia 45 seconds after occlusion of the proximal left anterior descending coronary artery *(left panel)*. Prolonged balloon inflation, protected by 60-cc/min hemoperfusion, did not result in any arrhythmia.

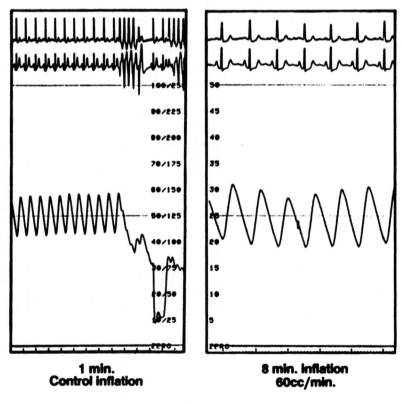

loon catheter are used for intake of blood and pressure.[21] These side holes communicate, distal to the balloon, with the end hole of the balloon catheter. The resistance in the hemoperfusion lumen (and its blood flow rates) depends on (1) the length of the channel (usually about 10 cm); (2) the design of the catheter (essentially, outer diameter, thickness of the catheter's walls, the collapsibility of the inner lumen by the inflated balloon pressure, and the size of the proximal side holes); (3) the presence of a guidewire (of which removal is usually recommended); and (4) blood viscosity (essentially, the hematocrit). Only one of these "autoperfusion" catheters, the Stack perfusion catheter (Advanced Catheter Systems, Santa Clara, Calif), is commercially available,[21] whereas two other similar systems have been developed by USCI (USCI, Bard, Inc., Billerica, Mass)[22] and Schneider (Schneider, Minneapolis) but have not yet been released.

In order to achieve "optimal" levels of hemoperfusion by the passive technique, the operator must accept the drawback of an enlarged deflated profile (for the Stack catheter, 0.056 to 0.062 in., according to the different balloon sizes) in order to achieve an enlarged inner lumen at the level of the balloon. The ten proximal side holes and the distal four side holes plus the end hole do not appear to be restrictive. The guidewire cannot be left in place because it leads to significant limitations in blood flow. Typically, just passing the balloon catheter over the guidewire through the stenotic segment causes ischemic manifestations. Such initial ischemia should be quickly relieved by pulling the guidewire after ensuring the positioning of the balloon at the lesion. If residual ischemia is encountered after this maneuver, autoperfusion will probably not be adequate. In fact, the deflated profile (or crossing profile) of 0.060 in. corresponds to 1.5 mm, which in a reference artery of 3 mm in diameter implies a 50% predilatation of the stenotic lesion diameter during the balloon engagement (Dotter effect).

The diameter of the proximal shaft in the Stack perfusion catheter is 4.5 F, which is obstructive for 8 F guiding catheters and impairs the qualities of aortic pressure monitoring and especially of angiographic flow. Obviously, because of the presence of side holes proximal to the balloon, distal pressure monitoring and contrast injection are impossible. Such limitations make it very difficult to establish the result of balloon angioplasty until the balloon catheter is pulled.

Notwithstanding such technical drawbacks, the Stack balloon catheter has demonstrated appreciable myocardial protection in selected clinical settings.[21–24] In general, autoperfusion will be more effective in patients with proximal stenosis, in those with vessels greater

than 3.0 mm in diameter, and in hypertensive patients. Flow rates are neither monitored nor adapted to the specific clinical conditions when autoperfusion catheters are used. In vitro studies[25] have revealed the blood flow rates reported in Figure 41–5. The original experiments by Advanced Catheter Systems were done with glycerol instead of blood, and the commercially reported flow rates (60 mL/min) do not appear to account for the peculiarity of the coronary circulation wherein blood flow is essentially diastolic. This is noteworthy since blood flow in the autoperfusion catheters is dra-

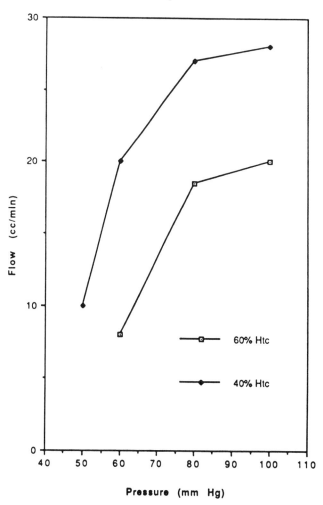

FIG 41–5.

In vitro, pressure gradient/blood flow graphs obtained with the Stack autoperfusion catheter.[25] A blood reservoir was kept at controlled pressure, in a steady-flow model, and blood collected at the end of the catheter. Increased hematocrit (60%) greatly reduces the effective blood flow with respect to a normal-to-low hematocrit. In vitro blood flows are 40% to 50% higher than expected in vivo because of increased intramural pressure. A typical transcoronary gradient of 80 mm Hg is expected to result in an in vivo flow of 15 cc/min.

matically affected by the aortic pressure and the hematocrit. Polycythemic patients will have less adequate blood flow than will anemic patients, although in the latter group O_2-carrying capacity will be decreased.

Current clinical experience has shown that autoperfusion catheters have become quite popular in the United States. The Stack catheter, however, is not used as a "routine" primary catheter. It is mostly used in cases in which clinicoangiographic parameters appear to be favorable for autoperfusion, in cases considered "high risk" for routine balloon catheters[23] (i.e., at high risk of hemodynamic/clinical deterioration during balloon inflation or abrupt reclosure after attempted dilatation), or for "bailout."[24]

Although it is not clear how many procedures performed with the use of Stack catheters could be effectively and safely accomplished with standard balloons, two issues appear to have been preliminarily proved in reported studies[23, 24] in which autoperfusion was successfully used to achieve prolonged inflation. First, the incidence of abrupt reclosure has decreased from an expected, to about 2%. Second, the clinical tolerance of abrupt reclosure seems to be greatly improved when an autoperfusion catheter is placed across the lesion while the patient is being transferred to surgery.

Autoperfusion catheters have also been employed to explore the theory that prolonged inflation results in a decreased restenosis rate at the 6-month follow-up. Preliminary results of one such study[23] have suggested that the recurrence rate is similar to that expected for routine balloon angioplasty, but significant factors could have adversely affected this conclusion. For example, the large deflated profile of the Stack catheter, by causing a preliminary Dotter effect, may establish a less favorable mechanism of initial dilatation, i.e., plaque disruption. Moreover, the selected cases in which autoperfusion catheters were utilized probably included patients at higher risk, not only for immediate complications but also for recurrence. Only prospective, randomized studies can reliably address this theory.

When abrupt reclosure occurs after failed angioplasty,[24] the autoperfusion catheter can be critically supportive, especially in patients with limited myocardial ischemia. If the abrupt reclosure jeopardizes large areas of myocardium or a great portion of the residual myocardium, the flow rate afforded by passive perfusion is normally inadequate for sustaining global heart function. If hypotension develops, the autoperfusion system becomes totally inadequate. Moreover, it may predispose the patient to local clotting in the absence of brisk flow.

Recent improvements in the Stack catheter design

have only addressed the problems that have arisen from the large proximal shaft diameter of 4.5 F by reducing it to 3.9 F. The distal catheter shaft remains the same (4.5 F).

Evaluation of autoperfusion flow by proximal (guiding catheter) angiography is inappropriate primarily because such an injection tends to significantly increase the "perfusion pressure" (a hand-held 10-cc syringe can easily generate 138 psi, which is more than 9 atm and more than 54 times greater than the aortic systolic pressure!). The forward flow demonstrated by such a maneuver is grossly misleading.

Retroperfusion (Coronary Sinus)

Since the 1940s, Beck and others[26] have tried, both experimentally and clinically, to establish an alternative route to the coronary arteries for supplying blood to the myocardium. With the recent advent of catheter interventions, this goal has been reestablished.[26, 27] The most recently developed retroperfusion device[27] involves pumping blood from an arterial cannula (at the femoral artery opposite to that being used for angioplasty) and phasic pumping by a mechanical pump into the coronary sinus. The coronary sinus needs to be cannulated by an 8.5 F balloon catheter introduced from the right jugular vein. The pump is R-triggered from an electrocardiographic signal in order to allow flow only during diastole, while a balloon at the catheter tip inflates and occludes the coronary sinus. Besides considering its complexity and cost, the system is limited by the fact that only the anterolateral and septal walls of the heart can be potentially protected. Preliminary evidence has suggested that the myocardial protection accomplished by this route of hemoperfusion is limited.[27] Because of the presence of venous communication with other cardiac veins and the absence of runoff in the arterial end of this closed hydraulic system, the pumped blood will establish limited flow but will mainly distend the most compliant segments of the circulation. This retroperfusion system has not been approved for clinical application.

Active Hemoperfusion (Prograde)

The focus of this section is our combined experimental and clinical experience with active hemoperfusion during the last 5 years.[18] In attempting to preserve prograde flow through the dilating catheter by the use of mechanical pumps, we encountered two technological problems[2, 3, 28–33]:(1) the need for a deflated balloon profile that would be compatible with routine usage of the catheter while allowing for sufficient blood flow through the inner lumen and (2) the need for a reliable pump that could deliver the high-pressure/low–blood flows typically required for protection of the dependent myocardial territory. Our initial findings with the use of pre-existing technology can be summarized as follows:

1. Most commercially available cardiovascular pumps[33] are essentially roller types, and even those most consistent with our aims, such as the "coronary" Olson pump, were found to be inadequate and unreliable. This was mainly due to slippage at the roller when the output pressure was higher than 80 psi.

2. Most commercially available balloon catheters now have lower profiles and thus are not feasible for hemoperfusion. These balloon catheters have an inner lumen of 0.020 in. or less, which is prohibitive for blood flow in the range of 30 to 60 cc/min. They would require backup pressures of more than 500 psi and create significant hemolysis.

In collaboration with Leocor, we have used the Corflo catheter/pump system and have found it to have innovative characteristics. These include[18] a coaxial double-lumen balloon catheter shaft made of nylon fibers (having a thinner wall than the typical polyethylene catheter) with a large proximal inner lumen (still having a 4.3 F outer diameter) that tapers shortly before the tip at the same time that it decreases its stiffness. The adoption of a polyester fiber for the balloon tissue allowed a deflated balloon profile within the range of most balloon catheters currently in use. The other feature consists of a piston pump specifically designed to produce pressures of up to 200 to 220 psi and capable of producing blood flows of up to 80 cc/min through the above catheters (Fig 41–6).

The Corflo pump was designed to be portable and battery powered for ease of operation in the catheterization laboratory and during transfer of patients to surgery. In our experience with the Corflo catheter, we have tested its capacity to pass and dilate routine coronary obstructions in randomly chosen patients. Of 395 lesions attempted in 240 patients among 10 centers,[19] the success rate of these catheters in passing and dilating the obstructions was 92% (363 lesions), which only increased by 4% (to 96%) when secondary catheters were used after the initial attempt failed.

The Corflo pump was used in an initial series of 110 patients[28] whose selection was based on their inability to tolerate at least 3 minutes of inflation because of symptoms, electrocardiographic changes, or hemodynamic deterioration (Tables 41–1 to 41–3). Flow rates were set according to a presumed 50% of the expected nor-

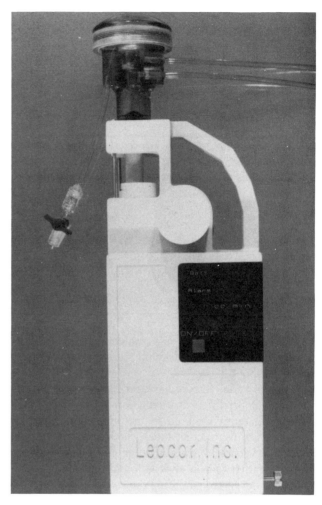

FIG 41–6.
Coronary Corflo (Leocor) pump. This pump is capable of generating up to 80 cc/min of blood flow through the inner lumen of a Leocor balloon catheter.

mal resting blood flow and raised as high as to 70 cc/min only when persistent ischemic changes occurred. Table 41–2 compares the tolerated inflation times in the absence of and during hemoperfusion. The investigators were monitoring symptoms of angina, the ST segments in the most significant three leads,[34] systemic blood pressure, and rhythm.

In 49 cases, the operator elected to test the possibility of protecting the myocardium beyond 10 minutes (maximum, 45 minutes). In the majority of the patients, however, the aim was to prolong inflation beyond 5 minutes or at least to double the control time without hemoperfusion. Only in 2 patients was the inflation terminated before planned because of persistent significant ischemic manifestations. The reason for less-than-optimal protection in these cases was always found to be re-

TABLE 41-1.
Clinical Data From the First 110 Patients Treated With
Hemoperfusion-Supported Angioplasty (Corflo Pump)

Category	N (%)
Gender	
Men	86 (78)
Women	24 (22)
History	
Prior myocardial infarction	49 (45)
Prior procedures	
Coronary artery bypass grafting	16 (15)
Percutaneous transluminal coronary angioplasty	23 (21)
Symptoms	
Unstable angina	62 (56)
Extent of disease	
Single-vessel	65 (59)
Multivessel	45 (40)
NYHA* functional class	
III	39 (35)
IV	55 (50)

*NYHA = New York Heart Association.

lated to the presence of side branches, which were located close to the treated lesion and blocked off by the inflated balloon.

The only side effect of hemoperfusion was found in 2 of 39 cases of right coronary dilation in which hemoperfusion apparently resulted in the unheralded onset of complete atrioventricular block. Such arrhythmias were quickly reversible, however, after hemoperfusion was stopped (rather than after deflation of the balloon alone) and were not observed during the routine controlled inflation. The impression of the investigators was that atrioventricular block resulted from neurogenic reflex from wall stimulation by the jet of blood at the end of the catheter, as suggested by the onset of localized spasm (Fig 41-7). To avoid such problems, keeping a demand pacemaker in place could be routinely recommended in cases of right coronary artery dilatation with hemoperfusion.

In this clinical study, neither significant hemolysis, ventricular arrhythmias, spasm, myocardial damage (by creatine kinase isoenzyme [CPK-MB] elevation), embo-

TABLE 41-2.
Perfusion Data*

Perfusion	CP† Score (0-4)	ST Score (0-4)	Inflation Time (min)
Preperfusion	2.9 ± 1	2.6 ± 1	1.3 ± 0.9
Hemoperfusion	1.4 ± 1	0.7 ± 1	7.1 ± 4.4
P value	< .005	.001	<.01

*Comparison of symptoms and ST elevation during the maximally tolerated control inflation and hemoperfusion-supported inflation.
†CP = chest pain

lism of clots or air, nor vessel injury was ever recognized as a result of hemoperfusion. The free plasma hemoglobin content increased only slightly, even after long (>10 minutes) inflation (mean, 5.5 mg/dL; control normal, 0 to 4), even though blood collected from the end of the balloon catheter after the procedure revealed moderate local levels of hemolysis (mean, 39 mg/dL).

The T wave on the surface electrocardiogram usually inverts quickly after hemoperfusion is begun, even without balloon inflation, and tends to normalize over the next 3 to 5 minutes. This phenomenon is believed to result from a mild level of local hypothermia caused by the extracorporeal circuitry. Such changes do not correlate with angina or with echocardiographic deterioration of local wall motion.

Currently, we have follow-up data for 82 patients from the initial population. All were followed at least 2 months after angioplasty (95% compliance). According to their symptoms and results from stress tests, all of which were positive before PTCA and negative early after, 18 patients underwent follow-up angiography. The others were asymptomatic and had a negative stress test. We documented 15 cases of restenosis (18.3%). We recognize that this follow-up is limited since angiography was not routinely done in all patients; however, the results are promising.

Our initial experience with the Corflo pump/catheters may be interpreted to show that (1) effective and adaptable flow rates can be achieved through coronary angioplasty balloon catheters, (2) no significant side effects will occur, (3) levels of blood flow between 30 and 60 cc/min will usually be effective in relieving myocardial ischemia manifestations during prolonged coronary occlusion, and (4) side branches at the level of the balloon are the only significant limitation in myocardial protection.

Other important questions to be asked, after hemoperfusion has been demonstrated as feasible, focus mainly on the indications for performing angioplasty with hemoperfusion protection. The potential uses for hemoperfusion include the following:

1. The remolding process of the occlusive lesion could become more favorable and allow for stable plastic reshaping in place of fracturing or elastic distension if inflation times could be prolonged without restrictions. Randomized trials currently underway are dedicated to demonstrating whether a single, slow, progressive-onset, prolonged inflation (>10 minutes) could result in better initial angiographic results (larger residual lumen, lower incidence of intimal flap/dissection, lower incidence of abrupt reclosure) and decrease the late recurrence rate.

TABLE 41-3.

Perfusion Data*

		Inflation Time		Flow Rate (Range)	Perfusion Time
Vessel†	(n)	Preperfusion	Hemoperfusion	cc/min	(min)
LAD	74	1.43	7.0	43(17–70)	9.4
RCA	39	1.3	5.5	39(17–70)	9.3
LCx	9	1.08	6.4	36(22–50)	7.9
Vein grafts	15	1.36	5.2	41(25–60)	8.3

*Technical data related to hemoperfusion-supported angioplasty from four vessels. The duration of inflation was usually not limited by ischemic manifestations, but by the operator's decision (see the text).

†LAD = left anterior descending; RCA = right coronary artery; LCx = left circumflex.

2. Hemoperfusion could offer a critical means of support for patients at high risk of developing complications during angioplasty, thus making it an acceptable procedure in these patients.

3. Hemoperfusion support could decrease the ischemic manifestations of abrupt reclosure (after failed angioplasty) during urgent or emergency surgery. The hemoperfusion extracorporeal circulation could be used to prevent ischemia during transport to surgery and to prepare for ischemic arrest. It is anticipated that the hemoperfusion circuitry could be used during surgery for the subselective administration of cardioplegic solution, which otherwise cannot be effectively provided by an aortic or venous route when there is a total occlusion with absence of collateral flow.

4. (Hemo)perfusion could be used with a modified perfusate (blood based or not), which should be useful for addressing the "no-reflow" phenomenon after acute myocardial infarction, as well as the problem of reperfusion injury.[35]

5. Hemoperfusion offers an opportunity for realizing topical administration of drugs directed at preventing restenosis. At present, restenosis after angioplasty with any technique appears to result in biological "scarring," which could possibly be prevented or suppressed by pharmacologic interventions[36, 37] and would be prohibitively expensive and/or toxic if it occurred systemically. Preliminary experiments are aimed at isolating a coronary segment while preserving blood flow through a modified balloon catheter and topically infusing small doses of drugs in a closed arterial segment.

Oxygen Carriers

Because of the high viscosity of blood and the limited flow rates allowed by balloon catheters, it has been suggested that low-viscosity blood substitutes — or oxygen carriers — be used during balloon angioplasty. The Food and Drug Administration recently approved perfluorocarbon emulsions, i.e., Fluosol (Alpha

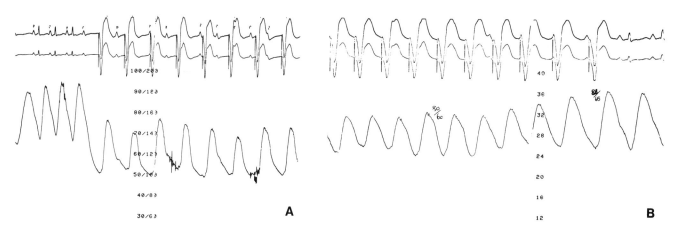

FIG 41-7.
Electrocardiographic and pressure tracings (**A** and **B**) from a patient with a right coronary obstruction who underwent hemoperfusion-supported angioplasty. The early and sudden onset (at 60 seconds) of complete atrioventricular block is shown (**A**) in the absence of chest pain and ST changes during hemoperfusion (40 cc/min). During ventricular pacing, the systemic blood pressure drops until hemoperfusion is stopped and sinus rhythm returns (**B**) in 30 seconds.

(Continued.)

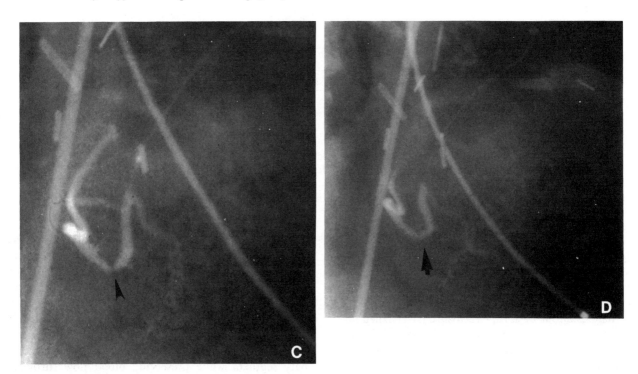

FIG 41–7   (cont.).
Distal balloon catheter angioplasty shows the presence of localized nonocclusive spasm *(arrow)* at a curve **(C)**. Intracoronary nitroglycerin (100 μg) resulted in quick resolution of the spastic obstruction **(D)** *(arrow)*.

Therapeutic Corporation), for this purpose.[38–40] Low-viscosity blood substitutes do allow higher flow rates at lower pressures. Unfortunately, their oxygen-carrying capacity is not ideal and thus results in only limited protection.[38–40] When this less-than-satisfactory substitute for blood is coupled with complexity in its preparation, high cost, and the limited total quantity that can be infused, this does not appear to be a competitive alternative to hemoperfusion.

Recently, some authors have reported experimental evidence suggesting that Fluosol DA, 20%, could be useful in preventing or limiting reperfusion injury during acute myocardial infarctions.[35] A lower-viscosity, leukocyte-free perfusate could have a favorable effect with respect to blood perfusion, but clinical evidence is needed to substantiate this claim.

Intra-aortic Balloon Pump

Intra-aortic balloon counterpulsation has been used for several years to support critically ill patients and was attempted in the early clinical experience with coronary angioplasty.[41] The capacity of this technique for increasing diastolic aortic pressure — the primary determinant of coronary blood flow — and decreasing the work of the heart suggested that it might be used to support critically ill patients during balloon angioplasty, espe-

cially those with acute myocardial infarction or unstable angina.

Clinical experience has demonstrated that intra-aortic counterpulsation offers poor protection for the dependent myocardial territory during balloon inflation but greatly helps in stabilizing critical patients.[42, 43]

Percutaneous Cardiopulmonary Support

The temptation to perform balloon coronary angioplasty in the surgical suite with total extracorporeal circulatory support was obvious to early interventionalists. Such a modification in the procedure would, in effect, have transformed a basic catheter technique into a complex and costly surgical procedure. Bard, Inc., has recently made available a "portable" extracorporeal circulation system for use in emergencies outside the cardiovascular suite. Such technology involves the use of a centrifugal pump, a polypropylene hollow-fiber membrane oxygenator, and a heat exchanger. It requires full heparinization (activated clotting time above 350 seconds) and the introduction of two large cannulas in a femoral vein and artery (18 to 20 F in size). Such introduction has been done recently by a percutaneous technique,[44, 45] which is preferred over surgical cutdown. Under the supervision of a perfusion technologist, the extracorporeal system is primed with 1,400 cc of crystalloid solution. The use of such a technique in the catheterization laboratory has been proposed[44, 45] in order to protect patients during "high-risk" coronary angioplasty.

Current experience with percutaneous cardiopulmonary support[46] has shown that a patient can be effectively supported with 3.5 L/min of artificial circulation even in the absence of spontaneous cardiac function (cardiac standstill or ventricular fibrillation). Unfortunately, cardiopulmonary support predominantly deals with preservation of global cardiac function but not with the ischemia in the myocardial area being affected by balloon angioplasty. Local mechanical and biochemical deterioration of the myocardium does occur, even though the onset of angina and electrocardiographic changes appear to be significantly delayed.[44, 45]

Indeed, cardiopulmonary support appears to make coronary angioplasty a viable option for patients who would otherwise be intolerant to even short balloon inflations because of their critically compromised myocardial state. It is obvious, however, that not all "high-risk" patients can or should have cardiopulmonary support for several reasons: (1) the high cost, increased procedural complexity, and significant complication rate[46] (especially the need for blood transfusions and surgical repair of the entry sites) discourage extensive use of the system; (2) the protection afforded is temporary, is only applicable for global cardiac function, and does not increase the likelihood that angioplasty will be successful in complicated coronary type "C lesions"[47] (i.e., long, diffuse, clot-complicated, ulcerated lesions, especially those located at a tight bend); and (3) the support is temporarily limited to 3 to 6 hours before circuit exchange is required (especially for the membrane oxygenator) and causes an increasing probability of side effects (bleeding, hemolysis, "pump-lung" syndrome). After angioplasty, if the patient has a dissection or an elastic clot with the inherent high probability that reclosure will occur during the next several hours or days, then cardiopulmonary support by itself will be inadequate.

Perhaps we have been influenced by our favorable experience with the simpler Corflo hemoperfusion system; nonetheless, we tend to limit the usage of cardiopulmonary support to patients with unusual problems who are not surgical candidates but have conditions that could be improved by a revascularization procedure. We use cardiopulmonary support when the baseline hemodynamic state is quite compromised (pulmonary edema, shock, severe hypotension) and/or multiple-vessel angioplasty of difficult lesions needs to be done. In cases of single-vessel angioplasty, especially with type A or B lesions,[47] routine angioplasty with standby usage of the

Corflo hemoperfusion system appears to be quite effective and safe even when large segments of the functional myocardium are compromised by balloon inflation.

When coronary angioplasty is unsuccessful and emergency surgery is required, the cardiopulmonary system may be a source of significant complications during the transfer (large apparatus that has to travel with the patient), during the surgical procedure itself (frequently, the surgeon prefers to switch to the traditional cardiac cannulation and extracorporeal circulation system), and after surgery (increased bleeding and local complications at the groin). Also, the direct cost of using cardiopulmonary support is approximately $4,000 (excluding additional costs for the occurrence of complications).

CONCLUSION

Clinical experience suggests that only a few of the proposed techniques are effective for supporting patients undergoing coronary angioplasty. The reasons for this vary. Percutaneous cardiopulmonary support in the catheterization laboratory simulates the support required for cardiac surgery, i.e., support of total-body systems, and is effective when cardiac pumping is absent, but is only adequate for maintaining global cardiopulmonary function. Active hemoperfusion through the balloon catheter seems to offer a simplified solution for achieving local myocardial protection during angioplasty. The combination may be ideal in some complex cases.

The indications for using the new technologies described here have not yet been established, but they may range from extending the application of balloon angioplasty to critically ill patients to improving patient comfort during the procedure, preventing complications, and enhancing the success rate, both immediately and at the 6-month follow-up.

REFERENCES

1. King SB III, Douglas JS, Grüntzig AR: Percutaneous transluminal coronary angioplasty, in King SB III, Douglas JS (eds): *Coronary Arteriography and Angioplasty.* New York, McGraw-Hill, 1985, pp 433–460.
2. Meier B, Grüntzig AR, Brown JE: Percutaneous arterial perfusion of acutely occluded coronary arteries in dogs (abstract): *J Am Coll Cardiol* 1984; 3:505.
3. Anderson HV, Leimgruber PP, Robin GS, et al: Distal coronary artery perfusion during percutaneous transluminal coronary angioplasty. *Am Heart J* 1985; 110:720–726.
4. Grüntzig AR, Myler RK, Hanna ES, et al: Coronary transluminal angioplasty. *Circulation* 1977; 55(suppl 3):84.

5. Holmes DR, Holubkov R, Vliestra RE, et al: Comparison of complications during percutaneous transluminal coronary angioplasty from 1977 to 1981 and from 1985 to 1986: The National Heart, Lung, and Blood Institute Percutaneous Transluminal Coronary Angioplasty Registry. *J Am Coll Cardiol* 1988; 12:1149–1155.

6. Kent KM. Restenosis after percutaneous transluminal coronary angioplasty. *Am J Cardiol* 1988; 61(suppl G):67–70.

7. Hartzler GO, Rutherford BD, McConahay DR, et al: "High-risk" percutaneous transluminal coronary angioplasty. *Am J Cardiol* 1988; 61(suppl G):36–37.

8. Sinclair N, McCabe CH, Sipperly ME, et al: Predictors, therapeutic options and long-term outcome of abrupt reclosure. *Am J Cardiol* 1988; 61(supply G):61–66.

9. Kaltenbach M, Beyer J, Walter S et al: Prolonged application of pressure in percutaneous transluminal coronary angioplasty. *Cathet Cardiovasc Diagn* 1984; 10:213–219.

10. Hodes ZI, Rothbaum DA, Linnemeier TJ, et al: Use of the ACS Stack perfusion dilatation catheter in PTCA to avoid coronary bypass surgery (abstract). *J Am Coll Cardiol* 1989; 13(suppl):15.

11. Quigley PJ, Perez JA, Mikat EM, et al: Effects of prolonged balloon inflation on arterial hyperplasia in rabbits (abstract). *Circulation* 1987; 76:184.

12. Bansol A, Choksi NA, Levine AB, et al: Determinants of arterial dissection during PTCA: Lesion type versus inflation rate (abstract). *J Am Coll Cardiol* 1989; 13(suppl A):229.

13. Remetz MS, Cabin HS, McConnell S, et al: Gradual balloon inflation protocol reduces arterial damage following percutaneous transluminal coronary angioplasty (abstract). *J Am Coll Cardiol* 1988; 11(suppl A):131.

14. Gould KL: *Coronary Artery Stenosis.* New York, Elsevier, 1991.

15. Velican C, Velican D: *Natural History of Coronary Atherosclerosis.* Boca Raton, FA, CRC Press, 1989.

16. Stein PD, Marzilli M, Sabbah HN, et al: Systolic and diastolic pressure gradients within the left ventricular wall. *Am J Physiol* 1980; 238:625–630.

17. Vatner SF: Correlation between acute reductions in myocardial blood flow and function in conscious dogs. *Circ Res* 1980; 47:201–207.

18. Angelini P: Preventing ischemia during angioplasty via mechanical hemoperfusion. *J Myocardial Ischemia* 1990; 2:81–100.

19. Angelini P, DiSciascio G, Brinker J, et al: Prolonged (>5 min) hemoperfusion supported PTCA (abstract) *Circulation* 1990; 82(suppl 3):681.

20. Erbel R, Clas W, Busch U, et al: New balloon catheters for prolonged percutaneous transluminal coronary angioplasty and bypass flow in occluded vessels. *Cathet Cardiovasc Diagn* 1986; 12:116–123.

21. Stack RS, Quigley PJ, Collins G, et al: Perfusion balloon catheter. *Am J Cardiol* 1988; 61(suppl G):77–80.

22. Campbell CA, Rezkalla S, Kloner RA, et al: The autoperfusion balloon angioplasty catheter limits myocardial ischemia and necrosis during prolonged balloon inflation. *J Am Coll Cardiol* 1989; 14:1045–1050.

23. Quigley PJ, Kereiakes DJ, Abbotsmith CW, et al: Prolonged autoperfusion angioplasty: Immediate clinical outcome and angiographic follow-up. *J Am Coll Cardiol* 1989; 13(suppl A):155.

24. Sundram P, Harvey JR, Johnson RG, et al: Benefit of the perfusion catheter for emergency coronary artery grafting after failed percutaneous transluminal coronary angioplasty. *Am J Cardiol* 1989; 63:282–285.

25. Angelini P, Wijay B: Effective blood flow through the Stack autoperfusion catheter. In vitro experiments. Data on file at Texas Heart Institute.

26. Corday E, Meerbaum S, Drury JK: The coronary sinus: An alternative channel for administration of arterial blood and pharmacological agents for protection and treatment of acute cardioischemia. *J Am Coll Cardiol* 1986; 7:711–714.

27. Berland J, Farcot JC, Barrier A, et al: Coronary venous synchronized retroperfusion during percutaneous transluminal angioplasty of left anterior descending coronary artery. *Circulation* 1990; 81(suppl 4):35–42.

28. DiSciascio G, Angelini P, Brinker J, et al: Reduction of ischemia with a new flow-adjustable hemoperfusion pump during coronary angioplasty. *J Am Coll Cardiol* 1992; 19:657 – 62.

29. Busch UW, Pfeiffer U, Kursawe U, et al: Technical and biological aspects of selective coronary perfusion through PTCA catheters (abstract). *Circulation* 1985; 72(suppl 3):470.

30. Angelini P, Heibig J, Leachman R: Distal hemoperfusion during percutaneous transluminal coronary angioplasty. *Am J Cardiol* 1986; 58:252–255.

31. Timmis AD, Crick JCP, Griffen B, et al: Arterial blood infusion for myocardial protection during PTCA (abstract). *J Am Coll Cardiol* 1986; 7(suppl A):105.

32. Angelini P, Leachman R, Heibig J: Flow characteristics of coronary balloon catheters. *Tex Heart Inst J* 1986; 13:213.

33. Heibig J, Angelini P, Leachman R, et al: Use of mechanical devices for distal hemoperfusion during balloon catheter coronary angioplasty. *Cathet Cardiovasc Diag* 1988; 15:143–149.

34. Bush HS, Angelini P, Ferguson JJ: 12-Lead electrocardiogram evaluation of myocardial ischemia during PTCA and its correlation with acute reocclusion (abstract). *J Am Coll Cardiol* 1991; 17:312.

35. Schaer GL, Karas SP, Santoian EC, et al: Reduction in reperfusion injury by blood-free reperfusion after experimental myocardial infarction. *J Am Coll Cardiol* 1990; 15:1385–1393.

36. Jonasson L, Holm J, Hansson GK: Cyclosporine A inhibits smooth muscle proliferation in the vascular response to injury. *Proc Natl Acad Sci USA* 1988; 85:2302–2306.

37. Libby P, Warner SJC, Friedman GR: Interleukin 1: mitogen for human vascular smooth muscle cells that induces the release of growth-inhibitory prostanoids. *J Clin Invest* 1988; 81:487–498.

38. Cleman M, Jaffe C, Wohlgelernter D: Prevention of ischemia during percutaneous transluminal coronary angioplasty by transcatheter infusion of Fluosol DA 20%. *Circulation* 1986; 74:555–562.

39. Jaffe CC, Wohlgelernter D, Cabin H, et al: Preservation of left ventricular ejection fraction during percutaneous transluminal coronary angioplasty by distal transcatheter coronary perfusion of oxygenated Fluosol DA 20%. *Am Heart J* 1988; 115:1156–1164.

40. Kent MK, Cleman M, Cowley M, et al: Reduction of

ischemia during percutaneous transluminal coronary angioplasty (PTCA) with oxygenated Fluosol (abstract). *Circulation* 1987; 76(suppl 4):27.

41. Alcan KE, Stertzer SH, Wallsh E, et al: The role of intraortic balloon counterpulsation in patients undergoing percutaneous transluminal coronary angioplasty. *Am Heart J* 1983; 105:527–530.

42. Voudris V, Marco J, Morice MC et al: "High-risk" percutaneous transluminal coronary angioplasty with preventive intraortic balloon counterpulsation. *Cathet Cardiovasc Diagn* 1990; 19:160–164.

43. Murphy DA, Craver JM, Jones EL, et al: Surgical management of acute myocardial ischemia following percutaneous transluminal coronary angioplasty. Role of the intraaortic balloon pump. *J Thorac Cardiovasc Surg* 1984; 87:332–339.

44. Shawl FA, Domanski MA, Punja S, et al: Percutaneous cardiopulmonary support in high risk patients undergoing percutaneous transluminal coronary angioplasty. *Am J Cardiol* 1989; 64:1258–1263.

45. Vogel RA, Tommaso CL, Gundry SR: Initial experience with coronary angioplasty and aortic valvuloplasty using elective semi-percutaneous cardiopulmonary support. *Am J Cardiol* 1988; 62:811–813.

46. Vogel RA, Shawl F, Tommaso C, et al: Initial report of the national registry of elective cardiopulmonary bypass supported coronary angioplasty. *J Am Coll Cardiol* 1990; 15:23–29.

47. Ryan TJ, Faxon DP, Gunnar RM, et al: Guidelines for percutaneous transluminal coronary angioplasty. A report of the American College of Cardiology/American Heart Association Task Force on Assessment of Diagnostic and Therapeutic Cardiovascular Procedures. *Circulation* 1988; 78:486–502.

42

Autoperfusion Balloon Angioplasty

Alan N. Tenaglia, M.D.

Christopher E. Buller, M.D.

Harry R. Phillips, M.D.

Percutaneous transluminal coronary angioplasty (PTCA) has become a standard treatment for coronary artery disease but still faces the problems of acute occlusion, restenosis, and limited applicability because of complex plaque morphology and total occlusion. The use of gradual and prolonged balloon inflations may help overcome these problems. Such an approach may reduce vessel trauma during PTCA and result in fewer dissections and acute occlusions.[1-5] Reduced nutrient flow to the vasa vasorum and desiccation of the plaque may reduce intimal hyperplasia and restenosis.[6] Prolonged inflation may also allow angioplasty to be performed safely and successfully on lesions previously felt to be unsuitable.[7]

The ability to perform prolonged inflations is limited by the resultant ischemia. Previous attempts to extend balloon inflation times have included pharmacologic methods using β-blockers, calcium blockers, or nitrates; perfusion techniques using antegrade perfusion with fluorocarbons or autologous blood; or retrograde perfusion from the coronary sinus.[8, 9] A practical solution is provided by perfusion balloon catheters (PBC), which allow passive blood flow to the distal myocardium during balloon inflation. This chapter will describe the development of the Stack Perfusion coronary dilation catheter (Advanced Cardiovascular Systems [ACS] Inc., Santa Clara, Calif), its current use and limitations, and future directions in the field.

DEVELOPMENT AND EARLY USE

In 1984, the Interventional Cardiovascular Program of Duke University Medical Center, in conjunction with Dr. John Simpson and ACS, developed a simple intracoronary reperfusion catheter that could be placed across an area of occlusion to maintain myocardial perfusion while patients were transferred to surgery after failed PTCA.[10, 11] The catheter contains 30 holes in its distal 10 cm that allow blood to enter proximally and exit distally to the occlusion.

An extension of this work led to the development of the Stack Perfusion coronary dilatation catheter (Fig 42–1).[12] The catheter shaft has side holes along its distal 10 cm (ten proximal and four distal to the balloon segment) such that during balloon inflation, blood enters proximally, travels through a central lumen, and exits distally. This allows passive perfusion of the myocardium distal to the the inflated balloon. Specifications, including flow rates, are shown in Table 42–1.

Animal studies have shown that using the PBC allows prolonged balloon inflation with attenuation of ischemia. In the canine coronary artery, standard balloon inflation for 3 minutes resulted in marked ischemia as indicated by ST elevation on electrocardiography (ECG), ventricular arrhythmias, and ventricular wall motion abnormalities. In contrast, balloon inflation with the perfusion catheter was tolerated for a mean of 37 minutes without any evidence of ischemia.[12, 13] More recent animal studies have shown adequate myocardial blood flow throughout a 90-minute inflation period, as documented by radio labeled microspheres.[14] When the balloon inflation time was extended to 6 hours, myocardial necrosis was reduced from 84% of the area at risk with standard balloon inflation to 25% in the PBC group.[15]

Studies in humans have also demonstrated attenuation of ischemia during balloon inflation.[16] In 11 pa-

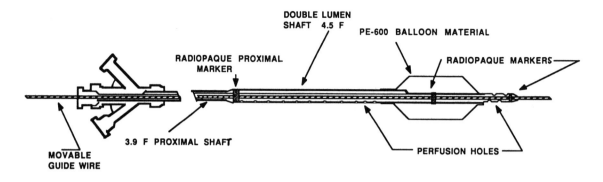

FIG 42–1.
ACS Stack Perfusion coronary dilatation catheter.

tients undergoing routine PTCA, an initial dilatation was performed with the use of a conventional angioplasty catheter (Simpson-Robert), with balloon inflation maintained until the development of severe chest pain (7 on a scale of 0 to 10), >4-mm ST elevation, a widened QRS complex, arrhythmias, or hypotension. The mean inflation time was 107 seconds. Next, dilatation was performed by use of the perfusion catheter; the mean inflation time increased to 513 seconds before the development of the same end points. To exclude a role for "fading ischemia," in which subsequent occlusions are better tolerated, possibly owing to recruitment of collaterals, a third dilatation was performed with the standard catheter, which again was tolerated for a mean of only 139 seconds. The difference in inflation time between the standard balloon and the PBC was statistically highly significant ($P < .001$).

The safety of prolonged inflations was tested in 50 patients undergoing routine PTCA with perfusion balloon dilatation for an average of 15 minutes. There was no evidence of myocardial damage as measured by ECG, ventriculography, or cardiac enzymes and no evidence of hemolysis as measured by plasma hemoglobin, serum haptoglobin, and lactic dehydrogenase levels.[17]

TABLE 42–1.
Specifications of the ACS Stack Perfusion Coronary Dilatation Catheter

Balloon Size (mm)	Shaft Diameter (F)	Profile (in.)	In Vitro Flow Rate* (mL/min)
2.5	3.9	0.057	67.7
3.0	3.9	0.058	65.2
3.5	3.9	0.060	59.2

*Flow rates measured with the use of 38% glycerol, a perfusion pressure of 80 mm Hg, and an inflation pressure of 60 psi.

These early studies proved the safety of prolonged dilatation with the PBC, and the device was approved by the Food and Drug Administration for general use on January 11, 1989. The original Stack Perfusion catheter (SP1, ACS) was replaced by a lower-profile PBC (SP2, also from ACS) on February 27, 1990, and remains the only such device approved for clinical use in the United States. Other autoperfusion balloon catheters are also under development.[18–22]

In addition to the original coaxial-design PBC, a perfusion balloon with a short guidewire lumen (Rx design) has also been developed and was recently released, for marketing (Fig 42–2). This design may allow more rapid placement of the PBC.

TECHNIQUE FOR AUTOPERFUSION ANGIOPLASTY

All patients are premedicated with aspirin, 325 mg daily, before the procedure. Angioplasty is performed via the femoral approach with an 8 F arterial sheath and guilding catheter. Twelve thousand units of heparin is given at the beginning of the procedure, and further intravenous heparin is administered as needed to maintain the activated clotting time at greater than 300 seconds. After arteriography of the target lesion in two orthogonal views, the autoperfusion catheter with a balloon-to-artery ratio of 1 to 1.1 is prepared and advanced across the lesion over a 0.018-in. high-torque floppy guidewire. In a minority of cases predilatation of the lesion with a standard 2.0-mm balloon is necessary to allow placement of the somewhat larger-profile autoperfusion catheter. The balloon is inflated gradually to 6 atm over a period of 3 minutes. Once the balloon is inflated, the guidewire is pulled back proximal to the side

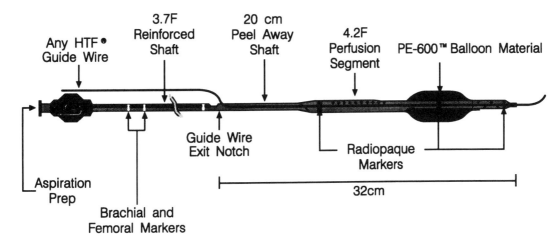

FIG 42–2.
Rx perfusion balloon catheter.

holes, and the rate of flow is documented by contrast injection with the balloon inflated. The guide catheter is then withdrawn slightly from the coronary ostium (0.5 to 1 cm) to facilitate entry of blood into the proximal side holes. Additional heparin is administered through the central lumen at a rate of 1,000 units every 3 minutes. After dilatation is completed, the guide catheter is reseated and the guidewire reinserted, with care taken not to pass the wire out the side holes, and the balloon is deflated. The balloon is then withdrawn into the aorta, and arteriography is repeated. If the initial inflation is unsuccessful (persistent stenosis, thrombosis, filling defect, large dissection, etc.), the balloon is passed across the lesion again, and further dilatations at higher inflation pressures (to a maximum of 8 atm) or for longer durations are performed. Slightly oversized balloons may successfully treat some dissections that cannot be tacked down with standard balloon-to-artery ratios. If successful PTCA cannot be performed due to persistent occlusive dissection, the deflated PBC catheter is left in place across the lesion while preparations are made for coronary artery bypass grafting (CABG).

The use of the Rx PBC differs slightly from the technique described above for the over-the-wire PBC. As with the other PBC, the guidewire is pulled back during balloon inflation to allow entry of blood into the proximal side holes. However, the operator must be careful not to pull the wire back so far that it exits from the catheter. In addition, during balloon inflation, heparin is administered via the guide catheter.

CURRENT INDICATIONS

The perfusion balloon catheter may be useful in four situations: for routine PTCA, for PTCA in high-risk cases, to salvage failed PTCA, and as a bridge to emergency CABG.

Perfusion Balloon Catheters for Routine PTCA

The results of PTCA using prolonged inflation with the PBC have been reported in 122 patients undergoing routine angioplasty at Duke University and Christ Hospital in Ohio.[23] A preliminary dilatation with a 2.0-mm standard balloon was used in 48% of patients, many as part of the protocol and in a minority necessary to allow placement of the PBC across particularly severe stenoses. Autoperfusion angioplasty was performed for a mean duration of 14 minutes. Acute success was achieved in 98% of patients. One patient required emergency bypass surgery for occlusive dissection, and another had in-hospital reocclusion. Of 67 patients eligible for 6-month angiographic follow-up at the time of the initial report, 94% underwent catheterization, and restenosis (>50% luminal diameter narrowing) was found in 30%. Since this report, the remainder of the patients have reached the 6-month follow-up date, and the final restenosis rate is 42%.[24] This is similar to the 43% rate in a large simultaneously acquired group of 2,191 patients undergoing standard PTCA at Duke who had a similar high rate of recatheterization (84%).[25]

To test the hypothesis that primary use of gradual prolonged dilatation will reduce the incidence of important dissections and to further evaluate restenosis, a large multicenter trial is under way. Patients with suitable lesions are randomly assigned to short (two 60-second inflations at 6 atm) vs. long (gradual inflation to 6 atm with a total inflation time of 15 minutes) inflations. All patients are followed with clinical evaluation, exercise treadmill tests, and outpatient cardiac catheterization at 6 months. End points will be acute success, myocardial infarction, death, repeat PTCA, bypass surgery, and angiographic restenosis.

Perfusion Balloon Angioplasty for High-Risk Lesions

Although there are no studies yet available in the literature, the PBC may extend the indications for angioplasty to include patients with high-risk lesions by allowing distal perfusion during balloon inflation. When compared with other angioplasty protection techniques, use of the perfusion balloon catheter is straightforward and employs familiar angioplasty skills. It is safer to use than other techniques such as intra-aortic balloon pumping or percutaneous cardiopulmonary support. It is also relatively inexpensive, especially when it can be used as the primary balloon catheter. If necessary, use of the PBC can also be combined with other protection techniques such as pharmacologic methods, intra-aortic balloon pumping, and cardiopulmonary support. Situations in which the PBC may be useful are listed in Table 42–2.

TABLE 42–2.

Situations in Which Use of the PBC May Reduce the Risk of PTCA

Lesions in coronary arteries that supply collaterals
Lesions in coronary arteries that jeopardize large amounts of myocardium
Reduced ventricular function
Patients intolerant of standard balloon inflations (severe pain, hypotension, arrhythmia)
Acute myocardial infarction

An example of the use of the PBC for high-risk angioplasty is shown in Figure 42–3. The patient was an 85-year-old woman with postinfarction angina and severe chronic obstructive pulmonary disease. At cardiac catheterization she was found to have an ejection fraction of 30%, with moderate to severe mitral regurgitation, total obstruction of the right coronary artery, and a 95% lesion in the left anterior descending artery, which also supplied collaterals to the right coronary. The patient underwent successful angioplasty without complications, and her clinical status improved.

Salvage of Failed PTCA by Perfusion Balloon Angioplasty

Currently, a major use of the perfusion balloon catheter is for salvage of failed standard PTCA in which a

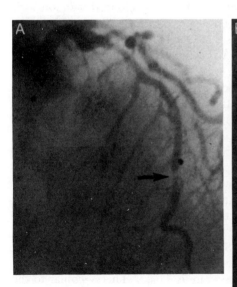 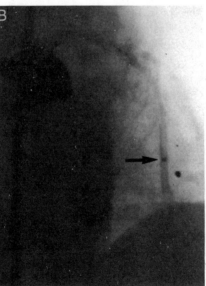 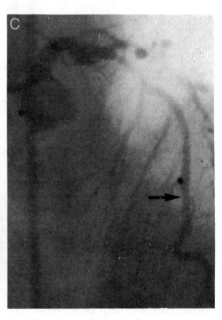

FIG 42–3.
Perfusion balloon catheter for high-risk angioplasty. **A,** a pre-PTCA stenosis in the left anterior descending artery *(arrow)* is shown in a right anterior oblique projection. **B,** perfusion balloon inflated across the lesion *(arrow)*. **C,** final result revealing nearly normal luminal diameter.

major dissection results in total or subtotal occlusion. By allowing prolonged inflation, the perfusion balloon can often "tack up" the dissection and avoid the need for emergency bypass surgery. In 28 patients who had occlusive dissections despite maximally tolerated prolonged inflations with standard balloons, prolonged inflations (21.4 ± 9.3 minutes) with the perfusion balloon resulted in successful procedures in 16 patients (57%) who otherwise would have required bypass surgery.[26] Two of the 16 patients had in-hospital reocclusion, but 14 were asymptomatic when discharged from the hospital. In the unsuccessful group, 10 underwent bypass surgery.

It appears that prolonged inflations using PBC can salvage at least half of failed PTCA cases after other attempts prove unsuccessful. In the majority of cases, attempts should be made to seal occlusive dissections with the PBC before employing more complex technology such as coronary stenting, atherectomy, or thermal angioplasty.

Use of Perfusion Balloon Catheters as a Bridge to Emergency Surgery

The PBC can be left across the coronary lesion in cases of persistent occlusion requiring coronary bypass surgery. In this way, distal perfusion is maintained while preparations are made for surgery. Previous studies with the simple reperfusion catheter show that this approach can result in safer surgery.[27, 28] When this approach is used, there is less risk of myocardial necrosis, and the patient is usually adequately stabilized to allow the cardiac surgeon to employ the mammary artery for grafting.

A unique indication for the PBC is in the management of coronary artery perforations that occur during an interventional procedure. By inflating the perfusion balloon across the area of perforation, the leak is sealed while antegrade perfusion is maintained.

LIMITATIONS

Not all lesions are suitable for PTCA using the perfusion balloon. The long distal tip of the device has the potential to damage the vessel and makes angulated or tandem lesions unsuitable. In lesions close to major side branches, balloon inflation will occlude these vessels and produce ischemia. Lesion characteristics that may preclude the use of the perfusion balloon are listed in Table 42–3.

Owing to the relatively high profile of the perfusion balloon catheter, it is more difficult to place across tight, rigid lesions than in the case of standard catheters

TABLE 42–3.

Lesion Exclusion Criteria for Use of the Perfusion Balloon Catheter

Narrowing proximal to the target lesion, which would compromise passive perfusion
Target lesion longer than the balloon (1.8 mm)
Tandem lesions within 2 cm (relative exclusion)
Major side branch within 1 cm of the target lesion
Sharp angulation within 2 cm distal to the target lesion

and may require predilatation with a smaller standard balloon. We have found, however, that with increased operator experience the number of lesions that require predilatation decreases to only a small minority.

The guidewire must be retracted back proximal to the side holes to allow adequate distal perfusion during balloon inflation. Rarely, guidewire reinsertion may be unsuccessful and result in a loss of distal access following balloon deflation.

Perfusion of the distal coronary bed through the PBC is dependent on driving pressure. Therefore, its usefulness is reduced when systemic blood pressure is low.

FUTURE DIRECTIONS

Low-Profile Perfusion Balloon Catheters

As noted above the relatively high profile of the currently available PBC (SP2) may limit its clinical utility. Lower-profile PBC devices would allow more lesions to be treated with autoperfusion angioplasty as well as reduce the need to predilate some very tight stenoses.

Profile reduction of autoperfusion balloon catheters is constrained by two factors. First, a direct relationship exists between the diameter of the autoperfusion lumen and the flow delivered. Second, excessive thinning of the catheter shaft may lead to a collapse of the autoperfusion lumen from extrinsic compression during balloon inflation. Despite these problems, a new perfusion catheter is being developed that has a lower profile than the existing design without sacrificing in vivo autoperfusion flow rates (SP4, ACS).

Thermal Perfusion Balloon Catheters

The combination of thermal and perfusion technologies may improve the results of angioplasty. A thermal perfusion balloon catheter (TPBC) is currently under development at Duke in conjunction with ACS.[29]

In contrast to other thermal catheters, the perfusion platform allows prolonged treatment with moderate temperatures to achieve the desired thermal effect. Preliminary animal experiments with the TPBC suggest that the device is safe and has the potential to reduce elastic recoil and prevent major dissections. It is hoped that the ability to control both duration and intensity of heating will allow the optimal thermal treatment of coronary artery disease.

CONCLUSIONS

The PBC allows safe performance of angioplasty with prolonged inflation times and results in high procedural success rates. It has an important role in salvaging failed angioplasty and as a bridge to emergency bypass surgery. In addition, the catheter is often of benefit in performing angioplasty of high-risk lesions. Whether prolonged inflation will be of benefit for routine angioplasty is currently under study in a randomized protocol. New devices with lower profiles and thermal capability should further expand the indications for perfusion balloon angioplasty.

REFERENCES

1. Kaltenbach M, Kober G: Can prolonged application of pressure improve the results of coronary angioplasty (TCA)? *Circulation* 1982; 66(suppl 3):123.
2. Kaltenbach M, Beyer J, Walter S, et al: Prolonged application of pressure in transluminal coronary angioplasty. *Cathet Cardiovasc Diagn* 1984; 10:213–219.
3. Palazzo A, Gustafson GM, Santilli E, et al: Unusually long inflation times during percutaneous transluminal coronary angioplasty. *Cathet Cardiovasc Diagn* 1988; 14:154–158.
4. Remetz MS, Cabin HS, McConnel S, et al: Gradual balloon inflation protocol reduces arterial injury following percutaneous transluminal coronary angioplasty (abstract). *J Am Coll Cardiol* 1988; 11:131.
5. Arie S, Checchi H, Coehlo WMC, et al: Coronary angioplasty — Unstable lesions and prolonged balloon inflation time. *Cathet Cardiovasc Diagn* 1990; 19:77–83.
6. Shani J, Gelbfish J, Rivera M, et al: Percutaneous transluminal coronary angioplasty: Relationship between restenosis and inflation times (abstract). *J Am Coll Cardiol* 1987; 9:64.
7. Guermonprez JL, Funck F, Pagny JY, et al: Use of coronary perfusion balloon catheter (PBC) as elective attempt in 24 cases of high risk PTCA: Clinical and ECG modifications during PTCA. *Circulation* 1990; 82(suppl 3):340.
8. Lasala JM, Cleman MW: Myocardial protection during percutaneous transluminal coronary angioplasty. *Cardiol Clin* 1988; 6:329–343.
9. Zalewski A, Goldberg S: Protection of the ischemic myocardium during coronary angioplasty. *Cardiovasc Clin* 1988; 19:79–98.
10. Hinohara T, Simpson JB, Phillips HR, et al: Transluminal catheter reperfusion: A new technique to reestablish blood flow after coronary occlusion during percutaneous transluminal coronary angioplasty. *Am J Cardiol* 1986; 57:684–686.
11. Hinohara T, Simpson JB, Phillips HR, et al: Transluminal intracoronary reperfusion catheter: A device to maintain coronary perfusion between failed coronary angioplasty and emergency coronary bypass surgery. *J Am Coll Cardiol* 1988; 11:977–982.
12. Stack RS, Quigley PJ, Collins G, et al: Perfusion balloon catheter. *Am J Cardiol* 1988; 61:77–80.
13. Collins GJ, Ramirez NM, Hinohara T, et al: The perfusion balloon catheter: A new method for safe prolonged coronary dilatation (abstract). *J Am Coll Cardiol* 1987; 9:106.
14. Christensen CW, Lassar TA, Daley LC, et al: Regional myocardial blood flow with a reperfusion catheter and an autoperfusion balloon catheter during total coronary occlusion. *Am Heart J* 1990; 119:242–248.
15. Zalewski A, Berry C, Kosman ZK, et al: Myocardial protection with autoperfusion during prolonged coronary artery occlusion. *Am Heart J* 1990; 119:41–46.
16. Quigley PJ, Hinohara T, Phillips HR, et al: Myocardial protection during coronary angioplasty with an autoperfusion balloon catheter in humans. *Circulation* 1988; 78:1128–1134.
17. Muhlestein JB, Quigley PJ, Phillips HR, et al: Does myocardial damage or hemolysis occur during prolonged perfusion balloon angioplasty (abstract) *J Am Coll Cardiol* 1990; 15:250.
18. Erbel R, Clas W, Busch U, et al: New balloon catheter for prolonged percutaneous transluminal coronary angioplasty and bypass flow in occluded vessels. *Cathet Cardiovasc Diagn* 1986; 12:116–123.
19. Turi ZG, Campbell CA, Gottimukkala MD, et al: Preservation of distal coronary perfusion during prolonged balloon inflation with an autoperfusion angioplasty catheter. *Circulation* 1987; 75:1273–1280.
20. Turi ZG, Rezkalla S, Campbell CA, et al: Amelioration of ischemia during angioplasty of the left anterior descending coronary artery with an autoperfusion catheter. *Am J Cardiol* 1988; 62:513–517.
21. Campbell CA, Rezkalla S, Kloner RA, et al: The autoperfusion balloon angioplasty catheter limits myocardial ischemia and necrosis during prolonged balloon inflation. *J Am Coll Cardiol* 1989; 14:1045–1050.
22. White CJ, Ramee SR, Banks AK, et al: New passive perfusion PTCA catheter. *Cathet Cardiovasc Diagn* 1990; 19:264–268.
23. Quigley PJ, Kereiakes DJ, Abbottsmith CW, et al: Prolonged autoperfusion angioplasty: Immediate clinical outcome and angiographic follow-up (abstract). *J Am Coll Cardiol* 1989; 13:155.
24. Quigley P, Tenaglia A, Kereiakes D, et al: Immediate and long-term outcome following gradual and prolonged inflation using an autoperfusion angioplasty catheter: Results of a multicenter trial. (Submitted for publication) 1991.
25. Tcheng JE, Fortin DF, Frid DJ, et al: Conditional probabilities of restenosis following coronary angioplasty. *Circulation* 1990; 82:111.
26. Smith JE, Quigley PJ, Tcheng JE, et al: Can prolonged perfusion balloon inflations salvage vessel patency after failed angioplasty? *Circulation* 1989; 80(suppl 2):373.

27. Sundram P, Harvey JR, Johnson RG, et al: Benefit of the perfusion catheter for emergency coronary artery grafting after failed percutaneous transluminal coronary angioplasty. *Am J Cardiol* 1985; 63:282–285.

28. Ferguson TB Jr, Hinohara T, Simpson JB, et al: Catheter reperfusion to allow optimal coronary bypass grafting

following failed transluminal coronary angioplasty. *Ann Thorac Surg* 1986; 42:399–405.

29. Buller CE, Davidson CJ, Sheikh KH, et al: Real-time transvenous intravascular ultrasound assessment of thermal and conventional perfusion balloon angioplasty. *Circulation* 1990; 82(suppl 3):460.

43

Left Ventricular Assist Devices Available to the Cardiologist: Indications, Techniques, and Early and Late Results

Richard W. Smalling, M.D., Ph.D.

Reversible ischemic dysfunction after a 2-hour coronary occlusion followed by reperfusion was described first in detail by Theroux and colleagues.[1] In chronically instrumented animals they discovered that after a 2-hour coronary occlusion, regional myocardial function gradually recovered after reperfusion. However, the time course was prolonged and required up to 3 weeks for full recovery.[1] Braunwald and Kloner later termed this phenomenon *myocardial stunning*.[2] We reported, in humans, late return of left ventricular function after successful reperfusion that was apparently not affected by surgical revascularization. This improvement in left ventricular function persisted at the 6-month follow-up and was not observed in patients with acute myocardial infarction who had not undergone successful reperfusion.[3] Thus, the concept has emerged that acute ischemic dysfunction may be reversible with timely reperfusion of the infarct-related artery. Nonetheless, the possibility remains that reperfusion injury might also exist and profound circulatory failure might occur after reperfusion prior to recovery of contractile function. Lee and colleagues reported that coronary angioplasty in the setting of cardiogenic shock secondary to acute myocardial infarction may improve survival both with and without left ventricular assistance using intra-aortic balloon counterpulsation.[4] Survival in successful angioplasty patients approached 69% but remained at 20% in patients without successful angioplasty.

Multiple techniques are in the process of evaluation in an attempt to minimize reperfusion injury. Allen and colleagues have demonstrated, in an animal model, that in hearts with reperfusion alone an infarct resulted in 44% of the risk region, whereas in hearts that had been arrested with cardioplegia during cardiopulmonary bypass with left ventricular venting, the infarct size was reduced substantially to 12% of the risk region.[5] The authors hypothesized that reducing oxygen consumption at the time of reperfusion was an essential ingredient in addition to left ventricular decompression. Failure to decompress the left ventricle resulted in an infarct size of 25% of the risk region. These data therefore suggest that left ventricular assist devices in the setting of coronary reperfusion may actually produce improved infarct salvage in addition to supporting the failing circulation.

Unfortunately, few experimental data exist regarding the optimal methods of left ventricular support. In a rather rigorous animal preparation, McDonnell and colleagues suggested that aortic counterpulsation resulted in a 17% decrease in oxygen consumption in the normal ventricle as compared with a greater than 50% decrease in oxygen consumption achieved by total left ventricular bypass. These data suggested that intra-aortic balloon counterpulsation was only 30% to 40% as effective as total left heart bypass.[6] Similarly, Takanashi and colleagues suggested that left heart bypass resulted in a 30% improvement in infarct salvage when compared with intra-aortic counterpulsation.[7]

There is no satisfactory agreement, however, on which patients are candidates for application of cardiopulmonary bypass or cardiac assist. Norman and colleagues suggested a scoring methodology incorporating cardiac index, pulmonary capillary wedge pressure, systemic vascular resistance, and urine output that seemed to predict survival with and without cardiac assist.[8] In patients with a cardiac index greater than 2 L/min/m^2 and a systemic vascular resistance less than 2,000 dyne-sec-cm^{-5}, survival was attained in 100% of patients. With institution of intra-aortic balloon counterpulsation, they found an increase in cardiac output of approximately 0.2 L/min with a decrease in pulmonary capillary wedge pressure of 5 mm Hg.

Which devices then are available to the cardiologist for left ventricular support? Lincoff and associates have published a good overview of devices currently under investigation or in routine use during supported coronary angioplasty. These include intra-aortic balloon counterpulsation, antegrade perfusion through angioplasty catheters, coronary sinus retroperfusion, cardiopulmonary support system, the Hemopump, and partial left heart bypass.[9] For the purposes of practicality the discussion of support devices will be limited to those capable of supporting arterial pressure and reducing left ventricular filling pressures during circulatory collapse without requiring left atrial cannulation. The devices currently available or under investigation include the intra-aortic balloon pump, the cardiopulmonary support system, and the Hemopump.

The ideal left ventricular assist device would be able to do the following:

1. Support the acutely failing circulation. Optimally, this would require an active form of pumping effectively bypassing the left ventricle.

2. Decrease the oxygen consumption of the left ventricle. In most instances, acute left ventricular failure is an ischemic event, and in the absence of reperfusion, ongoing ischemia usually persists. With limited inflow into the ischemic zone, tissue might be salvaged if the ischemic area oxygen consumption could be significantly reduced.

3. Improve collateral blood flow into ischemic myocardium. In the presence of continued restriction of antegrade blood flow into ischemic areas, an ideal device should result in improved collateral blood flow into the region at risk, thus limiting ischemic damage.

4. Decrease wall stress of the failing ventricle. There is some evidence that suggests that progressive dilatation of ischemic tissue occurs but may be prevented by vigorous left ventricular decompression.

The above concepts should be considered while reviewing each of the following modes of left ventricular assistance.

INTRA-AORTIC BALLOON COUNTERPULSATION

The intra-aortic balloon pump has been studied for many years and is familiar to virtually all interventional cardiologists. It has been refined through the years by progressive miniaturization and adaption for percutaneous vessel entry combined with over-the-wire guidance. The device is the simplest of the left ventricular assist modalities that will be discussed. Briefly, it utilizes a 40-cc elongated balloon coupled to a dual-lumen shaft. The balloon is usually inflated with helium gas in a controlled fashion. The timing/pumping console contains adjustments for the degree of balloon inflation as well as the number of cardiac cycles per balloon inflation and the timing of onset and offset of balloon inflation with regard to the QRS on the electrocardiographic (ECG) tracing. The balloon is driven to abruptly expand, acutely displacing 40 cc of blood at the end of left ventricular ejection (timed at the dicrotic notch of the arterial pressure waveform). This, in effect, increases blood pressure during diastole, theoretically improving coronary perfusion. Just prior to the onset of ejection the balloon is abruptly evacuated to create a relative decrease in intra-aortic blood volume of 40 cc. Thus, the ejecting ventricle sees an abrupt decrease in afterload that reduces the amount of work necessary to eject blood.

Physiology

Degree of Support

Due to the nature of the mechanism of left ventricular assistance, there is no active pumping from the left ventricle or left artrium into the systemic circulation. Blood is simply displaced within the aorta proper to produce a relative passive augmentation of blood flow. Due to the complexities of autoregulation in intact preparations, it is difficult to ascertain the true effective improvement in forward blood flow with the intra-aortic balloon pump. Norman and colleagues[8] have suggested that cardiac output increases by approximately 0.2 L/min. Other investigators have felt that the intra-aortic balloon produces as much as a liter-per-minute forward blood flow depending on vascular resistance and other considerations.

Degree of Left Ventricular Unloading

Although most cardiologists have observed a fall in left ventricular filling pressures and pulmonary capillary wedge pressures with counterpulsation, this finding is difficult to corroborate in the literature. McDonnell et al. have suggested that counterpulsation in acutely ischemic animals produces a fall in left ventricular end-diastolic pressure from 11.8 to 10.8 mm Hg, a change that is not statistically significant. Norman and colleagues, however, demonstrated a small but significant decrease in pulmonary capillary wedge pressure of 5 mm Hg with balloon counterpulsation[9] in humans.

Improvement in Regional Myocardial Blood Flow

There is some controversy as to the potential for improvement in regional myocardial blood flow during ischemia with intra-aortic balloon counterpulsation. Willerson and colleagues.[10] suggested that intra-aortic balloon pumping in combination with intravenous administration of mannitol improved collateral blood flow by up to 46%. Kerber et al., however, suggested that there was no change in collateral blood flow as measured by microspheres and furthermore that left ventricular end-diastolic pressure did not decrease although there was a slight decrease in left ventricular end-diastolic diameter.[11]

Reduction In Myocardial Oxygen Consumption

There are a few reports of actual measurements of myocardial oxygen consumption with intra-aortic balloon counterpulsation. McDonnell and colleagues[6] suggested that oxygen consumption fell during counterpulsation by up to 17% from 9.2 to 7.6 mL 0^2/min/100 g tissue. The data therefore suggest that intra-aortic balloon counterpulsation produces little change in myocardial oxygen consumption and ischemic bed coronary blood flow.

Indications

The indications for intra-aortic balloon counterpulsation are largely based on clinical impression. There are no controlled studies firmly establishing indications for use of this device. Nonetheless, an extensive amount of clinical experience combined with reports of uncontrolled trials have suggested the following indications:

Unstable Angina

The rapid evolution of interventional techniques in cardiology, including coronary angioplasty and thrombolysis, have produced more direct techniques for treating unstable angina currently. There is, however, a subset of patients who have unsuitable anatomy for angioplasty or who are not candidates for thrombolysis but who, in general, are felt to benefit from balloon pumping prior to elective surgical revascularization. It is felt by most that balloon pumping without definitive revascularization has little benefit in any setting. Gold and colleagues have reported that chest pain during unstable angina abated with balloon pumping in most patients. With interruption of balloon pumping, however, a significant number of patients demonstrated recurrence of

chest pain within 15 minutes that was abolished by reinstatement of counterpulsation.[12] Clearly, however, pharmacologic therapy including intravenous nitroglycerine, heparin, and aspirin, as well as β-blockers and calcium channel blockers, has reduced the number of patients who might otherwise have been considered candidates for counterpulsation for this indication.

Acute Myocardial Infarction

In general, in the era of thrombolysis and acute angioplasty for myocardial infarction, intra-aortic balloon counterpulsation is usually relegated to those patients with hemodynamic compromise after successful infarct artery reperfusion. DeWood and associates reported that balloon counterpulsation was useful in patients presenting in cardiogenic shock within 16 hours of the onset of symptoms. The majority of the patients in the study of DeWood et al. underwent coronary bypass surgery acutely. Institution of intra-aortic balloon counterpulsation late in the course of acute myocardial infarction complicated by shock was apparently much less efficacious.[13] Scheidt and associates reviewed a number of reports of small studies totaling 337 patients treated with intra-aortic balloon counterpulsation without surgery in cardiogenic shock. The survival rate in this patient population was 23% as compared with 81 patients treated with counterpulsation and coronary bypass operation with a survival rate of 47%. These data underscore the clinical impression that counterpulsation alone is much less helpful than reperfusion (particularly early reperfusion) coupled with counterpulsation.[14]

Failure to Wean From Cardiopulmonary Bypass

The use of intra-aortic balloon counterpulsation in patients who did not readily come off cardiopulmonary bypass after cardiac surgery is fairly routine. This hemodynamic failure usually occurs when support on cardiopulmonary bypass drops below 1 to 2 L/min. After institution of pharmacologic therapy some surgeons favor balloon pumping over high doses of pressors. Nonetheless, the requirement for intra-aortic balloon counterpulsation in the operating room is associated with approximately a 50% mortality rate.[8] Profound circulatory failure in this setting will usually not respond to intra-aortic balloon counterpulsation. Frequent ventricular arrhythmias and an intermittent need for cardiac pacing also complicate the situation and make intra-aortic counterpulsation less attractive.

Bridge to Cardiac Transplantation

Intra-aortic balloon counterpulsation can be utilized for a prolonged period of time. In compliant patients who are able to keep their leg straight (to prevent kinking of the balloon shaft) and who have fairly stable rhythms, balloon pumps have been left in place for at least a month. The chief limitations are vascular complications, which can be minimized with appropriate patient selection, use of a low-profile device, adequate anticoagulation, and prevention of infection, which may be aided by meticulous wound care and prophylactic antibiotics. There are no data available as to the efficacy of prolonged counterpulsation as a bridge to cardiac transplantation in chronic, severe refractory heart failure.

Contraindications

Intra-aortic balloon counterpulsation is contraindicated in patients with aortic insufficiency. The etiology of the low-output state should be clearly cardiac prior to the institution of intra-aortic balloon counterpulsation. Patients with septic shock or hypovolemia, especially from bleeding, are not candidates for this technique.

Method of Insertion

The device is typically inserted percutaneously over a guidewire through the common femoral artery by utilizing a 10 to 12 F sheath. The tip of the intra-aortic balloon is positioned just distal to the left subclavian artery. The balloon lumen is then coupled to an actuator device that is timed to the patient's ECG (or occasionally blood pressure). Balloons used in adults are most commonly 40 cc; however, some manufacturers make smaller and larger devices. The central lumen may be used for arterial pressure monitoring after guidewire removal. It is important to measure blood pressure proximal to the intra-aortic balloon because distal pressure (femoral artery pressure) may be significantly different from central aortic pressure and will not adequately reflect the amount of augmentation that occurs with counterpulsation.

Complications

The main complications of intra-aortic balloon counterpulsation with percutaneous delivery are vascular. Loss of distal pulses and the need for arterial exploration or repair occur in 22% of patients. Thrombosis and emboli occur in 14%, and local infections occur in 8% of patients treated. The most feared complication is profound leg ischemia resulting in amputation, which occurs in fewer than 1% of patients. With the new de-

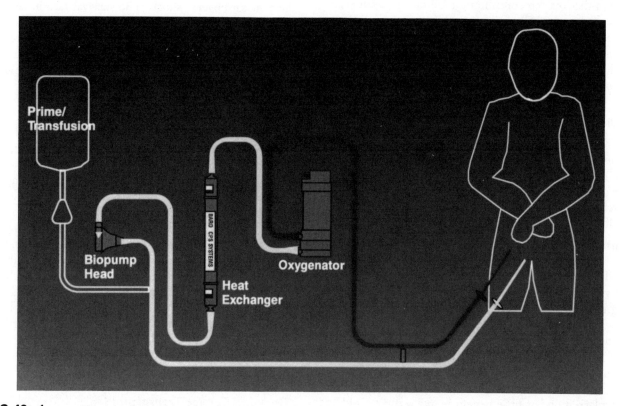

FIG 43–1.
System schematic for the BARD cardiopulmonary support system. Blood is aspirated via an 18 F cannula from the middle of the right atrium. It sequentially enters the oxygenator, heat exchanger, and Biomedicus pump prior to being returned to the common femoral artery cannula.

velopments in interventional techniques, including iliac angioplasty if necessary, lower-profile devices, and more sophisticated skills in device delivery, complications with intra-aortic balloon insertion are relatively minimal.[15]

CARDIOPULMONARY SUPPORT SYSTEM

The device described in this section is called the BARD cardiopulmonary support (CPS) system. There are other manufacturers who produce similar devices; however, the literature deals almost entirely with this particular device. The CPS system is quite simply a femoro-femoral bypass device as outlined in the schematic diagram depicted in Figure 43–1. A large venous cannula (see Fig 43–2) is inserted via the femoral vein into the middle of the right atrium. A similar arterial cannula is positioned in the common iliac artery via percutaneous entry of the femoral artery. After suitable priming, the system then aspirates blood from the middle of the right atrium through the femoral vein; the blood is then passed through an oxygenator, a heat exchanger, and finally a Biomedicus centrifugal pump, which then returns the blood to the patient via the arte-

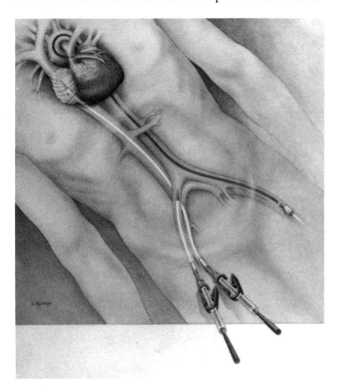

FIG 43–2.
This illustrates the cannula positions prior to instituting cardiopulmonary support. The venous cannula aspirates blood from the middle of the right atrium, and the arterial cannula returns blood to the common iliac.

rial cannula. This device, then, is a total cardiac bypass device and functions independently of left or right heart activity.

Physiology

Degree of Support

The average flow produced by this device is 4.9 L/min and ranges between 0.5 and 5.2 L/min. This device is capable of total support of the circulation[16, 17] independent of heart rhythm, right heart function, or pulmonary vascular resistance.

Degree of Left Ventricular Unloading

There are few reports of hemodynamics when this device is used and no reports of simultaneous direct left ventricular and arterial pressure measurements. However, Shawl and colleagues have reported decreases in pulmonary capillary wedge pressure from the mid-20s to 0 to 2 mm Hg during CPS.[16] Direct left ventricular venting has not been utilized with this device, although techniques are being developed to make this possible. If the data reported by Allen et al. for traditional cardiopulmonary bypass are correct, then left ventricular venting is probably critical for significant infarct salvage.[5]

Improvement in Regional Myocardial Blood Flow/Reduction and Oxygen Consumption

There are no studies reporting regional myocardial blood flow determinations with the device, nor are there direct studies of oxygen consumption with the CPS system. It is likely, however, with significant reductions in observed filling pressures as well as a decreased return to the left ventricle that oxygen consumption and myocardial work will be substantially reduced.

Indications

Acute Myocardial Infarction With Shock

Since the CPS system is limited to approximately 6 hours of support, its use in acute myocardial infarction with shock should be limited to those patients experiencing essentially total circulatory collapse prior to successful reperfusion of the infarct-related artery. Shawl and colleagues have reported using this device in eight patients presenting within 3 hours of the onset of symptoms of myocardial infarction. Two patients were in full cardiac arrest at the time of insertion of the cannulas and institution of support. Seven of the eight had successful angioplasty of the infarct-related vessels. The remaining patient had unsuitable anatomy and died. The remaining seven patients were alive at up to 8.8 months.[16] Survival in these patients was remarkably good in view of the fact that half of the vessels treated were right coronary arteries, which often have a poor outcome secondary to right ventricular dysfunction.

Acute Closure in PTCA

Shawl and colleagues have also reported their experience in three patients undergoing hemodynamic collapse in the setting of abrupt closure during coronary angioplasty.[17] All three patients survived the episodes, and two of the three subsequently underwent emergency coronary artery bypass surgery, with the third undergoing repeat dilatation of a closed right coronary artery. The time from onset of cardiac arrest to institution of CPS ranged from 10 to 25 minutes with a range of mean arterial pressure from 75 to 110 mm Hg on left ventricular support. The circulation was supported by using this device despite severe electrical instability including ventricular fibrillation. Once again, successful revascularization was a key to survival in this subgroup of patients.

Supported Elective PTCA and Valvuloplasty

Vogel et al. and Tomasso and colleagues have reported the concept of utilizing CPS in order to perform very high-risk angioplasty or valvuloplasty.[18–22] Due to a fairly high complication rate with this procedure in patients who subsequently underwent relatively uncomplicated dilatations, investigators have suggested that a standby approach for CPS may be advantageous.[22] In the standby support group of angioplasty patients (i.e., those with left ventricular ejection fractions less than 25% or target vessels supplying greater than 50% of the myocardium) 5 F sheaths were inserted into the contralateral artery and vein, and the CPS system was readied for subsequent cannulation and institution of bypass. They suggested that active CPS plus angioplasty be reserved for patients who have a history of prior hemodynamic collapse during invasive procedures, for those in whom the angioplasty procedure is aimed at the only patent vessel, or in those with very poor (ejection fraction less than 15%) left ventricular function.

Method of Insertion

In the absence of an emergency insertion, pelvic angiography is routinely employed to ascertain whether the aorto-ileo-femoral system will accept the 18 to 20 F cannulas. Occasionally it has been necessary to predilate the iliofemoral vessels prior to placement of the arterial cannula. Initially, 8 F sheaths are placed in the left femoral artery and vein followed by systemic heparinization of the patient with 300 units/kg of body weight. Following this an 8 F long dilator is introduced over an 0.038-in. flexible guidewire. The flexible guidewire is then replaced by a stiff 0.038-in guidewire with sequential dilatations over the stiff guidewire by using 12 and 14 F

dilators. Subsequently, the 18 to 20 F arterial cannula is inserted, and a 20 F cannula is inserted in the femoral vein with the tip of the cannula just above the junction of the right atrium and inferior vena cava. After successful cannula placement, the previously primed CPS system is moved to the field and the cannulas attached to the support system. As bypass is instituted, it is frequently necessary to give large quantities of crystalloid to support systemic pressure. Following the procedure the cannulas may be removed by using percutaneous techniques (with a C clamp) or by surgical repair.[16, 20]

Duration of Assistance

Percutaneous cardiopulmonary bypass is a short-term support measure. The longest reported duration of support is 8.5 hours.[17] Conceivably, with the development of improved oxygenators the support time may be lengthened.

Complications

The difficulties in using CPS are nontrivial. Up to 3% of patients treated with this device die secondary to the device use itself. Blood loss requiring transfusion occurred in 43% of patients, and over 40% of patients had

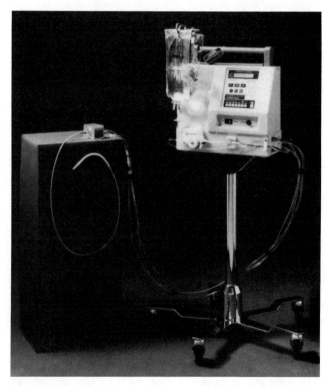

FIG 43–3.
Hemopump cardiac assist system with a 7-mm-diameter Silastic cannula, 9 F drive shaft electromagnetic motor, purge fluid tubing, and control console with support stand.

complications other than the need for transfusion. It is this rather significant morbidity associated with device use that has led to the development of the term *standby supported angioplasty.*[22]

TRANSVALVULAR LEFT VENTRICULAR ASSIST DEVICE: THE HEMOPUMP

The Hemopump lies somewhere between the intra-aortic balloon pump and the CPS system in its ability to support the circulation. In general, it is a 25-cm-long, 7-mm-diameter Silastic cannula attached to an axial-flow turbine that is powered by a 9 F drive shaft. The device was designed by Dr. Richard Wampler, initially constructed by the NIMBUS Corporation, and is currently manufactured by Johnson & Johnson. It is coupled electromechanically to an electromagnetic drive motor and control console. The turbine spins at up to 25,000 rpm, and produces a flow of up to 3.5 L/min.[23] The device is illustrated in Figure 43–3. The console is relatively compact for ease in mounting on the bed rail or gurney. The drive shaft requires a lubricant solution

of 40% dextrose and water ($D_{40}W$) to maintain the pump seal and reduce heating of the unit. The patient receives approximately 200 cc of $D_{40}W$ per day.

Physiology

Degree of Support and Left Ventricular Unloading

As previously stated, the Hemopump can produce up to 3.5 L of blood flow per minute depending on left ventricular filling pressure and mean arterial pressure or systemic vascular resistance. We have demonstrated in dogs that the device produces significant reduction in developed peak left ventricular systolic pressure and left ventricular end-diastolic pressure during regional ischemia. Similar changes occur in the absence of ischemia, although these are less marked.[24] Similar findings are also observed in humans as illustrated by Figure 43–4 and Table 43–1. Figure 43–4 illustrates tracings obtained in a 36-year-old man who was recovering from an acute anterior myocardial infarction complicated by cardiogenic shock. With the Hemopump on, left ventricular systolic pressure was reduced from approximately 55 to 35 mm Hg. Pulmonary artery end-diastolic

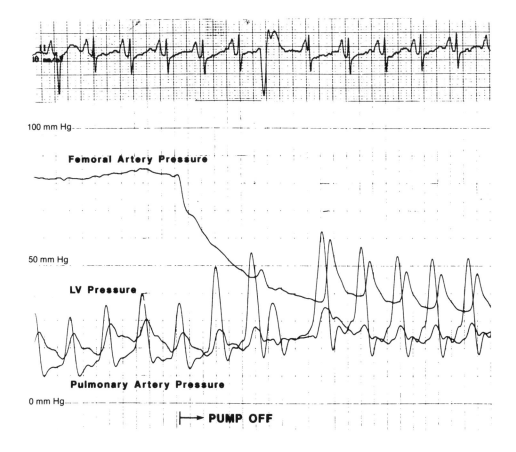

FIG 43–4.

Simultaneous pressures obtained in a 36-year-old man in cardiogenic shock supported by the Hemopump. As support is discontinued, there is an abrupt rise in left ventricular systolic pressure and pulmonary artery end-diastolic pressure with a significant fall in femoral artery pressure. During pump support, pulsatile arterial flow is absent.

TABLE 43–1.

Hemodynamics in Nine Patients With Cardiogenic Shock From Acute Myocardial Infarction Before, During, and After Hemopump Insertion

Parameter	Preinsertion	24 hr Postinsertion	72 hr Postinsertion
Cardiac output (L/min)	3.4	4.7*	5.8*
Pulmonary capillary wedge pressure (mm Hg)	26	15.7*	17*
Mean arterial pressure (mm Hg)	54	76*	86*

*Significant change from preinsertion.

pressure similarly decreased from 25 to 17 mm Hg. Simultaneously, mean arterial pressure increased from approximately 40 to 75 mm Hg. Table 43–1 depicts similar findings in nine patients with cardiogenic shock secondary to acute myocardial infarction. Significant increases in cardiac output and mean arterial pressure were observed with significant decreases in pulmonary capillary wedge pressure.

Improvement in Regional Myocardial Blood Flow and Reduction in Oxygen Consumption

We have demonstrated, in animals, that regional myocardial blood flow decreases slightly during Hemopump support at the same time a reduction in regional myocardial function is observed. This is presumed to be secondary to effective left ventricular unloading producing a reduction in the Starling effect

and a secondary reduction in contraction. This should produce a reduction in regional blood flow secondary to downregulation of coronary blood flow due to decreased demand.[24] To date there are no reports of direct measurements of oxygen consumption when the Hemopump is used. During regional myocardial ischemia in dogs, however, we have observed an increase in regional myocardial blood flow from 13% ± 8.7% to 26% ± 19%[24] of control. This suggests that collateral blood flow to the ischemic region is significantly increased during Hemopump support despite the fact that the epicardial vessel remained occluded in the risk region.

Indications

Of the three devices reported in this chapter the Hemopump is the only one remaining in investigational status at the present time. Therefore precise indications are as yet undetermined.

Acute Myocardial Infarction With Shock

The most promising data with this device have been generated in patients with acute myocardial infarction and secondary cardiogenic shock. Wampler and colleagues have reported on 53 patients treated with the Hemopump. Of the 53, the best outcome was observed in patients with acute myocardial infarction, where the survival rate was 41.2%. The cardiac index in all patients improved from 1.6 to 2.28 L/min at 24 hours, and similarly, the mean arterial pressure improved signifi-

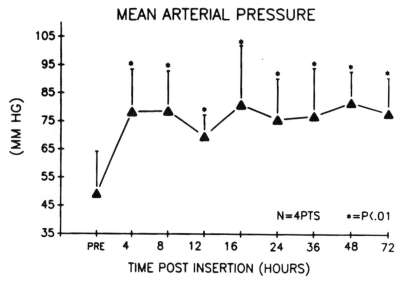

FIG 43–5.
Mean arterial pressure in four patients with cardiogenic shock. There is an abrupt increase in pressure with institution of left ventricular assistance that persists throughout the period of support.

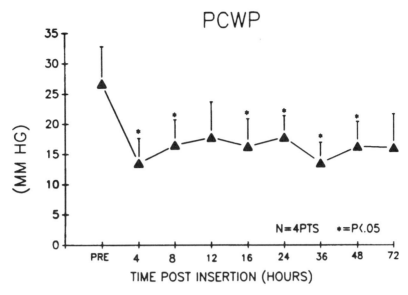

FIG 43-6.
Pulmonary capillary wedge pressure *(PCWP)* tracings obtained in four patients supported by the Hemopump. There is an abrupt fall in filling pressures from supraphysiologic to physiologic levels.

cantly from 57 to 65.3 mm Hg with a simultaneous reduction in vasopressor doses.[25] In our series of nine patients with shock secondary to acute myocardial infarction, direct pressure measurements were available in four as illustrated in Figures 43–4 to 43–6. As illustrated in Figure 43–4 mean arterial pressure rises abruptly after insertion of the device and allows discontinuation or reduction of vasopressor drug therapy. The

mean arterial pressure stabilizes and is maintained. Similarly, as illustrated in Figure 43–6, the pulmonary capillary wedge pressure falls abruptly and remains low during support and at device removal. However, as shown in Figure 43–7, cardiac output gradually recovers, consistent with the concept of slow recovery from myocardial stunning in the setting of an acute ischemic insult.

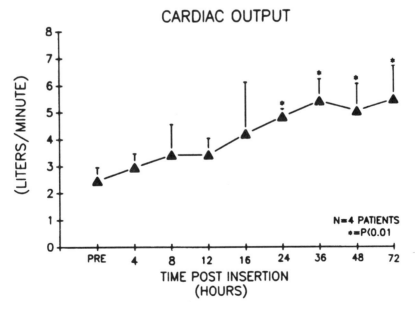

FIG 43-7.
Cardiac output measurements in four patients recovering from cardiogenic shock secondary to acute myocardial infarction. There is a gradual increase in cardiac output consistent with recovery from myocardial stunning after reperfusion.

Supported Angioplasty/Acute Closure in PTCA

In the United States use of this device was restricted by the Food and Drug Administration to patients in cardiogenic shock. However, in France, Loisance and colleagues have used the Hemopump as a support device during high-risk angioplasty.[26] In their experience they observed an increase in cardiac index of 23% and fall in pulmonary capillary wedge pressure of 17% with Hemopump support. Several patients developed severe electrical instability during the angioplasty procedure but remained conscious with good blood pressure during Hemopump-supported angioplasty. Since insertion of the device requires a cutdown on the femoral artery, widespread use of supported angioplasty has not been reported. We and others have successfully used the Hemopump to achieve hemodynamic stability prior to rescue angioplasty in acute myocardial infarction.

Failure to Wean From Cardiopulmonary Bypass

In the report of Wampler and associates, the patients entered into the protocol for failure to wean from cardiopulmonary bypass had a relatively dismal outcome. This was felt to be largely secondary to late institution of the device after prolonged attempts at coming off cardiopulmonary bypass with conventional methods.[25]

It is conceivable that earlier use of the Hemopump in this setting might produce an improved outcome.

Adjunct in the Treatment of Acute Cardiac Transplant Rejection

Frazier and colleagues[27, 28] have reported use of the Hemopump in acute rejection after cardiac transplantation. They reported successful implantation of the device in three patients ranging in age from 9 to 61 years. All patients survived their acute rejection episodes. The Hemopump supported the circulation while antirejection modalities were employed for up to 6 days. This particular indication may represent a unique role for the Hemopump.

Bridge to Cardiac Transplantation

Protocols for Hemopump use initially specifically excluded its use as a bridge to cardiac transplantation. However, as the indications were expanded, patients with refractory cardiogenic shock were included. We have treated one such patient for a total of 17 days. During this time, the patient's liver and renal function improved significantly, and he was switched to balloon pump support with normal liver and renal function for the remainder of his bridge period. During the initial

HEMOPUMP PLACEMENT
FEMORAL INTRODUCTION

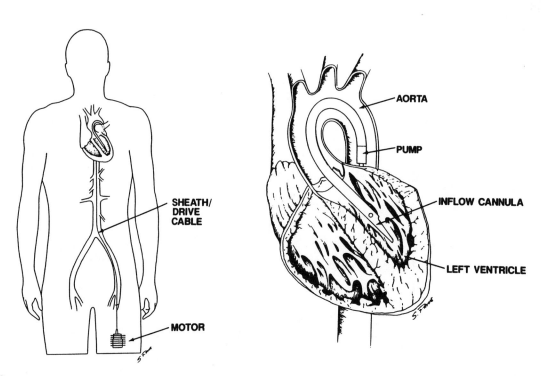

FIG 43–8.
Schematic illustrations of the Hemopump in place via the femoral artery demonstate the drive shaft exiting from the common femoral artery and the pumping cannula tip in the left ventricular outflow tract with the turbine exit port in the descending aorta.

phase of support, however, intra-aortic balloon pump support would have been ineffective due to severe left ventricular and atrial dysrhythmias subsequently controlled on propafenone and mexiletine.

Method of Insertion

Due to the substantial size of the Hemopump (7-mm diameter) introduction via the femoral vessels is commonly nontrivial. As in the case of the CPS system, it may be necessary to predilate the vessels prior to insertion. Various insertion techniques were described in detail by Duncan et al.[29] In general, a cutdown is performed over the common femoral artery. A tourniquet is placed on the common femoral artery at the level of the inguinal ligament while the superficial femoral and the profunda branches are clamped distally. Prior to clamping the vessels the patient must be systemically heparinized. A 12-mm woven Dacron graft is preloaded on to the drive shaft of the Hemopump, and a short segment of Penrose drain is attached over the exit of the turbine by utilizing no.2 silk ligatures. If the Hemopump does not readily pass into the descending aorta, the iliofemoral vessels may be dilated with a 10-mm angioplasty balloon over a 0.35-in. J-wire. After dilatation of the vessels the cannula is quickly inserted into the common femoral artery, the tourniquet is re-leased, the cannula is advanced to the level of the turbine, and the tourniquet is reapplied while the Penrose drain is quickly removed. The cannula is then rapidly advanced into the ascending aorta across the aortic arch and prolapsed across the aortic valve in a similar manner to catheterization of the left ventricle with a standard pigtail catheter. The 12-mm Dacron graft is then sutured to the arteriotomy and a small slotted Silastic plug inserted into the graft and tied by using the no.2 silk. The graft is then buried in the wound and the wound closed in layers. The drive shaft must be maintained relatively straight to prevent drive shaft fracture secondary to excessive flexing. If the iliac vessels are totally occluded, a retroperitoneal incision is made over the distal segment of the abdominal aorta with anastomosis of the Dacron graft directly to the descending abdominal aorta above the bifurcation of the iliacs. Figure 43–8 demonstrates in a schematic fashion a general overview of the insertion of the Hemopump device and the position of the Hemopump cannula tip and turbine within the left ventricle and aorta. In Figure 43–9 a radiographic image obtained in the cardiac catheterization laboratory illustrates the correct position of the Hemopump. The turbine is in the descending aorta, and the cannula tip is across the aortic valve and rests in the left ventricular chamber. Transthoracic insertion of the Hemopump has been accomplished by using a special short cannula; however, at the present time this method of insertion has been discontinued.

Duration of Assistance

Originally the pump was tested in animals for only 2 weeks.[23] During this period of time the experimental animals did not develop excessive hemoglobinuria, anemia, or thrombocytopenia. As previously stated, we have had the device in place for up to 17 days without significant adverse effects. The precise potential duration of support is as yet to be determined. Improvements in drive shaft fatigue life have made it possible to anticipate support periods of at least a month.

Contraindications and Complications

Patients with severe aortic stenosis and/or aortic insufficiency should not be considered for this device since it requires insertion across the aortic valve. Similarly, patients with prosthetic, mechanical aortic valves are not candidates for the device, although patients with porcine prosthetic aortic valves could conceivably undergo successful Hemopump insertion. The device actively aspirates blood from the left ventricular cavity, and hence in patients with documented left ventricular thrombus, it may pose undue risk for systemic embolization. In patients with severe right-sided failure or

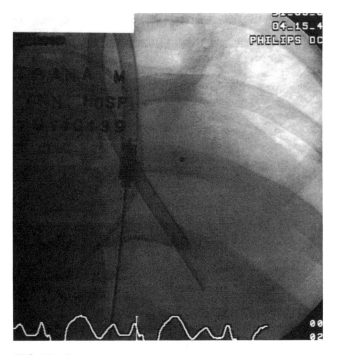

FIG 43–9.
A radiographic image obtained from a patient after successful Hemopump insertion demonstrates the cannula tip well within the left ventricular cavity and the turbine resting in the descending thoracic aorta.

TABLE 43-2.

Performance Characteristics of Left Ventricular Assist Devices

Characteristic	Intra-Aortic Balloon Pump	Hemopump	Cardiopulmonary Support System
Access site	Femoral artery (percutaneous)	Femoral artery (cutdown)	Femoral artery and vein (percutaneous or cutdown)
Size of cannula/sheath	10-12 F	7 mm by 25 cm with a 9 F drive shaft (requires a 12-mm Dacron graft)	18-20 F arterial and venous cannulas
Level of support	Passive displacement of blood, approx. 0.2-1 L/min forward flow	Active pumping from the LV* up to 3.5 L/min	Active pumping from the RA* through the oxygenator up to 5.2 L/min
Duration of support	Days to weeks	Days to weeks (17 days longest reported support)	Up to 8.5 hr
Anticoagulation requirement	Moderate	Minimal to moderate	Full heparinization required (ACT,* 350-400 sec)
LV decompression	Minimal	Excellent	Minimal to moderate
Stable cardiac rhythm required	Yes	No	No

*LV = left ventricle; RA = right atrium; ACT = activated clotting time.

dramatically increased pulmonary vascular resistance, the Hemopump may not be beneficial because it exclusively pumps blood from the left ventricle to the aorta. If forward flow through the right-sided circulation is severely impaired, then the Hemopump may be of little assistance.

The major complication has been a failure to insert the device, usually on the basis of severe peripheral atherosclerosis or difficulty in crossing the aortic valve.[25] Other complications include thrombocytopenia in 7.3%, dysrhythmias in 27% (not associated with hemodynamic sequelae), and peripheral embolism after pump removal in 2.4%. Interestingly, leg ischemia has been rare with this device.

SUMMARY

Tables 43-2 and 43-3 summarize the performance characteristics and complications associated with the left ventricular assist devices available to cardiologists. The intra-aortic balloon pump is the least invasive but also offers the least amount of support and, most important, requires synchronization with the cardiac rhythm, which ideally should be relatively slow and regular. The Hemopump offers an additional level of support up to 3.5 L/min but is considerably more invasive and requires femoral artery cutdown. It does decompress the left ventricle to a significant extent and is not totally dependent on cardiac rhythm. The CPS system offers the

TABLE 43-3.

Incidence of Complications of Left Ventricular Assist Devices

Complication	Intra-aortic Balloon Pump	Hemopump	Cardiopulmonary Support System
Loss of distal pulses, arterial repair	22%	All patients require arterial repair for device removal	12%-20%
Thrombosis/emboli	14%	2.4%	9%
Amputation	0.4%	0%	0%
Neurologic (foot drop etc.)	4%	4.8%	2%
Local infection	8%	2.4%	8%
Bleeding	13%	Minimal (not reported)	43%
Thrombocytopenia	Minimal	Minimal to moderate	Minimal to moderate
Hemolysis	Minimal	Minimal to moderate	Minimal to to moderate
Mortality secondary to device use	<1%	<1%	3%
Arrythmia	No	Yes	No
Insertion failure	5%	23%	Not reported

most support, up to 5.2 L/min, and can be inserted percutaneously in the majority of cases. Unfortunately, it is only suitable for supporting the circulation for up to 8.5 hours.

All of the left ventricular support devices are associated with significant complications. Perhaps the most benign device, again, is the intra-aortic balloon pump. The Hemopump has relatively few complications, however, it is associated with an insertion failure of approximately 23% at the present time. The CPS system had an exceedingly high complication rate, especially given its limited period of support.

Despite the excess of complications associated with the CPS system, it truly can totally support the circulation, which may be necessary in cardiac catheterization "crashes." Since the Hemopump is still investigational and requires the skills of both a surgeon and cardiologist (in most cases), use of this device is less attractive for catheterization laboratory "crashes." Despite the fact that the balloon pump requires synchronizaion with the cardiac rhythm and is not a very powerful circulatory support device, at the present time it remains the workhorse of ventricular support devices utilized by cardiologists. If a version of the Hemopump could be developed that was small enough to be inserted percutaneously and had the ability to track over a guidewire, use of the Hemopump might be substantially increased. The complication rate associated with the CPS system will most assuredly progressively diminish as technology and experience with the device continue to progress.

REFERENCES

1. Theroux P, Ross J Jr, Franklin D, et al: Coronary arterial reperfusion. III. Early and late effects on regional myocardial function and dimensions in conscious dogs. *Am J Cardiol* 1976; 38:599–606.
2. Braunwald E, Kloner RA: The stunned myocardium: Prolonged, postischemic ventricular dysfunction. *Circulation* 1982; 66:1146–1149.
3. Smalling RW, Fuentes F, Matthews MW, et al: Sustained improvement in left ventricular function and mortality by intracoronary streptokinase administration during evolving myocardial infarction. *Circulation* 1983; 68:131–138.
4. Lee L, Erbel R, Brown TM, et al: Multicenter registry of angioplasty therapy of cardiogenic shock: Initial and long-term survival. *J Am Coll Cardiol* 1991; 17:599–603.
5. Allen BS, Okamoto F, Buckberg GD, et al: Studies of controlled reperfusion after ischemia. XIII. Reperfusion conditions: Critical importance of total ventricular decompression during regional reperfusion. *J Thorac Cardiovasc Surg* 1986; 92:605–612.
6. McDonnell MA, Kralios AC, Tsagaris TJ, et al: Comparative effect of counterpulsation and bypass on left

7. ventricular myocardial oxygen consumption and dynamics before and after coronary occlusion. *Am Heart J* 1979; 97:78–88.
7. Takanashi Y, Campbell CD, Lass J, et al: Reduction of myocardial infarct size in swine: A comparative study of intraaortic balloon pumping and transapical left ventricular bypass. *Ann Thorac Surg* 1981; 32:475–485.
8. Norman JC, Cooley DA, Igo SR, et al: Prognostic indices for survival during postcardiotomy intra-aortic balloon pumping. Methods of scoring and classification, with implications for left ventricular assist device utilization. *J Thorac Cardiovasc Surg* 1977; 74:709–720.
9. Lincoff AM, Popma JJ, Ellis SG, et al: Percutaneous support devices for high risk or complicated coronary angioplasty. *J Am Coll Cardiol* 1991; 17:770–780.
10. Willerson JT, Watson JT, Platt MR: Effect of hypertonic mannitol and intraaortic counterpulsation on regional myocardial blood flow and ventricular performance in dogs during myocardial ischemia. *Am J Cardiol* 1976; 37:514–519.
11. Kerber RE, Marcus ML, Ehrhardt J, et al: Effect of intra-aortic balloon counterpulsation on the motion and perfusion of acutely ischemic myocardium. An experimental echocardiographic study. *Circulation* 1976; 53:853–859.
12. Gold HK, Leinbach RC, Buckley MJ, et al: Refractory angina pectoris: Follow-up after intraaortic balloon pumping and surgery. *Circulation* 1976; 54(suppl 3):41–46.
13. DeWood MA, Notske RN, Hensley GR, et al: Intraaortic balloon counterpulsation with and without reperfusion for myocardial infarction shock. *Circulation* 1980; 61:1105–1112.
14. Scheidt S, Collins M, Goldstein J, et al: Mechanical circulatory assistance with the intraaortic balloon pump and other counterpulsation devices. *Prog Cardiovasc Dis* 1982; 25:55–76.
15. Kantrowitz A, Wasfie T, Freed PS, et al: Intraaortic balloon pumping 1967 through 1982: Analysis of complications in 733 patients. *Am J Cardiol* 1986; 57:976–983.
16. Shawl FA, Domanski MJ, Hernandez TJ, et al: Emergency percutaneous cardiopulmonary bypass support in cardiogenic shock from acute myocardial infarction. *Am J Cardiol* 1989; 64:967–970.
17. Shawl FA, Domanski MJ, Wish MH, et al: Emergency cardiopulmonary bypass support in patient with cardiac arrest in the catheterization laboratory. *Cathet Cardiovasc Diagn* 1990; 19:8–12.
18. Vogel RA, Tommaso CL, Gundry SR: Initial experience with coronary angioplasty and aortic valvuloplasty using elective semipercutaneous cardiopulmonary support. *Am J Cardiol* 1988; 62:811–813.
19. Vogel JHK, Ruiz CE, Jahnke EJ, et al: Percutaneous (nonsurgical) supported angioplasty in unprotected left main disease and severe left ventricular dysfunction. *Clin Cardiol* 1989; 12:297–300.
20. Vogel RA: The Maryland experience: Angioplasty and valvuloplasty using percutaneous cardiopulmonary support. *Am J Cardiol* 1988; 62:11–14.
21. Vogel RA, Shawl F, Tommaso C, et al: Initial report of the national registry of elective cardiopulmonary bypass supported coronary angioplasty. *J Am Coll Cardiol* 1990; 15:23–29.

22. Tommaso CL, Johnson RA, Stafford JL, et al: Supported coronary angioplasty and standby supported coronary angioplasty for high-risk coronary artery disease. *Am J Cardiol* 1990; 66:1255–1257.

23. Wampler RK, Moise JC, Frazier OH, et al: In vivo evaluation of a peripheral vascular access axial flow blood pump. *Am Soc Artif Intern Organs* 1988; 34:450–454.

24. Merhige ME, Smalling RW, Cassidy D, et al: Effect of the Hemopump left ventricular assist device on regional myocardial perfusion and function. Reduction of ischemia during coronary occlusion. *Circulation* 1989; 80 (suppl 3):158–166.

25. Wampler RK, Frazier OH, Lansing A, et al: Treatment of cardiogenic shock with the Hemopump left ventricular assist device. *Ann Thorac Surg* 1991; 52:506–513.

26. Loisance D, Dubois-Randé JL, Deleuze Ph, et al: Prophylactic intraventricular pumping in high-risk coronary angioplasty. Lancet 1990; 335:438–440.

27. Frazier OH, Wampler RK, Duncan JM, et al: First human use of the Hemopump, a catheter-mounted ventricular assist device. *Ann Thorac Surg* 1990; 49:299–304.

28. Frazier OH, Macris MP, Wampler RK, et al: Treatment of cardiac allograft failure by use of an intraaortic axial flow pump. *J Heart Transplant* 1990; 9:408–414.

29. Duncan JM, Frazier OH, Radovancevic B, et al: Implantation techniques for the Hemopump. *Ann Thorac Surg* 1989; 48:733–735.

PART VIII

Mechanisms of Restenosis

A Paradigm for Restenosis Based on Cell Biology: Clues for the Development of New Preventive Therapies

James S. Forrester, M.D.

Michael Fishbein, M.D.

Richard Helfant, M.D.

James Fagin, M.D.

The central hypothesis of this chapter is that restenosis is the unique vascular expression of the systemic wound healing response. To support this unproven hypothesis, we will begin by defining the time course and the histopathology of coronary restenosis in man. We will then relate these data to a substantial body of relevant research in oncology, atherogenesis, and wound healing. From these correlations, we will develop a hypothetical schema for the pathogenesis of restenosis and conclude by discussing the possibilities for its prevention.

THE TIME COURSE OF RESTENOSIS

Although coronary angiography has little predictive value for restenosis of individual lesions,[1-6] serial angiography has defined its time course. Nobuyoshi et al. repeated coronary angiography in 229 patients at 1, 3, 6, and 12 months after successful coronary angioplasty.[3] The actuarial restenosis rate was 13% at 1 month, 43% at 3 months, and 53% at 1 year. They concluded that restenosis develops between the first and third month after coronary angioplasty. This conclusion has been confirmed by Serruys et al., who performed quantitative coronary angiography at a single predetermined follow-up time of 1, 2, 3, or 4 months in 342 patients.[4] Like Nobuyoshi et al., they found that the most sub-

stantial change in lumen diameter occurred between the second and third months. Serruys et al. also made the important observation that "almost all lesions deteriorate to some extent by 120 days post coronary angioplasty." Thus, whereas prior angiographic studies used categorical cutpoints to define restenosis as present or absent, these data suggest that restenosis is a response that "almost always" occurs but is of sufficient variation in magnitude that it is only detected by clinical or routine angiographic methods in 25% to 55% of patients.[1-6] This seemingly semantic distinction may be critical to our understanding of restenosis, as will be described below.

THE IMMEDIATE AND LATE CONSEQUENCES OF CORONARY ANGIOPLASTY

The rapidity of its development puts restenosis in the category of syndromes of accelerated atherosclerosis induced by injury.[7, 8] Because angiography is a relatively insensitive method for detecting intimal injury,[9] angioscopy has recently been used before, during and after balloon angioplasty. Uchida et al. found that whereas 64% of coronary angioplasty sites appeared angiographically normal immediately after coronary angioplasty, all had angioscopic evidence of intimal trauma,[10] a finding confirmed by Mizuno et al.[11] These angioscopic data are concordant with postmortem studies of patients dying within 30 days of coronary angioplasty, which consistently show that even after angiographically successful angioplasty there is a high incidence of intimal dissection, hemorrhage and thrombus formation.[12–25] The largest single study, by Potkin and Roberts, found that 95% of angiographically successful angioplasties had evidence of extensive intimal damage.[19] The distending force of the balloon also frequently injures the vascular media,[16–19] sometimes actually tearing it apart. Postmortem fixation obscures the stretching effect of balloon dilation because the normal segment of an eccentric lesion contracts during fixation.[26] Thus we can conclude that coronary angioplasty routinely causes

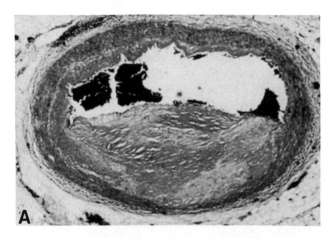

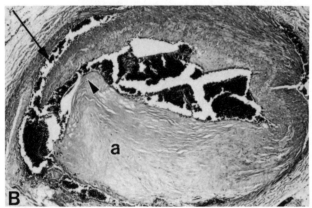

FIG 44–1.
Segments of right coronary artery from a patient who died after emergency percutaneous transluminal coronary angioplasty (PTCA) followed by bypass surgery for massive myocardial infarction. **A,** proximal nontreated segment. **B,** segment from a balloon angioplasty site showing separation of atheroma *(a)* from adjacent normal arterial wall *(arrowhead)* with dissection of blood through the disrupted media *(arrow)* (hematoxylin-eosin [HE] stain, ×25).

substantial injury to both the intimal surface and the media that is not detectable by angiography (Fig 44–1).

DENUDING AND STRETCHING: STIMULI FOR HYPERPLASIA

To examine the hypothesis that restenosis is the local vascular manifestation of the general biological response to injury we need to define its histologic appearance. At 1 to 3 months after coronary angioplasty, when coronary angiography indicates that restenosis is developing, histologic studies consistently show intimal hyperplasia. The intimal hyperplasia is not confined to the atheromatous segment of the vessel circumference and is often prominent over the normal segment. This is important because both intimal denuding[27, 28] and medial stretching injury[29, 30] are potent stimuli to intimal hyperplasia of normal vessels in animal studies. Thus, post–coronary angioplasty angiographic narrowing and intimal hyperplasia of *both* the normal and atherosclerotic segments suggest that restenosis is a generalized response to vascular injury that is not dependent upon the presence of atherosclerosis.

This concept is supported by in vivo human studies. There have now been a number of patients who developed restenosis after their first atherectomy and in whom the procedure was repeated.[31] Examined microscopically, these tissue samples of restenosis are quite striking. There is often a sharp linear demarcation between the residual atheroma and a newly formed layer of intimal hyperplasia. Histologically this tissue is indistinguishable from post–coronary angioplasty intimal hyperplasia. Furthermore, tissue with this same histologic appearance also develops on the inner surface of isolated Dacron grafts in the first 3 months after placement (Fig 44–2).[32] Taken together, we may use the foregoing to infer that the histologic basis of restenosis after coronary angioplasty is intimal hyperplasia and, further, that the response is neither specific to balloon injury nor even to angioplasty.

If restenosis is the vascular manifestation of a general biological response to tissue injury, then studies of the molecular and cell biology of wound healing[33] become potentially relevant to its pathogenesis. Wound healing is a generalized biological response that has been most extensively studied in the skin and the eye. Healing has been described in three overlapping phases[33]: inflammation, granulation and matrix formation (Fig 44–3). We will first review these three phases and then apply this information to develop a hypothetical construct of restenosis. This construct will then be used to examine potential strategies for preventing restenosis.

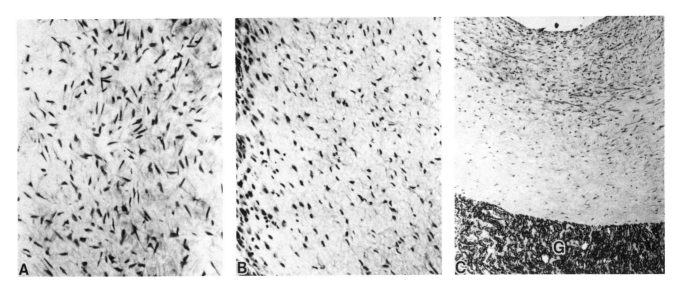

FIG 44–2.
Photomicrographs of intimal hyperplasia. **A,** after balloon angioplasty. **B,** in a dermal scar. **C,** (shown at lower magnification) on a synthetic (Gortex) vascular graft *(G)*. Note the histologic similarity of the proliferation (**A** and **B** ×100, **C** ×40).

THE INFLAMMATORY PHASE OF WOUND HEALING: CELLS AND GROWTH FACTORS

The *inflammatory* phase of wound healing begins with coagulation of blood and soluble serum fibronectin to form an extracellular matrix. Fibronectin has binding domains for both inflammatory cells and biologically active substances that appear in the early phases of wound healing. At the same time, platelets aggregate on the wound surface. The activated platelets release substances that promote local vasoconstriction and thrombus formation, as well as growth factors that activate

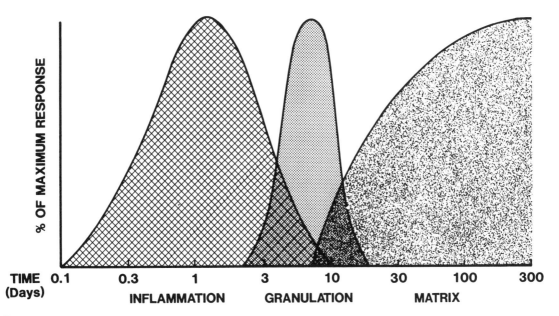

FIG 44–3.
The three phases of wound healing. The inflammatory phase begins at the instant of injury and persists for several days. Predominant features of this phase are platelet aggregation, deposition of the fibronectin extracellular matrix, and infiltration of inflammatory cells. The granulation phase overlaps with both the end of the inflammatory phase and the beginning of the matrix remodeling phase. The granulation phase lasts for 1 to 2 weeks and consists predominantly of modulation, migration, and proliferation of mesenchymal cells adjacent to the wound site. The matrix remodeling phase persists for months. It consists predominantly of proteoglycan deposition, followed by conversion of the extracellular matrix to collagen and elastin.

mesenchymal cells in the vicinity of injured tissue. Within a few hours monocytes also appear and increase in number over the first few days. Like platelets, monocytes secrete growth factors capable of initiating and promoting local tissue mesenchymal cell migration.

Although their specific roles are incompletely understood, there is little doubt that the combined action of several growth factors released in the inflammatory phase play an important role in the second and third phase of wound healing.[33-37] Topically applied growth factors, e.g., epidermal growth factor,[34] markedly accelerate wound healing in man. Growth factors have many different cellular sources, more than one biological action, and overlapping functions, and they serve to potentiate (or inhibit) each other's effects.[35, 36] With the caveat that the field is quite complex and the table may be incomplete, we have listed growth factors that may play an important role in wound healing and their most important potential roles in restenosis (Table 44-1). Platelet-derived growth factor released from the alpha granules of platelets is a potent stimulus to smooth muscle cell migration and proliferation.[38, 39] Conversely, fibroblast growth factor has a similar effect on endothelial cells.[40] Platelet-derived growth factor and fibroblast growth factor do not act alone, however, after tissue injury. Platelet-derived growth factor and fibroblast growth factor make cells "competent" to be acted upon by a second class of growth factors that cause "progression" to actual DNA synthesis. Prominent among these "progression" factors are epidermal growth factor and insulin-like growth factor.[40-43] Epidermal growth factor and insulin-like growth factor-1 also stimulate mesenchymal cell proliferation,[41, 42] and epidermal growth factor competes with heparin for the same cellular binding site.[42] Finally, transforming growth factor β is the most important growth factor in the regulation of extracellular matrix production.[44-47] Transforming growth factor β activates gene expression of proteoglycans and collagen, decreases the synthesis of proteolytic enzymes that degrade matrix proteins, and increases the synthesis of cell receptors for matrix protein.[44] Synthesis of chondroitin sulfate, the dominant extracellular matrix protein early in intimal hyperplasia, is increased 20-fold by transforming growth factor β.[45, 46]

It is tempting to visualize these growth factors as acting sequentially in wound healing. In fact, however, the temporal sequence of growth factor expression during wound healing is not yet defined. We found a twofold increase in platelet-derived growth factor B-chain mRNA and a ninefold induction of insulin-like growth factor-1 mRNA expression beginning at day 3 after injury, peaking at day 7, and returning to baseline at 2 weeks.[48] Cromack et al. have found a substantial increase in transforming growth factor β in healing tissue during the same time period.[49] Thus, the local tissue level of at least three growth factors is markedly increased during wound healing. While both the cell sources and the details of the interactions among these factors and other cytokines remain to be defined, we can reasonably infer that locally produced growth factors are a major stimulus for mesenchymal cell migration, proliferation, and extracellular matrix production in wound healing.

THE GRANULATION PHASE OF WOUND HEALING: CELLULAR PROLIFERATION

The beginning of local tissue cell migration into the wound site is a convenient marker for the onset of the *granulation* phase of wound healing (so called because large numbers of newly formed capillaries on the wound surface impart a granular appearance). The fibronectin extracellular matrix facilitates the migration of epithelial or endothelial cells from the wound margin and fibroblasts or smooth muscle cells from adjacent tissue. Both cell types proliferate. The epithelial or endothelial cells cover the wound surface; the fibroblast and/or smooth muscle cells synthesize new extracellular matrix components, particularly hyaluronic acid and proteoglycans.

The most prominent cell in intimal hyperplasia is the smooth muscle cell. Control of smooth muscle cell proliferation is determined by the actions of mitogens (e.g., platelet-derived growth factor, insulin-like growth factor-1) and the opposing effects of inhibitors (e.g., transforming growth factor β). Viewed microscopically, the smooth muscle cell has two phenotypes. The contractile phenotype predominates in the normal vascular media. It is a quiescent cell with numerous myofilaments, and it provides both vasomotion and structural support to the

TABLE 44-1..

Potential Role of Growth Factors in Restenosis

Growth Factor*	Potential Action in Restenosis
PDGF	Stimulates SMC* migration and proliferation
FGF	Stimulates endothelial cell and fibroblast proliferation
EGF	Replaces heparin on the cell surface; promotes SMC proliferation
IGF	Promotes SMC proliferation and extracellular matrix production
TGF	Regulates matrix remodeling; possibly regulates other growth factors

*PDGF = platelet-derived growth factor; FGF = fibroblast growth factor; EGF = epidermal growth factor; IGF = insulin-like growth factor; TGF = transforming growth factor; SMC = smooth muscle cell.

vessel. The synthetic phenotype is closely related to the fibroblast (hence often called a myofibroblast by electron microscopists). It has abundant synthetic organelles (e.g., free ribosomes, Golgi apparatus, rough endoplasmic reticulum). This phenotype is secretory; in particular, it produces extracellular matrix proteoglycan and collagen. Contractile-phenotype smooth muscle cells in cell culture are unresponsive to growth factors, whereas appropriately treated synthetic-phenotype cells are responsive.[50-53] When tissue is injured, nearby fibroblasts and/or synthetic-phenotype smooth muscle cells migrate into the injured area and then proliferate. This stage of cellular migration and proliferation in response to injury lasts roughly a week. It begins to terminate as the surface of the wound is covered by migrating cells, and the third phase of healing begins.

THE MATRIX REMODELING PHASE OF WOUND HEALING: PROTEOGLYCAN SYNTHESIS

The third phase, *extracellular matrix deposition and remodeling*, continues for months. When the wound surface is covered by a cell layer, the mesenchymal cells that migrated into the wound area slow their proliferation and begin to produce large amounts of proteoglycan that replaces fibronectin as the major extracellular matrix component. Proteoglycans are a diverse group of structurally related macromolecules that are found in the extracellular matrix and in association with the basement and plasma membrane of cells. The common structural elements are a protein backbone to which are attached one or more linear glycosaminoglycans. Although proteoglycans constitute only about 5% of the normal vessel dry weight, they are prominent in the extracellular matrix of intimal hyperplasia.

Three major connective tissue proteoglycans are chondroitin sulfate (CSPG), dermatan sulfate (DSPG), and heparin sulfate (HSPG). Fibroblasts and synthetic phenotype smooth muscle cells synthesize CSPG and DSPG, which are the predominant proteoglycans in the extracellular matrix of the healing wound. CSPG and DSPG are central to wound healing because they promote cell migration and proliferation.[54] Their secretion is regulated by transforming growth factor β.[55] In contrast, endothelial cells synthesize predominantly HSPG, which is not controlled by transforming growth factor β.[56] Heparin is a potent inhibitor of mesenchymal cell proliferation. Its antiproliferative effect may be due to its ability to potentiate the biologic activity of transforming growth factor β by dissociating it from its carrier protein, which normally renders it inactive.[57] Although antiprolif-

erative, heparin also markedly stimulates the synthesis of proteoglycans by smooth muscle cells.[54]

As the remodeling phase progresses to termination, the CSPG and DSPG proteoglycans are replaced by large fibrous bundles of type I collagen and elastin. The histologic appearance of wounds in the remodeling phase is proliferating fibroblasts scattered through abundant extracellular matrix. The process of wound healing is variable in duration but largely complete at 90 to 120 days.

THE MECHANISM OF RESTENOSIS: TESTABLE HYPOTHESES

We have reasonable inferential evidence to justify placing restenosis into this wound healing schema. Angioscopy and postmortem studies establish that vascular injury is common and often extensive after balloon angioplasty.[10-15] The serial angiography studies of Nobuyoshi et al. and Serruys et al. establish that restenosis appears during the third phase of wound healing, i.e., extracellular matrix formation and remodeling.[3,4] Autopsy and atherectomy histology show that the restenotic tissue consists of synthetic smooth muscle cells distributed within a large mass of extracellular matrix.[12,31] Special histologic stains show that much of the extracellular matrix is CSPG (Fig 44–4). We also know that growth factors are expressed at the vascular injury site and that these factors stimulate smooth muscle cell proliferation and extracellular matrix synthesis. Thus although the mechanism of vascular restenosis is not known, we can construct a hypothesis for the temporal sequence of restenosis by using these data (Fig 44–5).

Day 1.—Balloon inflation denudes the endothelial surface and exposes myointima. Since the atheroma is inelastic, much of the dilating force of the balloon is transmitted to the normal segment of the vascular circumference. When the dilating force exceeds the limit of the normal segment to stretch, tearing begins. Often this occurs at the junction between normal and atherosclerotic tissue, and the atheroma itself develops fissures.[13,19] The internal elastic lamina and media may be torn apart.[16-18] Platelets aggregate at these sites of vascular injury. The platelets release a plethora of substances, among which are growth factors[58] and an endoglycosidase that cleaves heparin proteoglycan from the surface of endothelial and smooth muscle cells.[51,52] Removal of heparin makes the cell receptive to the action of growth factors.[50,53] The heparin released into the extracellular space also avidly binds platelet-derived growth factor, epidermal growth factor, and fibroblast growth factor[58] increasing the local concentration of

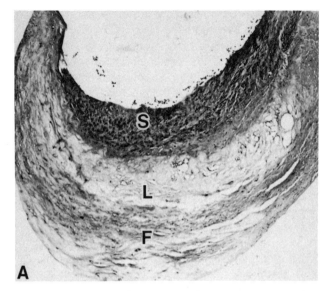

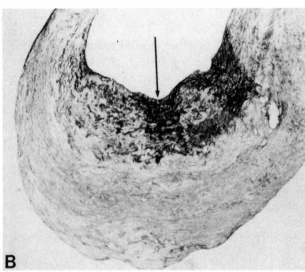

FIG 44–4.
Atherectomy specimen from the femoral artery of a patient who developed restenosis after balloon angioplasty. **A,** HE-stained specimen showing three zones: *S,* a superficial zone of smooth muscle cell proliferation (restenosis); *L,* the aceullar lipid core of the plaque; and *F,* the deeper fibrous region. **B,** Alcian blue/periodic acid–Schiff (PAS) stain showing localization of acid mucopolysaccharide material (proteoglycan) to the region of intense smooth muscle cell proliferation *(arrow)* (×40).

growth factors. Fibronectin released from plasma forms an early extracellular matrix that, with coagulated blood, fills the fissured areas on the vessel surface.[33]

Days 2 to 4.—On day 2 a proportion of the smooth muscle cells in the media begin to increase DNA synthesis and change to the synthetic phenotype.[59] Platelet-derived growth factor, transforming growth factor, and other growth factors released early from platelets and later from macrophages,[35] may induce this transformation. Smooth muscle cells proliferate first in the media.[50] By day 4, the smooth muscle cells begin to migrate to the injured area, and endothelial cells migrate from the lateral edge of the damaged blood vessel surface.[53, 59] A principal growth factor for endothelial migration is fibroblast growth factor.[40] The migration of cells induced by growth factors is facilitated by fibronectin and hyaluronic acid in the extracellular matrix.[60–62]

Days 5 to 10.—In extensive injury about 30% of the local smooth muscle cells migrate from the media to the intima, but only about half of the cells that migrate to the wound area proliferate.[63] Once in the myointimal space, the smooth muscle cells begin to produce CSPG and DSPG.[62] These proteoglycans gradually replace the fibronectin as the dominant component of the extracellular matrix.[62] By day 5, transforming growth factor β, the most potent of the growth factors regulating extracellular matrix formation,[45] begins to increase substantially in the injured tissue.[49] Depending on the area of denudation, endothelial cells cover the injured surface by about day 7.[63, 64] If the area of denudation is small (e.g., less than 1 cm long), intimal hyperplasia does not ensue.[65] Thus, there is probably a critical time (5 to 7 days) or critical lesion size in which endothelial coverage can precede maximum smooth muscle cell proliferation. Conversely, larger areas can remain chronically devoid of endothelial cells.[66]

Days 10 to 120.—As the endothelial cells cover the injured blood vessel surface, they cease proliferating and begin to synthesize heparin proteoglycan.[54] Adjacent smooth muscle cells avidly bind the heparin (quiescent smooth muscle cells bind ten times more heparin than do proliferating cells).[52] The smooth muscle cells become unresponsive to the proliferative effects of growth factors.[51] Since smooth muscle cell proteoglycan synthesis is independent of migration and proliferation, however, extracellular matrix production does not necessarily cease.[56] Restoration of blood vessel surface integrity sharply reduces the loss of proteoglycan from the injured surface,[67] and proteoglycan rapidly accumulates in the myointimal space.

By 2 weeks the synthetic smooth muscle cells in the extracellular matrix have begun to revert back to the contractile phenotype.[53, 66] There is, however, a striking difference in behavior depending upon their physical location: intimal smooth muscle cells adjoining a deendothelialized surface have 50 times the proliferation rate of those adjacent to a reendothelialized surface.[59] By 6 weeks the volume of myofilaments as a percentage of

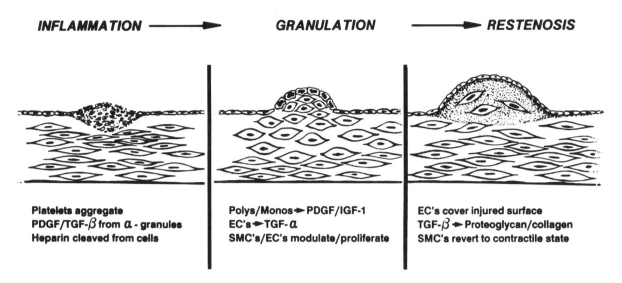

FIG 44–5.
A hypothetical schema for restenosis following injury to the vascular surface. The names of the phases of wound healing have been retained to support the analogy between the two phenomena. *PDGF* = platelet-derived growth factor; *TGF*-β = transforming growth factor β; *EC* = endothelial cell; *SMC* = smooth muscle cell.

cytoplasmic volume (an index of the contractile phenotype) is midway in its return to its value in the resting state.

Depending on the magnitude of injury and possibly other factors, intimal hyperplasia reaches a peak at 4 to 12 weeks.[68–71] The curve depicting the rate of intimal hyperplasia following vascular injury in animals bears a striking resemblance to that depicting the rate of appearance of angiographic restenosis in man.[3] As smooth muscle cell proliferation diminishes while proteoglycan synthesis continues, the volume of intimal hyperplasia mass occupied by the smooth muscle cell diminishes.[69] The injured blood vessel thus develops the histologic appearance of intimal hyperplasia: proliferating smooth muscle cells scattered through a loose extracellular matrix.[31]

By several months the return to a contractile phenotype is paralleled by a change in the extracellular matrix: proteoglycan is gradually replaced by collagen.[72] In the relatively normal segments of the vessel, this fibrotic remodeling and the restoration of responsiveness to vasoconstrictive stimuli[73, 74] may contribute to the angiographic phenomenon of narrowing in the normal segment proximal to the diseased segment as described by Serruys et al.[4]

Days 120 to 135.—By 180 days the relative percentage of contractile-phenotype smooth muscle cells has returned to the resting state level,[53, 75] and the restenotic response is probably largely complete. In the small minority of blood vessels with areas of chronic endothelial denudation, however, smooth muscle proliferation con-

tinues at levels many times that of the resting state (6% per day vs. resting cells at 0.1% per day).[59] This explains the observation of Nobuyoshi et al. that in a small percentage of lesions restenosis becomes evident between 6 and 12 months.[3]

POTENTIAL DIRECTIONS FOR THE PREVENTION OF RESTENOSIS

The preceding hypothetical construct suggests that there are many rate-limiting steps in the development of intimal hyperplasia and, by inference, a number of sites for its potential prevention. Some of these rate-limiting steps have already been tested in clinical trials; no intervention has so far been sufficiently successful to warrant widespread use. Before discussing possible interventions, however, we need to critically examine several potential limitations of previous clinical trials.

1. The relationship of dose and duration of the agent delivered at the injury site may have been inappropriate. For instance, thrombocytopenia substantially inhibits intimal hyperplasia in animals,[76] yet antiplatelet agents have been ineffective in man. Since the half-time for platelet aggregation after injury is measured in hours,[77] it is possible that a brief, intravenous infusion of a platelet antagonist in this period would be more effective than lower-dose, long-term oral administration.

2. The timing of drug administration may have been inappropriate. For instance, heparin inhibits intimal hyperplasia in animals but has not prevented restenosis in

man. Heparin binds growth factors at the injury site early after injury and could thereby facilitate cell migration and proliferation and thus enhance subsequent intimal hyperplasia. Since heparin also inhibits smooth muscle cell proliferation in the third phase of wound healing, however, later administration of heparin could inhibit intimal hyperplasia. Thus, continued heparin administration may be much more effective than brief intravenous therapy immediately after injury.

3. It is not always immediately apparent what therapeutic effect is desirable. For instance, given that growth factors accelerate wound healing through stimulation of mesenchymal cell proliferation, it is not clear whether this effect should be facilitated or inhibited.

Within these limitations, potential therapies and their rationale are listed in Table 44–2.

THE INFLAMMATORY PHASE: PLATELET INHIBITORS AND ANTI-INFLAMMATORY AGENTS

The biological rationale for platelet antagonists is strong. Platelets initiate the healing response to injury[76–78] by a release of growth factors (including platelet-derived growth factor and transforming growth factor β) from their alpha granules. In addition, they are the source of the endoglycosidase that cleaves heparin from the smooth muscle cells, a potentially critical step in smooth cell phenotypic modulation. Further, thrombocytopenia inhibits intimal hyperplasia after vascular injury in atherosclerotic animals, possibly through reduced smooth muscle migration to the injury site.[79] Carefully conducted clinical trials of aspirin and dipy-

ridamole, however, have been unsuccessful. Schwartz et al. reported a randomized, blinded, placebo-controlled study of long-term oral aspirin and dipyridamole (330 mg aspirin and 75 mg dipyridamol three times daily) combined with a 24-hour interval of intravenous dipyridamole in 376 patients. At 4 to 7 months after coronary angioplasty, follow-up angiography showed that 38% of treated patients and 39% of placebo patients had restenosis.[80] Thornton et al. compared long-term oral aspirin, 325 mg, with a warfarin (Coumadin) dose sufficient to maintain 2 to 2.5 times the control value. The restenosis rate in the 126-patient, aspirin-treated cohort was 27%, a level not different from the Coumadin-treated group and within the range of currently reported restenosis rates.[81] In addition to the aforementioned limitations of dose and duration, it is possible that these negative results reflect the dual effect of aspirin on thromboxane and prostacyclin metabolism. Thromboxane A_2 receptor antagonists could circumvent this limitation. Finally, newly developed monoclonal antibodies to platelet receptors such as the IIb/IIIa receptor for fibrinogen produce transient and potent antihemostatic effects. Platelet aggregation can be effectively eliminated, with a return over a 48-hour period, in a dose-dependent manner.[78] The potential value of such therapies has not been tested in man.

The rationale for use of anti-inflammatory agents is that they inhibit both cell accumulation and/or activation at the injury site. Reduction of the number of activated cells could decrease the expression of growth factors, thereby inhibiting the subsequent sequence of smooth muscle cell phenotypic modulation, migration, proliferation, and extracellular matrix formation. Cortisol inhibits smooth muscle cell protein synthesis and proliferation in cell culture,[82] and the combination of

TABLE 44–2.
Potential Therapies in Restenosis

Target	Examples	Action
Inflammatory phase		
Platelets	Aspirin, dipyridamole	Inhibit adhesion and aggregation
	Sulotroban	Block thromboxane receptor
	Monoclonal antibodies	Block IIa/IIIb fibrinogen receptor
Inflammatory cells	Steroids	Inhibit accumulation and activation
	Fish oil	Inhibit activation
	Cyclosporine A	Inhibit T lymphocytes
Granulation phase		
SMC*	Vincristine/actinomycin	Destroy SMCs
SMC receptor	Heparin	Inhibit SMC modulation
	Trapidil	Antagonize PDGF* action
Matrix remodeling phase		
Synthetic SMC	Colchicine, DSMO*	Reduce secretory organelles
Mesenchymal cells	Retinoids	Reduce matrix synthesis

*SMC = smooth muscle cell; PDGF = platelet = derived growth factor; DMSO = dimethyl sulfoxide.

steroids with heparin inhibits smooth muscle cell proliferation in animals.[83] Liu et al., however, report that the administration of steroids for 1 week after coronary angioplasty did not reduce the restenosis rate.[84] Cyclosporine A inhibits T lymphocyte activation. These cells may regulate the expression of growth factors by smooth muscle cells after vascular injury.[85] Cyclosporine A produces a highly significant reduction in both smooth muscle cell number and extracellular matrix production in the denuded rat endothelium.[85] Omega 3 fatty acids, which have both anti-inflammatory and anti-platelet actions, have been reported to reduce restenosis in some clinical trials but not in others.[86-90] The potential value of anti-inflammatory agents therefore remains entirely unresolved.

THE GRANULATION PHASE: CYTOTOXICS AND GROWTH FACTOR ANTAGONISTS

The rationale for the use of cytotoxics is that some can destroy smooth muscle cells. A logical choice in this category might be agents shown to be effective in myosarcomas. The combination of actinomycin and vincristine is quite effective in destroying proliferating malignant smooth muscle cells. Barath et al. used this combination to destroy proliferating smooth muscle cells after balloon denudation in animals.[91] There have been no clinical trials of cytotoxic agents in restenosis.

The rationale for the use of growth factor antagonists is that they could inhibit smooth muscle cell modulation, migration, or proliferation. Proliferating smooth muscle cells at 2 weeks after balloon injury produce ten times the amount of platelet-derived growth factor as do nonproliferating cells,[39] and messenger RNA tissue concentrations of its competence factor, insulin-like growth factor-1, are equally increased in injured areas.[48] Monoclonal antibodies and antagonists to receptors for various growth factors inhibit cell growth in vitro,[92] but none have yet been tested in animals or man. Heparin is particularly promising because it effectively prevents smooth muscle cell proliferation in cell culture and intimal hyperplasia in animals.[93, 94] Nevertheless heparin is also a potent stimulus to extracellular matrix production. The antiproliferative and anticoagulant domains of heparin are different, so it is possible to construct an antiproliferative, nonanticoagulant form of heparin.[95] Thus, although heparin has not yet been shown to be effective in preventing restenosis in man,[96] it is possible that ongoing clinical trials with higher doses of nonanticoagulant heparin may prove to be effective. Finally, angiotensin converting enzyme inhibitors have recently been re-

ported to prevent myointimal proliferation after vascular injury in rats,[97] presumably through their ability to block angiotensin II–mediated induction of platelet-derived growth factor-A gene expression in aortic smooth muscle cells.[98] Their potential role in humans remains to be defined.

THE EXTRACELLULAR MATRIX PHASE: ANTISECRETORY AGENTS

There are a variety of unrelated agents that are capable of inhibiting the synthesis of extracellular matrix. Both colchicine[99] and dimethyl sulfoxide (DMSO)[100] reduce the number of secretory organelles in smooth muscle cells. This effect is associated with a significant reduction in extracellular matrix production. Retinoids also inhibit extracellular matrix production in the animal model[101, 102] and are being tested in fibroproliferative disorders such as keloid formation.[102] Possibly because the preeminent role of extracellular matrix synthesis in restenosis has not been recognized, the antisecretory agents have not yet been formally tested for the prevention of restenosis. Finally, there are a number of agents that may prevent intimal hyperplasia through actions that are not clearly understood. Lovastatin, prostaglandin, and calcium antagonists, for instance, all inhibit smooth muscle cell proliferation and/or migration.[103-108]

CLINICAL IMPLICATIONS OF THE WOUND HEALING–RESTENOSIS HYPOTHESIS

Viewing restenosis as a local manifestation of the systemic wound healing process may resolve some questions and create others. The apparent absence of clinical/angiographic evidence of restenosis in about half the patients is explicable as the result of both a variable magnitude of injury and the subsequent magnitude of intimal hyperplasia. To paraphrase Serruys, we suggest that intimal hyperplasia "almost always" occurs after angioplasty; hence, depending on the angiographic criteria chosen, virtually all patients have some degree of restenosis. Second, the increased restenosis rate in certain anatomic configurations may be the result of an increased magnitude of injury (long lesions, disrupted lesions, etc.) or an accelerated hyperplastic response (at bends and bifurcations).[109] Third, an implication of the wound healing hypothesis is that restenosis will be independent of the *mechanism* of vascular injury. Thus vascular injury induced by atherectomy or laser treatment would also be expected to have similar or possibly even greater rates of restenosis if the injury is circumferential. Preliminary clinical trial data support this anticipated result. Finally, we anticipate that inhibition of intimal hyperplasia may only eliminate restenosis when the residual lumen remains large despite the restoration of vascular tone ("recoil") that gradually occurs in the remodeling phase. Thus it is possible that prevention of restenosis in some cases will require either prevention of recoil by stents or removal of atheroma mass in combination and in addition to potent local inhibition of intimal hyperplasia (Fig 44–6).

SUMMARY

The early and late histologic appearance of the angioplasty site is now established. Immediately after angioplasty, there is substantial evidence of vascular injury: the intimal surface is denuded, the atheroma has fissures, and the normal segment of the vessel circumference is stretched. When restenosis develops at 1 to 4 months, the histologic appearance of the restenotic lesion is intimal hyperplasia. Given this end point, we may theorize that the proximate cause of restenosis is denuding and stretching vascular injury. Since wound healing has been studied extensively in other tissues, we can hypothesize that the major milestones in the temporal sequence of restenosis are platelet aggregation, inflammatory cell infiltration, release of growth factors, medial smooth muscle cell modulation and proliferation, proteoglycan synthesis, and extracellular matrix remodeling. At each of these steps there are potential inhibitors. If restenosis is due to gradual narrowing of the residual lumen by intimal hyperplasia, then its prevention will require both creation of the largest possible residual lumen and substantial inhibition of intimal hyperplasia. For this reason, it is possible that restenosis will only be resolved by attention to multiple factors, including but not limited to appropriate timing of a potent inhibitor, its local delivery in high concentration,

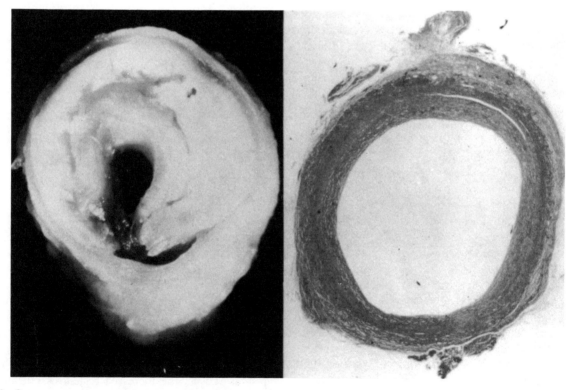

FIG 44–6.
Differences in mechanisms of recanalization. **A,** cross section of a coronary artery removed at autopsy following balloon angioplasty. The atheroma is disrupted at the junction between the relatively normal and atheromatous segments, and there is a dissection with thrombus formation at the site. **B,** cross section of an occluded saphenous vein bypass graft removed at reoperation and subsequently recanalized by excimer laser angioplasty. The atheromatous material has been largely removed. It is possible that resolution of the problem of restenosis will require a combination of approaches: a potent inhibitor of intimal hyperplasia, local delivery of the agent, and either partial removal of the atheroma or vascular stenting to create a large residual lumen. (**A** from Potkin BN, Roberts WC: *Am J Cardiol* 1988; 62:41–50. Used by permission. **B,** courtesy of Jacob Segalowitz, M.D.).

partial removal of atheroma mass, and prevention of late recoil.

Acknowledgement

The authors would like to express their gratitude for the superb secretarial/word processing assistance of Ms. Dwana Williams.

REFERENCES

1. Bertrand ME, Lablanche JM, Fourrier JL, et al: Relation to restenosis after coronary angioplasty to vasomotion of the dilated coronary arterial segment. *Am J Cardiol* 1989; 63:277–281.
2. Holmes DR, Vlietstra R, Smith H, et al: Restenosis after coronary angioplasty (PTCA): A report from the PTCA Registry of the National Heart, Lung and Blood Institute. *Am J Cardiol* 1984; 53:77–81.
3. Nobuyoshi M, Kimura T, Noksaka H, et al: Restenosis after successful coronary angioplasty: Serial angiographic follow-up of 229 patients. *J Am Coll Cardiol* 1988; 12:616–623.
4. Serruys PW, Luijten HE, Beatt KJ, et al: Incidence of restenosis after successful coronary angioplasty: A time related phenomenon. A quantitative angiographic study in 342 consecutive patients at 1, 2, and 3 months. *Circulation* 1988; 77:361–372.
5. Val PG, Bourassa MG, David PR, et al: Restenosis after successful coronary angioplasty: The Montreal Heart Institute Experience. *Am J Cardiol* 1987; 60:50–55.
6. Ellis SG, Roubin GS, King SB, et al: Importance of stenosis morphology in the estimation of restenosis risk after elective coronary angioplasty. *Am J Cardiol* 1989; 63:30–34.
7. Ip JH, Fuster V, Badimon L, et al: Syndromes of accelerated atherosclerosis: Role of vascular injury and smooth muscle cell proliferation. *J Am Coll Cardiol* 1990; 1:1667–1687.
8. Barnhart GR, Pascoe EA, Mills SA, et al: Accelerated coronary arteriosclerosis in cardiac transplant recipients. *Transplant Rev* 1987; 1:31–46.
9. Forrester JS, Litvack F, Grundfest W, et al: A perspective of coronary disease seen through the arteries of living man. *Circulation* 1987; 75:505–513.
10. Uchida Y, Hasegawa K, Kawamura K, et al: Angioscopic observation of the coronary luminal changes induced by coronary angioplasty. *Am Heart J* 1989; 117:769–776.
11. Mizuno Y, Miyamoto A, Shibuya T, et al: Changes of angioscopic macromorphology following coronary angioplasty (abstract) *Circulation* 1988; 77(suppl 2):289
12. Austin GE, Ratliff NB, Hollman J, et al: Intimal proliferation of smooth muscle cells as an explanation for recurrent coronary artery stenosis after coronary angioplasty. *J Am Coll Cardiol* 1985; 6:369–375.
13. Block P, Myler R, Stertzer S, et al: Morphology after transluminal angioplasty in human beings. *N Engl J Med* 1981; 305:382–385.
14. Giraldo AA, Esposo OM, Meis JM: Intimal hyperplasia as a cause of restenosis after coronary angioplasty. *Arch Pathol Lab Med* 1985; 109:173–175.
15. Ueda M, Becker AE, Fujimoto T: Pathologic changes induced by repeated coronary angioplasty. *Br Heart J* 1987; 58:635–643.
16. Gravanis MB, Roubin GS: Histopathologic phenomena at the site of coronary angioplasty. *Hum Pathol* 1989; 20:477–485.
17. Saner HE, Gobel FL, Salmonowitz E, et al: The disease-free wall in coronary atherosclerosis: Its relation to degree of obstruction. *J Am Coll Cardiol* 1985; 6:1096–1099.
18. Waller BF: Morphologic correlates of coronary angiographic patterns at the site of coronary angioplasty. *Clin Cardiol* 1988; 11:817–822.
19. Potkin BN, Roberts WC: Effects of coronary angioplasty on atherosclerotic plaques and relation of plaque composition and arterial size to outcome. *Am J Cardiol* 1988; 62:41–50.
20. Kochi T, Takebayashi S, Block PC, et al: Arterial changes after coronary angioplasty: Results at autopsy. *J Am Coll Cardiol* 1987; 10:592–599.
21. deMorais CF, Lopes EA, Checchi H, et al: Coronary angioplasty – histopathological analysis of nine necropsy cases. *Virchows Arch [A]* 1986; 410:195–202.
22. Soward AL, Essed CE, Serruys PW: Coronary arterial findings after accidental death immediately after successful coronary angioplasty. *Am J Cardiol* 1985; 56:794–795.
23. Schneider J, Grüntzig A: Coronary angioplasty: Morphological findings in 3 patients. *Pathol Res Pract* 1985; 180:348–352.
24. Mizuno K, Kurita A, Imazeki N: Pathological findings after coronary angioplasty. *Br Heart J* 1984; 52:588–590.
25. Bruneval P, Guermonprez JL, Perrier P, et al: Coronary artery restenosis following transluminal coronary angioplasty. *Arch Pathol Lab Med* 1986; 110:1186–1187.
26. Waller B: "Crackers, breakers, stretchers, drillers, scrapers, shavers, burners, welders, and melters" – the future treatment of atherosclerotic coronary artery disease? A clinical-morphologic assessment. *J Am Coll Cardiol* 1989; 13:969–987.
27. Sanborn TA, Faxon, DP, Haudenschild C, et al: The mechanism of transluminal angioplasty: Evidence for formation of aneurysms in experimental atherosclerosis. *Circulation* 1983; 68:1136–1140.
28. Steele PM, Chesebro JH, Stanson AW, et al: Balloon angioplasty: Natural history of the pathophysiologic response to injury in a pig model. *Circ Res* 1985; 57:105–112.
29. Leung DY, Glagov S, Mathews MB: Cyclic stretching stimulates synthesis of matrix components by arterial smooth muscle cells in vitro. *Science* 1976; 191:475–477.
30. Clowes AW, Clowes MM, Fingerle J, et al: Kinetics of cellular proliferation after arterial injury V. Role of acute distension in the induction of smooth muscle proliferation. *Lab Invest* 1989; 60:360–364.
31. Simpson JB, Selmon MR, Robertson GC, et al: Transluminal atherectomy for occlusive peripheral vascular disease. *Am J Cardiol* 1988; 61:96–101.
32. Greisler HP, Ellinger J, Schwarz TH, et al: Arterial regeneration over polydioxanone prostheses in the rabbit. *Arch Surg* 1987; 122:715–721.
33. Clark RAF: Overview and general considerations of

wound repair, in Clark RAF, Henson PM, (eds): *The Molecular and Cellular Biology of Wound Repair.* New York, Plenum, 1988.

34. Brown GL, Nanney LB, Griffen J, et al: Enhancement of wound healing by topical treatment with epidermal growth factor. *N Engl J Med* 1989; 321:76–79.

35. Barbul A, Pines E, Caldwell M, (eds): Growth factors and other aspects of wound healing: Biological and clinical implications. *Prog Clin Biol Res* 1988; 266:161–175.

36. Hjelmeland LM, Harvey AK: Growth factors: Soluble mediators of wound repair and ocular fibrosis. *Birth Defects* 1988; 24:87–102.

37. Knighton DR, Fiegel VD, Austin LL, et al: Classification and treatment of chronic nonhealing wounds. *Ann Surg* 1986; 204:322–330.

38. Ross R, Raines EW, Bowen-Pope DF: The biology of platelet-derived growth factor. *Cell* 1986; 46:155–169.

39. Walker LN, Bowen-Pope DF, Ross R, et al: Production of platelet-derived growth factor — like molecules by cultured arterial smooth muscle cells accompanies proliferation after arterial injury. *Proc Natl Acad Sci USA* 1986; 83:7311–7315.

40. Folkman J, Klagsbrun M: Angiogenic factors. *Science* 1987; 235:442–447.

41. Stiles CD, Capone GT, Scher CD, et al: Dual control of cell growth by somatomedins and platelet-derived growth factor. *Proc Natl Acad Sci USA* 1979; 76:1279–1283.

42. Waterfield MD: Epidermal growth factor and related molecules. *Lancet* 1989; 1:1243–1246.

43. Spencer EM, Skover G, Hunt TK: Somatomedins: Do they play a pivotal role in wound healing? In *Growth Factors and Other Aspects of Wound Healing Biological and Clinical Implications.* New York, Alan R Liss, 1988, pp 103–116.

44. Roberts AB, Flanders KC, Kondaiah P, et al: Transforming growth factor beta: Biochemistry and roles in embryogenesis, tissue repair and remodeling and carcinogenesis. *Recent Prog Horm Res* 1988; 44:157–197.

45. Sprugel KH, McPherson JM, Clowes AW, et al: The effects of different growth factors in subcutaneous wound chambers, in *Growth Factors and Other Aspects of Wound Healing: Biological and Clinical Implications.* New York, Alan R Liss, 1988.

46. Chen JK, Hoshi H, McKeehan WL: Transforming growth factor type beta specifically stimulates synthesis of proteoglycan in human adult arterial smooth muscle cells. *Proc Natl Acad Sci USA* 1987; 84:5287–5291.

47. Ignotz RA, Massague J: Transforming growth factor-beta stimulates the expression of fibronectin and collagen and their incorporation into the extracellular matrix. *J Biol Chem* 1986; 261:4337–4345.

48. Cercek B, Fishbein MC, Forrester JS, et al: Induction of insulin-like growth factor-1 m-RNA in rat aorta after balloon denudation. *Circ Res* 1990; 66:1755–1760.

49. Cromack DT, Sporn MB, Roberts AB, et al: Transforming growth factor beta levels in rat wound chambers. *J Surg Res* 1987; 42:622–628.

50. Campbell GR, Campbell JH, Manderson JA, et al: Arterial smooth muscle: A multifunctional mesenchymal cell. *Arch Pathol Lab Med* 1988; 112:977–986.

51. Castellot JJ, Wright TC, Karnovsky MJ: Regulation of vascular smooth muscle cell growth by heparin and heparin sulfates. *Semin Thromb Hemost* 1987; 13:489–503.

52. Castellot JJ, Addonizio ML, Rosenberg RD, et al: Cultured endothelial cells produce a heparin-like inhibitor of smooth muscle cell growth. *J Cell Biol* 1981; 90:372–379.

53. Campbell JH, Campbell GR: Endothelial cell influences on vascular smooth muscle phenotype. *Annu Rev Physiol* 1986; 48:295–306.

54. Wight TN: Cell biology of arterial proteoglycans. *Arteriosclerosis* 1989; 9:1–20.

55. Bassols A, Massague J: Transforming growth factor beta regulates the expression and structure of extracellular matrix chondroitin/dermatan sulfate proteoglycans. *J Biol Chem* 1988; 263:3039–3045.

56. Kinsella MG, Wight TN: Modulation of sulfated proteoglycan synthesis by bovine aortic endothelial cells during migration. *J Cell Biol* 1986; 102:678–687.

57. McCaffrey TA, Falcone DJ, Brayton CF, et al: Transforming growth factor-beta activity is potentiated by heparin via dissociation of the transforming growth factor beta/alpha$_2$–macroglobulin inactive complex. *J Cell Biol* 1989; 109:441–448.

58. Lobb RR: Clinical applications of heparin-binding growth factors. *Eur J Clin Invest* 1988; 18:321–336.

59. Clowes AW, Reidy MA, Clowes MM: Kinetics of cellular proliferation after arterial injury. I. Smooth muscle growth in the absence of endothelium. *Lab Invest* 1983; 49:327–333.

60. Holund B, Clemmensen K, Junker P, et al: Fibronectin in experimental granulation tissue. *Acta Pathol Microbiol Immunol Scand* 1982; 90:159–165.

61. Anseth A: Glycosaminoglycans in corneal regeneration. *Exp Eye Res* 1961; 1:122–127.

62. Bently JP: Rate of chondroitin sulfate formation in wound healing. *Ann Surg* 1967; 165:186–191.

63. Clowes AW, Schwartz SM: Significance of quiescent smooth muscle migration in the injured rat carotid artery. *Circ Res* 1985; 56:139–145.

64. Fishman JA, Ryan GB, Karnovsky MJ: Endothelial regeneration in the rat carotid artery and the significance of endothelial denudation in the pathogenesis of myointimal thickening. *Lab Invest* 1975; 32:339–351.

65. Reidy MA, Schwartz SM: Endothelial regeneration III. Time course of intimal change after small defined injury to rat endothelium. *Lab Invest* 1981; 44:301.

66. Clowes AW, Clowes MM, Reidy MA: Kinetics of cellular proliferation after arterial injury. III. Endothelial and smooth muscle growth in chronically denuded vessels. *Lab Invest* 1986; 54:295–303.

67. Alvai M, Moore S: Glycosaminoglycan composition and biosynthesis in the endothelium-covered neointima and de-endothelialized rabbit aorta. *Exp Mol Pathol* 1985; 42:389–400.

68. Stemerman MB, Spaet TH, Pitlick F, et al: Intimal healing: The pattern of reendothelialization and intimal thickening. *Am J Pathol* 1977; 7:125–137.

69. Clowes AW, Reidy MA, Clowes MM: Mechanisms of stenosis after arterial injury. *Lab Invest* 1983; 49:208–215.

70. Schwartz SM, Campbell GR, Campbell JH: Replication of smooth muscle cells in vascular disease. *Circ Res* 1986; 58:427–444.

71. Clowes AW, Kirkman TR, Riedy MA: Mechanisms of

arterial graft healing. Rapid transmural capillary ingrowth provides a source of intimal endothelium and smooth muscle in porous PTFE prostheses. *Am J Pathol* 1986; 123:220–230.

72. Diegelmann RF, Rothkopf LC, Cohen IK: Measurement of collagen biosynthesis during wound healing. *J Surg Res* 1975; 19:239–243.

73. Consigny PM, Tulenko TN, Nichosia RF: Immediate and long term effects of angioplasty–balloon dilation on normal rabbit iliac artery. *Arteriosclerosis* 1986; 6:265–276.

74. Castaneda-Zuniga WR, Laerum F, Rysavy J, et al: Paralysis of arteries by intraluminal balloon dilation. *Radiology* 1982; 144:75–76.

75. Manderson JA, Mosse PRL, Safstrom JA, et al: Balloon catheter injury to rabbit carotid artery I. Changes in smooth muscle phenotype. *Arteriosclerosis* 1989; 9:289–296.

76. Minar E, Ehringer H, Ahmadi R, et al: Platelet deposition at angioplasty sites and its relation to restenosis in human iliac and femoropopliteal arteries. *Radiology* 1989; 170:767–772.

77. Wilentz JR, Sanborn TA, Haudenschild CC, et al: Platelet accumulation in experimental angioplasty: Time course and relation to vascular injury. *Circulation* 1989; 75:636–642.

78. Harker LA: Role of platelets and thrombosis in mechanisms of acute occlusion and restenosis after angioplasty. *Am J Cardiol* 1989; 60:20–28.

79. Fingerle J, Johnson R, Clowes AW, et al: Role of platelets in smooth muscle cell proliferation and migration after vascular injury in rat carotid artery. *Proc Natl Acad Sci USA* 1989; 86:8412–8416.

80. Schwartz L, Bourassa MG, Lesperance J, et al: Aspirin and dipyridamole in the prevention of restenosis after coronary angioplasty. *N Engl J Med* 1988; 318:1714–1719.

81. Thornton MA, Grüntzig AR, Hollman J, et al: Coumadin and aspirin in prevention of recurrence after transluminal coronary angioplasty: A randomized study. *Circulation* 1984; 69:721–727.

82. Jarvelainen H, Halme T, Ronnemaa T: Effect of cortisol on the proliferation and protein synthesis of human aortic smooth muscle cells in culture. *Acta Med Scand* 1982; 660(suppl):114–122.

83. Gordon JB, Berk BC, Bettman, et al: Vascular smooth muscle proliferation following balloon injury is synergistically inhibited by low molecular weight heparin and hydrocortisone. *Circulation* 1987; 76(suppl 4):213.

84. Liu MW, Roubin GS, King SB: Research on coronary artery stenosis. Restenosis after coronary angioplasty. Potential biological determinants and role of intimal hyperplasia. *Circulation* 1989; 79:1374–1387.

85. Jonasson L, Holm J, Hansson GK: Cyclosporin A inhibits smooth muscle proliferation in the vascular response to injury. *Proc Natl Acad Sci USA* 1988; 85:2303–2306.

86. Grigg LE, Kay T, Manolas EG, et al: Does Max-EPA lower the risk of restenosis after PTCA: A prospective randomized trial. *Circulation* 1987; 76(suppl 4):214.

87. Reis GJ, Boucher TM, Sipperly ME, et al: Randomised trial of fish oil for prevention of restenosis after coronary angioplasty. *Lancet* 1989; 2:177–181.

88. Dehmer GJ, Popma JJ, Van den Berg EK, et al: Reduction in the rate of early restenosis after coronary angioplasty by a diet supplemented with n-3 fatty acids. *N Engl J Med* 1988; 391:733–740.

89. Slack JD, Pinkerton CA, Van Tassel J, et al: Can oral fish oil supplement minimize restenosis after coronary angioplasty (abstract)? *J Am Coll Cardiol* 1987; 9(suppl):64.

90. Milner MR, Gallino RA, Leffingwell A, et al: High dose omega-3 fatty acid supplmentation reduces clinical restenosis after coronary angioplasty. *Circulation* 1988; 78(suppl 2):634.

91. Barath P, Arakawa K, Cao J, et al: Low dose of antitumor agents prevents smooth muscle cell proliferation after endothelial injury (abstract). *J Am Coll Cardiol* 1989; 13:252.

92. Danielpour D, Dart LL, Flanders KC, et al: Immunodetection and quantitation of the two forms of transforming growth factor-beta (transforming growth factor beta$_1$ and transforming growth factor-beta$_2$) secreted by cells in culture. *J Cell Physiol* 1989; 138:79–86.

93. Clowes AW, Clowes MM: Kinetic of cellular proliferation after arterial injury: II. Inhibition of smooth muscle growth by heparin. *Lab Invest* 1985; 52:611–616.

94. Reidy MA: Biology of disease. A reassessment of endothelial injury and arterial lesion formation. *Lab Invest* 1985; 53:513–520.

95. Paul R, Herbert JM, Maffrand JP, et al: Inhibition of vascular smooth muscle cell proliferation in culture by pentosan polysulphate and related compounds. *Thromb Res* 1987; 46:793–801.

96. Ellis SG, Roubin GS, Wilenz J, et al: Results of a randomized trial of heparin and aspirin vs aspirin alone for prevention of acute closure and restenosis after angioplasty (PTCA). *Circulation* 1987; 76(suppl 4):213.

97. Powell JS, Clozel JP, Muller RKM, et al: Inhibitors of angiotensin-converting enzyme prevent myointimal proliferation after vascular injury. *Science* 1989; 245:186–188.

98. Naftilan AJ, Pratt RE, Dzau VJ: Induction of platelet-derived growth factor A-chain and c-*myc* gene expressions by angiotensin II in cultured rat vascular smooth muscle cells. *J Clin Invest* 1989; 83:1419–1424.

99. Chaldakov GN, Vankov VN: Morphological aspects of secretion in the arterial smooth muscle cell, with special reference to the Golgi complex and microtubular cytoskelton. *Atherosclerosis* 1986; 61:175–192.

100. Katsuda S, Okada Y, Nakanishi I, et al: Inhibitory effect of dimethyl sulfoxide on the proliferation of cultured arterial smooth muscle cells: Relationship to the cytoplasmic microtubules. *Exp Mol Pathol* 1988; 48:48–58.

101. Daly TJ, Weston WL: Retinoid effects on fibroblast proliferation and collagen synthesis in vitro and on fibrotic disease in vivo. *J Am Acad Dermatol* 1986; 15:900–902.

102. Panabiere-Castaings MH: Retinoic acid in the treatment of keloids. *J Dermatol Surg Oncol* 1988; 14:1275–1276.

103. Sahni R, Maniet AR, Voci G, et al: Prevention of restenosis by lovastatin (abstract). *Circulation* 1989; 80(suppl 2):65.

104. Morisaki N, Kanzaki T, Motoyama N, et al: Cell cycle–dependent inhibition of DNA synthesis by prostaglandin I$_2$ in cultured rabbit aortic smooth muscle cells. *Atherosclerosis* 1988; 71:165–171.

105. Nilsson J, Olsson AG: Prostaglandin E$_1$ inhibits DNA

synthesis in arterial smooth muscle cells stimulated with platelet-derived growth factor. *Atherosclerosis* 1984; 53:77–82.

106. Nomoto A, Hirosumi J, Sekiguchi C, et al: Antiatherogenic activity of FR 34235 (nilvadipine), a new potent calcium antagonist: Effect on cuff induced intimal thickening of rabbit carotid artery. *Atherosclerosis* 1987; 64:255–261.

107. Nilsson J, Sjolund M, Palmberg L, et al: The calcium antagonist nifedipine inhibits arterial smooth muscle proliferation. *Atherosclerosis* 1985; 58:109–122.

108. Betz E, Hammerle D, Viele D: Ca^{2+}-entry blockers and atherosclerosis. *Int Angiol* 1984; 3:33.

109. Davies PF, Remuzzi A, Gordon EJ, et al: Turbulent fluid shear stress induces vascular endothelial cell turnover in vitro. *Proc Natl Acad Sci USA* 1986; 83:2114–2117.

Arterial Angioplasty: Injury, Mural Thrombus, and Restenosis

James H. Chesebro, M.D.

Juan J. Badimon, Ph.D.

Lina Badimon, Ph.D.

Valentin Fuster, M.D., Ph.D.

Quantitative measurement of the minimal lumen diameter by angiography before and immediately after coronary angioplasty documents mean improvement from approximately 0.8 to 1.5 mm after balloon dilation, to 2.25 mm after atherectomy, and to 2.0 to 2.5 mm after laser angioplasty. All of these procedures have a common "Achilles heel" 3 to 6 months later when the minimum lumen diameter decreases to 1.3 to 1.4 mm. By conventional criteria (loss of 50% of the acute gain) this represents restenosis in more than 40% of patients in all groups.[1, 2] Thus even though newer methods of angioplasty have achieved larger minimal lumen diameters acutely, the high incidence of restenosis after the acute injury negates the acutely larger luminal opening.

Each of the methods of angioplasty produces diffuse injury to the arterial wall and is not capable of targeting removal or destruction of an eccentric or focal plaque on the mural circumference. Tears with balloon dilation presumably occur at the region with lowest tensile strength, and this may be in a normal portion of the artery in the case of an eccentric plaque. Thus newer devices are needed to remove or destroy eccentric plaque while sparing normal regions of artery.

Mechanisms of restenosis appear to involve acute arterial injury with dilation, stretch, cellular destruction, and possible recoil, mural thrombosis (intraluminal and intramural), organization of thrombus, a fibromuscular proliferation of smooth muscle cells and fibroblasts, production of extracellular matrix by fibroblasts and smooth muscle cells, reactive vasoconstriction, and accelerated progression of atherosclerosis.[3, 4] This chapter will focus on the relationship of thrombosis to proliferation and restenosis and discuss risk factors for thrombosis and restenosis, the pathology of restenosis, the pathogenesis of arterial thrombosis, the high thrombogenicity of mural thrombus, the role of thrombin, the phases and pathogenesis of smooth muscle cell proliferation and migration, and principles and directions of future studies.

CONGRUENT RISK FACTORS FOR THROMBOSIS AND RESTENOSIS

There are similar risk factors for thrombosis and restenosis that include unstable angina, smoking, diabetes, arterial dissection, and eccentric plaque; these may relate to arterial substrate or systemic effects for thrombosis. Other risk factors such as the preangioplasty and immediate postangioplasty minimum lumen diameter, long lesion of greater than 10 mm, acute bend in an artery, and proximal segment of the left anterior descending coronary artery involve the rheology of blood flow.[2, 5–13] More platelets are deposited with higher shear force (small diameter, high flow, or turbulence). El-Tamimi and colleagues found positive exercise test results 3 days after angioplasty in 79% of patients who later had angiographic restenosis or compared with 18%

of patients who had no restenosis at follow-up.[14] This suggests that subocclusive mural thrombus may form early and decrease coronary flow reserve as a marker and risk factor in patients who later develop restenosis.

ANGIOSCOPY, ATHERECTOMY SPECIMENS, AND AUTOPSIES IN RESTENOSIS

Coronary *angioscopy* performed immediately after angioplasty shows tears and fissures into the plaque and associated mural thrombus (not identifiable by angiography) in 70% to 80% of patients who receive standard doses of heparin and common platelet inhibitors.[15-17] Thus subocclusive mural thrombus occurs in the majority of patients in spite of current anticoagulant and platelet inhibitor therapy. These human observations are consistent with experimental studies in pigs that also show that heparin with or without common platelet inhibitors does not totally prevent subocclusive mural thrombus after balloon angioplasty.[18, 19]

Atherectomy specimens of restenotic lesions taken within the first 15 to 30 days after arterial angioplasty showed the presence of thrombus in 65% of patients (a large amount of thrombus that was more than 20% of the specimen was found in 25% of patients) and intimal smooth muscle cell hyperplasia in 75% of patients. There was no relationship between the presence of thrombus and the type of antithrombotic therapy administered.[20] Immunohistochemical staining also showed primitive mesenchymal cells (positive staining for vimentin) that had not yet differentiated into fibroblasts, or smooth muscle cells. In specimens from patients with restenosis and prior angioplasty performed more than 30 days before atherectomy, more collagen and extracellular matrix, presumably synthesized by fibroblasts and smooth muscle cells, were observed.

Autopsy specimens from patients who died at variable times and of variable causes after angioplasty showed fissures, tears, and dissections into or around the plaque, into normal arterial wall (usually opposite an eccentric plaque), and through the internal elastic lamina into the tunica media, as well as associated subocclusive intraluminal and intramural thrombus. Thrombus was associated with breaks or tears into plaque or into normal regions of arterial wall. With balloon dilation there was incomplete displacement and incomplete resolution of plaque and residual eccentric and serpiginous lumina.[21-30] These variable lumina presumably promoted turbulent blood flow, flow at high or low shear, or stasis of blood, all of which may promote associated thrombosis.

PATHOGENESIS OF ARTERIAL THROMBOSIS

Thrombus begins to form within milliseconds of arterial injury and is grossly visible overlying the region of deep injury (type III, tear through the internal elastic lamina into the tunica media or into plaque) within minutes. Thrombin is pivotal for arterial thrombus formation, as will be discussed. Arterial thrombus is platelet-rich and often whitish and thus greatly differs from clotted whole blood or a venous or stasis thrombus. We have calculated that as much as 5% of the intravascular platelet pool may be present in a single occlusive arterial thrombus after deep injury in pigs (unpublished data, W.G. Owen and J.H. Chesebro). The amount of thrombus formed after angioplasty appears in great part to be related to the surface area of deep injury (assuming arteries of similar type, caliber, and vasoconstriction) since platelet-rich thrombus covers the entire surface of deeply injured artery (Fig 45–1). Mural thrombus may form in at least 70% to 80% of cases of deep arterial injury and may lead to acute occlusion after deep injury of normal arteries. Mural thrombus may undergo a process of organization with fibromuscular proliferation and arterial stenosis within a month after angioplasty (Figs 45–2 and 45–3).[3, 18, 31-35]

The thrombogenic *substrates* in the arterial wall and the *rheology* of blood flow are the major influences in arterial thrombosis. Less potent systemic factors such as serum cholesterol, lipoprotein (a), lipoprotein-associated coagulation inhibitor (LACI), factor VII, plasma fibrinogen, catecholamines, and modifiers of thrombolysis (such as plasminogen activator inhibitor, [PAI-1]) modify the two major influences as recently reviewed.[36]

Arterial substrates for thrombosis after deep injury are similar in the normal tunica media and intimal plaque. The thrombogenic substrates are collagen types I and III, tissue thromboplastin, loss of endothelium and its antithrombotic protection, decreased prostacyclin, and phospholipid in cell membranes for the formation of activator complexes within the coagulation cascade.[3, 4, 36] After injury mural thrombus is fixed to the deep arterial structures and protrudes into the lumen (Fig 45–1). After mild injury or endothelial denudation, less thrombogenic collagen (types IV and V) is exposed to flowing blood and leads to only a single layer of platelet deposition.[31, 33]

The rheology of blood flow is measured in part by shear force and is a major influence on vascular thrombosis. Shear force is related directly to blood flow and inversely to the third power of the lumen diameter. At high shear force red cells force platelets to the periphery and increase adenosine diphosphate (ADP) concentra-

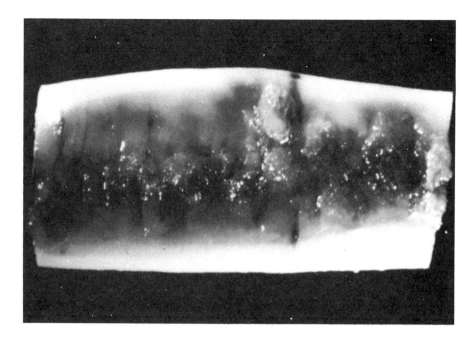

FIG 45−1.
Segment of porcine carotid artery dilated to 6 atmo by balloon angioplasty. The animal was euthanized 20 minutes later, the artery flushed with saline and fixed in situ with 4% paraformaldehyde, and the arterial segment opened longitudinally and photographed with a 2× magnifier. Platelet-rich mural thrombus overlies a deep arterial (type III) injury. Note that thrombus tracks along the deep arterial tear. Thus the extent of thrombus reflects the surface area of deep injury. (From Chesebro JH, Webster MWI, Zoldelyi P, et al: *Circulation* 1992, in press. Used by permission.)

tions on the cell membrane. Vasoconstriction may increase shear force and thus may increase platelet deposition. Increased platelet deposition may further increase vasoconstriction. Maximal platelet deposition is within the minimal lumen diameter of the stenosis. The thrombus becomes less platelet-rich, more red colored from red cell incorporation, and more fibrin-rich distal

to the stenosis.[3, 4, 34, 36–39] The risk of occlusion and restenosis is increased in high-shear arteries such as those with small lumen diameters or inadequately dilated arteries after percutaneous transluminal coronary angioplasty (PTCA).[1, 5–11]

Mural thrombus is markedly more thrombogenic than deeply injured arterial wall.[40] This results in a 6% to

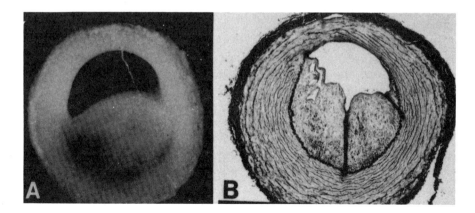

FIG 45−2.
A, a cross section of the common carotid artery at the site of balloon angioplasty 30 days after the procedure macroscopically shows a significant stenotic lesion in an artery that had previously been normal. **B,** a histologic section of same lesion as in **A** shows that the obstruction is due to organized mural thrombus (Lason's elastic−van Gieson stain, ×10). From Steele PM, Chesebro JH, Stanson AW, et al: *Circ Res* 1985; 57:105–112. Used by permission.)

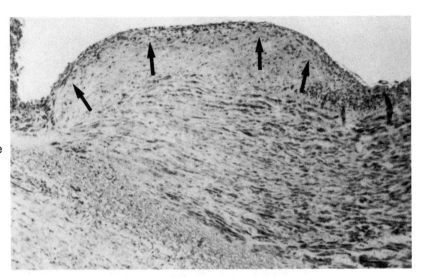

FIG 45–3.
A histologic cross section of the common carotid artery 2 weeks after balloon angioplasty shows the fibromuscular organization of a mural thrombus with a subendothelial cap and rim of smooth muscle cells *(arrows).* Immunohistochemical actin stain with aminoethylcarbazol (AEC) chromogen and background staining with Schmitt's hematoxylin, ×25.

68% risk of acute occlusion or restenosis after PTCA in patients with unstable angina or myocardial infarction after thrombolysis.[10, 41–44] In patients with unstable angina, mural thrombus also accounts for the increased risk of myocardial infarction, refractory angina, and death because of the high thrombogenicity of mural thrombus.[36, 40, 45] This marked thrombogenicity appears to be due to active thrombin that is adsorbed to fibrin within the thrombus by a site on thrombin that is near the C-terminal end and separate from the catalytic site.[46–53] Thrombin adsorbed to fibrin is internalized as the thrombus grows and is acutely exposed to flowing blood after breakage by the catheter, spontaneous embolization, or lysis. Platelets are exquisitely sensitive to activation by thrombin.[18, 33, 53] Thus thrombin at the surface of a thrombus activates more platelets for local deposition, which results in the growth of thrombus. Additional substances secreted by these activated platelets such as thromboxane A_2, serotonin, and ADP also cause additional platelet deposition.[53, 54]

The *pivotal role of thrombin* has been demonstrated in vivo.[18, 33] In vitro activation and aggregation of platelets can be initiated by thromboxane A_2, serotonin, ADP, collagen, epinephrine, thrombin, and other substances.[54] However, inhibition of in vitro aggregation does not predict the in vivo response to inhibitors of these substances.[33, 55] Inhibition of receptors to thromboxane A_2, serotonin, or both did not decrease platelet deposition after deep arterial injury but did decrease the severity of injury-associated vasoconstriction.[55]

Heparin inhibits thrombin (factor IIa) and factor Xa. To test whether heparin is effective in vivo, we administered six different ascending doses of unfractionated heparin starting immediately before angioplasty. High doses of unfractionated heparin up to 500 units/kg over the hour of the procedure reduced quantitative platelet and fibrinogen deposition but did not totally prevent mural thrombus after deep arterial injury.[18] Low–molecular-weight heparin (CY216), which has a greater anti–factor Xa effect, was no better than unfractionated heparin in reducing mural thrombosis, platelet deposition, or fibrinogen deposition. A reduced incidence of mural thrombosis correlated better with the antithrombin rather than the anti–factor Xa effect.[56]

The pivotal role of thrombin for in vivo thrombosis after deep arterial injury was documented by studies in pigs.[18, 33] Hirudin is the anticoagulant of the European leech *Hirudo medicinalis* and a specific and tight-binding ($K_d = 10^{-14}$) thrombin inhibitor. It inhibits platelet aggregation to thrombin but not to serotonin, thromboxane A_2, ADP, epinephrine, or collagen. At lower doses (mean activated partial thromboplastin time [aPTT] 1.7 times control) recombinant hirudin (CGP 39393) reduces fibrinogen deposition. At higher doses (aPTT two to three times control) hirudin completely prevents mural thrombosis and reduces platelet deposition to less than a single layer in vivo after deep arterial injury (Fig 45–4).[33] A bolus of heparin plus low-dose aspirin, 1 mg/kg/day or plus aspirin, 20 mg/kg/day, and dipyridamole was better than placebo in reducing the incidence and size of mural thrombosis but still left mural thrombosis in 25% to 48% of deeply injured arteries.[19] Thus hirudin as a thrombin inhibitor sets a new standard of treatment and therapeutic goal, namely, the complete prevention of mural thrombus in the lumen after deep arterial injury by angioplasty.

Different degrees of thrombin inhibition are required for different pathogeneses of thrombosis and against different actions of thrombin. Hirudin binds 1:1 with thrombin. Thus the plasma levels of hirudin necessary to completely prevent thrombosis in vivo are an index of the *thrombin content* of each pathogenic etiology of

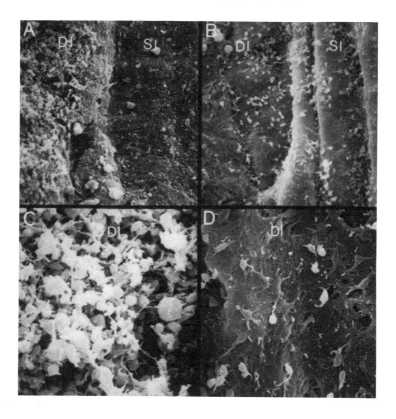

FIG 45–4.
Scanning electron photomicrograph of the injured luminal surface of the common carotid artery (original magnification, ×1,000) from animals treated with placebo **(A)** and 1.0 mg/kg hirudin **(B)**. The right side of each panel has subendothelial injury *(SI)*, and the left side has deep injury *(DI)*. **C,** a higher magnification (×3,000) of the platelet thrombus covering the area of deep injury in **A** (placebo). **D,** higher magnification (×3,000) of the area of deep injury from **B** (hirudin treated) with very few adherent platelets, similar to areas of subendothelial injury. (From Heras M, Chesebro JH, Webster MWI, et al: *Circulation* 1990; 82:1476–1484. Used by permission.)

thrombosis. Without arterial injury, five times higher plasma levels of hirudin are necessary to prevent platelet vs. fibrin thrombi in the lungs during disseminated intravascular coagulation.[57] Thus platelets are exquisitely sensitive to thrombin. The *thrombin content* of arteries with deep injury is eight to ten times greater than that of arteries with mild (deendothelialized) or type II injury.[33, 57–59] A second method of demonstrating the increased *thrombin content* and increased thrombogenicity of deeply injured arteries is by immunohistochemical staining of thrombus in a totally occluded artery. Immunohistochemical staining is positive for thrombin in thrombus adjacent to deep injury but not in thrombus adjacent to mild injury or within the center of the lumen.[59]

The *thrombin content* of a deeply injured artery appears to further *increase with a metallic stent* at the injury site since a previously effective dose of hirudin no longer completely prevents mural thrombus at the site of deep injury and a metallic stent.[60] This concept is supported by the fact that high-dose potent thrombin

inhibition can completely prevent thrombus formation within a metallic stent placed within a Gortex graft.[61]

Thrombin remains active and binds to arterial subendothelial matrix (especially to dermatan sulfate).[62] Generation of thrombin is accelerated 278,000 times by formation of the activator complex (prothrombinase complex) as compared with thrombin generation from a single factor alone.[63] The prothrombinase complex is the assembly of Ca^{2+} and factors Va and Xa on a phospholipid membrane such as the platelet or smooth muscle cell membrane. Whether additional thrombin is present (bound or generated) in the matrix of a deeply injured artery is currently under study in our laboratory.

THERAPEUTIC GOALS IN ANTITHROMBOTIC THERAPY

Antithrombotic therapy may be anticoagulant, antifibrin, antiplatelet, antithrombotic, or a combination of these depending on the type of therapy, the dosage, and the underlying pathogenesis of thrombosis. No single therapy of those on the market today produces all of these effects. For example, the thrombus largely due to stasis in venous thrombosis is similar to an in vitro blood clot, is predominantly fibrin, and requires antifibrin therapy, which also has an anticoagulant effect. Heparin is an antifibrin (inhibits the conversion of fibrinogen to fibrin) and an anticoagulant but must be administered to prolong the aPTT to >1.5 times control to prevent further growth of venous thrombus.

Antithrombotic therapy differs for arterial thrombosis. Heparin has very weak antiplatelet effects at usual doses and even at huge doses (500 units/kg over the first hour) cannot completely prevent mural thrombosis after deep injury.[18, 33] Aspirin is specifically antiplatelet in action, reduces the incidence of arterial thrombosis, but cannot completely prevent mural thrombosis after deep arterial injury.[19] Potent, specific, high-affinity antithrombin therapy with hirudin during deep arterial injury is antifibrin at low doses (aPTT 1.7 times control) and antiplatelet and antithrombotic (completely prevents mural thrombus) at a slightly higher but sharply defined anticoagulant dose producing an aPTT of 2.0 times control or greater in pigs. The human antithrombotic-antiplatelet dosage needs a definition. The in vivo response is not predicted by in vitro tests such as inhibition of platelet aggregation (which is very sharply defined with an all-or-none effect by thrombin).[33] Thus before clinical trials in humans are initiated, the dose-antithrombotic activity-response needs to be defined in vivo. This is first done in large animals, then in humans using the same mechanism of thrombosis as in the human trial. This stepwise approach will save time and money (and thus eventual cost to the patient) for drug development, reduce the number of patients required and the risk of study, and reduce the number of negative clinical trials usually involving large numbers of patients.

THROMBOSIS AND CELLULAR PROLIFERATION AND MIGRATION

Proliferation and migration of smooth muscle cells follow acute arterial injury, are independent processes, and can be divided into three phases from experimental data. Phase I is the first wave of proliferation and hypertrophy and peaks at 48 hours in medial smooth muscle cells. Phase II is the intermediate phase of smooth muscle cell proliferation and spans about 4 to 14 days. Smooth muscle cells migrate from the media to the intima, and approximately half proliferate within the intima. The late or phase III of smooth muscle cell prolif-

eration is 2 weeks and beyond. There is decreasing proliferation and predominately hypertrophy and production of extracellular matrix.[35, 64–66]

Medial smooth muscle cell proliferation in *phase I* is related to arterial injury or stretch of the media and not to the presence or absence of platelets. After endothelial denudation without medial injury or stretch only small increases in proliferation occur in spite of significant platelet deposition.[64, 67–71] The amount of stretch in atmospheres of balloon inflation pressure appears to influence medial smooth muscle cell injury and necrosis and correlates with the proportion of proliferating smooth muscle cells in the tunica media 48 hours after injury. The degree of medial smooth muscle cell proliferation did not correlate with deep or mild injury or quantitative ^{111}In-labeled platelet deposition.[67] Thus phase I proliferation appears to correlate with arterial stretch and cellular injury but not platelet deposition.

Medial proliferation in phase I appears to be related to basic fibroblast growth factor (bFGF) since smooth muscle cells of the rat express messenger (m) RNA for bFGF, and bFGF ligand was found by immunoblot analysis. Infusion of bFGF after gentle endothelial denudation increases medial proliferation. Infusion of anti-bFGF antibody decreases medial smooth muscle cell proliferation. Uninjured arteries without endothelial denudation do not respond to an intravenous infusion of bFGF.[68–71]

Other growth factors such as platelet-derived growth factor (PDGF), transforming growth factor β_1 (TGF-β_1), or thrombin may provide additional stimuli or helper functions in phase I. In neonatal rat smooth muscle cells thrombin appears to be mitogenic, but in the adult rat thrombin stimulates protein but not DNA synthesis (hypertrophic but not mitogenic). Thrombin also activates several transmembrane signaling pathways common to PDGF, which may also induce chemotaxis of smooth muscle cell.[72–74] TGF-β_1 is released from platelets and is also mitogenic.[75, 76] Thus thrombin, TGF-β_1, and PDGF costimulate with bFGF. Since cells migrate from the media to the intima in phase II, proliferation in phase II may be influenced by proliferation in phase I.

Intimal thickening in *phase II*, the intermediate phase, depends on both proliferation and migration of smooth muscle cells from the media to the intima.[77–83] Chemotaxis of smooth muscle cells is predominately due to PDGF (and other factors released from platelets including TGF-β_1[83]), but proliferation is due to several growth factors such as bFGF, PDGF, epidermal growth factor insulin growth factor, and TGF-β_1.[75, 76, 80, 81, 83, 84] These growth factors may be released from or regulated by platelets, smooth muscle cells, endothelial cells, monocytes, macrophages, or thrombus.[83-86]

Migration of smooth muscle cells does not depend on proliferation.[87,88] Approximately 50% of intimal smooth muscle cells migrate but do not proliferate.[89] In the rat, peak proliferation of smooth muscle cells in the intima occurs at 96 hours.[64] In pigs, new intimal smooth muscle cells are present by 4 to 7 days, and 48% are proliferating by 1 week after injury with 6 atm of balloon dilation.[35] A cap of smooth muscle cells forms just below the regenerated endothelium overlying mural thrombus by 2 weeks after injury and is associated with significant intimal cellular proliferation (see Fig 45–3).[31,35] This subpopulation of neointimal smooth muscle cells may also be present in the rat where subintimal cells had a different pattern of gene expression (strongly positive for PDGF-A and PDGF-B receptor transcripts).[65]

Mural thrombi have been related to neointimal fibromuscular proliferation, platelet antigens, and bands of fibrin in experimental and human plaque.[31,35,85,90-96] Fibromuscular plaque formation can result from distal extension of thrombus to a distal uninjured segment or after pulmonary embolization; these fibromuscular plaquelike lesions are rich in lipids and connective tissue in the absence of lipid feeding.[90] Antiplatelet serum that lowers the platelet count to less than 10,000 markedly reduces intimal proliferation in the rabbit aorta after injury with an indwelling polyethylene cannula or a balloon catheter.[85,96] In rats thrombocytopenia prevents intimal lesions 1 week after balloon injury.[68] Neointimal smooth muscle cells in rats contain large amounts of PDGF β-receptor mRNA; thus the studies with thrombocytopenia suggest that PDGF-BB from platelets plays a major role in the formation of neointima.

Platelet-rich, mural thrombus after deep injury leads to increased delivery of growth factors from platelets to the arterial wall. However, mild injury leads to only a single layer of platelets and markedly decreased fibrin, thrombin, and delivery of growth factors to the arterial wall.[31,53,83] These facts may largely account for the increased proliferative response after deep vs. mild arterial injury.[31,35] As discussed above, increased thrombin content is associated with deep arterial injury. In addition, the extent of secretion of factors by platelets correlates with the number of thrombin molecules activating platelets.[53] Thrombus also attracts monocytes and macrophages, which contain growth factors. Thus thrombus, platelets, and the associated cellular secretory products appear to play a significant role in phase II, or the intermediate phase, of smooth muscle cell proliferation (Fig 45–5).

In *phase III* smooth muscle cell proliferation de-

creases, but intimal cellular hypertrophy and extracellular matrix production from smooth muscle cells increase, presumably by factors that affect smooth muscle cells including TGF-β_1.[66,97,98] In arterial segments chronically denuded of endothelium, intimal thickening progressively increases via continued proliferation and matrix formation. In reendothelialized segments, proliferative activity usually returns to baseline in about 4 weeks, and matrix production continues out of proportion to proliferation but also decreases over a period of 4 to 6 weeks.[66,99] This may differ in species and with altered lipids.[100,101] With complete endothelial denudation, there is only partial ingrowth from healthy endothelial borders.[99]

Endothelial cells may also regulate the proliferation of smooth muscle cells. In injured and cultured endothelial cells, synthesis and secretion of a PDGF-like protein (PDGF$_c$) are increased.[102] Production and release of PDGF$_c$ by endothelial cells may be stimulated by tumor necrosis factor, TGF-β_1 (platelets contain large quantities), thrombin (induces dose-dependent PDGF$_c$ secretion), factor Xa, and agents that injure endothelial cells such as bacterial endotoxin phorbol esters.[83,102-107] Thrombin is adsorbed to fibrin that is within thrombi and intimal lesions and appears to be active from histochemical studies using fluorogenic substrates.[46-52,108,109] Thus thrombin from intimal lesions could stimulate the production and release of PDGF$_c$ by endothelial cells. Endothelial cells are regrown and functional by 1 week after balloon injury in the pig.[31,110] Thus the production of growth factors or inhibitors may be closely regulated in vivo by endothelial cells.

Other factors from endothelium may also stimulate the proliferation of smooth muscle cells.[111] Endothelium contains abundant bFGF, a cell-associated mitogen that is released by agents injurious to endothelial cells, appears to be important in the maintenance of endothelial cells, and stimulates the proliferation of smooth muscle cells and fibroblasts.[71] Porcine vascular cells produce a PDGF-like mitogen, and smooth muscle cells respond to purified porcine PDGF with a proliferative response.[112] Other factors such as interleukin-1, angiotensin converting enzyme (which may induce PDGF-A expression in smooth muscle cells), and insulin growth factor may also contribute to cellular proliferation after arterial injury.[113-116] These may act alone or synergistically with PDGF and bFGF.

FUTURE DIRECTIONS

Since 70% to 80% of arteries have asymptomatic mural thrombi immediately after angioplasty, the first and probably pivotal step for reducing the incidence of

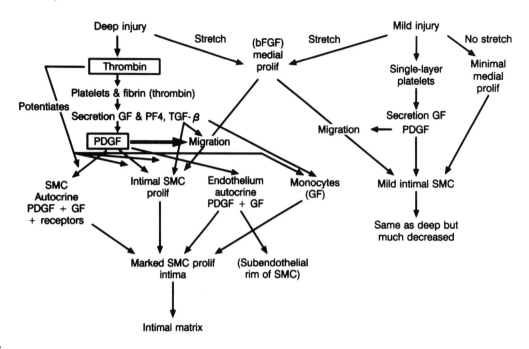

FIG 45–5.
Proposed mechanisms of the role of thrombus in smooth muscle cell *(SMC)* proliferation. Phase I, or the first wave of proliferation due to arterial stretch or direct injury, peaks at 48 hours, appears to be directly related to basic fibroblast growth factor *(bFGF, center),* and is independent of platelet deposition. Lack of stretch results in minimal phase I proliferation *(right).* Similar mechanisms are present after deep (into plaque or through internal elastic lamina) injury *(left)* or mild (endothelial denudation only) injury *(right).* The degree of phase II intimal proliferation of SMC at 1 to 2 weeks after arterial injury is considerably greater after deep injury. The reasons for this are presumably due to increased amounts of thrombin, which stimulates platelet and fibrin deposition, platelet secretion of platelet-derived growth factor *(PDGF),* transforming growth factor *(TGF-β),* other growth factors *(GF),* oncogene activation, and potentiation of other GF that may originate from platelets, monocytes, macrophages, endothelium, or smooth muscle cells. PDGF appears to play a pivotal role in the migration of SMC from the media to the intima (and is enhanced by TGF-β and other platelet-derived substances) and presumably is also an important GF in phase II intimal proliferation (see the text). Other secretory products from platelets such as platelet factor 4 *(PF4)* may be chemotactic to monocytes; TGF-β may contribute to proliferation and migration of SMC. Similar mechanisms are present after mild injury *(right)* but occur to a lesser degree. bFGF = basic fibroblast growth factor. (Adapted from Chesebro JH, et al: In Schwartz RS (ed): *Coronary Restenosis.* Boston, Blackwell, 1992.)

restenosis appears to be complete prevention of mural thrombus after angioplasty. A large amount of intraluminal and intramural thrombus and a hugh dose of growth factors need to be eliminated and the outcome observed. It appears that this can be accomplished with thrombin inhibition but that local delivery will be required to eliminate intramural thrombi. In addition, the duration of therapy requires detailed study. Details of delivery, dosage, and duration are under study in animals. These principles can then be applied to humans. The human dosage to eliminate intraluminal thrombus is also critical and is being evaluated. Without knowledge of these details human trials in restenosis will waste money, unwisely use investigator time, and place patients into premature studies and uncertain and unnecessary risks.

Investigations should involve small and then large animal studies with injury to reproduce the human situation, quantitation of thrombosis by documented techniques, steady-state therapy to judge the appropriate antithrombotic dose, evaluation of intraluminal and intramural thrombi, duration of therapy, mechanisms affecting these, and effect on neointimal proliferation. Fissures and tears with associated intramural thrombus are a normal occurrence with balloon angioplasty. Intravenous hirudin completely prevents intraluminal[18, 19, 33] but not intramural thrombi (unpublished data). Thus with this and future therapies the location of the thrombus also needs to be investigated, depending upon the goals of therapy, the pathogenesis of the disease, and mechanisms of the particular interventional therapy.

Alternate antithrombotic therapy may be considered. Inhibition of glycoprotein platelet membrane receptors such as glycoprotein IIb/IIIa does not appear promising since antibodies to the receptor are not effective at low shear (a situation that may be produced after successful angioplasty); additional adjunctive anticoagulation is required for inhibition.[117] Heparin does not block the growth of mural thrombus, but hirudin totally blocks growth at both high and low shear.[118]

Alternate antithrombotic therapy may also involve inhibition of thrombin generation at a more proximal level in the coagulation cascade. This approach may be equally or more effective than hirudin and perhaps safer since systemic anticoagulation may be avoided; evaluation is needed.

Mechanisms of cellular proliferation require continued study. Inhibitors of specific growth factors should be evaluated in animal models of arterial injury that reproduce the human injury as closely as possible (stretch, tears with deep injury, mural thrombosis, fibromuscular response) and should be tried with and without maximally effective antithrombotic therapy. After starting with smaller animal models, quantitative studies in each of the three phases of proliferation should be carried out in the pig or primate since these appear to be most predictive of results in humans.[119]

REFERENCES

1. Rogers J, Garratt KN, Kaufmann UP, Restenosis after atherectomy vs PTCA: Initial experience (abstract). *J Am Coll Cardiol* 1990; 15:197.
2. Chesebro JH, Webster MWI, Reeder GS, et al: Coronary angioplasty: Antiplatelet therapy reduces acute complications but not restenosis (abstract). *Circulation* 1989; 80(suppl 2):64.
3. Ip JH, Fuster V, Badimon L, et al: Syndromes of accelerated atherosclerosis: Role of vascular injury and smooth muscle cell proliferation. *J Am Coll Cardiol* 1990; 15:1667–1687.
4. Ip JH, Fuster V, Israel D, et al: The role of platelets, thrombin and hyperplasia in restenosis after coronary angioplasty. *J Am Coll Cardiol* 1991; 17(suppl):77–88.
5. Holmes DR, Vlietstra RE, Smith HC, et al: Restenosis after percutaneous transluminal coronary angioplasty (PTCA): A report from the PTCA registry of the National Heart, Lung, and Blood Institute. *Am J Cardiol* 1984; 53:77–81.
6. Mata LA, Bosch X, David PR, et al: Clinical and angiographic assessment 6 months after double vessel percutaneous transluminal coronary angioplasty. *J Am Coll Cardiol* 1985; 6:1239–1244.
7. Kaltenbach M, Kober G, Scherer D, et al: Recurrence rate after successful coronary angioplasty. *Eur Heart J* 1985; 6:276–281.
8. Levine S, Ewels CJ, Rosing DR, et al: Coronary angioplasty: Clinical and angiographic follow-up. *Am J Cardiol* 1985; 55:673–676.
9. Wijns W, Serruys PW, Reiber JHC: Early detection of restenosis after successful percutaneous transluminal coronary angioplasty by exercise redistribution. *Am J Cardiol* 1985; 55:357–361.
10. Leimgruber PP, Roubin GS, Hollman J, et al: Resteno-sis after successful coronary angioplasty in patients with single-vessel disease. *Circulation* 1986; 73:710–717.
11. Guiteras VP, Bourassa MG, David PR, et al: Restenosis after successful percutaneous transluminal coronary angioplasty: The Montreal Heart Institute experience. *Am J Cardiol* 1987; 60(suppl B):50–55.
12. Dehmer GJ, Popma JJ, van den Berg EK, et al: Reduction in the rate of early restenosis after coronary angioplasty by a diet supplemented with n-3 fatty acids. *N Engl J Med* 1988; 319:733–740.
13. Schwartz L, Bourassa MG, Lesperance J, et al: Aspirin and dipyridamole in the prevention of restenosis after percutaneous transluminal coronary angioplasty. *N Engl J Med* 1988; 318:1714–1719.
14. El-Tamimi H, Davies GJ, Hackett D, et al: Very early prediction of restenosis after successful coronary angioplasty: Anatomic and functional assessment. *J Am Coll Cardiol* 1990; 15:259–264.
15. Mizuno K, Miyamoto A, Sakurada M, et al: Evaluation of coronary thrombi after PTCA by angioscopy (abstract). *Circulation* 1989; 80(suppl 2):523.
16. Uchida Y, Hasegawa K, Kawamura K, et al: Angioscopic observation of the coronary luminal changes induced by percutaneous transluminal coronary angioplasty. *Am Heart J* 1989; 117:769–776.
17. Yanagida S, Mizuno K, Miyamoto A, et al: Comparison of findings between coronary angiography and angioscopy (abstract). *Circulation* 1989; 80(suppl 2):376.
18. Heras M, Chesebro JH, Penny WJ, et al: Effects of thrombin inhibition on the development of acute platelet-thrombus deposition during angioplasty in pigs: Heparin versus recombinant hirudin, a specific thrombin inhibitor. *Circulation* 1989; 79:657–665.
19. Lam JYT, Chesebro JH, Steele PM, et al: Antithrombotic therapy for arterial injury by angioplasty: Efficacy of common platelet-inhibitors versus thrombin inhibition in pigs. *Circulation* 1991; 84:814–820.
20. Johnson DE, Hinohara T, Selmon MR, et al: Primary peripheral arterial stenoses and restenoses excised by transluminal atherectomy: A histopathologic study. *J Am Coll Cardiol* 1990; 15:419–425.
21. Block PC, Myler RK, Stertzer S, et al: Morphology after PTCA in human beings. *N Engl J Med* 1981; 305:382–385.
22. Essed CE, van der Braud M, Becker AE: Transluminal coronary angioplasty and early restenosis: Fibrocellular occlusion after wall laceration. *Br Heart J* 1983; 49:393–396.
23. Austin GE, Ratliff NB, Hollman J, et al: Intimal proliferation of smooth muscle cells as an explanation for recurrent coronary artery stenosis after percutaneous transluminal coronary angioplasty. *J Am Coll Cardiol* 1985; 6:369–375.
24. Colavita PG, Ideker RE, Reimer KA, et al: The spectrum of pathology associated with percutaneous transluminal coronary angioplasty during acute myocardial infarction. *J Am Coll Cardiol* 1986; 8:855–860.
25. Kohchi K, Takebayashi S, Block PC, et al: Arterial changes after percutaneous coronary angioplasty: Results at autopsy. *J Am Coll Cardiol* 1987; 10:592–599.
26. Ueda M, Becker AE, Fujimoto T: Pathological changes induced by repeated percutaneous transluminal coronary angioplasty. *Br Heart J* 1987; 58:635–643.

27. O'Hara T, Nanto S, Asada S, et al: Ultrastructural study of proliferating and migrating smooth muscle cells at the site of percutaneous transluminal coronary angioplasty as an explanation for restenosis (abstract). *Circulation* 1988; 78(suppl 2):290.

28. Solymoss BC, Gote G, Leung TK, et al: Pathology of percutaneous transluminal coronary angioplasty complications (abstract). *Circulation* 1988; 78(suppl 2):445.

29. Potkin BN, Roberts WC: Effects of percutaneous transluminal coronary angioplasty on atherosclerotic plaques and relation of plaque composition and arterial size to outcome. *Am J Cardiol* 1988; 62:41–50.

30. Farb A, Virmani R, Atkinson JB, et al: Plaque morphology and pathologic changes in arteries from patients dying after coronary balloon angioplasty. *J Am Coll Cardiol* 1990; 16:1421–1429.

31. Steele PM, Chesebro JH, Stanson AW, et al: Balloon angioplasty: Natural history of the pathophysiologic response to injury in a pig model. *Circ Res* 1985; 57:105–112.

32. Heras M, Chesebro JH, Penny WJ, et al. Importance of adequate heparin dosage in arterial angioplasty in a porcine model. *Circulation* 1988; 78:654–660.

33. Heras M, Chesebro JH, Webster MWI, et al: Hirudin, heparin and placebo during deep arterial injury in the pig: The in vivo role of thrombin in platelet-mediated thrombosis. *Circulation* 1990; 82:1476–1484.

34. Lam JYT, Chesebro JH, Steele PM, et al: Is vasospasm related to platelet deposition? Relationship in a porcine preparation of arterial injury in vivo. *Circulation* 1987; 75:243–248.

35. Webster MWI, Chesebro JH, Grill DE, et al: Influence of deep and mild injury on smooth muscle cell proliferation after angioplasty. *Circulation* 1991; 84(suppl 2):296.

36. Fuster V, Badimon L, Badimon JJ, et al: Coronary artery disease and acute coronary syndromes. *N Engl J Med* 1992; 326:242–250, 310–318.

37. Lam JYT, Chesebro JH, Fuster V: Platelets, vasoconstriction, and nitroglycerin during arterial wall injury: A new antithrombotic role for an old drug. *Circulation* 1988; 78:712–716.

38. Badimon L, Badimon JJ, Galvez A, et al: Influence of arterial damage and wall shear rate on platelet deposition. Ex vivo study in a swine model. *Arteriosclerosis* 1986; 6:312–320.

39. Badimon L, Badimon JJ: Mechanism of arterial thrombosis in non-parallel streamlines: Platelet growth at the apex of stenotic severely injured vessel wall. Experimental study in the pig model. *J Clin Invest* 1989; 84:1134–1144.

40. Badimon L, Lassila R, Badimon J, et al: Residual thrombus is more thrombogenic than severely damaged vessel wall (abstract). *Circulation* 1988; 78(suppl 2):119.

41. Califf RM, Topol EJ, George BS: Characteristics and outcome of patients in whom reperfusion with intravenous tissue-type plasminogen activator fails. *Circulation* 1988; 77:1090–1099.

42. Baim DS, Diver DJ, Knatterud GL: PTCA "salvage" for thrombolytic failures — implications from TIMI II-A. *Circulation* 1988; 78(suppl 2):112.

43. Mabin TA, Holmes DR, Smith HC, et al: Intracoronary thrombus: Role in coronary occlusion complicating percutaneous transluminal coronary angioplasty. *J Am Coll Cardiol* 1985; 5:198–202.

44. Chesebro JH, Lam JYT, Badimon L, et al: Restenosis after arterial angioplasty: A hemorrheologic response to injury. *Am J Cardiol* 1987; 60:10–16.

45. Theroux P, Ouimet H, McCans J, et al: Aspirin, heparin, or both to treat acute unstable angina. *N Engl J Med* 1988; 319:1105–1111.

46. Seegers WH, Nieft M, Loomis EC: Note of the absorption of thrombin on fibrin. *Science* 1945; 101:520–521.

47. Liu CY, Nossel HL, Kaplan KL: The binding of thrombin by fibrin. *J Biol Chem* 1979; 254:10421–10425.

48. Francis CW, Markham RE Jr, Barlow GH: Thrombin activity of fibrin thrombi and soluble plasmic derivatives. *J Lab Clin Med* 1983; 102:220–230.

49. Kaminski M, McDonagh J: Studies on the mechanism of thrombin: Interaction with fibrin. *J Biol Chem* 1983; 258:10530–10535.

50. Berliner LJ, Sugawara Y: Human α-thrombin binding to nonpolymerized fibrin-Sepharose: Evidence for an anionic binding region. *Biochemistry* 1985; 24:7005–7009.

51. Kaminski M, McDonagh J: Inhibited thrombins: Interactions with fibrinogen and fibrin. *Biochem J* 1987; 242:881–887.

52. Vali Z, Scheraga HA: Localization of the binding site on fibrin for the secondary binding site of thrombin. *Biochemistry* 1988; 27:1956–1963.

53. Shuman MA: Thrombin-cellular interactions. *Ann N Y Acad Sci* 1986; 485:228–239.

54. Mruk JS, Chesebro JH, Webster WMI: Platelet aggregation with the coagulation system: Implications for antithrombotic therapy in arterial thrombosis. *J Coronary Artery Dis* 1990; 1:149–158.

55. Lam JYT, Chesebro JH, Badimon L, et al: Serotonin and thromboxane A$_2$ receptor blockade decrease vasoconstriction but not platelet deposition after deep arterial injury. *Circulation* 1986; 74(suppl 2):97.

56. Heras M, Chesebro JH, Webster MWI, et al: Antithrombotic efficacy of low molecular weight heparin in deep arterial injury. *Arteriosclerosis Thromb* 1992; 12:250–255.

57. Markwardt F, Kaiser B, Novak G: Studies on antithrombotic effects of recombinant hirudin. *Thromb Res* 1989; 54:377–388.

58. Ambler J, Butler KD, Kerry R, et al: Comparative effects of selective thrombin inhibition by hirudin on coagulation and thrombosis. *Circulation* 1989; 80(suppl 2):316.

59. Chesebro JH, Webster MWI, Zoldhelyi P, et al: Antithrombotic therapy in the progression of coronary artery disease. *Circulation* 1992, in press.

60. Garratt KN, Heras M, Holmes DR Jr, et al: Platelet deposition and thrombosis in arterial stents: Effect of hirudin compared with heparin plus antiplatelet therapy (abstract). *J Am Coll Cardiol* 1990; 15(suppl):209.

61. Krupski WC, Bass A, Kelly AB, et al: Heparin-resistant thrombus formation by endovascular stents in baboons: Interruption by a synthetic antithrombin. *Circulation* 1990; 81:570–577.

62. Bar-Shavit R, Eldora A, Vlodavsky I: Binding of throm-

bin to subendothelial extracellular matrix. *J Clin Invest* 1989; 84:1096–1104.

63. Mann KG, Tracy PB, Nesheim MW: Assembly and function of prothrombinase complex on synthetic and nature membranes, in Oates JA, Harwiger J, Ross R (eds): *Interaction of Platelets With Vessel Wall.* Washington, DC, American Physiologic Society, 1985, pp 47–57.

64. Clowes AW, Reidy MA, Clowes MM: Kinetics of cellular proliferation after arterial injury. I. Smooth muscle growth in the absence of endothelium. *Lab Invest* 1983; 49:327–333.

65. Majesky MW, Reidy MA, Bowen-Pope DF, et al: PDGF ligand and receptor gene expression during repair of arterial injury. *J Cell Biol* 1990; 111:2149–2158.

66. Snow AD, Bolender RP, Wright TN, et al: Heparin modulates the composition of the extracellular matrix domain surrounding arterial smooth muscle cells. *Am J Pathol* 1990; 137:313–330.

67. Webster MWI, Chesebro JH, Heras M, et al: Effect of balloon inflation on smooth muscle cell proliferation in the porcine carotid artery (abstract). *J Am Coll Cardiol* 1990; 15:188.

68. Fingerle J, Johnson R, Clowes AW, et al: Role of platelets in smooth muscle cell proliferation and migration after vascular injury in rat carotid artery. *Proc Natl Acad Sci USA* 1989; 86:8412–8416.

69. Fingerle J, Au WPT, Clowes AW, et al: Intimal lesion formation in rat carotid arteries after endothelial denudation in absence of medial injury. *Arteriosclerosis* 1990; 10:1082–1087.

70. Capron L, Bruneval P: Influence of applied stress on mitotic response of arteries to injury with a balloon catheter: Quantitative study in rat throracic aorta. *Cardiovasc Res* 1989; 23:941–948.

71. Lindner V, Lappi DA, Baird D, et al: Role of basic fibroblast growth factor in vascular lesion formation. *Circ Res* 1991; 68:106–113.

72. Berk BC, Taubman MB, Griendling KK, et al: Thrombin-stimulated events in cultured vascular smooth muscle cells. *Biochem J* 1991; 274:799–805.

73. Berk BC, Taubman MB, Gragoe EJ, et al: Thrombin signal transduction of mechanisms in rat vascular smooth muscle cells. *J Cell Biol* 1990; 265:17334–17340.

74. Huang C-L, Ives HE: Growth inhibition by protein kinase C late in mitogenesis. *Nature* 1987; 329:849–850.

75. Majesky MW, Lindner V, Twardzik DR, et al: Production of transforming growth factor B$_1$ during repair of arterial injury. *J Clin Invest* 1991; 88:904–910.

76. Battegay EJ, Raines EW, Seifert RA, et al: TGF-beta induces bimodal proliferation of connective tissue cells via complex control of an autocrine PDGF loop. *Cell* 1990; 63:515–524.

77. Hassler O: The origin of the cells constituting arterial intima thickening: An experimental autoradiographic study with the use of H3-thymidine. *Lab Invest* 1970; 22:286–293.

78. Webster WS, Bishop SP, Geer JC: Experimental aortic intimal thickening. *Am J Pathol* 1974; 76:245–260.

79. Thorgeirsson G, Robertson AL, Cohen DH: Migration

80. Grotendorst GR, Seppa HEJ, Kleinman HK, et al: Attachment of smooth muscle cells of collagen and their migration toward platelet-derived growth factor. *Proc Natl Acad Sci USA* 1981; 78: 3669–3672.

81. Ihnatowycz IO, Winocour PD, Moore S: A platelet-derived factor chemotactic for rabbit arterial smooth muscle cells in culture. *Artery* 1981; 9:316–317.

82. Nakao J, Ooyama T, Chang WC, et al: Platelets stimulate aortic smooth muscle cell migration in vitro. *Atherosclerosis* 1982; 43:143–150.

83. Bell L, Madri JA: Effect of platelet factors on migration of cultured bovine aortic endothelial and smooth muscle cells. *Circ Res* 1989; 65:1057–1065.

84. Ferns GAA, Raines EW, Sprugel KH, et al: Inhibition of neointimal smooth muscle accumulation after angioplasty by an antibody to PDGF. *Science* 1991; 253:1129–1132.

85. Moore S, Friedman RJ, Singal DP, et al: Inhibition of injury induced thromboatherosclerotic lesions by antiplatelet serum in rabbits. *Thromb Haemost* 1976; 35:70–81.

86. Libby P, Warner SJC, Salomon RN, et al: Production of platelet-derived growth factor–like mitogen by smooth-muscle cells from human atheroma. *N Engl J Med* 1988; 318:1493.

87. Bernstein LR, Antantoniades H, Zetter BR: Migration of cultured vascular cells in response to plasma and platelet-derived factors. *J Cell Sci* 1982; 56:71–82.

88. Weinstein R, Stemerman MB, Maciag T: Hormonal requirements for growth of arterial smooth muscle cells in vitro: an endocrine approach to atherosclerosis. *Science* 1981; 212:818–820.

89. Clowes AW, Schwartz SM: Significance of quiescent smooth muscle migration in the injured rat carotid artery. *Circ Res* 1985; 56:139–145.

90. Woolf N: Interaction between mural thrombi and underlying artery wall. *Haemostasis* 1979; 8:127–141.

91. Woolf N, Carstairs KC: Infiltration and thrombosis in atherogenesis: A study using immunofluorescent techniques. *Am J Pathol* 1967; 51:373–386.

92. Woolf N, Carstairs KC: The survival time of platelets in experimental mural thrombi. *J Pathol* 1969; 97:595–601.

93. Woolf N, Bradley JWP, Crawford T, et al: Experimental mural thrombi in the pig aorta. The early natural history. *Br J Exp Pathol* 1968; 49:257–264.

94. Woolf N, Davies MJ, Bradley JPW: Medical changes following thrombosis in the pig aorta. *J Pathol* 1971; 105:205–209.

95. Woolf N, Crawford T: Fatty streaks in the aortic intima studied by an immuno-histochemical technique. *J Pathol Bacteriol* 1960; 80:405–408.

96. Friedman RJ, Stemerman MB, Wenz B, et al: The effect of thrombocytopenia on experimental atherosclerotic lesion formation in rabbits. *J Clin Invest* 1977; 60:1191–1201.

97. Chen JK, Hoshi H, McKeehan WL: Transforming growth factor type-β specifically stimulates synthesis of proteoglycan in human adult arterial smooth muscle cells. *Proc Natl Acad Sci USA* 1987; 84:5287–5291.

98. Liau G, Chan LM: Regulation of extracellular matrix

RNA levels in cultured smooth muscle cells: Relationship to cellular quiescence. *J Biol Chem* 1989; 264:10315–10320.

99. Clowes AW, Clowes MM, Reidy MA: Kinetics of cellular proliferation after arterial injury. III. Endothelial and smooth muscle growth in chronically denuded vessels. *Lab Invest* 1986; 54:295–303.

100. Clowes AW, Reidy MA, Cloes MM: Mechanisms of stenosis after arterial injury. *Lab Invest* 1983; 49:208–215.

101. Minick CR, Stemerman MB, Insull W Jr: Role of endothelial and hypercholesterolemia in intimal thickening and lipid accumulation. *Am J Pathol* 1979; 95:131–158.

102. Fox PL, DiCorleto PE: Regulation of production of a platelet-derived growth factor–like protein by cultured bovine aortic endothelial cells. *J Cell Physiol* 1984; 121:298–308.

103. Hajjarka KA, Hajjarka DP, Silverstein RL, et al: Tumor necrosis factor–mediated release of platelet-derived growth factor from cultured endothelial cells. *J Exp Med* 1987; 166:235–245.

104. Daniel TO, Gibbs VC, Milfay DF, et al: Agents that increase cAMP accumulation block endothelial c-*sis* induction by thrombin and transforming growth factor-beta. *J Biol Chem* 1987; 262:11893–11896.

105. Daniel TO, Gibbs VC, Milfay DF, et al: Thrombin stimulates c-*sis* gene expression in microvascular endothelial cells. *J Biol Chem* 1986; 261:9579–9582.

106. Gajdusek C, Carbon S, Ross R, et al: Activation of coagulation releases endothelial cell mitogens. *J Cell Biol* 1986; 103:419–428.

107. Harlan JM, Thompson PJ, Ross RR, et al: Alpha-thrombin induces release of platelet-derived growth factor–like molecule(s) by cultured human endothelial cells. *J Cell Biol* 1986; 103:1129–1133.

108. Oka K, Tanaka K: Histochemical demonstration of thrombin using fluorogenic substrate. *Thromb Res* 1980; 19:125–128.

109. Tam WS, Fenton JW, Detwiler TC: Dissociation of thrombin from platelets by hirudin. *J Biol Chem* 1979; 254:8723–8725.

110. Webster MWI, Chesebro JH, Heras M, et al: Acetylcholine infusion identifies regrowth after porcine coronary endothelial denudation. *Circulation* 1989; 80(suppl 2):648.

111. Koo EWY, Gottlieb AI: Endothelial stimulation of intimal cell proliferation in a porcine aortic organ culture. *Am J Pathol* 1989; 134:497–503.

112. Johnson C, et al: Porcine cardiac valvular subendothelial cells in culture: Cell isolation and growth characteristics. *J Mol Cell Cardiol* 1987; 19:1185–1193.

113. Clinton SK, Dinarello CA, Cannon JG, et al: Induction in vivo of interleukin-1 (IL-1) gene expression in rabbit aortic tissue. *Circulation* 1988; 78(suppl 2):65.

114. Powell JS, Clozel JP, Muller RKM, et al: Inhibitors of angiotensin-converting enzyme prevent myointimal proliferation after vascular injury. *Science* 1989; 245:186.

115. Naftilan AJ, Pratt RE, Dzau VJ: Induction of platelet-derived growth factor A-chain and c-*myc* gene expression by angiotensin II in cultured rat vascular smooth muscle cells. *J Clin Invest* 1989; 83:1419.

116. Ross R, Raines EW, Bowen-Pope DF: The biology of platelet-derived growth factor. *Cell* 1986; 46:155.

117. Badimon L, Badimon JJ, Cohen M, et al: Thrombosis formation in stenotic and laminar flow conditions: Effect of an antiplatelet GPIIb/IIIa monoclonal antibody fragment. *Circulation* 1989; 80(suppl 2):422.

118. Badimon L, Badimon J, Lassila R, et al: Thrombin regulation of platelet interaction with damaged vessel wall and isolated collagen type I at arterial flow conditions in a porcine model: Effect of hirudin, heparin, and calcium chelation. *Blood* 1991; 78:423–434.

119. Ferrell M, Fuster V, Gold HK, et al: A dilemma for the 1990's: Choosing the appropriate experimental animal model for the prevention of restenosis. *Circulation* 1992; 85:1630–1631.

Platelet-Derived Growth Factor: Future Directions in the Prevention of Restenosis

W. Michael Kavanaugh, M.D.

This volume reports impressive technological advances in the mechanical treatment of occlusive atherosclerotic disease. Although these new methods significantly expand the therapeutic options we can offer patients, they do not address the underlying process of plaque formation and therefore can benefit patients only after their disease has reached a very advanced stage. Moreover, despite this explosion in technology, restenosis following therapy remains a major impediment to long-term success in a significant proportion of patients. These facts have lead to the increasing involvement of basic scientists in the development of new therapeutic strategies for the treatment of atherosclerosis and related diseases.

Atherogenesis is fundamentally a disorder of cellular proliferation and therefore is likely to involve the local release and action of growth factors. Histologically, this abnormal cell growth is particularly obvious when examining restenotic lesions in native coronary arteries, as well as atherosclerosis in the coronaries of transplanted hearts and in saphenous vein bypass grafts. Considerable evidence supports a "response-to-injury" model for the pathogenesis of these diseases.[1] This hypothesis proposes that vessel wall injury initiates lesion development, whether caused by hemodynamic, metabolic, immune, or mechanical insults. Subsequently, smooth muscle cells in the vessel wall are exposed to growth factors and other biologically active substances released from platelets, immune cells, endothelial cells, and perhaps smooth muscle cells themselves. This local release of growth factors at sites of endothelial injury could account for the migration and proliferation of smooth muscle cells that is so characteristic of these lesions. An

important implication of this model is that inhibition of growth factor action may prevent the proliferative response to injury that is ultimately responsible for vessel occlusion and clinical sequelae.

The experimental support for this theory originally came in large part from studies of cultured cells. Table 46–1 is a partial list of growth factors that have been reported to affect smooth muscle cell proliferation in vitro. This chapter will focus on platelet-derived growth factor (PDGF) as a model for how new approaches to therapy may be based on an understanding of the molecular biology of growth factors. Although PDGF is likely to be a crucial mediator of atherogenesis,[1, 2] it is not likely, however, to be the only growth factor involved. Control of cell growth in the vessel wall in vivo is a complex process involving multiple growth factors and interrelated regulatory mechanisms. For example, PDGF and its receptor have multiple isoforms that can be independently regulated and can be induced by other growth factors. Any growth factor–based therapy will have to take this complexity into account.

Figure 46–1 is a simplified depiction of the response-to-injury hypothesis as it applies to PDGF. PDGF is a basic glycoprotein that is not normally present in plasma but is released from activated platelets. Other cellular components of the vessel wall, including macrophages, endothelial cells, and smooth muscle cells, may also produce PDGF with the appropriate stimuli. Responses to PDGF are mediated by the PDGF receptor, a membrane glycoprotein that is expressed on the surface of mesenchymal cells such as smooth muscle cells in culture. Endothelial cells do not express PDGF receptor in vitro and are therefore unre-

TABLE 46–1.

Growth Factors Reported to Affect Smooth Muscle Cell
Proliferation In Vitro

Platelet-derived growth factor
Fibroblast growth factor
Interleukin-1
Insulin-like growth factor-1
Epidermal growth factor
Transforming growth factor-β
Endothelin

sponsive to PDGF. The PDGF receptor binds PDGF
with high affinity and initiates the intracellular signaling
process that ultimately culminates in cell division.

In vitro, PDGF triggers a variety of events in smooth
muscle cells, including proliferation, chemotaxis, contraction, and elaboration of extracellular matrix. It is
precisely these properties that make PDGF an attractive
candidate for an atherogenic substance. Recent in vivo
studies also support a role for PDGF in vascular cell
proliferation. Expression of both PDGF and its receptor
can be detected in native atherosclerotic plaques and in
experimental models of arterial injury.[3, 4]

BLOCKING THE EFFECTS OF PLATELET-DERIVED GROWTH FACTOR

To develop methods for preventing the effects of
PDGF, several approaches may be taken. First, the production of PDGF or its receptor could be blocked, either at the level of messenger RNA expression (transcription) or at the level of protein synthesis
(translation/secretion). Second, competitive antagonists
could be developed for PDGF, analogous to the way
"β-blockers" are used for the β-adrenergic receptor.
Third, one could interfere with the mechanisms by
which the PDGF receptor signals intracellularly in the
responsive cell. Finally, one could look for natural inhibitors of cellular proliferation. In Dr. Lewis T. Williams' laboratory at the University of California, San
Francisco, we have focused on two of these approaches:
developing competitive antagonists and interfering with
intracellular signaling.[5–9]

Figure 46–2 shows the PDGF receptor to be a single
molecule composed of three domains: an extracellular
domain, which is responsible for binding PDGF; a
transmembrane region that anchors the receptor to the
plasma membrane; and an intracellular domain, which is
responsible for transducing the PDGF stimulus to the
interior of the cell. The intracellular domain contains a
region that confers on the PDGF receptor the ability to
phosphorylate cellular proteins on tyrosines. This ty-

rosine kinase activity is essential for receptor signaling.
In the PDGF receptor, the tyrosine kinase domain is
split into two portions by a sequence known as the kinase insert (Ki) region. The Ki region is probably involved in targeting and regulation of signaling by the
receptor kinase.

The first step in PDGF stimulation of a responsive
cell is binding of PDGF to the receptor. Competitive
antagonists for this step could be developed in several
ways. First, thousands of compounds could be screened
more or less randomly for their ability to interfere with
PDGF binding. Alternatively, compounds might be ra-
tionally designed on the basis of the three-dimensional
structure of PDGF and its receptor. X-ray crystallogra-
phy studies necessary to solve the three-dimensional

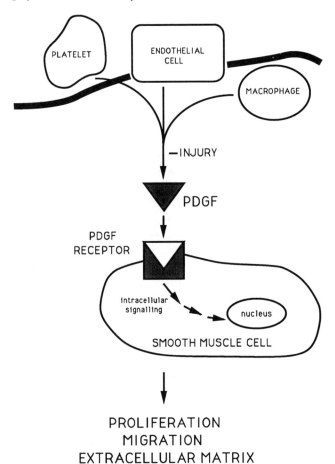

FIG 46–1.

The "response-to-injury" hypothesis of atherogenesis as it
may apply to PDGF. Vascular injury stimulates the release
of PDGF from activated platelets as well as from endothelial
cells and macrophages, which in turn stimulate neighboring
smooth muscle cells to proliferate and migrate to the neointima. The action of PDGF is mediated by the PDGF receptor, which initiates the signaling cascade to the nucleus of
the smooth muscle cell.

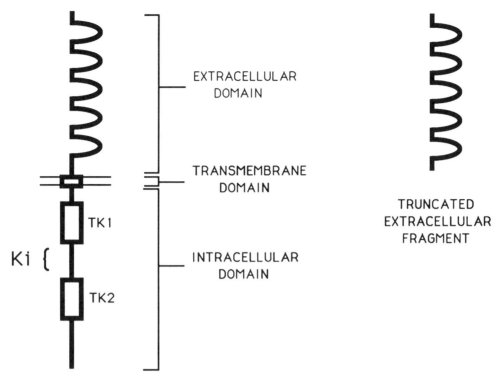

FIG 46–2.
The PDGF receptor. The extracellular domain binds PDGF, the transmembrane domain anchors the receptor to the membrane, and the intracellular domain contains the tyrosine kinase, which is split into two portions *(TK1* and *TK2)* by the kinase insert *(Ki)* sequence. The receptor fragment used as a PDGF antagonist (see the text) is depicted on the *right.*

structures are currently under way. This laboratory has also taken another approach. Competitive antagonists may work either by binding the receptor on the cell surface or by binding PDGF in the surrounding media. Dr. Roxanne Duan cloned and expressed a soluble fragment of the PDGF receptor that represents only the extracellular domain and lacks the transmembrane and intracellular portions (Fig 46–2).[7] This extracellular receptor fragment can be expressed and purified in large quantities and retains its ability to bind PDGF with high affinity. However, because it lacks a membrane anchor or an intracellular region, this fragment would not be expected to be able to transduce PDGF signals. When added to cell cultures, this fragment can block subsequent PDGF stimulation of mitogenesis, presumably by binding and sequestering all the available PDGF in the media. Because a portion of the receptor itself is used as an antagonist, inhibition of proliferation is specific for PDGF.

As mentioned, another way of blocking PDGF action is to interfere with signaling by the receptor. Following binding of PDGF, the PDGF receptor becomes activated by a series of processes that include dimerization and autophosphorylation (Fig 46–3).[5,6] Dimerization

occurs when receptor molecules associate in pairs. The tyrosine kinase of each receptor in the pair may then phosphorylate its partner on its intracellular portion, a process called autophosphorylation. We have taken advantage of the dependence of signaling on dimerization and autophosphorylation to develop another method for blocking PDGF effects. Dr. Hikaru Ueno has used a mutant PDGF receptor that contains normal extracellular and transmembrane domains but has an intracellular domain that lacks the essential tyrosine kinase. If a cell that expresses the normal PDGF receptor is made to express this mutant receptor as well, then when stimulated with PDGF, three types of dimers are expected to form (Fig 46–3): a homodimer containing two normal receptors, a homodimer containing two mutant receptors; and a heterodimer containing one mutant and one normal receptor. The normal dimer would signal normally, while the dimers containing one or more mutant receptors would be unable to autophosphorylate and thus would be incapable of transducing PDGF signals. When the mutant receptor is expressed in excess, most of the normal receptors will be tied up with a mutant receptor in inactive, heterodimeric complexes. In this way, a cell that contains the PDGF receptor and is normally re-

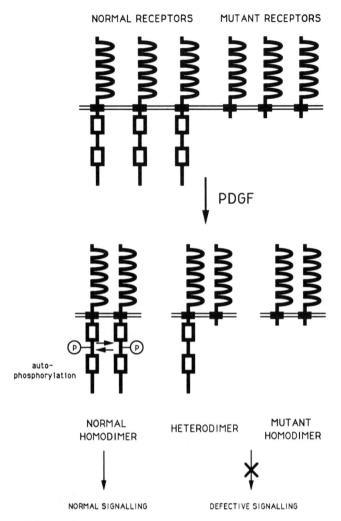

NORMAL RECEPTORS   MUTANT RECEPTORS

PDGF

auto-
phosphorylation

NORMAL
HOMODIMER   HETERODIMER   MUTANT
HOMODIMER

NORMAL SIGNALLING   DEFECTIVE SIGNALLING

FIG 46–3.
Dominant negative mutants of the PDGF receptor. When the normal receptor and a mutant receptor are expressed in the same cell, PDGF stimulation leads to the formation of three types of receptor dimers (see the text). In the normal homodimer, each receptor in the pair is capable of phosphorylating its partner (depicted with *arrows*). The other dimeric forms would be defective in autophosphorylation and signaling.

sponsive to PDGF can be made unresponsive to PDGF by introducing an excess of mutant receptors. Dr. Ueno has successfully used this "dominant negative mutant" approach to block PDGF signaling in amphibian and mammalian cell systems.[8]

Following PDGF binding, receptor dimerization and autophosphorylation, and a conformational change in the receptor, the receptor is said to be "activated." In this activated state, the receptor physically associates with and phosphorylates several cytoplasmic molecules involved in signal transduction (Fig 46–4).[5, 6] These cy-

toplasmic molecules, called second messengers, are presumably activated as a result of their interaction with the receptor and then continue the signaling cascade. One of these proteins is an enzyme called phosphatidylinositol-3-kinase, or PI3 kinase. PI3 kinase phosphorylates a phospholipid in the membrane; the precise role of this reaction in signaling is unknown. However, this enzyme appears to be necessary for proper signaling by several growth factor receptors.

Upon PDGF stimulation, PI3 kinase binds to the PDGF receptor at a specific sequence in the Ki region of the intracellular domain (Fig 46–4). We reasoned that blocking PI3 kinase binding to the PDGF receptor may also block the ability of the receptor to promote cell proliferation when activated by PDGF. Drs. Jaime Escobedo and David Kaplan in Dr. Williams' laboratory synthesized small peptides whose amino acid sequence corresponded to the region of the PDGF receptor involved in PI3 kinase binding (see Fig 46–4).[9] These peptides blocked the ability of the receptor to associate with PI3 kinase in vitro, presumably by competing for the available enzyme. Currently we are studying whether these peptides can block PI3 kinase/receptor interactions inside a cell and, if so, whether PDGF-stimulated proliferation is also blocked, as might be expected.

FUTURE STUDIES

Developing methods for interfering with growth factor action may lead to new approaches to the prevention of restenosis. First, PDGF effects in cell culture can be blocked by using an extracellular fragment of the PDGF receptor as a competitive antagonist. Future studies with this receptor fragment include its use in an animal model of vascular injury. Such studies may be extremely valuable in identifying the importance of PDGF in the vascular response to injury, as well as in characterizing the pharmacology of using this protein as a drug. Because this receptor fragment is a large and complicated molecule, further structure/function studies will attempt to identify simpler, active versions that may be easier to use in a clinical setting. Second, a mutant PDGF receptor can be used to block the function of the normal receptor in a cell. This dominant negative mutant approach will be most useful in studies of the role of PDGF in development in transgenic animals, where receptor gene expression can be manipulated. Finally, associations between the PDGF receptor and cytoplasmic second-messenger molecules can be disrupted in vitro by using small synthetic peptides derived from the receptor. If this approach proves to be effective in vivo,

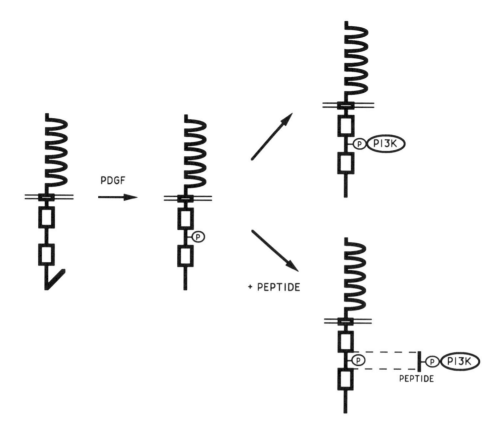

FIG 46–4.
Blocking PI3 kinase binding to the PDGF receptor with peptides. Upon PDGF stimulation, the receptor becomes activated by dimerization (not shown), autophosphorylation, and a conformational change in the receptor *(middle figure)*. In this activated state, the receptor binds cytoplasmic signaling molecules, one of which is PI3 kinase *(PI3K, upper right)*. PI3 kinase binding involves the Ki region of the receptor and one or more of the autophosphorylated tyrosine residues (denoted by a *"P"*). A synthetic peptide corresponding to this region can prevent PI3 kinase association with the receptor, probably by competing with the receptor for the available enzyme *(lower right)*.

the challenge will then be to develop stable versions of these molecules that can gain access to the cytoplasm of vascular smooth muscle cells in order to block PDGF receptor signaling.

It should be emphasized that these are only a few of the possible approaches to develop growth factor–based therapy and that significant obstacles remain. For example, it is unknown which of the isoforms of PDGF are more important in proliferative vascular disease. The extracellular receptor fragment described here blocks only one isoform of PDGF, and similar molecules effective for other isoforms of PDGF may have to be developed. Moreover, as mentioned above, attention to the involvement of multiple growth factors and complex regulatory mechanisms may influence the ultimate success of this therapeutic strategy. Finally, future studies will have to address the obvious issues of methods of drug delivery, the pharmacodynamics and kinetics of these agents, their immunogenicity, side effects, the timing and duration of therapy, etc. However, given the

extraordinary power and pace of research in molecular biology today, we can expect novel therapies based on growth factor biology to be available in the very near future.

Acknowledgment

I am indebted to Dr. Lewis T. Williams, to Drs. Roxanne Duan, Hikaru Ueno, Jaime Escobedo, and David Kaplan, and to Michael Pazin and Heather Colbert, whose work at the Howard Hughes Medical Institute and the University of California, San Francisco is described in this chapter. This manuscript was supported by National Institutes of Health grant 1 K11 HL02410-01.

REFERENCES

1. Ross R: The pathogenesis of atherosclerosis — An update. *N Engl J Med* 1986; 314:488–500.

2. Ross R, Bowen-Pope DF, Raines EW: Platelet-derived growth factor and its role in health and disease. *Trans R Soc Lond* 1990; 327:155–69.

3. Wilcox JN, Smith KM, Williams LT, et al: Platelet-derived growth factor mRNA detection in human atherosclerotic plaques by *in situ* hybridization. *J Clin Invest* 1988; 82:1134–1143.

4. Majesky MW, Reidy MA, Bowen-Pope DF, et al: PDGF ligand and receptor gene expression during repair of arterial injury. *J Cell Biol* 1990; 111:2149–2158.

5. Williams LT: Signal transduction by the platelet-derived growth factor receptor. *Science* 1989; 243:1564–1570.

6. Williams LT: Signal transduction by the platelet-derived growth factor receptor involves association of the receptor with cytoplasmic molecules. *Clin Res* 1989; 37:564–568.

7. Duan D-SR, Pazin MJ, Fretto LJ, et al: A functional soluble extracellular region of the platelet-derived growth factor (PDGF) β-receptor antagonizes PDGF-stimulated responses. *J Biol Chem* 1991; 266:413–418.

8. Ueno H, Colbert H, Escobedo JA, et al: Inhibition of PDGF Beta Receptor Signal Transduction by Coexpression of a Truncated Receptor. *Science* 1991; 252:844–847.

9. Escobedo JA, Kaplan DR, Kavanaugh WM, et al: A phosphatidylinositol-3 kinase binds to platelet-derived growth factor receptors through a specific receptor sequence containing phosphotyrosine. *Mol Cell Biol* 1991; 11:1125–1132.

Cell Biology of Restenosis: Role of Angiotensin II in Neointimal Cell Proliferation

Bradford C. Berk, M.D., Ph.D.

RESPONSE OF THE VASCULAR SMOOTH MUSCLE CELL TO INJURY

Temporal Pattern of Vascular Smooth Muscle Cell Response

In the normal coronary artery vascular smooth muscle cells (VSMC) exist in a growth-arrested, quiescent state. In this state, the VSMC express a characteristic phenotype oriented toward contraction and maintenance of vessel tone. However, this cell type is extremely plastic in its growth potential; it has the ability to migrate, proliferate, and/or undergo hypertrophy, depending on the situation. As a general feature of the cardiovascular system, VSMC hypertrophy in response to an increase in vascular load. This is a normal adaptive response that, for example, maintains constant wall stress in the presence of increased pressure. Hypertrophy is also adaptive in the sense that it is reversible. In contrast, VSMC proliferation is necessary for wound repair, yet it is maladaptive in that there is no regression of cell number after proliferation. Thus, the consequence of repeated proliferative responses is plaque formation and a resultant increase in cell mass that may obstruct the vessel. In disease states such as coronary atherosclerosis, the VSMC are frequently in this phenotypically modulated growth-activated mode. Further injury to the vessel, as occurs during angioplasty, triggers a response in cells that are already primed to proliferate. In particular, alterations in VSMC growth state may render the cells growth responsive to agonists that are not normally mitogenic, such as angiotensin II, serotonin, and α-thrombin.

The triggering of VSMC proliferation by balloon inflation involves several factors. The stretch imposed on the vessel wall by balloon inflation has been shown to increase calcium entry, activate growth factor gene expression, and stimulate VSMC growth and proliferation in vitro.[1, 2] It is also likely that there is immediate cell death (of both VSMC and endothelial cells) with release of growth factors and proteases. There is an almost immediate binding of inflammatory cells. VSMC, endothelial cells, and inflammatory cells secrete proteases that dissolve the extracellular matrix and allow smooth muscle cell migration.[3] Several cell types in the injured artery release factors that are chemotactic for smooth muscle cells, including serotonin, platelet-derived growth factor (PDGF), fibroblast growth factor (FGF), and a variety of prostaglandins and leukotrienes.[4] The initial insult triggers the migration of smooth muscle cells, particularly those in the proliferative mode, that already express receptors for these chemotactic factors. Recent data suggest that PDGF is the dominant chemotactic factor[5] while FGF may be the dominant mitogenic factor.[6]

When VSMC migrate from the media into the intima, they undergo a process known as phenotypic modulation.[7, 8] As a result, cells are converted from a contractile phenotype (characterized by expression of a large number of myosin fibers) to a synthetic phenotype (characterized by the synthesis of matrix proteins and growth factors). The process of phenotypic modulation during establishment of tissue culture has been well studied, and it is clear that as a part of the process, VSMC-specific contractile proteins such as α_1-actin are no longer expressed and that the ratio of proteins such as vimentin to desmin is significantly altered.[9] Thus, phenotypic modulation is a consequence of a genetic program that results in a cell committed to proliferation. Activation of this "growth" program is critical to the formation of restenotic plaque because proliferation and matrix deposition by these phenotypically modulated cells are critical factors in the subsequent hemodynamic dysfunction of the vessel.

Once VSMC have migrated and undergone phenotypic modulation in the neointima, they begin to proliferate. It has been shown by Clowes et al.[10] that approximately three rounds of division occur in the rat carotid following balloon injury. This proliferative phase involves both exogenous and endogenous growth factors. Exogenous factors include platelet-derived factors (PDGF and epidermal growth factor [EGF]), endothelial-derived factors (PDGF and FGF), matrix-derived factors (FGF), and inflammatory cell–derived factors (including macrophage-derived growth factor).[11, 12] In human coronary arteries it is unclear at what time maximal proliferation occurs and how long the proliferative phase lasts. In the rat model, it begins within 3 to 4 days following injury and reaches a maximum at approximately 14 days.[10, 13] Thereafter, there is a decrease in the rate of DNA synthesis as measured by ^{3}H-thymidine incorporation.

Finally, the VSMC enter a quiescent phase in which the proliferative rate decreases dramatically. The mechanisms responsible for initiating and maintaining this quiescent state are unclear but presumably include reestablishment of a normal endothelial layer that prevents platelet deposition and inhibits VSMC growth. It is also likely that the VSMC themselves cease to produce autocrine growth stimuli.

Features of Vascular Smooth Muscle Cell Growth Critical to Restenosis and Therapy

Targeting therapy to prevent restenosis will clearly require multiple approaches. An effort to inhibit VSMC proliferation would be an excellent approach since this proliferation reoccludes the blood vessel. Furthermore, VSMC proliferation involves a specialized cell that is actively proliferating, and it occurs over a sufficiently long time period to allow for successful pharmacologic therapy. Several features of this growth response have been established that might guide therapy. First, it is clear that many of the same events occur in the smooth muscle cell that are part of the initial development of the blood vessel; thus, migration, proliferation, and formation of matrix are all normal developmental responses as well as normal responses to injury. It is also

clear that the nature of the VSMC response is determined by the proteins necessary for growth. Thus, expression of growth factor receptors such as the PDGF receptor enables the smooth muscle cell to respond to PDGF. In addition, VSMC are able to establish an autocrine growth process by synthesis of their own PDGF. Of interest, it appears that the dominant PDGF receptor expressed in VSMC is for the PDGF B-chain, while the dominant growth factor synthesized endogenously is the PDGF A-chain.[8, 14] However, it seems probable that the A-chain has effects on other cell types or has effects on other functions in smooth muscle cells, such as matrix formation.

The neighboring cells in the matrix play an important, but as yet poorly defined, role in the VSMC proliferative response. For example, Hedin et al.[15] have shown that plating primary cultures of VSMC onto fibronectin or the adhesion molecule binding sequence RGDS peptide accelerates the transition from a contractile to a synthetic phenotype. It seems, then, that the nature of the extracellular matrix is critical to the state of VSMC growth. Endothelial cells maintain a balance between VSMC growth stimulation and growth inhibition. Endothelial cell substances such as heparin and endothelial-derived relaxing factor appear to inhibit growth,[6, 16] while endothelial-derived factors such as endothelin, PDGF, and FGF appear to promote growth. Transforming growth factor β (TGF-β) is a multifunctional growth factor made by a variety of cell types in the vessel.[17, 18] At low concentrations TGF-β has been shown to stimulate the proliferation of VSMC, while at high concentrations it inhibits their growth.[19]

It is clear that the smooth muscle cell itself maintains a complex intracellular balance between growth and quiescence. VSMC can synthesize autocrine growth factors, such as PDGF A-chain, but also can synthesize growth inhibitors. For example, the proliferative response to angiotensin II of VSMC from the spontaneously hypertensive rat aorta is mediated by secretion of PDGF A-chain.[20] Conversely, VSMC from Sprague-Dawley rats exhibit a hypertrophic response to angiotensin II.[21, 22] However, anti–TGF-β antibody converts this to a proliferative response.[23] Thus, a variety of matrix-cell, cell-cell, and intracellular interactions determine the nature of the VSMC growth response.

THE RENIN-ANGIOTENSIN SYSTEM WITHIN THE VESSEL

There is increasing evidence that the renin-angiotensin system may act as an in vivo paracrine system for vessel wall growth.[21, 22] Dzau and Gibbons[24] suggested that activation of the renin-angiotensin system locally in the vascular wall could be a mechanism by which certain forms of hypertension develop. These investigators and others have shown that many components of the renin-angiotensin system are present in vessels. While it appears that renin may be taken up into the vessel wall from the plasma, the mRNAs for angiotensinogen are present in the periaortic fibroblast cells, as well as in brown fat cells.[25, 26] Recent data suggest that both angiotensinogen and angiotensin converting enzyme (ACE) may also be expressed in neointimal cells.[27] Although the nature of these cells is unclear they appear to be phenotypically modulated VSMC. Thus, the vessel wall itself has the capacity to synthesize angiotensin II locally. The localization and regulation of the other components of the renin-angiotensin system, such as the angiotensin II receptor, remain to be elucidated.

Several provocative studies suggest that angiotensin II may play an important role in neointimal proliferation. In a recent report, Powell and coworkers[28] showed that ACE inhibition in the rat was able to block the formation of neointima following balloon injury. These investigators demonstrated that this was characteristic of several ACE inhibitors. Daemen et al.[29] found that angiotensin II infusion in a rat balloon injury model increased DNA synthesis in both aortic and carotid VSMC. Interestingly, the proliferative effect of angiotensin II appeared to depend on the pre-existing growth status of the VSMC. Neointimal VSMC showed a labeling frequency of 20% over 2 weeks, while there was a labeling frequency of only 5% in the normal vessel wall of a similar group of animals treated with angiotensin II. This phenomenon may be species specific because unpublished reports suggest that ACE inhibitors are much less effective in primate models of arterial injury than in the rodent model. All of these studies suggest that a complex relationship among local generation of angiotensin II, expression of receptors for angiotensin II, and the growth state of the VSMC in the wall combines to yield the proliferative response. The direct growth effects of angiotensin II in vivo remain unclear; indirect effects such as increased blood pressure, release of other neurohumoral mediators, and stimulation of the adrenergic nervous system may be important.

ROLE OF ANGIOTENSIN II AS A VASCULAR SMOOTH MUSCLE CELL GROWTH FACTOR

There is strong evidence to support a role for angiotensin II in hypertrophy of VSMC. Both my laboratory and the laboratory of Owens[21, 22] have shown that, in vitro, angiotensin II stimulates an increase in VSMC protein synthesis and protein content, without a change in cell number. Similarly, in the Goldblatt two-kidney one-clip model of hypertension, angiotensin II plays an important role in the increased medial mass due to VSMC hypertrophy.[30] Although there is no change in cell number in the Goldblatt model, there is an increase in DNA content in the deoxycorticosterone acetate hypertensive model, or in the spontaneously hypertensive rat.[31] This is explained by the appearance of polyploid VSMC in the thoracic aorta of these animals. It should be noted that in the aortic coarctation model, VSMC DNA synthesis occurs without polyploidy. Thus it appears that in a variety of models, angiotensin II can clearly cause hypertrophy. It may also cause hyperplasia under the right circumstances.

The findings of Daemen et al.[29] and Powell et al.[28] suggest that, in vivo, angiotensin II can play an important role in smooth muscle proliferation. In both cases, however, the effects of angiotensin II appear to be dependent on a pre-existing injury state. This suggests that alterations in VSMC phenotype underlie the effect of angiotensin II on VSMC growth. Alternatively, there may be alterations in the local renin-angiotensin system following injury that make angiotensin II a mitogen. Among the attractive possibilities are synergism between angiotensin II and factors present during injury, coupling of angiotensin II receptors to mitogenic signal pathways, increased expression of angiotensin II receptors in the neointimal cells, and expression of a different angiotensin II receptor.

The intracellular signaling events stimulated by angiotensin II may provide insights into its role in restenosis. Several laboratories have defined the early events stimulated by angiotensin II (for a review see Griendling et al.[32]). Angiotensin II binds to a high-affinity receptor that is present at concentrations between 30 and 350 fmol/mg protein on VSMC. Following binding to its receptor, phospholipase C is activated via a G protein–coupled cellular event. Activation of phospholipase C results in hydrolysis of the polyphosphoinositides to generate inositol phosphates and diacylglycerol. Inositol trisphosphate then stimulates the release of calcium from sarcoplasmic reticulum. Release of calcium activates a series of enzyme cascades involving calcium/calmodulin-dependent kinases with activation of the myosin light-chain kinase and contractile events. This series of events activates protein kinase C and exerts synergistic effects on a variety of transport functions. Protein kinase C is synergistically activated by calcium and diacylglycerol, and phosphorylates a variety of intracellular factors. Several of these have been shown to be involved in growth, including the Na^+/H^+ exchanger[33] and a variety of proto-oncogenes, including c-*fos* and c-*myc*. Taubman et al.[34] showed that angiotensin II could rapidly stimulate c-*fos* expression in cultured VSMC. Induction of c-*fos* was dependent upon protein kinase C. Thus, angiotensin II stimulates many of the early gene events involved in VSMC growth.

It has also become clear that there may be autocrine growth mechanisms induced by angiotensin II. Naftilan et al.[35] showed that angiotensin II stimulated expression of the PDGF A-chain mRNA in cultured VSMC and that PDGF A-chain was secreted by VSMC into the medium. The exact nature of the mitogenic events stimulated by the PDGF A-chain are unclear. In culture, the mitogenic effects of interleukin-1 on VSMC have been shown to be due to PDGF A-chain.[36] Yet, in the neointima, it appears that the primary receptor expressed is the PDGF B-chain receptor rather than the PDGF A-chain receptor.[14] It is certainly possible, however, that the PDGF A-chain may play an important role in VSMC proliferation via its effects on other cell types. Gibbons[23] has shown that TGF-β mRNA is induced by stimulation with angiotensin II. TGF-β has recently been shown by Battegay et al.[19] to have potent effects on mesenchymal cell growth. At low concentrations (0.1 to 1 ng/mL), TGF-β promotes VSMC growth, while at higher concentrations it inhibits this growth. The levels of TGF-β present in the vessel wall are unknown at this time. Thus, stimulation of autocrine growth mechanisms such as PDGF and TGF-β may account for the growth-promoting effects of angiotensin II.

The fact that increases in VSMC DNA synthesis occur in models of hypertension with differing etiologies suggests that the effect of angiotensin II may be the result of a common denominator such as hypertension rather than a direct effect of angiotensin II itself. Among the indirect effects of angiotensin II are those in the sympathetic nervous system. Faber and Brody[37] showed that almost 50% of the rise in blood pressure in angiotensin II–dependent hypertension was mediated by sympathetic activity. Thus, α-adrenergic stimulation may play an important role in smooth muscle cell growth. In fact, it has been shown by Majesky et al.[38] that α_1-adrenergic receptor stimulation increases PDGF A-chain mRNA expression in vivo. It is also possible that angiotensin II, by stimulating large increases in intracellular calcium, may synergize with mitogens that fail to do this and thereby activate the growth program. For example, FGF does not increase calcium levels in cultured VSMC, and the presence of angiotensin II might be synergistic with this factor to stimulate growth.

POTENTIAL THERAPEUTIC EFFORTS TO INHIBIT THE RENIN-ANGIOTENSIN SYSTEM

Angiotensin Converting Enzyme Inhibitors

The role of the local angiotensin system in the vascular response to balloon injury was investigated by Powell and coworkers,[28] who administered the angiotensin converting enzyme cilazapril to normotensive rats in which the carotid artery had been injured by balloon catheterization. As discussed above, balloon injury causes a migration of the VSMC from the media into the intima, synthesis of extracellular matrix with marked thickening of the intima, and an increase of approximately 100% in the ratio of neointima to media. Administration of cilazapril at 10 mg/kg of body weight per day for 14 days after balloon injury caused a greater than 50% reduction in the neointimal area. This appears to be a general feature of other ACE antagonists, including captopril.[28] Other agents such as verapamil (100 mg/kg/day) had no effect on neointimal proliferation in normotensive rats. From the findings of Powell et al. it appears likely that decreased angiotensin II formation is the mechanism for inhibition of neointimal proliferation by the converting enzyme inhibitors. Although converting enzyme inhibitors also block the enzymes that metabolize bradykinin, it seems unlikely that this is the mechanism for suppression of neointimal proliferation. In general, bradykinin appears to have a role in promoting proliferation, and inhibiting its conversion would have the opposite effect from that observed. Clinical trials of these angiotensin antagonists will be important. It should be noted that the effort to document similar inhibition of neointimal proliferation in primate and porcine models has been unsuccessful. This suggests that the interactions among platelets, endothelium, and VSMC are quite different in different species and that the true clinical value of a particular therapeutic approach can only be determined in humans and closely related primates.

ANGIOTENSIN II PEPTIDE ANTAGONISTS

For several years multiple angiotensin II receptor subtypes have been postulated from functional responses to angiotensin II, especially in the kidney and liver. Recently, peptide antagonists that discriminate between two angiotensin II receptor classes have been prepared (for a review see Timmermans et al.[39]). Dup 753 specifically blocks the AT_1 receptor, which is highly expressed in VSMC and the adrenal cortex. This receptor

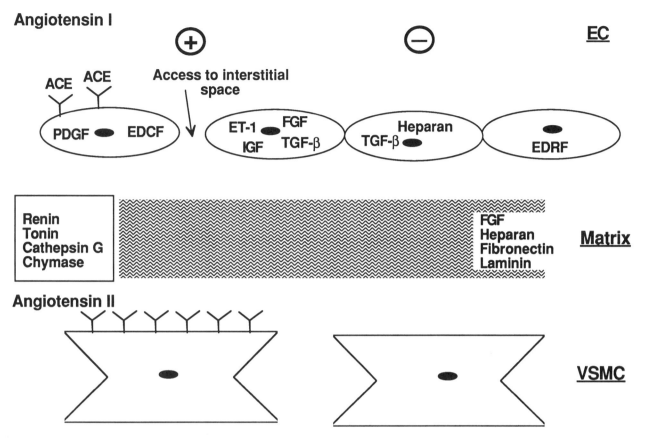

FIG 47–1.
Endothelial cell–vascular smooth muscle cell interactions during injury: role of angiotensin II. Depicted diagrammatically are the positive and negative growth influences present in the endothelium that may be altered during vascular injury. Among growth-promoting events are release or secretion of mitogens such as endothelin *(ET-1)*, FGF, PDGF, insulin-like growth factor *(IGF)*, and endothelial-derived constricting factors *(EDCF)*. Increased access to the interstitial space may allow lipoproteins and other plasma-derived materials to come in contact with VSMC. Emphasis is placed on increased expression of angiotensin converting enzyme *(ACE)* in the endothelial cells and the neointima to generate increased angiotensin II. There may also be metabolism of angiotensinogen and angiotensin I by a variety of endothelial cells, VSMC, and inflammatory cell-derived enzymes such as renin, tonin, cathepsin G, and chymase, Conversely, growth-inhibitory substances may include heparan and endothelial-derived relaxing factor (EDRF). TGF-β may have both positive and negative growth effects. Finally there may be liberation of growth-promoting and -inhibitory substances present in the extracellular matrix.

type is coupled to phospholipase C and appears to be responsible for the VSMC growth effects of angiotensin II (unpublished results). PD 123177 as well as EXP 655 and CGP 42112A selectively block the AT_2 receptor, which is highly expressed in the adrenal medulla, uterus, and brain. The use of these selective antagonists will allow more specific blockade of angiotensin II than the ACE inhibitors and may provide a new class of therapeutic agents for the treatment of restenosis.

In summary, the process of restenosis following angioplasty should be viewed in the context of the cell biology of the vessel wall response to injury. As shown in Figure 47–1, many growth-promoting events are necessary for satisfactory vessel repair and remodeling. The goal of future therapy will be to allow these repair mechanisms to occur while simultaneously preventing sustained VSMC proliferation and matrix accumulation. Our ever-increasing knowledge of the cellular events that occur during arterial injury offers hope that we will succeed in this effort.

REFERENCES

1. Laher I, Bevan JA: Stretch of vascular smooth muscle activates tone and $^{45}Ca^{2+}$ influx. *J Hypertens* 1989; 7:S17–S20.
2. Leung DYM, Glagov S, Mathews MB: Cyclic stretching stimulates synthesis of matrix components by ar-

terial smooth muscle cells in vitro. *Science* 1976; 191:475–477.

3. Clowes AW, Clowes MM, Au YPT, et al: Smooth muscle cells express urokinase during mitogenesis and tissue-type plasminogen activator during migration in injured rat carotid artery. *Circ Res* 1990; 67:61–67.

4. Bell L, Madri JA: Effect of platelet factors on migration of cultured bovine aortic endothelial and smooth muscle cells. *Circ Res* 1989; 65:1057–1065.

5. Fingerle J, Johnson R, Clowes AW, et al: Role of platelets in smooth muscle cell proliferation and migration after vascular injury in rat carotid artery. *Proc Natl Acad Sci USA* 1989; 86:8412–8416.

6. Linder V, Majack RA, Reidy MA: Basic fibroblast growth factor stimulates endothelial regrowth and proliferation in denuded arteries. *J Clin Invest* 1990; 85:2004–2008.

7. Chamley-Campbell J, Campbell R: What controls smooth muscle phenotype? *Atherosclerosis* 1981; 40:347–357.

8. Sjolund M, Hedin U, Sejersen T, et al: Arterial smooth muscle cells express platelet-derived growth factor (PDGF) A chain mRNA, secrete a PDGF-like mitogen, and bind exogenous PDGF in a phenotype- and growth state–dependent manner. *J Cell Biol* 1988; 106:403–413.

9. Blank RS, Owens GK: Platelet-derived growth factor regulates actin isoform expression and growth state in cultured rat aortic smooth muscle cells. *J Cell Physiol* 1990; 142:635–642.

10. Clowes AW, Reidy MA, Clowes MM: Kinetics of cellular proliferation after arterial injury: I. Smooth muscle growth in the absence of endothelium. *Lab Invest* 1983; 49:327–333.

11. Liebovich SJ, Ross RA: Macrophage-dependent factor that stimulates the proliferation of fibroblasts in vitro. *Am J Pathol* 1976; 84:501–513.

12. Libby PS, Warner JC, Friedman GB: Interleukin-1: A mitogen for human vascular smooth muscle cells that induces the release of growth-inhibitory prostanoids. *J Clin Invest* 1988; 81:487–498.

13. Clowes AW, Clowes HM, Reidy MA: Kinetics of cellular proliferation after arterial injury. III. Endothelial and smooth muscle growth in chronically denuded vessels. *Lab Invest* 1986; 54:295–303.

14. Wilcox JN, Smith KM, Williams LT, et al: Platelet-derived growth factor mRNA detection in human atherosclerotic plaques by in situ hybridization. *J Clin Invest* 1988; 82:1134–1143.

15. Hedin U, Bottger BA, Forsberg E, et al: Diverse effects of fibronectin and laminin on phenotypic properties of cultured arterial smooth muscle cells. *J Cell Biol* 1988; 107:307–319.

16. Campbell JH, Campbell GR: Endothelial cell influences on vascular smooth muscle phenotype. *Annu Rev Physiol* 1986; 48:295–306.

17. Antonelli-Orlidge A, Saunders KB, Smith S, et al: An activated form of transforming growth factor-beta is produced by co-cultures of endothelial cells and pericytes. *Proc Natl Acad Sci USA* 1989; 516:4544–4568.

18. Assoian RK, Sporn MB. Type β transforming growth factor in human platelets: Release during platelet degranulation and action on vascular smooth muscle cells. *J Cell Biol* 1986; 102:1217–1223.

19. Battegay EJ, Raines EW, Seifert RA, et al: TGF-β induces bimodal proliferation of connective tissue cells via complex control of an autocrine PDGF loop. *Cell* 1990; 63:515–524.

20. Scott-Burden T, Resink TJ, Baur U, et al: Epidermal growth factor responsiveness in smooth muscle cells from hypertensive and normotensive rats. *Hypertension* 1989; 13:295–304.

21. Berk BC, Vekshtein V, Gordon HM, et al: Angiotensin II–stimulated protein synthesis in cultured vascular smooth muscle cells. *Hypertension* 1989; 13:305–314.

22. Geisterfer A, Peach MJ, Owens GK: Angiotensin II induces hypertrophy, not hyperplasia of cultured rat aortic smooth muscle cells. *Circ Res* 1988; 62:749–756.

23. Gibbons GH, Pratt RE, Dzau VJ: Transforming growth factor-beta (TGF-β) expression modulates the bifunctional growth response of vascular smooth muscle cell (VSMC) to angiotensin II (AII) (abstract). *Clin Res* 1990; 38:287.

24. Dzau VJ, Gibbons GH: Autocrine-paracrine mechanisms of vascular myocytes in systemic hypertension. *Am J Cardiol* 1987; 60:I99–I103.

25. Campbell DJ, Habener J: Cellular localization of angiotensinogen gene expression in brown adipose tissue and mesentery: Quantification of messenger ribonucleic acid abundance using hybridization in situ. *Endocrinology* 1987; 121:1616–1626.

26. Cassis LA, Lynch KR, Peach MJ: Localization of angiotensinogen messenger RNA in rat aorta. *Circ Res* 1988; 62:1259–1262.

27. Rakugi H, Jacob HJ, Ingelfinger JR, et al: Evidence for local renin-angiotensin activation in the neointima after vascular injury (abstract): *Clin Res* 1991; 39:152.

28. Powell JS, Clozel J-P, Muller RKM, et al: Inhibitors of angiotensin-converting enzyme prevent myointimal proliferation after vascular injury. *Science* 1989; 245:186–188.

29. Daemen MJAP, Lombardi DM, Bosman FT, et al: Angiotensin-II induces smooth muscle cell proliferation in the normal and injured rat arterial wall. *Circ Res* 1991; 68:450–456.

30. Owens GK, Schwartz S: Vascular smooth muscle cell hypertrophy and hyperploidy in the Goldblatt hypertensive rat. *Circ Res* 1983; 53:491–501.

31. Owens GK: Control of hypertrophic versus hyperplastic growth of vascular smooth muscle. *Am J Physiol* 1989; 257:H1755–H1765.

32. Griendling KK, Berk BC, Ganz P, et al: Angiotensin II stimulation of vascular smooth muscle phosphoinositide metabolism. State of the art lecture. *Hypertension* 1987; 9(suppl 3):181–185.

33. Berk BC, Aronow MS, Brock TA, et al: Angiotensin II–stimulated Na$^+$/H$^+$ exchange in cultured vascular smooth muscle cells: Evidence for protein kinase C dependent and independent pathways. *J Biol Chem* 1987; 262:5057–5064.

34. Taubman MB, Berk BC, Izumo S, et al: Angiotensin II induction of c-*fos* mRNA in aortic smooth muscle involves Ca^{2+} mobilization and protein kinase C activation. *J Biol Chem* 1989; 264:526–530.

35. Naftilan A, Pratt R, Dzau V: Induction of c-*fos*, c-*myc* and PDGF A-chain gene expressions by angiotensin II in cultured vascular smooth muscle cells. *J Clin Invest* 1989; 83:1419–1424.

36. Raines EW, Dower SK, Ross R: Interleukin-1 mitogenic activity for fibroblasts and smooth muscle cells is due to PDGF-AA. *Science* 1989; 243:393–396.

37. Faber JE, Brody MJ: Central nervous system action of angiotensin during onset of renal hypertension in awake rats. *Am J Physiol* 1984; 247:H349–H360.

38. Majesky MW, Daemen MJAP, Schwartz SM: α₁-Adrenergic stimulation of platelet-derived growth factor A-chain gene expression in rat aorta. *J Biol Chem* 1990; 265:1082–1088.

39. Timmermans PBMWM, Wong PC, Chiu AT, et al: Nonpeptide angiotensin-II receptor antagonists. *Trends Pharmacol Sci* 1991; 12:55–62.

Inhibitors of Vascular Smooth Muscle Cell Proliferation as Therapy for Restenosis Following Percutaneous Transluminal Coronary Angioplasty: Current Agents and Approaches

Jai Pal Singh, Ph.D.

Keith L. March, M.D.

Proliferation of smooth muscle cells is an intrinsic response to vascular injury as a part of the tissue repair process. Studies in experimental animals have shown that injury to the vessel wall invariably results in a rapid induction of smooth muscle cell proliferation.[1–10] Under normal conditions, cell proliferation declines over time and reaches the basal level within weeks after injury.[3, 4, 8, 9] As a part of the repair program, smooth muscle cell proliferation probably occurs in most patients undergoing reperfusion of occluded arteries by percutaneous transluminal coronary angioplasty (PTCA). However, in a significant number of patients, smooth muscle cell proliferation seems to occur overtly and for a prolonged period. Deposition of smooth muscle cells and newly formed fibrous matrix at the luminal side of the arterial wall along with the residual atheromatous plaque greatly reduces vessel luminal diameter within 3 to 6 months following PTCA. At the present time the occurrence of this delayed restenosis represents a major complication following successful PTCA. Other devices such as atherectomy catheters and lasers have been developed in the hope that with controlled injury, removal of loose plaque material and a better postangioplasty luminal geometry may reduce the incidence of restenosis.

However, the rate of restenosis with these new devices has not been significantly lowered. Similarly, the use of implantable devices such as stents has not been proved to greatly reduce the incidence of restenosis. Since proliferation of smooth muscle cells is one of the major contributors to the pathogenesis of restenosis, it is thought that inhibition of smooth muscle cell proliferation may prove to be a useful pharmacologic approach to reduce restenosis. This chapter outlines the current understanding of the role of smooth muscle cell proliferation, the stimuli involved in induction of the proliferative response, and the agents that have been found to inhibit smooth muscle cell proliferation in vitro and in vivo. Some mechanism-based approaches to inhibit smooth muscle cell proliferation are also discussed.

SMOOTH MUSCLE CELL PROLIFERATION IN RESPONSE TO VASCULAR INJURY

A variety of animal experiments have demonstrated that injury to the vessel wall, including the perturbation of luminal endothelium, leads to smooth muscle cell proliferation. Intimal or medial damage by the balloon catheter in the rat,[4] pig,[5] rabbit,[6-9] and dog[10] has been shown to greatly increase cell proliferation. Similarly, vascular injury inflicted by luminal air drying[11] or perivascular placement of endotoxin-embedded thread[12] or an irritant plastic cuff[8] induces proliferation of smooth muscle cells. As illustrated in Figure 48–1, even a mild form of injury produced by placement of a blood clot perivascularly in the rabbit carotid artery[13] leads to smooth muscle cell proliferation and intimal thickening. Smooth muscle cell proliferation thus appears to be a common vascular response to injury irrespective of the method of injury or the type of vessel involved. In most of the injury models, the high level of proliferation observed initially declines rapidly, and cell proliferation is close to the preinjury level within 8 to 10 weeks.[3, 4, 8, 9] If other complicating factors are superimposed over injury, proliferation is more pronounced and prolonged. For example, in normocholesterolemic animals, injury to arteries induces cell proliferation and intimal thickening, which declines to a normal level after 6 to 8 weeks. A similar injury to hypercholesterolemic animals produces a proliferative response that is greater initially than in normocholesterolemic animals and persists for at least 12 weeks (unpublished data). Extrapolation of these animal model observations to humans would suggest that proliferation of smooth muscle cells occurs in most patients undergoing PTCA. Recent data derived from autopsy samples lends support to this notion. Histologic analysis of tissue samples derived from 20 patients at various time points after PTCA have shown that smooth muscle cell proliferation occurred in 83% to 100% of the patients.[14] Why then only about a third of the patients clinically manifest reocclusion is not precisely understood. It is possible that prolonged and overt proliferation leading to restenosis occurs due to the perturbation of normal repair processes, perhaps by additional complicating biological factors. Thus, an understanding of the cellular and molecular events during the normal tissue repair process as well as the repair responses in restenotic patients is critical to determine the underlying causes of restenosis.

FACTORS STIMULATING SMOOTH MUSCLE CELL PROLIFERATION

Smooth muscle cells maintained in tissue culture can be stimulated to undergo DNA synthesis and mitosis by several polypeptide growth factors and vasoactive hormones. The tissue culture approach has been instrumental in the identification of several of these activities and their cellular sources. Nevertheless, the relevance of tissue culture findings to the in vivo activity and actual availability at the injured site need to be considered. At the injured site, platelets are probably the early source of growth factors. Initial studies suggested that a polypeptide growth factor (platelet-derived growth factor [PDGF]) released by aggregating platelets plays a key role in vascular smooth muscle cell proliferation.[1, 15] Now it is known that PDGF-like molecules are also produced by macrophages[16] and vascular endothelial[17, 18] and smooth muscle[19, 20] cells. PDGF consists of two polypeptide chains arbitrarily termed A and B. The two polypeptide chains are linked by disulfide bonds generating three PDGF isoforms: AA homodimer, BB homodimer, and AB heterodimer. All three forms of PDGF can be found at the site of vascular injury. Recent studies indicate that there may be some functional differences in the three forms of PDGF.[21-23] In addition to growth stimulation, PDGF also stimulates smooth muscle cell migration[24] and production of arachidonic acid metabolites in mesenchymal cells.[25, 26] The prostanoids (prostaglandin E_2 or I_2 [PGE_2, PGI_2]) generated in response to PDGF may play important roles in the vessel wall, including inhibition of smooth muscle cell proliferation,[27] macrophage production of cytokines,[28] and platelet aggregation.[29] These effects of

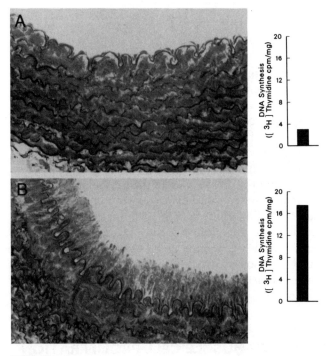

FIG 48–1.
Intimal thickening and DNA synthesis in a rabbit carotid artery in response to injury. **A,** carotid artery from a control rabbit. **B,** carotid artery from a rabbit subjected to perivascular blood clot–induced injury. Histology and DNA synthesis were determined at 2 weeks postinjury.

PDGF on vascular cells and the fact that PDGF is readily produced at the site of injury strongly suggest that PDGF is one of the important mediators of vascular response to injury.

Monocytes/macrophages infiltrate the vessel wall in response to injury and are commonly found in atherosclerotic plaque. Unlike platelets, which are deposited transiently at the injury site, macrophages can accumulate in the injured vessel and in atherosclerotic plaque for extended periods. These cells may thus represent a continuous source of growth stimulators and therefore may be of greater significance to the pathogenesis of proliferative restenosis. Several studies have produced evidence suggesting that monocytes/macrophages can serve as an important source of growth mediators, including the PDGF-BB homodimer.[16] Besner et al.[30] have recently isolated a heparin-binding growth factor from human mononuclear cells that appears to be different from PDGF and the heparin-binding fibroblast growth factor (FGF). Our studies have demonstrated that activated human monocytes produce a smooth muscle cell mitogen that is different from PDGF, FGF, or transforming growth factor α (TGF-α).[31] Furthermore, in situations where other growth factors such as PDGF are present, the macrophage-derived cytokine interleukin-1 (IL-1) also potentiates smooth muscle cell proliferation.[27]

In addition to platelets and infiltrating monocytes, cells of the vessel wall themselves may play an active role in growth regulation in a paracrine and autocrine manner. Vascular endothelial cells[17, 18] and smooth muscle cells[19, 21] in culture produce PDGF, FGF, and IL-1. Chronic production of these factors may contribute to pathogenesis. Endogenous inhibitors of smooth muscle cell proliferation have also been identified. Locally produced factors such as TGF-β,[32] heparin,[33] and PGI$_2$[34] may act as negative regulators of smooth muscle cell growth.

That multiple growth factors stimulate smooth muscle cell proliferation is illustrated in Figure 48–2. Induction of cell proliferation by various growth factors has been previously demonstrated by using cells derived from different animal species and under varying experimental conditions. From these studies it is difficult to evaluate the relative potency of these growth factors. The results presented in Figure 48–2 show the growth-stimulating activity of several growth factors under identical experimental conditions with smooth muscle cells derived from rabbit aorta. PDGF-BB was a potent stimulator of DNA synthesis. PDGF-AA, on the other hand, produced only a small effect on DNA synthesis when used at very high concentrations. Previous studies have shown that PDGF-AA stimulates the growth of fibroblasts and is produced in the arterial wall.[35] However, in light of the poor mitogenic activity on cultured smooth muscle cells, its role in smooth muscle proliferation needs further investigation. Monocyte-derived growth factor (MDGF) was also a potent stimulator for smooth muscle cell proliferation in vitro. Heparin-binding FGF stimulated rabbit aorta smooth muscle cells in vitro. These data show that the potency of FGF was slightly higher than that of PDGF-BB. In general, the

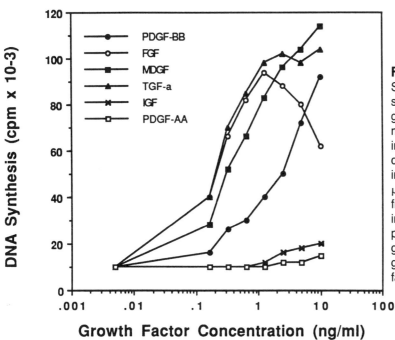

FIG 48–2.
Stimulation of DNA synthesis in rabbit aorta smooth muscle cells by various polypeptide growth factors. Quiescent cultures of smooth muscle cells in 96-well microtiter plates were incubated in Dulbecco's modified Eagle medium containing 1% human platelet-poor plasma, indicated concentration of growth factors, and 5 μCi (^{3}H)thymidine. After 24 hours, cells were fixed in methanol, and (^{3}H)thymidine incorporation in DNA was determined. *PDGF* = platelet-derived growth factor; *FGF* = fibroblast growth factor; *MDGF* = macrophage-derived growth factor; *TGF-α* transforming growth factor-α; *IGF* = insulin-like growth factor.

maximum stimulation of DNA synthesis was higher for PDGF-BB than for FGF. Other studies have shown that human vascular smooth muscle cells in culture express FGF and undergo DNA synthesis in response to exogenously added FGF.[36, 37] Furthermore, it was recently shown that systemic administration of FGF to deendothelialized rat carotid artery produced increased cell proliferation in vivo.[38] Another factor that may be important in smooth muscle cell proliferation but has not yet been widely discussed is (TGF-α). TGF-α is related to the epidermal growth factor (EGF) family of polypeptide growth factors and binds to the EGF receptor. A recent study by Castellot et al.,[37] showed that EGF stimulated the growth of calf and human smooth muscle cells. The results presented in Figure 48–2 show that when tested under identical conditions, TGF-α or EGF (data not shown) was a two- to five-fold more potent growth stimulator than PDGF-BB. Although the potency of TGF-α appears greater than that of PDGF-BB, the maximum level of (^{3}H)thymidine incorporation attained in response to TGF-α was slightly lower than PDGF-BB. In vivo, TGF-α may be derived from macrophages infiltrating the vessel wall following injury.[39]

Other growth-promoting factors such as Insulin-like growth factor (IGF), serotonin, and IL-1 may not directly induce cell proliferation but can potentiate cell growth when added in the presence of other mitogens. IGF-1 or serotonin have been shown to promote cells growth in conjunction with PDGF.[40, 41] The smooth muscle cell growth-promoting activity of IL-1 is illustrated in Figure 48–3. The addition of IL-1 alone did not significantly stimulate DNA synthesis in rabbit aorta smooth muscle cells. However, in the presence of PDGF, IL-1 produced a three- to six-fold stimulation of DNA synthesis. In addition, IL-1 induces the synthesis of prostanoids (PGE$_2$/PGI$_2$)[42] and FGF,[43] which in turn affect smooth muscle cell proliferation.

These studies suggest that multiple growth factors may participate in the generation of proliferative response at the site of vascular injury. Each of the cell types present at the injured site (platelets, mononuclear cells, and the vascular endothelial and smooth muscle cells) following balloon angioplasty could be a potential source of growth-stimulating activities. Thus, multiple factors from multiple cellular sources may be involved in smooth muscle cell proliferation in vivo. These considerations are important for the development of specific inhibitors of smooth muscle cell proliferation that demonstrate maximum efficacy in the treatment of restenosis.

FIG 48–3.
Effect of IL-1 alone and IL-1 plus PDGF on DNA synthesis in vascular smooth muscle cells. Stimulation of DNA synthesis was determined by (^{3}H)thymidine incorporation as described previously[27] and in Figure 48–2.

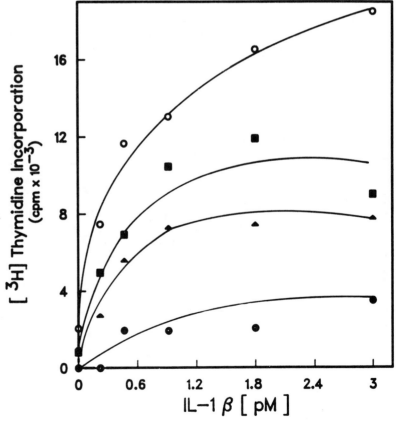

CELLULAR AND MOLECULAR EVENTS INDUCED BY GROWTH FACTORS

The factors stimulating smooth muscle cell proliferation discussed above mediate growth by initial binding to cell surface receptors. Specific, high-affinity receptors on smooth muscle cells have been demonstrated for PDGF, FGF, and EGF. Receptors for MDGF have not yet been characterized. Our studies have shown that MDGF does not compete with PDGF, FGF, or EGF for receptor binding, which suggests that separate receptors exist for MDGF.[31] In response to growth factors, quiescent cells in the G_0/G_1 phase traverse through G_1 into DNA synthesis "S" phase and then to mitosis (Fig 48–4). Although, the biochemical pathways involved in these various phases of the cell division cycle are not yet fully defined at the present time, recent findings on growth factor–induced signal transduction and growth factor–inducible cellular genes have provided important insights into some of the biochemical events associated with cell proliferation. For smooth muscle cells, PDGF receptors and the intracellular signaling system have been studied more extensively than the other mitogens mentioned above. We will therefore use the PDGF system as an example to illustrate the signal transduction cascade involved in growth factor action.

There are two types (α and β) of cell surface receptors for PDGF isoforms. PDGF-BB and PDGF-AB isoforms bind to both α- and β-receptors with high affinity, while the PDGF-AA form binds to α-receptors with high affinity. PDGF binding initiates a cascade of membrane-associated events, including receptor dimerization and autophosphorylation of receptor at tyrosine residues. Protein phosphorylation and dephosphorylation by membrane-associated and intracellular protein kinases and phosphatases are considered important postreceptor regulatory steps controlling cell proliferation. A major recent finding on PDGF signal transduction has been the demonstration of an essential role of the tyrosine kinase activity of the receptor.[44] Using cells containing mutated PDGF receptors, Williams and his associates have shown that receptors deficient in tyrosine kinase activity do not mediate growth in response to PDGF, even though these receptors exhibit high-affinity binding for PDGF.[44] Thus, the protein tyrosine kinase activity of the receptor is required for induction of cell growth. In addition to receptor autophosphorylation, several receptor-associated proteins become phosphorylated within minutes after PDGF treatment. Some of these recently identified receptor-associated proteins that become phosphorylated and participate in the generation of second messenger include phospholipase C-γ

Growth Factor Induced Signaling Pathway

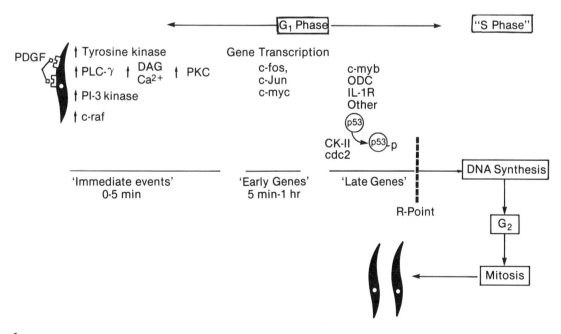

FIG 48–4.
Some of the known cellular events induced by platelet-derived growth factor (PDGF). *PLC*-γ = phopholipase C-γ; *PI-3 kinase* = phosphatidylinositol-3 kinase; *DAG* = diacylglycerol; *PKC* = protein kinase C; *ODC* = ornithine decarboxylase; *CK-II* = casein kinase-II.

(PLC-γ), guanosine triphosphatase (GTPase) activator protein (GAP), phosphatidylinositol-3-kinase (PI-3 kinase), and raf-1 protein. PLC-γ is an important enzyme in the generation of second-messenger phosphatidyl inositols and leads to an increase in cytosolic Ca^{2+} and activation of protein kinase C.[45] Coughlin et al.[46] have shown that deletion of the PI-3 kinase binding domain from the PDGF receptor leads to a loss of DNA synthesis in response to PDGF. Although these studies indicate the importance of the PDGF receptor domain to which PI-3 kinase binds, a direct involvement of PI-3 kinase activity in cell growth is not yet established. Also, FGF and EGF stimulate smooth muscle cell proliferation, apparently without requiring PI-3 kinase activation, and conversely, IGF stimulates PI-3 kinase[47] but has little effect on smooth muscle cell proliferation (see Fig 48–2), which suggests that further studies are needed to clarify the role of PI-3 kinase in cell growth regulation.

Signals from the cell membrane are ultimately transmitted to the nucleus, and transcription of new genes can be detected within 5 minutes of PDGF stimulation. Important growth-controlling steps reside in the G_1 phase of the cell cycle before the commitment of cells to DNA replicative "S" phase (Fig 48–4). Among the notable cellular genes induced shortly after PDGF stimulation ("early genes") are the proto-oncogenes c-*fos*, c-*myc*, and c-*jun*.[48, 49] These genes encode for proteins that function in cell division. Proteins products of c-*fos* and c-*jun* bind specific sequences of DNA and activate transcription of other genes ("late genes") directly involved in DNA replication and control of mitosis. Other "late genes" such as c-*myb* are not directly involved in DNA replication but play essential roles in the progression of cells from G_1 to S phase.[50] In addition to the genes associated with the transduction of positive signals for growth, genes exerting negative effects on cell growth are also expressed or their protein products modified in the G_1 phase of the cell cycle. The products of retinoblastoma, RB gene, and P^{53} gene, have been shown to act as suppressors: they produce cell growth arrest in the late G_1 phase.[51] The suppressor gene P^{53} is a substrate for protein kinase cdc-2[52] and casein kinase-II (CK-II).[53] Phosphorylation by these enzymes may play a role in modulation of P^{53} function and hence entry of cells into S phase. As discussed below, some of these signal transduction steps could be potential targets for drug intervention for restenosis.

PHARMACOLOGIC APPROACHES TO TREATMENT OF RESTENOSIS

Several pharmacologic agents have been tested in humans for their potential application in the prevention of restenosis following PTCA (Table 48–1). Initially, the rationale for using some of these agents was not necessarily related to smooth muscle growth inhibition. A few of the agents have been found to inhibit smooth muscle cell proliferation in vitro. However, their other pharmacologic actions prohibit long-term use in the treatment of restenosis. For example, ciprostene and trapidil inhibit smooth muscle cell proliferation in vitro, but their continuous infusion at concentrations sufficient to affect restenosis will also produce a vasodilatory effect. Similarly, although anti-inflammatory steroids, calcium channel blockers, and low–molecular-weight heparin have demonstrated utility in cell culture and animal models, human trials have not shown efficacy, most likely due to the inability to attain adequate therapeutic concentrations while avoiding systemic side effects. Recently, attention has been directed toward agents that inhibit smooth muscle cell proliferation. Listed in Table 48–1 are a number of agents that have been shown to inhibit smooth muscle cell proliferation in culture. However, many of these agents also lack specificity (for example, protein kinase C inhibitors) and therefore may not be ideal for clinical use.

In order to formulate new strategies for the treatment of restenosis, considerations of available data concerning the mechanisms involved in cell growth regulation can provide a rational framework for the identification of successful approaches to the prevention of restenosis. Several requirements for an "ideal" therapeutic approach may be tentatively put forth: (1) the activity should be specifically targeted to smooth muscle either by the use of smooth muscle cell–specific agents or by local delivery, (2) the effect should be predominantly cytostatic rather than cytotoxic so as not to destroy arterial media and its normal functions, (3) the agent should be effective/present during a "critical" time, and (4) the agent should be limited in its systemic effects. For each selected target, it is helpful to evaluate the currently available and future agents or methods in terms of their fulfillment of these criteria.

The first level at which the restenotic response to PTCA could conceivably be forestalled is that of the cell-cell interaction involved in platelet adherence and aggregation, as well as monocyte infiltration and activation. Attempts have been made to inhibit platelet aggregation by using antiplatelet drugs such as aspirin and dipyridamole, thrombin inhibitor, hirudin, and antibodies directed against platelet glycoprotein IIb-IIIa receptors. Studies with the antiplatelet agents thus far have shown little promise in restenosis, which suggests that blocking platelets alone may not be sufficient to prevent restenosis.[57–62] It was initially thought that in addition to their beneficial antithrombotic effects, antiplatelet agents would reduce growth stimuli such as PDGF at

TABLE 48–1.

Agents Tested for Restenosis/Smooth Muscle Cell Growth Inhibition*

Agent	In Vitro	In Vivo	In Clinic	Reference
Omega-3 fatty acid	−	−	+	54
Corticosteroid	+	+	−	55
Cyclosporine A	+	+	NA	56
Ciprostene	+	NA	−	57
Trapidil	+	+	NA	58–60
Dipyridamole	+	+	−	61, 62
Ticlopidine	NA	NA	−	62
Heparin/low–molecular weight heparin	+	+	−	63–65
Pentosan polysulfate	+	NA	NA	66
Dextran sulfate	+	+	NA	67
Colchicine	+	+	−	68
Vincristine	+	+	NA	69
Methotrexate	+	−	NA	70
Staurosporine	+	NA	NA	71, 72
H-7	+	NA	NA	71, 72
Diltiazem	+	+	−	73
Verapamil	+	+	−	74, 75
Nifedipine	+	+	NA	74, 76
Nitrendipine	+	NA	NA	77
HA-1077	+	NA	NA	78
Photofrin	+	NA	NA	79
Lovastatin	+	+	NA	80
Captopril	−	+	NA	81
Angiopeptin	−	+	NA	82
Ketanserin	+	−	−	83
Hirudine	−	+	NA	84
Sulotroban	−	NA	−	85
Terbinafine	+	NA	NA	86
Tyrosine kinase Inhibitors	NA	NA	NA	72, 87–90

*+ = positive effect; − = not effective; NA = data not available or not tested.

the injured site and may therefore reduce cell proliferation. However, it is now known that not only platelets but also macrophages and the cells of the vessel wall produce growth factors. Therefore, inhibition of platelet deposition may not be sufficient to limit the growth-stimulating factors at the injury site post-PTCA. Similarly, the use of anti-inflammatory steroids to limit growth stimuli from inflammatory cells has not proved efficacious.[55]

Inhibition of the initial interaction of growth factors with their receptors has been an attractive goal but has suffered from a lack of available antagonist molecules. Also, since multiple growth factors can stimulate smooth muscle cell proliferation (see Fig 48–2), a receptor antagonist directed against a single growth factor is likely to be insufficient to block growth in vivo. An additional concern raised by blockade of growth factor receptors is the elimination of beneficial distal responses unrelated to proliferation such as release of vasodilatory and antithrombotic prostaglandins. Finally, the receptor antagonists are likely to be peptide in nature and pose

additional difficulties relative to the delivery mechanisms. Notwithstanding these objections, receptor antagonists or soluble receptors of PDGF and FGF are likely to become available in the very near future and will be examined for their potential use in restenosis.

The next level of potential modulation is that of intracellular signal transduction steps described in the previous section. Tyrosine kinase, PI-3 kinase, and protein kinase C play roles in smooth muscle cell proliferation. Protein kinase C inhibitors such as staurosporine and H-7 have been shown to inhibit smooth muscle cell proliferation in vitro.[71, 72] Such compounds are characterized by relatively low specificity at the present time, although further structural information promises to lead to the development of a higher degree of specificity. Several classes of compounds inhibiting tyrosine kinase activity have been described. Although the tyrosine kinase inhibitors described initially suffered from a lack of specificity, the more recently described compounds such as (hydroxy)-phenylcarboxylates,[87] cinnamic acid derivatives,[88–90] and thiazolidine-diones[91] are clearly more selective for tyrosine kinase. The biological activity of these compounds is yet to be tested in smooth muscle cell assays in vitro or in animal models of restenosis.

An interesting target site for inhibition of cell proliferation is the late G_1 phase of the cell cycle before commitment to DNA synthesis. Inhibition of cell cycle progression in this part may allow growth inhibition in response to multiple growth factors and will avoid blocking of the early beneficial activities (e.g., PGI_2 generation) of growth factors. Evidence suggests that important regulatory steps reside in the G_1 phase of the cell cycle. A higher degree of selectivity may thus be achieved by inhibiting growth-regulatory steps than by inhibiting the general cellular processes. These observations are supported by in vivo and in vitro inhibition of smooth muscle cell growth by heparin.[92] It has been shown that some of the growth-inhibitory mechanisms of heparin reside in the late G_1 phase.[37] More importantly, heparin displays cell selectively with respect to growth inhibition. For example, heparin inhibits smooth muscle cells but does not have similar growth-inhibitory effects on endothelial cells.[93] An understanding of the mechanism of heparin action in G_1 phase may allow development of low–molecular–weight heparin mimetics acting at such an intracellular signal transduction step.

Inhibition of the activity or function of a key protein by small organic molecules has been a general approach to finding therapeutic agents. As described above, inhibition of cell proliferation can be achieved by small molecules such as inhibitors of a certain protein kinase required for cell growth. An alternate approach to specifically inhibit cellular mechanism that has recently become possible is to inhibit the synthesis of the protein/enzyme in question. An emerging technology that uses an antisense oligonucleotide to inhibit synthesis of a specific protein allows selective inhibition of cell growth. For example, antisense nucleotide probes designed to bind sequences necessary for the activation of transcription or translation of genes, e.g., proto-oncogenes c-*myc* or c-*myb*, have been shown to inhibit cell growth.[94, 95] Since local delivery of drugs is a promising option for restenosis, the use of antisense DNA for inhibition of cell proliferation is not only an attractive novel approach but also a feasible approach.

THE ACHIEVEMENT OF SPECIFICITY

The specificity of a compound is an important consideration for its therapeutic application. It is more so in the case of restenosis because of the intrinsically localized nature of the restenosis process and its involvement of smooth muscle and other cells that are by no means unique to the area of restenosis. As discussed above, a certain level of specificity is achieved by targeting specific cellular mechanisms for drug intervention. Further specificity can be achieved by local application of the pharmacologic agent. Local therapy offers the combined advantages of enhanced agent concentration at the desired site and diminished systemic concentration. Local application of therapeutic agents as an approach to the treatment of restenosis is potentially practical because of its prospectively identifiable location and time of onset correlating with the time of PTA and thus vascular access. Several possible approaches to local delivery are shown in Figure 48–5, which highlights an expected role for methods combined with devices. The illustrated devices are broadly divisible into those in which catheters deliver desired preparations onto or into the vascular wall and those in which permanent or temporary stents coated with or containing the desired preparations are affixed to the wall at the site of PTCA. A "combined" approach has also been described in which a balloon catheter such as that shown in Figure 48–5, part d, is used to place and shape a matrix that subsequently solidifies in situ to form a "paving" stent.[96] This stent could also incorporate an active pharmacologic agent to be released to the vascular wall as described.

A system in which a brief proximal infusion of a high concentration of agent into a particular vascular distribution could be performed with subsequent drainage distal to the capillary bed would achieve containment in terms of systemic levels. In Figure 48–5, part a, is a catheter able to temporarily contain a drug between its balloons for infusion into the arterial wall at elevated pressure. This design for intramural delivery is not ideal for application in vessels with frequent branches due to the expected pressure leaks into any branch enclosed between the balloons. Such a mechanism has been utilized, however, for delivery of marker proteins[97] as well as endothelial cells.[98] A "weeping" or "sprinkling" catheter (Fig 48–5, parts c or d) avoids the branch-leak difficulty by the placement of multiple small exit orifices in a balloon inflated to directly contact the vessel wall, and it has been used for the intramural infusion of several agents[99, 100] as well as DNA.[101] Considerations for all these catheters clearly include the amount of distal drug runoff, the residence time of the drug at the desired site, and the presence and degree of vessel injury caused by the infusion procedure. Such points are the topic of intense investigation at present.

Stents such as that shown in Figure 48–5, part e, have been adapted to carry genetically modified endothelial cells,[102] and trials of the in vivo effects of cellular stents expressing elevated levels of tissue-type plasminogen activator (t-PA) are presently under way. Stents may

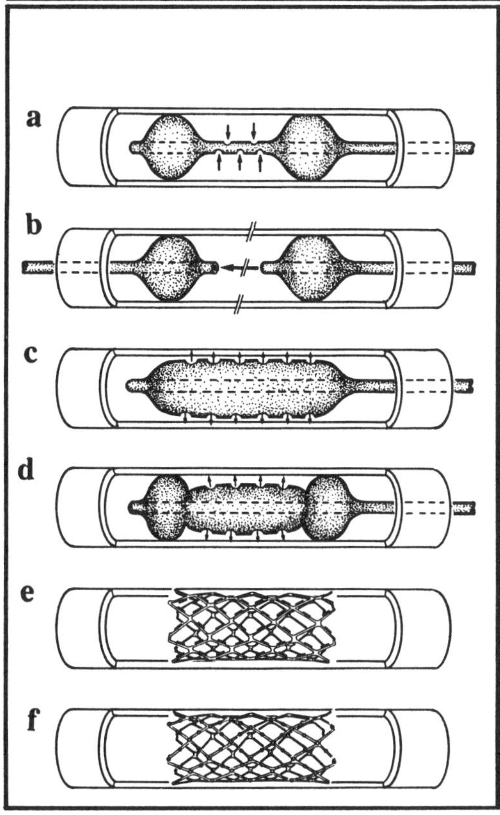

		GENERAL PROCEDURE	DELIVERY LOCATION	AGENT CONTACT TIME	LUMINA NEEDED
a		INFUSE AND DRAIN AGENT LOCALLY	INTRALUMINAL	MODERATE	3 – 4
b		INFUSE AGENT AND DRAIN DISTALLY	INTRALUMINAL	SHORT	2 x 2
c		INFUSE AGENT UNDER PRESSURE	INTRAMURAL	PROLONGED	1 – 2
d		COMPRESS AGENT AFTER INFUSION	ENDOLUMINAL	PROLONGED	3 – 4
e		STENT IS COATED WITH AGENT	ENDOLUMINAL	PROLONGED	–
f		STENT CONTAINS AGENT	ENDOLUMINAL	PROLONGED	–

FIG 48–5.

Approaches to transluminal local delivery of therapeutic agents. *a,* Catheter allowing localized irrigation and delivery between two balloons; *b,* catheter allowing selection of an entire perfusion bed; *c* and *d,* incorporation of multiperforated balloons while reducing branch and distal runoff; *e,* stent coated with a therapeutic agent; *f,* stent containing an agent either incorporated in a porous matrix or in hollow cavity.

also be constructed to contain drug within a hollow core for intramural infusion, again through outwardly facing orifices (Fig 48–5, part f), and finally, drugs can be incorporated in biodegradable substances for gradual release.

REFERENCES

1. Ross R, Glomset J: The pathogenesis of atherosclerosis. *N Engl J Med* 1976; 295:369–377, 420–425.
2. Ross R: The pathogenesis of atherosclerosis. *N Engl J Med* 1986; 314:448–500.
3. Goldberg ID, Stemerman MB, Schnipper LE, et al: Vascular smooth muscle kinetics: A new assay for studying patterns of cellular proliferation in vivo. *Science* 1979; 205:920–922.
4. Clowes AW, Reidy MA, Clowes MM: Kinetics of cellular proliferation after arterial injury. *Lab Invest* 1983; 83:327–333.
5. Steel PM, Chesebro JH, Stanson AW, et al: Balloon angioplasty: Natural history of pathophysiological response to injury in a pig model. *Circ Res* 1985; 57:105–112.
6. Wilentz JR, Sanborn TA, Haudenschild CC, et al: Platelet accumulation in experimental angioplasty: Time course and relation to vascular injury. *Circulation* 1987; 75:636–642.
7. Sanborn TA, Faxon DP, Haudenschiled CC, et al: The mechanism of transluminal angioplasty: Evidence for formation of aneurysms in experimental atherosclerosis. *Circulation* 1983; 68:1136–1140.
8. Hirosumi J, Nomoto A, Yoshitaka O, et al: Inflammatory responses in cuff-induced atherosclerosis in rabbits. *Atherosclerosis* 1987; 64:243–254.
9. Hanke H, Strohscneider T, Oberhoff M, et al: Time course of smooth muscle cell proliferation in the intima and media of arteries following experimental angioplasty. *Circ Res* 1990; 67:651–659.
10. Orlandi C, Singh JP, Bell FP, et al: Proliferative and lipid metabolism response to balloon angioplasty in ca-

nine renal arteries. *J Am Coll Cardiol* 1990; 15:1394–1400.

11. Richardson M, Hatton MWC, Buchanan MR, et al: Wound healing in the media of the normolipemic rabbit carotid artery injured by air drying or by balloon catheter deendothelialization. *Am J Pathol* 1990; 137:1453–1465.

12. Prescott MF, McBride CK, Court M: Development of intimal lesions after leukocyte migration into the vascular wall. *Am J Pathol* 1989; 135:835–846.

13. Nishizawa EE, Della-Colette AA: A new animal model for the study of drug on platelet thrombosis and atherosclerosis. *Thromb Haemost* 1985; 54:280.

14. Nobuyoshi M, Kimura T, Ohishi H, et al: Restenosis after percutaneous transluminal coronary angioplasty: Pathologic observation in 20 patients. *J Am Coll Cardiol* 1991; 127:433–439.

15. Ross R, Raines EW, Bowen-Pope DF: The biology of platelet-derived growth factor. *Cell* 1986; 46:155–169.

16. Shimokado K, Rains EW, Madtes DK, et al: A significant part of macrophage-derived growth factor consists of at least two forms of PDGF. *Cell* 1985; 43:277–286.

17. DiCorleto PE, Bowen-Pope DF: Cultured endothelial cells produce a platelet-derived growth factor like protein. *Proc Natl Acad Sci USA* 1983; 80:1919–1923.

18. Barrett TB, Gajdusek CM, Schwartz SM, et al: Expression of the *sis* gene by endothelial cells in culture and in vivo. *Proc Natl Acad Sci USA* 1984; 81:6772–6774.

19. Seifert RA, Schwartz SM, Bowen-Pope DF: Developmentally regulated production of platelet-derived growth factor–like molecules. *Nature* 1984; 311:669–671.

20. Nilsson J, Sjolund M, Palmberg L, et al: Arterial smooth muscle cells in primary culture produce a platelet-derived growth factor like protein. *Proc Natl Acad Sci USA* 1985; 82:4418–4422.

21. Barrett TB, Benditt EP: *sis* (Platelet-derived growth factor B chain) gene transcript levels are elevated in human atherosclerotic lesions compared to normal artery. *Proc Natl Acad Sci USA* 1987; 84:1099–1103.

22. Kazlauskas A, Bowen-Pope DF, Seifert R, et al: Differential effects of homo- and heterodimers of platelet-derived growth factor A and B chains on human and mouse fibroblasts. *EMBO J* 1988; 7:3727–3735.

23. Nister M, Hammacher A, Mellstrom K, et al: A glioma-derived PDGF A chain homodimer has different functional activities from a PDGF AB heterodimer purified from human platelets. *Cell* 1988; 52:791–799.

24. Grotendorst GR, Seppa HEJ, Kleinman HK, et al: Attachment of smooth muscle cells to collagen and their migration toward platelet-derived growth factor. *Proc Natl Acad Sci USA* 1981; 78:3669–3672.

25. Habenicht JR, Goerig M, Grulich J, et al: Human platelet-derived growth factor stimulates prostaglandin synthesis by activation and by rapid de novo synthesis of cyclooxygenase. *J Clin Invest* 1985; 75:1381–1387.

26. Chiou WJ, Bonin PD, Singh JP: Obligatory action of polypeptide growth factors for the interleukin-1 (IL-1) mediated prostaglandin E_2 production in fibroblasts. *J Immunol* 1990; 145:2155–2160.

27. Bonin PD, Fici GJ, Singh JP: Interleukin-1 promotes proliferation of vascular smooth muscle cells in coordination with PDGF or a monocyte derived growth factor (MDGF). *Exp Cell Res* 1989; 181:474–482.

28. Kunkel SL, Chensue SW, Phan SH: Prostaglandin as endogenous mediators of interleukin-1 production. *J Immunol* 1986; 136:186.

29. Kroll MH, Schafer AI : Biochemical mechanisms of platelet activation. *Blood* 1989; 74:1181–1195.

30. Besner G, Higashiyama S, Klagsbrun M: Isolation and characterization of a macrophage-derived heparin-binding growth factor. *Cell Reg* 1990; 1:811–819.

31. Singh JP, Bonin PD: Purification and biochemical properties of a human monocyte derived growth factor. *Proc Natl Acad Sci USA* 1988; 85:6374–6378.

32. Moses ML, Yang EY, Pietenpol JA: TGF-β stimulation and inhibition of cell proliferation:New mechanistic insights. *Cell* 1990; 63:245–247.

33. Clowes AW, Karnowsky MJ: Suppression by heparin of smooth muscle cell proliferation in injured arteries. *Nature* 1977; 265:625–626.

34. Morisaki N, Kanzaki T, Motoyama N, et al: Cell cycle dependent inhibition of DNA synthesis by prostaglandin I_2 in cultured rabbit smooth muscle cells. *Atherosclerosis* 1988; 71:165–171.

35. Barrett TB, Benditt EP: Platelet-derived growth factor gene expression in human atherosclerotic plaque and normal artery wall. *Proc Natl Acad Sci USA* 1988; 85:2810–2814.

36. Winkles JA, Friesel R, Burgess WH, et al: Human vascular smooth muscle cells both express and respond to heparin-binding growth factor I (endothelial cell growth factor). *Proc Natl Acad Sci USA* 1987; 84:7124–7128.

37. Castellot JJ Jr, Pukac LA, Caleb BL, et al: Heparin selectively inhibits a protein kinase C–dependent mechanism of cell cycle progression in calf aortic smooth muscle cells. *J Cell Biol* 1989; 109:3147–3155.

38. Linder V, Lappi DA, Baird A, et al: Role of basic fibroblast growth factor in vascular lesion formation. *Circ Res* 1991; 68:106–113.

39. Madtes DK, Rains EW, Sakariassen KS, et al: Induction of transforming growth factor-α in activated human alveolar macrophages. *Cell* 1988; 53:285–293.

40. Banskota NK, Taub R, Zellner K, et al: Insulin, insulin-like growth factor 1 and platelet-derived growth factor interact additively in the induction of the protooncogene c-*myc* and cellular proliferation in cultured bovine aortic smooth muscle cells. *Mol Endocrinol* 1989; 3:1183–1190.

41. Nemecek GM, Coughlin SR, Handley DA, et al: Stimulation of aortic smooth muscle cell mitogenesis by serotonin. *Proc Natl Acad Sci USA* 1986; 83:674–678.

42. Breviario F, Proserpio P, Bertocchi F, et al: Interleukin-1 stimulates prostacyclin production by cultured human endothelial cells by increasing arachidonic acid mobilization and conversion. *Atherosclerosis* 1990; 10:129–134.

43. Gray CG, Winkles JA: Interleukin-1 regulates heparin-binding growth factor 2 gene expression in vascular smooth muscle cells. *Proc Natl Acad Sci USA* 1991; 88:296–300.

44. Williams LT: Signal transduction by platelet-derived growth factor receptor. *Science* 1989; 243:1564–1570.

45. Majerus PW, Ross TS, Cunningham TW, et al: Recent insights in phosphatidylinositol signaling. *Cell* 1990; 63:459–465.

46. Coughlin SR, Escobedo JA, Williams LT: Role of

phosphatidylinositol in PDGF receptor signal transduction. *Science* 1989; 243:1191–1194.

47. Ruderman NB, Kapeller R, White MF, et al: Activation of phosphatidylinositol 3-kinase by insulin. *Proc Natl Acad Sci USA* 1990; 87:1411–1415.

48. Bravo R: Growth factor–responsive genes in fibroblasts. *Cell Growth Diff* 1990; 1:305–309.

49. Travali S, Koniecki J, Petralia S, et al: Oncogenes in growth and development. *FASEB J* 1990; 4:3209–3214.

50. Gewirtz AM, Anfossi G, Venturelli D, et al: GI/S transition in normal T lymphocytes requires the nuclear protein encoded by c-*myb. Science* 1989; 245:180–183.

51. Marshell CJ: Tumor supressor genes. *Cell* 1991; 64:313–326.

52. Bischoff JR, Friedman PN, Marshak DR, et al: Human P^{53} is phosphorylated by P^{60}-cdc2 and cyclin B-cdc2. *Proc Natl Acad Sci USA* 1990; 87:4766–4770.

53. Meek DW, Simon S, Kikkawa U, et al: The P^{53} tumour suppressor protein is phosphorylated at serine 389 by casein kinase II. *EMBO J* 1990; 9:3253–3260.

54. Dehmar GJ, Popma JJ, van der Berg EK, et al: Reduction in the rate of early restenosis after coronary angioplasty by a diet supplemented with n-3 fatty acids. *N Engl J Med* 1988; 319:734–740.

55. Pepine CJ, Hirshfeld JW, et al: A controlled trial of corticosteroids to prevent restenosis after coronary angioplasty. *Circulation* 1990; 81:1753–1761.

56. Jonasson L, Holm J, Hansson GK: Cyclosporine A inhibits smooth muscle proliferation in the vascular response to injury. *Proc Natl Acad Sci USA* 1988; 85:2303–2306.

57. Raizener A, Hollman J, Demke D: Beneficial effects of ciprostene in PTCA: A multicenter, randomized controlled trial. *Circulation* 1988; 78(suppl 2):290.

58. Ebrahimi R, Khorsandi M, Dimayuga P, et al: Trapidil inhibits vascular smooth muscle cell proliferation in vitro and in vivo (abstract). *Atherosclerosis* 1990; 10:815.

59. Liu MW, Roubin GS, Robinson KA, et al: Trapidil in preventing restenosis after balloon angioplasty in the atherosclerotic rabbits. *Circulation* 1990; 81:1089–1093.

60. Shinya O, Masaaki I, Morimichi S, et al: Trapidil (triazolopyrimidine), a platelet derived growth factor (PDGF) antagonist in preventing restenosis after percutaneous transluminal coronary angioplasty. *Circulation* 1990; 82(Suppl 3):428.

61. Schwartz L, Bourassa MA, Lesperance J, et al: Aspirin and dipyridamole in the prevention of restenosis after PTCA. *N Engl J Med* 1988; 318:1714–1719.

62. White CW, Knudson M, Schmidt D, et al: Neither ticlopidine nor aspirin- dipyridamole prevent restenosis post PTCA: Results from a randomized placebo-controlled multicenter trial. *Circulation* 1987; 76(suppl 4):213.

63. Lehmann KG, Doria RJ, Feuer JM, et al: Paradoxical increase in restenosis rate with chronic heparin use (abstract). *J Am Coll Cardiol* 1991; 17:181.

64. Pow TK, Currier JW, Minihan AC, et al: Low molecular weight heparin reduces restenosis after experimental angioplasty. *Circulation* 1989; 80(suppl 2):64.

65. Clowes AW, Karnowsky MJ: Suppression by heparin of smooth muscle cell proliferation in injured arteries. *Nature* 1977; 265:625–626.

66. Smith SG, Guyton JR, Woolbert SC, et al: Pentosan polysulfate inhibits vascular smooth muscle cell proliferation in vitro (abstract). *Atherosclerosis* 1990; 10:847.

67. Seewaldt-Becker E, Hallermayer G: Effect of dextran sulfate and dextran on injury-induced atherosclerosis in rats (abstract) *Atherosclerosis* 1990; 10:972.

68. O'Keefe JH, McCallister BD, Bateman TM, et al: Colchicine for the prevention of restenosis after coronary angioplasty (abstract) *J Am Coll Cardiol* 1991; 17:181.

69. Barath P, Arakawa K, Cao J, et al: Low dose of antitumor agents prevents smooth muscle cell proliferation after endothelial injury (abstract) *J Am Coll Cardiol* 1989; 13:252.

70. Murphy JG, Schwartz RS, Edwards WD, et al: Methotrexate and azathioprine fail to inhibit porcine coronary restenosis. *Circulation* 1990; 82(suppl 3):429.

71. Takagi Y, Hirata Y, Takata S, et al: Effect of protein kinase inhibitors on growth factor–stimulated DNA synthesis in cultured rat vascular smooth muscle cells. *Atherosclerosis* 1988; 74:227–230.

72. Matsumoto H, Sasaki Y: Staurosporine, a protein kinase C inhibitor interferes with proliferation of arterial smooth muscle cells. *Biochem Biophys Res Commun* 1989; 158:105–109.

73. Corcos T, David PR, Val PG, et al: Failure of diltiazem to prevent restenosis after percutaneous transluminal angioplasty. *Am Heart J* 1985; 109:926–931.

74. Jackson CL, Bush RC, Bowye D: Inhibitory effects of calcium antagonists on balloon catheter–induced arterial smooth muscle cell proliferation and lesion size. *Atherosclerosis* 1988; 69:115–122.

75. El-Sanadiki M, Cross KS, Mikat EM, et al: Verapamil therapy reduces intimal hyperplasia in balloon injured rabbit aorta. *Circulation* 1987; 76(suppl 4):314.

76. Whitworth HB, Roubin GD, Hollman J, et al: Effect of nifedipine on recurrent stenosis after percutaneous transluminal angioplasty. *J Am Coll Cardiol* 1986; 8:1271–1276.

77. Crockett L, Warshaw DM: Effect of nitrendipine on growth activity in cultured vascular smooth muscle cells. *J Cardiovasc Pharmacol* 1988; 12(suppl):153.

78. Shirotani M, Yui Y, Takahashi M, et al: A new intracellular calcium antagonist, HA-1077, an isoquinoline derivative, inhibits quiescent bovine arterial smooth muscle cell proliferation (abstract). *J Am Coll Cardiol* 1989; 13:153.

79. Dartsch PC, Ischinger T, Coppenath K, et al: Effect of photofrin II on growth of cultured human smooth muscle cells from non-atherosclerotic arteries and atheromatous plaques: Implication for photodynamic laser therapy of vascular stenoses. *Eur Heart J* 1989; 10:151.

80. Gellman J, Ezekowitz MD, Sarembock IJ, et al: Effect of lovastatin on intimal hyperplasia after balloon angioplasty: A study in an atherosclerotic rabbit. *J Am Coll Cardiol* 1991; 17:251–259.

81. Powell JS, Clozel JP, Muller RKM, et al: Inhibition of angiotensin-converting enzyme prevent myointimal proliferation after vascular injury. *Science* 1989; 245:186–188.

82. Marcus H, Trowbridge R, Foegh M: Effect of delayed angiopeptin treatment on myointimal hyperplasia following angioplasty (abstract). *J Am Coll Cardiol* 1991; 17:181.

83. Klein W, Eber B, Fluch N, et al: Ketanserin prevents acute occlusion but not restenosis after PTCA (abstract). *J Am Coll Cardiol* 1989; 13:44.

84. Sarembock IJ, Gertz SD, Gimple LW, et al: Angiographic and pathologic study of the effect of recombinant desulphatohirudin on restenosis following balloon angioplasty in rabbits. *Circulation* 1990; 82(suppl 3):338.

85. Finci L, Hoflong B, Ludwig B, et al: Sulotroban during and after coronary angioplasty: A double blind placebo control study. *C Kardiol* 1989; 78:50–54.

86. McCarty L, Van Valen RG, Denny IH, et al: Terbinafine: Effects on platelet-derived growth factor–stimulated smooth muscle cells in vitro and myointimal proliferation in vivo. *Faseb J* 1989; 3:A556.

87. Shechter Y, Yaish P, Chorev M, et al: Inhibition of insulin-dependent lipogenesis and anti-lipolysis by protein tyrosine kinase inhibitors. *EMBO J* 1989; 8:1671–1676.

88. Isshiki K, Imoto M, Sawa T, et al: Inhibition of tyrosine protein kinase by synthetic erbstatin analogs. *J Antibiot (Tokyo)* 1987; 40:1209–1210.

89. Yaish P, Gazit A, Gilon C, et al: Blocking of EGF-dependent cell proliferation by receptor kinase inhibitors. *Science* 1988; 242:933–935.

90. Lyall RM, Ziberstein A, Gazit A, et al: Tyrophostins inhibits epidermal growth factor (EGF)-receptor tyrosine kinase activity in living cells and EGF-stimulated cell proliferation. *J Biol Chem* 1989; 246:14503–14509.

91. Geissler JF, Traxler P, Regenass U, et al: Thiazolidinediones: Biochemical and biological activity of a novel class of tyrosine protein kinase inhibitors. *J Biol Chem* 1990; 2645:22255–22261.

92. Hoover RL, Rosenberg R, Haering W, et al: Inhibition of rat arterial smooth muscle proliferation by heparin. *Circ Res* 1980; 47:578–583.

93. Castellot JJ Jr, Addonizio ML, Rosenberg R, et al: Cultured endothelial cells produce inhibitors of smooth muscle cell growth. *J Cell Biol* 1981; 90:372–379.

94. Holt JT, Redner RL, Nienhus AW: An oligomer complementary to c-*myc* mRNA inhibits proliferation of HL-60 promyelocytic cells and induces differentiation. *Mol Cell Biol* 1988; 8:963–973.

95. Gewirtz AM, Calabretta B: A c-*myb* antisense oligodeoxynucleotide inhibits normal human hematopoiesis. *Science* 1988; 242:1303–1306.

96. Slepian MJ: Polymeric endoluminal paving and sealing: Therapeutics at the crossroads of biomechanics and pharmacology in Topol EJ (ed), *Textbook of Interventional Cardiology*. 1990, pp 647–670.

97. Goldman B, Blanke H, Wolinsky H: Influence of pressure on permeability of normal and diseased muscular arteries to horseradish peroxidase. *Atherosclerosis* 1987; 65:215–225.

98. Nabel EG, Plautz G, Boyce FM, et al: Recombinant gene expression in vivo within endothelial cells of the arterial wall. *Science* 1989; 244:1342–1344.

99. Wolinsky H, Thung SN: Use of a perforated balloon catheter to deliver concentrated heparin into the wall of the normal canine artery. *J Am Coll Cardiol* 1990; 15:475–481.

100. Muller DWM, Topol EJ, Abrams G, et al: Intramural methotrexate therapy for the prevention of intimal proliferation following porcine carotid balloon angioplasty. *Circulation* 1990; 82(suppl 3):429.

101. Nabel EG, Plautz G, Nabel GJ: Site-specific gene expression in vivo by direct gene transfer into the arterial wall. *Science* 1990; 249:1285–1288.

102. Dichek DA, Neville RF, Zwiebel JA, et al: Seeding of intravascular stents with genetically engineered endothelial cells. *Circulation* 1989; 80:12347–1353.

Pharmacologic Therapy in the Prevention of Restenosis After Percutaneous Transluminal Coronary Angioplasty

Walter R.M. Hermans, M.D.

Benno J. Rensing, M.D.

Pim de Feyter, M.D.

Patrick W. Serruys, M.D.

Percutaneous transluminal coronary angioplasty (PTCA) is an accepted form of treatment for providing relief of angina pectoris in patients with single-vessel and multivessel disease. Increased experience and advances in technology have resulted in a higher primary success rate (90% to 95%) and a lower acute complication rate (4% to 5%). Despite the therapeutic success of coronary angioplasty, the exact mechanisms of dilation remain speculative and involve multiple processes, including endothelial denudation, with rapid accumulation of platelet and fibrin; cracking, splitting or disruption of the intima and atherosclerotic plaque; dehiscence of the intima and plaque from the underlying media; and stretching or tearing of the media, with persistent aneurysmal dilation of the media and adventitia.[1, 2] The major limitation of PTCA is its high incidence of restenosis, which limits the long-term benefit of the procedure. Restenosis is the angiographic renarrowing at the site of PTCA, frequently accompanied by recurrence of symptoms of angina. The incidence of restenosis varies between 17% and 40%, a consequence of whether there has been complete angiographic follow-up as well as the way that restenosis is defined.[3-6] Over the past 10 years we have been unable to significantly influence the rate of this late complication. Although many of the risk factors for restenosis have been identified (Table 49–1)[5-40] most of these are difficult to influence, and we are unable to predict which patients or vessel segments will develop restenosis. Until now we have not found a pharmacologic solution. Also the use of one of the new interventional devices (directional atherectomy catheter,[41] the excimer laser,[42] stent,[43] or the rotational atherectomy[44]) has not prevented restenosis from occurring. The reason that a clinically significant restenosis occurs in only a minority of the dilated vessels remains an enigma. It seems that the solution to the restenosis problem depends on an understanding of the controlled healing process, which occurs in 60% to 80% of the vessels dilated.

POSSIBLE MECHANISMS OF RESTENOSIS AFTER PTCA

Besides the pathology of the dilated vessels of patients who died shortly or later on after PTCA,[45-47] it has become possible, with the use of the transluminal atherectomy device, to remove and examine primary and restenotic lesions.[48-50] Primary stenosis consisted in the majority of cases of atherosclerotic plaque (com-

TABLE 49–1.

Variables Associated With Higher Restenosis Rates in Patients With Follow-up Angiography

First Author	Year	Patients	Clinical	Hemodynamic or Procedure Related	Lesion Related
Scholl[7]	1981	45	Variant angina		Eccentric or calcified lesion
Dangoisse[8]	1982	31	Variant angina	> 9 inflations	
David[9]	1984	191	Variant angina		Pre-PTCA DS* > 90%
					Post-PTCA DS > 50%
					Eccentric stenosis
					Diffuse disease
					Absence of parietal dissection
Dorros[10]	1984	46			Proximal graft > body or distal
Holmes[5]	1984	557	Male sex	Pre-PTCA TSG* > 40 mm Hg	Pre-PTCA DS > 70%
			Canadian class III–IV	Post-PTCA TSG ≥ 20 mm Hg	PTCA on CABG*
			No previous MI*		
			Angina onset < 2 mo		
			Diabetes mellitus		
Marantz[11]	1984	73		Post-PTCA TSG > 18 mm Hg	Irregular lesion pre-PTCA
				> 7 atm	Large change in DS
Margolis[12]	1984	216	Diabetes mellitus (insulin)		
Schmitz[13]	1984	86		Larger balloon size, less restenosis	
Kaltenbach[6]	1985	333	Medication?		Second PTCA
					PTCA on CABG
Levine[14]	1985	100		Inflation pressure < 8 atm	Post-PTCA DS > 30%
					Delta DS < 55%
Mata[15]	1985	60		Balloon artery ratio ≤ 0.9	LAD or LCX > RCA*
					Calcified stenosis
					Post-PTCA DS > 40%
Probst[16]	1985	94		Collaterals pre-PTCA	
				Occlusion pressure > 45 mm Hg	
Serruys[17]	1985	28†			PTCA for total occlusion
Bertrand[18]	1986	229			"Dynamic" coronary stenosis (spontaneous or provoked spasm)
Clark[19]	1986	124†		More inflations	
				Higher inflation pressure	
Hollman[20]	1986	536	Diabetes mellitus		Multivessel PTCA
					Pre-PTCA DS ≥ 90%
					Post-PTCA DS > 40%
					Absence of intimal tear
Leimgruber[21]	1986	998	Old age	Post-PTCA TSG 15 mm Hg	LAD > RCA > LCX
			Unstable angina		Post-PTCA DS > 30%
			Angina onset < 2 mo		Absence of dissection
Powelson[22]	1986	50			Presence of intimal disruption‡
Roubin[23]	1986	411			Multi-lesion PTCA in one vessel
Uebis[24]	1986	100			Length of pre-PTCA stenosis > 2 mm
Hirshfeld[25]	1986	209			LAD > LCX or RCA
					Minimal luminal diameter < 0.64 mm
					Normal diameter < 3.0 mm
					Short-duration heparin therapy
Guiteras[26]	1987	100	Hypertension		Residual stenosis
					Eccentricity of lesion
Myler[27]	1987	164§	Diabetes mellitus	Inflation pressure > 10 atm	Pre-PTCA DS > 95%
			Hypercholesterolemia		
			New-onset angina		
			Current smoking		

(Continued).

Variables Associated With Higher Restenosis Rates in Patients With Follow-up Angiography—cont'd

First Author	Year	Patients	Clinical	Hemodynamic or Procedure Related	Lesion Related
Rapold[28]	1987	178	Variant angina		Post-PTCA > 45% Multivessel disease
Simonton[29]	1987	123	Diabetes mellitus History prior MI	Slow distal flow	Difficulty crossing lesion
Urban[30]	1987	91	CWP* ≥ 30 mm Hg		
Vandormael[31]	1987	129§	Male gender Diabetes mellitus		Proximal LAD disease Increased length stenosis (≥ 10 mm)
De Feyter[32]	1988	158¶			Presence of collaterals Multivessel disease LAD disease Transient ST-depression
Galan[33]	1988	160	Continuing smoker		
Lambert[34]	1988	119§	Diabetes mellitus		High-grade stenosis pre-PTCA Large residual stenosis
Weinstein[35]	1988	54			Dilatation of both bifurcation lesions
Bertrand[36]	1989	437			Presence of ergonovine-induced spasm before and after PTCA
Ellis[37]	1989	308			Stenosis at bend point of coronary artery
Uebis[38]	1989	272		≥ 3 Inflations	
Renkin[39]	1990	111	Recurrence of angina		Post-PTCA luminal diameter
Rupprecht[40]	1990	473	Unstable angina	Prolonged single inflation	Large residual stenosis post-PTCA High-grade stenosis pre-PTCA

*DS = diameter stenosis; CABC = coronary artery bypass graft; TSG = transstenotic gradient; MI = myocardial infarction; LAD = left anterior descending; LCX = left circumflex; RCA = right coronary artery; CWP = coronary wedge pressure.
†Patients with total occlusion.
‡Early restenosis (≤ 2 days).
§Patients with multiple lesions.
¶Patients with unstable angina.

posed of dense fibrous tissue and variable amounts of fatty atheromatous debris); however, in a small group only intimal hyperplasia was seen, histologically identical to restenotic lesions. Restenotic lesions showed in most cases intimal hyperplasia (characterized by proliferation of smooth muscle cells of the synthetic type with abundant extracellur matrix chiefly composed of proteoglycans), and in a minority, only atherosclerotic plaque was seen. Smooth muscle cell proliferation seems to play a pivotal role in the restenosis process.

The process that results in restenosis is initiated at the time that the disruptive action of the inflated balloon on the endothelium, intima, and/or media takes place. Since intact endothelium prevents platelet aggregation, a superficial endothelial injury leads to local platelet and leukocyte adhesion, but most of the platelets do not undergo a release action. However, in the case of a deep endothelial injury (as with a successful angioplasty) the hemostatic system is activated. Blood is exposed to collagen and other substances of the subintima that are potent stimuli for platelet aggregation mediated by the release of adenosine diphosphate (ADP), serotonin, thromboxane A_2 (TXA_2), fibrinogen, fibronectin, thrombospondin, and von Willebrand factor (Fig 49–1). These substances activate neighboring platelets via different metabolic pathways (thromboxane A_2, ADP, and platelet activating factor) and promote the formation of intramural thrombus, which could cause restenosis.[51, 52] (Fig 49–1).

Concomitantly several growth factors including platelet-derived growth factor (PDGF), epidermal growth factor (EGF), and transforming growth factor β (TGF-β) are released from thrombocytes, smooth muscle cells, endothelium, and macrophages. In this way they stimulate smooth muscle cells and fibroblasts to proliferate and migrate from the medial layer into the intima of the vessel wall. In some patients this response is excessive and is associated with abundant amounts of

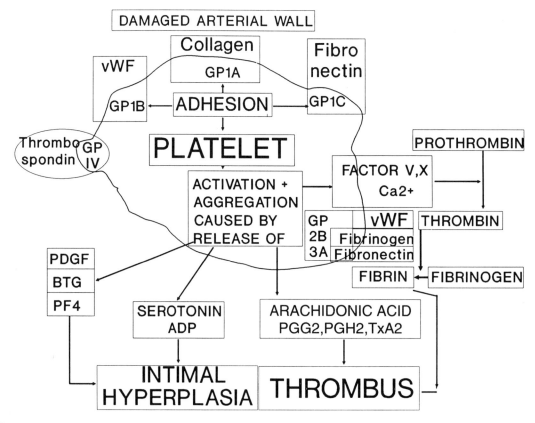

FIG 49-1.
Simplified schematic presentation of platelet adhesion, activation, and aggregation. Vascular injury with endothelial denudation exposes subendothelial collagen to circulating blood and induces platelets to adhere by using glycoprotein receptors *(GP)*. This adhesion is stimulated by von Willebrand factor *(vWF)*; fibronectin and thrombospondin bind to other glycoprotein receptors of the platelets. This adhesion leads to activation and aggregation with release of adenosine diphosphate *(ADP)*, serotonin, Ca^{2+}, thromboxane A_2, platelet-derived growth factor *(PDGF)*, (/) β-thromboglobulin *(BTG)*, and platelet factor 4 *(PF4)*, which could lead to intimal hyperplasia and thrombus formation. (Adapted from Essed CE, van den Brand M, Becker AE: *Br Heart J* 1983; 49:393–396.)

connective tissue formation. This results in hyperplasia of the intima with a reduction in luminal diameter and causes restenosis[53–55] (Fig 49–1).

Each of these steps could be sites of intervention that may halt the restenosis process[56] (Fig 49–2). The drugs that could reduce or prevent restenosis in the animal model are listed in Table 49–2. In this review we will concentrate on the drugs that have been tested for prevention of restenosis in the animal model (Table 49–3) and in postangioplasty patients (Table 49–4 and Fig 49–2).

ANIMAL MODEL

Lack of a practical animal restenosis model has limited the ability to investigate potential therapies. It is difficult to create arterial stenoses in animals that ex-

actly resemble human coronary artery disease. The dimensions of the arteries in the animal model should be similar to these of human beings, the development of the lesions should occur in an accelerated fashion, the lesions must produce high-grade including total, angiographically detectable luminal diameter narrowing, and the histologic composition of the lesions should be similar to the complex lesions that are typical of human atherosclerosis.[116]

At least four different species (pigs/swine, rats, dogs, rabbits) have been used to test new drugs for their ability to prevent restenosis[117] (see Table 49–3). There is no consensus as to the way that the stenosis should be created (inflated balloon, infused air, electrical stimulation); it is also undecided whether an atherogenic diet should be added since there is no animal with identical atherosclerotic disease to humans. The vessel that is the target for the experiment (iliac, carotid, or coronary ar-

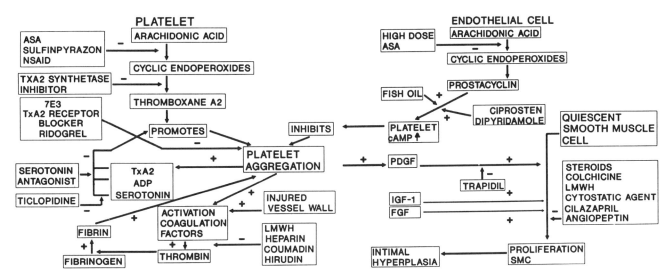

FIG 49–2.
Simplified schematic presentation of how the different drugs act on the different processes involved in the restenosis process. *ASA* = acetylsalicylic acid; *NSAID* = nonsteroidal anti-inflammatory drugs; TXA_2 = thromboxane A_2; *cAMP* = cyclic adenosine monophosphate; *PDGF* = platelet-derived growth factor; *IGF* = insulin-like growth factor; *FGF* = fibroblast growth factor; *LMWH* = low–molecular-weight heparin; *SMC* = smooth muscle cell; *QCA* = quantitative coronary angioplasty. (Adapted from Austin GE, Ratliff NB, Hollman J, et al: *J Am Coll Cardiol* 1985; 6:369–375.)

teries; aorta) is also different. The way that restenosis is assessed differs among the different models. Some use the degree of platelet deposition at the site of arterial injury; others use the percentage of intimal mitosis seen in the damaged arteries[118, 119] (see Table 49–3). Angiography is frequently used to assess restenosis, although some use visual evaluation and others use a computer-assisted technique to assess restenosis. Finally, no consensus has been reached as to the definition of restenosis that should be used when a new drug is tested (Fig 49–3).

TABLE 49–2.
Drugs to Prevent Restenosis Mechanisms

Thrombosis
  Heparin, hirudin, warfarin (Coumadin), acetylsalicylic acid, dipyridamole, sulfinpyrazone, dextran, thromboxane A_2 synthetase inhibitor, thromboxane A_2 receptor blocker, ticlopidine, prostacyclin, ciprostene, prostaglandin E_1, glycoprotein IIb/IIIa antibody (7E3), fish oil, nonsteroidal anti-inflammatory drugs
Cell proliferation
  Low-molecular-weight heparin, platelet-derived growth factor antagonist (trapidil), angiotensin converting enzyme inhibitor (cilazapril), colchicine, cytostatic agents, serotonin antagonist (ketanserin), angiopeptin, thiol protease inhibitor, calcium-calmodulin antagonist
Inflammation
  Corticosteroids, nonsteroidal anti-inflammatory drugs
Coronary vasospasm
  Nifedipine, diltiazem
Lipid
  Fish oil, lovastatin

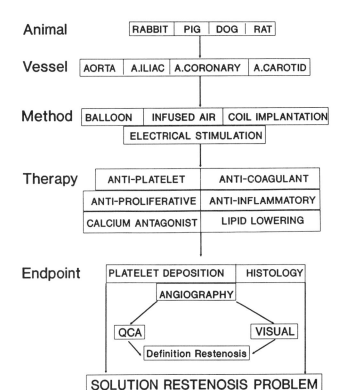

FIG 49–3.
Schematic presentation of the different animals, vessels, methods, therapy, and end points used to induce atherosclerotic narrowings and to assess the effect of different drug regimens.

TABLE 49–3.
The Effect of Drug Therapy in the Animal Model for Prevention of Restenosis

First Author	Year	Model	Drug	Dose	Animals Total	Fup*	Method	Effect
Clowes[57]	1977	Rat A. carotis	Heparin Placebo	5–14 days	45	7 days	Histology	Myointimal thickening, less with heparin
Gordon[58]	1987	Rabbit aorta	LMWH* Hydrocortison (H) LMWH + H Placebo (P)	2.5 mg/kg/day 1 mg/kg/day	16	2 wk	Histology	Ratio intimal/media thickness of LMWH and H separately and synergistically lower than placebo.
Pow[59]	1989	Rabbit A. iliaca	LMWH Placebo (P)	10 mg/kg/day	21	4 wk	Angiography Histology	ΔLD (Post-PTCA)-(Fup) = 1.1 mm P P and 0.3 mm LMWH ($P < .001$)
Oberhoff[60]	1990	Rabbit	LMWH Placebo	2.5 mg/kg/day	31	3, 7 or 28 days	Histology	Intimal mitosis ↓ ($P <. 05$) Intimal wall thickness ↓
Heras[61]	1989	Pig A. carotis	Hirudin Heparin	1 mg/kg/hr 6 dif* dose	55		Platelet deposition (PD)	Less PD in hirudin than heparin
Faxon[62]	1984	Rabbit A. iliaca	ASA* + dipyridamole (D) Sulfinpyrazone Placebo	32–25 mg/day 100 mg/day	25	4 wk	Angiography Histology	ASA + D and sulfinpyrazone reduce restenosis
Franklin[63]	1990	Rabbit	Warfarin (W) + ASA Placebo	1.5 normal PTT* 60 mg/day	22	~1 wk to 4 wk	Angiography	W + ASA: 80% less restenosis than placebo
Sanborn[64]	1986	Rabbit	TXA$_2$ synth inhibit* Heparin ASA	1 mg/kg/hr 500 U/kg 10 mg/kg	70	30 min	Platelet deposition	Less platelet accumulation using TXA$_2$ synth inhibit
Leung[65]	1990	Rabbit aorta	Antithrombin agent by infusion catheter	Dif dosage	25	30 min	Platelet deposition	Less platelet deposition with antithrombin agent
Liu[66]	1990	Rabbit A. iliaca	Trapidil Placebo	60 mg/kg/day	17	4 wk	Arteriography Histology	Intimal thickness decreases with trapidil

	Year	Model	Drug	Dose	n	Duration	Arteriography (QCA) O* Histology EM*	Comment
Currier[67]	1989	Rabbit A. iliaca	Colchicine (C₁) Colchicine (C₂) Placebo (P)	0.2 mg/kg 0.02 mg/kg	34	4 wk	Arteriography (QCA) O* Histology EM*	ΔLD (Post-PTCA)−(Fup) = 0.6 mm = 0.8 mm = 1.1 mm
Barath[68]	1989	Rabbit aorta	Vincristine + actinomycin Placebo	0.075 mg/kg + 0.015 mg/kg	36	3 days	EM*	Selective damage of proliferating smooth muscle cells
Müller[69]	1990	Minipigs	Methotrexate ASA + heparin	6.25 mg/ml	7	28 days	Histology	No effect on intimal smooth muscle or inflammatory cell infiltration
Murphy[70]	1990	Pigs	Methotrexate Azathioprine Placebo	Different dose 25 mg/day	NR*	28 days	Histology	No difference in intimal proliferation and restenosis
Powell[71]	1989	Rat A. carotis	Cilazapril Placebo	10 mg/kg 5 dif duration	127	14 days	Histology	Intimal hyperplasia decreased with 70% given days −6 to 14
Müller[72]	1990	Rat A. carotis	Captopril Hydralazine Verapamil	100 mg/kg/day 8 mg/kg/day 100 mg/kg/day	43	NR	Histology	Captopril superior vs. others in reduction of intimal hyperplasia
Lam[73]	1990	Pig A. carotis	Cilazapril	20 mg/kg/bid	16	4 wk	Morphology	No differences in atherosclerotic changes in the 2 groups
Bilazarian[74]	1991	Rat A. carotis	Cilazapril Placebo	5 mg/kg/day	9	−7 to 28 days	Angiography	Less restenosis with cilazapril vs. placebo
Foegh[75]	1989	Rabbit cardiac transplant	Angiopeptin Placebo	NR	20	6 wk	Histology	Intimal hyperplasia decreased by angiopeptin
Conte[76]	1990	Rabbits	Angiopeptin	20 µg/kg/day for 2 or 6 days	NR	21 days	Histology	Intimal thickening was decreased in both groups
Wilensky[77]	1991	Rabbit A. femoralis	Thiol protease inhibitor (TPI)	Perfusion catheter 50 µM for 45 sec	12	2 wk	Angiography Histology	Less reduction in MLD* in TPI-treated artery
Faxon[78]	1984	Rabbit	Nifedipine (N) Placebo (P)	40 mg/day	18	4 wk	Angiography Histology	Δ(Post-PTCA)−(Fup) = 0.9 mm (N) = 1.2 mm (P)
Gellmann[79]	1991	Rabbit A. femoralis	Lovastatin Placebo	6 mg/kg/day	30	39 days	Arteriography Histology	Intimal hyperplasia was decreased by lovastatin

*Fup = follow-up; LMWH = low−molecular-weight heparin; dif = different; ASA = acetylsalicylic acid; PTT = partial Thromboplastin time TXA₂ synth inhibit = thromboxane A₂ synthetase inhibitor; EM = electron microscopy; NR = not reported; QCA = quantitative coronary angiography; MLD = minimal lumen diameter.

TABLE 49–4.

The Effect of Drug Therapy on Restenosis per Patients After Successful Coronary Angioplasty With Follow-up Angiography and/or

Author	Year	Drug	Dose	Patient Total	Fup*
Hirshfeld[80]	1987	Heparin	Different duration	209	NR*
Ellis[81]	1989	Heparin (18–24 hr)	< 2.5 nor PTT*	416	61%
		Dextrose			
Lehmann[82]	1991	Heparin (daily)	10,000 units/day	30	77%
Thornton[83]	1984	ASA*	325 mg/day	248	72%
		Coumadin	2–2.5 nor PTT		
Urban[84]	1988	Coumadin + verapamil	> 2.5 nor PTT	110	77%
		Verapamil	NR		
Dyckmans[85]	1988	ASA	1,500 mg/day	203	40%
		ASA	320 mg/day		
Mufson[86]	1988	ASA	1,500 mg/day	453	37%
		ASA	80 mg/day		
Schanzenbacher[87]	1988	ASA	1,000 mg/day	79	100%
		ASA	100 mg/day		
Kadel[88]	1990	ASA	1,400 mg/day	188	92%
		ASA	350 mg/day		
Finci[89]	1988	ASA	100 mg/day	40	73%
		Placebo			
Schwartz[90]	1988	ASA + dipyridamole (D)	990 (ASA), 225 (D) mg/day	249	100%
		Placebo			
Chesebro[91]	1989	ASA + D	975 (ASA), 225 (D) mg/day	207	85%
		Placebo (P)			
White[92]	1987	ASA + D	650 (ASA), 225 (D) mg/day	236	75%
		Ticlopidine (Tic)	750 mg/day		
		Placebo			
Yabe[93]	1989	TXA$_2$ synth inhibit*	600 mg/day	33	100%
		Placebo			
Serruys[94]	1991	TxA$_2$ receptor blocker	40 mg/day	650	89%
		Placebo (P)			
Kitazume[95]	1988	ASA	300 mg/day (ASA)	280	100%
		ASA + Tic	+ 200 mg/day (Tic)		
		ASA + Tic + nicorandil (N)	+ 30 mg/day (N)		
Bertrand[96]	1990	Tic	500 mg/day	266	93%
		Placebo			
Knudtson[97]	1990	Prostacyclin (P) + ASA + D*	5 ng/kg/min (P) +	270	93%
		ASA + D	325 (ASA) + 225 (D) mg/day		
Gershlick[98]	1990	Prostacyclin	4 ng/kg/min	132	80%
		Placebo			
Raizner[99]	1988	Ciprostene	120 ng/kg/min max. 48 hr	311	80%
		Placebo			
Okamoto[100]	1990	Trapidil	600 mg/day	64	NR
		ASA + D	300 + 150 mg/day		
Klein[101]	1989	Ketanserin	0.1 mg/min for 24 hr	43	100%
O'Keefe[102]	1991	Colchicine	1.2 mg/day	197	74%
		Placebo			
Corcos[103]	1985	Diltiazem (Dil) + ASA + D	270 mg/day	92	100%
		ASA + D	650–225 mg/day		
O'Keefe[104]	1991	Dil + ASA + D	325 (Dil) +	201	60%
		ASA + D	325 (ASA) + 225 (D) mg/day		
Whitworth[105]	1986	Nifedipine + ASA	40 mg/day	241	82%
		ASA	325 mg/day		
Hoberg[106]	1990	Verapamil (V) + ASA + D	480 (V) +	196	88%
		ASA + D	660 (ASA) + 330 (D) mg/day		
Slack[107]	1987	Fish oil	2.4 g/day	162	85%
		Placebo			

(Continued.)

Clinical Follow-up

Time	Definition of Restenosis	Restenosis (%)			Risk Ratio†	95% CI‡
		Drug	Placebo	Sign*		
4-12 mo	> 50% DS* Fup (visual)	Longer heparin, less restenosis				
3-9 mo	> 50% DS Fup (visual)	41%	37%	NS*	1.1	0.8-1.5
NR	NR	82%	33%	P < .05	2.5	0.8-7.8
6-9 mo	loss > 50% gain Stress test − → +	27%	36%	NS	0.7	0.5-1.1
5 mo	> 50% DS Fup	29%	37%	NS	0.8	0.4-1.4
6 mo	> 50% DS Fup	21%	31%	NS	0.7	0.4-1.5
3-8 mo	> 50% DS Fup (visual)	51%	47%	NS		
6 mo	Clinical (re-PTCA, CABG*)	21%	17%	NS	1.2	0.5-2.9
4-6 mo	NR	31%	21%	NS	1.5	0.9-2.5
6 mo	> 50% DS Fup (visual)	33%	14%	NS	2.3	0.5-10.1
4-7 mo	> 50% DS Fup (QCA)	38%	39%	NS	1.0	0.7-1.3
5 mo	ΔMLD (post-PTCA) − (Fup) (QCA)	0.18 mm (P) 0.14 mm (ASA + D)		NS		
6 mo	> 70% DS Fup (visual)	18% (ASA + D) 20% (T) 20% (P)		NS	0.9 1.4	0.4-1.9 0.8-12.8
> 3 mo	loss > 50% gain	22%	53%	NS	0.3	0.0-1.4
6 mo	Δ MLD(post-PTCA) MLD (Fup)	0.31 ± 0.53 0.30 ± 0.54	TxA₂ P	NS		
6 mo	> 50% DS Fup	38% 27% 16%		P = .002		
6 mo	Loss > 50% gain	50%	41%	NS	1.3	1.0-1.8
6 mo	> 50% DS Fup Loss > 50% gain (caliper)	27%	32%	NS	0.9	0.6-1.3
5-7 mo	Loss > 50% gain	31%	34%	NS	0.8	0.5-1.4
6 mo	> 50% DS Fup (visual)	41%	53%	NS	0.8	0.6-1.0
	Clinical (MI,* re-PTCA,* CABG,* death)	17%	41%	P < .01	0.5	0.3-0.8
6 mo	Loss > 50% gain	20%	44%	P < .05	0.6	0.3-1.5
4-6 mo	NR (QCA)	33%	29%	NS	1.1	0.4-2.8
NR	Return ≥ 70% DS and loss of ≥ 50% gain	22%	22%	NS		
5-10 mo	> 70% DS Fup (visual)	15%	22%	NS	0.7	0.3-1.7
12 mo	≥ 70% AS* and loss of ≥ 50% gain	36%	32%	NS	1.1	0.7-1.9
6 mo	Loss > 50% of gain >50% DS Fup	29%	33%	NS	0.9	0.5-1.4
5 mo	Loss of ≥ 50% gain	56% 38%	62% 63%	Unstable Stable	0.9 0.6	0.6-1.3 0.4-1.0
6 mo	Clinical	16%	33%	P < .05	0.5	0.2-1.0
	Stress test − → +	67%	58%	NS	1.2	0.7-1.8

TABLE 49-4 (cont.).

Author	Year	Drug	Dose	Patient Total	Fup*
Reis[108]	1989	Fish oil	6.0 g/day	186	100%
		Placebo			
Milner[109]	1989	Fish oil	4.5 g/day	194	23%
		Placebo			100%
Dehmer[110]	1988	Fish oil	3.2 g/day	82	100%
		Placebo			
Grigg[111]	1989	Fish oil	3.0 g/day	108	94%
		Placebo			
Sahni[112]	1989	Lovastatin	20-40 mg/day	157	50%
		Placebo			
Rose[113]	1987	Steroid	48 mg/day	66	88%
		Placebo			
Stone[114]	1989	Steroid for restenosis	125 mg/mp*/day 240 mg p*/wk	102	53%
Pepine[115]	1990	Steroid	1.0 g mp	722	71%
		Placebo			

*Fup = follow-up (percentage of successful PTCA); Sign = significance; NR = not reported; DS = diameter stenosis; nor PTT = normal prothrombin time; NS = not significant; ASA = acetylsalicylic acid; CABG = coronary artery bypass grafting; TXA_2synth inhibit = thromboxane A_2synthetase inhibitor; dipyridamole; MI = myocardial infarction; AS = area stenosis; mp = methylprednisolone; P = prednisolone.

†Risk ratio with 95% confidence intervals (CI). A risk ratio less than 1 means that a lower restenosis rate is seen among the patients treated with the new drug vs. those who received placebo. A statistically significant ($P < .05$) lower restenosis rate is seen in those studies where the 95% confidence intervals do not cross a risk ratio of 1. A risk ratio of more than 1 indicates a higher restenosis rate among the patients treated with the new drug.

Recently a model for human restenosis was developed in the domestic crossbred swine fed a standard, nonatherogenic diet.[120] Metallic foreign bodies were implanted percutaneously in porcine coronary arteries with oversized PTCA balloons inflated to high pressure. Histologic examination of lesions revealed a marked proliferation of medial smooth muscle cells. The histopathologic features of the proliferative response were identical to those observed in human cases of restenosis after angioplasty (material obtained from patients for the treatment of restenosis by directional coronary atherectomy). This animal model may be useful in understanding the development of restenotic lesions and to test restenosis prevention drugs since this model seems to more closely resemble the response in human restenosis.

ANIMAL EXPERIMENTAL WORK AND HUMAN STUDIES

Anticoagulants

Heparin

For many years heparin administration has been an integral aspect of the PTCA procedure since it binds reversibly with antithrombin III (AT), which leads to a conformational change and an increased rate of thrombin inactivation. Heparin has additional antithrombotic actions, largely mediated through the formation of the same complex but involving precursor elements such as factor Xa.[121, 122] Because early discontinuation of heparin treatment after angioplasty is associated with acute occlusion of the dilated arterial segment, anticoagulation seems to be important in the early stages after PTCA. However, the optimal duration of heparin therapy is still unknown.

A prospective trial conducted by the M-HEART study group in 209 patients showed an inverse relationship between the duration of heparin therapy and the incidence of restenosis.[80] This was not confirmed in a randomized trial with 416 patients (469 stenoses) in Atlanta.[81] No differences in acute closure and restenosis were found in patients (all were without dissection) randomized to placebo or 18 to 24 hours of heparin therapy post-PTCA (all patients received acetylsalicylic acid [ASA] for 6 months). Restenosis was defined as a narrowing of more than 50% of the diameter at the time of follow-up angiography, which was performed in only 58.4% of the patients with heparin and 64.5% of the patients with placebo. More bleeding complications were seen in the group of patients who were treated with heparin (8.2% vs. 3.8%). Acute total closure was seen more frequently in the placebo group (2.4%) than in the group of patients treated with heparin (1.8%), and restenosis occurred in 41.2% (heparin) and 36.7% (placebo).

Recently Lehmann et al.[82] found in (only) 23 patients randomized to daily administration of 10,000 units of

Time	Definition of Restenosis	Restenosis (%)			Risk Ratio†	95% CI‡
		Drug	Placebo	Sign*		
6 mo	> 70% DS Fup	34%	23%	NS	1.5	0.9–2.5
6 mo	> 50% DS Fup	18%	27%	NS		
Clinical	Stress test − → +	22%	35%	*P* < .04	0.6	0.4–1.0
6 mo	> 50% DS Fup (visual)	19%	46%	*P* < .007	0.4	0.2–0.8
3–5 mo	Loss > 50% of gain (caliper)	34%	33%	NS	1.1	0.6–1.8
2–10 mo	> 50% DS Fup	14%	47%	*P* < .001	0.3	0.2–0.6
3 mo	> 50% DS Fup	33%	33%	NS		
6 mo	> 50% DS Fup	59%	56%	NS	1.1	0.7–1.7
4–8 mo (caliper)	> 50% DS Fup	43%	43%	NS	1.0	0.8–1.2

subcutaneous heparin (the exact duration of heparin therapy was not reported) or usual care that 82% of the heparin-treated patients suffered restenosis (14 out of 17) and 33% (2 out of 6) in the placebo group. Restenosis was defined by quantitative angiographic analysis. Thus chronic heparin use after successful angioplasty paradoxically increases the likelihood of angiographic restenosis and an adverse clinical outcome. Perin et al.[123] retrospectively compared baseline and post-heparin activated clotting times (ACT) between 76 patients with angiographic restenosis and 18 patients without restenosis. Patients with restenosis had significantly lower post-heparin ACTs than did patients without restenosis. Thus there appears to be a relationship between the procedural response to a bolus dose of heparin and the subsequent development of restenosis.

Low–Molecular-Weight Heparin

Since low–molecular-weight heparin (LMWH) affects platelet aggregation and platelet-dependent thrombin generation to a lesser extent than "regular" heparin does, it has fewer side effects, and yet both forms are known to inhibit the proliferation of vascular smooth muscle cells (dose dependent) and thrombosis after endothelial injury in the rat.[57, 124] However, the mechanism of this inhibition is not clear.[58] Recently, LMWH has been used after transluminal angioplasty of rabbit iliac arteries.[59] Two groups were studied: the first group (*n* = 9) received LMWH (10 mg/kg/day subcutane-

ously) immediately prior to transluminal angioplasty until follow-up angiography 1 month later, while the second group (*n* = 12) received a placebo. After 4 weeks all rabbits in the placebo group and 3 out of 9 rabbits in the group treated with LMWH had a loss of more than 50% of the gain in diameter after transluminal angioplasty. Histology revealed reduced intimal hyperplasia and no formation of thrombus in the LMWH-treated group.

Oberhoff et al.[60] showed a significant reduction in the extent of intimal mitosis the first 7 days after balloon angioplasty and only a moderate increase in intimal thickness after 28 days in 16 rabbits treated with LMWH as compared with 15 rabbits in the control group. They concluded that migration and proliferation of smooth muscle cells can be reduced by early treatment with LMWH after balloon angioplasty and that further clinical investigation is advocated.

At this moment several multicenter double-blind control trials with LMWH are currently ongoing in the United States and Europe. These will provide important information as to whether long-term administration of LMWH can decrease the restenosis rate in post-PTCA patients.

Hirudin

A new anticoagulant drug is *recombinant hirudin*. Hirudin prevents fibrinogen clotting and thrombin-catalyzed activation of factors V, VIII, and XIII and thrombin-induced platelet activation. Hirudin has been shown to be more effective in preventing thrombosis than heparin is (by quantifying the deposition of platelets and fibrinogen with the method of Dewanje in a swine model). This latter effect is probably due to the fact that hirudin is a more potent and specific thrombin antagonist.[61, 125] Trials designed to tests the efficacy of hirudin on early and late complications of PTCA have just started to recruit patients in Europe and the United States.

Warfarin (Coumadin)

In the early 1980s, warfarin (Coumadin) (vitamin K antagonist inhibiting thrombin formation) was administered to patients after PTCA to prevent acute and late complications. After a beneficial effect of antiplatelet drugs in preventing thrombosis in venous bypass grafts was shown, this new drug regimen was tested in a trial[83] in which 248 patients were randomized to either 325 mg ASA daily or Coumadin at a dose that resulted in a prothrombin time of 2 to 2.5 the normal value. In the ASA-treated group (126 patients) restenosis was angiographically documented in 27% of the patients vs. 36% of the patients treated with Coumadin. Restenosis criteria were a loss of >50% of the gain achieved at the time of PTCA, an increase of the stenosis more than 30% (National Heart, Lung and Blood Institute [NHLBI] IV), or the development of positive (for ischemia) exercise test findings if no angiogram was available. The results favored the ASA strategy, but the difference was only significant for a subgroup of patients with a long history of chest pain (> 6 months). In poorly compliant patients, restenosis rates were 32% in the Coumadin-treated group vs. 20% in the ASA-treated group.

In London, a more recent randomized trial[84] with 110 patients investigated the effect of a combination of warfarin (Coumadin) with verapamil as compared with verapamil alone. The incidence of restenosis was 25% by lesion and 29% by patient in the group treated with Coumadin and 33% and 37% in the control group (the NHLBI IV criterion was used). Although the incidence of angiographic restenosis tended to be lower with Coumadin, none of the differences were significant.

A randomized trial to evaluate the efficacy of warfarin (Coumadin) in restenosis prevention should be performed that would ensure adequate medication compliance with reliable and safe prothrombin time monitoring.

Antiplatelet Agents

Platelets play an important role in the development of restenosis after PTCA.[62] To prevent platelet deposi-

tion (which occurs within minutes of the procedure) and the associated release of smooth muscle cell mitogenic factors, antiplatelet therapy appears to be a logical approach.

Acetylsalicylic Acid

ASA is a "popular drug" in the restenosis prevention trials. In the animal model it reduces platelet-thrombus deposition in a dose of 1 mg/kg/day when given in addition to heparin.[123] ASA has the ability to inhibit platelet TXA_2 synthase and subsequent platelet activation by irreversibly blocking the enzyme cyclo-oxygenase, which is responsible for the conversion of arachidonic acid to TXA_2. At high doses, ASA may be less effective since it inhibits endothelial cells from producing prostacyclin (PGI_2), which prevents platelet aggregation.[126] However, it only partially inhibits platelet aggregation induced by ADP, collagen, or thrombin. Consequently, the effect of PDGF and other mitogens on smooth muscle cell proliferation may still occur[51] (see Fig 49–1).

Four Trials Comparing Different Dosages of Acetylsalicylic Acid.—In a trial in Homburg/Saar, 203 patients were randomized to either 1,500 or 320 mg/day. In a preliminary report they had restudied 25% of these patients (6 months after PTCA). Follow-up angiography showed restenosis (>50% diameter stenosis) in 13 of 44 (31%) patients in the lower-dose group vs. 9 of 42 patients (21%) in the group with the higher dose.[85]

However, in a randomized trial in Atlanta with 495 patients, the effectiveness of two doses of ASA (80 mg vs. 1,500 mg ASA daily started the day before PTCA) in the prevention of restenosis and acute complications after PTCA was compared.[86] Follow-up angiography was only available in 166 patients (34%). In the group with low-dose ASA, 47% of the patients had restenosis (>50% diameter stenosis in one or more sites) as compared with 51% in the group with the high dose. There were no differences in success or acute complication rates. Thus, restenosis was not favorably influenced by the use of a higher dose of ASA.

A smaller trial compared the effect of ASA, 100 mg/day vs. 1,000 mg/day started 1 day before PTCA until 6 months post-PTCA.[87] In addition, all patients received calcium channel blockers and long-acting nitrates. Restenosis (clinically significant stenosis requiring re-PTCA or a bypass operation) occurred in 7 of the 40 patients in the group with 100 mg ASA (18%) and in 8 of the 39 patients in the group with 1,000 mg ASA (21%). The authors concluded that restenosis is not favorably influenced by the use of high-dose ASA vs. low-dose ASA.

Kadel et al. found no significant differences regarding the rate of restenosis (and of side effects) in 200 patients randomized to 1,400 mg or 350 mg aspirin daily.[88] Thus no advantage can be seen for high-dosage aspirin vs. the standard dosage of 350 mg.

Aspirin vs. Placebo.—Finci et al.[89] designed a trial to compare 100 mg ASA with placebo; however, it was stopped prematurely after 40 patients (single blind) were enrolled because of reports showing the benefit of ASA (combined with dipyridamole) in preventing acute thrombosis in dilated vessels and the need for urgent bypass surgery.[127] Follow-up angiography at 6 months (95% of the patients) in this particular trial showed an incidence of restenosis (> 50% diameter stenosis) that was two times higher in the group treated with ASA (33%) as compared with the placebo-treated group (14%). Although the difference seems impressive, it was not statistically significant due to the small numbers.

Aspirin/Dipyridamole vs. Placebo.—In a well-designed trial at the Montreal Heart Institute and Toronto General Hospital,[90] 376 patients were randomized to ASA (990 mg daily) and dipyridamole (225 mg daily) or to placebo starting the day before the PTCA until follow-up angiography 4 to 7 months later. More acute complications were seen in the placebo-treated group, including 13 periprocedural myocardial infarctions in the placebo group vs. 3 in the treated group ($P < .05$). However no differences were observed in the restenosis rate (increase of diameter stenosis from <50% post-PTCA to >50% at follow-up): 39% (127 patients) in the placebo group vs. 38% (122 patients) in the treated group. All patients received heparin until 12 hours after the procedure (500 units/hr) and diltiazem until follow-up angiography.

Chesebro et al. randomized 207 patients (297 stenosis) to either ASA (975 mg/day) and dipyridamole (225 mg/day) or to placebo from the day before PTCA until 6 months later.[91] There was no difference in the restenosis rate defined in a linear model based on the minimum lumen diameter obtained by quantitative angiography. There were fewer acute complications (occlusion, myocardial infarction, re-PTCA, coronary artery bypass grafting [CABG] in less than 48 hours) in the group treated with ASA and dipyridamole (11% vs. 20% in the placebo group), thus confirming the results of the Montreal/Toronto trial.

It is clear from the above clinical data that although ASA does not influence the incidence of restenosis it definitely has a positive influence on acute complications during or directly after angioplasty. However, in recent work in the atherosclerotic rabbit, ASA (60 mg/day) and warfarin (Coumadin) (1.5 times the normal prothrombin time) were given as combination therapy starting 7 days before iliac transluminal angioplasty un-til final angiography at 4 weeks in 10 atherosclerotic rabbits. Restenosis (defined as a loss of half of the initial post–transluminal angioplasty gain) was seen in 2 of 10 rabbits treated with ASA and Coumadin vs. 12 of 12 rabbits in the control group. This suggest that early combination therapy can reduce restenosis in this model and that an interaction of thrombosis and platelet activation is a key element in restenosis.[63]

Dipyridamole

In a rabbit model, treatment with ASA and dipyridamole decreased platelet-thrombus deposition and restenosis after transluminal angioplasty.[62] The mechanisms by which dipyridamole has been suggested to inhibit platelet function are through (1) the inhibition of the phosphodiesterase enzyme in platelets, which results in an increase in intraplatelet cyclic adenosine monophosphate (cAMP) levels and the consequent potentiation of the platelet-inhibiting actions of PGI_2; (2) direct stimulation of the release of this eicosanoid by vascular endothelium; or (3) inhibition of the cellular uptake and metabolism of adenosine, thereby increasing its concentration at the platelet-vascular interface. Finally, in addition to such direct effects, dipyridamole may augment the platelet-inhibiting action of aspirin through pharmacokinetic interaction.[128] However, in clinical trials[90–92] no effect has been shown on the restenosis rate after angioplasty.

Sulfinpyrazone

In contrast to ASA, sulfinpyrazone is a competitive (reversible) inhibitor of platelet cyclo-oxygenase, but the exact mechanism of its antithrombotic activity is not well understood. Faxon et al. have shown a reduction in restenosis in the rabbit model.[62] There is no clinical evidence to date to support a role for sulfinpyrazone in preventing restenosis after coronary angioplasty.

Dextran

Dextran interferes with platelet activity by changing membrane function or by interacting with the von Willebrand factor–factor VIII complex. Although it has been shown to be efficacious during PTCA, there is no role established for dextran in restenosis prevention.[129, 130]

Thromboxane A₂

TXA_2 is a potent aggregational agent and vasoconstrictor. A specific synthetase inhibitor or receptor blocker of TXA_2 can antagonize these actions while at the same time leaving prostacycline production of the vascular endothelium unaffected.

Thromboxane A$_2$ Synthetase Inhibitor.—In rabbits it was shown that a selective thromboxane synthetase inhibitor was more effective than heparin or ASA in inhibiting platelet deposition after balloon angioplasty.[64] Another TXA$_2$ synthetase inhibitor was tested in a small number of patients to prevent restenosis after PTCA.[93] It was given a minimum of 5 days before the PTCA and continued until follow-up angiography (>3 months later). Restenosis was defined as a >50% loss of initial gain in luminal diameter. The results showed that 4 of the 18 patients (22%) with the TXA$_2$ synthetase inhibitor had restenosis vs. 8 of the 15 patients (53%) in the placebo group.

Thromboxane A$_2$ Receptor Blocker.—GR32191, a new TXA$_2$ receptor blocker, has been shown to completely inhibit prostaglandin endoperoxide and TXA$_2$-induced platelet aggregation, serotonin secretion, and β-thromboglobulin secretion without any effect on the actions of PGI$_2$.[131] Because of the inhibitory action of GR32191 on platelet aggregation, mural thrombus formation, and platelet protein storage granule secretion, a trial was conducted to assess its effect in preventing restenosis after coronary angioplasty. This trial, called CARPORT (Coronary Artery Restenosis Prevention On Repeated Thromboxane-Antagonism), randomized 697 patients in six clinics in Europe to a TXA$_2$ receptor blocker, 80 mg intravenously before PTCA and 40 mg orally for 6 months, or 250 mg of intravenous aspirin before PTCA and placebo for 6 months.[94] No difference was observed between the mean difference in diameter between post-PTCA and follow-up angiograms: -0.31 ± 0.53 in the control group and -0.30 ± 0.54 in the treatment group. Also no difference was observed in clinical events (death, CABG, re-PTCA, non-fatal myocardial infarction) between the two groups. Thus no benefit was shown of long-term TXA$_2$ receptor blockade with GR32191B used as single pharmacologic regimen against restenosis.

Soon results will be available from the GRASP (Glaxo Restenosis and Symptoms Project) trial (in the United States) with the same TXA$_2$ receptor blocker and a similar design.

Ticlopidine

The mechanism of action of ticlopidine is not exactly known, but it is a potent platelet inhibitor. The optimal effect occurs 3 days after the first administration and lasts for at least several days. In a multicenter trial in the United States, patients were randomized to ticlopidine (750 mg/day), to a combination of ASA (650 mg/day) and dipyridamole (225 mg/day), or to placebo. Restenosis was defined as a diameter obstruction of 70% or more at follow-up angiography (6 months). There was no difference in the restenosis rate; in the 65 patients who received the ticlopidine the restenosis rate was 29% as compared with 18% of the 57 patients who received ASA and dipyridamole. Of the 54 patients receiving placebo there was a restenosis rate of 20%. There was also no difference in the acute complication rate.[92]

In Japan, data collected retrospectively showed a lower restenosis rate when patients received a combination of ticlopidine (200 mg/day), nicorandil (30 mg/day), and aspirin (300 mg/day).[95]

In a recently finished trial in France, the TACT study, no benefit of therapy with ticlopidine (500 mg/day) vs. placebo in 266 patients randomized for the prevention of restenosis (defined as a loss of 50% of the gain achieved at PTCA) was shown. However, acute closure was significantly reduced in the ticlopidine-treated group.[96]

Prostacyclin or Prostacyclin Analogue

PGI$_2$ is a potent naturally occurring platelet inhibitor and vasodilator. In a Canadian trial 270 patients were randomized to placebo (136 patients) or to PGI$_2$ intravenously (5 to 7 mg/min) (134 patients) just prior to PTCA and up to 48 hours after PTCA.[97] All patients received 325 mg ASA and 225 mg dipyridamole starting before angioplasty until follow-up angiography 6 months later. Short-term administration of PGI$_2$ did not significantly lower the risk of restenosis: 27% in the treated group vs. 32% in the placebo group. Restenosis was defined as 50% or more narrowing at follow-up angiography or more than 50% loss of the immediate gain after angioplasty. Acute vessel closure and ventricular tachyarrhythmias were more common in the control group than in patients who received PGI$_2$.

In London 132 patients were randomized to either PGI$_2$ (4 ng/kg/min) or placebo infusion for 36 hours after PTCA. Patients were followed for 6 months and then restudied. No benefit was seen in the prevention of restenosis (defined as a loss of 50% of the gain achieved at PTCA).[98]

Ciprostene.—Ciprostene is a chemically stable analogue of PGI$_2$. To study the effect of ciprostene during PTCA, 311 patients were randomized shortly before PTCA (40 ng/kg/min) to ciprostene until 48 hours after PTCA (120 ng/kg/day) or to placebo. Acute closure occurred in 3 patients in the placebo group and none in the ciprostene-treated group. Restenosis, defined as a diameter stenosis of 50% or more at the time of follow-up angiography, was present in 52 of the 126 patients (41%) treated with ciprostene and in 65 of the 122 patients (53%) in the placebo group. The clinical end points of this trial included death, myocardial infarction, re-PTCA, or CABG. In 30 of the 149 patients (20%) treated with ciprostene, one of these clinical end points was observed as compared with 55 of the 147 patients (33%) in the placebo group. Although the clinical results favored ciprostene, there was no effect on the incidence of angiographic restenosis.[99]

Prostaglandin E₁

Since the deposition of platelets postangioplasty in porcine carotid arteries was reduced significantly more after infusion with prostaglandin E₁ (PGE₁) than with PGI₂ or dipyridamole, a study was attempted to determine the effect of intracoronary followed by intravenous PGE₁ on restenosis. Eighty patients were randomized to an infusion of 20 to 40 ng/kg/min 12 hours before PTCA or to placebo. Clinical follow-up showed abrupt occlusion in 3 of 40 patients in the placebo group as compared with none in the PGE₁ group. An additional re-PTCA was necessary in 4 of 40 vs. none in the PGE₁-treated group. No angiographic study has assessed the effect of PGE₁ on restenosis.[132]

New Anticoagulant and/or Antiplatelet Drugs.—

With the use of a new infusion balloon catheter the effect of local delivery of a new potent *antithrombin* agent on platelet deposition was tested at the site of balloon angioplasty in an ex vivo whole-artery perfusion model.[65] Platelet deposition was significantly reduced with the use of this new antithrombin agent vs. the control model.

Antiplatelet GPIIb/IIIa (7E3) antibody appears to be safe during PTCA with inhibition of platelet functions in a dose-response fashion and may be useful in preventing abrupt closure and possible restenosis.[52, 133]

Ridogrel is a new antiplatelet drug that eliminates almost all TXB₂ with a concomitant increase in 6-keto-PGF₁ₐ in serum. It was tested recently in combination with heparin in a PTCA setting. It appeared to be safe, and further studies seems to be warranted to study its effectiveness in preventing early and late restenosis.[134]

These new drugs need to be tested further to determine their efficacy in the treatment of patients during and after coronary angioplasty and for the prevention of restenosis.

Antiproliferative Drugs

Platelet-Derived Growth Factor Antagonist

Proliferation of vascular smooth muscle cells occurs during the development of atherosclerosis and is frequently observed in restenosis patients after coronary angioplasty. One of the possible signals that initiate abnormal growth is PDGF. Smooth muscle cells from dis-

eased human arteries are known to secrete mitogenic activity, and these cells express the gene for the PDGF A-chain selectively. In this way it could play an important role in the development of restenosis.[135–137]

Trapidil (triazolopyrimidine) has been shown to inhibit both cellular proliferation induced by PDGF in cell culture and intimal thickening in damaged carotid arteries. In an atherosclerotic model, rabbits were assigned to (1) placebo ($n = 8$) or (2) trapidil (60 mg/kg/day) ($n = 9$). The medication was started 2 days before balloon dilatation of the external iliac artery and continued for 4 weeks. Follow-up angiography showed a greater luminal reduction in the control group than in the trapidil-treated group ($P < .001$) with similar baseline values. Histology showed significantly less intimal hyperplasia in the trapidil-treated group vs. placebo.[66]

Okamoto et al. randomized 64 patients to trapidil (600 mg/day, started 1 week before PTCA and until 6 months after PTCA) or to ASA (300 mg/day) and dipyridamole (150 mg/day). Restenosis (defined as a loss of 50% of the initial gain) occurred in 6 of 30 patients in the trapidil-treated group and in 11 of 34 patients in the control group. Thus trapidil was shown to be effective in preventing restenosis after PTCA in this small group of patients.[100]

Serotonin Antagonist

Serotonin, like PDGF, is released during platelet degranulation at the time of vessel injury and appears to directly stimulate smooth muscle cell proliferation in addition to potentiating the effects of PDGF.[138] Therefore, the administration of a serotonin antagonist such as ketanserin may inhibit smooth muscle cell proliferation.

Klein et al.[101] looked at the effect of ketanserin on the incidence of early and late restenosis. Ketanserin was administered intravenously (0.1 mg/min) for 24 hours after PTCA to 21 patients (control group). After 24 hours, 3 patients in the placebo group had an occlusion vs. none in the control group. Follow-up angiography 4 to 6 months later showed no difference in restenosis rate: 29% in the placebo group and 33% in the ketanserin-treated group.

A large multicenter interventional trial (Post-Angioplasty Restenosis Ketanserin [PARK]) with ketanserin has recruited more than 600 patients to elucidate the question of whether a longer administration (6 months) has a beneficial effect on the incidence of restenosis. This study was negative.

Colchicine

Colchicine inhibits the proliferation and migration of smooth muscle cells and the release of chemotactants by leukocytes.[67] To study the effect of colchicine on restenosis, atherosclerotic rabbits with >50% diameter stenosis underwent iliac transluminal angioplasty. Colchicine was started 2 days before transluminal angioplasty (0.02 mg/day or 0.2 mg/day) until follow-up angiography at 4 weeks. The high-dose colchicine significantly decreased the diameter stenosis at follow-up, although no effect was seen with the low dose.

O'Keefe et al. randomized 197 patients (2:1) to colchicine, 1.2 mg/day, vs. placebo within 24 hours of PTCA until 6-month follow-up angiography. Due to side effects (diarrhea, dyspepsia), there was a 6.6% dropout of colchicine-treated patients. The restenosis lesion rate (defined as a return to >70% stenosis and loss of 50% of the initial gain) was 22% in both groups. Thus colchicine seems to be ineffective for the prevention of restenosis after PTCA.[102]

Cytostatic Agents

After the disruptive action of balloon dilatation a change in differentiation of smooth muscle cells (with a shift from the contractile to synthetic phenotype) is observed and accompanied by cell proliferation and extracellular matrix production, which is the basis for the restenosis process. Barath et al.[68] have hypothesized that cytostatic agents may prevent restenosis by selective injury to active and proliferating smooth muscle cells without damaging the normal smooth muscle cells. In their study rabbits were divided into four groups: the first group was a control group, the second group had only a balloon dilatation of the aorta, the third group received the cytostatic agents (vincristine, 0.075 mg/kg, and actinomycin D, 0.015 mg/kg), and the fourth group had balloon dilatation and cytostatic agents. All rabbits were sacrificed 3 days later. Electron microscopy revealed that the cytostatic agents prevented smooth muscle cell proliferation without damaging the "normal" smooth muscle cells. The principal concern about these agents is the potential for serious side effects because they are capable of damaging other rapidly dividing cells, e.g., gastrointestinal tract, bone marrow, and the reproductive system.

Müller et al.[69] used an infusion balloon catheter with methotrexate for local delivery in carotid arteries following balloon angioplasty in 10 Yucatan minipigs. No difference was observed in intimal proliferation in the animals treated with methotrexate or with placebo.

Murphy et al.[70] used methotrexate (1.25 mg 5 days per week or 20 mg intramuscularly or azathioprine (25 mg/day) in porcine coronary arteries where stenoses were created by implantation of oversized metallic coils. They found no difference in stenosis size (measured by histology) in the different groups.

As yet, there seems to be no role for cytostatic agents in the prevention of restenosis.

Angiotensin-Converting Enzyme Inhibitors

Several organs contain local ACE systems.[139] It appears that both the production of angiotensin II and its interaction with specific angiotensin II receptors (e.g., on medial smooth muscle cells) occur in these tissues apparently independently of the plasma renin-angiotensin system.[139] In the hypertensive rat model the formation of a neointima (smooth muscle cell proliferation) in aging rats is accelerated, and ACE inhibition can reduce medial hypertrophy.[140] It has been postulated that the local ACE system also plays an important role in the remodeling process after arterial injury.[71] There is also evidence to support the role of angiotensin II as a mitogen responsible for intimal hyperplasia after PTCA.[141] In rats, neointima formation was reduced by 80% 14 days after balloon dilatation of the left carotid artery when an ACE inhibitor was given either 6 days before or 1 hour before or 2 days after angioplasty and continued until 14 days after angioplasty. This effect seems to be dose dependent and is synergistic with the heparin effect. There was no effect with the administration of a single dose or when it was stopped 2 days after balloon dilatation.[71] Further study has shown that captopril (100 mg/kg/day) also reduces intimal hyperplasia to almost the same extent. Two other vasodilators, verapamil and hydrazaline, demonstrated a lesser effect.[72] These results indicate that hemodynamic effects on the vascular wall may influence the formation of intimal hyperplasia after balloon catheterization and that ACE inhibitors may reduce intimal hyperplasia through additional mechanisms related to inhibition of the angiotensin system. However Lam et al. found no effect on atherosclerotic changes after balloon angiography of the carotid artery in 3-months-old pigs despite adequate plasma ACE activity inhibition.[73]

In contrast Bilazarian et al. showed in a hypercholesterolemic rabbit atherosclerotic model of balloon angioplasty that cilazapril started 1 week prior to angioplasty of the iliac artery until final angiography gave less reduction in diameter when compared with the placebo group.[74]

Brozovich et al.[142] retrospectively analyzed the records of 322 patients with successful angioplasty and separated them into two groups: 36 patients with a drug regimen including ACE inhibition (hypertension or heart failure) and 286 with a drug regimen without ACE inhibition. Restenosis (defined as a return of the symptoms of angina with significant stenosis on the angiogram) occurred in 30% in the patients without ACE inhibition vs. 3% in the group with ACE inhibition. Thus it appears that inhibition of ACE may significantly reduce the incidence of restenosis after successful PTCA.

Currently, a large multicenter randomized trial in Europe (Multicenter European Research Trial with Cilazapril after Angioplasty to prevent Transluminal coronary Obstruction and Restenosis [MERCATOR]) has been completed to determine the effect of cilazapril on the incidence of restenosis. More than 700 patients have been randomized to cilazapril or placebo starting 4 to 6 hours after PTCA in addition to the standard therapy of 160 to 250 mg of ASA. After 6 months (or earlier if indicated by symptoms) a follow-up angiogram is performed. A similarly designed trial (MARCATOR) has recruited more than 1,000 patients in the United States and Canada but uses a different dosage schedule. Preliminary results are the same with both trials, showing no benefit in reducing restenosis.

Angiopeptin

It has been known for a long time that hypophysectomy inhibits neointimal (plaque) formation in response to endothelial injury.[143] This suggests that an endocrine factor may be involved in neointima formation. Insulin-like growth factor (IGF-1; somatomedin C) has been shown to be involved in the repair of the intima in injured arteries. Besides that, like PDGF, it is a potent mitogen for porcine aortic smooth muscle cells, and when added together to quiescent cultures, their effects are synergistic.[144, 145] Recently the effect of a newly synthesized class of pituitary growth hormone–inhibiting agents has been investigated on vascular smooth muscle cell hyperplasia following endothelial cell injury in vivo. These compounds are peptide analogues of somatostatin, have a high affinity for somatostatin receptors on pituitary cells, and inhibit pituitary growth hormone release. One of these agents, angiopeptin, was shown to inhibit vascular smooth muscle cell proliferation in response to a variety of vascular injuries. This seems to be due to a local effect directly on smooth muscle cells.[75] This new group of agents is currently undergoing investigation as an inhibitor of several variants of "accelerated atherosclerosis" (after angioplasty, cardiac transplantation, and coronary bypass surgery).

Conte et al.[76] showed that angiopeptin (20 μg/kg/day) given 1 day before injury to the iliac artery and aorta for 2, 6, or 21 days in male rabbits significantly reduces intimal thickness. Thus angiopeptin acts on an early mechanism of hyperplasia.

In the United States and in Scandanavian countries trials with angiopeptin are currently under way and will answer the question of whether it is effective in the prevention of restenosis.

New Antiproliferative Drugs.—Using a Wolinsky porous infusion catheter, Wilensky et al. injected a solution of a *thiol protease inhibitor (TPI)* into atherosclerotic rabbit femoral arteries immediately following angioplasty to evaluate the effect on restenosis. They found a smaller reduction in minimal luminal diameter after 2 weeks in the TPI-treated group than in the control group. They hypothesized that the process of vascular remodeling after angioplasty is significantly modified by TPI.[77]

Betz et al. used a *calcium-calmodulin antagonist* and found it to be effective in inhibiting smooth muscle cell proliferation after application of artherogenic stimuli in a dose-dependent manner. The results suggest that these new drugs could be used for inhibiting stenosis of intimal proliferation.[146]

Calcium Antagonist

Coronary spasm is frequently seen during and shortly after PTCA and may have a role in the pathogenesis of restenosis.[147] Calcium antagonists may reduce restenosis by inhibiting vasospasm. In an animal model[78] and in three randomized trials[103–105] calcium antagonists have not been shown to influence the incidence of restenosis. However, verapamil was shown to be effective in patients with stable angina pectoris.[106] Besides this, nifidepine and nicardipine are effective in progression/regression trials, so there may still be a role for calcium antagonists in preventing restenosis or the development of new atherosclerotic lesions.[148, 149]

Diltiazem

In a study from the Montreal Heart Institute,[103] 92 patients received diltiazem (270 mg) for 3 months, and all underwent recatherization 5 to 10 months after balloon angioplasty or earlier if symptoms returned. All patients also received ASA (650 mg) and dipyridamole (225 mg) for 6 months. Patients treated with diltiazem had a restenosis rate of 15% vs. 22% of the patients without diltiazem (restenosis was defined as a stenosis of 70% or more at the time of the follow-up angiography). The average decrease in diameter during follow-up was 4% in the diltiazem-treated group and 7% in the control group. It was concluded that diltiazem had no effect on restenosis and that coronary spasm is not a major mechanism of restenosis.

In a recently reported trial of O'Keefe et al.[104] a total of 201 patients were randomized to high-dose diltiazem (started 1 day before PTCA at a mean dose 329 mg/day) or to placebo to evaluate its usefulness in patients who undergo PTCA. Repeat angiography at 1 year was obtained in 60% of the patients. Restenosis was assessed by quantitative angiographic techniques and was defined as a return to $\geq 70\%$ of the luminal area stenosis and a loss $\geq 50\%$ of the initial gain with angioplasty. No difference in procedural complications (6 of 102 patients in the diltiazem-treated group and 8 of the 99 patients in the placebo group) or restenosis rate (36% vs. 30%) could be observed.

Nifedipine

In a 6 month follow-up trial at Emory University in Atlanta[105] 241 patients were randomized to either nifedipine (40 mg/day) or placebo. All patients also received ASA (325 mg/day). Restenosis was defined as a loss of more than 50% of the gain achieved at the time of the PTCA. In patients who were compliant and underwent follow-up angiography (84 patients in both groups) there was no difference in restenosis: 29% in the nifedipine-treated group and 33% in the placebo group.

Verapamil

Recently a trial of 196 patients randomized to verapamil (480 mg/day) in combination with ASA (660 mg/day) and dipyridamole (150 mg/day) or the combination without verapamil showed that a high dose of verapamil prevents restenosis (defined as a loss of 50% of the initial gain) after successful PTCA in stable patients.[106] No difference was found in the group with unstable angina before PTCA.

Lipid-Lowering Drugs

Fish Oils

Epidemiologic trials have shown that a diet rich in (n-3) polyunsaturated fatty acids (present in high concentrations in most saltwater fish) may account for the low incidence of coronary disease seen in Eskimos. Animal research has shown that these polyunsaturated fatty acids inhibit atherosclerosis in general. This can be partly explained through a lowering of serum lipid concentrations and decreased aggregation of platelets by altering the balance between PGI_2 and thromboxane, although many other effects of fish oil fatty acids has been described.[150] In the last few years several trials have studied the effect of n-3 fatty acids in the prevention of restenosis after PTCA.

Slack et al.[107] showed that adding 2.4 g of fish oil each day (rich in eicosapentanoic acid [EPA] to the usual post-PTCA regimen of calcium channel blocker, nitrates, ASA, and dipyridamole could reduce the incidence of clinical restenosis in patients with single-vessel disease (33% in the placebo group vs. 16% in the fish oil–treated group). In 49 patients with multivessel disease, no influence could be shown.

Reis et al.[108] showed that supplementing the normal diet with 6.0 g of fish oil daily starting just before the PTCA until 6 months later had no influence on the restenosis rate in 186 patients with successful PTCA. Angiographic restenosis (70% diameter stenosis at a site previously dilated to less than 50%) was present in 34% of the fish oil–treated group and 23% of the control group. However, repeat angiography was performed in only 68 patients (37%); almost all patients had recurrence of chest pain, which contributed to a selection bias in follow-up angiography.

Milner et al.[109] found that adding of 4.5 g of fish oil each day to a normal diet of 194 patients had a positive influence on clinical restenosis, with 19% (16 of the 84 patients) in the fish oil–treated group vs. 35% (35 of the 99 patients) in the placebo group experiencing a return of chest pain. However, in the first week, 11 of the 95 patients stopped taking the medication because of side effects.

In Dallas[110] 82 patients were randomized to ASA and dipyridamole with and without 3,200 mg (18 capsules!) EPA. Treatment was started 7 days before PTCA and was stopped 6 months after PTCA. In all 82 patients a second angiogram (on average 3 to 4 months after PTCA) was performed. Restenosis was defined as 50% or more narrowing of the dilatation site at follow-up angiography. Restenosis was seen in 36% in the placebo group and 16% in the treatment group. This trial suggests that n-3 fatty acids may effectively reduce restenosis in high-risk patients provided that they are compliant and are pretreated starting 7 days before PTCA.

In Melbourne[111] 108 patients were randomized to 10 capsules of fish oil or placebo. Medication was started the day before angioplasty and continued until 4 months after angioplasty. All patients also received ASA and verapamil. Restenosis was defined as a loss of >50% of the gain in luminal diameter at angioplasty (using caliper measurement). No difference in angiographically defined restenosis was observed: 34% in the fish oil–treated group vs. 33% in the control group.

It is clear that a consensus cannot be reached. These conclusions are in part related to differences in the design of the individual studies. Although all studies were randomized, only in two studies were patients and investigators blinded to n-3 supplementation. Different dosages and formulations were used, and patient compliance varied in the studies. There were also differences in the timing of initiation of therapy and variable methods (coronary angiography, stress test, symptoms) for the detection of restenosis.

To come to a final conclusion about the effect of fish oil in the prevention of restenosis after PTCA, the National Institutes of Health has just started a trial.

Cholesterol-Lowering Drugs

Hypercholesterolemia is a well-known risk factor for ischemic heart disease. Lipid modification is an important goal in secondary prevention in halting the progression of atherosclerosis in general. Also, there seems to be a relationship between the cholesterol/high-density lipoprotein (HDL) cholesterol ratio post-PTCA and the risk for restenosis.[151]

Recently it was shown that lovastatin reduces intimal hyperplasia following balloon angioplasty in hypercholesterolemic rabbits.[79] However, two trials in postangioplasty patients in which the effect of lipid lowering on the incidence of restenosis[112, 152] after PTCA was tested gave conflicting results.

In the first trial[112] 157 patients were randomized to lovastatin or to placebo for an unstated period of time. Only 50% of the patients had follow-up angiography at an average of 4 months after the PTCA (50 patients in the lovastatin-treated group and 29 patients in the follow-up group). Restenosis was defined as a narrowing of 50% or more at follow-up angiography. Restenosis was seen in 14% of the sites in the lovastatin-treated group and 47% in the placebo group, which suggests a beneficial effect of lovastatin in this selected group.

In the second trial,[152] aggressive treatment was used in 55 consecutive patients to lower the cholesterol level, including diet, colestipol, and lovastatin starting the day of PTCA. After 2 weeks cholesterol was reduced 50%. To date, 44 of the 45 patients have been restudied, with a restenosis rate of 34%. There was no difference in cholesterol levels between patients with and without restenosis.

Inhibitors of Inflammation

Corticosteroids

Corticosteroids have been suggested as a potential restenosis inhibitor.[153] Hydrocortisone is able to inhibit vascular smooth muscle growth in culture.[58] However, in a randomized trial where patients received placebo or corticosteroids from 48 hours before until 5 days after PTCA, there was no difference in restenosis (in both groups, 33%).[113] The same result was achieved when steroids were given as treatment for 102 patients with restenosis after PTCA.[114] Besides ASA, dipyridamole, and a calcium antagonist, patients received 125 mg methylprednisolone intramuscularly 1 day before the re-PTCA and 240 mg prednisone for 1 week. Only the 54 patients with follow-up angiography were analyzed. Restenosis was defined as a >50% diameter narrowing at the site. Restenosis was found in 36% of the steroid-treated group as compared with 40% in the standard treatment group.

In a recent multicenter trial in the United States[115] 850 patients were randomized to methylprednisolone or to placebo 2 to 24 hours before PTCA. In 71% of the patients follow-up angiography was performed. There was no difference between the two groups in the incidence of restenosis (defined as >50% diameter stenosis): 40% in the methylprednisolone-treated group vs. 39% of the patients in the placebo group.

These trials showed that the administration of corticosteroids has no influence on the incidence of restenosis.

Nonsteroidal Anti-inflammatory Drugs

Ibuprofen is known to decrease platelet-thrombus deposition in Gore-tex arterial grafts. In a study of normal porcine common carotid arteries pretreated with heparin, balloon angioplasty was performed and followed by a bolus (12.5 mg/kg) and infusion (75 to 100 μg/kg/min) of ibuprofen or placebo. Quantitative ^{111}In-labeled autologous platelet deposition at the site of angioplasty was significantly reduced by ibuprofen.[154] Whether this will affect the risk of late restenosis is unknown.

FUTURE DIRECTIONS

Molecular biology has provided us with detailed information about an important family of "peptide cell regulators factors" (PRF).[136, 137, 155–158] Although it seems to be far away from the bedside of the patient, this "new family" could lead to drugs that prevent restenosis after PTCA. In recent years it has become clear that cell proliferation and differentiation are controlled by many peptides and other agents through their interactions with cell surface receptors that send signals to the cell interior. Among the important signals that have been implicated in these processes are the phosphorylation of tyrosine residues on proteins and changes in the intracellular concentrations of the messenger molecules cAMP, diacylglycerol, inositol-1,4,5-triphosphate (IP3), and Ca^{2+}, which directly or indirectly exert most of their regulation on the phosphorylation and dephosphorylation of serine and threonine residues of particular proteins.[155]

Recent studies have demonstrated that mitogens such as PDGF and thrombin rapidly induce the hydrolysis of phosphatidylinositol biphosphate (PIP2) by phospholipase C and result in the formation of IP3 and diacylglycerol.[155]

IP3 mobilizes Ca^{2+} from intracellular calcium stores, and diacylglycerol stimulates protein kinase C activity. These signaling pathways have been considered to play

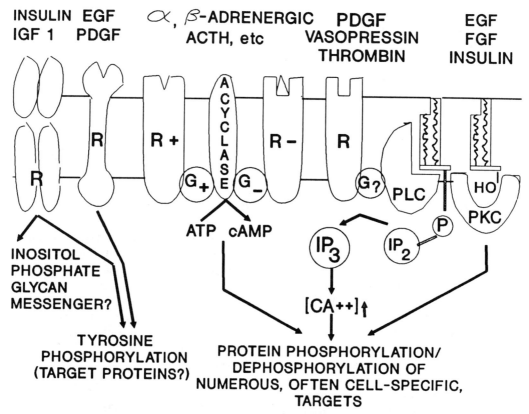

FIG 49–4.
See the text for an explanation.

important roles in cellular response. Unfortunately, it is not the sole signal transduction system. Other factors such as fibroblast growth factor (FGF), EGF, and insulin generate other signals independent of PIP2 hydrolysis.

A Japanese group has developed a monoclonal antibody against PIP2. Microintracellular injection of the antibody into the transformed cells causes a reversible and dose-dependent decrease in DNA synthesis and in the rate of cell proliferation and reverted the cell morphology to that of the untransformed cells, the normal phenotype. As predicted from the proposed scheme for growth factor transduction, microinjection and overproduction of phospholipase C or protein kinase C also can substitute for exogenous mitogens, whereas antibody to 1.4 inositol diphosphate or protein kinase C prevents proliferation (Fig 49–4). Thus, development and local release of new agents that inhibit inositolphospholipid metabolism may be useful for the treatment of human restenosis.

FUTURE DEVELOPMENTS

Despite 13 years of clinical experience and research in the field of restenosis after PTCA, there has been no major breakthrough in pharmacologic interventions. Besides that, assessment of the value of drug trials that have been performed in the past is extremely difficult because of differences in the selection of patients, methods of analysis, and the definition of restenosis. Recently our group has reviewed the influence of these three factors on the outcome and conclusion of restenosis studies.[159] Although there is no scientific proof that the tested drugs are effective, many clinicians continue to prescribe them to "prevent restenosis."

However, some positive results in selected patients have been reported by the use of fish oil, trapidil, and verapamil in postangioplasty patients. In addition, we seem to have found an animal model that more closely mimics the restenotic lesion of the patient.[120] In the near future the results will be known of ongoing multicenter trials with ACE inhibition, serotonin antagonist, hirudin, LMWH, angiopeptin, and other promising drugs such as inhibitors of thrombin production, growth factor blockers, PGI_2 analogues, and monoclonal antibodies against the platelet membrane receptors (GPIIb/IIIa) and the von Willebrand factor, and the outcome of these trials may bring us closer to solving the restenosis problem.

CONCLUSION

Clinical and experimental research must continue to look for the elusive *"magic bullet"* that can prevent aggregation of thrombocytes, prevent spasm, prevent proliferation of smooth muscle cells, and prevent atherosclerosis without any side effects and, if possible, in only 1 tablet! Moreover, the cost of this potential drug solution must be less expensive than repeating PTCA in 30% of all patients. It is clear that this magic drug has not been found, and in the meantime we will continue (re)dilating while we search for a pharmacologic or technical solution for the restenosis problem.

Acknowledgment

We thank E. Murphy, M.D., and B. Strauss, M.D., for their critical comments and corrections.

REFERENCES

1. Waller BF: Crackers, breakers, stretchers, drillers, scrapers, shavers, burners, welders and melters. The future treatment of atherosclerotic coronary artery disease? A clinical-morphologic assessment. *J Am Coll Cardiol* 1989; 13:969–987.
2. McBride W, Lange RA, Hillis LD: Restenosis after successful coronary angioplasty. Pathophysiology and prevention. *N Engl J Med* 1988; 318:1734–1737.
3. Serruys PW, Luijten HE, Beatt KJ, et al: Incidence of restenosis after successful coronary angioplasty: A time-related phenomenon. A quantitative angiographic study in 342 consecutive patients at 1, 2, 3 and 4 months. *Circulation* 1988; 77:361–371.
4. Nobuyoshi M, Kimura H, Nosaka H, et al: Restenosis after successful percutaneous transluminal coronary angioplasty: Serial angiographic follow-up of 299 patients. *J Am Coll Cardiol* 1988; 12:616–623.
5. Holmes DR, Vlietstra RE, Smith HC, et al: Restenosis after percutaneous transluminal coronary angioplasty (PTCA): A report from the PTCA Registry of the National Heart, Lung, and Blood Institute. *Am J Cardiol* 1984; 53:77–81.
6. Kaltenbach M, Kober G, Scherer D, et al: Recurrence rate after successful coronary angioplasty. *Eur Heart J* 1985; 6:276–281.
7. Scholl JM, David PR, Chaitman BR, et al: Recurrence of stenosis following percutaneous transluminal coronary angioplasty (abstract). *Circulation* 1981; 64(suppl 4):193.
8. Dangoisse V, Guiteras Val, David PR, et al: Recurrence of stenosis after successful percutaneous transluminal coronary angioplasty (PTCA) (abstract). *Circulation* 1982; 66(suppl 2):331.
9. David PR, Renkin J, Moise A, et al: Can patient selection and optimization of technique reduce the rate of restenosis after percutaneous transluminal coronary angioplasty (abstract). *J Am Coll Cardiol* 1984; 3:470.
10. Dorros G, Johnson WD, Tector AJ, et al: Percutaneous transluminal coronary angioplasty in patients with prior coronary artery bypass grafting. *J Thorac Cardiovasc Surg* 1984; 87:17–26.
11. Marantz T, Williams DO, Reinert S, et al: Predictors of restenosis after successful coronary angioplasty (abstract). *Circulation* 1984; 70(suppl 2):176.
12. Margolis JR, Krieger R, Glemser E: Coronary angioplasty: Increased restenosis rate in insulin dependent diabetics (abstract). *Circulation* 1984; 70(suppl 2):175.
13. Schmitz HJ, von Essen R, Meyer J, et al: The role of balloon size for acute and late angiographic results in coronary angioplasty (abstract). *Circulation* 1984; 70 (suppl 2):295.
14. Levine S, Ewels CJ, Rosing DR, et al: Coronary angioplasty: Clinical and angiographic follow-up. *Am J Cardiol* 1985; 55:673–676.
15. Mata LA, Bosch X, David PR, et al: Clinical and angiographic assessment 6 months after double vessel percutaneous coronary angioplasty. *J Am Coll Cardiol* 1985; 6:1239–1244.
16. Probst P, Zangl W, Pachinger O: Relation of coronary arterial occlusion pressure during percutaneous transluminal coronary angioplasty to presence of collaterals. *Am J Cardiol* 1985; 55:1264–1269.
17. Serruys PW, Umans V, Heyndrickx GR, et al: Elective PTCA of totally occluded coronary arteries not associated with acute myocardial infarction; short-term and long-term results. *Eur Heart J* 1985; 6:2–12.
18. Bertrand ME, LaBlanche JM, Thieuleux FA, et al: Comparative results of percutaneous transluminal coronary angioplasty in patients with dynamic versus fixed coronary stenosis. *J Am Coll Cardiol* 1986; 8:504–508.
19. Clark DA, Wexman MP, Murphy MC, et al: Factors predicting recurrence in patients who have had angioplasty [PTCA] of totally occluded vessels (abstract). *J Am Coll Cardiol* 1986; 7(suppl A):20.
20. Hollman J, Galan K, Franco I, et al: Recurrent stenosis after coronary angioplasty (abstract). *J Am Coll Cardiol* 1986; 7(suppl A):20.
21. Leimgruber PP, Roubin GS, Hollman J, et al: Restenosis after successful coronary angioplasty in patients with single-vessel disease. *Circulation* 1986; 73:710–717.
22. Powelson S, Roubin G, Whitworth H, et al: Incidence of early restenosis after successful percutaneous transluminal coronary angioplasty (PTCA) (abstract). *J Am Coll Cardiol* 1986; 7:63.
23. Roubin G, Redd D, Leimgruber P, et al: Restenosis after multilesion and multivessel coronary angioplasty (PTCA) (abstract). *J Am Coll Cardiol* 1986; 7(suppl A):22.
24. Uebis R, von Essen R, vorn Dahl J, et al: Recurrence rate after PTCA in relationship to the initial length of coronary artery narrowing (abstract). *J Am Coll Cardiol* 1986; 7(suppl A):62.
25. Hirshfeld JW Jr, Goldberg S, MacDonald R, et al: Lesion and procedure-related variables predictive of restenosis after PTCA – a report from the M-HEART Study (abstract). *Circulation* 1986; 76(suppl 4):215.
26. Guiteras P, Masotti M, Crexells C, et al: Determinants of restenosis after successful percutaneous transluminal coronary angioplasty (PTCA) (abstract). *Eur Heart J* 1987; 8(suppl 2):247.
27. Myler RK, Topol EJ, Shaw RE, et al: Multiple vessel coronary angioplasty: Classification, results and patterns

of restenosis in 494 consecutive patients. *Cathet Cardio-vasc Diagn* 1987; 13:1–15.

28. Rapold HJ, David PR, Guiteras VP, et al: Restenosis and its determinants in first and repeat coronary angioplasty. *Eur Heart J* 1987; 8:575–586.

29. Simonton CA, Mark DB, Hinohara T, et al: Restenosis following successful coronary angioplasty: A multivariable analysis of patient, procedure and coronary lesion-related risk factors (abstract). *J Am Coll Cardiol* 1987; 9:184.

30. Urban P, Meier B, Finci L, et al: Coronary wedge pressure in relation to spontaneously visible and recruitable collaterals. *Circulation* 1987; 75:906–913.

31. Vandormael MG, Deligonul U, Kern M, et al: Multilesion coronary angioplasty: Clinical and angiographic follow-up. *J Am Coll Cardiol* 1987; 10:246–252.

32. De Feyter PJ, Suryapranata H, Serruys PW, et al: Coronary angioplasty for unstable angina: Immediate and late results in 200 consecutive patients with identification of risk factors for unfavorable early and late outcome. *J Am Coll Cardiol* 1988; 12:324–333.

33. Galan KM, Deligonul U, Kern MJ, et al: Increased frequency of restenosis in patients continuing to smoke cigarettes after percutaneous transluminal coronary angioplasty. *Am J Cardiol* 1988; 61:260–263.

34. Lambert M, Bonan R, Cote G, et al: Multiple coronary angioplasty: A model to discriminate systemic and procedural factors related to restenosis. *J Am Coll Cardiol* 1988; 12:310–314.

35. Weinstein JS, Baim DS, Sipperly ME, et al: Salvage of branch vessels during bifurcation lesion angioplasty: Acute and long-term follow-up (abstract). *Circulation* 1988; 78(suppl 2):632.

36. Bertrand ME, LaBlanche JM, Fourrier JL, et al: Relation to restenosis after percutaneous transluminal coronary angioplasty to vasomotion of the dilated coronary arterial segment. *Am J Cardiol* 1989; 63:277–281.

37. Ellis SG, Roubin GS, King SB, et al: Importance of stenosis morphology in the estimation of restenosis risk after elective percutaneous transluminal coronary angioplasty. *Am J Cardiol* 1989; 63:30–34.

38. Uebis R, Schmitz E, vom Dahl J, et al: Single versus multiple balloon inflations in coronary angioplasty: Late angiographic results and recurrence (abstract). *J Am Coll Cardiol* 1989; 13:58.

39. Renkin J, Melin J, Robert A, et al: Detection of restenosis after successful coronary angioplasty: Improved clinical decision making with use of a logistic model combining procedural and follow-up variables. *J Am Coll Cardiol* 1990; 16:1333–1340.

40. Rupprecht HJ, Brenneke R, Bernhard G, et al: Analysis of risk factors for restenosis after PTCA. *Cathet Cardiovasc Diagn* 1990; 19:151–159.

41. Serruys PW, Strauss BH, Beatt KJ, et al: Angiographic follow-up after placement of a self-expanding coronary artery stent. *N Engl J Med* 1991; 324:13–17.

42. Margolis JR, Krauthamer D, Litvack F, et al: Six month follow-up of excimer laser coronary angioplasty registry patients (abstract). *J Am Coll Cardiol* 1991; 17:218.

43. Buchbinder M, Warth D, O'Neill W, et al: Multi-Center registry of percutaneous coronary rotational ablation using the rotablator (abstract). *J Am Coll Cardiol* 1991; 17:31.

44. Simpson JB, Baim DS, Hinohara T, et al: Restenosis of de novo lesions in native coronary arteries following directional coronary atherectomy: Multicenter experience (abstract). *J Am Coll Cardiol* 1991; 17:346.

45. Essed CE, van den Brand M, Becker AE: Transluminal coronary angioplasty and early restenosis: Fibrocellular occlusion after wall laceration. *Br Heart J* 1983; 49:393–396.

46. Austin GE, Ratliff NB, Hollman J, et al: Intimal proliferation of smooth muscle cells as an explanation for recurrent coronary artery stenosis after percutaneous transluminal angioplasty. *J Am Coll Cardiol* 1985; 6:369–375.

47. Nobuyoshi M, Kimura T, Ohishi H, et al: Restenosis after percutaneous transluminal coronary angioplasty: Pathologic observations in 20 patients. *J Am Coll Cardiol* 1991; 17:433–439.

48. Johnson DE, Hinohara T, Selmon MR, et al: Primary peripheral arterial stenoses excised by transluminal atherectomy: A histopathologic study. *J Am Coll Cardiol* 1990; 15:419–425.

49. Safian RD, Gelbfish JS, Erny RE, et al: Coronary atherectomy. Clinical, angiographic, and histological findings and observations regarding potential mechanisms. *Circulation* 1990; 82:69–79.

50. Garett KN, Holmes DR, Bell MR, et al: Restenosis after directional coronary atherectomy: Differences between primary atheromatous and restenosis lesions and influence of subintimal tissue resection. *J Am Coll Cardiol* 1990; 16:1665–1671.

51. Stein B, Fuster V, Israel DH, et al: Platelet inhibitor agents in cardiovascular disease: An update. *J Am Coll Cardiol* 1989; 14:813–836.

52. Coller BS: Platelets and thrombolytic therapy. *N Engl J Med* 1990; 322:33–42.

53. Clowes AW, Schwartz SM: Significance of quiescent smooth muscle migration in the injured rat carotid artery. *Circ Res* 1985; 56:139–145.

54. Ross R: The pathogenesis of atherosclerosis — an update. *N Engl J Med* 1986; 314:488–500.

55. Liu MW, Roubin GS, King SB III: Restenosis after coronary angioplasty. Potential biologic determinants and role of intimal hyperplasia. *Circulation* 1989; 79:1374–1387.

56. Forrester JS, Fishbein M, Helfant R, et al: A paradigm for restenosis based on cell biology: Clues for the development of new preventive therapies. *J Am Coll Cardiol* 1991; 17:758–769.

57. Clowes AW, Karnowsky MJ: Suppression by heparin of smooth muscle cell proliferation in injured arteries. *Nature* 1977; 265:625–626.

58. Gordon JB, Berk BC, Bettmann MA, et al: Vascular smooth muscle proliferation following balloon injury is synergistically inhibited by low molecular weight heparin and hydrocortisone (abstract). *Circulation* 1987; 76(suppl 4):213.

59. Pow TK, Currier JW, Minihan AC, et al: Low molecular weight heparin reduces restenosis after experimental angioplasty (abstract). *Circulation* 1989; 80(suppl 2):64.

60. Oberhoff M, Hanke H, Hanke S, et al: Experimental balloon angioplasty: Inhibition of intimal smooth muscle cell proliferation by low molecular weight heparin (abstract). *Circulation* 1990; 82(suppl 3):428.

61. Heras M, Chesebro JH, Penny WJ, et al: Effects of thrombin inhibition on the development of acute platelet-thrombus deposition during angioplasty in pigs. Heparin versus recombinant hirudin, a specific thrombin inhibition. *Circulation* 1989; 79:657–665.

62. Faxon DP, Sanborn TA, Haudenschild CC, et al: Effect of antiplatelet therapy on restenosis after experimental angioplasty. *Am J Cardiol* 1984; 53:72–76.

63. Franklin SM, Currier JW, Cannistra A, et al: Warfarin/aspirin combination reduces restenosis after angioplasty in atherosclerotic rabbits (abstract). *Circulation* 1990; 82(suppl 3):427.

64. Sanborn TA, Ballelli LM, Faxon DP, et al: Inhibition of ^{51}Cr-labelled platelet accumulation after balloon angioplasty in rabbits: Comparison of heparin, aspirin, and CGS 13080, a selective thromboxane synthetase inhibitor (abstract). *J Am Coll Cardiol* 1986; 7:213.

65. Leung WH, Kaplan AV, Grant GW, et al: Local delivery of antithrombin agent reduces platelet deposition at site of balloon angioplasty (abstract). *Circulation* 1990; 82(suppl 3):428.

66. Liu MW, Roubin GS, Robinson KA, et al: Trapidil in preventing restenosis after balloon angioplasty in the atherosclerotic rabbit. *Circulation* 1990; 81:1089–1093.

67. Currier JW, Pow TK, Minihan AC, et al: Colchicine inhibits restenosis after iliac angioplasty in the atherosclerotic rabbit (abstract). *Circulation* 1989; 80(suppl 2):66.

68. Barath P, Arakawa K, Cao J, et al: Low dose of antitumor agents prevents smooth muscle cell proliferation after endothelial injury (abstract). *J Am Coll Cardiol* 1989; 13:252.

69. Müller DWM, Topol EJ, Abrams G, et al: Intramural methotrexate therapy for the prevention of intimal proliferation following porcine carotid balloon angioplasty (abstract). *Circulation* 1990; 82(suppl 3):429.

70. Murphy JG, Schwartz RS, Edwards WD, et al: Methotrexate and azathioprine fail to inhibit porcine coronary restenosis (abstract). *Circulation* 1990; 82(suppl 3):429.

71. Powell JS, Clozel JP, Müller RKM, et al: Inhibitors of angiotensin-converting enzyme prevent myointimal proliferation after vascular injury. *Science* 1989; 245:186–188.

72. Müller RKM, Kuhn H, Powell JS: Converting enzyme inhibitors reduce intimal hyperplasia after balloon catheter induced vascular injury (abstract). *Circulation* 1989; 80(suppl 2):63.

73. Lam JYT, Bourassa MG, Blaine L, et al: Can cilazapril reduce the development of atherosclerotic changes in the balloon injured porcine carotid arteries (abstract)? *Circulation* 1990; 82(suppl 3):82.

74. Bilazarian SD, Currier JW, Haudenschild C, et al: Angiotensin converting enzyme inhibition reduces restenosis in experimental angioplasty (abstract). *J Am Coll Cardiol* 1991; 17:268.

75. Foegh ML, Khirabadi BS, Chambers E, et al: Inhibition of coronary artery transplant atherosclerosis in rabbits with angiopeptin, an octapeptide. *Atherosclerosis* 1989; 78:229–236.

76. Conte J, Foegh M, Wallace R, et al: Effect of short term treatment with angiopeptin, an octapeptide, on vascular myointimal hyperplasia (abstract). *Eur Heart J* 1990; 11(suppl):127.

77. Wilensky RL, March KL, Hathaway DR: Restenosis in an atherosclerotic rabbit model is reduced by a thiol protease inhibitor (abstract). *J Am Coll Cardiol* 1991; 17:268.

78. Faxon DP, Sanborn TA, Gottsman SB, et al: The effect of nifedipine on restenosis following experimental angioplasty (abstract). *Circulation* 1984; 70(suppl 2):175.

79. Gellman J, Ezekowitz MD, Sarembock IJ, et al: Effect of lovastatin on intimal hyperplasia after balloon angioplasty: A study in an atherosclerotic hypercholesterolemic rabbit. *J Am Coll Cardiol* 1991; 17:251–259.

80. Hirshfeld JW Jr, Goldberg S, MacDonald R, et al: Lesion and procedure-related variables predictive of restenosis after PTCA — a report from the M-HEART study (abstract). *Circulation* 1987; 76(suppl 4):215.

81. Ellis SG, Roubin GS, Wilentz J, et al: Effect of 18-24 hour heparin administration for prevention of restenosis after uncomplicated coronary angioplasty. *Am Heart J* 1989; 117:777–782.

82. Lehmann K, Doris RJ, Feuer JM, et al: Paradoxical increase in restenosis rate with chronic heparin use: Final results of a randomized trial (abstract). *J Am Coll Cardiol* 1991; 17:181.

83. Thornton MA, Grüntzig AR, Hollman J, et al: Coumadin and aspirin in the prevention of recurrence after transluminal coronary angioplasty: A randomized study. *Circulation* 1984; 4:69:721–727.

84. Urban P, Buller N, Fox K, et al: Lack of effect of warfarin on the restenosis rate or on clinical outcome after balloon angioplasty. *Br Heart J* 1988; 60:485–488.

85. Dyckmans J, Thönnes W, Ozbek C, et al: High vs low dosage of acetylic salicylic acid for prevention of restenosis after successful PTCA. Preliminary results of a randomized trial (abstract). *Eur Heart J* 1988; 9(suppl):58.

86. Mufson L, Black A, Roubin G, et al: A randomized trial of aspirin in PTCA: Effect of high vs low dose aspirin on major complications and restenosis (abstract). *J Am Coll Cardiol* 1988; 11:2:236.

87. Schanzenbacher P, Grimmer M, Maisch B, et al: Effect of high dose and low dose aspirin on restenosis after primary successful angioplasty (abstract). *Circulation* 1988; 78(suppl 2):99.

88. Kadel C, Vallbracht C, Weidmann B, et al: Aspirin and restenosis after successful PTCA: Comparison of 1400 mg vs 350 mg daily in a double blind study (abstract). *Eur Heart J* 1990; 11(suppl):368.

89. Finci L, Meier B, Steffenino G, et al: Aspirin versus placebo after coronary angioplasty for prevention of restenosis (abstract). *Eur Heart J* 1988; (suppl):156.

90. Schwartz L, Bourassa MG, Lespérance J, et al: Aspirin and dipyridamole in the prevention of restenosis after percutaneous transluminal coronary angioplasty. *N Engl J Med* 1988; 318:1714–1719.

91. Chesebro JH, Webster MWI, Reeder GS, et al: Coronary angioplasty antiplatelet therapy reduces acute complications but not restenosis (abstract). *Circulation* 1989; 80(suppl 2):64.

92. White CW, Knudson M, Schmidt D, et al: Neither ticlopidine nor aspirin-dipyridamole prevents restenosis post PTCA: Results from a randomized placebo-controlled multicenter trial (abstract). *Circulation* 1987; 76(suppl 4):213.

93. Yabe Y, Okamoto K, Oosawa H, et al: Does a thromboxane A$_2$ synthetase Inhibitor prevent restenosis after PTCA (abstract). *Circulation* 1989; 80(suppl 2):260.

94. Serruys PW, Rutsch W, Heyndrickx G, et al: Effect of long term thromboxane A$_2$ receptor blockade on angiographic restenosis and clinical events after coronary angioplasty. The Carport study (abstract). *J Am Coll Cardiol* 1991; 17:283.

95. Kitazume H, Kubo I, Iwama T, et al: Combined use of aspirin, ticlopidine and nicorandil prevented restenosis after coronary angioplasty (abstract). *Circulation* 1988; 78(suppl 2):633.

96. Bertrand ME, Allain H, LaBlanche JM, et al: Results of a randomized trial of ticlopidine versus placebo for prevention of acute closure and restenosis after coronary angioplasty (PTCA). The TACT study (abstract). *Circulation* 1990; 82(suppl 3):190.

97. Knudtson ML, Flintoft VF, Roth DL, et al: Effect of short-term prostacyclin administration on restenosis after percutaneous transluminal coronary angioplasty. *J Am Coll Cardiol* 1990; 15:691–697.

98. Gershlick AH, Timmis AD, Rothman MT, et al: Post angioplasty prostacyclin infusion does not reduce the incidence of restenosis (abstract). *Circulation* 1990; 82(suppl 3):497.

99. Raizner A, Hollman J, Demke D, et al: Beneficial effects of ciprostene in PTCA: A multicenter, randomized, controlled trial (abstract). *Circulation* 1988; 78(suppl 2):290.

100. Okamoto S, Inden M, Setsuda M, et al: Trapidil (triazolopyrimidine), a platelet derived growth factor (PDGF) antagonist in preventing restenosis after percutaneous transluminal coronary angioplasty (abstract). *Circulation* 1990; 82(suppl 3):428.

101. Klein W, Eber B, Fluch N, et al: Ketanserin prevents acute occlusion but not restenosis after PTCA (abstract). *J Am Coll Cardiol* 1989; 13:44.

102. O'Keefe JH, McCallister BD, Bateman TM, et al: Colchicine for the prevention of restenosis after coronary angioplasty (abstract). *J Am Coll Cardiol* 1991; 17:181.

103. Corcos T, David PR, Val PG, et al: Failure of diltiazem to prevent restenosis after percutaneous transluminal coronary angioplasty. *Am Heart J* 1985; 109:926–931.

104. O'Keefe JH, Giorgi LV, Hartzler GO, et al: Effects of diltiazem on complications and restenosis after coronary angioplasty. *Am J Cardiol* 1991; 67:373–376.

105. Whitworth HB, Roubin GS, Hollman J, et al: Effect of nifedipine on recurrent stenosis after percutaneous transluminal coronary angioplasty. *J Am Coll Cardiol* 1986; 8:1271–1276.

106. Hoberg E, Schwarz F, Schomig A, et al: Prevention of restenosis by verapamil. The verapamil angioplasty study (VAS) (abstract). *Circulation* 1990; 82(suppl 3):428.

107. Slack JD, Pinkerton CA, VanTassel J, et al: Can oral fish oil supplement minimize re-stenosis after percutaneous transluminal coronary angioplasty (abstract)? *J Am Coll Cardiol* 1987; 9(suppl):64.

108. Reis GJ, Boucher TM, Sipperly ME, et al: Randomised trial of fish oil for prevention of restenosis after coronary angioplasty. *Lancet* 1989; 2:177–181.

109. Milner MR, Gallino RA, Leffingwell A, et al: Usefulness of fish oil supplements in preventing clinical evidence of restenosis after percutaneous transluminal coronary angioplasty. *Am J Cardiol* 1989; 64:294–299.

110. Dehmer GJ, Popma JJ, van den Berg EK, et al: Reduction in the rate of early restenosis after coronary angioplasty by a diet supplemented with n-3 fatty acids. *N Engl J Med* 1988; 319:733–740.

111. Grigg LE, Kay TWH, Valentine PA, et al: Determinants of restenosis and lack of effect of dietary supplementation with eicosapentanoic acid on the incidence of coronary artery restenosis after angioplasty. *J Am Coll Cardiol* 1989; 13:665–672.

112. Sahni R, Maniet AR, Voci G, et al: Prevention of restenosis by lovastatin (abstract). *Circulation* 1989; 80(suppl 2):65.

113. Rose TE, Beauchamp BG: Short term high dose steroid treatment to prevent restenosis in PTCA (abstract). *Circulation* 1987; 76(suppl 4):371.

114. Stone GW, Rutherford BD, McConahay DR, et al: A randomized trial of corticosteroids for the prevention of restenosis in 102 patients undergoing repeat coronary angioplasty. *Cathet Cardiovasc Diagn* 1989; 18:227–231.

115. Pepine CJ, Hirshfeld JW, Macdonald RG, et al: A controlled trial of corticosteroids to prevent restenosis after coronary angioplasty. *Circulation* 1990; 81:1753–1761.

116. Gal D, Rongione AJ, Slovenkai GA, et al: Atherosclerotic Yucatan microswine: An animal model with high-grade, fibrocalcific, nonfatty lesions suitable for testing catheter-based intervention. *Am Heart J* 1990; 119:291–300.

117. LeVeen RF, Wolf GL, Villanueva TG: New rabbit atherosclerosis model for the investigation of transluminal angioplasty. *Invest Radiol* 1982; 17:470–475.

118. Steele PM, Chesebro JH, Stanson AW, et al: Balloon angioplasty; natural history of the pathophysiological response to injury in a pig model. *Circ Res* 1985; 57:105–112.

119. Wilentz J, Sanborn T, Haudenschild C, et al: Platelet accumulation in experimental angioplasty: Time course in relation to vascular injury. *Circulation* 1987; 75:636–642.

120. Schwartz RS, Murphy JG, Edwards WD, et al: Restenosis after balloon angioplasty. A practical proliferative model in porcine coronary arteries. *Circulation* 1990; 82:2190–2200.

121. Bettmann MA: Anticoagulation and restenosis after percutaneous transluminal coronary angioplasty. *Am J Cardiol* 1987; 60:17–19.

122. Ockelford P: Heparin 1986. Indications and effective use. *Drugs* 1986; 31:81–92.

123. Perin EC, Turner SA, Ferguson JJ: Relationship between the response to heparin and restenosis following PTCA (abstract). *Circulation* 1990; 82(suppl 3):497.

124. Majesky MW, Schwartz SM, Clowes MM, et al: Heparin regulates smooth muscle S-phase entry in the injured rat carotid artery. *Circ Res* 1987; 61:296–300.

125. Heras M, Chesebro JH, Webster MWI, et al: Hirudin, heparin and placebo during deep arterial injury in the pig. The in vivo role of thrombosis in platelet-mediated thrombosis. *Circulation* 1990; 82:1476–1484.

126. Oates JA, Fitzgerald GA, Branch RA, et al: Clinical implications of prostaglandin and thromboxane A$_2$ formation (Part I and II). *N Engl J Med* 1988; 319:689–698, 761–767.

127. Barnathan ES, Schwartz JS, Taylor L, et al: Aspirin and dipyridamole in the prevention of acute coronary thrombosis complicating coronary angioplasty. *Circulation* 1987; 76:125–134.

128. Fitzgerald GA: Dipyridamole. *N Engl J Med* 1987; 316:1247–1257.

129. Harker LA, Fuster V: Pharmacology of platelet inhibitors. *J Am Coll Cardiol* 1986; 8:21–32.

130. Swanson KT, Vlietstra RE, Holmes DR, et al: Efficacy of adjunctive dextran during percutaneous transluminal coronary angioplasty. *Am J Cardiol* 1984; 54:447–448.

131. Hornby EJ, Foster MR, McCabe PJ, et al: The inhibitory effect of GR32191, a thromboxane receptor blocking drug on human platelet aggregation, adhesion and secretion. *Thromb Haemost* 1989; 61:429–436.

132. See J, Shell W, Matthews O, et al: Prostaglandin E₁ infusion after angioplasty in humans inhibits abrupt occlusion and early restenosis. *Adv Prostaglandin Thromboxane Leukotriene Res* 1987; 17:266–270.

133. Ellis SG, Navetta FI, Tcheng JT, et al: Antiplatelet GPIIb/IIIa (7E3) antibody in elective PTCA: Safety and inhibition of platelet function (abstract). *Circulation* 1990; 82(suppl 3):191.

134. Timmermans C, Vanhaecke J, Vrolix M, et al: Ridogrel in the prevention of early acute reocclusion after coronary angioplasty (abstract). 1990; 82(suppl 3):190.

135. Libby P, Warner SJC, Salomon RN, et al: Production of platelet-derived growth factor like mitogen by smooth muscle cells from human atheroma. *N Engl J Med* 1988; 38:1493–1498.

136. Ross R: Platelet-derived growth factor. *Lancet* 1989; 1:1179–1182.

137. Majesky MW, Reidy MA, Bowen-Pope DF, et al: PDGF ligand and receptor gene expression during repair of arterial injury. *J Cell Biol* 1990; 111:2149–2158.

138. Nemecek GM, Coughlin SR, Handley DA, et al: Stimulation of aortic smooth muscle cell mitogenesis by serotonin. *Proc Natl Acad Sci USA* 1986; 83:674–678.

139. Dzau VJ: Circulating versus local renin-angiotensin system in cardiovascular homeostasis. *Circulation* 1988; 77(suppl 1):4–13.

140. Owens GK: Influence of blood pressure on development of aortic medial smooth muscle hypertrophy in spontaneously hypertensive rats. *Hypertension* 1987; 9:178–187.

141. Daemen MJAP, Lombardi DM, Bosman FT, et al: Angiotensin II induces smooth muscle cell proliferation in the normal and injured rat arterial wall. *Circ Res* 1991; 68:450–456.

142. Brozovich FV, Gottleib NB, Gottleib RS, et al: Prevention of restenosis after PTCA by angiotensin converting enzyme inhibitors (abstract). *J Am Coll Cardiol* 1991; 17:181.

143. Tiel ML, Stemerman MB, Spaet: The influence of the pituitary on arterial intimal proliferation in the rat. *Circ Res* 1978; 42:644–649.

144. Hansson H, Jennische E, Skottner A: Regenerating endothelial cells express insulin-like growth factor-1 immunoreactivity after arterial injury. *Cell Tissue Res* 1987; 250:499–505.

145. Clemmons DR: Exposure to platelet-derived growth factor modulates the porcine aortic smooth muscle cell response to somatomedin-C. *Endocrinology* 1985; 117:77–83.

146. Betz E, Fotev Z, Weidler R: Antiproliferative activity of a calcium-calmodulin-antagonist in experimentally induced atherosclerosis and cultures of artery wall cells (abstract). *Eur Heart J* 1990; 11(suppl):127.

147. David PR, Waters DD, Scholl JM, et al: Percutaneous transluminal coronary angioplasty in patients with variant angina. *Circulation* 1982; 66:695–702.

148. Lichtlen PR, Hugenholtz PG, Rafflenbeul W, et al: Retardation of angiographic progression of coronary artery disease by nifedipine. Results of the International Nifedipine Trial on Antiatherosclerotic Therapy (INTACT). *Lancet* 1990; 335:1109–1113.

149. Waters D, Lesperance J, Francetich M, et al: A controlled clinical trial to assess the effect of a calcium channel blocker on the progression of coronary atherosclerosis. *Circulation* 1990; 82:1940–1953.

150. Leaf A: Cardiovascular effects of fish oils. Beyond the platelet. *Circulation* 1990; 82:624–628.

151. Reis GJ, Silverman DI, Boucher TM, et al: Do serum lipid levels predict restenosis after coronary angioplasty (PTCA) (abstract)? *Circulation* 1990; 82(suppl 2):427.

152. Hollman J, Konrad K, Raymond R, et al: Lipid lowering for the prevention of recurrent stenosis following coronary angioplasty (abstract). *Circulation* 1989; 80 (suppl 2):65.

153. MacDonald RG, Panush RS, Pepine CJ: Rationale for use of glucocorticoids in modification of restenosis after percutaneous transluminal coronary angioplasty. *Am J Cardiol* 1987; 60:56–60.

154. Lam JYT, Chesebro JH, Dewanjee MK, et al: Ibuprofen: A potent antithrombotic agent for arterial injury after balloon angioplasty (abstract). *J Am Coll Cardiol* 1987; 9:64.

155. Michell RH: Post-receptor signalling pathways. *Lancet* 1989; 1:765–767.

156. Schneider MD, Parker TG: Cardiac myocytes as target for the action of peptide growth factors. *Circulation* 1990; 81:1443–1456.

157. Waterfield MD: Epidermal growth factor and related molecules. *Lancet* 1989; 1:1243–1246.

158. Green AR: Peptide regulatory factors: Multifunctional mediators of cellular growth and differentiation. *Lancet* 1989; 1:705–707.

159. Beatt KJ, Serruys PW, Hugenholtz PG: Restenosis after coronary angioplasty: New standards for clinical studies. *J Am Coll Cardiol* 1990; 15:491–498.

PART IX

Procedures for Valvular and Congenital Defects

Percutaneous Balloon Aortic Valvuloplasty: Update of Techniques, Results, and Indications in the Rouen Experience

Alain Cribier, M.D.

Lowell Gerber, M.D.

Brice Letac, M.D.

For the last 10 years, the use of balloon catheters has been considerably developed to provide nonsurgical treatment of vascular and valvular stenosis. In 1985, we investigated the use of balloon catheters for the treatment of severe calcific aortic valve stenosis in elderly patients considered to be poor or nonsurgical candidates for valve replacement because of both old age and associated comorbidities.[1] Our early experience demonstrated that the procedure was feasible and beneficial in most patients.[2, 3] This was confirmed in other centers.[4-9]

Since then, the technique has been refined and has become much simpler and safer.[10] With continued experience and the analysis of our large series of over 600 patients, the limits of the procedure have been clearly recognized and have led to a restricted patient selection. However, near 100 patients are still annually referred to our center for percutaneous balloon aortic valvuloplasty (BAV). The vast majority of these patients are octogenarians with severe left ventricular dysfunction and/or associated cardiac or noncardiac disease. The procedure is being used either as a "bridge to surgery" or as the ultimate therapeutic solution to improve the quality of the last months or years of life of very disabled patients.

Recently, the results of the U.S. Mansfield Multicenter Registry in which our group participated was reported in the literature.[11-18] The data of this registry were reviewed by the U.S. Food and Drug Administration, and the procedure was approved for nonsurgical patients.

EVOLUTION OF THE TECHNIQUE

The objective in performing BAV is to obtain the smallest transvalvular gradient and the largest aortic valve area. Our goal is to increase the valve area by at least 100% and achieve a valve area of nearly or above 1 cm². This is obtained by serially inflating balloons of increasing size across the valve.

In the first 506 patients of our series, whose clinical status are shown in Table 50-1, the peak-to-peak gradient was reduced from 71 ± 25 mm Hg to 29 ± 12 mm Hg, and the valve area was increased from 0.55 ± 0.2 cm² to 0.96 ± 0.32 cm². Figure 50-1 shows the valve area distribution before and after BAV. A valve area larger than 1 cm² could be obtained in 39% of the cases, whereas the technique failed to open the valve in 2% of the cases, a critical aortic valve stenosis persisted at the end of the procedure with a valve area below 0.5 cm².

Postmortem studies that we[19] and others[20] have done have allowed a good understanding of the mechanisms of BAV. These mechanisms involve separation of fused

TABLE 50-1.

Clinical Characteristics of the First 506 Patients of Our Series Who Underwent Balloon Aortic Valvuloplasty

Characteristic	Value
Patients	506
Male	239
Female	267
Mean age, yr	75 ± 11 (25 to 98)
≤70	143 (28%)
>70–<80	183 (36%)
≥ 80	180 (36%)
Etiology	
Unknown origin:	454 (90%)
Rheumatic	42 (8%)
Congenital	10 (2%)
Dyspnea (NYHA* class III or IV)	344 (68%)
Syncopal attacks	106 (21%)
Angina pectoris	253 (50%)
CHA* class III or IV	106 (21%)

*NYHA = New York Heart Association; CHA = Canadian Heart Association.

TABLE 50-2.

Technical Aspects of Balloon Valvuloplasty in the First 506 Patients of Our Series

Technical Aspect	
Catheter insertion:	
Femoral *(percutaneous)*	470 (94%)
Brachial *(cutdown)*	36 (6%)
Balloon catheter type	
Regular	262 (52%)
Double sized	244 (48%)
Largest balloon size used	
15 mm	18 (3%)
18 mm	58 (12%)
20 mm	280 (55%)
23 mm	125 (25%)
25 mm	10 (2%)
2 balloons	15 (3%)

commissures, fracture of calcific nodular deposits in the valve leaflets, and to a limited degree, stretching of the valve cusps to make the leaflets more pliable and mobile during systole. We emphasize that to be efficacious, the balloon has to be maximally inflated in order to exert an effective dilatation force. A lack of maximal inflation pressure might explain the unconvincing anatomic results in other hands.[21] We have shown that the 20-mm-diameter balloon does not always fully open the leaflets of the aortic valve. In the presence of a large aortic annulus, the use of two balloons side by side (as we did in our very early experience) or, preferentially, the use of a larger balloon size (23 mm or rarely 25 mm) may be required. Table 50-2 shows the distribution of the largest balloon sizes used in our overall experience.

Although we have found the larger diameters useful, we still recommend a step-by-step increase in balloon size in order to improve hemodynamic tolerance to inflation by large balloons, and to reduce the risk of seri-

ous complications such as massive aortic regurgitation or rupture of the aortic annulus.

We began our experience by using straight-tipped, single-sized balloon catheters designed for dilatation of the peripheral arteries and for congenital valve stenosis. Balloons 3 or 4 cm long with inflated diameters of 15, 18, or 20 mm were sequentially used. This early technique, which required several transcutaneous catheter exchange procedures, has become obsolete since the introduction of new devices. A specially designed aortic valvuloplasty catheter (Boston Scientific) has been used routinely in our laboratory for the last 3 years in a series of more than 300 patients. This device is a triple-lumen 9 F catheter with a 7 F tip shaped into a large pigtail-type curve (Fig 50-2). There is a distal lumen for pressure measurement and angiography. The proximal lumen located 10 cm above the balloon is used for continuous monitoring of the central aortic pressure. The balloon has a proximal segment 3 cm long and 20 or 23 mm in diameter when inflated. There is an abrupt taper to the distal segment, which is 2 cm long and 15 or 18 mm in diameter when inflated. When this catheter is used, it is possible to dilate first with the distal segment (15 or 18 mm) and then with the proximal segment (20 or 23 mm). Because of the length of the balloon and tip combined, one must be cautious when dilating with the proximal segment in patients who have a small left ventricular cavity. In such patients, a similarly constructed catheter with a single balloon size (15, 18, 20, or 23 mm) could be preferentially used. The low profile of the deflated balloon fits through a 14 F sheath, and the use of an arterial introducer has further decreased trauma to the femoral artery entry site.

The technique is now usually performed as follow: we routinely start the procedure by performing a right heart catheterization with a thermodilution balloon flo-

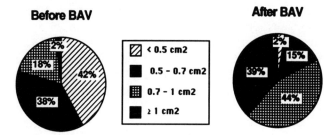

FIG 50-1.

Valve area distribution before balloon aortic valvuloplasty *(BAV)* and immediately after the procedure in the first 506 patients of our series.

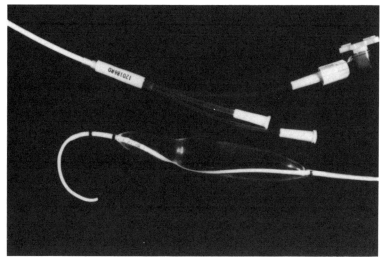

FIG 50–2.
Proximal and distal ends of the balloon aortic valvuloplasty catheter currently used in our institution. The balloon has a proximal diameter of 20 mm, a distal diameter of 15 mm, and a total length of 5.5 cm.

tation catheter, a supravalvular aortogram, and a coronary angiogram. Then the aortic valve is crossed with a 7 F Sones catheter over a 0.035-in. straight-tipped guidewire or (in about 20% of the cases) with a left coronary Amplatz catheter. Using this technique, we could always successfully cross the aortic valve in a minimal period of time (3 minutes on average). When the Sones catheter or a pigtail catheter exchanged over a long guidewire is used, a left ventricular angiogram is performed. A 0.035-in. extra stiff guidewire (Schneider Medintag) is then pushed into the left ventricle through the catheter. This guidewire has a very stiff core. Despite being very flexible, the distal end of the wire is systematically shaped into an exaggerated pigtail curve before use (Fig 50–3). The Sones and 8 F arterial sheaths are removed over the wire, and the femoral artery is catheterized with a 14 F sheath (Schneider-Metintag) whose hemostatic valve allows minimal blood leak during each necessary over-the-wire catheter exchange procedure. No groin compression is necessary throughout the procedure.

The 15- to 20-mm step-size balloon catheter is routinely used from the beginning. After being purged of air, it is introduced through the 14 F sheath and advanced over the wire until the pigtail end reaches the left ventricle. Two distal markers indicate its optimal position across the valve for accurate gradient measurement (Fig 50–4). The guidewire is removed, the mean gradient is recorded, the cardiac output is measured, and the valve area is calculated by computer with Gorlin's formula. The extrastiff guidewire is then readvanced up to the tip of the catheter, and the 15-mm distal segment is positioned across the valve. Balloon inflations are then performed with a hand-held syringe filled with a 50% contrast-saline mixture. Balloon inflation is started with a 20-cc syringe, and the balloon is

then rapidly and fully inflated with a 10-cc syringe. The stiff guidewire consistently prevents balloon unstability during inflation. Two inflations are usually performed and maintained for 20 to 40 seconds depending on the degree of decrease in aortic blood pressure and the clinical tolerance to reduced cardiac output. The balloon is then deflated, and its proximal 20-mm-diameter segment is placed across the valve. The same technique is then used for balloon inflation. Maximal balloon inflation must be obtained before deflation, and this is mainly judged by the balloon shape, which must appear slightly overdistended. Following each inflation or if the aortic blood pressure decreases to below 60 mm Hg, the

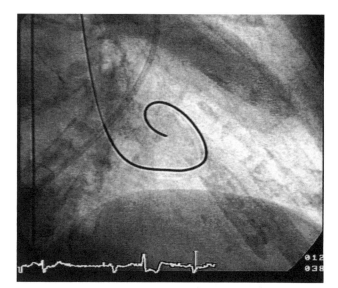

FIG 50–3.
The 0.035-in. backup exchange guidewire (Schneider-Medintag) in place in the left ventricle. The distal soft part of the guidewire has been shaped into an exaggerated curve. The extra stiff core prevents balloon instability during inflation.

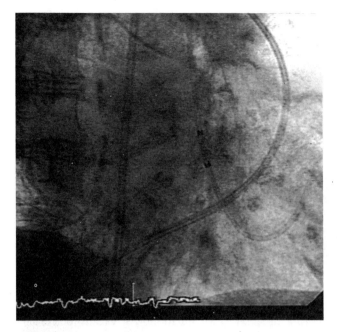

FIG 50–4.
The two distal markers of the valvuloplasty catheter in place across the aortic valve for accurate measurement of the transvalvular gradient.

pressure is simply released and the balloon pulled back into the aorta with the pigtail end left in the left ventricle. After a series of two to three inflations or in case of balloon rupture (always an innocuous event) the guidewire is removed and the transvalvular gradient and aortic valve area are measured. When the results are considered suboptimal, the balloon catheter is exchanged for a 23-mm balloon, and the same technique is applied (Fig 50–5 and Fig 50–6). After the final results have been recorded, a supravalvular aortogram is repeated with the same catheter for quantitation of aortic insufficiency.

The catheters and sheaths are removed at the end of the procedure. Patients remain supine in bed for 24 hours and are generally discharged 48 hours following the procedure.

PROCEDURE-RELATED COMPLICATIONS

Procedure-related complications in our overall series have been low despite the population of elderly and very sick patients (Table 50–3). Out of 506 patients, 5 died of electromechanical dissociation on the catheterization table during the procedure, and an additional 15 patients died in the hospital in the days following BAV. Nonlethal severe complications (stroke, pericardial tamponade, acute myocardial infarction, complete heart block, or massive aortic insufficiency) occurred in 4% of the cases. When the last 100 patients of this series are considered, the peri- and post-BAV hospital mortality rates were similar, but the nonlethal severe complication rate had decreased to 1% (1 isolated case of stroke).

We do not consider previous neurologic events or severe coronary disease (including a major lesion of the left main coronary artery) to be contraindications for BAV. However, we perform shorter balloon inflations in these cases to avoid any major drop in aortic blood pressure. Nevertheless, in spite of much experience with the procedure, there is still a risk of major complications when BAV is performed.[13, 18, 22]

FOLLOW-UP

It has been well recognized that dramatic clinical improvement usually follows successful BAV.[1–9, 23–25]

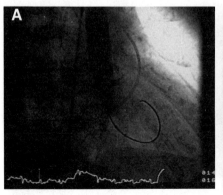
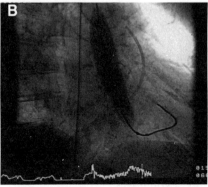
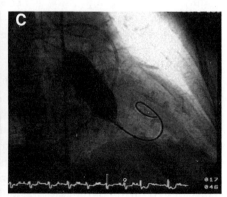

FIG 50–5.
Balloon aortic valvuloplasty in an 84-year-old woman. The 15- to 20-mm step-size catheter is first used. The valve is dilated with the 15-mm distal part of the balloon **(A)** and with the 20-mm proximal part of it **(B)**. Because of suboptimal results, a 23-mm single-size balloon is then used **(C).** The subsequent changes in valve hemodynamics are shown in Figure 50–6.

TABLE 50–3.

Procedure-Related Complications in the First 506 Patients of Our Series

Complication	No.	(%) of Patients
Death	20	(4.0)
Stroke	5	(1.0)
Pericardial tamponade	4	(0.8)
Massive aortic insufficiency	4	(0.8)
Acute myocardial infarction	2	(0.4)
Complete heart block	3	(0.6)
Femoral artery (whole series)	54	(11)
Femoral artery (last 100 patients)	5	(5.0)

The improvement of dyspnea and angina observed over a period of 16 ± 7 months in the first 156 patients of our series who survived without repeat BAV or valve replacement is shown in Figure 50–7.

However, the high restenosis rate is undoubtedly the limiting factor of the procedure.[3, 16, 23–26] Hemodynamic restenosis (defined as a 50% decrease in the gain in aortic valve area) was observed in 50% of our cases 7

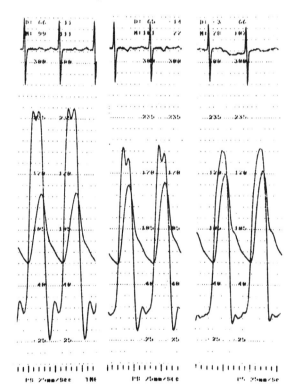

FIG 50–6.

Improvement in transvalvular gradient and valve area following balloon valvuloplasty (same patient as in Fig 50–5). The mean gradient decreased from 96 mm Hg *(left panel)* to 52 mm Hg after using the 20-mm balloon diameter *(middle panel)* and further decreased to 38 mm Hg after using the 23-mm balloon *(right panel)*. Subsequently, the valve area increased from 0.44 cm² to 0.78 cm² and to 0.90 cm².

months after BAV in our early series; the restenosis rate was 37% in a group of 65 patients who had systematic hemodynamic control 10 months post-BAV and 71% in a group of 31 patients whose repeat catheterization was done for clinical restenosis 6 months on average following the procedure. Restenosis is hardly predictable, but several factors such as old age, female gender, and adequacy of the BAV results have been shown to be related to the restenosis rate.[3, 12, 14, 23] However, it is a current observation that symptomatic improvement often persists several months in spite of signs of restenosis on echocardiography and Doppler controls.

When restenosis is associated with a recurrence of symptoms, BAV may be repeated when valve replacement remains too high a risk or is contraindicated.[17, 27, 28] In our experience, the results of a second procedure are comparable to those obtained after the first one (0.86 ± 0.18 cm² vs. 0.91 ± 0.32 cm² in our series of 77 patients in whom BAV was repeated 10 ± 6 months after the first procedure), and the risks of the second procedure are similar to those of the first one.

Survival curves after BAV could be established for the first 244 patients of our series. These curves demonstrated that patients' survival is related to the clinical status prior to BAV. The mortality rate at 1 year was 11% in patients up to 80 years of age with no associated disease or heart failure, whereas it was 46% in patients in whom surgery was definitely contraindicated. Patients who died were older and had more severe clinical impairment, more depressed left ventricular function, and more severe aortic stenosis. Similar findings were reported in the literature.[14, 23]

CURRENT INDICATIONS FOR BALLOON AORTIC VALVULOPLASTY

For the last 2 years, the procedure has been applied by us in a restricted and well-selected group of patients. The vast majority of this population involved elderly patients, most often octogenarians or even nonagenarians for whom surgery had been declined by the surgical team because of frailty, associated cardiac or noncardiac disease, or severe heart failure with major left ventricular dysfunction. In these very old patients, the goal of BAV is to improve the clinical status for the last months or years of life, whereas in some cases the hope is to sufficiently improve myocardial function and the clinical condition to enable a secondary valve replacement at an acceptably lowered risk.

With a large experience of more than 200 patients above the age of 80 years (mean, 85 ± 4) and with the technical improvements, the complication rate remains

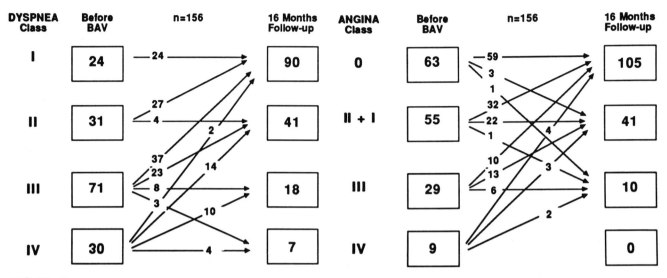

FIG 50–7.

Change in dyspnea (New York Heart Association classification) and angina pectoris (Canadian Heart Association classification) after balloon aortic valvuloplasty *(BAV)* in 156 patients followed over a mean period of 16 months.

acceptably low in this population despite the very old age and the poor clinical status of the patients. When the second half of this large series of patients was compared with the first half, the in-hospital mortality rate decreased from 6% to 1.3%, and the total complication rate, including minor complications at the femoral artery, improved from 23% to 9%. The rate of nonlethal severe complications remained similar (stroke, 2%; other complications, 1%). In these very old patients, the procedure ended with a mean transvalvular gradient of 26 mm Hg and a valve area of 0.98 cm² (73 mm HG and 0.46 cm², respectively, before BAV).

The actuarial mortality rate at 3 months, 1 year, and 2 years was 7%, 25%, and 50%, respectively. The mortality rate at 1 year was thus clearly below the death rate of similarly ill but 10-year-younger patients who were neither operated on nor submitted to BAV, as reported by O'Kieffe et al.[29] and Turina et al.[30] (mortality rates of 44% and 60%, respectively). Nevertheless, the most remarkable result of BAV is the marked clinical improvement obtained, with 60% of the surviving patients remaining improved at the 1-year follow-up and having returned to normal activities for their age. These results are obtained at the price of a procedure requiring only local anesthesia and a 5- or 6-day hospitalization stay. Thus, even short-term benefits make BAV a viable therapeutic option for elderly patients for whom no other modality of treatment exist.

Until the last 2 years, the surgical series on elderly patients rarely included octogenarians. The mortality rate for septuagenarians ranged from 3% to 18%.[31–33] Since 1990, we have been aware of five articles evaluat-

ing the surgical risk of cardiac surgery in patients above the age of 80 years. The perioperative death rate varied between 6% and 8%[34–36] and 28% and 30%.[37, 38] The mortality rate was doubled in the case of a lowered ejection fraction to below 40%.[35, 38] Associated coronary bypass grafting also markedly increased the risk.[34–36] Nonlethal major complications, particularly permanent debilitating neurologic events, occurred frequently in this elderly population (9.5% in the series of Levinson et al.[36]). Furthermore, most of the patients included in these surgical series were selected on the basis of their good preoperative clinical status, thus introducing a selection bias.[36, 37] As a matter of fact, because octogenarians are not a uniform group and because most of the patients submitted to BAV are those with a very high predicted risk for surgery, the results of BAV and those of aortic valve replacement are quite impossible to compare. Despite our extensive experience with BAV, octogenarians who are otherwise healthy and active are currently advised by us to have their valve replaced, whereas BAV is attempted as the first procedure in patients with frailty or comorbidities.

In patients with aortic stenosis and very depressed left ventricular function, suppressing mechanical obstacles to left ventricular ejection must urgently be considered, and surgical valve replacement remains the best therapeutic option. However, it is well documented that severe left ventricular dysfunction as well as advanced New York Heart Association functional class are important factors of perioperative death in patients who undergo valve replacement.[39–41] For this reason, BAV has been attempted early in our group[42, 43] as in other centers[44] as a possible way of improving myocardial function in order to subsequently lower the surgical risk. BAV has been shown in several reports to result in improved left ventricular function despite the fact that individual responses may vary considerably.[44] In 72 patients of our early series with an ejection fraction of 29% ± 5%, it increased to 34% ± 7% ($P < .001$) immediately after the procedure. In 11 patients of this group who had systematic hemodynamic control 5 months later, the ejection fraction that had increased from 29% ± 8% to 39% ± 10% after BAV had further increased to 52% ± 11%. However, the mortality of these patients remains high in the year following BAV despite transient dramatic improvement[42] because of both suboptimal valve enlargement and restenosis. Thus, performing BAV in such situations implies that both the physician and patient consider it to be a bridge to surgery. In our experience, it has sometimes been difficult to convince a patient to accept cardiac surgery after BAV, at a time of considerable functional improvement.

The interest of BAV as a bridge to surgery in the most severe situation is well illustrated by our short series of 10 moribund patients 54 to 78 years old who presented with cardiogenic shock when they were transferred to our laboratory. Due to their clinical condition and despite the catastrophic predictable short-term prognosis, surgery was declined, and BAV was attempted as a last-resort procedure. BAV was successfully and safely performed in all cases and resulted in a 100% increase in aortic valve area that reached 0.95 ± 0.3 cm² at the end of the procedure. Improvement in dyspnea was immediate and spectacular, and signs of shock disappeared within hours. One patient died in the days following the procedure because of early restenosis, and another patient died 3 weeks after hospital discharge because of intestinal bleeding. Six patients had successful valve replacement 6 days to 18 months after BAV. Before surgery, sustained marked clinical and hemodynamic improvement was confirmed in all cases. Two patients who were dramatically improved refused surgery and were still surviving with no symptoms 48 and 24 months, respectively, after BAV. Lifesaving emergency BAV in similar critical situations has also been reported by Desnoyer et al.[45]

In 1991, there is no discussion concerning the place of valve replacement in aortic stenosis, surgery being the gold standard treatment of the disease, with low-risk and excellent long-standing results for the vast majority of patients. In opposition, BAV is a palliative procedure that must be restricted to patients who have a high predictive risk for surgery, mainly because of advanced age or distressing clinical conditions. Despite affording only a partial reduction of the aortic stenosis and temporary clinical improvement, in many cases the procedure provides a reasonable and often the only therapeutic option for disabled patients.

REFERENCES

1. Cribier A, Savin T, Saoudi N, et al: Percutaneous transluminal valvuloplasty of acquired aortic stenosis in elderly patients. An alternative of valve replacement? *Lancet* 1986; 1:63–67.
2. Cribier A, Savin T, Berland J, et al: Percutaneous transluminal balloon valvuloplasty of adult aortic stenosis: Report of 92 cases. *J Am Coll Cardiol* 1987; 9:381–386.
3. Letac B, Cribier A, Koning R, et al: Results of percutaneous transluminal valvuloplasty in 218 adults with valvular aortic stenosis. *Am J Cardiol* 1988; 62:598–605.
4. McKay RG, Safian RD, Lock JE, et al: Balloon dilatation of calcific aortic stenosis in elderly patients in postmortem, intraoperative, and percutaneous valvuloplasty studies. *Circulation* 1986; 74:119–125.
5. Isner JM, Salem DN, Desnoyer MR, et al: Treatment of calcific aortic stenosis by balloon valvuloplasty. *Am J Cardiol* 1987; 59:313–317.
6. Drobinski G, Lechat P, Metzger P, et al: Results of percutaneous catheter valvuloplasty for calcified aortic stenosis in the elderly. *Eur Heart J* 1987; 8:322–328.
7. Jackson J, Thomas S, Monaghan M, et al: Inoperable aortic stenosis in the elderly: Benefit from percutaneous transluminal valvuloplasty. *Br Med J* 1987; 294:83–86.
8. Schneider JF, Wilson M, Gallant TE: Percutaneous balloon aortic valvuloplasty for aortic stenosis in elderly patients at high risk for surgery. *Ann Intern Med* 1987; 106:696–699.
9. Safian RD, Berman AD, Diver DJ, et al: Balloon aortic valvuloplasty in 170 consecutive patients. *N Engl J Med* 1988; 319:125–130.
10. Cribier A, Gerber L, Berland J, et al: Percutaneous balloon aortic valvuloplasty: The state of the art, a review of two years experience in Rouen. *J Intervent Cardiol* 1988; 1:237–250.
11. O'Neill WW: Seminar on balloon aortic valvuloplasty. *J Am Coll Cardiol* 1991; 17:187–188.
12. Holmes DR Jr, Nishimura RA, Reeder GS: In-hospital mortality after balloon aortic valvuloplasty: Frequency and associated factors. *J Am Coll Cardiol* 1991; 17:189–192.
13. O'Neill WW: Predictors of long-term survival after percutaneous aortic valvuloplasty: Report of the Mansfield Scientific Balloon Aortic Valvuloplasty Registry. *J Am Coll Cardiol* 1991; 17:193–198.
14. McKay RG: Overview of acute hemodynamic results and procedural complications. *J Am Coll Cardiol* 1991; 17:485–491.
15. Reeder GS, Nishimura RA, Holmes DR: Patient age and results of balloon aortic valvuloplasty: The Mansfield Scientific Registry Experience. *J Am Coll Cardiol* 1991; 17:909–913.
16. Bashore TM, Davidson CJ: Follow-up recatheterization after balloon aortic valvuloplasty. *J Am Coll Cardiol* 1991; 17:1188–1195.

17. Ferguson JJ, Garza RA: Efficacy of multiple balloon aortic valvuloplasty procedures. *J Am Coll Cardiol* 1991; 17:1430–1435.

18. Isner JM: Acute catastrophic complications of balloon aortic valvuloplasty. *J Am Coll Cardiol* 1991; 17:1436–1444.

19. Letac B, Gerber L, Koning R: Insights on the mechanism of balloon valvuloplasty of aortic stenosis. *Am J Cardiol* 1988; 62:1241–1247.

20. Safian RD, Mandell VS, Thurer RE, et al: Postmortem and intraoperative balloon valvuloplasty of calcific aortic stenosis in elderly patients: Mechanisms of successful dilation. *J Am Coll Cardiol* 1987; 9:655–660.

21. Robicsek F, Harbold NB, Daugherty HK, et al: Balloon valvuloplasty in calcified aortic stenosis: A cause for caution and alarm. *Ann Thorac Surg* 1988; 45:515–525.

22. Lembo NJ, King SB, Roubin GS, et al: Fatal aortic rupture during percutaneous balloon valvuloplasty for valvular aortic stenosis. *Am J Cardiol* 1987; 60:733–737.

23. Block PC, Palacios IF: Clinical and hemodynamic follow-up after percutaneous aortic valvuloplasty in the elderly. *Am J Cardiol* 1988; 62:760–763.

24. Lewin RF, Dorros G, King JF, et al: Percutaneous transluminal aortic valvuloplasty acute outcome and follow-up of 125 patients. *J Am Coll Cardiol* 1989; 4:1210–1217.

25. Holmes DR Jr, Nishimura RA, Reeder GS, et al: Clinical follow-up after percutaneous aortic balloon valvuloplasty. *Arch Intern Med* 1989; 149:1405–1409.

26. Meany BT, Spriging D, Chambers J, et al: Aortic valvuloplasty in the elderly: Is re-stenosis inevitable? *Circulation* 1988; 78(suppl 2):531.

27. Ross TC, Banks AK, Collins TJ, et al: Repeat balloon aortic valvuloplasty for aortic restenosis. *Cathet Cardiovasc Diagn* 1989; 18:96–98.

28. Letac B, Cribier A, Koning R, et al: Aortic stenosis in elderly patients aged 80 or older: Treatment by percutaneous balloon valvuloplasty in a series of 92 cases. *Circulation* 1989; 80:1514–1520.

29. O'Keefe JH, Vlietstra RE, Bailey KR, et al: Natural history of candidates for balloon aortic valvuloplasty. *Mayo Clin Proc* 1987; 62:976–991.

30. Turina J, Hess O, Sepulcri F, et al: Spontaneous course of aortic valve disease. *Eur Heart J* 1987; 8:471–483.

31. Bergdahl L, Bjork VO, Jonasso R: Aortic valve replacement in patients over 70 years. *Scand J Thorac Cardiovasc Surg* 1981; 15:123–129.

32. Santiga JT, Flora J, Kirsh M, et al: Aortic valve replacement in the elderly. *J Am Geriatr Soc* 1983; 31:211–215.

33. Blakeman BM, Pifarré R, Sullivan HJ, et al: Aortic valve replacement in patients 75 years old and older. *Ann Thorac Surg* 1987; 44:637–639.

34. Culliford AT, Galloway AC, Colvin SP, et al: Aortic valve replacement for aortic stenosis in patients aged 80 years and older. *Am J Cardiol* 1991; 67:1256–1266.

35. Bashour TT, Hanna ES, Myler RK, et al: Cardiac surgery in patients over the age of 80 years. *Ann Thorac Surg* 1990; 13:267–270.

36. Levinson JR, Akins CW, Buckley MJ, et al: Octogenarians with aortic stenosis: Outcome after aortic valve replacement. *Circulation* 1989; 80:149–156.

37. Edmunds LH Jr, Stephenson LW, Edie RN: Open-heart surgery in octogenarians. *N Engl J Med* 1988; 319:131–136.

38. Deleuze P, Loisance DY, Besnainou F, et al: Severe aortic stenosis in octogenarians: Is operation an acceptable alternative? *Clin Cardiol* 1990; 50:226–229.

39. Scott WC, Miller DC, Haverich A, et al: Determinants of operative mortality for patients undergoing aortic valve replacement. *J Thorac Cardiovasc Surg* 1985; 89:400–413.

40. Carabello BA, Green LH, Grossman W, et al: Hemodynamic determinants of prognosis of aortic valve replacement in critical aortic stenosis and advanced congestive heart failure. *Circulation* 1980; 62:42–48.

41. Smith N, McAnulty JH, Rahimtoola SH: Severe aortic stenosis with impaired left ventricular function and clinical heart failure: Results of valve replacement. *Circulation* 1978; 58:255–264.

42. Berland J, Cribier A, Savin T, et al: Percutaneous balloon valvuloplasty in patients with severe aortic stenosis and low ejection fraction. Immediate results and 1-year follow-up. *Circulation* 1989; 79:1189–1196.

43. Cribier A, Lafont A, Eltchaninoff H, et al: La valvuloplastie aortique percutanée réalisée en dernier recours chez les patients atteints de rétrécissement aortique en état critique. *Arch Mal Coeur* 1990; 83:1783–1790.

44. Safian RD, Warren SE, Berman AD, et al: Improvement in symptoms and left ventricular performance after balloon aortic valvuloplasty in patients with aortic stenosis and depressed left ventricular ejection fraction. *Circulation* 1988; 78:1181–1191.

45. Desnoyer MR, Salem DN, Rosenfield K, et al: Treatment of cardiogenic shock by emergency aortic balloon valvuloplasty. *Ann Intern Med* 1988; 108:833–835.

51

Percutaneous Balloon Mitral Valvotomy

Peter C. Block, M.D.

Percutaneous mitral valvotomy (PMV) using dilating balloon catheters is a therapeutic alternative to surgical mitral commissurotomy for selected patients with symptomatic mitral stenosis.[1-7] The procedure has appeal since it can be done in a cardiac catheterization laboratory percutaneously, without general anesthesia and with a relatively low risk. Patients usually leave the hospital 24 to 36 hours after the procedure.

TECHNIQUE OF DOUBLE-BALLOON PERCUTANEOUS MITRAL VALVOTOMY

A transseptal puncture is first performed by using standard techniques from the right femoral vein with a sheath, dilator, and modified Brockenbrough needle. The tip of the needle used to puncture the atrial septum is no. 22. The needle tip is advanced through the foramen ovale, care being taken not to advance the larger dilator and sheath until the operator is certain of a position within the left atrium. This is documented by pressure measurements as well as by oxygen saturation measured from the tip of the needle after puncture. If a satisfactory left atrial position is not documented, the needle should be retracted and the sequence repeated. Heparin should not be administered until the transseptal puncture has been completed safely and the Mullin sheath (8 F, USCI, Billerica, Mass) is positioned in the left atrium.

Biplane fluoroscopy is helpful in evaluating the position of the needle tip before and after transseptal puncture. A retrograde pigtail catheter in the ascending aorta helps to delineate the position of the aortic valve and avoid inadvertent aortic puncture. If the foramen ovale is difficult to engage with the Brockenbrough needle

tip, an echocardiogram in the catheterization laboratory can be helpful to document needle tip position.

A Mullin sheath is then advanced over a dilator into the left atrium. Heparinization is performed with 100 units/kg body weight given intravenously. A 7 F floating balloon-tipped catheter (Arrow International, Reading, Penn) is passed through the sheath antegradely across the mitral valve. Simultaneous pressures from the left ventricle and left atrium are then measured. An alternative method of measuring the gradient across the mitral valve is to advance the pigtail catheter from the aortic root into the left ventricle and then measure the left atrial pressure through the Mullin sheath before the Arrow catheter is advanced. Cardiac output is measured simultaneously (with either thermodilution or the Fick technique) to allow calculation of the mitral valve area.

The floating balloon catheter is then advanced with the help of a bent guidewire out the aortic valve and into the ascending aorta. Two 0.038-in. transfer wires can be advanced through the floating balloon catheter once the tip is placed in the descending aorta. The floating balloon catheter and Mullin sheath are then removed, with the two transfer wires left behind (Fig 51–1,A). The dilating balloon catheters are then advanced over each guidewire and placed in position to straddle the stenotic mitral valve. It is not always necessary to predilate the atrial septum with a small balloon catheter. If the foramen ovale has been punctured by the transseptal needle, dilating balloon catheters can frequently be advanced over the guidewires without the need for predilation of the atrial septum. If, however, the transseptal puncture has been made through the muscular portion of the atrial septum, predilation with a 5-mm dilating balloon catheter placed over one of the two transfer guidewires can be performed to allow eas-

583

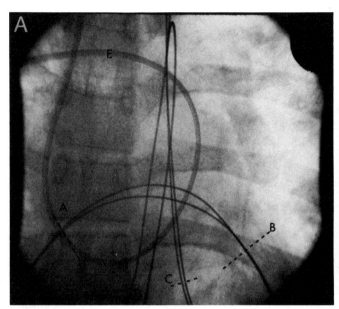 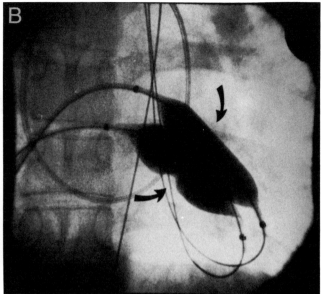

FIG 51–1.
A, two 0.038 in. transfer wire guides in place after the floating balloon catheter has been removed (see the text). *A* =atrial septum; *B* = plane of the mitral valve; *C* = plane of the aortic valve; *D* = descending aorta; *E* = Swan-Ganz catheter in the pulmonary artery. **B,** two dilating balloon catheters partially inflated across the stenotic mitral valve. Note the waist *(arrows)* produced by the valve before full inflation.

ier passage of the two dilating balloon catheters across the atrial septum and then the stenotic mitral valve.

Once in position the dilating balloon catheters are inflated. It is usually easier to inflate one balloon fully and then the second — the inflated first balloon holds the second balloon in place as the mitral valve is split. Balloon inflations are performed with a hand-held 60-mm Luer-Lok syringe containing a third contrast and two thirds saline. Frequently a "waist" can be seen in the balloons as they are inflated (Fig 51–1,B). If the balloons are correctly positioned across the mitral valve, the inflation obstructs left ventricular inflow and leads to transient hypotension. Rapid inflation/deflation cycles lasting no more than 20 seconds are imperative to avoid prolonged hypotension and syncope. After one or two inflations, the balloon dilating catheters are removed, but the transfer wires are left behind. The floating balloon catheter and transseptal sheath are replaced over one of the wires so that the sheath tip lies in the left atrium. The wire guide and transfer wire are removed. The retrograde pigtail catheter is advanced across the aortic valve again, and repeat pressure measurements are made in the left ventricle and left atrium with simultaneous cardiac output measurements to allow calculation of the mitral valve area after PMV. A ventriculogram is then performed through the 7 F catheter in the left ventricle to evaluate mitral regurgitation. After the catheters are withdrawn, an oxygen run is per-

formed with a Swan-Ganz catheter. If there is evidence of left-to-right shunting through the atrial septum, cardiac output determinations should be repeated by using the Fick technique.

CHOICE OF DILATING BALLOON CATHETERS

The effective balloon dilating area is an important determinant of the success of PMV and also influences postvalvotomy mitral regurgitation.[8] The optimal effect of an effective balloon dilating area-to-body surface area ratio for any given patient should be between 3.1 and 4.0 cm^2/m^2. In practice, combinations of either a 15-, 18-, or 20-mm dilating balloon catheter with a second dilating balloon catheter of one of the three sizes is usually used. Left atrial pressure should be lowered to less than 14 mm Hg (assuming normal left ventricular end-diastolic pressure [LVEDP]), and the mitral gradient should be 6 mm or less post-PMV. PMV should not be considered satisfactory unless the left atrial pressure is reduced to this level.

RESULTS

The initial experience with PMV included patients with many different kinds of mitral valve morphology

TABLE 51–1.

Results of Percutaneous Mitral Valvotomy

Variable	Pre-PMV	Post-PMV
Mitral gradient (mm Hg)	15±0.5	5±0.2*
Mitral valve area (cm^2)	0.9±0.1	2.0±0.1
*P < .0001		

TABLE 51–2.

Determination of Echocardiograph Score*

Variable	Minimal	Severe
Valve rigidity	1	4
Valve thickening	1	4
Calcification	1	4
Subvalvular thickening	1	4
Echocardiographic score total	4	16

*A score of 1 for each factor in minimal disease and a score of 4 for each factor in severe disease.

and severity of mitral valve stenosis. Recent experience seems much better than the initial experience since issues of the learning curve of the technique, technical problems with high-profile balloons, better choice of patients, etc., have made considerable differences in the results obtained.[9] In comparing the immediate outcome of one series of the first 150 patients with the last 161 patients undergoing PMV, there was no difference between the two groups in age, sex, New York Heart Association (NYHA) classification, presence of calcification, atrial fibrillation, degree of mitral regurgitation, mean pulmonary artery or left atrial pressures, cardiac output, pulmonary vascular resistance, mitral valve gradient, and mitral valve area before the procedure. There were, however, fewer patients in the early group with mobile, thin, noncalcified valves without severe valvular disease. A good result (defined as a mitral valve area of greater than 1.5 cm^2 post-PMV) was obtained in 77% in the early group and 75% in the later group (not significant). However, after PMV more than a 2+ increase in mitral regurgitation was present in 13% of the early group and only 6% of the later group. Left-to-right shunting was detected in 22% of the earlier group and only 11% of the later group (P = .0001). There were three deaths in the early group but no deaths in the later group. From these data it seems that improvements in technique, patient selection, and operator experience decreased mortality as well as left-to-right shunting and the development of significant mitral regurgitation. The high rate of success of PMV is maintained.

In general the mean mitral valve area increases from 0.9 ± 0.1 cm^2 to 2.0 ± 0.1 cm^2 (*P* <.0001) (Table 51–1). The mitral valve gradient falls from 15 ± 0.5 to 5 ± 0.2 mm Hg (*P* <.0001). Mean pulmonary artery pressure, left atrial pressure, and pulmonary arteriolar resistance all similarly fall significantly.

FACTORS INFLUENCING THE OUTCOME OF PERCUTANEOUS MITRAL VALVOTOMY

Experience with closed surgical mitral commissurotomy has shown that valve pliability, the degree of leaflet

thickening, and the severity of subvalvular fibrosis and agglutination have an important impact on the immediate outcome of the procedure.[10–12] One would therefore expect a similar experience with PMV. A "score" of four echocardiographic variables has been developed that provides information that may predict the outcome of PMV.[13] Leaflet rigidity, leaflet thickening, valvular calcification, and subvalvular fibrosis are scored from 0 to 4. Table 51–2 describes this scoring system. A higher score represents a calcified, immobile valve with extensive subvalvular thickening. The best outcome with PMV occurs in patients with echocardiographic scores of less than 8 (91% good results). The increase in mitral valve area is significantly greater in such patients than in patients with echocardiographic scores greater than 8. Of the four components of the echocardiographic score, valve thickening and mobility correlate best with the absolute change in mitral valve area.

The increase in mitral valve area is also related to the inflated dilating balloon size. Care should be taken in the selection of dilating balloon catheters so as to obtain a maximum final mitral valve area without changing or only minimally increasing mitral regurgitation.[8]

Patients without fluoroscopic calcium in the mitral valve have a greater increase in mitral valve area after PMV than do patients with calcified valves. Other factors adversely affecting the final mitral valve area post-PMV are the presence of atrial fibrillation, previous surgical mitral commissurotomy, and the severity of mitral regurgitation. It should be noted, however, that PMV can produce a good outcome in patients who have had previous surgical commissurotomy if the mitral valve morphology is favorable and the echocardiographic score is low.[13, 14] In one study, the post-PMV mean mitral valve area in 71 patients with previous surgical commissurotomy was 1.8 ± 0.1 cm^2 vs. a valve area of 2.1 ± 0.1 cm^2 in patients without previous surgical commissurotomy.

SELECTION OF PATIENTS FOR PERCUTANEOUS MITRAL VALVOTOMY

Patients with minimally calcified valves and maintenance of valvular mobility are the best candidates for PMV. Clinically, the presence of an opening snap is frequently the predictor of a good mitral split. Thus patients with minimally or noncalcified valves without severe subvalvular fibrosis and with good mobility and minimal thickening of the valve leaflets by echocardiography are the best candidates. Patients with a history of previous mitral commissurotomy done surgically, some valvular calcification, severe pulmonary hypertension, mild (no more than grade 2/4+) mitral regurgitation, or left ventricular dysfunction should not be excluded from consideration for PMV. The presence of insignificant other valvular disease that does not need repair and the presence of nonsurgical coronary artery disease or other associated disease states are not contraindications. Patients who have severe pulmonary hypertension secondary to mitral stenosis need careful monitoring during PMV to avoid hypovolemia, hypotension, and right-sided heart failure. All patients who are potential candidates for PMV should have a careful echocardiographic examination (Fig 51–2). An "echocardiographic score" can be generated by grading the four factors. Evaluation of the left ventriculogram gives information concerning the degree of mitral regurgitation and frequently shows severe subvalvular fibrosis when it cannot be seen on the echocardiogram. Contraindications to PMV are the following: high echocardiographic score (greater than 11), the presence of left atrial thrombus, a recent untreated thromboembolic event, severe associated coronary disease in a patient who is a candidate for combined mitral valve surgery and coronary bypass surgery, severe associated regurgitant disease of the aortic or mitral valve, and the presence of left ventricular thrombus (Table 51–3).

LONG-TERM RESULTS

Cardiac catheterization, echocardiographic analysis, and clinical evaluation of a cohort of 41 patients 2 years after PMV show that 41% of the patients are NYHA class I and 49% in addition are NYHA class II. Fifty-one percent of the patients remained improved by one

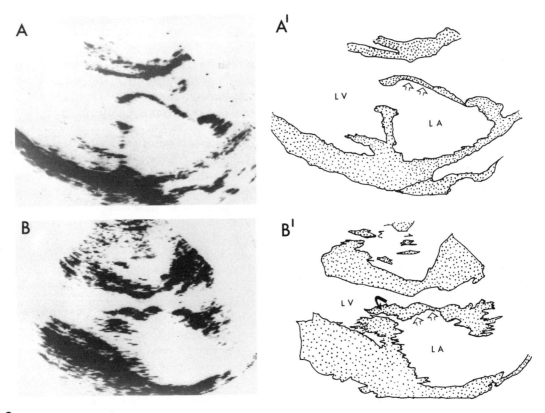

FIG 51–2.
Echocardiograms and outline diagrams of a mitral valve favorable for PMV (**A** and **A'**) and not favorable for PMV (**B** and **B'**). The favorable valve has thin, mobile leaflets (*arrows,* **A'**); the unfavorable valve has thick, rigid leaflets (**B'**), severe subvalvular thickening (*curved solid arrow,* **B'**), and calcification. LA = left atrium, LV = left ventricle.

TABLE 51–3.

Indications and Contraindications for Percutaneous Mitral Valvotomy

---

Factors favorable for PMV
  Echocardiographic score of 8 or less
  Young age
  Presence of opening snap
  Normal sinus rhythm
  No calcification of valve
Factors unfavorable for PMV
  Echocardiographic score of 10 or more
  Age greater than 70 yr
  No opening snap
  Atrial fibrillation (long-standing)
  Calcification of valve
  Severe subvalvular fibrosis
  Thickened atrial septum (>3 mm)
Contraindications to PMV
  Left atrial thrombus
  Recent (3 mon) thromboembolic event
  2+ or higher grade of mitral regurgitation
  Left ventricular thrombus
  Associated surgical coronary or other valve disease

NYHA class at the 2-year follow-up. Twenty-four percent were improved by two NYHA classes. Cardiac catheterization analysis shows that approximately 50% of the patients had no restenosis (restenosis defined as a loss of more than 50% of the gain in mitral valve area achieved at the time of PMV). However, a comparison of the cardiac catheterization data with simultaneously performed echocardiograms indicated that the immediate post-PMV cardiac catheterization data give a spurious calculation of the actual mitral valve area. This is due to the combination of left-to-right shunting producing a higher right-sided cardiac output measured by thermodilution techniques even in patients in whom oxymetry does not show a significant oxygen step-up as well as some venting of the left atrium through the atrial defect, which lowers left atrial pressure in the immediate post-PMV period. This combination of factors works in the same direction to maximize the calculated mitral valve area. Echocardiographic analysis of the same patients done immediately post-PMV shows that the immediate post-PMV mitral valve area is less than that calculated by cardiac catheterization data and that more than two thirds of patients have no restenosis at the 2-year follow-up. Hence, echocardiographic evaluation of the mitral valve area immediately post-PMV by planimetry and two-dimensional echocardiography may be the best way of following patients after mitral valvotomy.

At 2-year follow-up left ventricular cineangiography, 10% of patients had developed more mitral regurgitation in comparison to their immediate post-PMV status.

Possible explanations include mitral valve tearing or late chordal rupture. In 5% of the patients, however, the mitral regurgitation decreased more than two grades. The improvement in papillary muscle dysfunction, elastic recoil of the mitral annulus, and gradual fusion of the commissure, which produced mitral regurgitation at its junction with the mitral annulus, could all account for the improvement.

Clinical follow-up has been studied 4 years after PMV. The mean follow-up time was 20 ± 1 months (range, 0 to 49 months). The patients were divided into two groups according to the morphologic echocardiographic score. Two hundred ten patients had echocardiographic scores of less than 8, and 110 patients had scores greater than 8. Patients in the former group were older and had a higher incidence of atrial fibrillation and calcification under fluoroscopy. More in this group also had previous surgical commissurotomy. Freedom from total events (death, mitral valve replacement, and severe functional disability [NYHA classes III and IV]) at the 4-year follow-up was greater in patients in the group with low echocardiographic scores (80% $\pm$ 5% vs. 40% $\pm$ 10%; $P < .0001$). Similarly, survival rates were 99% $\pm$ 1% in the group with low echocardiographic scores vs. 75% $\pm$ 6% in the group with high echocardiographic scores ($P = .0001$). Thus patients with an echocardiographic score of less than 8 have an excellent 4-year clinical follow-up, and PMV should be the treatment of choice in this group of patients.

COMPLICATIONS OF PERCUTANEOUS MITRAL VALVOTOMY

There are many potential complications of PMV. They include the production of mitral regurgitation, thromboembolic events, problems related to transseptal catheterization (tamponade, creation of a left-to-right shunt through the atrial septum), and rhythm disturbances. However, overall mortality and morbidity with PMV is low and similar to surgical commissurotomy. PMV should have less than a 1% mortality rate. The incidence of thromboembolic episodes and stroke should be 1% or less. An increase in mitral regurgitation occurs in approximately 45% of patients. However, in most patients this increase is only mild and well tolerated clinically. Severe mitral regurgitation (4+) occurs in only 0.9% of patients. An undesirable increase in mitral regurgitation (greater than 2+) occurs in 12.5% of patients, but it is well tolerated in most. Unfavorable mitral valve anatomy (severe subvalvular stenosis, calcification, and scarring of the anterior leaflet) seems to be more likely associated with severe post-PMV mitral regurgitation. A transient heart block of less than 24 hours' duration occurs in fewer than 1% of patients. Pericardial tamponade is usually a complication of transseptal puncture and occurs in fewer than 1% of cases. If during the course of PMV persistent hypotension (not related to vagal tone or hypovolemia) occurs and is associated with a diminution in fluoroscopically visible cardiac pulsations, the first diagnosis should be pericardial tamponade. Treatment with pericardial drainage in the cardiac catheterization laboratory by using a pigtail catheter should be instituted immediately. Tamponade may occur from left ventricular apex perforation either by a wire guide or by the dilating balloons. This is usually a catastrophic complication and requires urgent cardiac surgery — even if the tamponade is initially controlled by pericardiocentesis.

PMV results in a 20% incidence of left-to-right shunting across the atrial septal defect as determined by oxymetry immediately after the procedure. The size of the defect is small (pulmonary-to-systemic flow ratio of less than 2:1 in the majority of patients). A greater percentage of patients have a left-to-right shunt that can be detected by transesophageal color-flow Doppler echocardiography. Clinical, echocardiographic, surgical, and hemodynamic follow-up of patients with a post-PMV left-to-right shunt shows that the defect closes in 59% of patients. Any persistent left-to-right shunt is usually well tolerated.

CONCLUSION

PMV is a safe and effective procedure and offers an alternative to surgical commissurotomy in selected patients with mitral stenosis. A careful echocardiographic evaluation and cardiac catheterization with left ventricular cineangiography should be done in each patient before commitment to PMV. Patients with an echocardiographic score of 8 or less (mobile valve, little calcium, little valve thickening, little subvalvular fibrosis) should have good results and have little or no restenosis at long-term follow-up. Patients with a higher echocardiographic score may have a good result, but the restenosis rate is higher, and the immediate results are less predictable. Nevertheless, the option of an attempt at PMV should be given to most patients who have symptomatic mitral stenosis that requires mechanical repair.

REFERENCES

1. Lock JE, Kalilullah M, Shrivastava S, et al: Percutaneous catheter commissurotomy in rheumatic mitral stenosis. *N Engl J Med* 1985; 313:1515–1518.
2. Inoue K, Owaki T, Nakamura F, et al: Clinical application of transvenous mitral commissurotomy by a new balloon catheter. *J Thorac Cardiovasc Surg* 1984; 87:394–402.
3. McKay RG, Lock JE, Safian RD, et al: Balloon dilatation of mitral stenosis in adult patients: Postmortem and percutaneous mitral valvuloplasty studies. *J Am Coll Cardiol* 1987; 9:723–731.
4. Palacios IF, Block PC, Brandi S, et al: Percutaneous balloon valvotomy for patients with severe mitral stenosis. *Circulation* 1987; 75:778–784.
5. Babic VV, Pejcic P, Djurisic Z, et al: Percutaneous transarterial balloon valvuloplasty for mitral valve stenosis. *Am J Cardiol* 1986; 57:1101–1104.
6. Zaibag M, Al Kasab S, Riberio PA, et al: Percutaneous double balloon mitral valvotomy for rheumatic mitral valve stenosis. *Lancet* 1986; 1:757–761.
7. Vahanian A, Michel PL, Cormier B, et al: Results of percutaneous mitral commissurotomy in 200 patients. *Am J Cardiol* 1989; 63:847–852.
8. Roth RB, Block PC, Palacios IF: Predictors of increased mitral regurgitation after percutaneous mitral balloon valvotomy. *Cathet Cardiovasc Diagn* 1990; 20:17–21.
9. Block PC, Palacios IF, Jacobs ML, et al: Mechanism of percutaneous mitral valvotomy. *Am J Cardiol* 1987; 59:179.
10. Commerford PJ, Hastie T, Beck W: Closed mitral valvotomy: Actuarial analysis of results in 654 patients over 12 years and analysis of preoperative predictors of long-term survival. *Ann Thorac Surg* 1982; 33:473–479.
11. Gross RI, Cunningham JN, Snively SL, et al: Long-term results of open radical mitral commissurotomy: Ten-year follow-up study of 202 patients. *Am J Cardiol* 1981; 47:821.
12. Kirklin JW, Barrett-Boyes BG: Mitral valve disease with or without tricuspid valve disease, in *Cardiac Surgery*. New York, Wiley, 1986.
13. Wilkins GT, Weyman AE, Abascal VM, et al: Percutaneous mitral valvotomy: An analysis of echocardiographic variables related to outcome and the mechanism of dilatation. *Br Heart J* 1988; 60:299–308.
14. Michel MSJ, Blackston EH, Kirklin JW, et al: Outcome probabilities and life history after surgical mitral commissurotomy: Implications for balloon commissurotomy. *J Am Coll Cardiol* 1991; 17:29–42.
15. Nakano S, Kawashima Y, Hirose H, et al: Reconsiderations of indications for open mitral commissurotomy based on pathologic features of the stenosed mitral valve — A fourteen year follow-up study in 347 consecutive patients. *J Thorac Cardiovasc Surg* 1987; 94:336–342.

52

Percutaneous Double-Balloon Valvotomy for Patients With Severe Mitral Stenosis: Five Years' Follow-up Experience

Carlos E. Ruiz, M.D., Ph.D.

He Ping Zhang, M.D.

Habib Gamra, M.D.

John W. Allen, M.D.

Francis Y.K. Lau, M.D.

In this chapter, we describe a methodology and personal experience in treating severe mitral stenosis by the percutaneous double-balloon valvotomy (PDBV) technique. Our experience, based on a series of over 600 procedures performed between September 1985 and February 1991, has led us to view PDBV as a safe, effective, less costly nonsurgical alternative for patients who have clinical indications for surgical mitral valvotomy.

HISTORY

Even though the incidence of rheumatic heart disease has markedly decreased in the United States and most industrialized nations,[1, 2] it continues to be the primary underlying cause of mitral stenosis. A high prevalence of mitral stenosis in developing nations is common,[3, 4] and some recent reports indicate that the incidence of rheumatic fever in the United States is beginning to increase.

Open mitral valve commissurotomy remains the popular treatment of choice for stenotic disease in many places around the world. An alternative procedure, nonsurgical balloon valvotomy, was first reported by Inoue et al.[5] Two major balloon techniques, single-balloon[5]

and double-balloon,[6] have been currently used. We have modified and simplified the technique in an attempt to minimize both the procedure time and the concomitant risks. We feel that there are theoretical reasons that make the double-balloon technique safer and more effective than the single-balloon approach to valvotomy.

PATIENT SELECTION

Appropriate patients for the PDBV are symptomatic, New York Heart Association (NYHA) functional class II or above, without any absolute contraindications for PDBV. Such contraindications would include an interrupted inferior vena cava, documented or suspected intracardiac clots, or a recent history of thromboembolism within the last 6 months.

In selecting the candidates for PDBV, two-dimensional echocardiography combined with color Doppler flow analysis should be used to assess the degree of mitral stenosis, the valve structure, and the degree of mitral regurgitation; transesophageal echocardiography (TEE) should be performed to detect left atrial clots in patients at high risk of emboli. Careful echocardiographic analysis by an experienced echocardiographer must be carried out in all patients prior to PDBV and can be used to evaluate the post-PDBV results as well as long-term changes.

In symptomatic patients with mitral stenosis, valve areas should be less than 1.5 cm^2 by two-dimensional planimetry and Doppler pressure half-time methods. A valve area of greater than 1.7 cm^2 should lead one to reassess the origin of the patient's symptoms before proceeding with PDBV. Two-dimensional echocardiography should be utilized to determine what portions of the mitral apparatus are involved: commissures, leaflets, and/or subvalvular structures. Evaluation of mitral morphology should include valve mobility, valve thickness, degree of calcification, and submitral involvement. Each factor plays an important role in the outcome of valvotomy. Previous investigators[7] have combined these four features into a valve echocardiographic score and used this as a global assessment of valve structure and function.

Another factor that requires assessment is the degree of mitral regurgitation. Patients with moderate to severe mitral regurgitation are not considered candidates for PDBV. Color-flow and pulsed Doppler are used to grade the degree of mitral regurgitation. It is important to assess the degree of mitral regurgitation in multiple planes while keeping in mind that the assessment of two-dimensional Doppler is a thin tomographic view of the ventricle.

An ideal candidate would have a minimal leaflet thickening, a generous doming motion free of significant submitral involvement, and a noncalcified or minimally calcified valve with commissural fusion and without mitral regurgitation. A marginal candidate may have severe leaflet stenosis, minimal reduction in transverse orifice diameter, heavy submitral involvement with marked fibrosis or calcification, and moderate mitral regurgitation. Our experience has suggested that marginal candidates may still achieve significant hemodynamic and clinical improvement following PDBV, but the ideal candidate would have better results and a less likelihood of developing restenosis. These factors must be considered in the risk-benefit assessment of each patient before the procedure.

At this time, there is no 100% sensitive diagnostic tool available to exclude patients with small atrial clots. TEE provides the best assessment for atrial thrombus (Fig 52–1) and should be considered prior to PDBV. This is the technique of choice to screen candidates for left atrial thrombi. Prior to TEE assessment, our identification of left atrial thrombi was very low. With TEE assessment, approximately 20% of patients are found to have left atrial thrombi.[8] Therefore, transthoracic echocardiography should not be considered an adequate

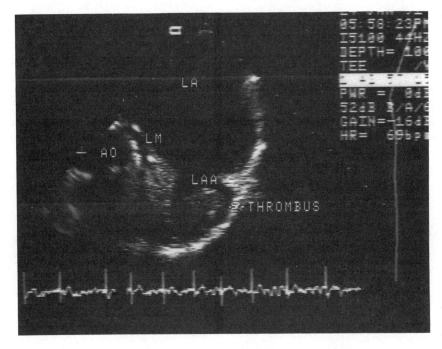

FIG 52–1.
Thrombus in the left atrial appendage *(LAA)* detected by transesophageal echocardiography and undetected by transthoracic echocardiography. *LA* = left atrium; *LM* = left main artery; *AO* = aorta.

screen for a left atrial thrombus. Additional advantages of TEE are further assessment of valve structure and mitral regurgitation. However, our experience suggests that a transthoracic study is adequate to assess valve structure and regurgitation and is the method of choice for planimetering the valve area to assess the degree of stenosis.

PERCUTANEOUS DOUBLE-BALLOON VALVOTOMY PROTOCOL

All patients and especially those with an enlarged left atrial cavity and/or chronic atrial fibrillation should be fully anticoagulated for at least 2 months before the procedure. Oral anticoagulant therapy is discontinued at least 48 hours prior to the procedure.

With the cardiac surgical theater on standby, patients are taken to the catheterization laboratory where both sides of the groin are surgically prepared and properly draped. An 8 F Hemaquet sheath (USCI, Billerica, Mass) is placed in the left femoral vein by the Seldinger technique. A thermodilution Swan-Ganz catheter is then advanced via the sheath, and pressures are obtained from the right atrium, the right ventricle, and the pulmonary artery. A 5 F or 6 F Hemaquet sheath is placed in the left femoral artery by the same technique, and a 5 F or 6 F pigtail catheter is advanced to the ascending aorta, where pressures are again recorded. With the same percutaneous approach, the right femoral vein is then cannulated to access the left atrium by the transseptal technique.

Transseptal catheterization is accomplished from the right femoral vein by using the standard technique with a modified Brockenbrough needle and an 8 F Mullins transseptal sheath-dilator (USCI). A biplane cinefluoroscopy x-ray unit rather than a single-plane unit is highly recommended to facilitate correct placement of the needle before the transseptal puncture and to thereby minimize the risks of cardiac perforation (Fig 52–2). We routinely stain the interatrial septum with contrast medium to facilitate placement of the septostomy balloon catheter in the middle of the septum. Once the transseptal needle has successfully crossed the interatrial septum, continuous pressure monitoring is done through the needle to obtain left atrial pressure readings. Before advancing the Mullins sheath, we obtain a blood sample to confirm the left atrial oxygen saturation values. Contrast medium is injected through the needle to determine the distance to the left atrial wall and to judge the space available to advance the sheath without perforating the atrial wall. At this point, the patient is fully anticoagulated with heparin (150 IU/kg).

Baseline hemodynamic measurements include systemic arterial, left ventricular, pulmonary artery, pulmonary capillary wedge, and left atrial pressures as well as a diagnostic oxygen saturation series. The mean gradient across the mitral valve is measured by using the Mullins sheath and the retrograde pigtail catheter, which has been advanced across the aortic valve into the left ventricular cavity. Simultaneous cardiac outputs are obtained by the thermodilution technique. When significant tricuspid insufficiency is present, the Fick technique is used.

After collecting the baseline hemodynamic data, the

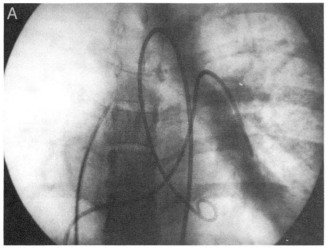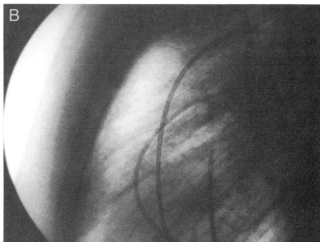

FIG 52–2.
Transseptal needle properly oriented against the interatrial septum before the puncture. **A,** straight anteroposterior view. **B,** lateral view.

Mullins transseptal sheath is advanced into the left ventricle by a slight pullback and counterclockwise manipulation while the sheath is advanced into the left ventricle. Care must be taken not to pull back too far; should the sheath accidentally be drawn into the right atrium, the patients' anticoagulation would preclude making a new puncture through the septum in most cases.

For this procedure, unlike other techniques, the guidewires are not advanced to the descending aorta because the size of the balloon catheter provides sufficient stability along the longitudinal axis of the left ventricle to secure both balloons across the mitral apparatus. Therefore the duration of the procedure and the patient's exposure to radiation are considerably shortened.

A 260-cm specially shaped (2½ turns) exchange wire with a 10-cm tapered inner core (Ruiz–Lau-up guidewire, Schneider Inc., Minneapolis) (Fig 52–3) is advanced and placed at the apex of the left ventricle via the Mullins transseptal sheath. A 7 F catheter (6 mm in diameter by 3 cm in length) with a dilating balloon (Medi-Tech, Inc., Watertown, Mass.) is advanced over the guidewire through the Mullins transseptal sheath to the left atrium. The sheath is then retracted from the shaft of the septostomy balloon catheter to allow expansion of the balloon. The balloon is then inflated across the septum until the waist in the balloon disappears (Fig 52–4) while the guidewire is maintained in the same position in the left ventricle. After septostomy, the Mullins sheath is readvanced into the left ventricle, and a second, identically shaped exchange wire is advanced and positioned next to the first one (Fig 52–5). The transseptal sheath is then withdrawn.

Valvotomy balloons are 5 cm in length by the appropriate diameter (Cook Co., Bloomington, Ind) and should be selected according to mitral annulus size as

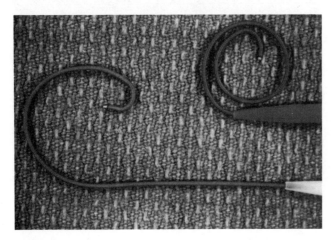

FIG 52–3.
Ruiz–Lau-up guidewire (Schneider, Inc., Minneapolis).

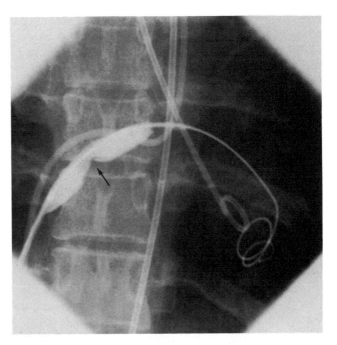

FIG 52–4.
Septostomy balloon catheter across the interatrial septum. Notice the indentation of the septum in the contour of the balloon *(arrow)*.

measured from two-dimensional echocardiography. The balloon annulus (B/A) diameter ratio was calculated as the balloon diameter divided by the annulus diameter. The double-balloon diameter is the sum of the two balloon diameters. A combination of catheters with a balloon length of 5.0 cm and a diameter of 18 to 20 mm (total diameter of 36 to 40 mm) is typically used in normal-sized adults (body surface area [BSA], > 1.5 m²) to achieve an oversizing of the annulus of between 10% to 30% (average oversize, 20%). In no instance should the mitral annulus be oversized more than 40%.

The first valvotomy balloon catheter is advanced over one of the wires and positioned across the mitral valve, with a large double loop of the preshaped wire extending out of the tip of the balloon catheter and positioned in the apex of the left ventricle. A second balloon dilatation catheter is advanced over the second wire and positioned parallel to the first one across the mitral valve. The two balloon catheters are then inflated by hand simultaneously (Fig 52–6,A and B) until the waist of the stenotic valve over the balloons' silhouette disappears (Fig 52–6,C and D). Inflation times range from 20 to 50 seconds. One or two inflations are usually done.

Immediately after the procedure, the balloon catheters are removed, and a pigtail catheter is advanced transseptally over the guidewire to the left ventricle. Pullback pressures are recorded from the left ventricle

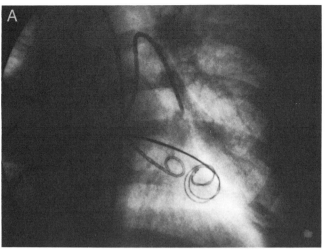 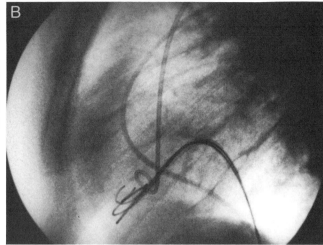

FIG 52–5.
Two specially shaped exchange guidewires already across and positioned at the apex of the left ventricle. **A,** anteroposterior view. **B,** lateral view.

to the left atrium. Simultaneous recordings of pressure are obtained from both cavities by using the retrograde left ventricular pigtail catheter and the transseptal left atrial pigtail catheter. Simultaneous cardiac output, pulmonary artery pressure, and systemic hemodynamic measurement are also recorded.

The procedure is routinely completed in about 1 hour, and most patients are discharged home within 24 hours.

METHODS OF ASSESSMENT

The mitral valve area is calculated before and after PDBV by using the Gorlin formula, the Doppler pressure half-time, and two-dimensional echocardiographic planimetry. The Gorlin mitral valve area is determined immediately after the procedure while the echo Doppler measurements are obtained within 24 hours after PDBV.

Results of valvotomy were considered optimal if the mitral valve area postvalvotomy was ≥ 1.50 cm^2 and the percent increase was $\geq 50\%$. The criteria were chosen on the basis of the following considerations: (1) patients with a mitral valve area ≥ 1.50 cm^2 are relatively asymptomatic and are considered to have a mild mitral stenosis;[9] (2) the second requirement was a 50% increase in mitral valve area after valvotomy because this would exclude an increase in mitral valve area due to measurement variability and atrial septal defect flow created during the procedure and because the Gorlin formula itself already overestimates the mitral valve area by up to 15% for mild mitral stenosis.[10]

The degree of valvular calcification is graded fluoro-

scopically from 0+ (no calcium) to 4+ (dense valvular and subvalvular calcium).

Left ventriculography is performed to evaluate the severity of mitral regurgitation, which is graded 0+ (no regurgitation) to 4+ (severe) according to the degree of opacification of the left atrium and pulmonary veins.[11, 12]

At the end of the procedure, samples to determine oxygen saturation are systematically drawn, and left atrial cineangiography in the cranial left anterior oblique projection is performed to detect and evaluate any left-to-right shunt.

RESULTS OF PERCUTANEOUS DOUBLE-BALLOON VALVOTOMY

In our series of over 600 cases (mean age, 46 ± 14 years; range, 17 to 85; 18% males and 82% females), significant overall hemodynamic improvement was achieved after balloon valvotomy. The mean mitral valve gradient decreased from 16 to 5 mm Hg, the cardiac output increased from 3.81 to 5.41 L/min, the mean pulmonary artery pressure decreased from 38 to 29 mm Hg, the mean left atrial pressure decreased from 27 to 16 mm Hg (Fig 52–7,A), and the mitral valve area by both the Gorlin and Doppler methods increased significantly from 0.88 to 2.39 cm^2 and from 0.96 to 2.05 cm^2, respectively (Fig 52–7,B). Optimal results by the Gorlin formula were obtained in 93% of the patients.

Multiple stepwise regression analysis was used to determine whether variables such as age, sex, valvular cal-

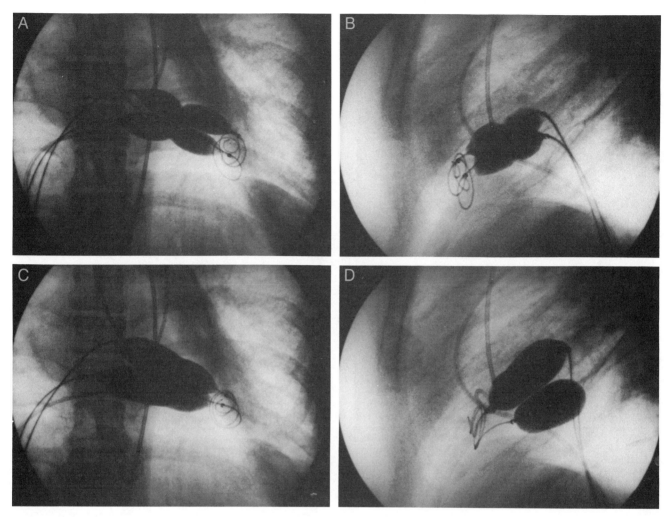

FIG 52–6.
View of two balloons during inflation. The balloons are parallel to each other and across the mitral valve. The exchange guidewires with a specially preshaped double loop extend out of the tip of the balloon catheters and are lodged at the apex of the left ventricle. During inflation the waist produced by the stenotic valve on the balloon silhouette is seen (**A,** anteroposterior view; **B,** lateral view). After full inflation of both balloons the fused commissures are cracked, and the waist on the balloon silhouette has disappeared (**C,** anteroposterior view; **D,** lateral view).

cification, prevalvotomy NYHA functional class, rhythm, prevalvotomy mitral valve area, and B/A diameter ratio would predict postvalvotomy and absolute increases in mitral valve area. Calcification, prevalvotomy mitral valve area, and the B/A diameter ratio were the significant predictors for postvalvotomy and absolute increases in mitral valve area as determined by both the Gorlin formula and Doppler method.

Before valvotomy, 70% of the patients were in NYHA functional class III or IV. After valvotomy, more than 86% of the patients were in functional class I and 13% in class II.

When patients were separated according to the degree of calcification, 55% of the patients had noncalci-

fied (0+) or minimally calcified (1+) valves (group 1), and 45% had moderately to heavily (2+ to 4+) calcified valves (group 2). Hemodynamic parameters and mitral valve area by both the Gorlin and Doppler methods were significantly improved in both groups. However, the absolute and percent increases in mitral valve area (Figs 52–8,A and 52–9,A) and the absolute and percent decreases in mean mitral valve gradient, mean pulmonary artery pressure, and mean left atrial pressure were significantly greater in group 1 (Figs 52–8,B and 52–9,B). The absolute and percent increases in cardiac output did not differ between the two groups (Figs 52–8,B and 52–9,B). When the Gorlin formula was used, optimal results were achieved in 98% of the pa-

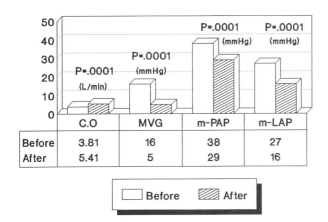

A.

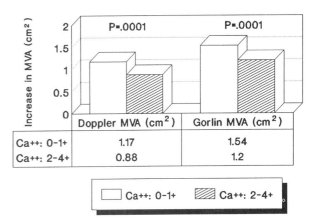

A.

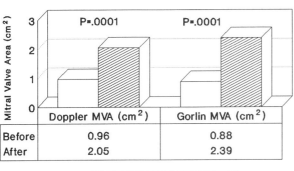

B.

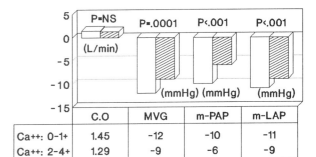

B.

FIG 52–7.
A, hemodynamic changes before PDBV and after PDBV. **B,** mitral valve area (both Doppler and Gorlin) changes before PDBV and after PDBV. *CO* = cardiac output; *MVG* = mitral valve gradient; *m-PAP* = mean pulmonary artery pressure; *m-LAP* = mean left atrial pressure.

FIG 52–8.
A, comparision of the absolute increase in mitral valve area (both Doppler and Gorlin) after PDPV according to the degree of calcification. **B,** comparision of absolute change in hemodynamic values after PDBV according to the degree of calcification. Abbreviations are as in Figure 52–7.

tients in group 1 and 85% in group 2 (P ≤ .001); with the echo Doppler method, optimal results were obtained in 86% in group 1 and 64% in group 2 (P ≤ .001). It therefore appears that valvular calcification is closely related to hemodynamic improvement and optimal results.

PROCEDURE TOLERANCE AND COMPLICATIONS

The procedure is performed with patients under local anesthesia and is generally well tolerated. The double-balloon technique allows sufficient hemodynamic support during balloon inflations, and blood flow has

been shown by color-flow Doppler analysis during balloon inflation to occur around the inflated balloons.

Several major complications can be associated with PDBV, including an increase in mitral insufficiency, left ventricular perforation, tamponade, large atrial septal defects, cerebrovascular accidents, transient ischemic attacks, and death (procedure related if within 6 weeks postvalvotomy). The creation of acute severe mitral insufficiency could happen by tearing the mitral valve leaflet or any of its delicate structures. Severe acute mitral regurgitation requires emergency surgery for repair (Fig 52–10). In our experience, 46% of the patients had at least a 1+ increase in mitral regurgitation; however, only 4% had a 2+ or more increase, including four patients who developed severe acute mitral regurgitation

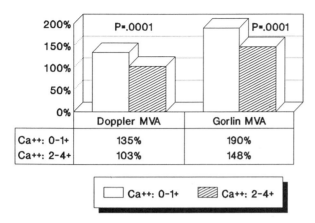

A.

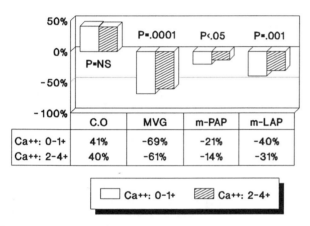

B.

FIG 52-9.
A, comparison of the percent increase in mitral valve area (both Doppler and Gorlin) after PDBV according to the degree of calcification. **B,** comparision of the percent change in hemodynamic values after PDBV according to the degree of calcification. Abbreviations are as in Figure 52-7.

requiring emergency surgery. There were two young patients, one of them status postpartum, who had no valvular calcification and in whom the anterior mitral leaflet was ruptured and required mitral valve replacement. Another patient with a heavily calcified valve developed severe mitral regurgitation and required mitral valve replacement for a torn anterior leaflet (Fig 52-11). A fourth patient who had end-stage mitral stenosis and developed 3+ mitral regurgitation but refused surgery remained in functional class IV and expired of pneumonia and sepsis 6 weeks postvalvotomy. In about 10% of the patients, the pre-existing mitral insufficiency improved or disappeared after PDBV.

Left ventricular perforations induced by the dilata-

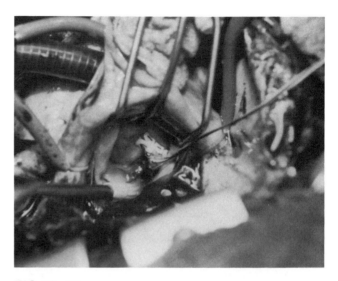

FIG 52-10.
Repaired anterior mitral valve leaflet after it was torn by one of the balloon valvotomy catheters.

tion balloon catheters occurred in six patients. Five of them were over 60 years of age, and three died. Two of them expired 5 and 6 weeks postprocedure, respectively. PDBV could be performed successfully 6 months later in one of the six patients. The rate of left ventricular perforation could be reduced by using pigtail balloon catheters[13] (Fig 52-12) or a guidewire with 2½ turns in the distal, soft, tapered-tip exchange wire.

Two patients developed pericardial tamponade during the procedure, including one young patient with a tear in the interatrial septum that extended down into the inferior vena cava and caused a sudden pericardial tamponade requiring surgical evacuation. At surgery the tear was small, and the bleeding stopped spontaneously.

A major potential risk of PDBV for patients who are in atrial fibrillation, who have a large left atrial cavity, and who have a calcific mitral valve is mobilization of a clot during the procedure, which could result in a catastrophic cerebrovascular embolic accident. In our experience we have had no major cerebrovascular accidents; however, three patients suffered mild transient ischemic attacks that occurred during the procedure in two patients and 18 hours after the valvotomy in one patient. All were resolved in less than 12 hours and left no neurologic deficits. Surprisingly, all three patients were in normal sinus rhythm and fully anticoagulated during the procedure. No embolic phenomena were detected in any of the patients who were in atrial fibrillation during the procedure. One patient had a cerebrovascular accident 3 days postprocedure with probable emboli. Therefore we advise anticoagulation with warfarin (Coumadin) for 3 months postprocedure.

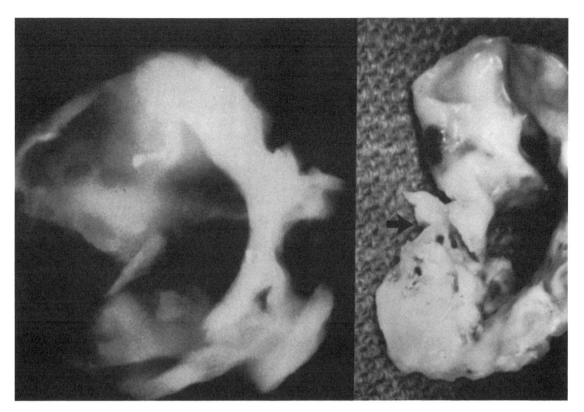

FIG 52–11.
Rupture of a calcified mitral valve (arrow) *(right)* and the same valve as seen by x-ray *(left)*.

A left-to-right shunt was detected by either oximetry or left atrial angiography in 12% of the patients. The pulmonary-to-systemic flow ratio (Qp/Qs) was found to be greater than 1.5:1 in only 2% of the patients.

Four patients developed traumatic pericardial effusion during the attempt to perform the transseptal approach, and the procedure was aborted. Two of the patients came back a week later and underwent uneventful

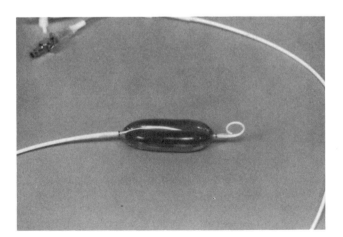

FIG 52–12.
Ballon valvotomy pigtail catheter.

PDBV of their mitral valve, a third one went to surgery, and in the fourth one the procedure was continued uneventfully without systemic anticoagulation. Technical failure such as an inability to cross the mitral valve or to inflate the balloon occurred in three patients in our early experience.

Atrial and ventricular arrhythmias induced by catheters, wires, and balloon dilating catheters were common in all patients but usually well tolerated.

We experienced four procedure-related deaths, three of them secondary to a large left ventricular perforation and one caused by a severe mitral regurgitation as previously described.

COMPARISON OF INOUE SINGLE-BALLOON VS. DOUBLE-BALLOON VALVOTOMY

We have 85 consecutive patients who underwent percutaneous mitral valvotomy with the Inoue single-balloon method. The hemodynamic results and mitral valve areas were compared between the Inoue single-balloon (IB) and the double-balloon techniques. The two groups were similar in age, gender, and calcification.

Before valvotomy, cardiac output, mean mitral valve gradient, mitral valve area by both the Gorlin and Doppler methods, left atrial pressure, and heart rate were not significantly different between the groups except for mean pulmonary artery pressure, which was higher in the PDBV group ($P \leq .05$) (Fig 52–13,A and B). After valvotomy, the PDBV group had a significantly larger valve area and cardiac output ($P \leq .0001$) (Fig 52–13,A and B).

The absolute value change, which may reflect a difference between the techniques more accurately because it does not depend on values before valvotomy, was also compared. The percent change in values before and af-

ter the procedure was compared between the groups. Figure 52–14,A shows that the absolute increase in mitral valve area and cardiac output and the absolute decrease in mitral valve gradient, mean pulmonary artery pressure, and mean left atrial pressure were greater in the PDBV group. Figure 52–14,B shows that the percent changes in mitral valve area and cardiac output were significantly greater in the PDBV group.

Optimal results were achieved in 76% of patients in the IB group and 93% of patients in the PDBV group ($P \leq .0001$) (Fig 52–15).

The mortality rate and need for emergency surgery

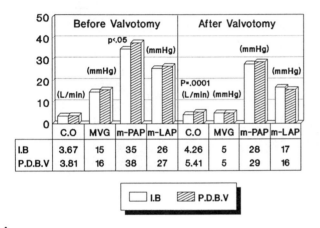

A.

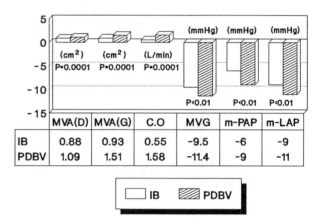

A.

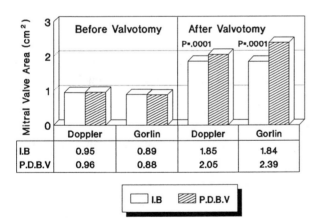

B.

FIG 52–13.
A, comparison of hemodynamic values before valvotomy and after valvotomy between the Inoue single-balloon and the double-balloon techniques. **B,** comparison of mitral valve area (both Doppler and Gorlin) before valvotomy and after valvotomy between the Inoue single-balloon and the double-balloon techniques. Abbreviations are as in Figure 52–7.

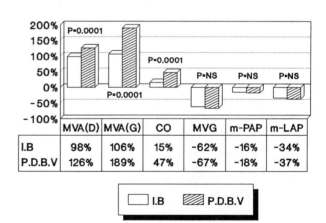

B.

FIG 52–14.
A, comparison of absolute change in hemodynamic values before and after valvotomy with the Inoue single-balloon vs. the double-balloon technique. **B,** comparison of the percent change in hemodynamic values when the Inoue single-balloon and the double-balloon techniques are used for percutaneous mitral valvotomy. MVA(D) = mitral valve area determined by Doppler; MVA(G) = mitral valve area determined by Gorlin; other abbreviations are as in Figure 52–7.

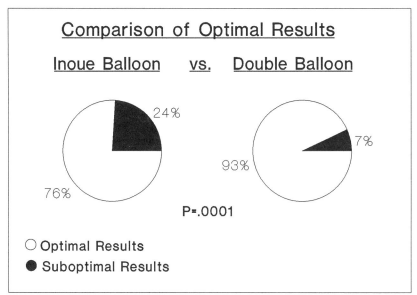

FIG 52–15.
Percentage of patients with optimal results as determined by the Gorlin formula.

were about the same with either technique. Angiography revealed that a left-to-right shunt developed in 5% of patients in the IB group and 12% in the PDBV group ($P \leq .05$). However, only 1.2% of the patients in the IB group had a left-to-right shunt with a Qp/Qs > 1.5:1 vs. 1.9% in the PDBV group (not significant). Emergency surgery was required in 3.6% of patients in the IB group and 3.4% in the PDBV group; 2.4% of patients in the IB group vs. 0.9% in the PDBV group required mitral valve replacement or repair due to severe mitral regurgitation. No left ventricular perforation developed with the single-balloon technique. Technical failure because of an inability to cross the mitral valve or to inflate the balloon occurred in two patients in the IB group and three in the PDBV group. However, 3

months later repeat attempts were successful in two patients, one in each group.

Fifty-two percent of the patients in the IB group had at least a 1+ increase in mitral regurgitation vs. 46% in the PDBV group (not significant). However, 19% in the IB group and 4% in the PDBV group had a 2+ or more increase in mitral regurgitation ($P \leq .001$) (Fig 52–16).

Clinical evaluation after valvotomy showed that the groups did not differ with regard to NYHA functional class: over 98% of patients in both groups improved their functional class to I or II.

The correlation between B/A diameter ratio and mitral valve area after valvotomy was examined in a person-to-person matched group. The rationale for matching groups was to minimize the factors that may

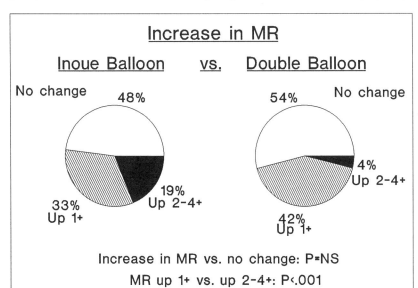

FIG 52–16.
Percentage of patients with an increase in mitral regurgitation *(MR)* after percutaneous balloon mitral valvotomy.

influence mitral valve area outcome with either procedure. The criteria for matching were (1) gender, exact match; (2) age, within 10 years; (3) calcification, 0+, exact match; 1 to 4+, match within 1+; and (4) mitral valve area before valvotomy, within 0.15 cm^2.

The postvalvotomy mitral valve area was significantly correlated with the B/A diameter ratio ($r = 0.62$, $P \leq .0001$). The trend is the larger the B/A diameter ratio used, the larger the mitral valve area. However, because the postvalvotomy mitral valve area may depend on the prevalvotomy mitral valve area, further analysis was performed to find a relationship between the absolute increase in mitral valve area and the B/A diameter ratio. Figure 52–17 shows that the trend remained: the larger the B/A diameter ratio, the greater the increase in mitral valve area ($r = 0.66$, $P \leq .0001$). The mean B/A diameter ratio was 45% larger in the PDBV group than in the IB group (1.16 ± 0.13 vs. 0.80 ± 0.10, respectively; $P \leq .0001$), and the mean increase in mitral valve area was 65% greater in the PDBV group than in the IB group (1.58 ± 0.55 vs. 0.93 ± 0.30 cm^2, respectively; $P \leq .0001$).

We have shown in a previous report[14] that if the total cross-sectional diameter of two circles (assuming that the diameter of the two circles are equal) is the same as the diameter of a single circle, the total surface area of two circles would be 50% smaller than the surface area of a single one (Fig 52–18,A and B). This allows one to safely use two simultaneously inflated balloons and oversize the annulus diameter by at least 25%. This is why a larger B/A diameter ratio may be used with the double-balloon technique. The predilection of the two balloons to fit into the commissures may be a reason for the greater efficiency of this technique in opening the stenotic valve, the mechanism of balloon valvotomy being commissural splitting.[15] Because the area occupied by the two expanded balloons does not exceed the valvular orifice area, the longitudinal diameter of the valvular apparatus can be safely overstretched, and more effective splitting of the fused commissures can be obtained (Fig 52–18,C). Furthermore, when two balloons are simultaneously inflated, tension applied to the plane of the mitral commissures is twice the tension applied vertically according to Laplace's law. Hence, there is more effective splitting of the fused commissures and less risk of rupturing or tearing the mitral leaflets, which are the weakest structures of the mitral valve apparatus; consequently, there is less risk of creating severe mitral regurgitation, and a larger mitral valve area is achieved. Since the double-balloon technique geometrically approaches the shape of the mitral annulus configuration without overoccupying the valvular orifice area, the free space between balloons allows continued flow of blood across the valve during maximum inflation and thus results in improved hemodynamic stability during inflation.

The greater mitral valve area postvalvotomy as determined by the Gorlin formula may be largely dependent on a higher cardiac output, which could be explained by the higher incidence of left-to-right shunting (12%) found in the PDBV group. The difference in mitral

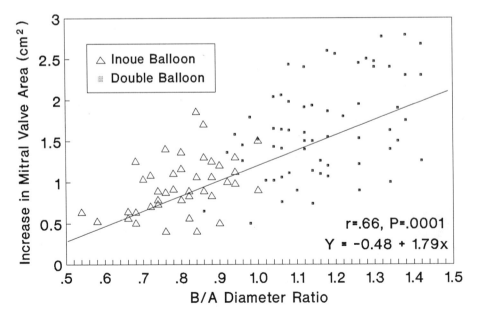

FIG 52–17.
Relationship between the increase in mitral valve area (Gorlin method) to the balloon/annulus *(B/A)* diameter ratio in a person-to-person matched group. See the text.

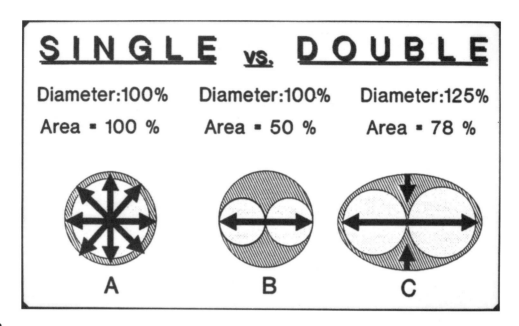

FIG 52–18.
A, for a given cross-sectional diameter a single circle generated from this diameter will have a 50% larger surface area. **B,** however, if from the same diameter we would generate two circles by using each radius as the diameter for each of the new circles, the total cross-sectional diameter would remain unchanged, while the total area generated by the sum of the two new circles would be 50% smaller than the original circle. **C,** therefore that allows us to oversize the longitudinal diameter of this stretchable ring by as much as 125% and it would still not occupy the total inner area of the original ring.

valve area postvalvotomy as calculated by the Doppler pressure half-time method between the groups was smaller than that calculated by the Gorlin formula. However, the mean of the mitral valve area as determined by the Doppler method was still significantly greater in the PDBV group, so the larger mitral valve area achieved with the double-balloon method is corroborated by both methods of calculation.

The double-balloon technique achieves greater immediate hemodynamic results and a larger mitral valve area postvalvotomy. However, long-term follow-up of both of our groups will eventually determine whether or not the immediate hemodynamic superiority of the double-balloon technique is clinically important.

REPEAT CATHETERIZATION AND ECHOCARDIOGRAPHIC DOPPLER FOLLOW-UP

The percutaneous balloon valvotomy technique achieves significant immediate hemodynamic results and clinical improvement, but little is known about its long-term outcome.[16] From our follow-up data during a 5-year period in 152 patients, we believe that the hemodynamic and clinical improvement was still significant. Although only a part of the patients during this period

had echo Doppler follow-up, the patients who were followed may still be considered a representative sample because their age, gender, degree of valvular calcification, NYHA functional class, cardiac rhythm, and prevalvotomy and postvalvotomy mitral valve areas were similar to those of the rest of our patient population.

The purposes of the study were (1) to evaluate the follow-up results following valvotomy, (2) to determine which factors influence mitral valve area and restenosis at follow-up, and (3) to compare the values of invasive and noninvasive techniques for measuring mitral valve area.

One hundred fifty-two patients had serial echo Doppler studies (mean, 15 ± 11 months; range, 1 to 51 months), and 40 of those also underwent repeat catheterization (mean, 21 ± 11 months; range, 3 to 51 months). Follow-up clinical evaluation and echo Doppler assessment were performed at 1, 3, 6, 9, and 12 months after valvotomy and every 6 months thereafter. Repeat catheterization studies were performed in selected patients, including 3 patients who underwent a second PDBV.

Restenosis was defined as (1) mitral valve area at follow-up ≥1.5 cm^2, a reduction $>50\%$ from the original gain, and a decrease of more than 1 SD (0.25 cm^2) of the individual variation of the echo Doppler valve area measurements in our laboratory; or (2) mitral valve area at follow-up <1.5 cm^2, a reduction $>20\%$ from the original gain, and a decrease greater than 1 SD. A mitral valve area ≥1.5 cm^2 at follow-up may not mean that no anatomic valve restenosis developed. If the valve area at follow-up decreased from the original gain by 50%, the area has clearly been reduced significantly, and the change does not represent just measurement variation. On the other hand, a mitral valve area <1.5 cm^2 at follow-up does not always indicate that restenosis has occurred. It might be a measurement error or a suboptimal result. A 20% loss from the original gain and a decrease greater than 1 SD in patients with a mitral valve area <1.5 cm^2 was chosen because it was considered a reasonable decrease that is out of the range of measurement error.

The follow-up results in 40 patients who underwent repeat catheterization and echo Doppler studies show that at follow-up the cardiac output decreased and the mean mitral valve gradient increased significantly from the immediate post-PDBV value but the mean pulmonary artery pressure remained about the same (Fig 52–19,A). At follow-up, the mitral valve area calculated by the Gorlin equation had a significant decrease; however, no evidence was seen of a significant decrease in mitral valve area measured by the echo Doppler method (Figs 52–19,B and 52–20). Figure 52–16, A also shows that all follow-up hemodynamic values were still significantly improved from prevalvotomy values. Mitral valve area as determined by the echo Doppler method or the Gorlin formula did not differ significantly before or at follow-up. The mean difference in mitral valve area (Gorlin area minus the Doppler area in each patient) was -0.06 cm^2 before valvotomy and 0.15 cm^2 at follow-up (not significant). However, the mean mitral valve area immediately after valvotomy was 0.53 cm^2 larger by the Gorlin formula ($P \leq .0001$) (Fig 52–20).

Simple and multiple stepwise regression analyses were used to determine whether age, sex, calcification, prevalvotomy NYHA functional class, rhythm, and postvalvotomy mitral valve area were associated with mitral valve area at follow-up. With multiple stepwise regression, the postvalvotomy mitral valve area and the degree of calcification were significantly associated with follow-up mitral valve area (both Gorlin and Doppler). With simple regression, the postvalvotomy mitral valve area, the degree of calcification, and age were the significant predictors for mitral valve area by both the Gorlin and echo Doppler methods at follow-up.

Since valvular calcification was found to be a significant factor influencing the immediate outcome of valvotomy as previously demonstrated and has been identified as an important factor in long-term results following surgical experience with closed mitral com-

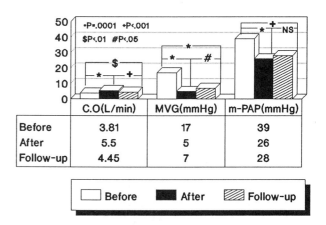

A.

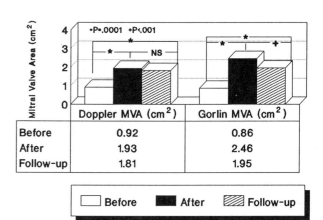

B.

FIG 52–19.
A, changes in hemodynamic values before valvotomy, after valvotomy, and at follow-up in patients who underwent repeat catheterization. **B,** changes in mitral valve area (both Doppler and Gorlin) before valvotomy, after valvotomy, and at follow-up in patients who underwent repeat catheterization. Abbreviations are as in Figure 52–7.

missurotomy,[17, 18] one might wonder whether it affects the long-term outcome following balloon mitral valvotomy. In order to answer this question, the patients who were recatheterized were separated into two groups: 20 patients in group 1 with noncalcified or minimally calcified valves and 20 patients in group 2 with moderately to heavily calcified valves. The mean age in group 2 was much older than group 1 (54 ± 12 vs. 35 ± 8 years, respectively). The mean Doppler mitral valve area was significantly larger in group 1 than in group 2 immediately postvalvotomy and at follow-up as well (Fig 52–21,A); the mean Gorlin mitral valve area was greater in group 1 at follow-up (Fig 52–21,B). The

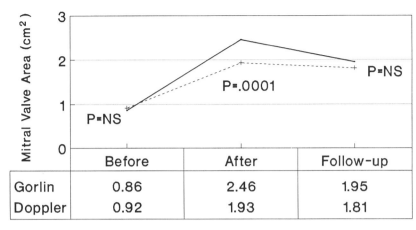

FIG 52–20.
Changes in mitral valve area before valvotomy, after valvotomy, and at follow-up as measured by the Gorlin formula and the echo Doppler method in patients who underwent repeat catheterization. The difference in mitral valve area estimated by the two methods was significant immediately after valvotomy but was not significant at late follow-up.

mean Doppler mitral valve area at follow-up was not significantly smaller than that immediately after valvotomy in either group; the mean Gorlin mitral valve area was significantly smaller in group 2. The trend toward a decrease at follow-up was parallel by both measurements between the two groups (Fig 52–21,A and B).

In 152 patients who underwent echo Doppler studies at follow-up, the mean mitral valve area decreased from 1.89 ± 0.42 cm^2 postvalvotomy to 1.78 ± 0.38 at follow-up ($P \leq .05$ by the t-test; not significant by the Wilcoxon rank-sum test); the mean decrease in mitral valve area was 0.11 ± 0.38 cm^2 ($P \leq .001$ by the paired t-test). Figure 52–22 shows that the pattern of decrease in mitral valve area in different follow-up periods was almost identical.

Regression analysis confirmed that the mitral valve area postvalvotomy, the degree of calcification, age, and NYHA functional class were the most significant factors influencing mitral valve area at follow-up.

After valvotomy, 86% of the patients were in NYHA functional class I, and 12% were in class II. At follow-up, 70% remained in NYHA functional class I, and 25% were in class II. The overall restenosis rate was 14% during the follow-up.

When those patients were separated according to the degree of calcification, 52% of the patients were in group 1 (noncalcified or minimally calcified valves), and 48% were in group 2 (moderately to severely calcified valves). Figure 52–23 shows that the mitral valve area (Doppler) was significantly larger postvalvotomy and at follow-up in group 1 than in group 2. The mitral valve area decreased in both groups, and the trend toward a decrease was parallel between the groups, as in the subgroup of the patients who underwent repeat catheterization at follow-up.

At follow-up, in group 1, 79% of the patients were in NYHA functional class I, and 20% were in class II; in group 2, 59% of the patients were in class I, 31% were in class II, and 10% were in class III or IV.

The restenosis rate can be determined more accurately by using the Kaplan-Meier method. The results showed that the restenosis rate was about 5% or lower in each 6-month period of follow-up. The cumulative percentage of patients free from restenosis was 77% at the 48-month follow-up (Fig 52–24). From Figure 52–25 it appears that valvular calcification is associated with a higher incidence of restenosis.

During 5 years of follow-up, although the mitral valve area decreased from immediately after the procedure, the increase from prevalvotomy values was still significant, and 70% of the patients remained in NYHA functional class I. The degree of calcification may relate to restenosis and clinical symptoms at follow-up. The mitral valve area immediately after valvotomy directly influenced the valve area at follow-up, i.e., the larger the valve area created by the valvotomy, the larger it remained at late follow-up.

Turi et al.[19] reported a prospective, randomized trial in 40 patients to compare percutaneous balloon mitral valvotomy and surgical closed commissurotomy. They showed that the hemodynamic improvement between balloon valvotomy and closed commissurotomy was comparable through 8 months of follow-up.

Most previous studies report a restenosis rate after closed commissurotomy of 25% to 28%.[20, 21] For example, Lyons et al.[20] found restenosis in 25% of their patients 5 years after successful closed mitral commissurotomy. Heger et al.[21] reported a 28% rate of restenosis in their 10- to 14-year follow-up study after successful closed commissurotomy and suspected that restenosis

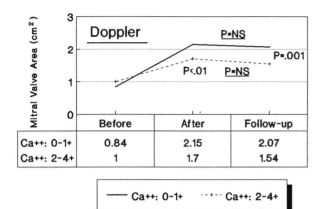

A.

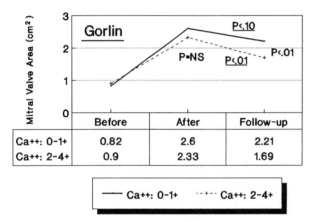

B.

FIG 52–21.
A, comparison of the echo Doppler mitral valve area before valvotomy, after valvotomy, and at follow-up according to the degree of calcification in patients who underwent repeat catheterization. The Doppler mitral valve area at follow-up had no significant decrease from immediate after the procedure in both groups. **B,** comparison of the Gorlin mitral valve area before and after valvotomy and at follow-up according to the degree of calcification in patients who underwent repeat catheterization. The Gorlin mitral valve area at follow-up had no significant decrease from immediately after procedure in the valvular calcium 0 to 1+ group but had a significant a decrease in the calcium 2 to 4+ group.

may have occurred in the early years after commissurotomy. Houseman et al.[22] reported that 16% of their patients who underwent open mitral commissurotomy had restenosis and required reoperation; 78% remained in NYHA functional class I or II at the follow-up study (mean, 46 months).

Our follow-up results showed that the restenosis rate

after balloon mitral valvotomy was lower than after closed commissurotomy and was close to open commissurotomy. However, the highest incidence of restenosis following surgical commissurotomy was observed around 8 to 10 years after the procedure. Therefore, the longer follow-up results still need to be compared between balloon mitral valvotomy and surgical commissurotomy. The previous investigators did not clearly identify restenosis until reoperation or autopsy. Our follow-up results indicate that restenosis does not always mean that the patient requires a repeat procedure; the patient with restenosis is sometimes free of symptoms. A large percentage of the patients in whom restenosis developed according to our strict definition were still in NYHA functional class I, which indicated that redilatation was not needed for these patients based on clinical symptoms. If restenosis requiring reoperation were the criterion used, the rate of restenosis in our study would be much lower.

Mitral valve area measured by noninvasive (echo Doppler) or invasive (Gorlin) methods did not differ significantly at follow-up. In our study, the differences between these two methods yielded significantly different results immediately after valvotomy, but these differences disappeared at follow-up. The valve area overestimation by the Gorlin formula immediately after valvotomy reflects the fact that many variables influence area calculation, primarily those affecting cardiac output determination such as valvular regurgitation, atrial septal defect, and acute changes in left atrial compliance. All of these factors can alter the estimation of valve area without changing the "true" area. However, the degree of valvular regurgitation and atrial septal defect diminished in a large percentage of the patients at late follow-up, so the cardiac output at follow-up is less affected by these acute events.[23–25] Another important reason for overestimation of mitral valve area immediately after valvotomy by the Gorlin formula is that the mitral valve gradient was too low or could not even be measured in a number of patients. Fluid-filled catheters are imprecise in measuring small gradients,[26] which would have greater impact on a calculation of mitral valve area. At follow-up, cardiac output decreased, and the mitral valve gradient increased significantly from immediately after valvotomy, which caused a significant decrease in the Gorlin-determined mitral valve area at follow-up; consequently, the significant difference between Gorlin- and Doppler-determined mitral valve area immediately after valvotomy disappeared at follow-up. Echo Doppler calculation is a less variable measurement of valve area than the Gorlin formula.[27, 28] Furthermore, repeat catheterization at follow-up costs $4,000 to

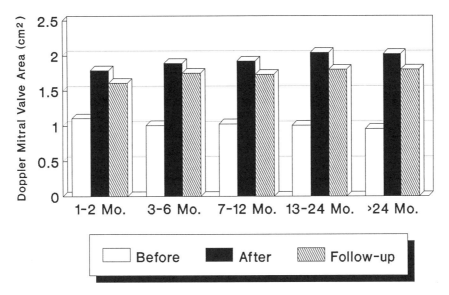

FIG 52–22.
Echo Doppler mitral valve area before valvotomy, after valvotomy, and at 5 different follow-up periods.

$5,000 in the United States, whereas the average cost for a two-dimensional color-flow Doppler study is about $800. Echo Doppler measurement, if carefully performed, is consistent and reliable. In addition, echo Doppler is better accepted by patients. Thus, the expense and discomfort of cardiac catheterization can be avoided at follow-up examination. Echo Doppler is the procedure of choice for follow-up evaluation, and invasive study is required only in selected patients to resolve discrepancies between clinical and echo Doppler findings after valvotomy.

CLINICAL IMPLICATIONS AND COST IMPACT

PDBV has three major advantages over surgical commissurotomy: (1) the procedure-related mortality rate is lower,[17, 18, 22, 29] (2) the restenotic valve can be more safely redilated,[25] and (3) PDBV is much less expensive. The average cost for surgical commissurotomy in the United States ranges from $20,000 to $40,000, primarily because of physician's fees, intensive care costs, and room charges. The average cost for PDBV is between $4,500 and $9,500. Although after 5 years of follow-up the results of PDBV are comparable to closed commis-

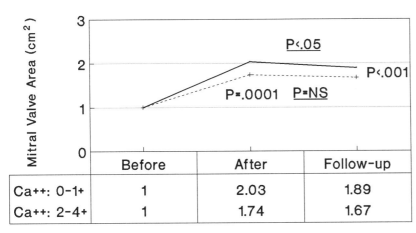

FIG 52–23.
Comparison of the Doppler mitral valve area before valvotomy, after valvotomy, and at follow-up according to valvular calcification.

	Before	After	Follow-up
Ca++: 0-1+	1	2.03	1.89
Ca++: 2-4+	1	1.74	1.67

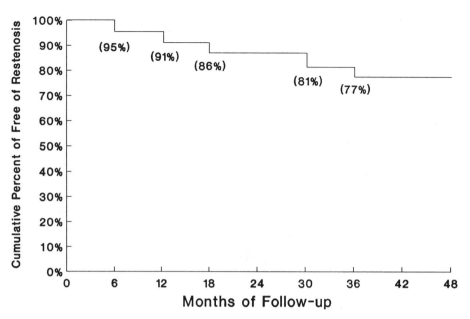

FIG 52–24.
Cumulative percentage of patients free of restenosis as determined by the Kaplan-Meier method in 152 patients following percutaneous balloon valvotomy.

surotomy, the cost-effectiveness on a long-term (10 to 20 years or longer) basis still needs to be determined. The patient's hospital stay is shorter, and the convalescent period before being able to return to work should also be much shorter. These economic advantages may be especially significant in countries where this kind of disease is common. The relatively high cost of each balloon catheter may not make these advantages apply in some developing countries where the cost of surgical closed commissurotomy is without a doubt less expensive than the price of the balloons.[19]

In conclusion, we believe that PDBV is a safe, effective, and palliative procedure for severe mitral stenosis; that the long-term results should not differ much from

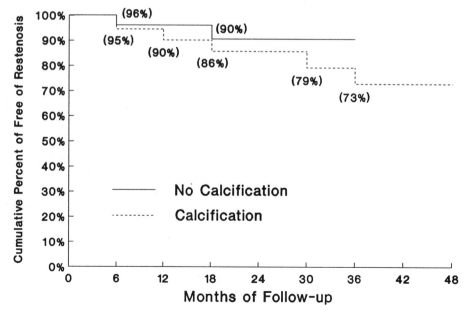

FIG 52–25.
Cumulative percentage of patients free from restenosis as determined by the Kaplan-Meier method between the noncalcified valve group and the calcified valve group following percutaneous balloon mitral valvotomy.

the results in patients who underwent closed surgical commissurotomies[19-21] and that the technique can be safely performed by interventional cardiologists familiar with transseptal cardiac catheterization. This procedure requires the coordinated efforts of the catheterization laboratory, the noninvasive laboratory, and cardiovascular surgery teams.

REFERENCES

1. Roberts WC: Morphologic features of the normal and abnormal mitral valve. *Am J Cardiol* 1983; 51:100.
2. Gordis L: The virtual disappearance of rheumatic fever in the United States; lessons in the rise and fall of disease. T. Duckett Jones Memorial Lecture. *Circulation* 1985; 72:1155.
3. Markowitz M: Observations on the epidemiology and preventability of rheumatic fever in developing countries. *Clin Ther* 1981; 4:240.
4. Community control of rheumatic heart disease in developing countries 1. A major health problem. *WHO Chron* 1980; 34:336.
5. Inoue K, Owani T, Nakamura T, et al: Clinical application of transvenous mitral commissurotomy by a new balloon catheter. *J Thorac Cardiovasc Surg* 1984; 87:394.
6. Al Zaibag M, Ribeiro PA, Al Kasab S, et al: Percutaneous double-balloon mitral valvotomy for rheumatic mitral-valve stenosis. *Lancet* 1986; 1:757.
7. Abascal VM, Wilkins GT, Choong CY, et al: Mitral regurgitation after percutaneous balloon mitral valvuloplasty in adults: Evaluation by pulsed Doppler echocardiography. *J Am Coll Cardiol* 1988; 11:257.
8. Kronzon I, Tunick PA, Glassman E, et al: Transesophageal echocardiography to detect atrial clots in candidates for percutaneous transseptal mitral balloon valvuloplasty. *J Am Coll Cardiol* 1990; 16:1320.
9. Abascal VM, Wilkins GT, O'Shea JP, et al: Prediction of successful outcome in 130 patients undergoing percutaneous balloon mitral valvotomy. *Circulation* 1990; 82:448.
10. Wranne B, Msee PA, Loyd D: Analysis of different methods of assessing the stenotic mitral valve area with emphasis on the pressure gradient half-time concept. *Am J Cardiol* 1990; 66:614.
11. Grossman W: Profiles in valvular heart disease, in Grossman W (ed): *Cardiac Catheterization and Angiography*, ed 3. Philadelphia, Lea & Febiger, 1985, p 359.
12. Sellers RD, Levy MJ, Amplatz K, et al: Left retrograde cardioangiography in acquired cardiac disease. Technique, indications and interpretation in 700 cases. *Am J Cardiol* 1964; 14:437.
13. Berland J, Gamra H, Rocha P, et al: Mitral valvuloplasty: Improvement in safety and efficacy by using the new pigtail balloons (abstract). *Circulation* 1988; 78(suppl II):II-490.
14. Ruiz CE, Boltwood CM Jr, Lau FYK: Percutaneous double balloon aortic valvuloplasty in an adult patient with calcific aortic stenosis and a Bjork-Shiley prosthetic mitral valve. *Cathet Cardiovasc Diagn* 1988; 15:265.
15. Block PC, Palacios IF, Jacobs ML, et al: Mechanism of percutaneous mitral valvotomy. *Am J Cardiol* 1987; 59:178.
16. Beekman RH: Percutaneous balloon valvuloplasty: Long-term studies are needed. *J Am Coll Cardiol* 1987; 9:732.
17. John S, Vashi VV, Jairaj PS, et al: Closed mitral valvotomy: Early results and long-term follow-up of 3724 consecutive patients. *Circulation* 1983; 68:891.
18. Ellis L, Singh JB, Morales DD, et al: Fifteen- to twenty-year study of one thousand patients undergoing closed mitral valvuloplasty. *Circulation* 1973; 48:357.
19. Turi ZG, Reyes VP, Raju BS, et al: Percutaneous balloon versus surgical closed commissurotomy for mitral stenosis: A prospective, randomized trial. *Circulation* 1991; 83:1179.
20. Lyons WS, Tompkins RG, Kirklin JW, et al: Early and late hemodynamic effects of mitral commissurotomy. *J Lab Clin Med* 1959; 53:499.
21. Heger JJ, Wann LS, Weyman AE, et al: Long-term changes in mitral valve area after successful mitral commissurotomy. *Circulation* 1979; 59:443.
22. Houseman LB, Bonchek L, Lambert L, et al: Prognosis of patients after open mitral commissurotomy. Actuarial analysis of late results in 100 patients. *J Thorac Cardiovasc Surg* 1977; 73:742.
23. Fields CD, Slovenkai BS, Isner JM: Atrial septal defect resulting from mitral balloon valvuloplasty: Relation of defect morphology to transseptal balloon catheter delivery. *Am Heart J* 1990; 119:568.
24. Roth RB, Block PC, Palacios IF: Predictors of increased mitral regurgitation after percutaneous mitral balloon valvotomy. *Cathet Cardiovasc Diagn* 1990; 20:17.
25. Chen CR, Hu SW, Chen JY, et al: Percutaneous mitral valvuloplasty with a single rubber-nylon balloon (Inoue balloon): Long-term results in 71 patients. *Am Heart J* 1990; 120:561-568.
26. Gorlin R: Calculations of cardiac valve stenosis: Restoring an old concept for advanced applications. *J Am Coll Cardiol* 1987; 10:920.
27. Fredman CS, Person AC, Labovitz AJ, et al: Comparison of hemodynamic pressure half-time method and Gorlin formula with Doppler and echocardiographic determinations of mitral valve area in patients with combined mitral stenosis and regurgitation. *Am Heart J* 1990; 119:121.
28. Smith MD, Handshoe R, Handshoe S, et al: Comparative accuracy to two-dimensional echocardiography and Doppler pressure half-time methods in assessing severity of mitral stenosis in patients with and without prior commissurotomy. *Circulation* 1986; 73:100.
29. Ruiz CE, Allen JW, Lau FYK: Percutaneous double balloon valvotomy for severe rheumatic mitral stenosis. *Am J Cardiol* 1990; 65:473.

APPENDIX

The following is a list of the equipment that we currently use to perform PDBV, as well as the manufacturers of such equipment.

- 5, 6, 7, or 8 F Hemaquet sheaths (USCI Division, C.R. Bard, Inc., Billerica, Mass)
- 8 F thermodilution Swan-Ganz catheter (American-Edwards, Santa Ana, Calif)

- 5, 6, or 7 F pigtail catheter (Cordis, Miami, Fla)
- Modified Brockenbrough transseptal needle (Cook Co., Bloomington, Ind)
- 8 F Mullins transseptal sheath (USCI Division, C.R. Bard, Inc., Billerica, Mass)
- 160 cm × 0.032 in. teflon-coated wire (Cook Co. Bloomington, Ind)
- Ruiz–Lau-up guidewire. A 260 cm × 0.038-in. 10-cm core taper, heavy duty (Schneider, Inc., Minneapolis)

- 7 F wedge catheter (Arrow International, Inc., Reading, Penn)
- 7 F Blue Max Medi-Tech catheter for the septostomy with a 3 × 6-mm balloon (Medi-Tech, Inc., Watertown, Mass)
- 8 F balloon dilatation catheters with 5.0 cm × 15-, 18-, or 20-mm balloon (Cook Co., Bloomington, Ind)

53

Long-Term Follow-up of Balloon Mitral Valvotomy: The Montreal Heart Institute Experience

Doria Scortichini, M.D.

Pascal Barraud, M.D.

Raoul Bonan, M.D.

Since the inception of percutaneous balloon valvotomy by Inoue et al. in 1984,[1] several investigators have demonstrated its effectiveness in the treatment of symptomatic severe mitral stenosis.[2-5] The best hemodynamic and clinical results are obtained in patients with thin, pliable, noncalcified valves in the absence of severe degrees of fibrosis and fusion of the subvalvular apparatus. More recently, the feasibility and success of this procedure in older patients with calcific valvular disease,[6] those with high echocardiographic scores,[7] and those at high risk for surgery[8] have also been demonstrated. The influence of mitral valve morphology on both the immediate and long-term outcome of closed and open mitral commissurotomy has been emphasized by past surgical series. Calcified, fibrotic, and immobile valves resulted in a higher operative mortality, earlier reoperation for restenosis, and decreased patient survival.[9, 10]

Both closed mitral commissurotomy and balloon dilatation of the mitral valve increase the valve area by similar mechanisms. Balloon dilatation produces complete or partial separation of the fused edges of either one or both commissures. It fractures nodular calcium within the mitral valve leaflets without tearing the leaflets, disrupting the valve ring, or releasing embolic material.[11]

Closed mitral commissurotomy results in long-term survival and lasting improvement in functional status in over 85% of patients at 15 years.[12] Although we have no reason to suspect that these outcomes will be different for balloon mitral valvotomy (BMV), the benefits of this intervention must be determined by close scrutiny of long-term follow-up data. The course of mitral regurgitation and atrial shunting, which by the very nature of the BMV technique become integral components of the result, must be delineated. Factors contributing to restenosis must be identified and modified in order to decrease the need for a second procedure. Lasting functional improvement and long-term event-free survival must be documented before BMV can compare favorably with surgical mitral commissurotomy in the treatment of certain subgroups of patients with mitral stenosis.

It is for this purpose that we are reporting the long-term clinical results of 146 patients who underwent BMV at the Montreal Heart Institute since 1987. From this large cohort, 50 patients were randomly and prospectively recatheterized at 6 months. Another 57 patients had serial echocardiographic examinations before, within 48 hours after, and at 6-month intervals after valvotomy. This was done to follow the evolution of atrial shunting, restenosis, and mitral regurgitation and to ascertain whether these factors had any impact on the patients' clinical course. The characteristics of these two subgroups of patients did not differ in any way from the rest of the study population.

PATIENT SELECTION

BMV was performed on 146 patients at the Montreal Heart Institute from March 1987 to October 1989. All patients were screened for the presence of a left atrial thrombus by transthoracic and more recently transesophageal echocardiography prior to BMV. The degree of mitral regurgitation was assessed by both transthoracic echocardiography and left ventriculography. Patients with a left atrial thrombus and greater than 2 + mitral regurgitation according to the criteria of Sellers et al.[13] were excluded from consideration for BMV. The echocardiographic score was used to grade the abnormal morphology of the mitral valve and its apparatus.[14] Patients with echocardiographic scores greater than 11, signifying moderate to severe distortion of the mitral valve and subvalvular structures, were referred for open heart surgery. Patients who were considered poor surgical risks even with a score greater than 11 had BMV. We have previously shown that their survival with BMV is statistically improved over that of surgical intervention. At the 6-month follow-up 80% of the survivors were in functional New York Heart Association (NYHA) class I or II. BMV-related deaths occurred in 9% as compared with an estimated operative mortality of 15%.[8]

The demographic characteristics of our patients are shown in Table 53–1. The mean age of the population was 53 ± 14 years but ranged from 23 to 80; 88% were

TABLE 53–1.
Patient Population

Patients	146 (March 87 to Oct 89)
Age (yr)	53 ± 14 (23–80)
Female sex	129 (88%)
Previous surgical commissurotomy	34 (23%)
Previous embolic episode	24 (16%)
Oral anticoagulants	67 (46%)
NYHA functional class	48 (33%)
II	
III–IV	98 (67%)
Mitral regurgitation (n = 144)	
0+	64 (44%)
1+	67 (47%)
2+	13 (9%)
Mitral calcification (fluoroscopy)	66 (45%)
Echocardiographic score*	8.5 ± 1.7
Echocardiographic score*	63 (45%)
> 8 (n = 141)	
LA† diameter (mm)	52 ± 8
LA† diameter ≥ 60	23 (16%)
* Wilkins echocardiographic score.[14]	
†Left atrium.	

female. Twenty-three percent had previous surgical commissurotomy, and 16% had a prior embolic episode. Forty-six percent were receiving oral anticoagulants at the time of BMV. Two thirds of our patients were in NYHA classes III and IV. The majority of patients had mild mitral regurgitation (0 to 1 +), while 9% had 2 + mitral regurgitation. An echocardiograph score of less than 8 was present in 55%; 84% had a left atrial size of 52 ± 8 mm.

TECHNIQUE

Before BMV right and left heart pressures, oximetric runs, and arteriovenous and venovenous indicator dilution curves (indocyanine green) were obtained by using a left femoral artery (pigtail 7 F) and left femoral venous approach (Goodale Lubin 8 F). Cardiac output was determined by the Fick method. Oxygen consumption was measured directly with a metabolic rate meter (Waters Instrument, Harrow, U.K.). Left atrial transseptal catheterization was performed by the right femoral venous approach with a standard Brockenbrough needle, an 8 F Mullins transseptal long sheath, dilatator (USCI, Billerica, Mass). Correct needle position in the left atrium was confirmed by pressure measurement. The sheath and dilatator were then advanced and the needle removed. After achieving left atrial access, 4,000 units of heparin was given intravenously. Mitral valve area was calculated by using the Gorlin formula. The mean transmitral pressure gradient was measured by planimetry from the simultaneous left atrial and left ventricular pressure recordings and averaged three consecutive beats if the patient was in sinus rhythm and ten if atrial fibrillation was present. Left ventriculography in the 30-degree right anterior oblique (RAO) projection was done, and mitral regurgitation was quantified according to the criteria of Sellers et al. After pre-BMV measurements, the dilatator was removed and a 7 F balloon-tipped end-hole catheter advanced from the sheath to the left ventricle in order to facilitate crossing the mitral valve and to avoid accidental passage of the guidewire between chordae. The long sheath was then advanced to the left ventricle, and a 0.038-in.-diameter, 260-cm long, "extra stiff" Teflon-coated guidewire was positioned at the apex of the left ventricle. The J tip of the guidewire was manually precurved in order to create a loop in the apex and prevent left ventricular damage. The 7 F balloon catheter and the sheath were removed, a 7 F, 6-mm angioplasty catheter balloon (Cook Inc., Bloomington, Ind) was passed over the guidewire to the level of the interatrial septum, and the septum was dilated. After removal of this catheter, a 12 F catheter with two balloons in a single shaft (Bifoil, Schneider, Zurich, Switzerland) or two 9 F separated balloons were positioned across the mitral valve. When a second catheter balloon was used, a second long exchange guidewire was placed in the left ventricle apex by using the long sheath catheter. Two to five inflations by hand were performed until the waist in the balloons caused by the mitral stenosis disappeared. The first inflation was performed at low pressure in order to remove air from the balloon catheter. Two separate balloons were used in 53% of cases, one Bifoil catheter balloon in 44%, and one single balloon in 3%. The most frequent balloon diameter combination was 19 + 19 mm (67%). To prevent additional damage to the interatrial septum, the dilatation catheters were removed only after several aspirations under negative pressure to obtain the thinnest profile and finally by adding rotation on its long axis during the pullback.

Immediately after BMV, hemodynamic measurements, left ventriculography, oximetric runs, and dye dilution curves were repeated.

IMMEDIATE RESULTS

Of our initial 146 patients who underwent BMV, 130, or 89%, were discharged without further need for intervention. Sixteen, or 11%, had in-hospital events. Five patients were considered technical failures. In 1

case transseptal catheterization could not be performed. In the remaining 4 patients, proper balloon catheter placement across the stenotic mitral valve was not possible. The left atrial diameters of these patients were 70, 61, 60, 72, and 55 mm respectively. Of these, 1 had a successful repeat BMV. Major complications occurred in 7 patients (4.8%). These included 4 valve ruptures, 1 cardiac tamponade secondary to left atrial perforation, and 2 large atrial-septal shunts. All 7 patients with the exception of 1 survived urgent mitral valve replacement. Elective mitral valve replacement was performed in 3 of 5 patients who were technical failures and in 1 patient who was considered an incomplete success. There were 4 deaths, which amounted to a mortality rate of 2.7%. Figure 53–1 shows the causes of death and summarizes the hospital course of the survivors.

Hemodynamic outcome following BMV can be discussed either in terms of changes in intracardiac pressures or as percentages of patients achieving a complete or incomplete success. After completion of BMV, most patients have significantly improved hemodynamic profiles. There are substantial decreases in left atrial pressure, mean mitral valve gradient, mean pulmonary artery pressure, and pulmonary arteriolar resistance, together with a dramatic increase in calculated mitral valve area. Complete success, defined as a greater than 25% increase in the pre-BMV mitral valve area and a

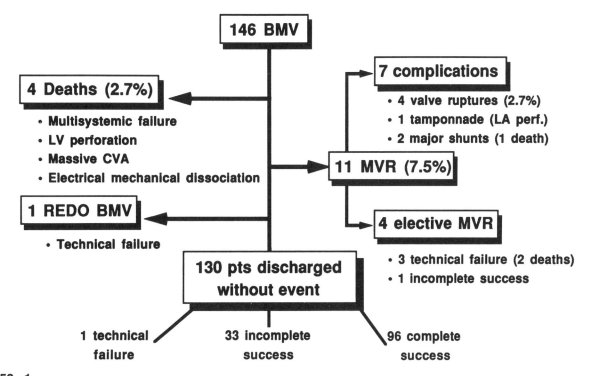

FIG 53–1.
Events during hospitalization. *BMV* = balloon mitral valvotomy; *LV* = left ventricle; *CVA* = cardiovascular accident; *LA* = left atrial; *MVR* = mitral valve replacement.

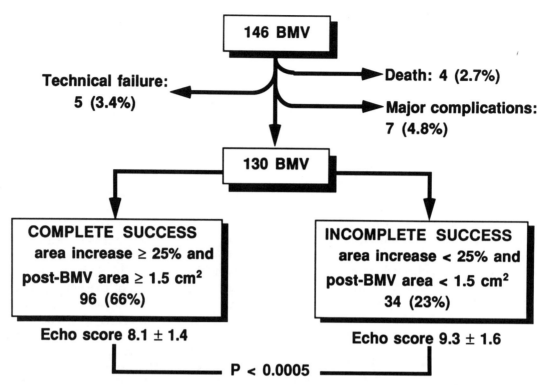

FIG 53–2.
Immediate results.

post-BMV mitral valve area greater than or equal to 1.5 cm², was demonstrated in two thirds of our patients.

Incomplete success, defined as an area increase of less than 25% and a post-BMV area less than 1.5 cm² occurred in 23% of our patients (Fig 53–2). With the use of multivariate analysis and stepwise logistic regression we identified several factors predictive of complete success. These include cardiac index (2.6 ± 0.7 vs. 1.9 ± 0.7 L/min/m², $P = .0001$), NYHA class <3 ($P = .002$), left atrial size (50 ± 8 vs. 56 ± 8 mm, $P = .05$), and echocardiographic score less than or equal to 8 ($P = .01$). This is not surprising since a lower cardiac index, a larger left atrium, more severe distortion of the mitral valve, and impaired functional status reflect more advanced and chronic disease, which is more difficult to correct with palliative therapies such as mitral surgical commissurotomy and BMV. Furthermore, the finding that valvular morphology is important in predicting the immediate and long-term success of mitral valvuloplasty parallels the results of prior surgical experience with closed mitral commissurotomy[15] and other centers performing BMV.[17–19]

LONG-TERM RESULTS

Of the 130 patients discharged from the hospital event free, 96 were complete successes, while 33 were incomplete successes. Five percent of the patients were lost to follow-up (1 technical failure, and 1 incomplete and 5 complete successes). Of the 123 remaining patients, there were 6 deaths, 3 cardiac and 3 noncardiac. Five patients required interventions for restenosis. Two necessitated a mitral valve replacement, 2 a second BMV and 1 an open commissurotomy. Mitral valve replacement was required for severe mitral regurgitation in 1 patient. In the 2 patients with suboptimal post-BMV mitral valve areas (i.e., incomplete success), 1 had a mitral valve replacement, and the other had a second BMV (Fig 53–3).

One hundred nine patients were followed for 20 ± 9 months. As shown in Figures 53–4 and 53–5, long-term clinical status is related to the initial outcome of BMV and the preprocedural echocardiographic score. At long-term follow-up, 90% of our complete successes were in NYHA classes I and II as compared with 82% of our incomplete successes. Similarly, 70% of the patients with an echocardiographic score less than 8 were in functional class I, while only 40% of the patients with echocardiographic scores greater than 8 were in this class at long-term follow-up. The overall 3-year survival rate was 86% (94% for patients with echocardiographic scores less than 8 vs. 72% for patients with scores greater than 8, $P = .03$) (Fig 53–6).

The echocardiographic score was a significant independent predictor of event-free survival. Eighty-four

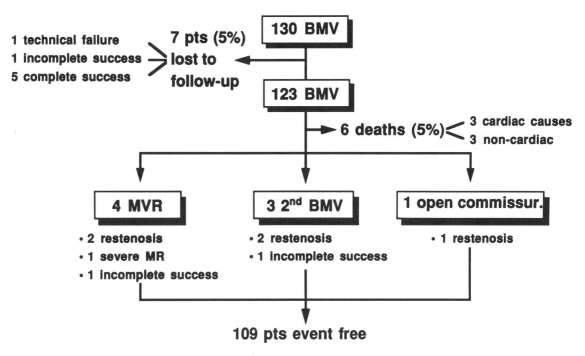

FIG 53–3.
Events during long-term follow-up. *MVR* = mitral valve replacement; *MR* = mitral regurgitation.

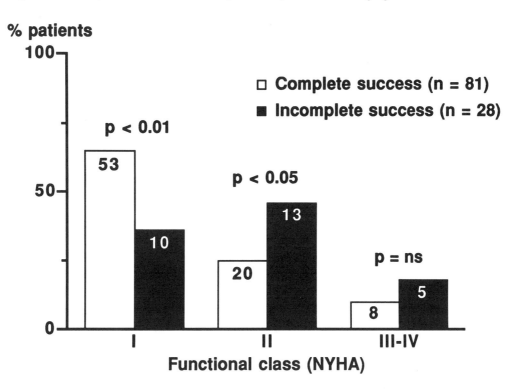

FIG 53–4.
Long-term clinical status related to results of BMV.

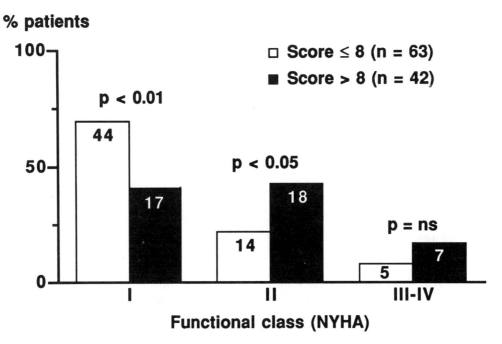

FIG 53–5.
Long-term clinical status related to echocardiographic score.

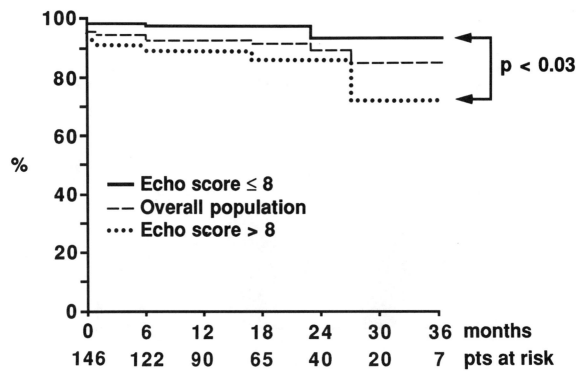

FIG 53–6.
Actuarial curves: overall mortality.

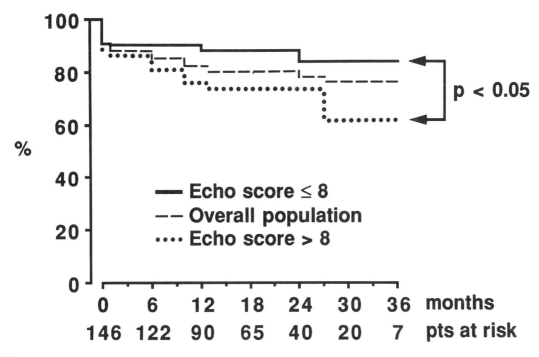

FIG 53–7.
Actuarial curves: absence of cardiac event (mortality, mitral valve replacement, second BMV).

percent of patients with an echocardiographic score less than or equal to 8 were event-free survivors at the 3-year follow-up. This figure decreased to 62% for patients with echocardiographic scores over 8 ($P < .05$) (Fig 53–7).

HEMODYNAMIC FOLLOW-UP

BMV is an effective treatment for mitral stenosis. Of the 109 patients cited above, 88% remained in functional NYHA classes I and II at the 20-month follow-up. Interestingly, these clinically successful outcomes often had evidence of atrial shunting, mitral regurgitation, and restenosis at a certain interval following the procedure. With knowledge of the natural history and predictors of these complications, patient selection and follow-up can be modified in order to achieve the best clinical results. To assess the incidence and long-term evolution of these three parameters, 50 patients were prospectively recatheterized at 6 months.

Atrial Shunting

The transvenous technique of BMV requires a transseptal approach to the left atrium. In order to facilitate passage of the valvulotomy balloon catheters, the interatrial septum is dilated with either a 6- or 8-mm balloon

catheter. An iatrogenically created atrial shunt may result as a consequence of these maneuvers.

The reported incidence of residual left-to-right atrial shunts detected by oximetry is in the 10% to 25% range.[20-24] However, this method lacks sensitivity.[25-27] We recently reported a 62% incidence of atrial shunting immediately following BMV with the use of the venovenous indicator dilution technique.[28] However, a more interesting issue is the long-term evolution of left-to-right shunting in patients post-BMV. For this, we used the catheterization data of the 50 patients mentioned above.

Prior to BMV no patient had evidence of an atrial shunt by either venovenous dilution curves or by oximetry. Immediately after BMV, venovenous dye dilution curves identified a left-to-right atrial shunt in 70% (35/50) of the patients, while oximetry detected only 36% (18/50). Shunts detected by oximetry were always present by venovenous indicator dilution curves. The mean Qp/Qs of the 50 patients was 1.23 ± 0.24. Only 10 (20%) patients had a sizable shunt with a Qp/Qs value greater than 1.5, and none had a shunt ratio greater than 2.

At the 6-month follow-up the atrial shunt resolved in 13 of 35 patients, or 37%, decreased in magnitude in 9 (26%), and was unchanged or increased in 13. The proportion of shunts recognized by indicator dilution curves decreased from 70% immediately following

BMV to 48% at the 6 month follow-up. Those detected by oximetric analysis were reduced from 36% to 18%. The Qp/Qs ratio also decreased from 1.23 ± 0.24 to 1.13 ± 0.2 by 6 months after valvuloplasty. A moderate shunt with a Qp/Qs greater than 1.5 persisted in 5 patients (10%). Of these 5, 3 had restenosis, and 1 was considered a hemodynamic failure.

Previously,[29] we found that the use of a Bifoil balloon catheter ($P < .005$), a smaller left atrium ($P < .01$), and mitral valve calcification ($P < .003$) were independent predictors of the presence of atrial shunting after BMV. In addition, cardiac output was the only independent predictor of a significant (Qp/Qs > 1.5) shunt after BMV. This is in agreement with the findings of Casale et al.[30] In their study of 150 patients, mitral valve calcification and a lower cardiac output before mitral valvotomy was identified as independent predictors of a left-to-right shunt immediately after valvuloplasty.

In conclusion, it appears that although atrial shunting commonly occurs post-BMV, over 60% of patients will have a reduction or total resolution of the shunt. In 40% the shunt will remain unchanged or minimally increased. Only 10% will be left with a significant shunt.

Mitral Regurgitation

Mitral regurgitation produced after BMV may be secondary to trauma to the valvular and subvalvular apparatus from the passage of large balloon dilating catheters. Injury to the papillary muscles and chordae tendinae may cause edema of these structures and result in permanent or transient dysfunction. The mitral annulus may be overstretched, and possible splitting of the commissures too close to this structure may cause mitral incompetence. Another explanation for regurgitation following valvotomy is related to the distorted anatomy of the mitral apparatus, and a lack of adequate leaflet coaptation due either to leaflet or chordae retraction probably contributes to postvalvotomy regurgitation. Immediately following BMV, increased or new mitral regurgitation is reported in up to 50% of patients. Fortunately, severe mitral regurgitation caused by either leaflet or chordal rupture is uncommon.

The changes in degree of mitral regurgitation were evaluated in 50 patients undergoing left ventriculography in the 30-degree RAO projection before, immediately after, and 6 months post-BMV. Mild mitral regurgitation (0 to 1+) was present in 47 (94%) patients prior to BMV. Three patients had 2+ mitral regurgitation, and no patient had 3+ mitral regurgitation prevalvotomy. Immediately following BMV, mitral regurgitation increased in severity in 32% of the patients. But in only 1 patient was the increase greater than 1 grade. In 68% of patients the mitral regurgitation remained unchanged.

Six months later, mitral regurgitation diminished in magnitude in 13, or 26%, and was unchanged in 27, or 54%. Mitral regurgitation increased in severity in 10 patients (20%). However, a moderate degree (3+ mitral regurgitation) developed in only 2 patients (4%). Mitral valve replacement was not necessary in any of these patients, and most remained improved and in functional NYHA class I or II at follow-up. No correlation had been found between the echocardiographic morphologic features of the mitral apparatus and mitral regurgitation after BMV. In contrast to the findings of Roth et al.[31] no technical factors such as the ratio of effective balloon dilating area to body surface area was predictive of an increase in mitral regurgitation after valvotomy. However, we identified a larger left atrial size (54 ± 9 mm vs. 49 ± 7 mm; $P = .005$) and absence of previous mitral regurgitation ($P = .02$) to be independent predictors of an increase in mitral regurgitation after BMV.

Restenosis

Restenosis of the mitral valve following valvotomy or valvuloplasty is most likely caused by progression of the rheumatic disease process.[32] After surgical mitral commissurotomy, despite excellent immediate hemodynamic and clinical results, up to 53% of patients will require a second intervention at the 12-year follow-up. The majority of these will be mitral valve replacements secondary to either residual stenosis or restenosis. Restenosis also occurs following BMV. Reported rates range from 0% to 27%.[34–37] As can be seen in Table

TABLE 53–2.

Follow-up Studies on Balloon Mitral Valvotomy

First Author	No. of Patients	Mean Age	Mean Follow-up (mo)	Restenosis Rate (%)
Zaibag[36]	41	26	12	0
Vahanian[38]	91	43	9	4
Abascal[37]	20	52	7.5	20
Palacios[35]	37	55	13	22
MHI*	41	47	6	27

*MHI = Montreal Heart Institute.

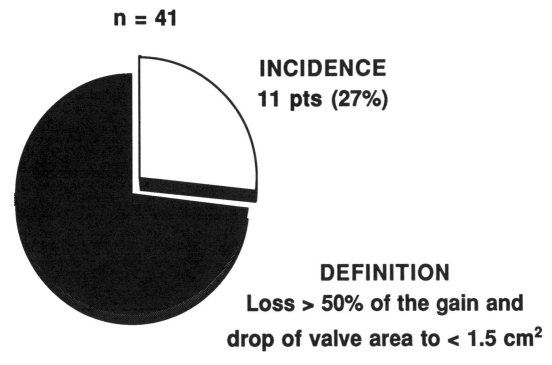

n = 41

INCIDENCE
11 pts (27%)

DEFINITION
Loss > 50% of the gain and
drop of valve area to < 1.5 cm²

FIG 53–8.
Hemodynamic restenosis at 6 months.

53–2, age differences between reported series may account for the variation in rates of restenosis. Age as a factor must also be considered when comparing restenosis rates between surgical series and valvotomy series.

Restenosis is defined as a loss of greater than 50% of the initial gain in valve area first obtained together with a final area of less than 1.5 cm² immediately following valvotomy. From our cohort of 50 patients who were recatheterized, 9 patients considered as incomplete successes or hemodynamic failures were excluded from our analysis of restenosis. Evidence of hemodynamic restenosis was shown in 11 of 41 patients (27%) at the 6-month follow-up (Fig 53–8). To determine whether any factors were predictive of restenosis, we analyzed 53 pre- and post-BMV variables and compared them in patients with and without restenosis. Patients with hemodynamic restenosis were older, had more morphologic change of the mitral apparatus (i.e., higher echocardiographic score), more commonly had radiographic evidence of mitral valve calcification and had less improvement in mitral valve area following BMV than did those without restenosis. Multiple stepwise logistic regression analysis identified the post-BMV mitral valve area (1.94 ± 0.34 vs. 2.76 ± 0.79; $P < .0001$) as the only independent predictor of recurrent mitral stenosis (Table 53–3).

Regardless of the 27% restenosis rate, 90% of the patients were improved by at least one NYHA class at the 6-month follow-up. Therefore the rate of "clinical restenosis" appears to be much less than the restenosis detected by hemodynamic follow-up.

TABLE 53–3.
Predictive Factors for Hemodynamic Restenosis 6 Months After Balloon Mitral Valvotomy

Predictor	Restenosis (n = 11)	No Restenosis (n = 30)	P
Age	55 ± 14	44 ± 11	.02
Calcification (x-ray)	7 (64%)	9 (30%)	.05
Leaflet mobility* score >2	5 (45%)	1 (3%)	.002
Leaflet calcific* score >2	4 (36%)	2 (6%)	.03
Echocardiographic score* ≥8	9 (82%)	10 (33%)	.02
Post-BMV valve area (cm²)	1.94 ± 0.34	2.76 ± 0.79	.002

*Wilkins echocardiographic score.[14]

ECHOCARDIOGRAPHIC FOLLOW-UP

Two-dimensional echocardiography is a useful, noninvasive tool that provides real-time images of cardiac structures and has proved invaluable in the diagnosis and assessment of the severity of both mitral stenosis and regurgitation.[39-41]

To evaluate the prevalence of echocardiographic atrial shunting, mitral regurgitation, and restenosis, a two-dimensional and Doppler echocardiographic examination was performed before, within 48 hours, at 6 months, and again at a mean of 19 ± 6 months (range 9 to 33 months) in 57 patients who had undergone a successful BMV.

Atrial Shunting

As mentioned previously, the venovenous dilution curve technique is very sensitive and detects atrial shunting in 70% of patients immediately post-BMV. With echo-Doppler, technically adequate evaluation of a left-to-right shunt was feasible in 93% (54/57) of cases. The echo-Doppler study succeeded in detecting an atrial shunt in 61% of the patients immediately after BMV. At the 19-month follow-up, 30% (16/54) of the patients still had evidence of a left-to-right shunt, including 5 patients with an initial shunt ratio greater than 1.5. Although the sensitivity and specificity of transthoracic color Doppler for shunt detection is 65% and 63%, respectively, all shunts with a Qp/Qs ratio greater than 1.5 are recognized by this technique.

Overall, the results of echocardiography are in close agreement with the venovenous dilution curve technique. Both demonstrate an initial prevalence of atrial shunting in the 60% to 70% range immediately after BMV. At the 6-month follow-up both reveal a total resolution or reduction in atrial shunting in over half the patients. More valuable is the 19-month echocardiographic follow-up which shows no increase in the degree of atrial shunting and even its disappearance in 3 of the 8 patients with an initial Qp/Qs ratio greater than 1.5. As shown in Table 53-4, the predictors of persistent atrial shunting at long-term follow-up include the immediate magnitude of the shunt, the size of the deflated balloon, the mitral valve area post-BMV, and the presence of restenosis.

Mitral Regurgitation

The evolution of mitral regurgitation was assessed by echocardiography and graded from $1+$ to $4+$ in severity by color Doppler according to the extension and width of the regurgitant jet within the left atrium. Fifty-seven patients were studied at specific time intervals af-

TABLE 53-4.
Predictors for Long-Term Persistence of Atrial Shunting

	Univariate Analysis		
Predictor	AS* (+) (n = 16)	AS (−) (n = 38)	P Value
Bifoil balloon (pts*)	7 (45%)	5 (14%)	<.01
Qp/Qs > 1.5 (pts)	5 (31%)	3 (8%)	<.03
MVA* post-BMV (cm²)	2 ± 0.6	2.5 ± 0.9	<.05
Restenosis (pts)	6 (38%)	6 (16%)	<.05
Duration of the procedure (min)	107 ± 29	124 ± 26	<.05

*AS = atrial shunting; pts = no. patients; MVA = mitral valve area.

ter valvuloplasty. Prior to BMV 12 patients had no evidence of mitral regurgitation, 40 had $1+$ mitral regurgitation and 5 had $2+$ mitral regurgitation. Immediately after valvuloplasty, mitral regurgitation remained unchanged in 42, or 74% of the patients. In 14 (24%) patients, mitral regurgitation increased by one grade and in 1 patient, by two grades. At an average of 19 months after BMV, mitral regurgitation was unchanged in 26 (46%) patients and increased by one grade in 12 (21%). In only 1 patient did mitral regurgitation increase by two grades. A decrease in the severity of mitral regurgitation was seen in 31% of patients. Table 53-5 demonstrates remarkably similar results obtained by either ventriculography or echocardiography for the evolution of mitral regurgitation after valvotomy. Of note is the fact that approximately 75% of patients have either improvement or no change in the degree of migurgitation at long-term follow-up an average of 19 months post valvotomy.

There have been several mechanisms offered for the decrease in mitral regurgitation accompanying mitral valvulotomy: reversal of mitral valve "stretching" incurred by BMV or recoil of the mitral apparatus, fibrosis and healing of the ends of the commissures excessively split to the mitral valve annulus by the balloon, and resolution of edema causing transient papillary muscle dysfunction.[35]

Worsening of mitral regurgitation after BMV is not related to technical aspects of the procedure, i.e., balloon size or the morphologic appearance of the subvalvular apparatus on echocardiography.[42]

Restenosis

Restenosis as previously defined developed in 12 of 57 patients (21%). Fifty-eight percent of patients with restenosis improved by at least one NYHA class as compared with 89% of those without echocardiographic evidence of restenosis. As shown in Table 53-6, age, a smaller post-BMV echocardiographic mitral valve area,

TABLE 53–5.
Mitral Regurgitation at Follow-up vs. Before Balloon Mitral Valvotomy

Mitral Regurgitation	Left ventriculography (n = 50)		Echo-Doppler (n = 57)	
	Post-BMV	6 mo	Post-BMV	Long-Term (19 ± 9 mo)
Unchanged	34 (68%)	27 (54%)	42 (74%)	26 (46%)
Increased by				
1+	15 (30%)	9 (18%)	14 (24%)	12 (21%)
2+	1 (2%)	1 (2%)	1 (2%)	1 (2%)
3+	—	—	—	—
Decreased	—	13 (26%)	—	18 (31%)

and a higher total echocardiographic score, especially when secondary to valve calcification or reduced valve mobility, are notable predictors of restenosis. The restenosis rate for patients older than 60 years is 40% in comparison to 11% in patients younger than 60 years. Restenosis occurred in 30% of patients with echocardiographic scores of 8 or greater as opposed to only 1 patient (5%) with an echocardiographic score less than

8. Palacios et al.[35] also reported significantly higher restenosis rates in the presence of higher echocardiographic scores. In their series of 27 recatheterized patients with a mean age of 55 years followed for 13.1 months, the rate of restenosis was 70% in those with an echocardiographic score greater than 8 and only 4% with a score of 8 or less.

Unlike atrial shunting and mitral regurgitation, restenosis appears to correlate with the severity of morphologic changes of the valve as reflected in the echocardiographic score. The past surgical literature is replete with reports of poor outcomes and short-lived results obtained with either closed or open mitral commissurotomy when the mitral valve was calcified, thickened, and immobile.[9, 44, 45]

COMPARISON OF SURGICAL COMMISSUROTOMY AND PERCUTANEOUS MITRAL BALLOON VALVOTOMY

Both surgical commissurotomy (open or closed) and BMV offer excellent functional improvement in patients with severe mitral stenosis. As can be seen in Table 53–7, which compares surgical and nonsurgical series of patients undergoing treatment for mitral stenosis, most patients are in class III or IV prior to their intervention, but the majority are dramatically improved and in class I or II at the last follow-up. The early mortality rate for each of the three procedures is comparable and ranges from 0% to 4% for BMV,[38] 1% to 4% for open commissurotomy, and 2% to 3.8% for closed commissurotomy. Similarly the late mortality rate is low and ranges from 1% to 5%. The 14% mortality rate reported by Rutledge et al.[46] includes patients who died of unknown and noncardiac causes. All three procedures are palliative. The rate of restenosis varies from 3% to 27%. In the case of BMV, restenosis is higher when the average age of the patients in the series is greater than 40 years (see Table 53–2). Reoperation for restenosis occurs at an average of

TABLE 53–6.
Predictive Factors for Restenosis by Univariate Analysis

Factor	No Restenosis (n = 45*)	Restenosis (n = 12)	P
Age (yr)	49 ± 14	62 ± 9	<.001
Valve area by echocardiography after dilatation (cm²)	2.5 ± 0.9	1.9 ± 0.6	<.05
Total echocardiographic score†	7.9 ± 1.4	8.9 ± 1.6	.05
Calcification (patients)†			
1	17	1	
2	18	5	.05
3	9	9	
Valve mobility (patients)†			
1	0	1	
2	38	5	<.005
3	6	6	
Valve thickening (patients)†			
1	4	0	
2	38	10	NS
3	2	2	
Subvalvular apparatus (patients)†			
1	10	2	
2	22	9	NS
3	12	1	
Valve area by catheterization after dilatation (cm²)	2.5 ± 0.9	1.9 ± 0.6	<.05
Pulmonary vascular resistance	184 ± 129	306 ± 263	<.05

*n = 44 for echocardiographic characteristics.
†Wilkins echocardiographic score.[14]

TABLE 53–7.

Comparison of Surgical Commissurotomy and Balloon Mitral Valvotomy

Series	No. Patients	Age (yr)	Mean Follow-up	Calcium	NYHA III–IV
Closed commissurotomy; John, 1983[12]	3,724	27.3	5 + yr (up to 20 yr)	18%	99%
Closed commissurotomy; Rutledge, 1982[46]	303	40	5 + yr (up to 15 yr)	18%	80%
Open commissurotomy; Housman, 1976[47]	100	42	46 mon	—	83%
Open commissurotomy; Breyer, 1985[48]	91	43	59 mon	—	66%
BMV; Vahanian, 1989[38]	300	43	9 mon	32%	79%
BMV; BVR,* 1988	309	56	—	13%	67%
BMV; MHI*	146	53	20 mon	47%	68%

Series	Mortality (%) Early	Mortality (%) Late	MVR* (%)	MR†	Restenosis Rate (%)	Class I–II‡
Closed commissurotomy; John, 1983[12]	3.8	4.3	0.9	8% (severe 0.3%)	(5 yr) 4.2	98
Closed commissurotomy; Rutledge, 1982[46]	2	14	18	2% severe	5	92
Open commissurotomy; Housman, 1976[47]	1	1	15	—	16	78
Open commissurotomy; Breyer, 1985[48]	4.3	5.4	12	4%	9	79
BMV; Vahanian, 1989[38]	0	—	2.6	—	3	—
BMV; BVR, 1988	4	5	—	—	—	—
BMV; MHI	2.7	3.4	7.5	2%	27	88

*BVR = Balloon Valvuloplasty Registry from the National Heart, Lung and Blood Institute; MHI = Montreal Heart Institute; MVR = mitral valve area;
†Percent increase in mitral regurgitation greater than two grades at follow-up.
‡Percentage at patients in classes I and II at follow-up.

6 to 10 years after surgical commissurotomy and has a higher operative mortality that ranges from 6.7% to 15%.[9, 12, 32, 47, 48] At reoperation an overwhelming majority of patients will undergo a mitral valve replacement with its associated high morbidity and reduced long-term survival rate: 60% survival rate at 10 years vs. over 90% for surgical commissurotomy.[49–51] We recently performed BMV on 27 patients on average of 14 years after previous commissurotomy. A complete or incomplete success was obtained in 21 patients. One death occurred for a mortality rate of 4%. Although long-term follow-up is still needed for this subgroup of patients, BMV may be a more beneficial alternative than mitral valve replacement. Another subgroup of patients who can benefit from BMV are those who are considered to be high surgical risks (estimated operative mortality rate greater than 15%) and have a high echocardiographic score. Balloon valvulotomy was performed on 34 such patients[8] with a mortality rate of 9%. Furthermore, at the 6-month follow-up 80% of the survivors were clinically improved and in functional class I or II.

CONCLUSION

That BMV is an effective palliative procedure for symptomatic, severe mitral stenosis was demonstrated not only by long-term clinical follow-up results but also by the inclusion of catheterization and serial echocardiographic data.

At an average follow-up of 19 months, significant functional improvement can be expected in over 88% of the patients undergoing the procedure. Mortality and morbidity are low and compare favorably with those of closed and open surgical mitral commissurotomy. Atrial shunting created secondary to the technique of transseptal puncture has no deleterious effects on a patient's clinical outcome. At the 19-month follow-up over 60% of patients demonstrate a decrease or total resolution of their left-to-right atrial shunt. Only 10% to 15% of patients have a residual shunt ratio greater than 1.5. Mitral regurgitation was present in up to 55% of the patients before BMV. At the 19-month follow-up over 75% of the patients had no change or a decrease in the severity of mitral regurgitation. Mitral regurgitation increased in severity by two grades in only 2% of our patients. Valve rupture at the time of the procedure occurred in 2.7% of the population. However, in the four patients in whom this event occurred, three survived urgent mitral valve replacement. Restenosis, defined as a 50% decrease in the initial gain obtained in mitral valve area and a final area of less than 1.5 cm^2, was demonstrated in 27% of patients by hemodynamic data at 6 months and in 21% of patients by echocardiographic criteria at 19 months. Clinically this did not result in any deterioration in functional status. In fact, 90% of the patients remained in class I or II despite evidence of restenosis.

The above results imply that BMV should be the procedure of choice for severe, symptomatic mitral stenosis in the proper patient population. Although closed mitral commissurotomy is a safe and effective procedure, it requires thoracotomy and will soon become obsolete for the treatment of mitral stenosis. Open mitral commissurotomy, however, is still indicated for patients who have a left atrial thrombus or a deformed valve and are good surgical candidates. A major disadvantage of the procedure is the requirement for cardiopulmonary bypass. Additionally, in 8% to 44% of patients who come to open mitral commissurotomy, the mitral valve is replaced.[47, 48, 52]

BMV is indicated in any patient with severe mitral stenosis and an echo cardiographic score less than 11. This includes patients with prior commissurotomy, whose operative mortality rate ranges from 6.7% to 15% for a repeat open heart procedure but is only 4% for BMV. BMV delays the requirement for cardiopulmonary bypass, thoracotomy, and valve surgery in a relatively young patient population who may eventually need surgery an average of 6 to 10 years after the initial intervention for mitral stenosis. In addition, this technique can be repeated without the attendant morbidity and mortality of a second open heart procedure. The benefits of BMV in the pregnant patient include the avoidance of general anesthesia and prolonged surgical recovery. This must be weighed against the low risks of fetal and maternal radiation exposure. The latter could be reduced to a minimum with proper lead shielding. As already mentioned, the subgroup of patients with echocardiographic scores greater than 11 who are high-risk surgical candidates secondary to concomitant serious medical conditions have a survival advantage with BMV and remain functionally improved up to 6 months following valvuloplasty.

Although the use of BMV for the treatment of mitral stenosis is becoming more widely accepted, especially in patients who have had a prior commissurotomy, research in this area of interventional cardiology is far from complete. Longer follow-up studies are needed before BMV can be recommended in certain subgroups of patients without reservation over open mitral commissurotomy or mitral valve replacement. Another issue that requires research is whether BMV can be repeated on multiple occasions without detrimental effects on the mitral valve and subvalvular apparatus. Research addressing the possible inflammatory mechanisms triggered by balloon valvotomy of the mitral valve may be useful in understanding and possibly deferring the process of restenosis. Finally, investigation into other interventional, nonoperative techniques such as laser valvuloplasty or the use of ultrasound to "crack" the mitral valve may warrant some attention.

REFERENCES

1. Inoue K, Owaki T, Nakamura T, et al: Clinical application of transvenous mitral commissurotomy by a new balloon catheter. *J Thorac Cardiovasc Surg* 1984; 87:394–402.
2. Lock J, Khalilullah M, Shrivastava S, et al: Percutaneous catheter commissurotomy in rheumatic mitral stenosis. *N Engl J Med* 1985; 313:1515–1518.
3. Zaibag M, Kasab S, Ribeiro PA, et al: Percutaneous double balloon mitral valvotomy for rheumatic mitral valve stenosis. *Lancet* 1986; 1:757–761.
4. McKay RG, Lock J, Keane JF, et al: Percutaneous mitral valvuloplasty in an adult patient with calcific rheumatic stenosis. *J Am Coll Cardiol* 1986; 7:1410–1415.
5. Palacios I, Block P, Brandi S, et al: Percutaneous transvenous balloon valvotomy for patients with severe mitral stenosis. *Circulation* 1987; 75:778–784.
6. Palacios I, Lock J, Keane J, et al: Percutaneous transvenous balloon valvotomy in a patient with severe calcific mitral stenosis. *J Am Coll Cardiol* 1986; 7:1416–1419.
7. Serra A, Bonan R, Lefèvre T, et al: Balloon mitral valvuloplasty in patients with high echocardiographic score (abstract). *Circulation* 1989; 80 (suppl 2):73.
8. Lefèvre T, Bonan R, Serra A, et al: Percutaneous mitral valvuloplasty in surgical high risk patients. *J Am Coll Cardiol* 1991; 17:348–354.
9. Commerford P, Hastie T, Beck W: Closed mitral commissurotomy: Actuarial analysis of results in 654 patients over 12 years and analysis of pre-operative predictors of long-term survival. *Ann Thorac Surg* 1982; 33:473–479.
10. Ellis L, Singh J, Morales D, et al: Fifteen to twenty-year study of one thousand patients undergoing closed mitral valvuloplasty. *Circulation* 1973; 48:357–364.
11. McKay R, Lock J, Safian R, et al: Balloon dilation of mitral stenosis in adult patients. Post mortem and percutaneous mitral valvuloplasty studies. *J Am Coll Cardiol* 1987; 9:123–131.
12. Johns S, Bashi V, Jairag P, et al: Closed mitral commissurotomy: Early results + long-term follow-up of 3724 consecutive patients. *Circulation* 1983; 68:891–896.
13. Sellers RD, Levy MJ, Amplatz K, et al: Left retrograde cardioangiography in acquired cardiac disease. Technical

indication and interpretations in 700 cases. *Am J Cardiol* 1964; 14:437–447.

14. Wilkins GT, Weyman AE, Abascal VM, et al: Percutaneous mitral valvotomy: An analysis of echocardiographic variables related to outcome and the mechanism of dilatation. *Br Heart J* 1988; 60:299–308.

15. Grantham R, Dagget W, Cosimi A, et al: Transventricular mitral valvotomy. Analysis of factors influencing operative and late results. *Circulation* 1974; 49 (suppl 2):200–212.

16. Deleted in proof.

17. Nobuyosh M, Hamasaki N, Kimura T, et al: Indications, complications and short-term clinical outcome of percutaneous transvenous mitral commissurotomy. *Circulation* 1989; 80:782–792.

18. Reid C, Chandraratna P, Kawanishi DT, et al: Influence of mitral valve morphology on double balloon catheter balloon valvuloplasty in patients with mitral stenosis—analysis of factors predicting immediate and 3 month results. *Circulation* 1989; 80:515–524.

19. Abascal V, Wilkins G, O'Shea JP, et al: Prediction of successful outcome of 130 patients undergoing percutaneous balloon mitral valvotomy. *Circulation* 1990; 82:448–456.

20. McKay CR, Kawanishi DT, Rahimtoola SH: Catheter balloon valvuloplasty (CBV) of the mitral valve in adults using a double balloon technique: Early hemodynamic results. *JAMA* 1987; 257:1753–1761.

21. McKay CR, Kawanishi DT, Kotlewski A, et al: Improvement in exercise capacity and exercise hemodynamics 3 months after double-balloon catheter balloon valvuloplasty treatment of patients with symptomatic mitral stenosis. *Circulation* 1988; 77:1013–1021.

22. Vahanian A, Michel PL, Slama M, et al: La commissurotomie mitrale percutanée. A propos de 130 cas. *Arch Mal Coeur* 1988; 81:755–762.

23. Come PC, Riley MF, Diver DJ, et al: Noninvasive assessment of mitral stenosis before and after percutaneous balloon mitral valvuloplasty. *Am J Cardiol* 1988; 61:817–825.

24. Palacios IF, Block PC: Atrial septal defect during percutaneous mitral valvotomy (PMV): Immediate results and follow-up (abstract). *Circulation* 1988; 78(suppl 2):529.

25. Wood EH: Diagnostic applications of indicator-dilution technique in congenital heart disease. *Circ Res* 1962; 10:531–569.

26. Grossman W: Shunt detection and measurement, in Grossman W (ed): *Cardiac Catheterization and Angiography*. Philadelphia, Lea & Febiger, 1986, pp 155–169.

27. Yang SS, Bentivoglio LG, Maranhao V, et al: *From Catheterization Data to Hemodynamic Parameters*. Philadelphia, FA Davis, 1988, pp 166–188.

28. Cequier A, Bonan R, Serra A, et al: Left-to-right atrial shunting after percutaneous mitral valvuloplasty. Incidence and long-term hemodynamic follow-up. *Circulation* 1990; 81:1190–1197.

29. Desideri A, Bonan R, Vanderperren O, et al: Incidence and predictors for long-term persistence of atrial shunting after percutaneous mitral valvuloplasty (abstract). *Clin Invest Med* 1990; 13:68.

30. Casale P, Block PC, O'Shea JP, et al: Atrial septal defect after percutaneous mitral balloon valvuloplasty: Immediate results and follow-up. *J Am Coll Cardiol* 1990; 15:1300–1304.

31. Roth RB, Block PC, Palacios IF: Predictors of increased mitral regurgitation after percutaneous mitral balloon valvotomy. *Cathet Cardiovasc Diagn* 1990; 20:17–21.

32. John S, Perianayagam JW, Abraham K, et al: Re-stenosis of the mitral valve: Surgical considerations and results of operation. *Ann Thorac Surg* 1978; 25:316–321.

33. Deleted in proof.

34. Vahanian A, Michel PL, Cormier B, et al: Results of percutaneous mitral commissurotomy in 200 patients. *Am J Cardiol* 1989; 63:847–852.

35. Palacios IF, Block PC, Wilkins GT, et al: Follow-up of patients undergoing percutaneous mitral balloon valvotomy. Analysis of factors determining restenosis. *Circulation* 1989; 79:573–579.

36. Zaibag AM, Ribeiro PA, Kasab SA, et al: One-year follow-up after percutaneous double balloon mitral valvotomy. *Am J Cardiol* 1989; 63:126–127.

37. Abascal VM, Wilkins GT, Choong CY, et al: Echocardiographic evaluation of mitral valve structure and function in patients followed for at least 6 months after percutaneous balloon mitral valvuloplasty. *J Am Coll Cardiol* 1988; 12:606–615.

38. Vahanian A, Michel PL, Cormier B, et al: Mitral valvuloplasty: The French experience, In Topol EJ (ed): *Interventional Cardiology*. Philadelphia, WB Saunders, 1990, pp 868–886.

39. Wann LS, Weyman AE, Dillon JC, et al: Determination of mitral valve area by cross-sectional echocardiography. *Ann Intern Med* 1978; 88:337–341.

40. Henry WL, Griffith JM, Michaelis LL, et al: Measurements of mitral valve orifice area in patients with mitral valve disease by real-time, two-dimensional echocardiography. *Circulation* 1979; 51:827–831.

41. Abbasi AS, Allen MW, DeCristofano D, et al: Detection and estimation of the degree of mitral regurgitation by range-gated pulsed Doppler echocardiography. *Circulation* 1980; 61:143–147.

42. Muller T, Petitclerc R, Lespérance J, et al: Mitral regurgitation assessed by echo-Doppler after percutaneous mitral valvuloplasty (abstract). *Circulation* 1989; 80(suppl 2):167.Deleted in proof.

43. Deleted in proof.

44. Ellis LB, Benson H, Harken DE: The effect of age and other factors on the early and late results following closed mitral valvuloplasty. *Am Heart J* 1968; 75:743–751.

45. Smith WM, Neutze JM, Barrett-Boyes BG, et al: Open mitral valvotomy. Effect of pre-operative factors on result. *J Thorac Cardiovasc Surg* 1981; 82:738–751.

46. Rutledge R, McIntosh CL, Morrow AG, et al: Mitral valve replacement after closed mitral commissurotomy. *Circulation* 1982; 66(suppl 1):162–166.

47. Housman LB, Bonchek L, Lambert L, et al: Prognosis after open mitral commissurotomy actuarial analysis of late results in 100 patients. *J Thorac Cardiovasc Surg* 1977; 73:742–745.

48. Breyer RH, Mills SA, Hudspeth AS, et al: Open mitral commissurotomy: Long-term results with echocardiographic correlation. *J Cardiovasc Surg* 1985; 26:46–52.

49. Teply JF, Grunkemeier GL, Sutherland HD, et al: The

ultimate prognosis after valve replacement: An assessment at 20 years. *Ann Thorac Surg* 1981; 32:111–119.

50. Karp RB, Cyrus RJ, Blackstone EH, et al: The Bjork-Shiley valve: Intermediate-term follow-up. *J Thorac Cardiovasc Surg* 1981; 81:602–614.

51. Borkon AM, McIntosh CL, Von Rueden TJ, et al: Mitral valve regurgitation with the Hancock bioprosthesis: 5 to 10 year follow-up. *Ann Thorac Surg* 1981; 32:127–137.

52. Roe BB, Edmundo LH, Fishman NH: Open mitral valvulotomy. *Ann Thorac Surg* 1971; 12:483–491.

54

Interventional Catheterization in the Treatment of Congenital Lesions

Michael R. Nihill, M.D.

Charles E. Mullins, M.D.

The era of interventional cardiology started in the mid-1960s with the work of Dotter and Judkins,[1] who dilated peripheral arterial stenoses with graded bougie catheters. At about the same time Rashkind and Miller[2] introduced a balloon catheter into the heart to enlarge the interatrial septal defect in children with transposition of the great arteries. Grüntzig and coworkers[3] combined Dotter's technique with the concept of a balloon catheter to dilate peripheral arterial, renal, and finally stenotic coronary arteries in the mid to late 1970s. These small balloons, up to 5 mm in diameter, were used to dilate peripheral and central vessel stenosis and even congenital pulmonary vein stenosis.[4] In 1979 Semb and colleagues[5] used an angiographic CO_2 inflated balloon catheter to relieve severe congenital pulmonary valve stenosis in a neonate. Shortly afterward Jean Kan and associates[6] converted the Grüntzig balloon design to a larger scale to dilate stenotic pulmonary valves. These techniques have now been applied to dilatation of congenital and acquired stenosis of every valve within the heart,[7-9] as well as dilatation for coarctation of the aorta,[10,11] pulmonary artery branches,[12] pulmonary veins,[4] venae cavae,[13] and even subvalvular aortic membranes.[14]

A large experience has rapidly accumulated since 1982 in the field of dilatation of congenital cardiovascular lesions. Although the length of follow-up of these first patients treated with balloon dilatation is relatively short, the initial excellent results have been enthusiastically received by both pediatric and adult cardiologists, and the technique has been applied to a variety of congenital and acquired stenotic lesions in the heart and great vessels. Short-term evaluation of up to 8 years has revealed maintenance of the initial good results; an ongoing review of the early results has led to an evolution of the technique of dilatation for various lesions.

VALVULOPLASTY

The results of balloon valvuloplasty depend on both the pathology of the lesion as much as the technique of dilatation. For instance, congenital pulmonary valve stenosis can be due to fusion of the commissures of a tricuspid or bicuspid valve, a pinhole opening in a membranous-like valve, or thick myxomatous leaflets. Valve stenosis may be associated with concomitant obstructive lesions such as a small pulmonary valve annulus, supravalvular pulmonary artery stenosis, subvalvular membranous obstruction, or congenital and acquired diffuse muscular infundibular stenosis. In the majority of patients with congenital pulmonary or aortic valve stenosis, the valve is mobile and domes in systole, and the annulus is cf normal size. These valves can be very effectively dilated by inflating one or two rigid balloons across the annulus. Judicious overdistension of the valve annulus can virtually abolish the gradient with no restenosis over the next 2 to 5 years.

PULMONARY VALVE STENOSIS

Technique

A right-heart catheterization is performed and a careful pullback recorded from the branch pulmonary arteries across the main pulmonary artery, pulmonary valve, and annulus to the subvalvular area and then to the right ventricular inflow tract. More than one area of stenosis may be identified in this fashion.

A Cardiomarker catheter (USCI Division of C.R. Bard, Inc., Billerica, Mass) is positioned in the right ventricular apex or outflow tract near the pulmonary annulus so that the 1-cm marks at the tip of the catheter are perpendicular to at least one plane of the biplane angiographic system. This catheter provides an intracardiac grid to measure the pulmonary annulus at the hinge points of the valve. We also perform a right ventricular angiogram in the anteroposterior (AP) and lateral projections with the catheter at the apex so that any infundibular stenosis may be identified. From the angiogram we also identify the level of the valve annulus and place a lead shot marker on the chest wall so that the middle of the balloon may be placed across the annulus during dilatation. The balloon diameter is selected to be 50% to 60% greater than the measured annulus diameter for pulmonary valve stenosis. When the annulus size is greater than 18 to 20 mm in diameter, the bulk of the balloon catheter on a 9 F shaft is usually too large to fit easily into the relatively small femoral veins of children less than 15 years of age; in these patients two balloons are chosen whose combined diameter is 50% greater than the annulus diameter.[9] We do not calculate effective dilatation areas or valve orifice areas since we have found empirically that a combined balloon diameter of 50% greater than the annulus diameter produces very effective relief of isolated pulmonary valve stenosis.

An end-hole catheter is passed across the pulmonary valve, preferably into the left lower lobe of the pulmonary artery. A 0.038-in. Teflon-coated exchange wire (USCI, Billerica, Mass; Argon Medical Corp., Athens, Tex) with a curve formed at the floppy end is passed through the catheter and lodged in the left lower lobe pulmonary artery. The end-hole catheter and sheath are withdrawn and the exchange wire left in place. A tightly furled balloon catheter (Mansfield Scientific, Inc., Mansfield, Mass; Medi-Tech, Inc., Watertown, Mass) is advanced percutaneously over the wire and positioned across the pulmonary annulus. If a single balloon is used, we advance another catheter from the opposite femoral vein into the right ventricle to monitor pressure during balloon inflation and to measure a pullback gradient after the inflations. When two balloons are used from each femoral vein, a third venous access line is obtained from the brachial or axillary vein to monitor right ventricular pressure and administer drugs if necessary.

The balloon catheter is inflated with a 1:5 diluted solution of contrast material. A "waist" should be seen in the midportion of the balloon, which should disappear with full inflation (Fig 54–1). During inflation the op-

erator must control the balloon position, for the balloon will tend to be ejected into the pulmonary artery during inflation. Likewise, when two balloons are used, one balloon may slide alongside the other into the pulmonary artery during inflation. After two to three inflations lasting 4 to 8 seconds, the balloons are withdrawn along the guidewires into the inferior vena cava. One of the balloon catheters is replaced with an end-hole catheter, and a pressure pullback is recorded from the main pulmonary artery, with a pause below the annulus and then resumption of measurement in the inflow portion of the right ventricle. In most patients with isolated pulmonary valve stenosis, there is almost complete abolition of the valve gradient; sometimes there is a residual gradient across the infundibular portion of the right ventricle that is caused by septal hypertrophy or congenital infundibular stenosis.

Patients are sedated during the balloon inflation; some older patients experience chest pain during inflation. There is often significant tachycardia after several balloon inflations because of a rebound from the systemic hypotension produced by occlusion of the pulmonary valve. The degree of systemic hypotension is significantly less when two balloons are used or when there is an atrial septal defect or a patent foramen ovale. Two balloons side by side allow a significant amount of blood to pass around them into the pulmonary circulation; for example, a combined balloon diameter 20% greater than the annulus diameter occludes only 70% of the annulus area. If there is significant tachycardia after balloon dilatation, we allow some time for the heart rate to turn to predilatation levels before measuring the residual gradient. Propranolol may be administered to reduce the tachycardia-induced infundibular narrowing.

Infants with critical pulmonary valve stenosis have a pinhole-sized opening in the pulmonary valve and a dilated right ventricle with severe tricuspid regurgitation. Attempts to pass a full-size balloon across this is usually not possible and, if successful, results in severe hypotension, bradycardia, and cardiac arrest. We use serial, graded dilatations starting with a small 4- to 5-mm balloon and perform progressive dilatations up to a balloon diameter 50% greater than the annulus. We also recommend placing these children under general anesthesia with endotracheal intubation for better control of hemodynamics and respiration.

Results

We have performed pulmonary valve dilatation in 136 patients ranging in age from 1 day to 76 years and with a mean age of 6.4 years; 20 patients were less than 1 year of age, and 3 patients were 51, 71, and 76 years

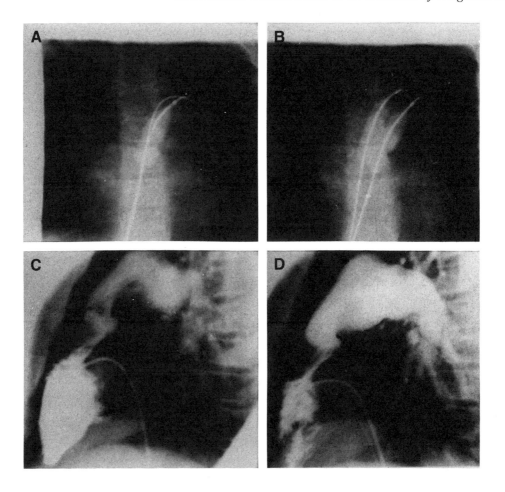

FIG 54–1.
Pulmonary valvuloplasty. **A,** a single balloon across the pulmonary valve shows a waist at the level of the valve. **B,** two balloons across the pulmonary valve in a 5-year old patient with pulmonary valve stenosis. **C,** right ventricular angiogram, lateral projection, showing a narrow jet passing through a doming pulmonary valve with moderate infundibular hypertrophy. **D,** right ventricular angiogram after valvuloplasty showing a broader jet through the pulmonary valve with the anterior leaflet flattened against the anterior wall. There is an increase in the infundibular contraction after valvuloplasty that is causing a residual gradient of 20 mm Hg across the infundibular region.

of age. The ratio of the balloon diameter to the annulus diameter averaged 1.31 with a range of 0.57 to 2.7. Seventy-five patients had a double-balloon dilatation with an annulus size of 5 to 35 mm (mean, 19.3 mm). These patients had a balloon-annulus ratio of 1.35, whereas those patients with a single-balloon dilatation had a balloon-annulus ratio of 1.17.

Right ventricular pressure ranged from 40 to 210 mm Hg before balloon dilatation (mean, 89.36 ± 31.1 mm Hg), with a gradient of 20 to 192 mm Hg (mean, 69.83 + 32.1 mm Hg). After balloon dilatation the right ventricular pressure ranged from 15 to 130 mm Hg, with a mean of 44.9 + 21.8 mm Hg. The gradient after balloon dilatation ranged from 0 to 124 mm Hg, with a mean of 22.9 + 21.9 mm Hg. The percent drop in gradient ranged from 2% to 100%, with an average drop of

68.25%. The residual gradient was between 0 and 20 mm Hg in 68% of the patients, between 21 and 40 mm Hg in 19%, and greater than 42 mm Hg in 13%.

The Valvuloplasty and Angioplasty of Congenital Anomalies (VACA) registry reported on 822 valvuloplasties performed between 1981 and 1986 from 26 institutions.[15] Thirty-five percent of the patients were less than 2 years of age, and there were 35 patients over 20 years of age. Most patients had a significant reduction in the transvalvular gradient, with the mean gradient falling from 71 ± 33 to 28 ± 21 mm Hg. Twenty-five percent had a residual gradient of less than 15 mm Hg; many of those having a higher gradient had residual infundibular hypertrophy that would be expected to regress over the following 4 to 6 weeks.[16] Balloon dilatation of dysplastic pulmonary valves has not been as successful as in isolated pulmonary valve stenosis[17] because of the greater thickness of the valve and the small size of the pulmonary annulus and main pulmonary artery associated with this anomaly; however, a significant reduction in the gradient may be achieved in many patients with dysplastic pulmonary valves,[18] but surgical enlargement of the annulus is usually required.

Complications

There were no deaths in our series of 136 patients. Complications were minor and consisted of blood loss requiring transfusion in three infants and episodes of hypotension and bradycardia in two infants who had critical pulmonary stenosis and tricuspid regurgitation. Major complications occurred in 0.6% of patients in the VACA registry report,[15] including 1 death, 1 patient with hemopericardium, and 2 patients with significant tricuspid regurgitation. Minor complications including venous thrombosis, apnea, and transient arrhythmias occurred in 11 patients.

Conclusion

Isolated congenital stenosis of the pulmonary valve can be effectively relieved by balloon dilatation and the gradient reduced by 70% to 90% if the balloon diameter is 50% greater than the annulus diameter. Residual gradients are usually due to infundibular hypertrophy, which regresses over the ensuing 3 to 6 weeks.[16] Follow-up studies with cardiac catheterization and Doppler echocardiography have shown no increase in the gradient.[19]

AORTIC STENOSIS

Balloon aortic valvuloplasty was first reported by La-babidi in 1983,[20] and the technique has been applied to a wide range of patients ranging from infants with critical aortic stenosis,[21] children and adolescents with congenital aortic valve stenosis, to octogenarians with calcific aortic stenosis.[22]

Patients and Methods

Balloon dilatation of congenital aortic valve stenosis has been carried out at Texas Children's Hospital in 67 patients ranging in age from 12 days to 27 years. Fifteen patients previously had surgical aortic valvotomy, 1 patient had a conduit from the left ventricular apex to the descending aorta because of a small aortic annulus, and 1 patient had a prosthetic Ionescu-Shiley valve.

Technique

After a right-sided heart catheterization, a Mullins transseptal sheath (USCI, Billerica, Mass) is placed in the left atrium and a catheter advanced through the sheath into the left ventricle to monitor pressure. Venting of the left ventricle during balloon inflation has not been found necessary. Angiograms are performed in the left ventricle in the right anterior oblique (RAO) and long-axial projections to rule out subvalvular and supravalvular stenosis. A Cardiomarker (USCI, Billerica, Mass) catheter is advanced retrogradely above the aortic valve for aortography or placed in the left ventricle in infants; the diameter of the annulus is calculated in two planes and measured at the base of the doming cusps in systole. We recommend using two balloons with a combined balloon diameter of 10% to 20% greater than the aortic annulus as measured at the base of the valves.

An end-hole catheter is advanced across the aortic valve into the left ventricle. Through this catheter, a 0.038-in. Teflon-coated exchange wire (USCI, Billerica, Mass, Argon Medical Corp., Athens, Tex) with a 180-degree curve formed at the soft end is passed into the left ventricle so that the apex of the curve is at the apex of the left ventricle and the tip of the wire facing the left ventricular outflow tract (Fig 54–2). A second end-hold catheter and wire are placed in a similar fashion in the apex of the left ventricle and a second exchange wire advanced. With the wires in position and a stable cardiac rhythm established, the catheters are withdrawn over the exchange wires and the percutaneous sheaths and catheters withdrawn. Tightly furled balloon catheters are inserted percutaneously over the guidewires and advanced to the aortic root. Long balloon catheters are used to dilate the aortic valve to avoid ejection of the partially inflated balloon. The length of the balloon is estimated to reach from the left ventricular apex to the midportion of the ascending aorta. The balloon catheters are advanced singly across the aortic valve and positioned to lie side by side with the midpoints at the previously marked aortic annulus. Both balloons are inflated simultaneously until the waist at the annulus disappears (Fig 54–2). Left ventricular pressure is monitored during inflation through the transseptal catheter, and in some patients systemic pressure is monitored by a radial or brachial artery line. Alternatively, an angiographic balloon catheter is inserted into the left ventricular transseptal sheath and floated out to the ascending aorta for continuous pressure monitoring and angiography. After an average of five inflations, both balloon catheters are withdrawn across the aortic valve and placed in the descending aorta so that the deflated balloon does not obstruct the carotid arteries, and the left ventricular pressure is remeasured. One of the balloon

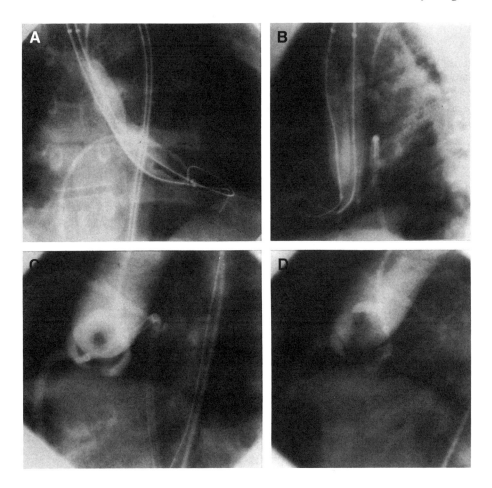

FIG 54–2.
Aortic valvuloplasty. **A** and **B,** two long balloons passed retrogradely into the left ventricle show a notch at the level of the aortic annulus. A transseptal sheath has been advanced to the left ventricle, and through this a balloon catheter has been floated out to the transverse aortic arch to measure simultaneous left ventricle and aortic pressures during and after valvuloplasty. **C** and **D,** orifice view of the aortic valve before **(C)** and after **(D)** valvuloplasty. The central black area in the left panel represents the aortic orifice in the center of the aortic annulus. After valvuloplasty this has become a linear slit extending from the left sinus of Valsalva to the right.

catheters is exchanged for an end-hold catheter that is advanced to the midportion of the ascending aorta to record simultaneous left ventricle and ascending aorta pressure. If there is a satisfactory reduction in gradient obtained, the second balloon catheter is withdrawn and a second angiogram obtained in the aortic root to estimate the degree of aortic regurgitation.

Results

Our initial two patients had dilatation with a single 4-cm-long balloon. This was quite successful in a 5-year-old patient with an annulus measuring 15 mm in diameter, but it was unsuccessful in a 10-year-old patient whose annulus measured 23 mm. A 12-day-old infant with congestive heart failure and critical aortic stenosis underwent balloon dilatation using the prograde

route through the foramen ovale, mitral valve, and left ventricular outflow tract. In the latter patient, the aortic annulus measured 7 mm. Initially a 4-mm and then a 6-mm balloon was advanced across the valve over a guidewire whose tip had been placed in the descending aorta. Sixty-one patients had dilatation with two balloons that were advanced retrogradely across the aortic valve. To facilitate crossing the aortic valve, carotid artery cutdown has been used to insert balloon catheters in infants with critical aortic stenosis.[21]

The left ventricle-to-aortic gradient was reduced from a mean of 71.2 mm Hg (range, 37 to 115 mm Hg) to a mean of 28.5 mm Hg (range, 0 to 75 mm Hg) after balloon dilatation.

Aortic regurgitation up to grade 3+ was present in 35 patients before dilatation and was present in 47 patients after balloon dilatation, but only 1 patient increased regurgitation by two grades. Two infants aged 12 days and 2 months were in heart failure before balloon dilatation but improved symptomatically, with a decrease in heart size and pulmonary edema and an increase in ejection fraction. One patient with a small aortic annulus and previous left ventricle-to-aortic conduit placement had an unsuccessful dilatation and underwent surgery to enlarge the aortic annulus. Valve dilatation with a single balloon was unsuccessful in our first patient, who had a 23-mm annulus; she underwent surgical valvotomy.

Other reports of balloon valvuloplasty for congenital aortic valve stenosis have shown similar good results.[20, 23] The VACA registry[24] reported on 204 children with a mean age of 10 years, 38 of whom were less than 1 year of age. Valvuloplasty was successful in 94% with a reduction in the peak systolic gradient from 77 ± 2 to 30 ± 1 mm Hg. A comparison between the use of single vs. double balloons revealed a reduction in the peak systolic gradient of 67% when two balloons were used vs. 43% with a single balloon.[25]

Complications

Blood loss requiring transfusion occurred in one patient. Femoral pulses were decreased in seven patients. Surgical exploration and embolectomy were required in one patient, and in the others the pulses returned with good peripheral circulation after the administration of heparin in three patients and intravenous streptokinase in three other patients. Transient left bundle-branch block occurred during balloon inflation in eight patients and lasted from 30 minutes to 24 hours. In the latter part of our experience, the number of balloon inflations decreased, and the incidence of left bundle-branch block became infrequent and transient. Midcavity obstruction after valvuloplasty was seen in three of our infants less than 2 years of age but disappeared by echocardiography within 6 months.[26] Follow-up studies by cardiac catheterization and echocardiography has demonstrated no restenosis in 98% of the patients over a period of 1 to 7 years.

Major complications occurred in 11 patients (5%) from the VACA registry.[24] Five patients, all less than 12 months of age, died, 1, 12 days after valvuloplasty. Other complications included a torn iliac artery and severe aortic regurgitation.

SUBAORTIC STENOSIS

Balloon dilation of membranous subaortic stenosis is successful if the obstruction is within a few millimeters of the aortic valve and the membrane is thin and not a fibromuscular ridge.

Lababidi and Walls[27] reported dilating subaortic lesions in 32 patients aged 10 weeks to 18 years. Membranous stenosis was present in 27 and fibromuscular stenosis in 4 patients. The balloon diameter was equal to or 2 mm less than the aortic annulus. When the obstruction was membranous, the gradient was reduced from a mean of 73 ± 34 to 17 ± 10 mm Hg and remained low over an average follow-up period of 4.5 years. Fibromuscular obstructions had higher initial gradients (average, 155 ± 15 mm Hg) and a smaller reduction to an average of 84 ± 37 mm Hg. A similar experience was reported by Suarez de Lezo et al.,[28] who dilated subaortic membranes in 27 patients with a mean age of 12 ± 9 years. The peak systolic gradient was reduced from an average of 71 ± 32 to 21 ± 13 mm Hg with no significant increase in the degree of aortic regurgitation. "Restenosis" was more common in children less than 12 years of age, and 6 of them underwent redilation with a further reduction in the gradient.

Conclusions

Balloon dilatation of congenital aortic valve stenosis can be achieved with excellent results comparable to those obtained by surgical valvotomy. There was a mild to moderate increase in the degree of aortic regurgitation after valvuloplasty that was well tolerated, and few patients have required surgery for aortic regurgitation. Infants and children with congestive heart failure caused by critical aortic stenosis can have successful palliation and improvement in left ventricular function by balloon valvuloplasty, and this makes them more suitable candidates for surgery if necessary to achieve further reduction of the gradient. Patients with thin, membranous subaortic stenosis close to the aortic valve can also have successful balloon dilation.

CONGENITAL MITRAL VALVE STENOSIS

Patients and Methods

At Texas Children's Hospital balloon dilatation of the mitral valve for congenital mitral stenosis has been undertaken ten times in eight patients whose ages ranged from 7 months to 36 years.[29] Five children had congenital mitral stenosis caused by fused commissures, two patients had parachute mitral valves, and one patient had a mitral arcade. Six of these patients had additional cardiac defects. The technique of mitral valve dilatation is similar to that used in adults and children with rheumatic mitral stenosis.[30,31] At Texas Children's

Hospital we use two long balloons to dilate the mitral valve; the combined diameter is selected to equal the mitral annulus diameter measured from an apical four-chamber echocardiogram or an RAO angiogram of the left atrium or left ventricle.

A transseptal puncture is performed and a transseptal sheath (USCI, Billerica, Mass) is advanced to the left atrium. Angiography with a 1-cm marker catheter is performed in the left atrium in the RAO and four-chamber projections to measure the mitral annulus and to visualize the valve leaflets and distal orifice. All patients are anticoagulated after the transseptal puncture. An end-hole catheter one French size less than the sheath is advanced across the mitral valve to the left ventricle to record simultaneous left atrial and left ventricular end-diastolic pressure. Left ventricular angiography is also performed with a retrograde pigtail cathe-

ter or a marker catheter through the transseptal sheath to estimate the degree of mitral regurgitation before the balloon dilatation.

A second transseptal puncture is performed from the opposite side of the groin, and each long sheath is advanced to the left atrium above the mitral valve. An end-hole Gudale-Lubin or balloon catheter is used to cross the mitral valve, and the tip is positioned near the apex of the left ventricle with care taken not to cross through any chordae. A Teflon-coated 0.035- or 0.038-in. exchange wire is prepared by making a U-shaped curve at the junction of the stiff core and the soft tip of the wire so that the curve is positioned at the left ventricular apex to prevent perforation by the rigid balloon catheter tip (Fig 54–3). The end-hole catheters and sheaths are removed and the long (6- to 8-cm) balloon catheters advanced across the mitral valve so that the

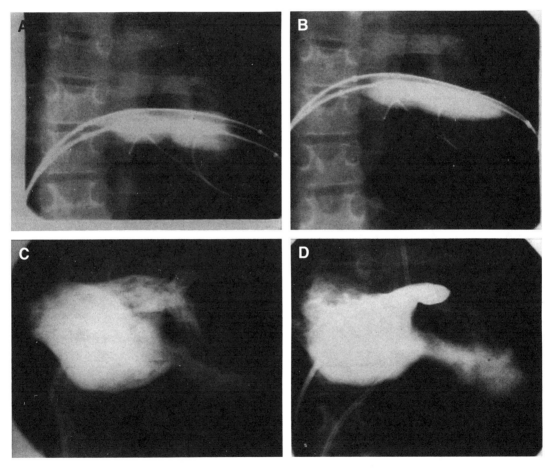

FIG 54–3.
Mitral valvuloplasty. **A** and **B,** two balloons inflated across the mitral annulus with a notch at the level of the distal leaflets. **C** and **D,** left atrial angiogram in an AP projection before **(C)** and after **(D)** valvuloplasty. The patient is a 5-year-old with congenital mitral valve stenosis and fusion of the commissures, a small annulus, and a small distal orifice of the mitral valve. After annuloplasty there is an increased excursion of the mitral leaflets with a reduction in the mean gradient from 13 to 5 mm Hg.

catheters point to the apex and not transversely across the short axis of the ventricle. Both balloons are inflated simultaneously, with the midportion of the balloon across the distal orifice of the valve leaflets, while making sure that none of the balloons are seated across the atrial septum. The balloons are inflated until the waist at the level of the leaflets disappears.

The balloons are replaced with end-hole and angiographic catheters to measure simultaneous left ventricular and left atrial pressures.

Results

The patients' ages ranged from 7 months to 36 years. Combined balloon sizes ranged from 10 mm up to 20 mm with a mean balloon-annulus ratio of 1.13 (range, 0.87 to 1.26). The left atrial a wave-to-left ventricle end-diastolic pressure gradient averaged 25 ± 6 mm Hg, with a range of 18 to 39 mm Hg before balloon dilatation, and fell to an average of 9.0 ± 3 mm Hg (range, 8 to 13 mm Hg) after dilatation. The mean pressure gradient decreased from an average of 18 ± 7 mm Hg (range, 13 to 32) to 8.0 ± 3 mm Hg (range, 5 to 13) after dilation. Mitral valve area increased from 0.8 ± 0.2 to 1.4 ± 0.3 cm^2/M^2. There was no correlation between the decrease in the mitral valve gradient and the balloon-annulus ratio or the number of inflations.

Complications

One patient with a parachute mitral valve and supravalve membrane developed significant mitral regurgitation (2+) that was well tolerated clinically. One polycythemic patient who was not anticoagulated developed a transient ischemic episode after catheterization. Another patient developed an acute hemopericardium that was evacuated uneventfully.

Long-Term Results

Six patients have been followed for 4 to 54 months with continued clinical improvement and only a slight decrease in mitral valve area by echocardiography from 1.4 ± 0.3 to 1.2 ± 0.2 cm^2/M^2. Two patients developed restenosis over the following 7 to 12 months. One patient had a repeat balloon dilation with larger balloon catheters and has had sustained improvement over the following 4 years; the second patient weighed 5.4 kg at her initial valvuloplasty and developed restenosis within the following 12 months. She was referred to surgery where extensive valve reconstruction was performed, but she died on the second postoperative day.

Conclusions

A significant reduction in the transvalvular gradient with a marked improvement in symptoms can be expected if the congenital mitral stenosis is caused by commissural fusion; patients with a parachute mitral valve and an associated supravalve ring will have less improvement in hemodynamics but may experience a temporary improvement in symptoms.

TRICUSPID STENOSIS

We have performed balloon dilatations for stenotic lesions of the right ventricular inflow tract five times. One patient had rheumatic tricuspid stenosis and previous replacement of aortic and mitral valves. His tricuspid valve was dilated on two occasions 1 year apart. Symptoms of restenosis occurred 9 months after the initial dilatation. Since the second dilatation, he has been asymptomatic for 12 months. Two patients with bioprosthetic valves in the tricuspid position underwent dilatation with relief of the gradient from the right atrium to the right ventricle. One was a 54-year-old woman with a 27-mm Ionescu valve and the other a 10-year-old boy with a 33-mm porcine valve. A 12-year-old child had a conduit placed from the right atrium to the right ventricle as part of a Fontan operation for tricuspid atresia. She developed intimal thickening and stenosis at the proximal end of the conduit, and this was successfully dilated with relief of right-sided heart failure.

Technique

End-hole catheters are inserted in each femoral vein and passed across the tricuspid valve to the main and left pulmonary arteries. Teflon-coated exchange wires (0.038 inch) are advanced to the left pulmonary artery and the catheters and sheaths withdrawn over the guidewires. Two balloons whose combined diameter equal the tricuspid annulus diameter are advanced over the guidewires, with the distal tip of the balloons lying in the right ventricular outflow tract and the midportion of the balloon lying across the annulus and tricuspid leaflets (Fig 54–4). Both balloons are inflated simultaneously. Elimination of the waist in the balloons is not possible with the prosthetic valves, but relief of the gradient occurs in both cases. When balloons are inflated across a rigid structure such as a prosthetic valve ring, balloon rupture may result in a circumferential tear of the balloon rather than the usual longitudinal tear. This may produce difficulties in withdrawing the balloon

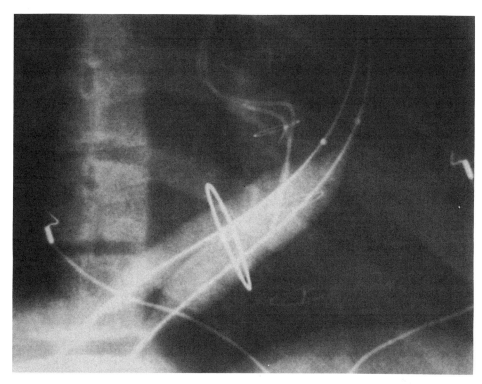

FIG 54–4.
Tricuspid valvuloplasty. Two exchange wires have been passed through the stenotic prosthetic Hancock tricuspid valve into the left pulmonary artery. Two balloons are advanced over the wires and inflated, with the midportions at the level of the tricuspid sewing ring.

through the femoral vein because the distal part of the balloon inverts and becomes bulky or even detaches from the catheter shaft.

COARCTATION OF THE AORTA

Native Coarctation

Technique

Biplane angiography is performed in both the posteroanterior (PA) and lateral projections and also in the RAO and left anterior oblique (LAO) projections if the anatomy of the coarctation repair is unusual. Usually a discrete ridge is best seen in the lateral projection (Fig 54–5). A 1-cm marker catheter (Cardiomarker, USCI, Billerica, Mass) is advanced to the transverse aortic arch and is used as an internal grid to measure the isthmus and coarctation area. At our institution we make a measurement at the base of the left subclavian artery; if this measurement is greater than 50% of the diameter of the midthoracic aorta, we proceed with the balloon dilation. An alternative route for angiography is to advance an angiographic balloon catheter from the left atrium to the left

ventricle and into the ascending aorta and transverse arch; this catheter is left there for pressure monitoring and postdilation angiography and obviates the need to pass a retrograde catheter across the area of dilation. The balloon catheter may be passed progradely across the coarctation in children with transposition of the great arteries or a ventricular septal defect.[32] In patients with transposition, an end-hole catheter is advanced from the right ventricle to the ascending aorta and down past the coarctation; an exchange wire is passed through this catheter and a balloon dilation catheter exchanged for the end-hole catheter. When there is a ventricular septal defect, an end-hole catheter can be manipulated across the defect to the ascending aorta. Care should be taken when advancing the bulkier balloon dilation catheter across the defect to avoid heart block.

The balloon diameter is chosen to be 100% to 110% of the isthmus measurement. Before inserting the balloon over the exchange wire, negative pressure is applied to the balloon to completely empty it of contrast material and form two even folds of the balloon on each side of the shaft. The folds are then wrapped around the balloon in a clockwise or counterclockwise direction de-

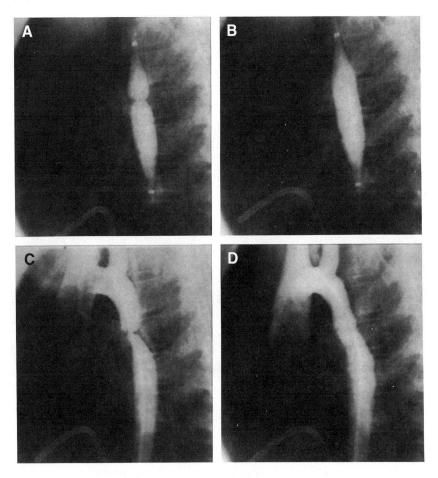

FIG 54–5.
Coarctation angioplasty. **A** and **B**, a balloon catheter has been passed retrograde to the area of coarctation and inflated, with disappearance of the waist. **C** and **D**, the discrete coarctation membrane is seen in **C**, and this is abolished after balloon angioplasty **(D).**

pending upon the natural lie of the folds. When the balloon is inserted through the skin, the balloon catheter is rotated in a similar direction to keep the "wings" of the balloon folded against the shaft. Similarly, when extracting the balloon from the artery over the wire, the balloon is rotated to refold the wings in the same direction used when inserting the balloon. For coarctation dilation, a short balloon 2 to 3 cm in length is sufficient; longer balloons will lie in the transverse aortic arch and block the carotids even when deflated.

Patients are heparinized with 50 units/kg of heparin, and an end-hole catheter is advanced into the left subclavian artery or the ascending aorta. A Teflon-coated exchange wire is advanced through the end-hole catheter with the tip of the wire in the ascending aorta or left subclavian artery, and the catheter is withdrawn. Having the wire and tip of the balloon catheter in the left subclavian artery reduces the risk of emboli into the cerebral circulation from the catheter or balloon. Sometimes

the distance from the subclavian artery to the area of coarctation is too short to allow the midportion of the balloon to be across the area of coarctation. In these cases the exchange wire is advanced to the ascending aorta.

At the present time balloons with a diameter of 10 mm or less can be mounted on 5 or 4.5 F catheters and can be advanced through a 6 or 7 F sheath into the femoral artery. This is advantageous in small infants where the balloon is not advanced percutaneously through the artery, which lessens damage to the artery. In newborns, the umbilical artery can be cannulated and can accept a 5-mm balloon on a 5 F shaft. With larger-size catheters the subcutaneous tissue is dilated with pointed forceps or a sheath introducer, and the balloon is advanced over the guidewire through the skin and into the artery without a sheath.

The midportion of the balloon is positioned across the area of coarctation. In most cases this is situated just above the left main bronchus in the PA projection. If the coarctation area is not in the usual place, a lead marker can be placed on the skin over the area of the coarctation as a guide for balloon positioning. The correct position of the balloon can be verified by partially inflating the balloon and observing the position of the waist.

The balloon is rapidly inflated while recording with biplane fluoroscopy and cineangiography to observe the presence and position of the waist in the balloon (Fig 54–5). The waist should be at the central straight part of the balloon between the two markers; if the waist disappears and there is a persistent gradient, then a larger-size balloon can be used to repeat the dilation. However, if the waist persists with full inflation, a larger-size balloon is not indicated. Coarctation membranes usually disappear with the first or second inflation with an appropriately sized balloon; only two to three dilations are necessary.

There may be some variability in the anatomy of the aortic isthmus in native coarctation. Intimal and medial tears are more likely to occur in native coarctation since there is not the protection afforded by the perivascular fibrosis that occurs with postoperative recoarctation. Although aneurysms at the site of dilation in native coarctation have been reported, there have not been any reported instances of acute dissection or rupture of the aorta at the coarctation site at the time of balloon dilation. However, there was one case report of a transverse tear of the ascending aorta in an infant[33] where the distal tip of the balloon catheter was positioned at the base of the innominate artery. Balloon catheters straighten as the balloon inflates, and if the balloon is curved around the aortic arch, it will tend to straighten and apply traction to the transverse arch against the aortic root.

After two to four dilations the balloon is deflated, and constant negative pressure is applied while the balloon is rotated and withdrawn so that the folds of the balloon rewrap before withdrawing it over a wire and out through the femoral artery puncture or sheath. The wire is left in place, and a sheath and dilator or sheath and catheter are advanced over the wire and inserted into the groin. An end-hole catheter is passed over the exchange wire proximal to the dilation area for pressure measurements and angiography. It is extremely important not to advance an unguarded catheter or wire across the area of a freshly dilated coarctation because the catheter wire may get caught in the intimal tears and provoke dissection or aneurysm formation.

Postdilation angiography should be performed in both the AP and lateral projections as well as ROA and LAO projections to profile any possible aneurysms that might occur at the site of dilation. After 2 to 3 minutes when the vasodilatory effects of the contrast material have abated, a pullback pressure recording is made from the aortic arch to the descending aorta to record any residual gradient. The catheter and exchange wire are withdrawn into the sheath, and the sheath is aspirated and flushed with heparin.

Results

At Texas Children's Hospital we have performed balloon dilation of native coarctation in 85 patients ranging in age from 1 day to 29 years with a mean age of 5.0 ± 3 years. The patients' weights ranged from 1.7 to 60.3 kg. A single balloon was used in all patients, and the balloon-isthmus ration ranged from 0.5 to 1.68 with an average of 1.13. The gradient across the coarctation ranged from 0 to 80 mm Hg, with a mean gradient of 43.5 ± 16.6; after dilation the gradient ranged from 0 to 65 with a mean of 11.12 ± 7.9 mm Hg. Residual gradients were less than 10 mm Hg in 62% of the patients, between 11 and 20 mm Hg in 22.4%, and greater than 21 mm Hg after dilation in 15%. If the isthmus diameter was less than 50% of the diameter of the midthoracic aorta, there was likely to be a residual gradient of greater than 20 mm Hg. These latter patients will probably need surgical enlargement of the isthmus area and coarctation. From the VACA registry,[34] 141 procedures were reported in 140 patients ranging in age from 3 days to 29 years; 31 of these patients were less than a year of age. Gradients across the coarctation averaged 48 ± 8.6 mm Hg, and after dilation the gradient averaged 12 ± 11.3 mm Hg. The coarctation diameter increased from a mean of 3.9 to 8.8 mm. Eighty-five percent of these patients had a residual gradient of less than 20 mm Hg. Other reports of smaller series have showed similar results.[35–37]

Complications of the procedure have been mainly related to femoral artery occlusions in the smaller patients.[38, 39] One death 25 hours after balloon dilation has been reported and was probably due to ventricular fibrillation; there was one report of rupture of the ascending aorta in an infant.[33] Most of the femoral artery occlusions resolved with the administration of heparin and/or streptokinase, and several patients have required surgical thrombectomy and repair of the femoral artery. The development of an aneurysm at the site of the balloon dilation has been reported in several instances,[11, 40] but the overall occurrence rate appears to be 4% to 5%. While some of these aneurysms have been reported to be quite large and surgery was recommended,[40] in our experience we have seen four patients who developed an aneurysm after balloon dilation, and these have remained stable over the ensuing 2 to 4 years and have not required surgery.[11]

Intermediate follow-up of up to 7 years after balloon dilation of native coarctation has shown that the residual gradient remains stable with a very low incidence of recoarctation in children over 1 year of age. A recurrence rate of 60% to 70% has been observed in infants undergoing balloon dilation of native coarctation who were less than 1 to 3 months of age.[41]

Conclusions

Ongoing review of the results of native coarctation angioplasty and longer-term follow-up will probably show that this technique can achieve long-lasting results with minimal residual gradient and no aneurysm formation in about 70% of children and adolescents. When there is hypoplasia of the isthmus, surgical repair of the isthmus and coarctation is preferred. There has not been a large experience with coarctation angioplasty in patients over the age of 25 years; progressive changes with age in the intima and media of the aorta proximal and distal to the coarctation may predispose to aneurysm formation or dissection.[42]

Further development of low-profile balloons with larger inflated diameters will minimize arterial complications. In some cases the use of an intraluminal stent may permit enlargement of a hypoplastic isthmus without too much disruption of the aortic media and subsequent aneurysm formation.

Recoarctation

Technique

The technique for balloon dilation of a recoarctation stenosis is similar to that of native coarctation. The balloon diameter is chosen to be 100% to 110% of the isthmus measurement. The appropriate balloon is prepared in the usual way. For recoarctation dilation, a longer balloon 3 to 5 cm in length may be necessary, depending upon the anatomy of the residual stenosis.

Recoarctation stenoses may require more prolonged and repeated dilations than native coarctation to eliminate the waist. If there is a persisting waist in an appropriately sized balloon, high–inflation pressure balloons (Blue Max, Meditech) can be used. These balloons can be inflated up to 16 atm and are suitable for dilating tough fibrous lesions.

Results

Fifty-six patients have undergone dilation of coarctation restenosis after various surgical operations for native coarctation at Texas Children's Hospital. The patients' ages ranged from 3 months to 21 years with a mean age of 7 years and they weighed from 3.3 to 68.5 kg with a mean weight of 25 kg. The balloon diameter averaged 125% greater than diameter of the isthmus at the base of the subclavian artery, with the balloon-isthmus ratio ranging from 0.5 to 2.5 times the isthmus diameter. The average gradient prior to dilation was 43.4 mm Hg, (range, 10 to 90) and decreased to an average of 13.7 mm Hg (range, 0 to 60). Fifty-three percent of our patients had a residual gradient of less than 35 mm Hg, 22% had a residual gradient of 10 to 20 mm Hg, and 23% had a residual gradient of greater than 21 mm Hg. The VACA registry reported on 200 patients who had recoarctation dilation at an average age of 7 years (range, 1 month to 26 years).[43] The gradient was reduced from a mean of 41.9 to 13.3 mm Hg with an increase in the coarctation diameter from 5.2 to 8.9 mm. Residual gradients of less 20 mm Hg were found in 79.4% of the patients.

Complications

In the combined VACA study, five patients died of complications due to the procedure. One patient had acute rupture of the coarctation segment, and two patients died suddenly 6 to 14 hours after dilation, apparently of ventricular fibrillation with no evidence of disruption of the aorta. One further patient died of a cerebral vascular accident possibly induced by occlusion of the carotid artery by the balloon in the transverse aortic arch; other neurologic complications occurred in three other patients. One further patient died with persistently low cardiac output after a successful dilation. Four patients developed postcoarctectomy syndrome with significant reactive hypertension. Femoral artery complications occurred in 17 patients (8.5%), including 11 with thrombosis and 6 with diminished femoral pulses.

PULMONARY ARTERY BRANCH STENOSIS

Stenosis of the pulmonary artery branches may be due to congenital discrete narrowing of bifurcation points or diffuse hypoplasia associated with pulmonary artery atresia and the tetralogy of Fallot. Stenoses may be associated with previous surgical shunts or grafts, with or without hypoplasia of the pulmonary artery. In either congenital or acquired pulmonary artery branch stenosis a combination of discrete and diffuse lesions may be seen. Proximal natural stenoses or stenoses associated with shunts are ideal lesions for balloon dilation with or without stent implantation.

Balloon dilation of proximal stenoses may be contraindicated if there are diffuse peripheral branch stenoses in the small tertiary branches of the pulmonary arteries because of the greater risk of rupture. Long hypoplastic segments of pulmonary arteries are not a contraindication since they can be adequately treated by balloon dilation.[44, 45]

Technique

Biplane angiography is carried out with a marker catheter to identify the site of stenosis and any peripheral branch stenoses that might be present. All measurements should be made during systole because in congenital pulmonary branch stenosis the systolic excursion of the pulmonary arteries can be quite wide and discrete stenoses may be apparent only during systole.

After angiography, pullback pressure recordings are made from the distal pulmonary arteries to the proximal branch and also to the main pulmonary artery.

An end-hole catheter is advanced into the pulmonary artery and passed distal to the narrowing. Access to the stenotic pulmonary artery branch involves a curved catheter course; a superstiff exchange wire is preferred so that the relatively stiff balloon catheters can make the curve from the main pulmonary artery to the right or left pulmonary artery branches.

The balloon size selected is 3 to 4 times the diameter of the stenotic diameter. Three to four prolonged dilations may be necessary to eliminate residual waists, and previously undetected narrowings may appear during balloon inflation.

Results

Balloon angioplasty of pulmonary branch stenosis has been overall disappointing in the reduction of gradients in spite of an apparently good dilation because of the elasticity of the pulmonary arteries (Fig 54–6). The VACA registry[46] reported on dilation of 182 arteries in 156 patients whose ages ranged from 0.22 to 46.2 years with an average age of 7.7 years. There was a mild but significant decrease in the average proximal pulmonary pressure from 69 ± 25 to 63 ± 22 mm Hg and a similar small decrease in the gradient across the stenotic artery from 49 ± 25 to 37 ± 26 mm Hg.

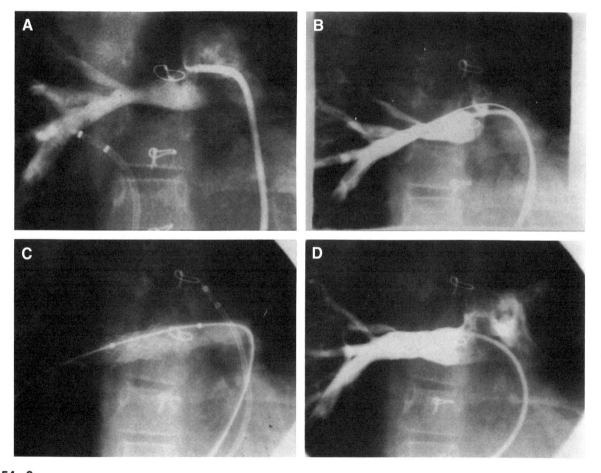

FIG 54–6.
Pulmonary branch angioplasty. **A,** an angiogram in the main pulmonary artery in the AP projection shows a waistlike stenosis at the distal portion of the right pulmonary artery in a patient who had repair of the tetralogy of Fallot and takedown of an ascending aorta-to-right pulmonary artery shunt. **B,** there is no significant change in the diameter of the stenotic pulmonary artery after dilation with a balloon catheter. **C,** inflation of an intra-arterial stent at the region of the pulmonary artery stenosis. **D,** significant enlargement of the pulmonary artery stenosis with reduction of the gradient after stent inflation to 15 mm.

A large series of 218 angioplasty procedures performed in 135 patients by Rothman et al.[47] reported a success rate of 58% as judged by an increase of greater than 50% of the predilation stenosis diameter, an increase of greater than 20% in flow to the affected lung, or a decrease of greater than 20% in the ratio of the systolic right ventricular pressure to the aortic pressure. Once again, the reduction in right ventricular aortic pressure was only modest and decreased from an average ratio of 84% ± 22% to 72% ± 21% after dilation in 84 patients.

In our own series of 31 patients with isolated pulmonary branch stenosis, the average proximal pressure decreased from a mean of 73.3 ± 30.65 mm Hg to 61.74 ± 25.87, and the gradient across the stenotic area decreased from a mean of 49.45 ± 34.7 to 31.74 ± 28.36 mm Hg.

These results have considerably improved with the use of intraluminal stents coupled with balloon dilation. At Texas Children's Hospital we have inserted stents in 14 patients with pulmonary branch stenosis; the proximal pulmonary artery pressure fell from a mean of 77.6 ± 47.2 to 50.6 ± 25.9 mm Hg, and the gradient across this stenotic area fell from a mean of 56.9 ± 47.98 to 14.4 ± 23.1 mm Hg. The initial results of a collaborative trial of the use of intravascular stents in pulmonary branch stenosis has confirmed our own initial results.[48]

Complications

From the VACA registry[45] complications were reported in 21 of 186 patients (11.3%) and included 5 deaths. Pulmonary artery rupture was associated with 2 deaths and low cardiac output; paradoxical embolus and sinus arrest occurred in the 3 other deaths. Other complication included perforation or rupture of the pulmonary artery in 9 patients, bleeding requiring transfusion in 3, and aneurysm formation in 2. Failure to dilate the pulmonary branch stenosis occurred in 4 patients due to an inability to pass the balloon catheter across the stenotic area.

Restenosis

Relatively short-term follow-up data are available from the report of Rothman et al.[47] Angiograms were performed to evaluate 57 of their 218 procedures 10 ± 11 months after dilation; of the 32 procedures initially considered successful, restenosis occurred in 5 (16%).

The initial experience with balloon dilation of pulmonary artery branch stenosis has shown a success rate of 49% to 60%. The ongoing evaluation of the use of intra-arterial stents in this lesion shows promise for an increased success rate and fewer instances of restenosis (Fig 54–6).[48]

PULMONARY VEIN STENOSIS

The site of stenosis of the pulmonary veins usually occurs at the entrance to the left atrium. This may be a congenital lesion or acquired after surgery to correct anomalous pulmonary venous connection. Selective pulmonary arteriography or pulmonary artery wedge angiography is necessary to identify the exact site of the stenosis. The right pulmonary veins are usually best visualized in a PA projection, while the left pulmonary veins may require a LAO projection to visualize the veins as they enter the left atrium.

Technique

If the atrial septum is intact, a transseptal puncture is required to enter the left atrium, and an end-hole catheter is passed through the long transseptal sheath to explore the pulmonary veins. A Teflon-coated exchange wire is passed through the catheter into the vein as far as possible into the lung. Selective angiography in the vein is carried out with the end-hole catheter to measure the size of the vein. It is usually difficult to pass even small balloon catheters through a long transseptal sheath; the balloon catheters may have to be advanced over an exchange wire through the hole made in the atrial septum with the transseptal sheath. The midportion of the balloon is positioned at the stenotic site, and several inflations are made until the waist disappears. The largest-size balloon should equal the diameter of the pulmonary vein proximal to the stenosis. The balloon length should be short to avoid dilating the atrial septum. This is especially important in the right pulmonary veins where approach to the veins across the atrial septum takes a curved course and long balloons will tend to pull out of the vein and/or enlarge the atrial septal puncture hole. Several balloon sizes may be needed to gradually enlarge the vein stenosis to an adequate size.

After dilation, an angiographic catheter is advanced into the vein, and selective angiograms with angled views are taken to measure the result.

Results

Balloon dilation of pulmonary vein stenosis was one of the first angioplastic procedures described for the treatment of congenital cardiovascular defects.[4] Although this initial report was not encouraging because of the high recurrence rate, we have continued to use this procedure for lack of a better alternative. Nine patients have undergone 13 pulmonary vein dilations at our institution since 1980, one patient having 5 dilations. Initially there was significant reduction in the pulmonary vein-to-left atrium gradient from a mean of 14.6 (range, 4 to 28 mm Hg) to 8.7 (range, 0 to 15 mm Hg). However, restenosis occurred in six patients; one patient had dilation of the left pulmonary veins five times. The VACA registry has reported pulmonary vein dilation in five patients with success in three.[49]

Complications of the procedure itself are minimal. Rupture of the pulmonary vein is a risk but has not been reported.

PATENT DUCTUS ARTERIOSUS OCCLUSION

Percutaneous closure of a patent ductus with a Teflon plug was first reported by Porstmann et al. in 1967.[50] A smaller collapsible umbrella for ductus occlusion was developed by Rashkind and Cuaso,[51] and after modifications to the delivery system by Mullins,[52] an extensive clinical trial revealed that within certain constraints of patent ductus size, most patent ducts could be closed with a catheter-delivered device.[53]

Technique

The diagnosis of patent ductus is established by cardiac catheterization with detailed biplane angiography of the ductus to determine the exact size and configuration of the ductus. In addition to the exact size and anatomy of the ductus, the adjacent landmarks such as tracheal air shadow and vertebral relationships are identified angiographically on straight AP and lateral angiocardiograms. The diameter of the narrowest portion of the ductus is accurately measured. Comparison with the known diameter of the angiography catheter is usually sufficient for this measurement. The ductus must be at least 2.5 mm in diameter to easily accommodate the 8 F delivery sheath for the occlusion and no more than 4.0 mm in diameter to obtain adequate fixation with the standard 12-mm occluding umbrella. A ductus over 4.0 mm in diameter will require the use of the larger (17-mm) occluding device. This is particularly so with very short "window"-type ductus.

Once the decision is made to occlude the ductus transvenously, a second venous line is introduced for rapid delivery of supplemental medications, especially sedation, during critical phases of the procedure. An arterial line should also be in place for monitoring of the patient's status or occasionally to advance an angiographic catheter retrogradely to a position adjacent to the ductus for test angiograms during implantation of the device. This is particularly important in patients with ductus of unusual configuration. Care must be

taken in these cases to keep this retrograde catheter away from the device during implantation.

The sheath in the Mullins transseptal set (USCI) comes with a 180-degree distal curve to facilitate passage from the left atrium to the left ventricle. This curve needs to be straightened slightly to better conform to the course of right ventricle to pulmonary artery to patent ductus arteriosus to aorta, i.e., a curve of approximately 90 degrees and usually of a smaller curve radius to conform to the particular patient's size. The distal end of the sheath with the contained dilator is immersed in sterile boiling water for 15 to 60 seconds. While still in the boiling water, the distal curve is gently reshaped to conform to the desired anatomy. The sheath and dilator are held in that curvature during removal from the boiling water and immediately immersed in sterile cold flush solution to fix the new curve. The dilator will have to be separately reformed in the boiling water back to its original straight or slightly curved configuration.

The 8 F long transseptal sheath and dilator are advanced over a wire to the area of the right atrium, and with the sheath tip at the low right atrium/inferior vena cava junction, the wire and dilator are removed. After clearing the sheath of air, a long 8 F end hole or angiographic catheter is introduced directly through this sheath into the right atrium and from there maneuvered through the right ventricle, main pulmonary artery, and ductus and into the descending aorta. The long sheath then is advanced over the catheter, also through the ductus to the descending aorta.

The catheter is withdrawn from the long sheath and the sheath left as a direct channel through the ductus. With the removal of the catheter from the long sheath, the sheath should immediately be capped with an 8 F side arm back-bleed valve to prevent excessive blood loss from the large sheath now directly in communication with the aorta. Once the proximal end of the sheath is capped, blood should be allowed to flow from the side arm on its own to ensure that there is no entrapped air within the system. The sheath is then attached to the pressure/flush system and thoroughly flushed.

As an alternative technique to manipulation of the catheter through the right heart and ductus via the long sheath (when the long sheath severely compromises easy manipulation of the catheter), an end-hole catheter is introduced through a standard venous sheath. The catheter is advanced through the right heart, through the ductus, and into the descending aorta. Once the end-hole catheter is in the descending aorta, an exchange, extrastiff 0.038-in. guidewire is passed through the catheter well into the descending aorta, the catheter removed, and the wire left in place through the ductus.

The prepared long sheath and dilator set are advanced over the exchange wire through the right heart and through the ductus to a point in the descending aorta several centimeters distal to the aortic end of the ductus. Occasionally, neither the catheter nor wire can be passed progradely from the pulmonary artery through the ductus into the aorta. In these cases, a retrograde end-hole catheter is advanced to the area of the ductus from a femoral artery. Either the catheter itself or a soft-tipped exchange-length guidewire passed through the catheter is then passed from the aorta through the ductus into the pulmonary artery. The soft end of the wire is allowed to lay free in the main pulmonary artery (MPA). A long sheath is then or has already been advanced into the MPA over a standard catheter from the femoral vein. A retrieval basket or snare is passed through the sheath, and the retrograde wire is grasped in the pulmonary artery and withdrawn out through the femoral vein. An alternate method is to manipulate the retrograde catheter or wire directly into the distal end of the sheath and back out of the femoral vein end of the sheath. An end-hole catheter is advanced over the venous end of the wire to the MPA and through the ductus. If an 8 F catheter can be used for this maneuver, then the long sheath can be advanced directly over this catheter.

Only after the sheath is in place through the ductus are the occluding device and delivery catheter opened and inspected for proper function of the components. A gentle curve is formed on the distal end of the delivery wire and attaching knuckle to correspond roughly to the course of right ventricle to pulmonary artery to the ductus. This will help prevent the delivery wire from springing away from the ductus as it is released. The curve should be formed so that the attaching knuckle is on the concave side of the curve. The ductus-occluding umbrella is then attached and locked onto the delivery system and loaded into the loading device. The umbrella should not be loaded prior to this time to reduce the duration of time that the spring legs of the umbrella must stay in the collapsed position. The side port of the delivery catheter is attached to a separate flushing system and flushed completely free of any air.

At this time, younger or uncooperative patients should be given a supplemental dose of sedation and should be precisely positioned for straight AP and lateral projections. A cineangiocardiogram using 1/2 to 1 cc/kg of contrast is performed by injecting directly through the sheath, which is still positioned in the descending aorta with the tip adjacent to the ductus (Fig 54–7). This will give exact last-minute anatomy and show any distortion of the ductus shape by the sheath. The sheath is then flushed, and the tip of the delivery pod is introduced through the back-bleed device into the proximal end of the sheath and advanced within the cardiac silhouette to a location approximately at the tricuspid valve. The delivery catheter and sheath are fixed in this position while the delivery wire is advanced. This delivers the still-folded umbrella out of the pod into the sheath. The wire is slowly advanced by moving the umbrella further through the sheath to a point just within the sheath tip in the dorsal segment of the aorta. With the sheath and delivery catheter fixed at this point against the patient's leg, the delivery wire alone is advanced several millimeters while carefully watching for the distal legs (only) of the umbrella to open completely in the aorta (Fig 54–7). During this maneuver the sheath may need to be withdrawn simultaneously several millimeters while holding the delivery catheter/wire in a fixed position to get the legs away from the posterior aortic wall and allow full opening of the distal legs to 90 degrees. The central hinge mechanism of the umbrella device should still be within the end of the sheath. The locking nut on the proximal delivery rod is advanced against the "Y" connector of the delivery catheter and locked. This prevents any separate movement of the delivery wire from the catheter.

The entire system with only the distal legs opened is withdrawn very slowly as a unit while watching for very slight flexing or bending of the distal legs as they begin to enter the narrower portion of the ductus. As the device is properly fixed within the ductus, the overall to-and-fro movement of the device and delivery catheter usually decreases. The hinge portion of the device should now approximate the narrowest portion of the ductus as determined by previous landmarks. The delivery wire and catheter are fixed in this position while the sheath alone is withdrawn several centimeters off of the proximal legs of the occluding device. With this maneuver, the proximal legs of the device should open on the pulmonary side of the ductus with fixation of the device within the ductus. The sheath is readvanced against the opened proximal legs of the device. This helps to keep the proximal legs forced open against the pulmonary end of the ductus. Even with new, very good imaging systems, these proximal legs are very difficult to see on the fluoroscope, so their opening is assumed with the knowledge that the sheath has been withdrawn several centimeters off of the proximal legs after the distal legs were fixed. Very gentle, minute, to-and-fro motion of the delivery wire is then carried out to more firmly fix the now opened occluding umbrella within the ductus and to simultaneously test for sufficient and accurate fixation. With the delivery sheath readvanced up against and buttressing the proximal legs of the device, very slight tension is applied to the delivery wire while the

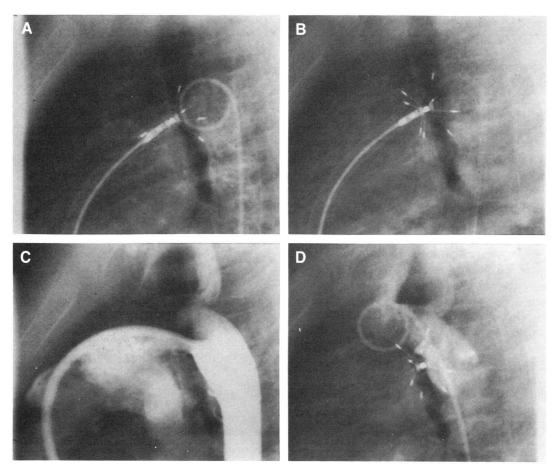

FIG 54–7.
Patent ductus arteriosus occlusion. **A,** the occlusion umbrella has been delivered through a long sheath into the descending aorta, and the distal legs have unfolded. The proximal legs are folded inside the sheath. The sheath and umbrella are pulled into the ductus. **B,** the sheath has been withdrawn so that the proximal legs unfold on the pulmonary artery side of the ductus. **C,** an aortogram in the lateral projection shows the pulmonary artery end of a 5-mm ductus at the anterior part of the tracheal column. **D,** aortic angiogram showing the umbrella in position with a minimal residual leak.

release mechanism at the proximal end of the catheter is activated to release the occluding device in the ductus. The umbrella usually moves slightly posteriorly away from the delivery catheter, and the delivery sheath may tend to spring anteriorly away from the device. Even when the sheath seems well away from the device, the delivery wire is slowly and gently withdrawn while closely observing the device on fluoroscopy. Once the delivery system is completely free of the device, the delivery system is withdrawn.

To verify the exact position of the device and to document the success of the occlusion after implantation of the device, a descending aorta angiocardiogram with contrast injected immediately adjacent to the device should be performed. It is imperative that the injection be close to the aortic end of the ductus and not in the left ventricle or even the ascending aorta. With dilution

of the contrast and loss of contrast material into the right subclavian and carotids from injections proximal to the ductus, small leaks through the occluding device will be missed. Positioning a catheter in the aorta adjacent to the ductus may be accomplished by either a retrograde catheter carefully positioned adjacent to the implanted device or by a balloon angiocatheter advanced, after transseptal puncture, from the left ventricle, out the ascending aorta, and around the arch to a position immediately adjacent to the ductus for a confirmatory angiocardiogram.

If the original ductus is greater than 4.0 mm in diameter or has a very short and broad aortic end or, on the other hand, is very long and tortuous, the 17-mm device should be utilized. This device requires the use of an 11 delivery sheath.

Once the 11 F sheath is in place, the procedure is

identical to that using the 12-mm device except that the larger device and delivery system are utilized. The larger occluding device is of heavier construction and "springier," which necessitates greater pull tension for loading. When it opens, the 17-mm device is also easier to visualize, and it offers more tactile sensation when being implanted. For these reasons it seems to become "fixed" more firmly, thus making the delivery portion of the procedure more precise.

Results

The umbrella occluding device began clinical trials in 1981. During the first 2 years of use there were problems with an inability to deliver the device to the ductus and embolization of the device during implantation. As a consequence, there were several significant changes in the device, the delivery system, and the technique. Since the last of these changes the results with the ductus occlusion device have been very good, although still not perfect. In the last 175 patients at Texas Children's Hospital, implantation of the device was successful in 96%. Nine percent of these patients were less than 1 year of age, and 20% weighed less than 10 kg. Thirteen patients had significant residual leaks and were reoccluded after 3 to 6 months. Total occlusion was accomplished in 89%, including these reocclusion patients. The remaining residual leaks were mostly infinitesimally small with no murmur and only detectable by high-quality Doppler/echocardiography.

ATRIAL SEPTAL DEFECT CLOSURE

The first report of atrial septal defect closure with a catheter-delivered device was in 1974 by Drs. King and Mills.[54] Although successfully used in several patients, this device never gained popularity because of its large-sized delivery system. A smaller device was developed by Rashkind and Cuaso in 1977;[55] this was a modification of the patent ductus arteriosus occlusion umbrella and consisted of a large single umbrella of polyurethane foam mounted on a single set of stainless steel arms. The distal ends of the arms had three tiny hooks attached to alternate arms that embedded the umbrella on the left side of the atrial septum. The delivery pod was 15 F in size and had a centering mechanism formed by three additional proximal arms in the pod. The umbrella devices were 25, 30, and 35 mm in diameter. Further modifications to this device have been carried out by Lock et al.[56, 57] who fashioned a double-umbrella "clamshell" device with two layers of fabric mounted on spring-jointed wires so that in the open position the umbrellas flex toward each other and grip the atrial sep-

tum between them without the use of hooks. This clamshell device has no centering mechanism, and the size of the device must be at least twice the size of the atrial septal defect. This limits the use of the device to defects in the fossa ovalis in the center of the atrial septum and to defects that are 20 mm or less in diameter. Larger devices may impinge upon the tricuspid and mitral valves or the pulmonary veins. The device can be delivered through an 11 F sheath.

Technique

Biplane angiography in RAO and four-chamber projections is carried out with a marker catheter in the right upper pulmonary vein. The four-chamber view will profile the atrial septal defect, and the size is measured with the marker catheter as an internal grid (Fig 54–8). However, it has been found that the size of the defect measured by shunt flow either by angiography or by echocardiography is somewhat smaller than the stretched size of the defect. Therefore a sizing balloon is used. These balloons range in inflated size from 15 to 24 mm. The deflated balloon is advanced into the left atrium, inflated to a predetermined size, and gently pulled across the atrial septum until it occludes the atrial septal defect. The occlusion is confirmed by transesophageal echocardiography and angiography with the marker catheter in the left atrium. The inflated size of the balloon is then confirmed with a caliper.

The clamshell umbrellas come in 17-, 23-, 28-, and 40-mm-diameter sizes, and all of them can be delivered through an 11 F sheath. An 8 F end-hole catheter is passed from the inferior vena cava across the atrial septal defect into the left atrium or left upper pulmonary vein. A 0.038-in. Teflon exchange wire is then advanced through this catheter into the left atrium and the catheter withdrawn. An 11 F sheath and dilator are passed over the exchange guidewire into the left atrium, and the dilator is withdrawn from the sheath. Prior to insertion, the sheath is molded with a gentle curve of about 45 degrees at its distal end so that it will lie perpendicular to the plane of the atrial septum. The clamshell occluder device is loaded in a similar manner to the ductus occlusion umbrella into a special delivery catheter and pod. This pod is then inserted into the sheath and advanced to the inferior vena cava–right atrial junction. The delivery rod is unlocked and advanced until the distal legs of the umbrella protrude from the sheath in the left atrium. The sheath and umbrella are withdrawn as a unit until resistance is felt against the atrial septum. The position of the distal legs on the left side of the atrial septum is confirmed by transesophageal echocardiography and also by angiography of the right atrium in the

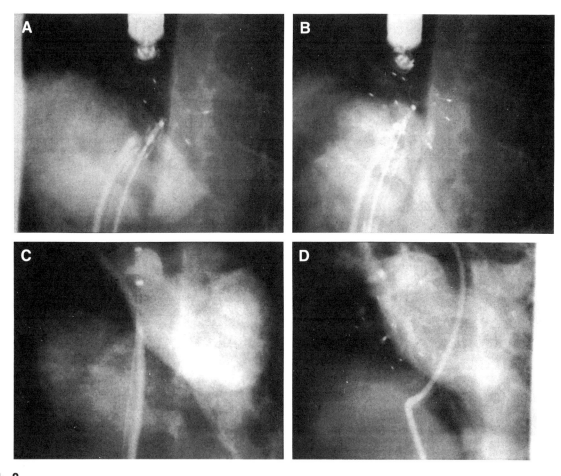

FIG 54–8.
Atrial septal defect occlusion. **A,** the clam shell device has been advanced into the left atrium and the distal legs have been released. A right atrial angiogram is performed and shows the distal legs on the left side of the septum while the proximal legs are still folded inside the long delivery sheath. At the top of the picture can be seen a transesophageal echocardiogram probe. **B,** the sheath has been further withdrawn, the proximal legs unfold on the right side of the septum, while the distal legs bend so that the tips grip the septum. A right atrial angiogram is performed to confirm the position of the proximal legs on the right side of the septum. **C,** left atrial angiogram showing a small (8-mm) atrial septal defect with left-to-right shunting. **D,** left atrial opacification on a right pulmonary angiogram, with the position of the clamshell device occluding the atrial septal defect.

four-chamber projection. Gentle traction is applied to the sheath and delivery wire so that the distal end of the umbrella flexes slightly against the atrial septum. The sheath is then withdrawn further so that the proximal umbrella legs open on the right atrial side of the atrial septum. Both the distal and proximal legs can usually be visualized by high-resolution image intensifiers. The sheath is then advanced against the proximal portion of the umbrella as a buttress during the release procedure. While applying gentle traction to the delivery rod and forward pressure with the sheath, the umbrella is released and the delivery wire withdrawn into the sheath. A final angiogram is performed with the catheter in the right atrium or a catheter in the right pulmonary artery. After recirculation, any residual leaks may be seen from the four-chamber projection. Transesophageal color echocardiography is also very useful in detecting even tiny residual leaks across the atrial septum after the umbrella has been implanted.

Results

At the present time, the clamshell atrial septal defect occluder device is under investigational protocol at several centers.[57] We have used this device in 52 patients whose ages ranged from 2 to 80 years. Implantation was successful in 49 patients. Residual shunting around the occluder may be detected by echocardiography for several days postimplantation but has usually disappeared by 1 week. In 3 of our patients the device was dislodged through a larger-than-anticipated defect. Since we have been using both transesophageal echo and balloon sizing of the atrial septal defect, no device embolizations have occurred. There have been three late deaths in older patients, 80, 76, and 65 years of age, 2 of whom had cancer and right-to-left shunting through a patent foramen ovale. One 56-year-old patient who also had cancer suffered a stroke after the catheterization.

VENTRICULAR SEPTAL DEFECT CLOSURE

Initial attempts to close ventricular septal defects in experimental animals were described by Rashkind and Cuaso in 1977[55] with his ductus occlusion device. Lock et al.[58] and O'Laughlin and Mullins[59] reported the use of the Rashkind umbrella to close ventricular septal defects in patients with postmyocardial infarction and congenital ventricular septal defects. Muscular defects in the trabecular septum are the preferred site for occlusion device insertion; the proximity of semilunar and atrioventricular valve tissue to defects in the perimembranous or inlet septum makes device insertion difficult and may interfere with valve function.

Technique

The occlusion device is delivered via a long sheath passed through the defect from the venous side. The delivery route of the occlusion device depends upon the location of the defect: midtrabecular and apical muscular defects are approached from the right jugular vein, while outflow anterior and posterior perimembranous defects can be accessed from the femoral approach. The ventricular septal defect is crossed more easily from the left ventricle with the blood flow because there are fewer trabeculations on the septum. Either from a transseptal or retrograde femoral approach, an end-hole balloon catheter is directed through the ventricular septal defect into the right ventricle. A long (400 cm) Teflon-coated exchange wire is advanced through the catheter into the right ventricle and then to the right atrium; this wire is snared and withdrawn through the jugular or femoral sheath. An 11 F sheath and dilator are advanced over the exchange wire from the venous side, and the tip of the sheath is passed into the left ventricle. After angiography to confirm the position of the sheath and the ventricular septal defect, the exchange wire is carefully withdrawn and any kinking of the sheath avoided. Transesophageal echocardiography is very helpful in confirming the position of the sheath and later the legs of the occlusion device.

The 17-mm ductus occlusion umbrella and its loading catheter are advanced through the long sheath until the distal legs open in the left ventricle (Fig 54–9); the sheath and device are withdrawn as a unit until the distal legs impinge upon the left ventricular endocardium. Echocardiography and further angiography through the sheath are repeated to confirm the position of the distal legs of the umbrella. If the position is satisfactory, the device is drawn into the defect so that the distal legs are flexed; the sheath is further withdrawn into the right ventricle until the proximal legs of the device open either on the right ventricular side of the defect or in the defect "tunnel." Further angiography can be performed through the sheath to confirm device placement in the ventricular septal defect; if the position is satisfactory, the device is released.

Results

Occlusion of congenital or postoperative ventricular septal defects has proved to be a feasible undertaking in selected cases.[58–60] While only 17 cases of closure of congenital defects have been reported this early, experience is encouraging; about 50% have had complete occlusion of the defect, while the rest have had a considerable reduction in the Qp:Qs ratio immediately after device placement. Long-term evaluation is needed to see whether late complete occlusion occurs.

CONCLUSION

Balloon valvuloplasty has proved to be a very effective and safe technique in patients who have congenital stenotic lesions of the pulmonary, aortic, mitral, and tricuspid valves. Balloon valvuloplasty is now the treatment of choice for isolated congenital pulmonary valve stenosis. The technique has a place as initial palliation for those children with congestive heart failure caused by severe pulmonary stenosis who have a small annulus. Likewise, balloon dilatation of stenotic valves in the tetralogy of Fallot or other complex lesions may serve as an alternative temporary palliation. In these more complex lesions, the results are limited by the size of the pulmonary annulus and associated lesions, such as infundibular, supravalvular, and branch pulmonary artery stenosis.

Palliation of congenital aortic valve stenosis is also amenable to balloon dilatation, with results comparable to those obtained by surgical valvotomy. Balloon dilatation of the aortic valve can also be performed with little increase in the degree of aortic regurgitation in those patients who have residual gradients after surgical valvotomy. Dilatation of membranous subaortic stenosis is possible if the subaortic membrane is thin and close to the aortic valve.

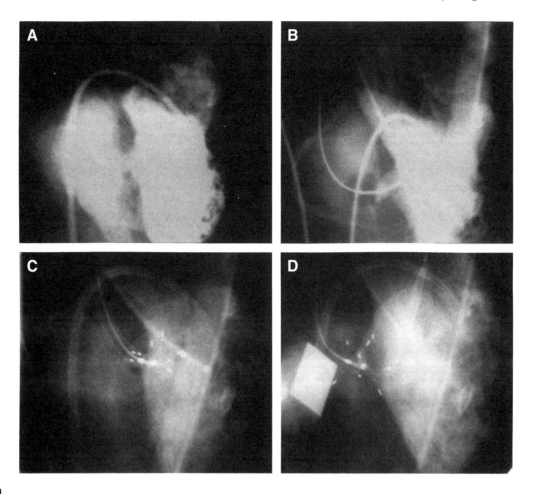

FIG 54-9.
Ventricular septal defect occlusion. **A,** a left ventricular angiogram in a long-axis projection shows a midmuscular ventricular septal defect. **B,** left ventricular angiogram showing a balloon inflated on the right side of the atrial septum and partially occluding the muscular ventricular septal defect. The balloon has been passed through a transseptal sheath over a wire that has been passed into the right ventricle and to the superior vena cava, where it has been retrieved with a snare. **C,** a ductus occlusion umbrella has been passed through a transseptal sheath, and the distal legs have been opened on the left ventricular side of the septum while the proximal legs remain in the long sheath. **D,** left ventricular angiogram showing the distal legs on the left ventricular side of the conical-shaped ventricular septal defect while the proximal legs have been opened on the right side of the septum with almost complete occlusion of the left-to-right shunt.

Congenital commissural fusion of the mitral valve is rare but has been relieved by balloon dilatation with two balloons. Rheumatic mitral stenosis in children should be readily relieved as it has been in older patients and would be the preferred method of palliation in small patients.

Bioprosthetic valves in children are notorious for undergoing degeneration and calcification resulting in stenosis and insufficiency. When these valves are used in conduits from the right ventricle to the pulmonary artery or from the right atrium to the right ventricle in a modified Fontan operation, early degeneration and obstruction of the valve may necessitate surgical removal

of an otherwise adequate conduit. Balloon dilatation of conduits obstructed by "intimal peel" may enable one to postpone surgery until a time when a larger conduit can be placed.

Balloon angioplasty of postoperative coarctation restenosis is now considered the preferred treatment when there is a significant gradient; while some controversy still exists about the use of balloon dilation to treat native coarctation, the accumulated experience from several large series indicates that this is an effective and safe procedure with a low incidence of aneurysm formation and restenosis.

After 5 years of trials and exploration, balloon dilatation techniques have been developed and modified to suit a variety of congenital and acquired stenotic lesions of cardiac valves, arteries, and veins. Some lesions, such as isolated pulmonary valve stenosis, will be exclusively treated by balloon dilatation, while others, such as pulmonary stenosis with a small annulus, may be initially palliated by balloon dilatation in order to improve ventricular function and cardiac output in preparation for surgical repair with cardiopulmonary bypass. Continued longitudinal follow-up and restudy of patients treated by balloon dilatation will allow guidelines to be formulated for optimal utilization of these techniques.

REFERENCES

1. Dotter CT, Judkins MP: Transluminal treatment of arteriosclerotic obstruction. *Circulation* 1964; 30:654–670.
2. Rashkind WJ, Miller WW: Creation of an atrial septal defect without thoracotomy: A palliative approach to complete transposition of the great arteries. *JAMA* 1966; 196:991–992.
3. Grüntzig AR, Senning A, Siegenthaler WE: Nonoperative dilation of coronary artery stenosis: Percutaneous transluminal coronary angioplasty. *N Engl J Med* 1979; 301:61–68.
4. Driscoll DJ, Hesslein PS, Mullins CE: Congenital stenosis of individual pulmonary veins: Clinical spectrum and unsuccessful treatment by transvenous balloon dilation. *Am J Cardiol* 1982; 49:1767–1772.
5. Semb BKH, Tjonneland S, Stake G, et al: "Balloon valvotomy" of congenital pulmonary valve stenosis with tricuspid valve insufficiency. *Cardiovasc Radiol* 1979; 2:239–241.
6. Kan JS, White RI, Mitchell SE, et al: Percutaneous balloon valvuloplasty: A new method for treating congenital pulmonary valve stenosis. *N Engl J Med* 1982; 307:540–542.
7. Lababidi Z, Wu RJ, Walls TJ: Percutaneous balloon aortic valvuloplasty: Results in 23 patients. *Am J Cardiol* 1984; 53:194.
8. Kveselis DA, Rocchini AP, Beekman R, et al: Balloon angioplasty for congenital and rheumatic mitral stenosis. *Am J Cardiol* 1986; 57:348–350.
9. Mullins CE, Nihill MR, Vick GW, et al: Double balloon technique for dilation of valvular or vessel stenosis in congenital and acquired heart disease. *J Am Coll Cardiol* 1987; 10:107–114.
10. Sperling DR, Dorsey TJ, Rowen M, et al: Percutaneous transluminal angioplasty of congenital coarctation of the aorta. *Am J Cardiol* 1983; 51:562–564.
11. Morrow WR, Vick GW, Nihill MR, et al: Balloon dilation of unoperated coarctation of the aorta: Short- and intermediate-term results. *J Am Coll Cardiol* 1988; 11:133–138.
12. Lock JE, Castenada-Zuniga WR, Fuhrman BP, et al: Balloon dilation angioplasty of hypoplastic and stenotic pulmonary arteries. *Circulation* 1983; 67:962–967.
13. Rocchini AP, Cho KJ, Byrum C, et al: Transluminal angioplasty of superior vena cava obstruction in a 15-month-old child. *Chest* 1982; 82:506–508.
14. Lababidi Z, Weinhaus L, Stoeckle H, et al: Transluminal balloon dilation for discrete subaortic stenosis. *Am J Cardiol* 1987; 59:426–425.
15. Stanger P, Cassidy SC, Girod DA, et al: Balloon pulmonary valvuloplasty: Results of the valvuloplasty and angioplasty of congenital anomalies registry. *Am J Cardiol* 1990; 65:775–783.
16. Fontes VF, Esteves CA, Sousa JEMR, et al: Regression of infundibular hypertrophy after pulmonary valvuloplasty for pulmonary stenosis. *Am J Cardiol* 1988; 62:977–979.
17. DiSessa TG, Alpert BS, Chase NA, et al: Balloon valvuloplasty in children with dysplastic pulmonary valves. *Am J Cardiol* 1987; 60:405–407.
18. Marantz PM, Huhta JC, Mullins CE, et al: Results of balloon valvuloplasty in typical and dysplastic pulmonary valve stenosis: Doppler echocardiographic follow-up. *J Am Coll Cardiol* 1988; 12:476–479.
19. McCrindle BW, Kan JS: Long-term results after balloon pulmonary valvuloplasty. *Circulation* 1991; 83:1915–1922.
20. Lababidi Z: Aortic balloon valvuloplasty. *Am Heart J* 1983; 106:751–752.
21. Fischer DR, Ettedgui JA, Park SC, et al: Carotid artery approach for balloon dilation of aortic valve stenosis in the neonate: A preliminary report. *J Am Coll Cardiol* 1990; 15:1633–1636.
22. Cribier A, Saoudi N, Berland J, et al: Percutaneous transluminal valvuloplasty of acquired aortic stenosis in elderly patients: An alternative to aortic valve replacement? *Lancet* 1986; 1:63–67.
23. Rao PS: Balloon aortic valvuloplasty in children. *Clin Cardiol* 1990; 13:458–466.
24. Roccini AP, Beekman RH, Ben Shacher G, et al: Balloon aortic valvuloplasty: Results of the valvuloplasty and angioplasty of congenital anomalies registry. *Am J Cardiol* 1990; 65:784–789.
25. Beekman RH, Rocchini AP, Crowley DC, et al: Comparison of single and double balloon valvuloplasty in children with aortic stenosis. *J Am Coll Cardiol* 1988; 12:480–485.
26. Ludomirsky A, O'Laughlin MP, Nihill MR, et al: Left ventricular mid-cavity obstruction after balloon dilation in isolated aortic valve stenosis in children. *Cathet Cardiovasc Diagn* 1991; 22:89–92.
27. Lababidi ZA, Walls JE: Balloon dilation of thin fixed subaortic stenosis. *Circulation* 1990; 82(suppl 3):583.
28. Suarez de Lezo J, Medina A, Pan M, et al: Long-term results after balloon dilation for discrete subaortic stenosis. *Circulation* 1990; 82(suppl 3):583.
29. Grifka RG, O'Laughlin MP, Nihill MR, et al: Double transseptal, double balloon valvuloplasty for congenital mitral stenosis. *Circulation* 1991; 85:123–129.
30. Alday L, Juaneda E: Percutaneous balloon dilation in congenital mitral stenosis. *Br Heart J* 1987; 57:479–482.
31. Spevak PJ, Bass JL, Ben-Shachar G, et al: Balloon angioplasty for congenital mitral stenosis. *Am J Cardiol* 1990; 66:472–476.
32. Al Yousef S, Khan A, Nihill M, et al: Perkutane transvenose antegrade Balloonangioplastie bei Aortenisthmusstenose. *Herz* 1988; 13:36–40.
33. Krabrill KA, Bass JL, Lucas RV, et al: Dissecting transverse aortic arch aneurysm after percutaneous translumi-

nal balloon dilation angioplasty of an aortic coarctation. *Pediatr Cardiol* 1987; 8:39–42.

34. Tynan M, Finley JP, Fontes V, et al: Balloon angioplasty for the treatment of native coarctation: Results of valvuloplasty and angioplasty of congenital anomalies registry. *Am J Cardiol* 1990; 65:790–792.

35. Lababidi ZA, Daskaloppulos DA, Stoeckle H: Transluminal balloon coarctation angioplasty: Experience with 27 patients. *Am J Cardiol* 1984; 54:1288–1291.

36. Rao PS, Thapar MK, Kutayli F, et al: Causes of recoarctation after balloon angioplasty of unoperated aortic coarctation. *J Am Coll Cardiol* 1989; 13:109–115.

37. Rao PS: Balloon angioplasty of aortic coarctation: A review. *Clin Cardiol* 1989; 12:618–628.

38. Rothman A: Arterial complications of interventional cardiac catheterization in patients with congenital heart disease. *Circulation* 1990; 82:1868–1871.

39. Burrows PE, Benson LN, Williams WG, et al: Iliofemoral arterial complications of balloon angioplasty for systemic obstructions in infants and children. *Circulation* 1990; 82:1697–1704.

40. Marvin WJ, Mahoney LT, Rose EF: Pathological sequelae of balloon dilation angioplasty for unoperated coarctation of the aorta in children (abstract). *J Am Coll Cardiol* 1986; 7:117.

41. Evans VL, Nihill MR, Al Yousef S: Balloon dilation angioplasty for native coarctation of the aorta in infants. (abstract) *J Am Coll Cardiol* 1986; 7:46.

42. Erbel R, Bednarczyk I, Pop T, et al: Detection of dissection of the aortic intima and media after angioplasty of coarctation of the aorta. An angiographic, computer tomographic, and echographic comparative study. *Circulation* 1990; 81:805–814.

43. Hellenbrand WE, Allen HD, Golinko RJ, et al: Balloon angioplasty for aortic recoarctation: Results of valvuloplasty and angioplasty of congenital anomalies registry. *Am J Cardiol* 1990; 65:793–797.

44. Lock JE, Castenada-Zuniga WR, Fuhrman BP, et al: Balloon dilation angioplasty of hypoplastic and stenotic pulmonary arteries. *Circulation* 1983; 67:962–967.

45. Rocchini AP, Kveselis D, Dick M, et al: Use of balloon angioplasty to treat peripheral pulmonary stenosis. *Am J Cardiol* 1984; 54:1069–1073.

46. Kan JS, Marvin WJ, Bass JL, et al: Balloon angioplasty-branch pulmonary artery stenosis: Results from the val-

vuloplasty and angioplasty of congenital anomalies registry. *Am J Cardiol* 1990; 65:798–801.

47. Rothman A, Perry SB, Keane JF, et al: Early results and follow-up of balloon angioplasty for branch pulmonary artery stenosis. *J Am Coll Cardiol* 1990; 15:1109–1117.

48. O'Laughlin MP, Perry SB, Lock JE, et al: Use of endovascular stents in congenital heart disease. *Circulation* 1991; 83:1923–1939.

49. Mullins CE, Latson LA, Neches WH, et al: Balloon dilation of miscellaneous lesions: Results of valvuloplasty and angioplasty of congenital anomalies registry. *Am J Cardiol* 1990; 65:802–803.

50. Porstmann W, Weirny L, Warnke H: Closure of persistent ductus arteriosus without thoracotomy. *Thoraxchirurgie* 1967; 15:199–201.

51. Rashkind WJ, Cuaso CC: Transcatheter closure of patent ductus arteriosus. Successful use in a 3.5 kilogram infant. *Pediatr Cardiol* 1979; 1:3–7.

52. Bash SE, Mullins CE: Insertion of patent ductus occluder by transvenous approach: A new technique. *Circulation* 1984; 70:285.

53. Rashkind WJ, Mullins CE, Hellenbrand WE, et al: Nonsurgical closure of patent ductus arteriosus: Clinical application of the Rashkind PDA occluder system. *Circulation* 1987; 75:583–592.

54. King TD, Mills NL: Nonoperative closure of atrial septal defects. *Surgery* 1974; 75:383–388.

55. Rashkind WJ, Cuaso CC: Transcatheter closure of atrial septal and ventricular septal defects in experimental animal. *Proc Assoc Eur Pediatr Cardiol* 1977; 14:8.

56. Lock JE, Rome JJ, Davis R, et al: Transcatheter closure of atrial septal defects: Experimental studies. *Circulation* 1989; 79:1091–1099.

57. Lock JE, Hellenbrand W, Latson L, et al: Clamshell umbrella closure of atrial septal defects: Initial results. *Circulation* 1989; 80(suppl 2):592.

58. Lock JE, Block PC, McKay RG, et al: Transcatheter closure of ventricular septal defects. *Circulation* 1988; 78:361–368.

59. O'Laughlin MP, Mullins CE: Transcatheter closure of ventricular septal defect. *Cathet Cardiovasc Diagn* 1989; 17:175–179.

60. Roth SJ, Bridges ND, Keane JF, et al: Transcatheter closure of ventricular septal defects (VSDs): Echocardiographic assessment. *Circulation* 1990; 82(suppl 3):582.

PART X

Pacing and Ablation

55

Optimal Pacing Therapy: Hemodynamics, Modes, and Devices

William H. Spencer III, M.D.

For several reasons, this would appear to be an appropriate time to describe optimal pacing therapy. Reliable dual chamber (DDD) pacemakers have been implanted for over a decade and have provided a source of long-term follow-up studies. Rate-responsive pacemakers have been available for research for almost a decade, and a large number of hemodynamic studies have been spawned. Finally, now that dual-chamber, sensor-driven, rate-responsive pacemakers have recently been approved for general clinical use, virtually all pacing modes are available.

Obviously, the primary goal of cardiac pacing should be the prevention of syncope or death from bradycardia. This goal was accomplished with the earliest and simplest of pacemaker systems. As more elaborate and capable pacemakers have evolved, the goal of maintaining or restoring more normal hemodynamic responses of a wide range of physiologic demands has emerged.

Optimal pacing therapy will be reviewed from several perspectives — hemodynamics of pacing, pacing modes, the latest devices, and finally, the latest implantation techniques.

HEMODYNAMICS OF PACING

There is an ever-enlarging body of literature regarding the hemodynamics of pacing. Because many of the studies involved small sample sizes and varying populations of patients (and their associated diseases) and failed to control all variables, often confusing results have been published. Despite all these obvious drawbacks, however, a consensus has emerged.

One must consider the hemodynamics of pacing from several different perspectives. For example, in patients with normal left ventricular function, the hemodynamic requirements at rest or with minimal exertion are quite different from those with more vigorous exertion. Also, patients with varying forms and severity of left ventricular dysfunction present special needs.

For optimal hemodynamic performance at rest in patients with normal left ventricular function, the provision of atrioventricular (AV) synchrony is of paramount importance, especially to prevent the pacemaker syndrome.[1-3] The provision of an appropriately timed atrial systole provides up to a 20% increase in cardiac output when compared with single-chamber pacing.[4, 5] Atrial systole provides an "atrial kick" that transiently elevates the left ventricular end-diastolic pressure above the mean left atrial pressure (Fig 55-1). Then in accordance with a familiar Starling principle of the heart, more left ventricular end-diastolic fiber length results in more left ventricular stroke work and more stroke volume[6] (Fig 55-2). Because changes in venous return are minimal at rest or with light activity, optimal cardiac performance is dependent upon atrial systole to preserve or restore appropriate hemodynamics.

With more vigorous exertion, the provision of an adequate rate response with or without AV synchrony is most important in increasing the cardiac output.[7, 8] The increase in cardiac output with exertion follows the following formula: cardiac output = rate × stroke volume.

HEMODYNAMICS OF LEFT VENTRICULAR PRESSURE

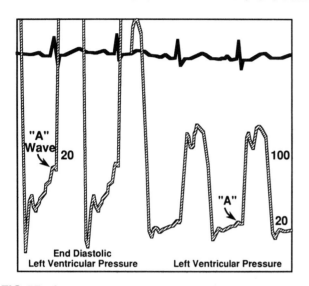

FIG 55–1.
Left ventricular pressure tracing showing the A wave or "atrial kick" at the end of diastole.

Whereas stroke volume may rise by as much as 50% with exercise, normal individuals may increase their heart rate by as much as 300% to 400% of the resting rate.[9] Because of the overwhelming magnitude of the increase in heart rate with exertion, rate responsiveness accounts for most of the increment in cardiac output at this time. Unfortunately, many patients who require pacemakers have chronotropic incompetence, the inability to increase the heart rate appropriately on demand, which deprives them of an important adapta-

tion.[10] When ventricular rate-responsive pacing (VVIR) is compared with fixed-rate ventricular pacing (VVI) in exercise testing, a greater than 30% increase in maximum heart rate, maximum work capacity, and maximum exercise time are seen.[11] In summary (Fig 55–3), at rest or with low-level exertion, the provision of AV synchrony is most important, but in order to increase the cardiac output with exercise, rate responsiveness is foremost.

Two special problems compromise the hemodynamics of pacing systems even in patients with normal left ventricular function and give emphasis and relevance to the preceding remarks — the pacemaker syndrome and chronotropic incompetence. The pacemaker syndrome is characterized by syncope, near-syncope, dizziness, or weakness in its most severe and, happily, rare forms and by palpitations, light-headedness, or precordial awareness in its milder and more common presentations.[2, 3] Although it has been reported with almost all forms of cardiac pacing under rare and sometimes bizzare circumstances,[12, 13] the pacemaker syndrome is almost always associated with single-chamber ventricular pacing.[2] The underlying pathophysiology is usually ventriculoatrial conduction or, more uncommonly, a simple loss of appropriate AV synchrony in susceptible individuals that results in abnormally high atrial pressures due to atrial contraction against closed AV valves, activation of atrial stretch receptors, and a vagally mediated peripheral vasodilatation.[14, 15] The accepted treatment of the symptomatic pacemaker syndrome is "upgrading" to dual-chamber pacing to provide appropriate AV synchrony with its attendant hemodynamic benefits and abolishment of ventriculoatrial conduction.[16]

Chronotropic incompetence, an inadequate or inap-

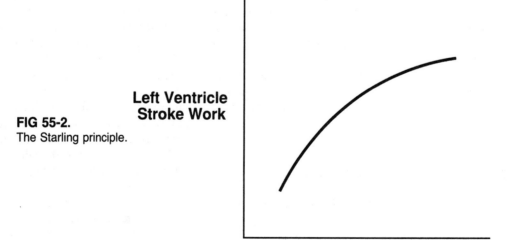

FIG 55-2.
The Starling principle.

AV SYNCHRONY AND RATE RESPONSIVENESS

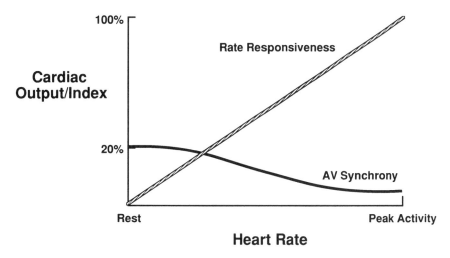

FIG 55–3.
The relative importance of atrioventricular *(AV)* synchrony and rate responsiveness from rest to peak exercise.

propriate heart rate response to exercise, limits the hemodynamic effectiveness of pacemaker systems, especially DDD pacing modes, by depriving these systems of rate responsiveness.[17]

While several diagnostic criteria have been proposed for chronotropic incompetence,[18, 19] the most practical and useful test appears to be a failure to achieve 75% of one's maximum predicted heart rate (MPHR by the As-

trand formula = 220 − age [years]) at peak exercise. Chronotropic incompetence is associated with AV block, sinus node disease, atrial fibrillation, heart transplantation, and antiarrhythmic drug therapy. Chronotropic incompetence may also be idiopathic, in which case there appears to be a considerable incidence of "silent myocardial ischemia".[20] Atrial chronotropic incompetence occurs in up to a third of patients with either

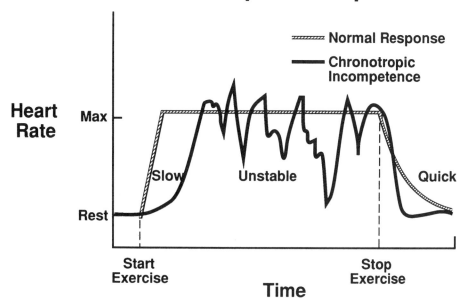

FIG 55–4.
The various forms of chronotropic incompetence (see the text).

sinus node disease, AV block, or both.[21, 22] Failure to appropriately increase the ventricular rate with exercise has been said to occur in up to 60% of pacemaker candidates with atrial fibrillation.[23] Chronotropic incompetence may take several forms (Fig 55–4): failure to achieve an adequate heart rate throughout exercise, a delayed rise in the heart rate with exercise, extreme fluctuations of the heart rate with bradycardia during exercise, or too rapid deceleration of the heart rate following exercise. Patients in the pacemaker population may also show a day-to-day variability in chronotropic incompetence; it may be present some days and absent others.[24] Because many pacing systems rely on a natural increase in the atrial or ventricular rate with exercise to provide rate responsiveness, chronotropic incompetence may seriously limit the hemodynamic capabilities of such systems.[17, 25]

In summary (Table 55–1), in patients with normal left ventricular function, VVI pacing provides the lowest cardiac output at rest, VVIR pacing adds nothing at rest, while DDD and DDDR pacing increase the resting cardiac output approximately 20% by providing AV synchrony. During exercise with VVI pacing, the cardiac output increases approximately 50% by utilizing an energy-expensive increase in stroke volume. By providing a pacing rate increase with exercise, VVIR pacing raises the cardiac output by 30% as compared with VVI pacing. Because of chronotropic incompetence, DDD pacing populations are able to raise their exercise cardiac output by only 25% when compared with the VVI group. By comparison, since DDDR pacing provides both rate responsiveness and AV synchrony, the cardiac

TABLE 55–1.

Comparison of the Average Cardiac Outputs Obtained in Various Pacing Modes With VVI Pacing at Rest and With Exercise as Zero

	VVI	VVIR	DDD	DDDR
Rest	0	0	+20%	+20%
Exercise	0	+30%	+25%	+35%

output with exercise rises an average of 35% more than in the VVI group.

Nowhere is the provision of optimal pacing therapy more important than in that segment of the pacing population with left ventricular dysfunction, which may be systolic, diastolic, or both. Rate-responsive pacing is especially important because most patients with left ventricular dysfunction cannot appreciably increase the stroke volume with exertion because rate-adaptive pacing can prevent compensatory ventricular dilatation[26] and because many patients with compromised ventricles have chronotropic incompetence. Colucci et al.[27] showed that patients with congestive heart failure have much lower heart rates at peak exercise when compared with normal controls (Fig 55–5) and attributed these lower peak heart rates to postsynaptic β-adrenergic desensitization. Provision of proper AV synchrony helps most patients with left ventricular dysfunction maintain or increase stroke volume at rest and with exertion in the face of increasing preload and heart rate. Since stroke volume is usually increased by increasing end-diastolic volume and maintaining or slightly increasing the ejection fraction, special attention must be given to

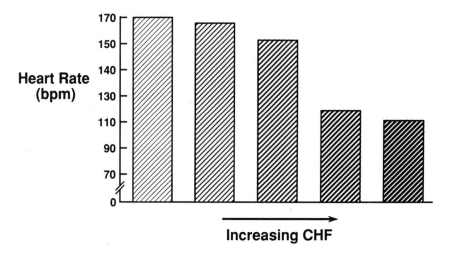

FIG 55–5.
Maximum heart rates attained at peak exercise vs. increasing severity of congestive heart failure *(CHF)*. (From Colucci WS, Riberio JP, Rocco MB, et al: *Circulation* 1989; 80:314–323. Used by permission.)

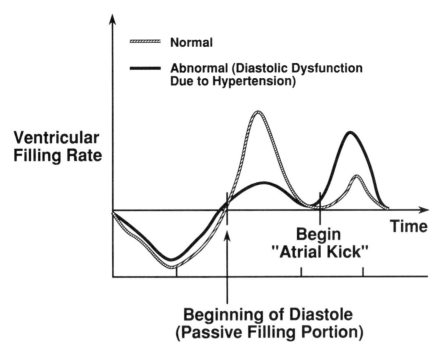

FIG 55–6.
Diastolic filling patterns in normal individuals *(hatched line)* and in patients with diastolic dysfunction *(solid line)*. (Courtesy of Medtronic, Inc.)

diastolic filling patterns, especially in patients with poor diastolic compliance. Patients with hypertension, valvular disease, coronary disease, and restrictive cardiomyopathy, even those elderly hearts whose left ventricular wall thickness (and presumably diminished diastolic compliance) increases with age,[28] have markedly altered diastolic filling patterns (Fig 55–6), with more filling occurring late in diastole and dependent on an atrial kick and less filling in the early passive phase of diastolic filling. An appropriately timed atrial systole allows more

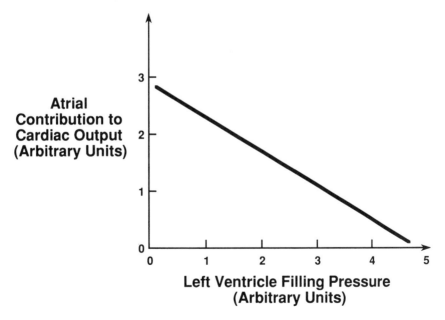

FIG 55–7.
The atrial contribution to the cardiac output is inversely related to the mean left ventricular filling pressure. (From Greenberg B, Chatterjee K, Parmley WP: *Am Heart J* 1979; 98:742–751. Used by permission.)

end-diastolic fiber stretch and helps avoid symptom-producing high filling pressures. However, the higher the mean left ventricular filling pressure, the lower the atrial contribution to cardiac output[29] (Fig 55–7). This observation is true probably because the left ventricle is maximally dilated by high passive filling pressures prior to atrial systole and the "atrial kick" is able to make very little additional contribution to increasing the end-diastolic fiber length. Nevertheless, it would appear that in pacemaker recipients with mild to moderate left ventricular dysfunction, the presence of appropriate AV synchrony plays an important role in maintaining or restoring stroke volume reserves.

Considerable attention of late has been given to optimizing the AV interval to maximize the cardiac output. From a practical standpoint, the optimal AV delay ranges around 150 ± 25ms. Because the AV delay begins with atrial capture during a paced beat and begins much later (approximately 30 to 40 ms) with a sensed P wave (the native impulse must travel from the sinoatrial node to the lead in the right atrial appendage and be sensed by the pacemaker amplifier), the effective AV delay (Fig 55–8) is considerably longer with sensed P waves. By electronically making both sensed and paced AV intervals equal to approximately 150 ms, a slight increase in cardiac output of patients with pacemakers is achieved that may be important in those patients with impaired ventricular function.[30] Also, electronically

shortening the AV delay with increasing heart rates during exertion in an attempt to mimic the normal PR interval shortening with exercise has led to a minimal improvement in cardiac output.[31] Finally it should be recalled that when AV intervals are short and necessitate ventricular pacing, the ventricular activation sequence is ectopic in origin. The left ventricular asynchrony that is produced by a paced beat originating in the apex of the right ventricle results in some minimal deterioration in the diastolic and probably systolic performance of the left ventricle.[32] If possible, normal AV conduction with a normal ventricular activation sequence should be encouraged.

Finally, as will be discussed further in the next section, the selection of dual-chamber pacing where possible in patients with left ventricular dysfunction results in a considerably lower incidence of atrial fibrillation. Atrial fibrillation deprives the heart of AV synchrony and produces inappropriate tachycardias and variable diastolic filling intervals, all of which detract from ventricular performance.

MODES OF PACING

As noted in the foregoing section, certain modes of cardiac pacing have hemodynamic advantages over others. Whether improved hemodynamics result in im-

PACED P WAVE - FIXED AV DELAY

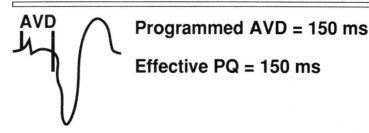

AVD   Programmed AVD = 150 ms

Effective PQ = 150 ms

SENSED P WAVE - FIXED AV DELAY

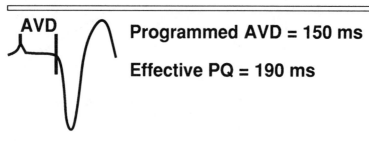

AVD   Programmed AVD = 150 ms

Effective PQ = 190 ms

FIG 55–8.
Paced and sensed AV delays showing that the sensed delay is longer. *AVD* = atrioventriculor defect.

proved clinical outcomes of patients with pacemakers is no longer a matter of debate. For years we have been taught that the prognosis and survival of patients with sick sinus syndrome treated with ventricular pacemakers is not generally different from the natural history of the disease itself.[33] However, several reports of late have pointed to a distinct advantage conferred by dual-chamber or atrial pacing vs. ventricular pacing in sinus node disease.[34–36] Also, similar results have been reported by Alpert et al. (Fig 55–9) in patients with chronic high-degree AV block with and without congestive heart failure; dual-chamber pacing conferred a statistically significant improvement in 5-year mortality when compared with ventricular pacing.[37] The preceding reports and many others in the recent pacing literature deal with retrospective, nonrandomized, noncontrolled studies, many of which were not conducted in a most scientific manner. Nevertheless, the overall results are striking and compelling. Table 55–2 shows a comparison of ventricular pacing (VVI) and dual-chamber or atrial pacing with percentages that are approximations of those found in the large body of literature. The comparisons are those of long-term (3 to 4 years) follow-up of patients paced for sinus node disorders. Similar but probably not as striking results might be expected with long-term follow-up studies involving the two pacing modes (VVI vs. DDD) in patients with advanced AV block. As can be seen, there are dramatic differences in the incidence of atrial fibrillation (40% vs. 6%) over the 3- to 4-year intervals. Also, there was a decidedly differ-

TABLE 55–2.
Relative Incidence of Atrial Fibrillation, Thromboembolism, New Congestive Heart Failure, and Mortality Over a 3- to 4-Year Period in DDD (AAI) and VVI Pacing Modes

Disorder	VVI	DDD(AAI)
Atrial fibrillation	40%	6%
Thromboembolism (CVA*)	23%	6%
Congestive heart failure	37%	15%
Mortality rate (4 yr)	19%	6%

*CVA = cardiovascular accident.

ent occurrence of thromboembolism, usually manifested as a cerebrovascular accident (23% VVI vs. 6% DDD [AAI]), over the follow-up period that is possibly related to the presence of atrial fibrillation. Ventriculoatrial (retrograde) conduction has also been implicated as a poor prognostic factor and a marker for potential atrial fibrillation and thromboembolism in patients with VVI pacing.[38] The development of new congestive heart failure is also more frequent (37% vs. 15%) in the ventricularly paced groups. Finally, the mortality of patients with physiologic pacing is lower than that of patients with ventricular inhibited pacemakers over a 3- to 5-year follow-up.[37, 39] With the above, then, it is evident that DDD (or AAI where possible) mode pacing considerably improves the clinical outcome and prognosis of pacemaker recipients, especially those with sinus node disorders.

When the VVI single-chamber, fixed-rate pacing

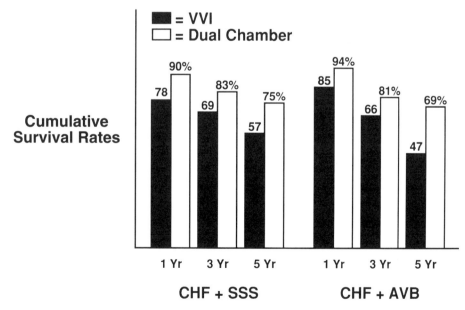

FIG 55–9.
Survival rates in patients with DDD and VVI pacemakers, sick sinus syndrome *(SSS)* or AV block *(AVB),* and congestive heart failure *(CHF).* (From Alpert MA, Curtis JJ, San Felippo JF, et al: *J Am Coll Cardiol* 1986; 7:925–932. Used by permission.)

mode is compared with the VVIR single-chamber, rate-responsive pacing mode, not only does one find a clear improvement in exercise capacity of approximately 30%,[11, 40] but also follow-up studies have shown a reduction in heart size and pressures with VVIR pacing.[26] It would appear, then, that when a ventricular pacemaker is indicated, VVIR pacing should be the choice in most instances.

We compared dual-chamber, sensor-driven, rate-responsive pacing (DDDR) with dual-chamber pacing (DDDD) by utilizing two consecutive 24-hour Holter monitors in a single-blind fashion.[41] When the maximum heart rates achieved in each 15-minute interval during the two 24-hour periods were compared, considerable rate augmentation was demonstrated for DDDR pacing vs. DDD pacing (Fig 55–10). Seven of the ten subjects tested preferred the sensor-driven, rate-responsive pacing mode, DDDR. Also, DDDR pacing did not result in more atrial arrhythmias than DDD pacing despite clear evidence of accelerated-rate atrial pacing and the potential for atrial competitive pacing.

AAI(R) mode pacing is rarely employed in the United States, generally less than 1% of the time.[42] Although it is usually used in patients with sinus node disorders, atrial pacing cannot be employed in all such patients since it is generally accepted that one must demonstrate 1:1 AV conduction at atrial pacing rates up to and greater than 120/min in order to ensure against

AV block. With such care, the yearly incidence of significant AV block in patients with atrial pacemakers is generally less than 1%.[43] As noted previously, the risk of subsequent development of atrial arrhythmias that would prevent atrial pacing is low.[34] Undoubtedly, the placement of an atrial pacing lead requires more care and skill than the placement of a ventricular lead and results in higher pacing thresholds and poorer sensing characteristics. Finally and possibly more importantly in this era of cost constraints, since it is a single-chamber, single-lead system, AAI(R) pacing is less costly than DDD(R) pacing and probably could be used in the majority of pacemaker candidates for sinus node disorders.

Now that data and discussions regarding the hemodynamics of pacing and comparisons between various modes of pacing have been presented, certain conclusions appear to be in order. First, VVI, single-chamber, fixed-rate ventricular pacing is almost obsolete. There are undoubtedly uncommon instances of invalidism or incapacity where only backup pacing is needed, in which case one might employ a VVI pacing system, but such a pacing system should not be used to treat patients with sinus node disorders and probably should not be used in high-grade AV block if the atria are in sinus rhythm. Second, the only clear-cut indication for sensor-driven, single-chamber ventricular pacing (VVIR) is atrial fibrillation (and other conditions where it is impossible to sense and pace the atrium) with some degree of AV

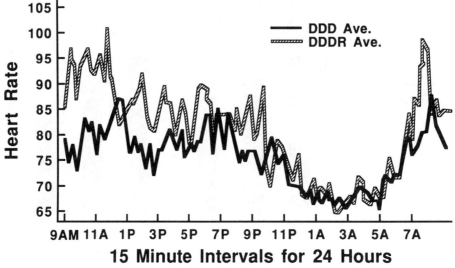

FIG 55–10.
Average maximum heart rates during 15-minute intervals of ten patients in DDDR pacing *(hatched line)* and DDD pacing *(solid line).* (From Spencer WH, Markowitz T, Alagona P: *PACE* 1990; 13:1847–1851. Used by permission.)

block. Like VVI pacing, VVI(R) pacing should not be used in patients with sinus node disorders. Third, where possible, atrial pacemakers, AAI(R), or dual-chamber pacemakers, DDD(R), should be implanted in all other patients requiring a pacemaker. Because of its flexibility and wide range of potential pacing modes, DDD(R) pacing would seem to be the best option unless economic issues prevail due to its higher cost.

DEVICES

A presentation of all the devices available for pacing therapy is beyond the scope of this chapter. Instead, only those sensor-driven devices currently available commercially in the United States along with a few models in the clinical evaluation phase will be discussed. Activity-sensing pacemakers providing rate responsiveness have been implanted for a number of years in the United States and are currently the most popular pacing system. Two single-chamber, later-generation activity-sensing devices (Legend, Medtronic, Inc., and Sensolog II, Pacesetter Systems) that utilize a piezoelectric crystal to detect body vibrations are currently available. Dual-chamber devices utilizing an activity-sensing mode (Elite, Medtronic, Inc., and Synchrony II, Pacesetter Systems) are also available. By sensing body vibrations these devices are capable of increasing the paced rate with exertion. These pacing devices have improved signal-processing algorithms to allow smoother and more complete heart rate increases with exertion. Acceleration and deceleration times (at the cessation of activity all input by the sensor disappears, which makes deceleration an arbitrarily determined procedure) are programmable to several different values. Differential AV intervals between paced and sensed atrial events and decreasing AV intervals with increasing heart rate are also available. Both systems allow analysis of the pacemaker's response to a given activity over a given period of time by the use of trend measurements and histograms, thus making optimal sensor settings easier. The generator size is smaller than previous models, yet the expected pacemaker life is longer. Despite drawbacks such as idiosyncratic responses to various activities such as higher heart rates while walking downstairs vs. walking up, vulnerability to extraneous environmental vibrations, and a lack of response to mental or emotional activities, activity pacing has proved to be very successful because of its stability, simplicity, reliability, and speed of response. Much of the success of these pacing systems is due to the fact that most activities of patients with pacemakers are short and transient and require only a prompt, modest increase in heart rate.

Also available commercially is a single-chamber pacing system that measures changes in transthoracic impedance between a bipolar pacing lead and the pacemaker can (Meta MV, Telectronics Inc., Englewood, Colo.). Changes in transthoracic impedance are an approximation of minute ventilation and provide a physiologic parameter for increasing the paced rate to meet metabolic demands.[44] To date, this pacing system has proved to be reliable and useful, but because it has an additional current drain related to the sensor, its size is slightly larger and its life expectancy shorter than other rate-responsive pacemakers. The dual-chamber version, Meta DDDR, is currently undergoing clinical evaluation and will feature a more rapid response time, a shorter time requirement for sensor programming, shortening of the AV interval and postventricular atrial refractory period with higher heart rates, and mode switching to VVI(R) during atrial arrhythmias.

Two devices currently undergoing clinical evaluation utilize unique sensor systems. By measuring the ventricular depolarization gradient (VDG), the electronic integral of the area under the paced QRS,[45] the Prism pacing system (Telectronics, Inc., Englewood, Colo) can potentially be a closed-loop autoprogramming system. Since the area under the VDG decreases with mental and sympathetic activity and increases with increasing heart rate, such a closed-loop system is possible.[46] The Precept pacemaker (CPI, Minneapolis) measures changes in intracardiac impedance via a special tripolar lead. The pre-ejection interval (PEI), or the interval between the paced stimulus or native QRS and the onset of right ventricular contraction, is measured by impedance changes in the right ventricle. Presumably, changes in the PEI are effected by sympathetic activity in much the same way as the sinoatrial node, which permits the pacing algorithm to increase the pacing rate appropriately.[47] Single- and dual-chamber models of the Precept pacemaker are undergoing clinical investigation.

The first pacemakers that utilized dual sensors to increase the paced rate were DDD(R) pacemakers, which sensed both the P wave and activity. In the near future, there will be more combinations of artificial sensors tested and marketed; already the prototype of an activity and QT interval pacemaker has been implanted in Europe.[48] Dual-sensor pacemakers may be designed to react in many different ways. The two obvious interactions of dual sensors would be either to have one sensor initiate a rate response and then have another sensor continue the rate response during further exercise or to have both sensors validate the other signal and produce a rate response. The first of these interactions would probably be employed initially by combining a rapidly

TABLE 55–3.
Suggested Sensor Combinations for Dual-Sensor Pacemakers

Activity/QT
Activity/MV*
VDG*/MV
Activity/So$_2$*

*MV = mitral valve; VDG = ventricular depolarization gradient; So$_2$ = oxygen saturation.

responding sensor, such as activity sensor, with a slower more "physiologic" sensor such as QT sensing or minute ventilation sensing. As can be seen in Table 55–3, there have been several suggested combinations for dual-sensor devices. Because of its rapid response, activity sensing is usually suggested as one member of the combination of sensors. As time and clinical evaluations pass, the question of whether dual sensors with complex algorithms and interactions will really prove better than a single sensor will be answered.

Finally, rate-responsive pacing systems that employ standard cardiac pacing leads would appear to have a long-term advantage over those systems requiring special-lead systems. Standard-lead devices can be used as replacement generators for an older fixed-rate system that has undergone generator depletion without adding an extra lead. For standard-lead devices, one can change from one rate-responsive pacing system to another without having to introduce a new lead. Special leads for rate-responsive pacemakers add a new level of complexity and larger size to pacemaker leads. Although one might in the future, no special-lead, rate-responsive pacemaker has yet stood the test of time. Because of their reliability and flexibility, it would appear better to utilize standard pacing leads with rate-responsive pacemakers.

In the future, pacemaker devices will continue to become smaller because advancing lead technology will make battery current drains much less. Standard leads and standard connectors will allow the interchange of various pacing systems. The systems themselves will have more autoprogramming or self-optimization to permit adaptations to changing clinical situations without a great deal of slow, time-consuming physician input. Most importantly, as a few sensors are selected and mass produced, pacemaker systems should cost less.

IMPLANTATION TECHNIQUES

In 1979, Littleford and Spector[49] described a technique and a device, a "peel-away" sheath, that allowed insertion of pacing electrodes in the subclavian vein without a venous cutdown. Over the next dozen years, a revolution took place, with pacemaker implantation moving from the operating room and surgeons to the cardiac catheterization laboratory and cardiologists. Presently, it is estimated that between 60% and 70% of pacemaker implantations are performed by cardiologists.[50] Still, with all its popularity, the subclavian percutaneous introducer technique has not been without its critics,[51] who are concerned about its safety. Parsonnet et al.[52] reported a 5.7% incidence of complications in 632 consecutive pacemaker implantations. The percutaneous introducer approach in the hands of infrequent implanters (fewer than 12 implants per year) contributed significantly to the observed complications. Still, it is evident that the percutaneous introducer method of pacemaker implantation can be safe and efficacious when performed by experienced, well-equipped physicians.[53] A very medial approach to the subclavian vein near the junction of the clavicle and first rib (Fig 55–11) is perhaps safer than the previously recommended more lateral approach near the middle third of the clavicle, but concerns about lead compression and disruption by the two bones may arise. Byrd[54] has de-

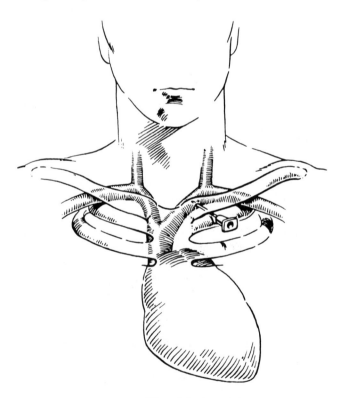

The subclavian window.

FIG 55–11.
The subclavian window provides a very medial approach to subclavian venous puncture. (From Belott PH: In Barold SS, Mugica J (eds): *New Perspectives in Cardiac Pacing* 2. Mt Kisco, NY, Futura, 1991, p 112. Used by permission.)

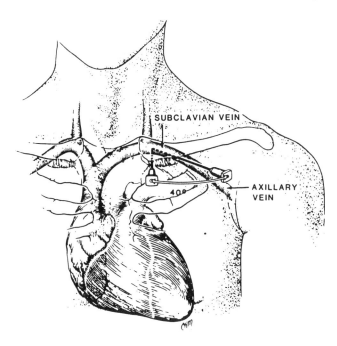

The safe zone.

FIG 55–12.
The "safe zone," the region between the first rib and the clavicle in a 40-degree arc extending laterally from the sternum. (From Belott PH: In Barold SS, Mugica J (eds): *New Perspectives in Cardiac Pacing 2.* Mt Kisco, NY, Futura, 1991, p 112. Used by permission.)

scribed a "safety zone" for cannulating the subclavian vein. The "safety zone" is defined as the region between the first rib and the clavicle in a 40-degree arc extending from the sternum laterally (Fig 55–12). When this technique is used, major complications such as pneumothorax and hemopneumothorax are prevented. Pacemaker implantation, then, can be performed by experienced well-trained cardiologists in the cardiac catheterization laboratory with safety and rapidity, provided that strict aseptic conditions are maintained.

Ambulatory or outpatient pacemaker implantation is steadily gaining popularity and acceptance. Reports have cited a very low, less than 1%, incidence of complications when outpatient pacemaker implantation is carried out in as many as 80% of patients requiring pacemakers.[55, 56] A 3- to 4-hour period of unmonitored observation and no antibiotic chemoprophylaxis have been utilized. The ambulatory approach to pacemaker implantation will probably continue to gain popularity and acceptance as the financial constraints of pacemaker implantation increase.

In conclusion, optimal pacing therapy for the present includes more dual-chamber (or AAI) pacing. Rate modulation should be provided along with AV syn-

chrony. Ambulatory, percutaneous implantation of pacing systems is safe and efficacious in experienced hands. Standard-lead systems should be employed on the most advanced devices. Finally, better patient prognosis and clinical outcomes can be provided by a judicious choice of pacing therapy.

REFERENCES

1. Erlebacher JA, Danner RL, Stelzer PE: Hypotension with ventricular pacing: Atrial vasodepressor reflex in human beings. *J Am Coll Cardiol* 1984; 4:550–555.
2. Ausubel K, Furman S: The pacemaker syndrome. *Ann Intern Med* 1985; 103:420–429.
3. Alicandri C, Fouad FM, Tarzir C, et al: Three cases of hypotension and syncope with ventricular pacing: Possible role of atrial reflexes. *Am J Cardiol* 1978; 42:137–142.
4. Samet P, Bernstein WH, Nathan DA, et al: Atrial contribution of cardiac output in complete heart block. *Am J Cardiol* 1965; 16:1–10.
5. Benchimol A, Duenas A, Liggett MS, et al: Contribution of atrial systole to the cardiac function at a fixed and at a variable ventricular rate. *Am J Cardiol* 1965; 16:11–21.
6. Linden RJ, Mitchell JH: The relation between left ventricular end diastolic pressure and myocardial segment length and observation on the contribution of atrial systole. *Circ Res* 1960; 8:1092–1099.
7. Fananapazir L, Bennett DH, Monks P: Atrial synchronized ventricular pacing; Contribution of the chonotropic response to improve exercise performance. *PACE* 1983; 6:601–608.
8. Karlof I: Hemodynamic effect of atrial triggered versus fixed rate pacing at rest and during exercise in complete heart block. *Acta Med Scand* 1975; 197:195–206.
9. Epstein SE, Beiser GD, Stampfer M, et al: Characterization of the circulatory response to maximal upright exercise in normal subject and patients with heart disease. *Circulation* 1967; 35:1049–1062.
10. Hammond HK, Froelicher VF: Normal and abnormal heart rate responses to exercise. *Prog Cardiovasc Dis* 1985; 27:271–296.
11. Benditt D, Mianmulli M, Fetters J: Single chamber cardiac pacing with activity-initiated chronotropic response: Evaluation by cardiopulmonary exercise testing. *Circulation* 1987; 75:184–189.
12. Wish M, Cohen A, Swartz J, et al: Pacemaker syndrome due to a rate-responsive ventricular pacemaker. *J Clin Electrophysiol* 1988; 2:504–507.
13. DenDulk K, Lindemans FW, Brugada P, et al: Pacemaker syndrome with AAI variable pacing: Importance of atrioventricular conduction properties, medication, and pacemaker programmability. *PACE* 1988; 11:1226–1233.
14. Ogawa S, Dreifus LS, Shenoy PN, et al: Hemodynamic consequences of atrioventricular and ventriculoatrial pacing. *PACE* 1978; 1:8–13.
15. Johnson AD, Laiken SL, Klein GJ: Hemodynamic compromise associated with ventricular atrial conduction following transvenous pacemaker placement. *Am J Med* 1978; 65:75–79.
16. Raza ST, Lajos TZ, Bhayana JN, et al: Improved cardio-

vascular hemodynamics with atrioventricular sequential pacing compared with ventricular demand pacing. *Ann Thorac Surg* 1984; 38:260–264.

17. Griffin JC, Spencer WH III, Cashion WR, et al: Exercise capability of patients receiving DDD pacemakers (abstract). *PACE* 1984; 7:460.

18. Wilkoff BL, Corey J, Blackburn G: A mathematical model of a cardiac chonotropic response to exercise. *J Electrophysiol* 1989; 3:176–180.

19. Holden W, McAnulty JH, Rahimtoola SH: Characterization of heart rate response to exercise in the sick sinus syndrome. *Br Heart J* 1978; 40:923–930.

20. Ellestad MHJ, Wan MKC: Predictive implications of stress testing. Follow-up of 2,700 subjects after maximal treadmill stress testing. *Circulation* 1975; 51:563–569.

21. Prior M, Masterson M, Blackburn G, et al: Critical identification of patients with sinus node dysfunction for possible sensor-driven pacing (abstract). *PACE* 1988; 11:512.

22. Daubert C, Mabo PH, Druelles PH: Dysfunction sinusale et anomalies de conduction auriculoventriculaire: *Stimucoeur* 1988; 16:206–210.

23. Corbelli R, Masterson M, Wilkoff BL: Chronotropic response to exercise in patients with atrial fibrillation. *PACE* 1990; 13:179–187.

24. Benditt DG, Ruetikofer J, Fetter J, et al: Variability of sino atrial rate-response during exercise testing in sinus node dysfunction (abstract). *PACE* 1988; 11:798.

25. Neumann G, Funke H, Kirchhoff PG, et al: Clinical experience with the universal DDD pacemaker, in Barold SS, Mugica J (eds): *The Third Decade of Cardiac Pacing.* Mt Kisco, NY, Futura 1982, p 225.

26. Faerestrand S, Ohm O: A time-related study by Doppler and M-mode echocardiography of hemodynamics, heart size, and AV valvular function during activity sensing rate responsive ventricular pacing. *PACE* 1987; 10:507–518.

27. Colucci WS, Riberio JP, Rocco MB, et al: Impaired chronotropic response to exercise in patients with congestive heart failure; role of postsynaptic beta adrenergic desensitization. *Circulation* 1989; 80:314–323.

28. Gerstenblith G, Frederiksen J, Frank C, et al: Echocardiographic assessment of a normal adult aging population. *Circulation* 1977; 56:273–278.

29. Greenberg B, Chatterjee K, Parmley WP, et al: The influence of left ventricular filling pressure on atrial contribution to cardiac output. *Am Heart J* 1979; 98:742–751.

30. Janosik D, Pearson A, Buckingham T: The hemodynamic benefit of differential AV delay intervals for sensed and paced atrial events during physiologic pacing. *J Am Coll Cordiol* 1989; 14:499–507.

31. Ritter P, Dauber C, Mabo P, et al: Hemodynamic benefit of rate adapted AV delays in dual chamber pacing. *Eur Heart J* 1989; 10:637–646.

32. Bedotto JB, Grayburn PA, Black WH, et al: Alterations in left ventricular relaxation during atrioventricular pacing in humans. *J Am Coll Cardiol* 1990; 15:658–664.

33. Shaw DB, Holman RR, Gowers JI: Survival in sinoatrial disorder (sick-sinus syndrome). *Br Med J* 1980; 280:139–141.

34. Alpert M, Curtis J, SanFelippo J, et al: Comparative survival following permanent ventricular and dual chamber pacing for patients with chronic symptomatic sinus node

dysfunction with and without congestive heart failure. *Am Heart J* 1987; 113:958–968.

35. Rosenqvist M, Brant J, Schuller H: Long-term pacing in sinus node disease: Effects of stimulation mode on cardiovascular morbidity and mortality. *Am Heart J* 1988; 116:16–22.

36. Sasaki Y, Shimotori M, Akahane K, et al: Long-term follow-up of patients with sick sinus syndrome: A comparison of clinical aspects among unpaced, ventricular inhibited paced, and physiologically paced groups. *PACE* 1988; 11:1575–1583.

37. Alpert MA, Curtis JJ, SanFelippo JF, et al: Comparative survival after permanent ventricular and dual chamber pacing for patients with chronic high-degree atrioventricular block with or without preexistent congestive heart failure. *J Am Coll Cardiol* 1986; 7:925–932.

38. Ebagosti A, Gueunoun M, Saadjian A, et al: Long-term follow-up of patients treated with VVI pacing with special reference of VA retrograde conduction. *PACE* 1988; 11:1929–1934.

39. Santini M, Alexidou G, Ansalone G, et al: Relation of prognosis in sick sinus syndrome to age, conduction defects, and modes of permanent cardiac pacing. *Am J Cardiol* 1990; 65:729–735.

40. Smedgard P, Kristensson BE, Kruse I, et al: Rate-responsive pacing by means of activity sensing versus single rate ventricular pacing: A double-blind cross-over study. *PACE* 1987; 10:902–915.

41. Spencer WH, Markowitz T, Alagona P: Rate augmentation and atrial arrhythmias in DDDR pacing. *PACE* 1990; 13:1847–1851.

42. Personal communication: TP Edery, Medtronic Inc, Minneapolis, Feb 27, 1991.

43. Rosenqvist M, Obel I: Atrial pacing and the risk for A-V block: Is there a time for change in attitude? *PACE* 1989; 12:97–101.

44. Lau CP, Antoniou A, Ward DE, et al: Initial clinical experience with a minute ventilation sensing rate modulated pacemaker: Improvements in exercise capacity and symptomatology. *PACE* 1988; 11:1815–1822.

45. Callaghan F, Volemann W, Livingston A, et al: The ventricular depolarization gradient: Effects of exercise, pacing rate, epinephrine, and intrinsic heart rate control on the right ventricular evoked response. *PACE* 1989; 12:1115–1130.

46. Paul V, Garratt C, Ward DE, et al: Closed loop control of rate adaptive pacing: Clinical assessment of a system analyzing the ventricular depolarization gradient. *PACE* 1989; 12:1896–1902.

47. Chirife R: Physiologic principles of a new method for rate responsive pacing using the pre-ejection interval. *PACE* 1988; 11:1545–1554.

48. Personal communication: AR Rickards, Munich, FRG, Oct 8, 1990.

49. Littleford PO, Spector D: Device for the rapid insertion of a permanent endocardial pacing electrode through the subclavian vein: Preliminary report. *Ann Thorac Surg* 1979; 27:265–269.

50. Personal communication: TP Edery, Medtronic Inc, Minneapolis, Feb 27, 1991.

51. Furman S: Subclavian puncture for pacemaker lead placement (editorial). *PACE* 1986; 9:467.

52. Parsonnet V, Bernstein AD, Lindsay B: Pacemaker implantation complication rates: An analysis of some contributing factors. *J Am Coll Cardiol* 1989; 13:917–921.
53. Belott PH: In Barold SS, Mugica J (eds): *New Perspectives in Cardiac Pacing 2*. Mt Kisco, NY, Futura, 1991, p 112.
54. Byrd CL: Safe introducer technique (abstract). *PACE* 1990; 13:501.
55. Zegelman M, Kreuzer J, Wagner R: Ambulatory pacemaker surgery — medical and economic advantages. *PACE* 1986; 9:1299–1303.
56. Zegelman M, Kreuzer J, Clossen SC, et al: Ambulatory implantation of rate adaptive pacemakers — A survey after 8 years (abstract). *PACE* 1990; 13:1216.

56

Recent Advances in Implantable Defibrillator Therapy

Roger A. Winkle, M.D.

Prior to the introduction of the automatic implantable cardioverter defibrillator (AICD), the long-term prognosis for patients with prior cardiac arrest or recurrent sustained ventricular tachycardia was very poor. Despite the introduction of serial electrophysiologic testing[1-3] for management of these patients and the availability of drugs such as amiodarone, only a minority of patients could have their arrhythmias controlled with drugs. The 2-year sudden death rate for patients not controlled with drugs as assessed by serial electrophysiologic testing was 39% ± 8%, and even for those patients whose arrhythmias were rendered noninducible by drugs, the sudden death rate remained an alarmingly high 16% ± 4%.[4]

The implantable defibrillator was introduced by Mirowski in the early 1980s.[5, 6] Initially, there were many who were skeptical about this radical new form of therapy, and it took several years to accumulate enough patient implants and long-term follow-up data to determine the impact of these devices on the rates of sudden cardiac death in patients who had survived cardiac arrest or hemodynamically compromising, sustained ventricular tachycardia. In an early paper, Mirowski et al.[7] estimated a predicted 52% 1-year mortality rate in patients receiving the device based on appropriate device discharges. This compared with an actual observed rate of 18%. In the largest single-center series Winkle and his colleagues have reported on long-term survival after 70, 273, and 555 patients received devices.[8-10] In their latest report the 1-, 5-, and 10-year actuarial survival rates for death due to all causes was 91.9%, 74.2%, and 59.1%. The sudden death rate remains approximately 1% per year over the 10 years of follow-up. Other smaller series reported by Tchou et al.[11] and Kelly et al.[12] have shown similar low rates of sudden death.

These remarkable survival data have resulted in the automatic implantable defibrillator and subsequent second- and third-generation devices becoming the "gold standard" therapy for patients with life-threatening arrhythmias in the 1990s. The number of new implants worldwide is growing at an exponential rate and will exceed 8,000 in 1991. These devices are no longer simply implantable automatic defibrillators. They now contain a variety of diagnostic features and therapeutic options that truly make them "implantable electrophysiology laboratories." This paper will review many of these new features.

BRADYCARDIA PACEMAKERS IN PATIENTS RECEIVING DEFIBRILLATORS

Nearly all patients with life-threatening arrhythmias have serious underlying cardiac disease. The single largest patient population is those patients with coronary heart disease, followed by patients with cardiomyopathies and valvular heart disease. Approximately 10% of all patients receiving implantable defibrillators require bradycardia pacemakers for the usual clinical indications of sick sinus syndrome or high-degree atrioventricular block.[9] At the present time these patients require two separate devices. The implantation of two separate devices requires special care in order to make certain that the defibrillator does not overcount pacemaker spikes and intrinsic QRS complexes or T waves during paced rhythm and falsely sense that a tachycardia is present.[13] Alternatively, the defibrillator must not sense pacemaker spikes occurring randomly during an episode of ventricular fibrillation and inappropriately determine that there is a slow intrinsic rhythm with failure to deliver lifesaving defibrillation shocks. In addition, the implantation of two separate devices results in a considerable amount of additional expense as well as the need for multiple ventricular leads.

It is often assumed that all patients dying suddenly with implantable defibrillators have a ventricular tachyarrhythmia as their terminal rhythm. We have, however, noted several patients with automatic implantable defibrillators (AICDs) who had recurrent cardiac arrest without delivery of a discharge from the device. Several of these arrests have been electrocardiographically proven to be due to a bradyarrhythmia. The presence of a backup bradycardia pacemaker in a patient who may have never previously experienced a bradyarrhythmia could result in additional lives being saved. In our patients receiving newer defibrillators with backup pacing, we have noted that 2% of patients without a history of bradycardias have subsequently been found to be pacemaker dependent at follow-up office visits.

ADVANTAGES OF LOW-ENERGY CARDIOVERSION

Low-energy cardioversion offers several advantages over high-energy shocks for the termination of ventricular tachyarrhythmias. Low-energy shocks can be delivered more rapidly since charge times are shorter for lower stored energies. For shocks below 1 to 2 J there is less discomfort to the patient than with higher-energy shocks. Because less energy is required, there is a saving in battery capacity for the device, which should result in less frequent generator changes. Several studies have shown the efficacy of shocks below 5 to 10 J to be 62% to 65%.[14-17] Most studies have shown that slower ventricular tachycardias are more easily converted with low-energy shocks than are faster ventricular tachycardias or ventricular fibrillation.

ANTITACHYCARDIA PACING FOR ARRHYTHMIA TERMINATION

Electrophysiologists have used antitachycardia pacing since the earliest days of electrophysiologic studies as a mechanism for terminating induced ventricular tachycardias.[18] In one study comparing antitachycardia pacing with cardioversion, there was no significant difference in arrhythmia termination, rates being approximately 80% for both techniques.[19] Antitachycardia pacing has the major advantage of being painless to the patient when compared with low- or high-energy shocks. Cardioversion has a higher rate of arrhythmia acceleration than antitachycardia pacing does.[19] Cardioversion results in a 23% incidence of the induction of atrial arrhythmias, whereas antitachycardia pacing virtually never results in the induction of atrial tachyarrhythmias.[19] Several early antitachycardia pacemakers were utilized as a treatment modality for patients with recurrent sustained ventricular tachycardia. Unfortunately, occasional arrhythmia acceleration resulting in hemodynamically unstable ventricular tachycardias and ventricular fibrillation severely limited the widespread use of these devices.

NEWER COMBINATION IMPLANTABLE DEVICES

At the present time several manufacturers are conducting clinical trials of multidimensional antiarrhythmic devices. These devices are fully programmable and offer single-chamber bradycardia pacing capabilities, antitachycardia pacing, low-energy cardioversion, and defibrillation therapy (Table 56–1). These devices give physicians a wide range of options for treating ventricular tachyarrhythmias. They can, in a single patient, deliver antitachycardia pacing therapy for extremely slow and hemodynamically well-tolerated ventricular tachycardia, low-energy cardioverting shocks for intermediate-rate ventricular tachycardias, and initial high-energy defibrillation shock for extremely rapid ventricular tachycardia and/or ventricular fibrillation. These devices are largely noncommitted for ventricular tachyarrhythmias. This means that they will not deliver therapy for short self-terminating episodes of ventricular tachyarrhythmias. They have widely programmable arrhythmia detection criteria, including a variable duration of arrhythmia before initial therapy is delivered as well as the capability to look for the sudden onset of a tachyarrhythmia or stability of heart rate during a tachycardia episode. These later features help to distinguish ventricular tachycardia from sinus tachycardia or atrial fibrillation. They offer the option to deliver progressively more aggressive antitachycardia therapy. For example, if antitachycardia therapy is programmed for a slower, well-tolerated ventricular tachycardia and fails to terminate the arrhythmia, the devices will then deliver low-energy or high-energy shocks to terminate the arrhythmia. Several devices have a "fail-safe" feature. If after a programmed period of time (usually 20 to 30 seconds) less aggressive therapy has not terminated ventricular tachycardia, the defibrillator will give a high-energy shock to "get the job done" before the patient experiences severe hemodynamic consequences.

These devices are all roughly the same size and weigh in the 200- to 220-g range. They deliver maximum energies in the 30- to 40-J range, which is well

TABLE 56–1.
Features Available in Newer Tiered Therapy Devices

Full programmability
Antitachycardia pacing
Low-energy cardioversion
Defibrillation
VVI bradycardia pacing
Noninvasive programmed stimulation
Advanced diagnostics
Stored electrograms

above the minimum energy required for terminating most ventricular tachyarrhythmias. Devices differ in types of delivered waveform, with different manufacturers utilizing monophasic, biphasic, sequential, or a combinations of these waveforms in their devices. These devices have a wide range of built-in diagnostics. They permit a determination of sensing and shocking lead impedances and measure battery voltage status for a determination of device end of life. Most are anticipated to have a 4- to 6-year battery life.

Delivery of therapy is recorded in internal memory by using a wide range of techniques. Some devices store the date and time of each shock. Others provide a sequence of RR intervals before and after therapy or give the mean cycle length during the tachycardia and after a return to normal rhythm. Other devices store electrograms of the entire arrhythmia episode. These newer defibrillators also vary with regard to types of sensing circuitry, with some devices requiring programming to optimize the arrhythmia sensing and others utilizing fully automatic gain control.

NONINVASIVE PROGRAMMED STIMULATION

Virtually all of the new implantable devices will include capabilities for performing noninvasive programmed stimulation. These devices can deliver single, double, and triple extra stimuli at a variety of drive cycle lengths. Some devices utilize the implanted device itself through its programmer, and others utilized "slaved induction" with an external programmed stimulator. Devices have a variety of burst and ramping functions for the induction of ventricular fibrillation. The ability to perform noninvasive program stimulation is a frequently used feature of these newer devices in patients with life-threatening arrhythmias. Patients frequently undergo changes in their clinical status (such as additional myocardial infarction, worsening left ventricular function) or changes in their antiarrhythmic regimen. All of these factors could result in a varying long-term pattern of ar-

rhythmia recurrence. The ability to easily induce a patient's tachyarrhythmia in order to assess the efficacy of the programmed antitachycardia therapy is extremely valuable. We generally place a radial arterial line and a peripheral intravenous line as safety precautions during the use of noninvasive program stimulation. These studies are well accepted by the patients when carried out under benzodiazepine sedation. They are often done on an outpatient basis. Full external resuscitation measures must be available, and we prefer to perform our "noninvasive" testing in the electrophysiology laboratory.

INCREASED COMPLEXITY OF NEWER DEVICES

The newer devices have functioned extremely well to date and in fact have relatively few serious shortcomings. There are, however, a number of logistic problems created by these devices. At the present time each manufacturer is utilizing a different shocking lead pin size for their devices, and some manufacturers now have more than one type of pin size available on their shocking leads. This results in the need for a number of converters and/or adapters. These create the potential for mechanical failure and add bulk to the patient's generator pocket.

The increased sophistication of these devices results in increasing complexity during long-term follow-up. With first-generation implantable defibrillators, follow-up could be performed in virtually any physician's office because the only parameter to be checked was battery status, which was determined indirectly by measurement of "charge time." A single AID Check device could evaluate all models of defibrillators available until approximately 2 years ago. Since that time almost every new device has its own programmer. A busy implant center now needs to have four or five different programmers to cover the spectrum of devices being implanted. Since these devices have far more programmable features than most bradycardia pacemakers, the level of programming sophistication is considerable. One must also have very detailed knowledge of each patient's induced and spontaneous ventricular tachyarrhythmias as well as the response of each tachyarrhythmia to antitachycardia pacing, cardioversion, and defibrillation before the device can be programmed properly. It is often difficult to evaluate all therapeutic modalities at a single electrophysiologic session. We frequently have patients return for at least one additional electrophysiologic study following hospital discharge in order to optimize device programming.

EXPANDING CLINICAL USES OF ADVANCED DEVICES

The improvements in newer implantable antitachycardia devices is resulting in increased numbers of patients for whom these devices can be utilized. Since antitachycardia pacing can painlessly terminate episodes of sustained ventricular tachycardia, these devices can now be utilized in patients with more frequent episodes of sustained ventricular tachycardia. It is not uncommon to see an entirely asymptomatic patient with 30 to 50 episodes of ventricular tachycardia terminations since the prior office visit. In the past, devices that only delivered high-energy shocks could not be implanted in these patients due to the discomfort and psychological impact of frequent defibrillator shocks. Because antitachycardia pacing utilizes relatively small amounts of energy from the device batteries, the overall battery drain is reduced despite increased frequency of arrhythmia termination.

In the past, implanted defibrillators could not be readily used in patients with ventricular tachycardia rates that overlapped with their sinus rates. The sudden-onset feature of the newer defibrillators should permit some crossover to exist between the maximum sinus rate and slowest ventricular tachycardia rate, although these patients remain difficult to deal with.

These newer devices are changing the way in which we utilize antiarrhythmic drugs in patients with implantable defibrillators. Many patients who were receiving antiarrhythmic drugs to suppress nonsustained episodes of ventricular tachyarrhythmia no longer need such drug therapy. The devices can be programmed to permit longer runs of self-terminating arrhythmia before activating. In addition, devices can abort therapy delivery during charging or at the end of charging if the arrhythmia has spontaneously terminated. Other patients are now given antiarrhythmic therapy who would not have received such therapy in past. The main reason for giving them drug therapy is to slow the rate of their ventricular tachycardia to make antitachycardia pacing or low-energy cardioversion more efficacious.

The newer devices are favored in patients with unexplained syncope and induced ventricular tachyarrhythmias. In such patients there is always a certain element of doubt as to whether or not a bradyarrhythmia or tachyarrhythmia was the cause of their syncope. The newer devices with their bradycardia pacemakers provide adequate treatment for both possible arrhythmic causes of syncope.

In the past frequent device discharges required repeated hospitalizations, prolonged ambulatory monitoring, or the use of external transtelephonic electrocardiographic (ECG) recording devices in order to document the cause of device discharge. The availability of stored electrograms and other advanced diagnostics in these devices permit the physician to rapidly determine the arrhythmia causing therapy delivery. This knowledge allows physicians to make appropriate programming adjustments in the antitachycardia regimen or in the patient's drug therapy to minimize the occurrence of these arrhythmias.

NONTHORACOTOMY LEAD SYSTEMS

Mirowski et al.[20] had initially wanted to utilize a transvenous defibrillation system in humans but ultimately changed to a spring-patch system because it was more reliable for defibrillation. They demonstrated that 5- to 15-J monophasic defibrillation shocks were able to successfully defibrillate patients intraoperatively following coronary artery bypass surgery. This early work was extended to a catheter that was designed to be used in conjunction with the first-generation implantable cardioverter/defibrillator. In a pilot study, up to two thirds of patients could be defibrillated with energies of 25 J or less.[21] The transvenous catheter system compared favorably with the spring-patch lead system in use in the early 1980s. This catheter system was further refined and is the Endotak lead system.[22] This system consists of a transvenous defibrillation catheter with superior vena caval and distal right ventricular apical electrodes that can be used alone or in conjunction with a subcutaneous patch. The initial catheter design was associated with mechanical problems in several patients. It has subsequently been redesigned. Approximately two-thirds of all patients who have undergone intraoperative testing with the new Endotak system have undergone permanent implantation of the catheter and/or catheter patch system. Limited long-term follow-up in a multicenter clinical trial has shown promising results. Medtronic has utilized several nonthoracotomy leads, including a right ventricular apical electrode, a superior vena caval electrode, a coronary sinus electrode, and a subcutaneous patch electrode. A number of patients have undergone chronic implantation with various combinations of these leads. Long-term follow-up is limited, but the system shows promise.

The ability to implant devices in more than half of all patients by utilizing nonthoracotomy approaches should result in increased acceptance by the patients and their physicians. However, due to problems with superior vena caval spring electrodes in the early 1980s, one would anticipate an increased incidence of lead migrations, lead fractures, and other mechanical problems related to these systems. To date, however, actual clinical practice has shown these problems to be relatively infrequent.

PROPHYLACTIC IMPLANTATION OF ANTITACHYCARDIA DEVICES

During the first decade of defibrillator therapy, these devices have been utilized exclusively in those patients who had already experienced an episode of life-threatening ventricular tachyarrhythmia or who have had syncope with an inducible ventricular tachyarrhythmia. A high percentage of these patients have experienced one or more out-of-hospital cardiac arrests. Only a minority of patients experiencing sudden cardiac death are fortunate enough to be successfully resuscitated. By utilizing assessment of left ventricular function, 24-hour Holter monitors, and signal-averaged ECG recordings it is now possible to identify a group of patients at very high risk for sudden cardiac death. Therapeutic efforts to date have focused on the use of β-blocking drugs, antiplatelet agents, calcium channel blocking drugs, and suppression of complex ventricular ectopy with antiarrhythmic therapy. Of these therapies, only β-blocking drugs have shown consistent reductions in sudden death and overall mortality.[23] The Coronary Artery Suppression Trial (CAST)[24] in fact showed an increased mortality rate in patients with ventricular ectopy treated with encainide, flecainide, and moricizine as compared with mortality in patients treated with placebo. Electrophysiologic testing can identify post–myocardial infarction patients at risk for arrhythmias,[25] and serial electrophysiologic testing in order to choose antiarrhythmic drug therapy may result in reduced rates of sudden death and recurrent life-threatening arrhythmias in those patients whose arrhythmias become noninducible on drug therapy.

Despite these advances there remains a large number of patients identified as being at high risk for whom no current therapy will have a significant impact on their sudden death risk. A number of investigators feel that the prophylactic use of implantable defibrillators in such patients will markedly reduce the number of sudden cardiac deaths. Several multicenter trials are underway to examine this possibility. One study, the Coronary Artery Bypass Graft (CABG) Patch, randomly assigns patients to receive a defibrillator at the time of clinically indicated coronary bypass surgery. Patients must have an ejection fraction below 35% and an abnormal signal-averaged ECG to qualify for randomization. Another study, the Multicenter Automatic Defibrillator Implantation Trial (MADIT), enrolls patients with complex ventricular ectopy, poor left ventricular function, and inducible, sustained, monomorphic ventricular tachycardia not suppressed by intravenous procainamide.

If these studies demonstrate the value of prophylactic device implantation, they will offer the potential for prolonged survival in a large number of patients who are at high risk for sudden cardiac death but have not yet experienced any clinical events.

REFERENCES

1. Mason JW, Winkle RA: Electrode-catheter arrhythmia induction in the selection and assessment of antiarrhythmic drug therapy for recurrent ventricular tachycardia. *Circulation* 1978; 58:971–985.
2. Mason JW, Winkle RA: Accuracy of the ventricular tachycardia–induction study for predicting long-term efficacy and inefficacy of antiarrhythmic drugs. *N Engl J Med* 1980; 303:1073–1077.
3. Horowitz LN, Josephson ME, Farshidi A, et al: Recurrent sustained ventricular tachycardia 3. Role of the electrophysiologic study in selection of antiarrhythmic regimens. *Circulation* 1978; 58:986–997.
4. Swerdlow CD, Winkle RA, Mason JW: Determinants of survival in patients with ventricular tachyarrhythmias. *N Engl J Med* 1983; 308:1436–1442.
5. Mirowski M: The automatic implantable cardioverter-defibrillator: An overview. *J Am Coll Cardiol* 1985; 6:461–466.
6. Mirowski M, Mower MM, Staewen WS, et al: Standby automatic defibrillator. An approach to prevention of sudden coronary death. *Arch Intern Med* 1970; 126:158–161.
7. Mirowski M, Reid PR, Winkle RA, et al: Mortality in patients with implanted automatic defibrillators. *Ann Intern Med* 1983; 98:585–588.
8. Echt DS, Armstrong K, Schmidt P, et al: Clinical experience, complications, and survival in 70 patients with the automatic implantable cardioverter/defibrillator. *Circulation* 1985; 71:289–296.
9. Winkle RA, Mead RH, Ruder MA, et al: Long-term outcome with the automatic implantable cardioverter-defibrillator. *J Am Coll Cardiol* 1989; 13:1353–1361.
10. Winkle RA, Mead RH, Ruder MA, et al: Ten year experience with implantable defibrillators (abstract). *Circulation*, in press.
11. Tchou PJ, Kadri N, Anderson J, et al: Automatic implantable cardioverter defibrillators and survival of patients with left ventricular dysfunction and malignant ventricular arrhythmias. *Ann Intern Med* 1988; 109:529–534.
12. Kelly PA, Cannom DS, Garan H, et al: The automatic implantable cardioverter-defibrillator: Efficacy, complications and survival in patients with malignant ventricular arrhythmias. *J Am Coll Cardiol* 1988; 11:1278–1286.
13. Epstein AE, Kay N, Plumb VJ, et al: Combined automatic implantable cardioverter-defibrillator and pacemaker systems: Implantation techniques and follow-up. *J Am Coll Cardiol* 1989; 13:121–131.
14. Ciccone JM, Saksena S, Shah Y, et al: A prospective randomized study of the clinical efficacy and safety of transvenous cardioversion for termination of ventricular tachycardia. *Circulation* 1985; 71:571–578.
15. Zipes DP, Jackman WM, Heger JJ, et al: Clinical trans-

venous cardioversion of recurrent life-threatening ventricular tachyarrhythmias: Low energy synchronized cardioversion of ventricular tachycardia and termination of ventricular fibrillation in patients using a catheter electrode. *Am Heart J* 1982; 103:789–794.

16. Yee R, Zipes DP, Gulamhusen S, et al: Low energy countershock using an intravascular catheter in an acute cardiac care setting. *Am J Cardiol* 1982; 50:1124–1129.

17. Waspe LE, Kim SG, Matos JA, et al: Role of a catheter lead system for transvenous countershock and pacing during electrophysiologic tests: An assessment of the usefulness of catheter shocks for terminating ventricular tachyarrhythmias. *Am J Cardiol* 1983; 52:477–484.

18. Fisher JD, Mehra R, Furman S: Termination of ventricular tachycardia with bursts of rapid ventricular pacing. *Am J Cardiol* 1978; 41:94–102.

19. Saksena SA, Chandran P, Shah Y, et al: Comparative efficacy of transvenous cardioversion and pacing in patients with sustained ventricular tachycardia: A prospective, randomized, cross-over study. *Circulation* 1985; 72:153–160.

20. Mirowski M, Mower MM, Gott VL, et al: Feasibility and effectiveness of low-energy catheter defibrillation in man. *Circulation* 1973; 47:79–85.

21. Winkle RA, Bach SM Jr, Mead RH, et al: Comparison of defibrillation efficacy in humans using a new catheter and superior vena cava spring–left ventricular patch electrodes. *J Am Coll Cardiol* 1988; 11:365–370.

22. Saksena S, Parsonnet V: Implantation of a cardioverter/defibrillator without thoracotomy using a triple electrode system. *JAMA* 1988; 259:69–72.

23. The Norwegian Multicenter Study Group: Timolol-induced reduction in mortality and reinfarction in patients surviving acute myocardial infarction. *N Engl J Med* 1981; 304:801–807.

24. Echt DS, Liebson PR, Mitchell LB, et al: Mortality and morbidity in patients receiving encainide, flecainide, or placebo. The Cardiac Arrhythmia Suppression Trial. *N Engl J Med* 1991; 324:781–788.

25. Bourke JP, Richards DAB, Ross DL, et al: Routine programmed electrical stimulation in survivors of acute myocardial infarction for prediction of spontaneous ventricular tachyarrhythmias during follow-up: Results, optimal stimulation protocol and cost-effective screening. *J Am Coll Cardiol* 1991; 18:781–788.

57

Transvenous Catheter Ablation of Cardiac Arrhythmias

Michael A. Ruder, M.D.

Roger A. Winkle, M.D.

Nellis A. Smith, M.D.

R. Hardwin Mead, M.D.

The goal of transvenous catheter ablation is to permanently and safely interrupt the tachycardia circuit responsible for a particular arrhythmia. In the previous edition of this book, the state of the art of catheter ablation in 1988 was presented. In the last 3 years, there have been tremendous advances in techniques. This chapter will review the status of catheter ablation of cardiac arrhythmias up to 1988 and address the question of how close we have come to achieving our goal since then.

HISTORICAL PERSPECTIVE

There are a number of clinical situations in which total interruption of atrioventricular (AV) conduction is desirable. Although it is usually used to control excessive ventricular rates during atrial fibrillation, any supraventricular tachyarrhythmia in which the AV node is an integral part of the tachycardia circuit could be controlled by ablation of the AV junction.

Previously, permanent ablation of the AV junction required surgical ligation, formalin injection, or direct cryoablation with thoracotomy and cardiopulmonary bypass. Gallagher et al.[1] and Scheinman et al.,[2] in an effort to avoid thoracotomy, pioneered percutaneous catheter ablation using high-energy shocks. In this technique, a standard electrode catheter, introduced via a femoral vein, is placed against the right atrial septum and positioned to record the best His bundle electrogram. A shock from a standard defibrillator is delivered with a chest wall patch serving as the current sink. The shock energy used is usually 200 to 300 J. A pacemaker, often rate adaptive, is then inserted.

The technique is highly successful and safe. Although the Percutaneous Cardiac Mapping and Ablation Registry (PCMAR), a collection of centers that chose to participate, suggested a success rate (defined as complete heart block) of 65%,[3] in experienced centers the success rate could approach 100%. For example, at Sequoia Hospital, we have used high-energy ablation to achieve complete heart block in 102 patients with a success rate on the initial attempt of 92% (Fig 57–1). Seven patients required a second attempt, and this was successful in all but 2. The complication rate was low. Although deaths due to ablation have been reported, we have seen transient hypotension in only 2 patients and pacemaker complications in 2 patients.

The disadvantages of the high-energy technique are that general anesthesia is required and that as many as 60% of patients after high-energy ablation do not have an "adequate" escape rate, that is, should pacemaker failure occur, the escape rate from the high junction or ventricle may be so slow that the patient might lose consciousness. In addition, high-energy ablation essentially delivers an "explosion" within the heart.[4] Standard defibrillators de-

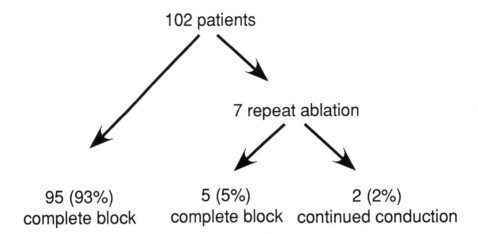

FIG 57–1.
Results of high-energy ablations to achieve complete blocks at Sequoia Hospital. After one (93%) or two (5%) attempts, 98% are in complete heart block.

liver energy over a period of 30 to 35 ms, and during this period of time, electrolysis of plasma into various gases occurs around the catheter tip, effectively insulating the catheter tip from the surrounding blood. Further buildup of electrical charge occurs on the catheter tip due to the long delivery time of energy. With enough charge buildup, arcing across the gas bubble occurs, and an actual fireball of several centimeters results. This frequently causes a sudden, localized pressure rise of as much as 80 atm in a period of milliseconds. The percussion wave generated by this sudden pressure rise, called barotrauma, is undesirable and is likely responsible for the infrequent complications seen with high-energy ablations.

However, it is clear that catheter ablation of the AV junction was a dramatic improvement over thoracotomy in those patients in whom total control of AV conduction was the only solution to arrhythmia control. Electrophysiologists then looked toward ablating patients with accessory pathways, AV node reentrant tachycardia, and other tachyarrhythmias.

Accessory Pathways

Given the success of ablation of the AV junction, attention was directed to the possibility of ablating accessory pathways. Work by Sealy et al. as early as 1968 showed that a wide surgical incision just above the AV annulus (through the accessory pathway) cured patients with the Wolff-Parkinson-White syndrome. The surgery is quite successful; for example, at Sequoia Hospital we have operated on over 150 patients since 1985 with a success rate greater than 98% and no deaths.

It seemed logical that a shock delivered via a catheter placed on the accessory pathway, just above the annulus, would also interrupt conduction across the accessory pathway. On the left side (which contains 50% of the accessory pathways), this area would be approached via the coronary sinus. Unfortunately, the thin-walled coronary sinus often could not safely withstand the barotrauma of the shock, and Fisher et al. reported rupture with subsequent pericardial tamponade in several patients.[5] More disappointing was the fact that at least on the left side this approach was uniformly unsuccessful. This appeared to be due to the fact that the distance between the coronary sinus and the ventricular summit was great enough that transmural necrosis at the actual annular level was not achieved with ablation and thus conduction from the atrium to the ventricle via the accessory pathway was still possible. Finally, it was known from animal work that higher energies delivered via the coronary sinus could cause lesions in the left circumflex coronary artery. For all of these reasons, this approach was abandoned.

However, the technique did prove successful for posteroseptal accessory pathways. These occur in the posterior portion of the septum and account for 25% of accessory pathways. The ablating catheter can be "anchored" in the coronary sinus and the ablating shock delivered just outside the coronary os. We, as have others,[6] have generally seen a success rate of 70% without major complications. Finally, about 25% of accessory pathways occur along the right free wall. High-energy shocks can be delivered above the tricuspid annulus, but there is a significant risk of damage to the right coronary artery, including coronary spasm as well as permanent damage to the media and intima.[7] At least one investigator has successfully delivered shocks here and reported success in a high number of patients with right free wall accessory pathways;[8] however, most electrophysiologists have avoided this approach. Since right free wall accessory pathways can also be surgically divided without placing the patient on cardiopulmonary bypass, the risk of high-energy catheter ablative techniques for right free wall accessory pathways becomes even more unacceptable. In summary, with high-energy shocks, posteroseptal pathways, but not those occurring along the right or left free wall, could be ablated.

Atrioventricular Node Reentrant Tachycardia

AV node reentrant tachycardia is probably the most common supraventricular tachycardia. The tachycardia circuit is thought to involve conduction down a "slow" pathway and up a "fast" pathway; the pathways may be either intranodal and perhaps functional, or they may be anatomically distinct, with the fast pathway located anteriorly and the slow pathway posteriorly. In 1985, Ross et al., in a revolutionary development, described a surgical technique consisting of dissection of the anteroseptum and possibly interruption of one of the pathways; here the tachycardia is cured but AV conduction is preserved.[9] The question immediately posed was whether this could be replicated by using a catheter technique. By delivering high-energy shocks near the AV node, a moderate degree of success (76%) was obtained, but unfortunately heart block was produced in a significant number (10%) of patients.[10] The clinical question facing electrophysiologists when confronted with a patient who required nonpharmacologic management of AV node reentrant tachycardia became whether to proceed with thoracotomy characterized by a high degree of success (95%)[11] and a low incidence of heart block (<5%) or opt for a catheter ablation with a 10% chance of heart block and subsequent need for a permanent pacemaker.

Ventricular Tachycardia

In terms of volume of patients, ventricular tachyarrhythmias are much more prevalent than supraventricular tachyarrhythmias. In the broadest sense, ventricular tachycardia/ventricular fibrillation is the leading cause of death in the United States.

The conceptual model for ventricular tachycardia in ischemic heart disease is that the border of a healed myocardial infarct consists of a zone of scar interdigitating with normal muscle. These islands of muscle separated by scar can result in reentry cycles and thus "reentry" ventricular tachycardia. With this model in mind, Harken et al. developed a surgical technique of per-

forming an aneurysmectomy and endocardial resection of the area responsible for the ventricular tachycardia.[12] Most electrophysiologists have also generously applied cryoablation at the time of endocardial resection. Surgery is successful in about 75% of operative survivors but is associated with at least a 5% to 10% mortality rate. Hartzler,[13] Morady et al.,[14] and others have attempted to replicate the surgical approach of endocardial resection and cryoablation with a catheter technique. High-energy shocks were applied transcutaneously to the area mapped to show earliest activation during ventricular tachycardia, presumably the site of reentry. Although ablation results were initially encouraging, a number of factors make catheter ablative techniques for recurrent ventricular tachycardia less attractive, including a low success rate (35% to 45%), a relatively high complication rate (10% to 15%), and increasing acceptance of automatic cardioverter defibrillators.[15]

Summary

Thus, as of 1988, we can say that catheter ablation of the AV junction in an attempt to achieve complete heart block was highly successful, although the need for general anesthesia and the generally poor infra-Hissan "escape" rhythms were disadvantages. Extranodal AV accessory pathways in the posteroseptal area were successfully ablated, but those in other areas, the right and left free walls, were not generally approached. AV node reentrant tachycardia could be modified, but with what some electrophysiologists regarded as an unacceptably high incidence of heart block. Modification of the AV node to control the rate during atrial fibrillation but with preserved AV conduction was not consistently achievable. It is probably fair to say that most investigators had become disenchanted with the idea of ablations for ventricular tachycardia except in special situations.

ENERGY SOURCES

The source of the ablating energy, high-energy direct-current shocks, was the origin of several of the problems facing high-energy ablation. As described above, the shock caused an explosion in the heart due to electrical arcing across the electrolyzed gases, which produced an insulating sphere surrounding the catheter tip. The high-energy shocks were necessarily imprecise and, because of barotrauma, potentially dangerous. A better energy source was necessary, and several possibilities have been examined (Table 57–1). At least one group of investigators has managed to avoid the problem with arcing during high-energy shocks by shorten-

TABLE 57–1.

Potential Modalities for Electrophysiologic Ablations

High-energy shocks
   Standard defibrillations
   Defibrillators with shortened energy delivery time
Radio frequency current
Cryotherapy
Laser
Mechanical (cutting)
Ultrasound
Chemical (ethanol, formalin)
Microwave

ing the duration of energy delivery; however, in the United States, this has not become popular. For our purposes, most of the discussion will focus on radio frequency (RF) energy.

RF energy is similar to electrocautery and is a sine wave of alternating current at 200 to 750 kHz. It is applied via a large tipped catheter to avoid the coagulation formation commonly seen when standard catheters with small tips are used. The use of RF energy has broadened the applications of catheter ablation considerably.

ATRIOVENTRICULAR JUNCTION

When RF energy is used, the same high success rate seen with high-energy ablation can be obtained but without the need for general anesthesia. More importantly, the escape rhythm is faster and more reliable, usually originating above the bundle of His (Figs 57–2 and 57–3). For example, in our series at Sequoia Hos-

pital, 73% of our first 25 patients had an escape rhythm at an average rate of 39 ± 12 beats per minute.

ACCESSORY PATHWAYS

The greatest advantage of RF energy is seen in the ablation of accessory pathways. Accessory pathways in any location are now potential "targets" for ablation. Initially, attempts at ablating accessory pathways consisted of applying RF energy to the atrial side of the AV groove, thus mimicking the surgical experience. This approach was generally disappointing, and satisfactory results were not obtained until Kuck et al. developed the revolutionary technique of applying energy to the ventricular insertion point of the accessory pathway.[16] These investigators have consistently reported close to a 98% success rate and essentially no complications. For left free wall pathways, the technique involves placing a large tipped semimaneuverable catheter retrogradely into the left ventricle and manipulating it against the mitral annulus under the mitral valve. Ideally, potentials from the accessory pathway are recorded. The time from the earliest recorded intraventricular signal to the onset of the delta wave is typically 25 to 35 ms. RF energy is delivered from this catheter to a chest wall patch (Figs 57–4 through 57–14).

With much the same technique, accessory pathways in all locations, including the septum and right free wall, are accessible to RF energy[17] ablation. After an initial "learning curve," it appears that many centers will be able to obtain a success rate in the range above 90%.

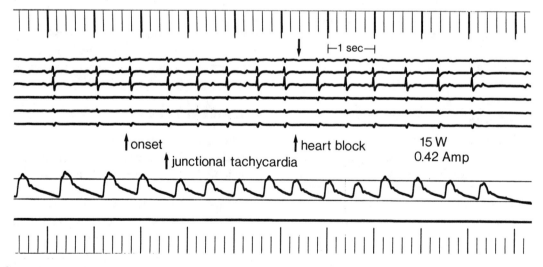

FIG 57–2.
In a 52-year-old man with refractory paroxysmal atrial fibrillation, RF energy is applied to the proximal perinodal region. Junctional tachycardia (presumably due to stimulation by the RF energy) ensures, followed by heart block. Surface leads only (I, II, III, aVR, aVL, aVF) are shown.

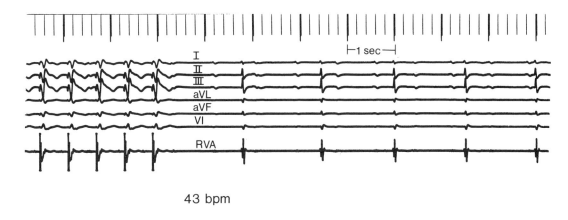

43 bpm

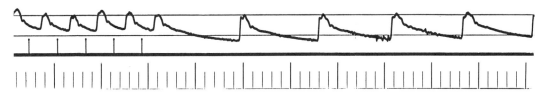

FIG 57–3.

In the same patient as in Figure 57–2, the escape rhythm is 43 beats per minute (bpm) with a narrow QRS complex when the pacemaker is inhibited. The escape rhythm is faster and more reliable after RF ablation as compared with high-energy shocks.

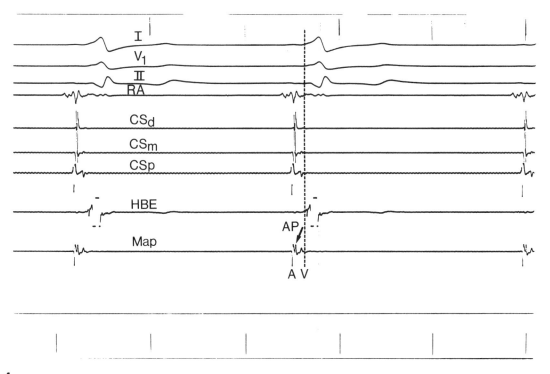

FIG 57–4.

A 24-year-old man with a left free wall accessory pathway. In the baseline tracing, there is obvious ventricular preexcitation on the surface electrocardiogram (I, VI, II). The mapping catheter has been placed retrogradely across the aortic valve and manipulated to lie near the accessory pathway. An electrical potential due to activation of the accessory pathway *(arrow)* is recorded in the mapping catheter. *RA* = right atrium; *CSd, CSm, CSp* = coronary sinus (distal, middle, and proximal, respectively); *HBE* = His bundle electrogram; *Map* = mapping and ablation catheter; *AP* = accessory pathway.

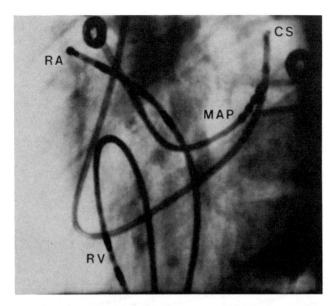

FIG 57–5.
A 60-degree left anterior oblique (LAO) projection of catheter placement in the same patient as in Figure 57–4. The mapping and ablation catheter *(MAP)* is in the left ventricle and positioned under the initial valve near the mitral annulus. Catheters are also in the coronary sinus *(CS)*, right ventricular apex *(RV)*, and the right atrium *(RA)*.

ATRIOVENTRICULAR NODE REENTRANT TACHYCARDIA

Just as the approach to accessory pathways initially mimicked that of surgery, with the RF energy being applied to the atrium above the annulus and subsequently being applied to the ventricle, so did the initial experience using RF energy for AV node reentry tachycardia follow the example of the surgical approach. That is, the catheter was manipulated anteriorly, and energy was delivered in such a fashion that the surgical, anterior dissection was simulated. The results were good, with cure obtained in 70% to 85% of patients and heart block in 5%.[18]

For years some investigators have postulated that the true theoretical construct for AV node reentrant tachycardia was that the "slow" pathway was not a functional pathway within the atrioventricular node but is physically removed from the node and lies posteriorly, near the coronary sinus os. Jackman et al. have examined the possibility of curing AV node reentrant tachycardia by applying RF energy posteriorly, where the "slow" pathway may lie, in the hope of avoiding heart block. As a matter of fact, there is a substantial body of evidence suggesting that AV node reentrant tachycardia is entirely intranodal. However, Jackman et al. have prelimi-

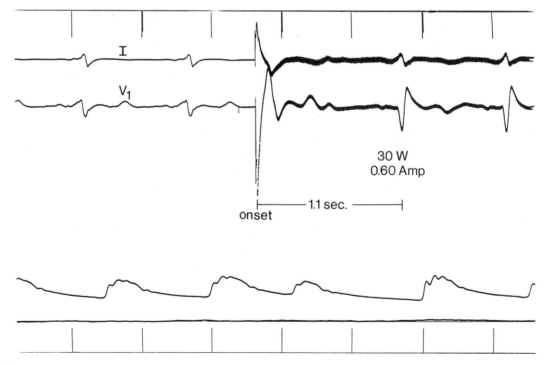

FIG 57–6.
Case 1. After 1.1 seconds of RF energy, the delta wave has disappeared (most evident in lead V1), thus signifying successful ablation of the accessory pathway.

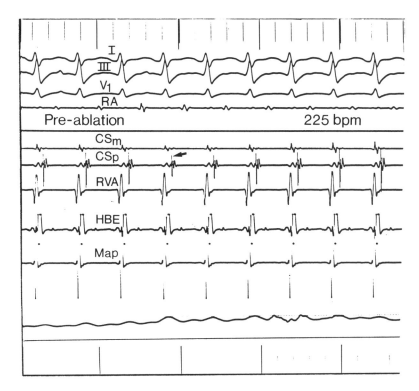

FIG 57–7.

Case 2. Orthodromic AV reentry tachycardia in an 11-year-old boy with a concealed left free wall accessory pathway. The earliest retrograde atrial activation is seen in the proximal coronary sinus. An accessory pathway potential *(arrow)* is recorded. The mapping catheter has been placed in the left ventricle near this site. Abbreviations are as in Figure 57–4.

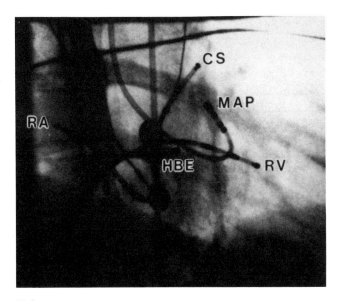

FIG 57–8.

Case 2. A 30-degree right anterior oblique (RAO) projection of catheters shows the large tipped mapping catheter *(MAP)* placed opposite the earliest recorded retrograde atrial activation in the coronary sinus *(CS)*. Catheters are also placed in the right atrium *(RA)*, in the right ventricle *(RV)*, and near the His bundle *(HBE)*.

narily reported impressive results when using this posterior technique and have avoided complete heart block. The thought of curing AV node reentrant tachycardia by ablating a structure so posterior is fascinating, and the success of the method offers insight into the pathophysiology of AV node reentrant tachycardia.

We have found a success rate of 100% (2 patients requiring two attempts) with 1 episode of complete heart block in our first 18 patients. A "posterior" approach was attempted in most of these patients and was successful in 4 (Fig 57–15); the other patients required ablations closer to the AV node.

Although further refinements in technique will lead to a lower incidence of heart block and greater insight into the tachycardia mechanism, it can be said that AV node reentrant tachycardia, the most common supraventricular tachycardia, can now be predictably cured by RF energy ablation.

VENTRICULAR TACHYCARDIA

In contrast to the clear advantages RF energy has over high-energy shocks in other arrhythmias, RF energy does not appear to offer much in ventricular tachy-

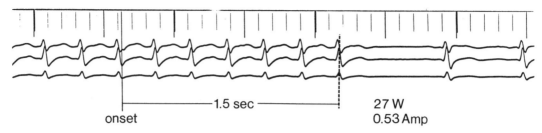

FIG 57–9.
Case 2. RF energy during AV reentry tachycardia stops the tachycardia.

cardia ablation. This clearly is an extremely important field, and patients with ventricular tachycardia outnumber those with supraventricular tachyarrhythmias. Progress has been made with bundle-branch reentry ventricular tachycardia, which appears to be a macro reentry tachycardia typically seen in patients with a dilated cardiomyopathy and baseline left bundle-branch block. The reentrant circuit consists of conduction down the right bundle branch, through diseased left ventricular muscle, and reentry back into the right bundle area near the His bundle.[19] This can be successfully cured by ablating the proximal right bundle, ideally by using RF energy (Fig 57–16). Although this particular entity is not common, electrophysiologists watch closely for any

evidence of bundle-branch reentry because of the vulnerability of the tachycardia to ablative techniques.

Not a great deal of progress has been made since 1988 in the general field of ablation of ventricular tachycardia. Surgery itself (involving large areas of resection and cryoablation) is wholly successful in fewer than 70% of cases, and catheter ablation would not be expected to be more successful. During surgical resections of aneurysms, we commonly find a large thrombus overlying the area of reentry; this thrombus would presumably prevent destructive energy from reaching the endocardium. Finally, the left ventricle is inherently difficult to map. These facts explain why catheter ablative techniques have not shown the same amount of success

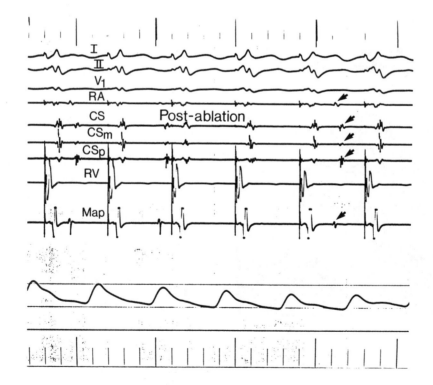

FIG 57–10.
Case 2. After the ablation, there is a block from the ventricle to the atrium during ventricular pacing. The *arrows* point to atrial activation, which is clearly unrelated to ventricular pacing. Thus, the concealed pathway has been ablated. See Figure 57–4 for abbreviations.

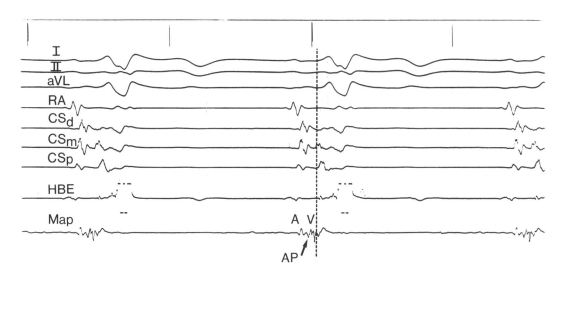

FIG 57–11.

Case 3. A 21-year-old woman with a posteroseptal accessory pathway. The earliest ventricular activation is seen in the posterior portion of the right ventricle, against the septum. A potential from the accessory pathway is recorded *(AP)*. Abbreviations are as in Figure 57–4.

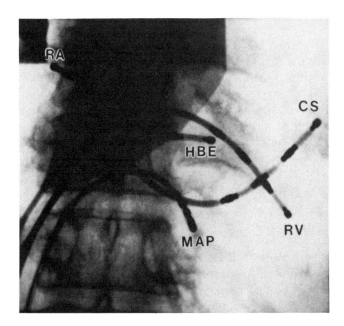

FIG 57–12.

Case 3. A 30-degree RAO projection of final catheter position. The large tipped ablation catheter *(MAP)* is just across the tricuspid valve, torqued against the septum. Catheters are in the coronary sinus *(CS)*, right ventricle *(RV)*, right atrium *(RA)*, and His bundle *(HBE)*.

in curing ventricular tachycardia as they have with supraventricular tachycardias. We have tended to restrict our ablation attempts to patients who are truly not surgical aneurysmectomy candidates and who are not candidates for more sophisticated antitachycardia pacing/defibrillator combinations. In those patients who do undergo catheter ablative techniques, we have found that an approach through the mitral valve via the atrial septum allows easier left ventricular mapping. It seems that the worldwide success rate has not improved dramatically since 1988.

An intriguing new concept is that of "chemical" ablation, primarily investigated by Brugada et al.[20] Central to this approach is the concept that ventricular tachycardia is associated with a "culprit" artery just as myocardial ischemia typically involves a culprit artery. That is, the micro reentry circuit responsible for post–myocardial infarction ventricular tachycardia is contained in the border zone between scar and viable myocardium in which islands of connective tissue interdigitate with myocardium. This area of the reentry circuit is fed by a particular artery, which may be identified by infusing an antiarrhythmic agent or iced saline via a suitably small angioplasty catheter and occluding the lumen of the artery with the angioplasty balloon to pre-

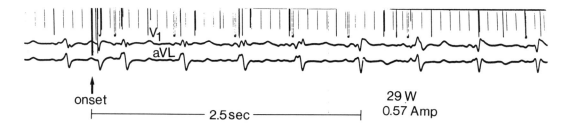

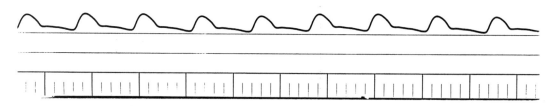

FIG 57–13.
Case 3. After 2.5 seconds of RF energy delivery, the delta wave was permanently ablated. This is more clearly seen in aVL.

vent backflow. If these agents reproducibly terminate induced ventricular tachycardia, the artery involved has been identified as the artery feeding the myocardium that is responsible for ventricular tachycardia, the "culprit" artery. One can then destroy this area permanently by infusing a toxic substance, typically absolute ethanol. The technique is promising but early in its investigational phase. It offers an intriguing insight into pathophysiology if it proves widely successful, and it presents an interesting collaboration between coronary and electrophysiology interventionalists.

ATRIOVENTRICULAR NODE MODIFICATION

Some 20% of patients older than 60 years have either paroxysmal or chronic atrial fibrillation. For those patients in whom maintenance of sinus rhythm is not possible, control of ventricular rate is achieved with AV nodal blockers such as digoxin, β-blockers, or calcium channel blockers. Although a "cure" of atrial fibrillation with catheter ablative techniques appears not to be possible (however, there is an intriguing suggestion that high-energy shocks delivered in the low right atrium might "cure" atrial flutter),[21] various attempts have been made to permanently modify AV conduction such that rapid conduction is eliminated but that normal conduc-

tion, for example fewer than 100 beats per minute, remains and a permanent pacemaker is avoided. Unfortunately, these attempts to consistently and safely alter AV conduction have thus far been unsuccessful.[22] It is clear that there are patients who have failed complete AV junction ablation either via catheters or at the time of open thoracotomy and whose rates during atrial fibrillation became slower than before the ablation. Thus it appears that it is theoretically feasible to consistently produce some sort of permanent control over the rapidity of AV conduction. If this can be consistently achieved, the benefits would be widespread in view of the prevalence of atrial fibrillation.

SUMMARY

In 1991, with RF energy the success rate for producing complete AV block approaches 100%. However, the goal of permanently modifying the rapidity of AV conduction during chronic atrial fibrillation and yet avoiding a permanent pacemaker remains elusive. Accessory pathways in all locations can now be safely ablated in a cost-effective manner,[23] and this may soon become the treatment of choice, preferable to drugs. Ablation now offers an effective and safe alternative to chronic medical therapy in the treatment of AV node reentrant tachycardia. Electrophysiologists will likely become

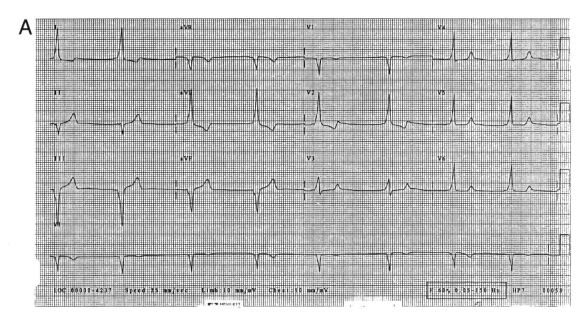

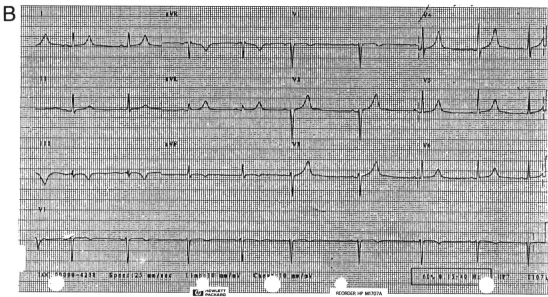

FIG 57–14.
Case 3. Electrocardiograms before **(A)** and after **(B)** ablation show the loss of delta waves.

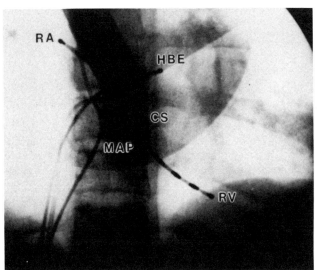

FIG 57–15.
Although AV node reentrant tachycardia is generally approached with ablation near the AV node (*HBE* in this 30-degree RAO projection), a posterior approach is sometimes effective, with a lower risk of heart block. Here, a burst delivered near the coronary sinus *(CS)* os via the large tipped mapping catheter *(MAP)* was effective. The concept of such physically distinct AV nodal pathways as the cause of AV node reentrant tachycardia is intriguing. Catheters are also in the right atrium *(RA)* and right ventricle *(RV)*.

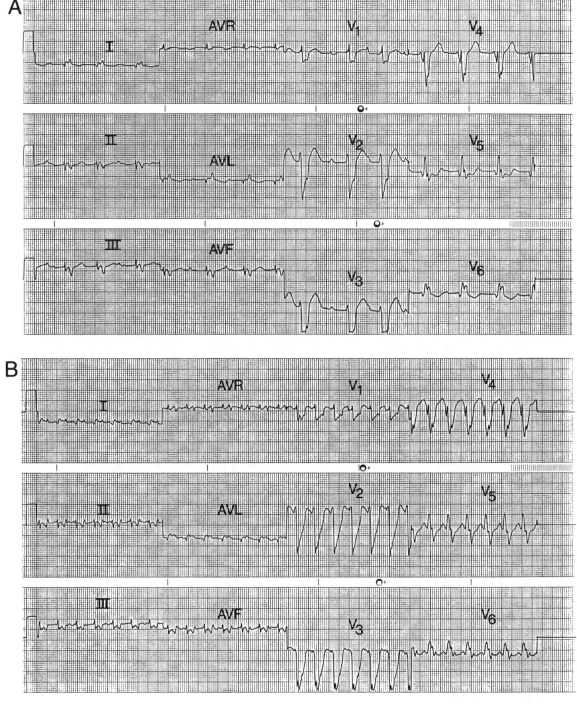

FIG 57–16.

A 72-year-old man with bundle-branch reentry ventricular tachycardia. The baseline electrogram **(A)** and that during ventricular tachycardia **(B)** are nearly identical and show left bundle-branch block. The macroreentrant tachycardia circuit appears to be conducting down the right bundle, through diseased and dilated left ventricle tissue, with reentry into the right bundle. Ablation of the right bundle (somewhat more distal than the bundle of His) is curative.

comfortable with the notion of performing an initial diagnostic electrophysiology study and curing the patient with catheter ablation in the same setting.[24] Finally, although ventricular tachycardia associated with bundle-branch reentry can now be reliably cured by interrupting the right bundle branch, most forms of ventricular tachycardia remain difficult to control by using catheter ablation techniques.

REFERENCES

1. Gallagher JJ, Svenson RH, Kasell JH, et al: Catheter technique for closed-chest ablation of the atrioventricular conduction system. *N Engl J Med* 1982; 306:194–200.
2. Scheinman MM, Morady R, Hess DS, et al: Catheter-induced ablation of the atrioventricular junction to control refractory supraventricular arrhythmias. *JAMA* 1982; 248:851–855.
3. Scheinman MM, Evans GT: Catheter electrical ablation of cardiac arrhythmias: A summary report of the Percutaneous Cardiac Mapping and Ablation Registry, in Brugada P, Wellens HJJ (eds): *Cardiac Arrhythmias: Where to Go From Here?* Mount Kisco, NY, Futura, 1987.
4. Bardy GH, Coltorti F, Ivey TD, et al: Some factors affecting bubble formation with catheter-mediated defibrillation pulses. *Circulation* 1986; 73:525–538.
5. Fisher JD, Brodman R, Kim SG, et al: Attempted nonsurgical electrical ablation of accessory pathways via the coronary sinus in the Wolff-Parkinson-White syndrome. *J Am Coll Cardiol* 1984; 4:685–694.
6. Ruder MA, Mead RH, Gaudiani V, et al: Transvenous catheter ablation of extranodal accessory pathways. *J Am Coll Cardiol* 1988; 11:1245–1253.
7. Ruder MA, Davis JD, Eldar M, et al: Effects of catheter-delivered electrical discharges near the tricuspid annulus in dogs. *J Am Coll Cardiol* 1987; 10:693–701.
8. Warin JF, Haissaguerre M, Lemetayer P, et al: Catheter ablation of accessory pathways with a direct approach: Results in 35 patients. *Circulation* 1988; 78:800–815.
9. Ross DL, Johnson DC, Denniss AR, et al: Curative surgery for atrioventricular junctional (AV nodal) reentrant tachycardia. *J Am Coll Cardiol* 1985; 6:1383–1392.
10. Haissaguerre M, Warin JF, Lemetayer P, et al: Closed-chest ablation of retrograde conduction in patients with atrioventricular nodal reentrant tachycardia. *N Engl J Med* 1989; 320:426–433.
11. Ruder MA, Mead RH, Smith NA, et al: Comparison of pre- and postoperative conduction patterns in patients surgically cured of atrioventricular node reentrant tachycardia. *J Am Coll Cardiol* 1991; 17:397–402.
12. Harken AH, Horowitz LN, Josephson ME: Comparison of standard aneurysmectomy and aneurysmectomy with directed endocardial resection for the treatment of recurrent sustained ventricular tachycardia. *J Thorac Cardiovasc Surg* 1980; 80:527–534.
13. Hartzler GO: Electrode catheter ablation of refractory focal ventricular tachycardia. *J Am Coll Cardiol* 1983; 2:1107–1113.
14. Morady F, Scheinman MM, DiCarlo LA Jr, et al: Catheter ablation of ventricular tachycardia with intracardiac shocks: Results in 33 patients. *Circulation* 1987; 75:1037–1049.
15. Winkle RA, Mead RH, Ruder MA, et al: Long-term outcome with the automatic implantable cardioverter-defibrillator. *J Am Coll Cardiol* 1989; 13:1353–1361.
16. Kuck KH, Kunze KP, Schluter M, et al: Ablation of a left-sided free-wall accessory pathway by percutaneous catheter application of radiofrequency current in a patient with the Wolff-Parkinson-White syndrome. *PACE* 1989; 12:1681.
17. Calkins H, Sousa J, Rosenheck S, et al: Catheter ablation of accessory atrioventricular pathways using radiofrequency energy (abstract). *J Am Coll Cardiol* 1991; 17:232.
18. Lee MA, Morady F, Kadish A, et al: Catheter modification of the atrioventricular junction with radiofrequency energy for control of atrioventricular nodal reentry tachycardia, *Circulation* 1991; 83:827–835.
19. Tchou P, Jazayeri M, Denker S, et al: Transcatheter electrical ablation of right bundle branch: A method of treating macroreentrant ventricular tachycardia attributed to bundle branch reentry. *Circulation* 1988; 78:246–257.
20. Brugada P, de Swart H, Smeets JLRM, et al: Transcoronary chemical ablation of ventricular tachycardia. *Circulation* 1989; 79:475–482.
21. Saoudi N, Atallah G, Kirkorian G, et al: Catheter ablation of the atrial myocardium in human type I atrial flutter. *Circulation* 1990; 81:762–771.
22. Engelstein ED, Duckeck W, Geiger M, et al: Clinical efficacy of AV nodal modulation versus ablation with radiofrequency current in atrial fibrillation/flutter (abstract). *J Am Coll Cardiol* 1991; 17:175.
23. de Buitleir M, Sousa J, Calkins H, et al: Dramatic reduction in medical care costs associated with radiofrequency catheter ablation of accessory pathways (abstract). *J Am Coll Cardiol* 1991; 17:109.
24. Morady F, Kadish A, Calkins H, et al: Diagnosis and immediate cure of paroxysmal supraventricular tachycardia (abstract). *Circulation* 1990; 82(suppl 3):689.

PART XI

Rational Application of Interventional Techniques

58

Percutaneous Balloon Pericardial Window

Peter C. Block, M.D.
Igor F. Palacios, M.D.

Definitive treatment of pericardial tamponade requires removal of compressing pericardial fluid by prompt pericardiocentesis and drainage.[1-8] In most patients with pericardial effusion and tamponade, percutaneous pericardial drainage with an indwelling pericardial catheter is adequate, and recurrence of pericardial effusion and tamponade is relatively uncommon. Pericardial fluid accumulation usually decreases over the first 24 to 48 hours after catheter drainage, and the catheter can then be removed safely. However, recurrence of effusion and cardiac tamponade is an indication for placement of a pericardial window.[2] Longer-lasting drainage of the pericardium is necessary in only 14% of patients with pericardial effusion and tamponade.[3] Several additional approaches are possible to prevent reaccumulation of pericardial fluid, including intrapericardial installation of sclerosing agents (tetracycline) and the use of chemotherapy and radiotherapy.[4-6] A surgically created pericardial window gives long-term drainage for pericardial effusion,[7, 8] but especially in conditions of malignant pericardial effusion, morbidity and late recurrence of symptoms are common.[9, 10] Therefore, particularly in patients with metastatic malignancy and a limited life span, it is desirable to avoid surgery and general anesthesia. Other causes of pericarditis with effusion may occasionally produce tamponade — inflammatory pericarditis, pericardial effusion associated with renal failure, and nonspecific pericarditis. A percutaneous balloon pericardial window may also avoid surgery and allow adequate drainage of pericardial effusion in these instances.[11]

TECHNIQUE

All patients with pericardial tamponade should first have standard pericardiocentesis via the subxiphoid approach. A standard 5.5 F pigtail catheter is placed in the pericardial space and, after all fluid is aspirated, is sutured and left in the pericardial space for ongoing drainage. The catheter can then be aspirated three or four times each day, and the amount of pericardial fluid that has reaccumulated is recorded. After each drainage of the pericardial space the pigtail catheter must be flushed with a small amount (1 mL) of heparinized saline to maintain patency. If after 3 days there is ongoing drainage of more than 100 cc/24 hr, placement of a pericardial window is indicated. The patient is taken to the cardiac catheterization laboratory and sedated with diazepam and morphine if appropriate. The subxiphoid area around the indwelling pericardial pigtail catheter is infiltrated with 1% Lidocaine (Xylocaine) for local anesthesia. Three or 4 cc of contrast medium is injected through the pigtail catheter into the pericardial space under fluoroscopy to identify the parietal pericardium (Fig 58–1). A 0.038-in. stiff (Cook, Inc.) transfer wire guide with a preshaped curlicue at the tip is advanced through the pigtail catheter and introduced well into the pericardium (Fig 58–2). The pigtail catheter is removed, the wire guide is left within the pericardial space, and a 20-mm-diameter, 3-cm-long dilating balloon catheter (Mansfield, Inc., Watertown, Mass) is advanced over the wire guide until it straddles the parietal pericardium. If it is difficult to advance the dilating balloon catheter, a 10 or 11 F dilator can first be advanced over the guidewire. It is important to advance the bal-

687

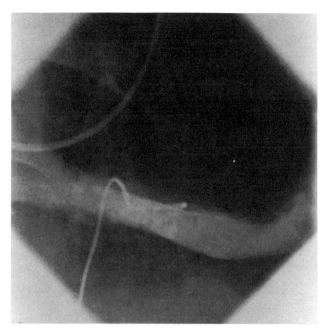

FIG 58–1.
Fluoroscopic view of the injection of contrast medium into the pericardial space outlining the parietal pericardium.

loon beyond the skin and subcutaneous tissues so as to avoid a pericardial-cutaneous fistula. The balloon is then inflated manually until the waist produced by the

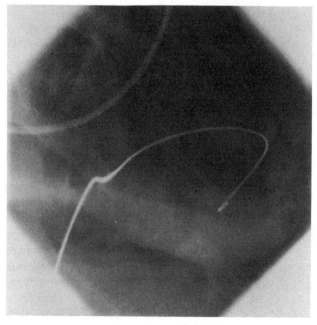

FIG 58–2.
The 5.5 F pigtail catheter is seen in the pericardial space. The 0.038-in. wire guide is through the pigtail catheter, and the tip is in the pericardial space.

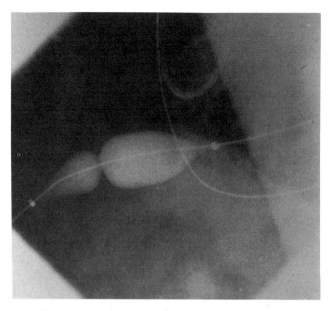

FIG 58–3.
The dilating balloon catheter has been advanced over the wire guide and straddles the parietal pericardium in the mid-portion of the inflated balloon.

parietal pericardium disappears (Figs 58–3 and 58–4). Two to three inflations are usually performed to ensure an adequate opening in the parietal pericardium. Lateral fluoroscopy is helpful in showing the indentation of the balloon. The balloon dilating catheter is then removed and the wire guide left in place. A new 5.5 F pigtail catheter is advanced over the wire guide into the peri-

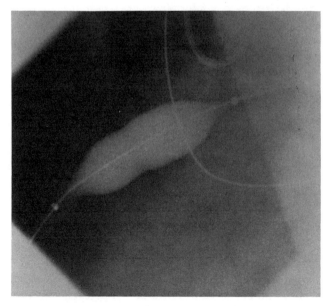

FIG 58–4.
The fully inflated balloon produces a pericardial window.

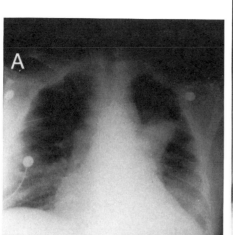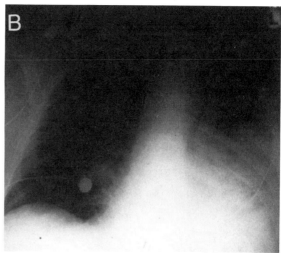

FIG 58–5.
A, chest x-ray film (posteroanterior) of a patient with malignant pericardial effusion on admission. Note the large cardiac silhouette. **B,** posteroanterior chest x-ray film of the same patient 3 days after percutaneous balloon pericardial window. Note the smaller cardiac silhouette and a new left pleural effusion.

cardial space for ongoing drainage if necessary. Contrast can be injected through the pigtail catheter to visualize drainage of the pericardial space. Daily pericardial drainage monitoring is continued as it was before the placement of the pericardial window. If there is less than 50 cc drainage per 48 hours over the next day or when there is evidence of a new or increasing pleural effusion (usually on the left) by chest x-ray, the pigtail catheter can be removed. Two-dimensional echocardiography may be used to monitor the amount of pericardial effusion after placement of the percutaneous balloon pericardial window. The radiologic development of a new pleural effusion or an increase in a pre-existing pleural effusion takes approximately 3 days.[11] The range is 2 to 5 days. Pleural effusion usually occurs on the left side but can be bilateral (Fig 58–5). The pleural effusion usually involves only a third to a half of the hemithorax. In the series reported no patient required thoracentesis for relief of symptoms of the pleural effusion. Recurrent pericardial tamponade or pericardial effusion is unlikely. In patients with inflammatory pericarditis and malignant pericardial effusion, a surgical window frequently closes. However, a repeat percutaneous pericardial window can be performed without anesthesia and the risk of surgery.

The number of patients treated with this technique so far is small. However, it does appear that the procedure can be performed successfully, particularly in patients with malignant pericardial effusion. The results seem to be similar to standard surgical pericardial window placement. The technique should not be used in patients with infectious pericarditis for fear of drainage of infected fluid into the mediastinum and pleural cavities. A small multicenter trial has confirmed the usefulness of this technique. Excessive pleural fluid may accumulate.

The presumed mechanism of a percutaneous balloon pericardial window is that balloon inflation produces a tear in the parietal pericardium. This leads to a communication of the pericardial space with the mediastinum and thence the pleural and possibly the abdominal cavity.

REFERENCES

1. Guberman BA, Fowler NO, Engel PJ, et al: Cardiac tamponade in medical patients. *Circulation* 1981; 64:633–640.
2. Fowler NO: Cardiac tamponade, in Fowler NO (ed): *The Pericardium in Health and Disease.* Mt Kisco, NY, Futura, 1985, pp 247–280.
3. Koperly SL, Callahan JA, Tajik AJ, et al: Percutaneous pericardial catheter drainage: Report of 42 consecutive cases. *Am J Cardiol* 1986; 58:633–635.
4. Davis S, Sharma SM, Blumberg ED, et al: Intrapericardial tetracycline for the management of cardiac tamponade secondary to malignant pericardial effusion. *N Engl J Med* 1978; 229:1113–1114.
5. Gregory JR, McMurtrey MJ, Mountain CF: A surgical approach to the treatment of pericardial effusion in cancer patients. *Am J Clin Oncol* 1985; 8:319–323.
6. Hankins JR, Satterfield JR, Aisner J, et al: Pericardial window for malignant pericardial effusion. *Ann Thorac Surg* 1980; 30:465–469.
7. Fontenelle LJ, Cuello L, Dooley BN: Subxiphoid pericardial window: A simple and safe method for diagnosing and treating acute and chronic pericardial effusions. *J Thorac Cardiovas Surg* 1971; 62:95–97.

8. Santos GH, Frater RWM: The subxiphoid approach in the treatment of pericardial effusion. *Ann Thorac Surg* 1977; 23:467–470.

9. Palatinos GM, Thurer RJ, Kaiser GA: Comparison of effectiveness and safety of operations on the pericardium. *Chest* 1985; 88:30–33.

10. Piehler JM, Pluth JR, Schaff HV, et al: Surgical management of effusive pericardial disease. Influence of extent of pericardial resection on clinical course. *J Thorac Cardiovasc Surg* 1985; 90:506–516.

11. Palacios IF, Tuzcu EM, Ziskind AA, et al: Percutaneous balloon pericardial window for patients with malignant pericardial effusion and tamponade. *Cathet Cardiovasc Diagn* 1991; 22:244–249.

59

Overview of New Technologies: The Bottom Line

Robert Ginsburg M.D.

From "simple" balloon angioplasty to gene transfection, the field of interventional cardiology continues to evolve at a rapid pace. Originally it was hoped that the balloon would increase the luminal size of arteries in a safe, cost-effective, and durable manner that would obviate the need for surgical bypass procedures. However, with time it was realized that this dream would not be fulfilled. Issues such as restenosis, diffuse disease, and abrupt closures would become significant medical problems. These issues stimulated the development of new, alternative techniques that in addition to cracking plaque would sand, cut, slice, and suck it away.

RATIONALE

The goal to developing alternatives to balloons is to prolong durability (i.e., prevent restenosis), increase safety, and treat otherwise impossible-to-treat lesions. Restenosis is a real phenomenon that occurs about 40% of the time with balloons, and as a result the overall impact on medical costs is of great concern. Although a nice annuity for cardiologists, repetitive angioplasty for the same lesion robs the health care system and is a major problem to those involved with cost containment. Therefore, enormous amounts of work are under way to understand and treat the phenomenon. Because it appears that restenosis is a natural response to injury, inhibiting the process will be and has proved to be extremely difficult to eliminate. A pharmacologic approach including agents such as steroids, angiotensin converting enzyme (ACE) inhibitors, colchicine, aspirin, heparin, warfarin (Coumadin), antimitotics, fish oils, etc., have all been tried without any uniform or convincing success. Mechanical approaches to decrease restenosis have

also been evaluated. Initially, the concept to device development was to remove enough plaque and to leave behind a rheologically benign surface that would not be a fertile nesting ground for platelets. Therefore the mechanical cutters, sanders, and slicers were developed. For the most part, these technologies have not changed restenosis. Much more interesting, however, has been the observations recently made with endovascular stents. In de novo stenoses, it was observed that in vessels larger than 3 mm the restenosis rate was very low in the 5% to 8% range — clearly very different from the experience with balloons. Additionally, the atherectomy data suggested that in large vessels with focal, de novo lesions the restenosis rate is very low. It appears from these observations that the process of intimal proliferation is a finite and self-limiting response to injury. Therefore, if the vessel is large enough and the lumen created is of sufficient size, then the resulting lumen, even after intimal proliferation, should remain of sufficient diameter to sustain a good clinical result. Thus, if one can eliminate acute clot formation and create a large luminal area, restenosis may be less of a problem.

The second rationale for developing new technologies is to decrease the incidence of acute complications. The recommendations from the American College of Cardiology and the American Heart Association task forces is that percutaneous transluminal coronary angioplasty (PTCA) should only be performed in centers with surgical backup. The reason for this is that even with the most experienced operators the rate of complications requiring some form of urgent surgery is 2% to 3%. However, every interventionist knows that even in the best of situations an operating room may not be available or some other kind of scheduling problem exists. Moreover, there are many catheterization laboratories around the country that are not in places with immediate access to cardiac surgeons, yet they have operators skilled in angioplasty. Therefore, what is needed are devices that do not rip and tear the atheromatous plaque but result in a more predictable and safe angioplasty result. Current results and clinical experience suggest that several of the newer devices such as the Simpson Atherocath. Rotablator, and the excimer laser have fewer complications than balloons do. However, it must be qualified that these devices are suitable for specific well-defined lesions and are not as versatile as balloons. Nonetheless, it suggests that safer devices are possible.

Additionally, if complications do occur, there are several devices that can support a patient until either transport to a surgical center or until an operating room is available. These include support devices such as intra-aortic balloon pumping, percutaneous cardiopulmonary support systems, perfusion catheters, and endovascular stents. In an acute crisis, the availability of cardiopulmonary support (CPS) and stents should make most mad dashes to the operating room very rare.

The final role for new technologies is the ability to foray into vessels that until now could not be treated by balloons. These include ostial lesions, vein grafts, calcified lesions, total occlusions, and diffuse disease. None of the newer devices can do it all, but each new method has found its respective niche. For example, the Simpson Atherocath is ideal for large, proximal ostial stenoses, and the excimer laser is effective for type B and C lesions. Whether or not the expansion of angioplasty indications is wise or prudent will require further evaluation and experience since the more complex the lesions treated the greater the potential risk of complications.

CLINICAL ASSESSMENT

During the past few years several devices have been approved by the Food and Drug Administration (FDA) and several have disappeared. The ones to never make it to the coronaries include the Laserprobe hot tip catheter, the Smart-Laser, and the Kensey catheter. The Simpson Atherocath and excimer laser have been approved, and the Rotablator and endovascular stents will also receive approval in the very near future.

Initially, the appeal of many of these new technologies was for marketing purposes — for both the hospital as well as one's own practice. As incredible pressure for cost containment as well as sobering clinical reports began to appear, only new technologies that actually improve upon balloons — not equivalents — were to be the survivors. Additionally, the FDA and the respective companies involved with these new devices realized that the old standard of "see one, do one, teach one" was no longer wise. Therefore beginning with the Atherocath and subsequently with the Palmaz stent, certifying didactic and practical courses were required.

The Simpson Atherocath is more expensive than standard balloons and more difficult to use. Additionally, in its present format the guiding catheters are larger than those used for balloon PTCA. The atherectomy catheter is not recommended for degenerated vein grafts, distal circumflex vessels, unprotected left main arteries, calcified aorta-ostial lesions, severely tortuous arteries, heavy calcification, diffuse lesions greater than 20 mm, and vessels smaller than 2.5 mm. Its specific indications and places where it has an advantage over balloons are in ostial lesions, eccentric stenoses in large proximal vessels, nondegenerated saphenous vein grafts, protected left main arteries, and ulcerated lesions. Some data suggests that in very focal stenoses in large vessels the restenosis rate is lower in de novo lesions when this device is used vs. balloons. In probably 10% to 15% of all angioplasty cases the atherectomy catheter may have a role. Although it could probably be used more often than that, the costs are not as yet justifiable.

Free-beam laser angioplasty utilizing catheters with concentric arrays of fibers is undergoing extensive evaluation. Two laser systems presently being evaluated include the excimer and holmium: YAG systems. The excimer laser system has been through the FDA panel and has been approved for specific indications. The excimer catheter should be competitively priced to balloons; however, the laser generators themselves are quite expensive. The laser systems appear to be better than balloons in type B and C lesions. The lasers work well in total occlusions once they are traversed by a guidewire, as well as in diffuse disease and calcified stenoses. They are not useful in tortuous or acutely angulated vessels, bifurcation lesions, thrombus, and vessels with flaps or dissections. The laser catheter is user friendly but requires some additional skills. The ablation rate of these systems is slow, and there is a tendency to advance the catheter too rapidly through a lesion, which can cause dissections. There is no evidence to date that restenosis is improved with this technology, and to avoid complementary balloon angioplasty, only vessels less than 2.5 mm should be treated. Therefore the laser systems in their present format are reserved for complex angioplasty.

The Rotablator is now available for the treatment of peripheral vascular disease and should be approved for the treatment of coronary artery disease. Because of the fixed burr size the device is ideally suited for vessels smaller than 2.5 mm. The Rotablator gives a very predictable result since it does not tear the vessel but rather sands the area of plaque. This may cause transient spasm, but abrupt closures or flaps are rare. The device will probably cost slightly more than balloons, and a control box is needed. The Rotablator is ideally suited for diffuse disease (<25 mm), calcified lesions, tortuous vessels, and lesions where guide support is a problem. The wire used with the device is not as flexible as one might be used to, and sometimes an exchange of wires may be necessary. There is no evidence as yet that it significantly alters restenosis.

The endovascular stent is approved for peripheral vascular applications but not as yet for the heart. The problem with the stent is that during acute placement there is the real possibility of thrombus formation. Once past this initial hurdle, however, the stent endothelializes, and the risk of thrombus dissipates. The stent has several specific roles. First, in de novo lesions in large vessels there is evidence that there is less restenosis. However, because of the expense, the inherent risks, and the fact that other devices may do as well in similar circumstances, the device is not a primary tool for this type of stenosis. The stent is very useful in complications from balloon angioplasty such as abrupt closure and flap formation. It can truly snatch victory from the jaws of defeat! It is not ideal in vessels loaded with thrombus because of its propensity to clot. In vessels that have recurrent restenosis the stent may be of some use, especially if the vessel is larger than 3 mm in diameter.

The transluminal extraction catheter, also approved for peripheral use, has a smaller coronary application niche than the above devices. The freely rotating blades in an unprotected environment, even with guidewire support, makes the risk of perforation or dissection real. The device excels in old vein grafts because of its vacuum waste removal system. It may be the only device suitable for older vein grafts, but further information and data are needed. Regarding the restenosis rate, it has no improvement over balloons, and because of the fixed tip size, treated vessels should be smaller than 3 mm in diameter.

MEDICAL-INDUSTRIAL INTERACTIONS

More so than at any other time in our lives are the issues of health costs and insurance for all being actively discussed at senior levels. Because of the need for urgent cost containment, Medicare is now determining the costs of new technologies in their decision of whether or not to approve a specific procedure. The physician reimbursements and hospital-reimbursements for angioplasty will decrease over the next few years. Therefore, there will be greater pressure on companies to decrease hardware costs and may make the integration of new technologies somewhat more difficult. The focus in industry research will be the development of cheaper and safer tools for angioplasty. Several questions will cross the table in marketing conference rooms: does one really need an ultrasonic picture of the inside of the vessel to perform successful angioplasty? How many combinations and permutations of balloons and wires are really needed in angioplasty? Do lasers, atherectomy catheters, and stents add enough to the procedure to justify their costs? Maybe we should just put our energies into transthoracic fiberoptic guided left internal mammary artery (LIMA) implantation! Will the catheter of the decade will be called Mr. Workhorse rather than Slinky, Skinny, MVP, Slalom, Shadow, Ace, or Orion?

THE BOTTOM LINE

Angioplasty as a procedure will continue to undergo constant scrutiny by the medical community as well as third-party payers. Is the procedure equivalent or better than medicine or surgery and in what situations? Can it improve morbidity or mortality in patients with coronary artery disease? Can it prevent myocardial infarction? Is it truly cost-effective? These and many more questions will be raised.

In the final decade of this century, interventional cardiology will continue to evolve. Advancements will be made on the basis of our knowledge of the underlying pathophysiology rather than the shotgun approach that worked so well in the past. Whether it be new pharmacologic agents, better mechanical devices, or genetic engineering, it will nonetheless be an exciting time.

60

A Multidevice, Lesion-Specific Treatment Strategy for Unfavorable Coronary Lesions

Martin B. Leon, M.D.

Augusto D. Pichard, M.D.

Kenneth M. Kent, M.D.

Lowell F. Satler, M.D.

Jeffrey J. Popma, M.D.

Pamela A. Shotts, R.N.

Kathleen M. Donovan, R.N.

Since the introduction of percutaneous coronary artery angioplasty (PTCA) by Andreas Grüentzig almost 15 years ago,[1] the use of applied mechanical barotrauma via catheter-based techniques has been fully integrated as an important therapeutic alternative in patients with coronary artery disease. Nevertheless, there has also been an enhanced recognition of the problems and limitations associated with PTCA, including (1) the management of unfavorable lesion morphologies (such as ostial lesions, diffuse disease, intracoronary thrombus, etc.); (2) abrupt closure syndrome (in 2% to 5% of cases); (3) treating high-"risk" patients (requiring mechanical or pharmacologic support); and (4) chronic restenosis at the treated lesion site. In an effort to effectively confront these limitations that render PTCA either less successful or more hazardous, a variety of new investigational angioplasty techniques have emerged over the past 5 years. Broadly, investigational angioplasty devices fall into one of three categories — laser angioplasty, atherectomy, and stent implantation. The ultimate clinical utility of these investigational angioplasty devices will depend upon the critical assessment of their indicated use patterns, efficacy and safety profile, user friendliness, and cost-effectiveness vs. conventional PTCA.[2, 3]

The purpose of this manuscript is to describe a large single-center experience with a variety of investigational angioplasty devices to develop use profiles in the management of unfavorable coronary lesions.[4] Upon careful review of these data, we have observed the emergence of a multidevice lesion-specific approach integrated with PTCA to optimize acute angiographic results in a variety of lesion subsets. The clear delineation of when new investigational angioplasty techniques should be applied will ultimately change the overall operating strategies of interventional cardiologists in the next many years.

METHODS

Investigational Angioplasty Devices

1. *Excimer laser coronary angioplasty (ELCA)*[5]: The 308-nm, pulsed-stretched (200 ns) excimer laser was used in all cases (Advanced Interventional Systems, Irv-

ine, Calif). Initially, the pulse energy density used was 35 to 40 mJ/mm² but later was increased to 45 to 60 mJ/mm.² This system was routinely operated at 20 Hz for 3-second bursts with slow antegrade movement (1 mm/sec) of the over-the-wire laser catheter. Laser catheters used included 1.3-, 1.6-, and 2.0-mm-diameter devices usually employing minimum dead space technology with several hundred, 50-μm optical fibers.

2. *Fluorescence-guided laser angioplasty (FGLA)*[6]: A dual-laser system (MCM Laboratories, Mountain View, Calif) incorporating a diagnostic laser for fluorescence spectroscopy coupled to a pulsed dye laser for tissue ablation was used in a small number of patients. A 1.5-mm over-the-wire laser catheter was employed after guidewire recanalization of severe lesions or chronic total occlusions.

3. *Laser balloon angioplasty (LBA)*[7]: The continuous-wave Nd:YAG system was operated with dedicated catheters (2.5 to 3.5 mm in diameter) for 20-second graded heat trains followed by 20-second cooling sequences with the balloon inflated and the laser off (USCI, Billerica, Mass). Single or multiple exposures were used depending on clinical circumstances.

4. *Directional coronary atherectomy (DCA)*[8]: The technique of directional atherectomy employing variable catheter sizes (5 to 7 F) matched to the vessel dimensions each containing a housing and cutting unit for tissue removal and retrieval (Devices for Vascular Intervention, Redwood City, Calif) was utilized in all patients. More recently, we have selectively used a lower-profile catheter system with a refined nose cone and polyethylene terephthalate (PET) balloon construction.

5. *Transluminal extraction atherectomy (TEC)*[9]: This front-end cutting and suction extraction device removes *macro* particulate matter through catheter sizes varying from 1.8 to 2.5 mm (InterVentional Technologies, San Diego).

6. *High-speed rotational ablation (ROTA)*[10]: Steel burrs (from 1.25 to 2.5 mm in diameter) mounted on flexible catheters that rotate at greater than 175,000 rpm remove plaque *micro* particulate matter with egress into the coronary microcirculation (Heart Technology, Bellevue, Wash). A "stepped" technique of slowly increasing catheter sizes, based upon lesion severity and vessel size, was utilized during the study.

7. *Stent implantation*[11]: Balloon-expandable, either tubular slotted stents made of stainless steel (Johnson & Johnson Interventional Systems, Warren, NJ) or coiled stents made of tantalum (Medtronic, San Diego), were utilized for all procedures. Predilatation with undersized balloon catheters was usually performed prior to stent implantation, and postdilatation was often required to optimize angiographic results.

Patient Population

This report encompasses all patients treated consecutively by one or more of the senior interventional operators between October 1, 1988, and December 1, 1991. A total of 1,604 lesions in 1,456 patients were treated by one of the aforementioned investigational angioplasty techniques (Table 60–1). The use of adjunct balloon angioplasty was at the discretion of the operator and varied during the course of the study. Initially, there was greater interest in attempting to achieve "stand-alone" results with each of the investigational angioplasty devices. After January 1, 1991, the more liberal use of adjunct balloon angioplasty was recommended in an effort to optimize initial angiographic results such that the largest, least disrupted lumen would be achieved at each treatment site.

Definition of Terms

Unfavorable Angioplasty Lesions.—The categories of unfavorable angioplasty lesions included in this report were chronic total occlusions, dissections (either de novo or PTCA induced), lesion eccentricity, intralesion or perilesion thrombus, saphenous vein graft pathology, diffuse disease (greater than 2-cm axial length), ostial lesions, and undilatable lesions (wire crosses the lesion but unable to cross with a balloon catheter, unable to dilate with a balloon catheter, or incessant recoil after dilatation).

Angiographic Success.—The final post-treatment lumen diameter stenosis was less than 50% of reference vessel segments, with or without adjunct balloon angioplasty.

Major Complications.—In-hospital death, Q wave myocardial infarction, or urgent coronary artery bypass graft surgery were major complications.

TABLE 60–1.
Investigational Angioplasty Devices, Washington Cardiology Center: 1,604 Lesions in 1,456 Patients Through 12/1/91

Device	Lesions Treated
Lasers	
Excimer laser angioplasty	229
Fluorescence-guided laser angioplasty	15
Laser balloon angioplasty	36
Atherectomy	
Directional atherectomy	584
Transluminal extraction atherectomy	65
High-speed rotational atherectomy	374
Stents	
JJIS	11
Wiktor	287
ACS temporary	3

Procedure Success.—Acute angiographic success without in-hospital major complications counted as procedural success.

RESULTS

Of the 1,604 lesions treated, 1,312 (81.7%) fulfilled criteria for unfavorable lesion characteristics (Fig 60–1). Lesion eccentricity was the most frequent unfavorable characteristic, but saphenous vein graft disease, diffuse lesions, and ostial stenoses were all present in more than 10% of the unfavorable lesions treated (Fig 60–2). The percentage of unfavorable lesions treated by each device varied from 56% for stents to 100% for TEC (Fig 60–3). Importantly, the vast majority of stent patients who did not fulfill unfavorable lesion characteristics were in a category of single or multiple restenosis episodes.

The primary angiographic success for all lesions treated with investigational angioplasty devices was 95.2% (Fig 60–4). The angiographic success was lowest in the treatment of lesion-related thrombus (80%) and in chronic total occlusions (87%). Success rates were surprisingly high in several lesion subsets including ostial lesions (91%), dissections (92%), diffuse disease (92%), saphenous vein grafts (96%), and undilatable lesions (98%) (Fig 60–4).

Angiographic success by device was lowest with TEC (86%), largely reflecting the high prevalence of intraluminal thrombus in patients treated with that device (Fig 60–5).

The frequency of major complications (by event) in the 1,456 patients treated included death in 1.3%, urgent bypass surgery, 2.5%; and Q wave myocardial infarction, 3.6% (Fig 60–6). Abrupt closure in the cathe-

terization laboratory or during hospitalization occurred in 3.9% of patients. The overall frequency of major complications by patient was 3.9%. Complications (death, myocardial infarction, bypass surgery, or abrupt closure) were more frequently noted in TEC patients and LBA patients (11% for each device) (Fig 60–7). Again, the increased frequency of complications was undoubtedly due to the high prevalence of intraluminal thrombus in TEC patients and of post-PTCA dissections in patients treated with LBA. The overall procedure success rate was reduced to 91.3% after considering the major complications described above.

When appropriate, adjunct balloon angioplasty was performed to assist in achieving optimal procedure results. In only 28% of procedures was the investigational device used as sole therapy (Fig 60–8). This varied from as high as 36% with DCA (usually pre-DCA dilatation of de novo severe stenoses) to as low as 8% with TEC. In rare instances did adjunct PTCA contribute to major complications when associated with investigational device treatment.

DISCUSSION

In this single-center analysis of acute results after multidevice investigational angioplasty treatment in a large cohort of patients with predominantly unfavorable coronary lesions, potential changes in future operating strategies have emerged. Previously, other than modest variations in balloon angioplasty technique, treatment approaches of markedly variable lesion subsets have become generalized and homogeneous. In retrospect, it seems unreasonable to assume that all coronary lesion morphologies should respond in a uniform manner to mechanical barotrauma. Intravascular ultrasound studies

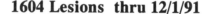

1604 Lesions thru 12/1/91

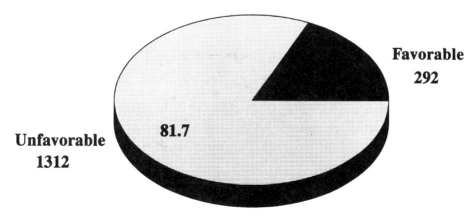

FIG 60–1.
Percentage of favorable and unfavorable lesions treated with investigational angioplasty devices.

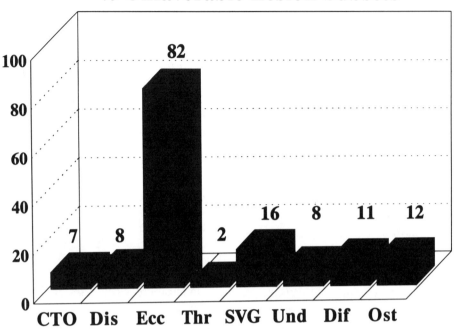

FIG 60–2.
Of the unfavorable lesions treated, the relative frequency of specific unfavorable lesion subsets. *CTO* = chronic total occlusions; *Dis* = dissections; *ECC* = eccentricity; *Thr* = thrombus; *SVG* = saphenous vein graft; *Und* = undilatable lesion; *Dif* = diffuse disease; *Ost* =ostial lesion.

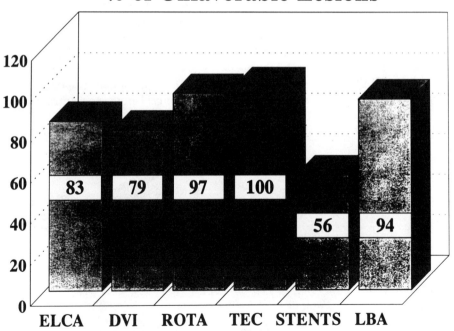

FIG 60–3.
Of all lesions treated, the percentage that had unfavorable characteristics treated by a given device. *ELCA* = excimer laser coronary angioplasty; *DVI* = pacemaker; *ROTA* = rotational ablation; *TEC* = transluminal extraction atherectomy; *LBA* = laser balloon angioplasty.

% Successful Treatment

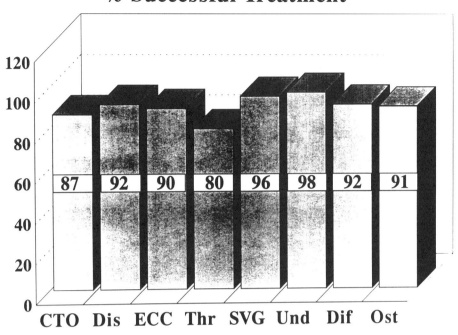

FIG 60–4.
Percent angiographic success after treatment of specific unfavorable lesion subsets with multiple investigational devices.

% Angiographic Success

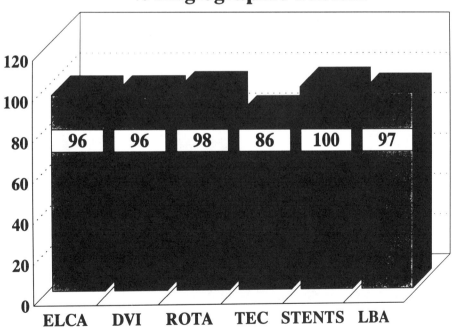

FIG 60–5.
Percent angiographic success for all unfavorable lesion subsets treated by specific investigational devices (abbreviations as in Fig 60–3).

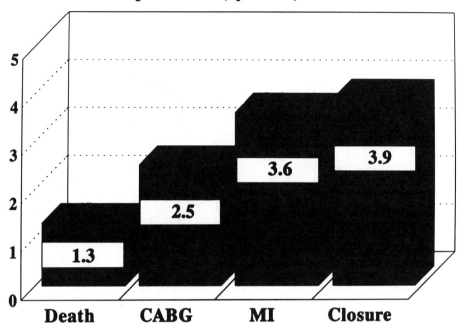

FIG 60–6.
Percent complications by event for the entire patient cohort. *CABG* = coronary artery bypass grafting; *MI* = myocardial infarction.

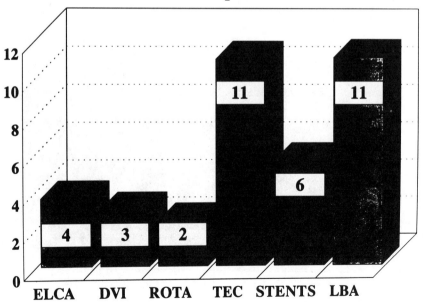

FIG 60–7.
Percentage of complications (death, MI, CABG, or abrupt closure) for the entire patient cohort treated with specific investigational angioplasty devices (abbreviations as in Fig 60–3).

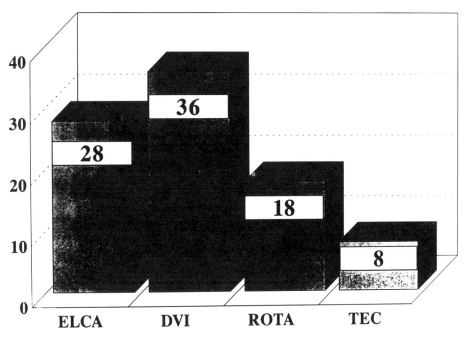

FIG 60–8.
Percentage of unfavorable lesions treated as "stand-alone" procedures (without associated balloon angioplasty) for specific investigational devices (abbreviations as in Fig 60–3).

have indicated that at the site of greatest lumen compromise, lesion morphology appears to favor more fibrocalcific components, which reduces lesion compliance and would diminish the efficacy and safety of mechanical expansion techniques.[12] From a mechanistic viewpoint, initial debulking of such noncompliant lesions by either laser angioplasty or atherectomy techniques, followed by balloon dilatation to achieve the largest vessel lumen, might increase efficacy as well as safety in many of the unfavorable lesion categories treated. The availability of these new devices provides exciting options to test these and other hypotheses.

The overall initial angiographic success rate with multiple investigational angioplasty devices in unfavorable PTCA lesions was greater than 95%. Importantly, this also includes evolution in device technology and operator learning curve experiences during the earlier phases of the study. Unfortunately, no direct comparisons can be made between devices for specific lesion subsets, and no definitive comparisons with PTCA would be appropriate from the current data set. However, historical comparisons with similar lesion cohorts treated with PTCA indicate that a multidevice lesion-specific approach may offer certain advantages. For instance, we achieved a 98% success rate in previously undilatable lesions with a combination of techniques used in this study. Similarly, initial success rates of greater

than 90% for diffuse disease, ostial lesions, and dissections would appear to be substantially improved when compared with conventional PTCA techniques.[13, 14] A particular area of concern is the relatively lower success rates in lesions with thrombus-containing elements. This has caused us to revise our strategy, which now favors more aggressive direct intraluminal and systemic pretreatment lytic therapy prior to catheter manipulation. There are also many prototype devices being developed that might facilitate the removal of thrombus in coronary arteries. Concepts including laser thrombolysis, suction thrombectomy, rheolytic thrombectomy, mechanical thrombectomy, and ultrasound thrombus ablation are all undergoing intensive evaluation at the present time.

The frequency of major complications observed during this study is similar to overall complications reported in large angioplasty series.[15–17] In view of the high-risk nature of the lesion subsets treated, the frequency of complications was acceptable, but direct comparisons with similar lesion subsets managed with PTCA alone are problematic. TEC and LBA procedures were associated with the highest major in-hospital complications (11%). In each case, the complication frequency appeared to reflect underlying clinical circumstances and not device-related problems. The high frequency of intraluminal thrombus associated with many of the vein grafts treated with the TEC device contributed to lower success, more frequent embolic sequelae, and occasional episodes of abrupt closure. LBA was used predominantly in situations of flow-limiting dissections, which inherently were higher-risk scenarios with frequent attendant complications. In many instances, subsequent PTCA was extremely helpful in aborting potential complications by improving initial suboptimal angioplasty results. Frequent vasospasm associated with ROTA could be treated effectively with low-pressure dilatations, and superficial disruption associated with the TEC device has been repaired during adjunct PTCA procedures.

A useful lesson derived as the study evolved was the importance of adjunct PTCA during investigational angioplasty procedures. The concept of "stand-alone" treatment appears to offer little advantages from the standpoint of acute angiographic outcome and may result in higher complications, especially with ELCA and TEC procedures. Relative "undersizing" by using ablative/atherectomy devices that partially remove the non-compliant fibrocalcific elements of the plaque may change lesion compliance and facilitate subsequent mechanical balloon expansion. This technique appears to reduce the frequency of flow-limiting dissections, minimizes deep vessel wall trauma, and may diminish subsequent adverse healing responses. The treatment goal was to provide the best opportunity for a smooth wide channel at the completion of the procedure. Therefore, the overall adjunct balloon angioplasty frequency of 72% should not be construed as a failure of investigational angioplasty techniques as sole definitive therapy but rather a recognition that the integration of investigational angioplasty with PTCA may be a more appropriate treatment strategy.

The purpose of this study was not to examine long-term outcome and restenosis after investigational angioplasty procedures. Thus far, follow-up in the various lesion subsets with the multiple devices is not sufficiently complete to justify conclusive statements. Clearly, additional work is required to determine whether multidevice profiled therapy in unfavorable angioplasty lesions has a beneficial impact on restenosis.

Strategic Device-Specific Use Patterns

After this large experience with most of the currently available investigational angioplasty devices, an appreciation for which unfavorable lesion subsets respond best to specific therapies can be clarified. ELCA appears most appropriate in situations of diffuse disease, recanalized chronic total occlusions, ostial lesions, and undilatable lesions. LBA is most effective for flow-limiting dis-

sections in clinical situations of threatened or true abrupt closure. DCA is best suited to larger (greater than 3 mm) straight vessel segments, usually in a proximal location, and in lesions with marked eccentricity or surface irregularity. DCA is also effective in certain saphenous vein graft lesions, ostial stenoses (especially in the left anterior descending coronary artery), some noncalcified undilatable lesions, and focal dissections. TEC is generally reserved for thrombus-containing lesions, especially in degenerated older saphenous vein grafts. ROTA appears better suited to smaller vessels (less than 3.0 mm) in straight or tortuous segments, proximal or midvessel location, and especially in regions of calcification. Rotational atherectomy also appears to be effective in diffuse disease, ostial lesions, and undilatable lesions. Stent implantation is an effective treatment modality for focal pathology in saphenous vein grafts, suboptimal PTCA results, lesions with marked eccentricity, and dissections (either de novo or PTCA induced). Surprisingly, there is relatively little direct overlap among devices for the specific unfavorable lesion characteristics tailored to each device's optimal use pattern.

Limitations of the Study

This large descriptive report represents a survey study providing useful general observations but little quantitative comparative analyses. More definitive statements can only be drawn from carefully planned prospective and retrospective assessments employing direct chart audit techniques, quantitative coronary angiography, and randomized clinical trials (between devices or device vs. PTCA). It is our expectation that such studies will be forthcoming in the near future.

CONCLUSIONS

From our observations of almost 1,500 patients treated with investigational angioplasty techniques we conclude the following: (1) a multidevice, lesion-specific approach appears to improve acute angiographic responses in patients with unfavorable coronary lesions; (2) complications in this patient cohort appear acceptable, especially given the high-risk nature of these lesions subsets; and (3) adjunct balloon angioplasty is often necessary to optimize angiographic results or treat procedure-related complications. Therefore, an integration of coronary angioplasty techniques with newer investigational angioplasty devices in a variety of unfavorable lesion subsets would appear to produce the most efficacious and safe procedural outcome. It is our expectation that these devices will find clinical application in a variety of situations, thus enhancing the interventional cardiologists' ability to manage more complex lesion subsets.

Acknowledgment

We wish to acknowledge the superb secretarial and administrative assistance of Jenene Reaves in the preparation of this manuscript and the expertise of Moshe Mehlman in coordinating graphic arts.

REFERENCES

1. Grúntzig AR: Transluminal dilatation of coronary artery stenosis (letter). *Lancet* 1978; 1:263.
2. Abele JE: Objective assessment of new technology. *Cardiovasc Diagn* 1991; 23:268–269.
3. Topol EJ: Promises and pitfalls of new devices for coronary artery disease. *Circulation* 1991; 83:689–694.
4. Leon MB, Kent KM, Satler LF, et al: A multidevice, lesion-specific approach for unfavorable coronary anatomy (abstract). *J Am Coll Cardiol* 1992; 19:93.
5. Litvack F, Grundfest WS, Papaioannou T, et al: Role of laser and thermal ablation devices in the treatment of vascular diseases. *Am J Cardiol* 1988; 61:81–86.
6. Bartorelli AL, Leon MB, Almagor Y, et al: In vivo human atherosclerotic plaque recognition by laser-excited fluorescence spectroscopy. *J Am Coll Cardiol* 1991; 17:160–168.
7. Spears JR, Reyes VP, Fromm BS, et al: Percutaneous coronary laser balloon angioplasty: Initial results of a multicenter experience. *J Am Coll Cardiol* 1990; 16:293–303.
8. Hinohara T, Robertson GC, Selmon MR, et al: Directional coronary atherectomy. *J Invasive Cardiol* 1990; 2:217–226.
9. Meany T, Kramer B, Knopf W, et al: Multicenter experience of atherectomy of saphenous vein grafts: Immediate results and follow-up (abstract). *J Am Coll Cardiol* 1992; 19:262.
10. Teirstein PS, Warth DC, Haq N, et al: High-speed rotational atherectomy for patients with diffuse coronary artery disease. *J Am Coll Cardiol* 1991; 18:1694–1701.
11. Schatz RA: A view of vascular stents. *Circulation* 1989; 79:445–457.
12. Douek PC, Bonner RF, Keren G, et al: Vessel wall responses to plaque in angiographically normal and functional stenotic coronaries (abstract). *Circulation* 1991; 84(suppl 2):677.
13. Black AJR, Namay DL, Niederman AL, et al: Tear or dissection after coronary angioplasty: Morphologic correlates of an ischemic complication. *Circulation* 1989; 79:1035–1042.
14. Topol EJ, Ellis SG, Fishman J, et al: Multicenter study of percutaneous transluminal angioplasty for right coronary artery ostial stenosis. *J Am Coll Cardiol* 1987; 9:1214–1218.
15. Cowley MJ, Dorros G, Kelsey SF, et al: Acute coronary events associated with percutaneous transluminal coronary angioplasty. *Am J Cardiol* 1983; 53:12–16.
16. Bredlau CE, Roubin GS, Leingruber PT, et al: In-hospital morbidity and mortality in patients undergoing elective coronary angioplasty. *Circulation* 1985; 72:1044–1052.
17. Detre K, Holubkov R, Kelsey S, et al: Percutaneous transluminal coronary angioplasty in 1985–1986 and 1977–1981. *N Engl J Med* 1988; 318:265–270.

Index

A

Abdominal aortic aneurysm, cardiopulmonary bypass support and, 439
Accessory pathways, catheter ablation
  with high-energy shocks, 672–673
  with radio frequency energy, 674–680
Acetylsalicylic acid, for restenosis prevention, 558–559
Activase, 379, 383 (see also Tissue plasminogen activator)
Acute coronary occlusion
  in angioplasty
    cardiopulmonary bypass support, 484
    Hemopump support, 488
    PTCA long-wire technique for, 97–99
  laser balloon angioplasty for, 268
  utilization considerations, 268–269
  transfusion catheters in, monorail system experience, 122–123
Acute coronary syndromes
  laser balloon angioplasty for, 269–270
  percutaneous transluminal coronary angioscopy in, 41–54

Acute coronary thrombosis, etiology and treatment, 273
Acute myocardial infarction
  angioplasty therapy, 359–373
    algorithm, 364
    application categories, 367, 368
    benefits and limitations, 365–366
    benefits and results, 367
    deficiencies of thrombolytic therapy, 360–362
    direct PTCA when thrombolysis is contraindicated, 369
    after failed lytic therapy, 370–371
    future research, 365
    historical perspective, 359–360
    limitations, 368
    lytic therapy vs., 367–369
    patient selection, 364–365
    review of major clinical series, 362–363
    speed of treatment, 369
    with thrombolysis contraindicated, 369
    with shock
      cardiopulmonary bypass support, 483–484
      Hemopump support, 485, 486–487
    thrombolysis in (see Thrombolysis, in acute myocardial infarction)

Aneurysm, abdominal aortic, cardiopulmonary bypass support and, 439
Angina
  changes after balloon aortic valvuloplasty, 580
  laser balloon angioplasty for, 266, 270
  unstable, intra-aortic balloon counterpulsation for, 481
Angiographic system, video mixer in, 38
Angiography
  classified by level of technical development, 53
  in coarctation angioplasty, 633
  ileofemoral, in cardiopulmonary bypass support, 437, 438
  for Palmaz-Schatz stent deployment, 322–323, 325, 326, 327
  in pulmonary branch angioplasty, 637
  quantitative coronary
    analysis for rotary ablation, 144–145
    automated, 19
    in Wallstent experience, 335, 336, 337, 339
  restenosis and, 495
  thrombolysis
    cineangiograms, case examples, 392, 395, 398–400, 404, 406

Angiopeptin, for restenosis prevention, 563
Angioplasty
  for acute myocardial infarction (see Acute myocardial infarction, angioplasty therapy)
  antegrade perfusion during, 426
  balloon (see Balloon angioplasty)
  coarctation, 633–636
  for congenital lesions (see Congenital lesions, interventional catheterization for)
  coronary bypass surgery vs. (see Emory Angioplasty vs. Surgery Trial)
  failed, stenting in, 302–304
  high-risk
    cardiopulmonary bypass support, 484
    factors defining patient risk, 425–426
    Hemopump support, 488
    perfusion balloon catheters for, 474
    prophylactic and standby circulatory support, 425–433
  immediate and late consequences, 495–496
  injury, mural thrombus, and restenosis, 509–520
  investigational devices, 695–696
  for unfavorable coronary lesions, 695–703

Angioplasty (*cont.*)
  laser (*see* Laser angioplasty;
    Laser angiosurgery;
    Laser balloon
    angioplasty)
  Magnum system (*see*
    Magnum system, for
    coronary angioplasty)
  percutaneous transluminal
    coronary (*see*
    Percutaneous
    transluminal coronary
    angioplasty)
  procedural mortality, 426
  supported (*see* Supported
    angioplasty)
  thrombolytic therapy and,
    361–362
  ultrasound (*see* Ultrasound
    angioplasty)
Angioplasty patients, exercise
  thallium scintigraphy in,
  10
Angioscopy
  catheter ultrasound imaging
    vs., 59
  in coronary interventions, 41
  percutaneous transluminal
    coronary (*see*
    Percutaneous
    transluminal coronary
    angioscopy)
  restenosis and, 495–496,
    510
Angioscopy system
  clinical experience, 33–40
  components, 34, 35
  discussion, 38–39
  observations, 36–38
  patients, 34–35
  protocol, 35–36
  risks and limitations, 38
  technical aspects, 33–34, 35
Angiotensin converting
  enzyme inhibitors, 530,
  562–563
Angiotensin II, in neointimal
  cell proliferation,
  527–533
Angiotensin II peptide
  antagonists, 530–531
Anisoylated plasminogen
  streptokinase activator
  complex (APSAC), 378,
  379
  left ventricular function and,
    381
  mortality and, 381–383
  patency of infarct-related
    artery and, 381
  results in acute myocardial
    infarction, 407
  streptokinase and t-PA vs.,
    400–402

Anticoagulants, for restenosis
  prevention
  heparin, 556–557
  hirudin, 557–558
  low-molecular-weight
    heparin, 557
  new drugs, 561
  warfarin (Coumadin), 558
Anti-inflammatory agents, for
  restenosis prevention,
  502–503, 565
Antimyosin antibody imaging,
  12–13
Antiplatelet agents, for
  restenosis prevention,
  558
  acetylsalicylic acid,
    558–559
  dextran, 559
  dipyridamole, 559
  new drugs, 561
  prostacyclin or prostacyclin
    analogue, 560–561
  prostaglandin E1, 561
  sulfinpyrazone, 559
  thromboxane A2, 559–560
  ticlopidine, 560
Antiproliferative drugs, for
  restenosis prevention
  angiopeptin, 563
  angiotensin-converting
    enzyme inhibitors, 530,
    562–563
  colchicine, 561–562
  cytostatic agents, 562
  new drugs, 563
  platelet-derived growth
    factor antagonist, 561
  serotonin antagonist, 561
Antisecretory agents, for
  restenosis prevention,
  503
Antitachycardia devices (*see*
  Implantable
  defibrillator)
Antithrombotic therapy (*see*
  Thrombolysis)
Aortic aneurysm, abdominal,
  cardiopulmonary bypass
  support and, 439
Aortic coarctation (*see*
  Coarctation of aorta)
Aortic stenosis
  echocardiographic
    assessment, 68, 70, 71,
    72
  interventional
    catheterization,
    628–630
  complications, 630
  patients and methods,
    628
  results, 629–630
  technique, 628–629

Aortic valvuloplasty (*see*
  Percutaneous balloon
  aortic valvuloplasty)
Aorto-ostial lesions
  balloon angioplasty for, 84,
    86
  excimer laser coronary
    angioplasty for, 227,
    228
APSAC (*see* Anisoylated
  plasminogen
  streptokinase activator
  complex)
APSAC Interventional
  Mortality Study
  (AIMS), 381, 382
Argon laser angioplasty, for
  peripheral and coronary
  vascular lesions,
  255–261
  centering balloon in, 2, 255
  early coronary experience,
    259–260
  methods, 255–256
  multicenter experience,
    257–259
  Park Nicollet Heart Center
    experience, 4, 256–257
Arrhythmias
  balloon inflation and, 460
  implantable defibrillator
    therapy (*see* Implantable
    defibrillator)
  after streptokinase therapy,
    390
  transvenous catheter
    ablation, 671–683
    accessory pathways,
      672–673, 674–680
    atrioventricular junction,
      671, 674
    atrioventricular node
      modification, 680
    atrioventricular node
      reentrant tachycardia,
      673, 676–677, 678,
      681
    energy sources, 673–674
    with high-energy shocks,
      results and
      disadvantages, 671–672
    historical perspective,
      671–672
    ventricular tachycardia,
      673, 677–680, 682
Arterial evaluation, 33–40
Arterial occlusion (*see*
  Occlusion)
Arterial size and angulation,
  directional coronary
  atherectomy and, 165,
  167
Arterial substrates for
  thrombosis, 510

Arterial wall, ultrasound
  plaque ablation and,
  287–288
Arteriography (*see also*
  Angiography),
  automated quantitative
  coronary, 19
Aspirin, in restenosis
  prevention, 502
Aspirin, for restenosis
  prevention, 502,
  558–559
Atherectomy
  coaxial, devices for, imaging
    and, 62
  directional coronary (*see*
    Directional coronary
    atherectomy)
  with Rotablator (*see*
    Percutaneous
    transluminal coronary
    rotary ablation, with
    Rotablator)
  specimens, in restenosis, 510
  transluminal extraction (*see*
    Transluminal extraction
    atherectomy)
AtheroCath, 61, 158–159,
  161–163, 164
Atherogenesis,
  response-to-injury
  hypothesis, 521–522
Atheroma, observation of, 36
Atherosclerotic plaque (*see*
  Plaque)
Atrial fibrillation, pacing
  modes and, 657
Atrial septal defects
  closure, 642
    results, 643–644
    technique, 642–643
  echocardiography and,
    71–72
Atrial shunting, after balloon
  valvotomy, 620
  echocardiographic follow-up,
    618
  hemodynamic follow-up,
    615–616
Atrioventricular junction,
  catheter ablation
  with high-energy shocks,
    671
  with radio frequency energy,
    674, 675
Atrioventricular node
  modification, 680
Atrioventricular node reentrant
  tachycardia, catheter
  ablation
  with high-energy shocks,
    673
  with radio frequency energy,
    676–677, 678, 681

Atrioventricular synchrony, in
pacing, 651–653
Autoperfusion, 459, 461–462
Autoperfusion balloon
angioplasty, 471–477
development and early use,
471–472
future directions, 475–476
indications, 473–475
limitations, 475
technique, 472–473
Autoperfusion catheters
low-profile, 475
monorail-type, 120–121
systems, 424, 427
Stack, 461, 462, 471–477
thermal, 475–476
Autopsy specimens, in
restenosis, 510

B

Balloon angioplasty
autoperfusion (*see*
Autoperfusion balloon
angioplasty)
development of alternatives
to, 1–3
graded inflation to achieve
full balloon expansion,
416
intravascular ultrasound and,
59–61
laser (*see* Laser balloon
angioplasty)
limitations, 457
Magnum system (*see*
Magnum system, for
coronary angioplasty)
matching technology to
lesions, 79–88
bifurcations, 79–80, 82,
83
calcification, 81
eccentricity, 82, 85
left main disease, 83, 86
ostial lesions, 84, 86
prior bypass surgery, 84,
86–87
thrombus, length, and
bend point, 80–81, 84,
85
total occlusion, 82–83
microwave (*see* Microwave
balloon angioplasty)
monorail system results,
126–127
myocardial protection (*see*
Myocardial protection,
in coronary angioplasty)
plaque fracture after, 60
problems, 81
Balloon catheters
for aortic valvuloplasty, 577

characteristics, 119
for laser angioplasty, 2, 255,
264
for pericardial window,
687–688
sliding rail, 120
monorail (*see* Monorail
system)
special applications,
120–122
for valvotomy, 581–582,
592, 597, 610–611
Balloon dilation, stent delivery,
323
Balloon inflation, vascular
injury from, 499
Balloon pump, intra-aortic, for
systemic circulatory
support, 427–428
Balloons, for monorail system,
116
results, 122
Balloon valvuloplasty (*see*
Catheter balloon
valvuloplasty;
Percutaneous balloon
aortic valvuloplasty)
Bard cardiopulmonary support
system
complications, 484–485
duration of assistance, 484
indications, 483–484
method of insertion, 484
performance characteristics,
490
physiology, 483
portable, 439, 441–442,
466–467
system schematic, 482
BARI (Bypass Angioplasty
Revascularization
Investigation), 137
Baxter-Edwards ultrasound
generator, 292
Bifurcations
balloon angioplasty for,
79–80, 82, 83
directional coronary
atherectomy for, 167
excimer laser coronary
angioplasty for,
237–238, 239
Blood flow and velocity (*see*
Myocardial blood flow;
Perfusion;
Transcatheter blood
flow measurement)
Blood pressure (systemic)
balloon angioplasty and, 459
elevated in cardiopulmonary
bypass support, 446
Bradycardia pacemakers, in
patients receiving
defibrillators, 665–666

Bypass Angioplasty
Revascularization
Investigation (BARI), 137
Bypass graft disease, stent
prosthesis for, 315
Wallstent experience, 334,
337, 338–339, 341,
344, 345
Bypass grafting
after failed PTCA, 416, 417
location of diseased arteries
after, 136
Bypass surgery
angioplasty vs. (*see* Emory
Angioplasty vs. Surgery
Trial)
prior, balloon angioplasty
and, 84, 86–87
survival rate for PTCA vs., 189

C

CABRI (Coronary Artery
Bypass
Revascularization
Investigation), 138
Calcification
balloon angioplasty and, 60,
81
directional coronary
atherectomy and, 62,
164–165
Calcium antagonists, for
restenosis prevention,
563
diltiazem, 563–564
nifedipine, 564
verapamil, 564
Cannulation, in
cardiopulmonary bypass
support, 437–439, 483
removal in elective group,
447–448
Cardiac arrest,
cardiopulmonary bypass
support and, 446, 447
Cardiac arrhythmias (*see*
Arrhythmias)
Cardiac transplantation
Hemopump support, 488–489
intra-aortic balloon
counterpulsation and,
481–482
Cardiogenic shock
cardiopulmonary bypass
support, 446
Hemopump support, 485,
486–487
Cardiopulmonary bypass
support (*see*
Percutaneous
femorofemoral
cardiopulmonary bypass
support)

Cardiopulmonary resuscitation,
thrombolytic therapy
and, 377
Cardioversion, low-energy,
advantages, 666
Catheter balloon valvuloplasty
for congenital lesions, 625
echocardiography
applications, 67–75
assessment of benefit
mechanism, 72
detection of associated
lesions, 68–69
detection of
complications, 71
evaluation of efficacy, 72
guidance for procedure,
71–72
quantitation of valve
stenosis, 67–68
suitability assessment for
procedure, 69–71
Catheter design, for ultrasound
imaging, 55–57
Catheter exchange, in PTCA
long-wire technique, 92
Catheterization, for congenital
lesions (*see* Congenital
lesions, interventional
catheterization for)
Catheters
in ablation of arrhythmias
(*see* Arrhythmias,
transvenous catheter
ablation)
autoperfusion (*see*
Autoperfusion catheters)
balloon (*see* Balloon
catheters)
in blood flow assessment (*see*
Transcatheter blood
flow measurement)
combined imaging and
therapeutic, ultrasound
imaging and, 63–64
for directional coronary
atherectomy, 158–159
Doppler, 27
intracoronary monorail,
121, 122
fluid-core, for laser
thrombolysis, 274–276,
277
for laser angioplasty,
215–216, 217–218,
264
with excimer laser, 226,
233–237
peripheral, 244
for laser angiosurgery,
179–180, 181
for laser angiosurgery II,
196–198
Magnarail, 121

Catheters *(cont.)*
  for Palmaz-Schatz stent
    deployment, 322
  for percutaneous balloon
    mitral valvotomy,
    581–582
  for percutaneous balloon
    pericardial window,
    687–689
  for percutaneous rotational
    thrombectomy, 172,
    173
  for percutaneous
    transluminal coronary
    angioscopy, 42, 44
    guiding catheter, 43–44
    insertion and flushing, 45
  transluminal
    extraction-endarterectomy
    (see Transluminal
    extraction-endarterectomy
    catheters)
Catheter ultrasound imaging
  (see Ultrasound
  imaging, intravascular)
Cell biology of restenosis
  angiotensin II in neointimal
    cell proliferation,
    527–533
  paradigm based on,
    495–508
Cellular proliferation, in
  wound healing,
  498–499 *(see also*
  Smooth muscle cells)
Cerebrovascular accident
  in balloon valvotomy, 596
  pacing modes and, 657
Cholesterol-lowering drugs,
  for restenosis
  prevention, 565
Chronotropic incompetence,
  652–654
Cineangiograms, streptokinase
  therapy case examples,
  392, 395, 398–400,
  404, 406
Ciprostene, for restenosis
  prevention, 560–561
Circulatory support, in
  high-risk coronary
  angioplasty *(see*
  Supported angioplasty)
CK-MB fraction, as
  reperfusion indicator,
  389, 390, 391
Classification of lesions, 415,
  416
Closed mitral
  commissurotomy, 609
Closure *(see* Occlusion)
Clot dissolution, by ultrasound
  angioplasty, 290–291

Coarctation of aorta *(see also*
  Aortic stenosis)
  native coarctation
    angioplasty results,
    635–636
  angioplasty technique,
    633–635
  recoarctation, 636
Colchicine, for restenosis
  prevention, 561–562
Color-flow mapping, in
  valvular regurgitation
  detection, 69
Comfort Disc, 447, 448
Commissurotomy
  closed mitral, 609
  surgical, balloon valvotomy
    vs., 619–620
Community hospital,
  thrombolyis in acute
  myocardial infarction
  in, 387–411
Compression disk, 447, 448
Computed tomography,
  SPECT ^{201}TI
  scintigraphy, 7, 8, 9
Congenital lesions,
  interventional
  catheterization for,
  625–647
  aortic stenosis, 628–630
  arterial septal defect closure,
    642–644
  coarctation of aorta,
    633–636
  mitral valve stenosis,
    630–632
  patent ductus arteriosus
    occlusion, 639–642
  pulmonary artery branch
    stenosis, 636–638
  pulmonary vein stenosis,
    638–639
  subaortic stenosis, 630
  tricuspid stenosis,
    632–633
  valvuloplasty, 625–628
  ventricular septal defect
    closure, 642–644
Congestive heart failure
  maximum heart rates at peak
    exercise in, 654
  pacing modes and, 657
Cook stent, 302
Corflo pump, 463–464
Coronary angioplasty *(see*
  Angioplasty)
Coronary angioscopy,
  percutaneous
  transluminal *(see*
  Percutaneous
  transluminal coronary
  angioscopy)

Coronary arteries *(see also*
  Arterial *entries*),
  locations of diseased,
  after PTCA and bypass
  graft, 136
Coronary artery bypass
  grafting *(see* Bypass
  grafting)
Coronary Artery Bypass
  Revascularization
  Investigation (CABRI),
  138
Coronary atherectomy *(see*
  Atherectomy)
Coronary blood flow and
  velocity, transcatheter
  assessment *(see*
  Transcatheter blood
  flow measurement)
Coronary blood flow decrease,
  segmental wall motion
  and, 458
Coronary bypass surgery *(see*
  Bypass surgery)
Coronary endothelium *(see*
  Endothelium)
Coronary lesions
  unfavorable, treatment
    strategy for, 695–703
  complications, 697, 700,
    701–702
  conclusions, 702–703
  definition of terms,
    696–697
  discussion, 697, 701–702
  investigational angioplasty
    devices, 695–696
  limitations of study, 702
  patient population, 696
  results, 697–701
  strategic device-specific
    patterns, 702
  vascular, argon laser
    angioplasty for, 255–261
Coronary occlusion *(see*
  Occlusion)
Coronary patency, after
  thrombolytic therapy,
  380–381
Coronary plaque *(see* Plaque)
Coronary stents *(see* Stents)
Coronary syndromes, acute *(see*
  Acute coronary
  syndromes)
Coronary thrombosis *(see*
  Thrombosis)
Corticosteroids, for restenosis
  prevention, 565
Coumadin, for restenosis
  prevention, 558
Creatine kinase, CK-MB
  fraction as reperfusion
  indicator, 389, 390, 391

Cyclosporine A, for restenosis
  prevention, 503
Cytostatic/cytotoxic agents, for
  restenosis prevention,
  502–503, 562

D

DCA *(see* Directional coronary
  atherectomy)
Defribillator, implantable *(see*
  Implantable
  defibrillator)
Dextran, for restenosis
  prevention, 559
Diastolic filling patterns,
  altered, 655
Diastolic/systolic velocity ratio,
  27–29, 31
Digital radiography, in blood
  flow assessment, 19
Diltiazem, for restenosis
  prevention, 563–564
Dipyridamole, for restenosis
  prevention, 502, 559
Dipyridamole ^{201}TI
  scintigraphy, 9–10
Directional coronary
  atherectomy (DCA),
  157–169, 696, 702
  advantages over dilatation,
    157
  case selection, 161–162
  catheter design, 158–159
  clinical results, 159–161
  complications, 160
  future directions, 169
  histology, 167, 168
  historical perspective,
    157–158
  indications, 168
  lesion characteristics and
    outcome, 160, 161
  procedure, 162–163
  restenosis, 167, 168
  as salvage technique for
    failed PTCA, 160–161,
    168
  vessel type and outcome,
    160
Directional coronary
  atherectomy (DCA),
  favorable and
  unfavorable lesions,
  163–167
DNA synthesis
  growth factors and, 537,
    538, 539, 540
  response to injury, 536
Doppler catheter and
  guidewire, for coronary
  blood flow
  measurement, 20–21

Doppler catheters, 27
  intracoronary monorail, 121, 122
Doppler echocardiography (*see* Echocardiography)
Doppler guidewire, 21, 27–32
Doppler ultrasound systems, catheter-based, 27
Doppler velocity measurements, in stenosis assessment, 68, 69
Doppler velocity spectral display, 28, 30–31
Dymed 3010 flashlamp-excited pulse dye laser, 274
Dyspnea, changes after balloon aortic valvuloplasty, 580

E

EAST (*see* Emory Angioplasty vs. Surgery Trial)
Eccentric lesions
  excimer laser coronary angioplasty for, 236–237, 238
  PTCA and, 82
Echocardiography
  in catheter balloon valvuloplasty (*see* Catheter balloon valvuloplasty, echocardiography applications)
  in valvotomy follow-up, 601–605, 618–619
  valvular regurgitation detected by, 68–69, 71, 72
Elderly, thrombolytic therapy for, 377
Electrocardiograms, streptokinase therapy case examples, 392–394, 396–398, 401–402, 405
Electrocardiography, thrombolytic therapy and, 376
Embolization, in excimer laser coronary angioplasty, 235–236
Eminase, 379 (*see also* Anisoylated plasminogen streptoki-nase activator complex)
Emory Angioplasty vs. Surgery Trial, 133–138
  baseline screening, 135–136
  comparison of randomized and eligible but not randomized patients, 136–137
  expectations, 137

follow-up status, 137
  other trials addressing selection, 137–138
  purpose and end points, 134–135
  structure, 133–134
Endothelium
  angioscopic definition, 47
  smooth muscle cell proliferation and, 515, 528, 531, 549–550
European Cooperative Group study/trial, 360, 370, 371
Excimer laser
  fluorescence, 225
  interaction with tissue, 224
  photochemical ablation, 225
  physical characteristics, 223
  thermal effect, 224–225
  xenon chloride, 223–224
Excimer laser coronary angioplasty (ELCA), 223–231, 695–696, 702
  ablation in vascular system, 225
  case selection, 230
  clinical protocol, 226–227
  fiber-optic delivery system and catheter design, 225–226
  future directions, 230–231
  initial clinical experience, 227–229, 230
  late restenosis after, 229
  potential indications, 230
  wire-guided techniques and trial results, 233–241
    discussion, 239, 241
    guide catheters, 236, 237
    laser catheters, 233, 234, 235
    lesions treated, 234–235
    methods, 233–234
    multicenter clinical sites, 234
    patient enrollment, 234–235
    potential indications, 241
    specific lesion recommendations, 236–239
    success and complications, 235–236
    technical guidelines learned, 236
Excimer laser peripheral angioplasty, 243–253
Exercise thallium scintigraphy, 6–9
  in coronary angioplasty patient, 10
Express catheter, 120

F

F-2-deoxyglucose (FDG) imaging, 8, 14
Femoral artery
  occlusion of, ultrasound recanalization for, 294
  prosthesis implantation in, 311–312
Femorofemoral cardiopulmonary bypass (*see* Percutaneous femorofemoral cardiopulmonary bypass support)
Femoropopliteal occlusions and stenoses, argon laser angioplasty for, 256, 257, 258
  ultrasound recanalization for, 293–295
Fiber-optics, in laser angioplasty, 225–226
Fibrinolytic drugs, success rates of, 273
Fibroblast growth factor, 498, 514, 516, 537–538
Fish oils, for restenosis prevention, 564
Flashlamp-excited pulsed dye laser, 274
Fluorescence, laser-induced, 183–184, 185, 225
Fluorescence-guided laser angioplasty, 696
Fluorescence spectroscopy, in laser angiosurgery II, 198–200
Fluorocarbon perfusion (Fluosol-DA), 424–427, 466
Frankfurt experience, with long-wire technique in PTCA, 89–100

G

German Angioplasty Bypass Intervention (GABI), 138
Gianturco-Roubin stent, 302
GISSI trial, 382, 383
Global Utilization of Streptokinase and Tissue Plasminogen Activator for Occluded Coronary Arteries (GUSTO), 383
Grafting (*see* Bypass grafting; Vein grafts)
Granulation phase of wound healing, 497, 498–499, 501
  restenosis prevention and, 503

Growth factor antagonists, in restenosis prevention, 503
Growth factor induced signaling pathway, 539
Growth factors
  cellular and molecular events induced by, 539–540
  in cellular proliferation in arterial injury, 514–515, 516, 521–522, 528, 536–538, 549
  in restenosis, 497–498, 499–500
Gruppo Italiano per lo Studio della Streptochinasi nell'Infarto Miocardico (GISSI), 382, 383
Guidewires
  for balloon valvotomy, 592, 593
  Doppler, 20–21, 27–32
  in monorail system, 113–117
GUSTO trial, 383

H

HARTS device
  deployment, 350–351
  left coronary arteriogram after stent delivery, 352
  materials and construction, 349–350
  pathologic studies, 351–353
  histologic changes after stenting, 354, 355
  potential clinical applications, 353–356
  recovery, 351, 352
  results, 351, 352
  vessel diameter after implantation and recovery, 353
Heart rate, at peak exercise, in congestive heart failure, 654
Heat-activated recoverable temporary stent (*see* HARTS device)
Hemodynamics of pacing, 651–656
Hemoperfusion
  active (prograde), 462–465
  passive, 459, 461–462
  retroperfusion (coronary sinus), 462
Hemoperfusion-supported angioplasty
  with Corflo pump, clinical data, 464
  ECG and pressure tracings, 465

Hemoperfusion-supported
  angioplasty *(cont.)*
  potential uses, 464–465
Hemopump, 485
  complications, 489–490
  contraindications, 489
  duration of assistance, 489
  illustration, 484
  indications, 486–490
  method of insertion, 488,
    489
  performance characteristics,
    490
  physiology, 485–486
Hemostasis, compression disk
  for, 447, 448
Heparin
  low-molecular-weight, for
    restenosis prevention,
    557
  in optimal thombolytic
    regimen, 383
  for restenosis prevention,
    503, 556–557
  in thrombin inhibition, 512
Hibernating myocardium, 4
  in dog model, 5
High-risk angioplasty *(see
  Angioplasty, high-risk)*
High-speed rotational ablation
  (ROTA), 696, 702
Hirudin
  for restenosis prevention,
    557–558
  in thrombin inhibition,
    512–513
Histology
  changes after HARTS
    device stenting, 354, 355
  of restenosis, 167, 496–497
  of tissue ablated by
    continuous-wave vs.
    pulsed lasers, 205
History of interventional
  cardiology, 625
Hi-Torque Floppy guidewire,
  162
Holmium:YAG laser, 216, 217
  infrared wavelengths, 217
Holmium:YAG laser
  angioplasty
  discussion and conclusion,
    219–220
  guidance, 216
Holmium:YAG laser
  angioplasty, clinical
    experience, 215–221
  complications, 219
  laser failure, 219
  patient selection, 216–217
  procedure, 217–218
  results, 218–219
Hot balloon, for monorail use,
  121

Hyperplasia, in restenosis,
  496–497, 501
Hypertension, thrombolytic
  therapy and, 377

I

Ileofemoral angiography, in
  cardiopulmonary bypass
  support, 437, 438
Ileofemoral arterial system,
  tortuous,
  cardiopulmonary bypass
  support and, 439, 440
Ileofemoral stenoses, critical,
  cardiopulmonary bypass
  support and, 439, 441
Iliac arteries, laser angioplasty
  of, 246, 248, 251
Imaging *(see* Nuclear
  cardiology techniques in
  myocardial assessment;
  Ultrasound imaging)*
Impedance catheter and
  guidewire, for coronary
  blood flow
  measurement, 21–25
Implantable defibrillator,
  therapeutic advances,
  665–670
  advantages of low-energy
    cardioversion, 666
  antitachycardia pacing for
    arrhythmia termination,
    666
  bradycardia pacemakers and,
    665–666
  expanding clinical uses of
    advanced devices, 668
  increased complexity of
    newer devices, 667
  newer combination devices,
    666–667
  noninvasive programmed
    stimulation, 667
  nonthoracotomy lead
    systems, 668–669
  prophylactic implantation,
    669
  results, 665
Infarct-avid imaging with
  radiolabeled
  myosin-specific
  antibody, 12–13
Infarct Survival Collaborative
  Group (ISIS),
  382–383
Inferior myocardial infarction,
  patient selection for
  thrombolytic therapy,
  375–376
Inflammation inhibitors, for
  restenosis prevention,
  502–503, 565

Inflammatory phase of wound
  healing, 497–498, 501,
  502–503
Inoue single-balloon
  valvotomy,
  double-balloon
  valvotomy vs., 597–601
Interleukin-1, DNA synthesis
  in vascular smooth
  muscle cells and, 538
Interventional cardiology
  history, 625
  new technologies, 691–693
Intra-aortic balloon pump,
  466, 480
  complications, 482–483
  contraindications, 482
  indications, 481–482
  method of insertion, 482
  performance characteristics,
    490
  physiology, 480–481
  for systemic circulatory
    support, 427–428
Intracardiac thrombi, detected
  by echocardiography, 69
Intracoronary diagnostic
  (pressure-monitoring)
  catheter, monorail-type,
  121
Intracoronary Doppler
  catheter, monorail-type,
  121, 122
Intravascular ultrasound
  imaging *(see* Ultrasound
  imaging, intravascular)*
Ischemia, recurrent, after lytic
  therapy, 370
Ischemia control, after failed
  PTCA, 420–421
ISIS (Infarct Survival
  Collaborative Group),
  382–383

L

Laser angioplasty
  advantages, 215
  argon *(see* Argon laser
    angioplasty)*
  delivery catheters, 215–216,
    217–218
  excimer *(see* Excimer laser
    coronary angioplasty)*
  fluorescence-guided, 696
  guidance and control of
    ablation, 216
  infrared *(see* Holmium:YAG
    laser angioplasty)*
  optimal laser wavelength,
    215
  peripheral *(see* Argon laser
    angioplasty; Peripheral
    laser angioplasty)*

pulsed laser ablation of
  plaque *(see* Plaque
  ablation, by pulsed laser)*
Laser angiosurgery (LAS),
  179–187
  catheter design, 179–180
  delivery scheme (schematic),
    181
  future directions, 186–187
  operating room, 182
  results, 183, 184
  target ablation, 180–183
  target recognition, 183–186
Laser angiosurgery (LAS) II,
  189–202
  catheter design, 196–198
  goals and method, 190
  optical fiber considerations
    and pulse stretching,
    194–196
  selection of ablation laser,
    191–194
    fluence, 192, 193
    irradiance, 192
    wavelength, 192–194
  spectroscopy and diagnostic
    algorithm, 198–200
  subsystems, 190, 191
  system control and
    operation, 200–201
Laser balloon angioplasty
  (LBA), 696, 702
  for acute closure, 268
    utilization considerations,
      268–269
  for acute coronary
    syndromes, 269–270
  concept, 263
  correlation of tissue effects
    and benefit, 267–269
  future of, 270–271
  for prevention of PTCA
    stenosis, 267–268
  for PTCA failure without
    acute closure or
    ischemia, 269
  technique, 263–264
  therapeutic mechanisms and
    clinical correlations,
    263–272
  tissue effects, 264–265
  desiccation, 267
  for total coronary
    occlusions, 269
  viscoelastic recoil reduced
    in, 266–267
Laser catheters, ultrasound
  imaging and, 62, 64
Laser-induced fluorescence,
  183–184, 185, 225
Laser light, restenosis and, 190
Lasers *(see also specific types)*
  comparison by parameters of
    ablation, 204

continuous-wave vs. pulsed, 203–206
interaction with tissue, 224
near-infrared, comparison of tissue absorption parameters, 217
pulsed, selective ablation of plaque vs. normal vessel wall, 210–211, 212
Laser thrombolysis, 273–280
background, 273
clinical studies, 277–279
with Dymed 3010 flashlamp-excited pulse dye laser, 274
fluid-core laser catheter, 274–276, 277
advantages, 274–275, 276
schematic drawings, 275, 276
implications, 279
preclinical studies, 277, 278
selective, 274
technique, 276–277
LAS (*see* Laser angiosurgery)
LBA (*see* Laser balloon angioplasty)
Left anterior descending artery, stenosis of, directional coronary atherectomy for, 166
Left coronary artery, arteriogram after stent delivery, 352
Left main coronary disease, balloon angioplasty for, 83, 86
Left ventricle, thrombolytic therapy and, 381
Left ventricular assist devices
cardiopulmonary support system, 482, 483–485
Hemopump, 484, 485–490
indications, techniques, and results, 479–492
intra-aortic balloon counterpulsation, 480–483
performance characteristics, 490
requirements of ideal, 480
Left ventricular dysfunction, pacing for, 654
Left ventricular function, after thrombolytic therapy, 381
Left ventricular pressure, hemodynamics, 651–652, 655
Left ventricular unloading
cardiopulmonary bypass support and, 483
Hemopump and, 485–486

intra-aortic balloon counterpulsation and, 480–481
Leriche syndrome, 251
Lesions
classification, 415, 416
congenital (*see* Congenital lesions)
coronary (*see* Coronary lesions)
exclusion criteria for perfusion balloon catheter, 475
high-risk, perfusion balloon angioplasty for, 474
length of, balloon angioplasty and, 81, 84, 85
ostial (*see* Aort-ostial lesions; Ostial lesions)
Lipid-lowering drugs, for restenosis prevention
cholesterol-lowering drugs, 565
fish oils, 564
Long-wire technique, in PTCA (*see* Percutaneous transluminal coronary angioplasty, long-wire technique)
Lytic therapy (*see* Thrombolysis)

M

Magnarail catheter, 121
Magnarail probing catheter, 121
Magnarail system, 103–104
Magnum system, for coronary angioplasty, 101–112
assessment and outlook, 109–111
chronic total coronary occlusions, instruction for recanalization, 102, 104
chronic total coronary occlusions, 101–102
results of recanalization, 104–106
results, 109, 111
routine angioplasty, 107–109
technique, 101
wire development, 101, 103
Matrix remodeling phase of wound healing, 497, 499
restenosis prevention and, 503

Mechanical transducers, in ultrasound imaging, 55–57
Medinvent stent, 302
Microwave balloon angioplasty, 281–285
angiography of iliac artery, 284
in rabbit models, 281–283
system illustrated, 282
thrombi and, 284–285
Mitral commissurotomy
balloon valvotomy vs., 619–620
closed, 609
Mitral regurgitation
after balloon valvotomy, 599, 616, 620–621
echocardiographic follow-up, 618, 619
hemodynamic follow-up, 616
detected by echocardiography, 71
Mitral stenosis
echocardiography in, 67–73
criteria for valvuloplasty, 70–71
treatment of congenital, 630–632
complications, 632
patients and methods, 630–632
results, 632
Mitral valve
area estimated with Doppler techniques, 68, 69
calcified, rupture of, 597
prolapse, balloon inflation and, 460
Mitral valvotomy (*see* Percutaneous balloon mitral valvotomy; Percutaneous double-balloon mitral valvotomy)
Monorail Doppler catheter, 121
Monorail mega catheter, 121
Monorail pressure catheter, 121
Monorail system, 113–131
applications
autotransfusion catheter, 120–121
hot balloon, 122
intracoronary diagnostic (pressure monitoring) catheter, 121
intracoronary Doppler catheters, 121, 122
other diagnostic and therapeutic devices, 122

perfusion catheter, 121
balloons, 116, 121
catheter shaft characteristics, 115
clinical experience, 122
acceptance, 124
Palmaz-Schatz stent, 123–124
related logistical developments, 124
results with monorail balloons, 122
transfusion catheters in acute coronary occlusion, 122–123
clinical results of balloon angioplasty, 126–127
description, 113–116
double-wire technique for branching stenosis, 124, 125
logistics, 124, 127, 130
in other devices, 127
procedure for PTCA, 116–117, 118
PTCA results in high-grade stenoses without total obstruction, 126
rationale of balloon catheter exchange, 124–125
steerability and contrast flow, 125–126
stenting, 123, 127, 128–129
technical development, 116–117
Monorail transfusion catheter, 121
Montreal Heart Institute, balloon valvotomy at, 609–623
Mortality
in hospital with supported angioplasty, 430
in PTCA vs. bypass grafting, 189
after thrombolytic therapy, 381–383
Mural thrombus (*see* Thrombus)
Myocardial blood flow
during angioplasty, 426–427
cardiopulmonary bypass support and, 483
Hemopump and, 486
intra-aortic balloon counterpulsation and, 481
Myocardial infarction
acute (*see* Acute myocardial infarction)
cardiogenic shock after, PTCA for, 372

Myocardial infarction (cont.)
  inferior, patient selection for
    thrombolytic therapy,
    375–376
  laser balloon angioplasty for,
    270
  plasminogen activators and,
    371
  rescue PTCA in, 371–372
Myocardial oxygen
    consumption
  cardiopulmonary bypass
    support and, 483
  Hemopump and, 486
  intra-aortic balloon
    counterpulsation and,
    481
  requirements, 457–459
Myocardial protection, in
    coronary angioplasty,
    457–469
  active hemoperfusion
    (prograde), 462–465
  intra-aortic balloon pump,
    466
  oxygen carriers, 465–466
  oxygen requirements,
    457–459
  passive hemoperfusion/
    autoperfusion, 459,
    461–462
  percutaneous
    cardiopulmonary
    support, 466–467
  retroperfusion (coronary
    sinus), 462
Myocardial viability, assessed
    by nuclear cardiology
    techniques, 3–18
Myocardium
  hibernating, 4
    in dog model, 5
  stunned, 3–4, 479
    in dog model, 5
Myosin-specific antibody,
    radiolabeled,
    infarct-avid imaging
    with, 12–13

N

Neodymium-YAG (Nd:YAG)
    laser, in laser
    angiosurgery II,
    191–196
Neodymium:YAG (Nd:YAG)
    laser, in laser balloon
    angioplasty, 263, 265
Nifedipine, for restenosis
    prevention, 563–564
Nonsteroidal
    anti-inflammatory
    drugs, for restenosis
    prevention, 565

Nuclear cardiology techniques
    in myocardial
    assessment, 3–18
  clinical decision making,
    15–16
  hibernating myocardium, 4
  infarct-avid imaging with
    radiolabeled
    myosin-specific
    antibody, 12–13
  noninvasive evidence of
    preserved viability, 4
  positron emission
    tomography, 13–15
  specific agents and
    techniques, 4–15
  stunned myocardium, 3–4
  technetium 99m myocardial
    perfusion agents,
    11–12, 13
  thallium 201 imaging, 4–10

O

Occlusion
  acute coronary (*see* Acute
    coronary occlusion)
  of atrial septal defect,
    642–644
  chronic, PTCA long-wire
    technique for, 92, 97
  chronic total
    balloon angioplasty for,
    82–83
    excimer laser coronary
    angioplasty for,
    238–239, 240
    excimer laser coronary
    angioplasty for, 227,
    229, 230
  chronic total occlusions,
    238–239, 240
  femoropopliteal
    argon laser angioplasty
    for, 256, 257, 258
    ultrasound recanalization
    for, 293–295
  of iliac arteries, laser
    angioplasty for, 246,
    248, 251
  patent ductus arteriosus,
    interventional
    catheterization
    treatment, 639–642
  reocclusion (*see* Reocclusion)
  stent prosthesis implantation
    for, 311–312
  of superficial femoral artery,
    laser angioplasty for,
    39, 245–250
  swine coronary model,
    174–175
  total
    angioplasty for, 259–260

laser balloon angioplasty
    for, 269
  ultrasound angioplasty for,
    in vivo animal studies,
    289–290
  of ventricular septal defect,
    644, 645
  in Wallstent experience,
    337, 338–339, 341
Opacification of stenosis, in
    PTCA long-wire
    technique, 90–92
Ostial lesions
  balloon angioplasty for, 84,
    86
  directional coronary
    atherectomy for, 164,
    166
  excimer laser coronary
    angioplasty for, 227,
    228
Oxygen carriers, in balloon
    angioplasty, 465–466

P

Pacemakers, 659–660
  bradycardia, in patients
    receiving defibrillators,
    665–666
  implantation techniques,
    660–661
  sensors in, 659–660
Pacing
  dual-chamber, 654, 657, 658
  dual-chamber,
    rate-responsive, 658,
    659
  fixed-rate ventricular, 652,
    654, 657, 658
  hemodynamics, 651–656
  modes, 656–659
  optimal therapy, 651–663
  ventricular rate-responsive,
    652, 654, 658
Palmaz-Schatz coronary stent,
    302, 319–331
  for acute closure, 417
  angiograms of treated
    lesions, 325, 326, 327
  background, 319
  complications, 324–328
  deployment technique,
    322–324
  design and delivery system,
    319–321
  monorail stenting with,
    123–124, 128–129
  patient selection,
    preparation, and
    management, 321–322
  restenosis with, 304–305
    in aortocoronary bypass
    grafts, 329

management, 329
    in native coronary
    arteries, 328–329
Park Nicollet Heart Center,
    argon laser angioplasty
    at, 4, 256–257
Patency of infarct-related
    artery, after
    thrombolytic therapy,
    380–381
Patent ductus arteriosus
    occlusion, interventional
    catheterization
    treatment, 639–642
Peptide cell regulators factors,
    for restenosis
    prevention, 565
Percutaneous balloon aortic
    valvuloplasty, 630–632
  catheter for, 577
  changes in dyspnea and
    angina pectoris after
    procedure, 580
  clinical characteristics of
    patients, 576
  complications, 578, 579
  evolution of technique,
    575–578
  follow-up, 578–579, 580
  improvement in
    transvalvular gradient
    and valve area, 579
  indications, 579–581
  Rouen experience, 575–582
  technical aspects, 576
  valve area distribution
    before and after
    procedure, 576
Percutaneous balloon mitral
    valvotomy, 583–588
  choice of dilating balloon
    catheters, 584
  clinical follow-up, 587
  complications, 587–588
  double-balloon technique,
    583–584
  double-balloon valvotomy
    (*see* Percutaneous
    double-balloon mitral
    valvotomy)
  factors influencing outcome,
    585
  Montreal Heart Institute
    experience, 609–623
  echocardiographic
    follow-up, 618–619
  follow-up studies, 616
  hemodynamic follow-up,
    615–617
  immediate results,
    611–612
  long-term results,
    612–615
  patient selection, 610, 621

surgical commissurotomy
vs., 619–620
technique, 610–611
patient selection, 586, 587
results, 584–585
long-term, 586–587
scoring system for
prognosis, 585
Percutaneous balloon
pericardial window,
687–690
Percutaneous double-balloon
mitral valvotomy,
589–608
assessment methods, 593
clinical implications and cost
impact, 605–607
hemodynamic values in, 595,
596, 598, 602
history, 589
Inoue single-balloon method
vs., 597–601
mitral valve area by degree
of calcification, 596,
604
patient selection, 589–591
procedure tolerance
complications, 595–597
protocol, 591–593
repeat catheterization and
echo Doppler
follow-up, 601–606
results, 593–595, 596
technique, 583–584
Percutaneous femorofemoral
cardiopulmonary bypass
support, 435–456,
466–467
Bard system for left
ventricular assist, 482,
483–485, 490
cannula removal in elective
group, 447–448
cannulation, 437–439, 483
cardiogenic shock and
cardiac arrest,
subsequent therapy in,
446
complications, 450–451, 453
contraindications, 436, 437
coronary perfusion with
separate roller pump, 454
discussion, 451–453
duration of clamp
compression, 452
equipment, 436
failure to wean from
Hemopump in, 488
intra-aortic balloon
counterpulsation in, 481
future directions, 453–454
in high-risk coronary
angioplasty, 427–428,
467

ileofemoral angiography,
437, 438
indications, 435–436
initiation, 443, 444–446
left ventricular venting, 454
limitations, 452
observation during elective
intervention, 448–450
orders after, 449
physiology, 442–443
portable system, 439,
441–442, 466–467
PTCA technique in elective
group, 443, 446
technical considerations,
439, 440
technique in elective group,
436
termination
elective group, 446–447
emergent group, 446–448
observation after, 450
Percutaneous rotational
thrombectomy (PRT)
as alternative to
thrombolysis, 171–176
catheter design and use, 172,
173
concept and theory, 171
coronary studies, 173–174
coronary thrombosis and
reocclusion, 174–175
initial work, 172–173
potential clinical use,
175–176
Percutaneous thrombolytic
coronary
revascularization (*see*
Thrombolysis)
Percutaneous transluminal
coronary angioplasty
(PTCA)
acute closure in, 435
cardiopulmonary bypass
support in, 484
Hemopump support in,
488
acute complications, 417
for acute myocardial
infarction (*see* Acute
myocardial infarction,
angioplasty therapy)
angioscopy after, 47–48
balloon angioplasty (*see*
Balloon angioplasty)
for cardiogenic shock after
myocardial infarction,
372
cardiopulmonary bypass
support and, 443–446,
484
catheterization events during
direct infarct
angioplasty, 417

complications, in-hospital,
421
coronary artery flow
evaluation in, Doppler
guidewire for, 27–32
demographics, 417
development for stenoses
and occlusions in
Frankfurt, 90
disadvantages of
conventional steerable
technique, 89
failure
salvaged by perfusion
balloon angioplasty,
474–475
therapy for, 421–422
without acute closure or
ischemia, laser balloon
angioplasty for, 269
graded inflation to achieve
full balloon expansion,
416
in hospitals without surgical
backup, 419–420
limitations, 149, 695
location of diseased arteries
after, 136
long-wire technique,
89–100
for acute occlusions after
angioplasty, 97–99
for branching stenoses,
92, 93–96
for chronic occlusions, 92,
97
exchange of balloon
catheters, 92
measurement of
peripheral coronary
pressures, 98
schematic diagram, 91
stenosis opacification and
dilatation, 90–92
multivessel, procedural
outcome after, 416
perfusion balloon catheters
for, 473–474
physician fees, 418
post-thrombolytic,
plasminogen activator
impact on outcome, 371
prior bypass surgery and, 84,
86–87
problems in, 81, 695
rescue, 371–372
restenosis after (*see*
Restenosis, after PTCA)
results, 263, 316, 319
sliding rail system for,
113–131
clinical results, 126–127
monorail technique,
116–117, 124

strategies, 80
surgical standby, 415–424
ACA/AHA published
guidelines, 415
avoiding trouble, 421–422
cost analysis, 418–419
intraprocedural factors,
415–418
ischemia control,
420–421
patient classification by
risk, 419
patient statistics, 418
preprocedural factors,
415, 416
specific guidelines,
422–423
strategies, 419
surveys of experience, 418
survival rate for bypass
grafting vs., 189
thrombolytic
revascularization vs.,
angioscopy in selecting,
42
Percutaneous transluminal
coronary angioscopy
(PTCAS)
assessment variables, 45
catheter models, 42
discussion, 48–53
failed, reasons for, 50
guiding catheter, 43–44
indications, 42
light and imaging units,
42–43
results, 45–48
angioscopy after
thrombolysis or PTCA,
47–48
catheter insertion and
flushing, 45
findings in acute coronary
syndrome, 46–47
success rates, 45–46
with routine contrast
arteriography,
requirements for, 49
safety, 52
study patients, 42
technical feasibility and
clinical benefits, 41–54
technique, 44–45
Percutaneous transluminal
coronary rotary
ablation, with
Rotablator, 141–147
burr size vs. size of residual
stenosis, 145
complications and
evaluation, 146
historical and experimental
studies, 141
instrument design, 141–142

Percutaneous transluminal
    (cont.)
  international registry results,
    143–144
  mechanism of action,
    145–146
  medications, 142–143
  procedure, 142
  quantitative coronary
    angiography, 144–145
Perfusion
  antegrade, during
    angioplasty, 426
  with separate roller pump,
    in cardiopulmonary
    bypass support, 454
Perfusion catheters
  balloon (*see* Autoperfusion
    balloon angioplasty)
  monorail-type, 121
Perfusion methods
  active hemoperfusion
    (prograde), 462–465
  passive hemoperfusion/auto-
    perfusion, 459, 461–462
  retroperfusion (coronary
    sinus), 462
Pericardial tamponade,
    percutaneous balloon
    pericardial window for,
    687–690
Peripheral coronary pressures,
    measured in PTCA
    long-wire technique, 98
Peripheral laser angioplasty,
    243–253
  with argon laser (*see* Argon
    laser angioplasty)
  discussion, 248–252
  methods and clinical
    material
    angiographic findings, 244
    follow-up, 244
    laser and laser catheters, 244
    patient population,
      243–244
    study inclusion criteria,
      243
    treatment protocol,
      244–245
  patency rates after, 249, 251
  results, 245
    complications, 246–247
    follow-up, 247–248
    iliac arteries, 246, 248, 251
    popliteal region, 246
    superficial femoral artery,
      245–250
Peripheral stent prosthesis
    implants
  results, 311–312
  technique of implantation,
    310–311

PET (positron emission
    tomography),
    myocardial viability
    assessed by, 13–15
Pharmacologic therapy, in
    restenosis prevention,
    547–571
  action mechanisms, 551
  animal experimental work
    and human studies,
    554–565
  animal model, 550–553, 556
  anticoagulants, 556–558,
    561
  antiplatelet agents, 558–561
  antiproliferative drugs,
    561–563
  calcium antagonists, 563–564
  drugs to prevent restenosis
    mechanisms, 551
  effects on animals, 552–553
  effects on humans, 554–557
  future developments and
    directions, 565–566
  inhibitors of inflammation,
    565
  lipid-lowering drugs,
    564–565
Photochemical ablation, 225
Physiology, of
    cardiopulmonary bypass
    support, 442–443
Piccolino monorail balloon
    catheter, 114, 118, 120,
    127, 128–129
Pigtail catheter, for
    percutaneous balloon
    pericardial window,
    687–689
Plaque
  angioscopic identification
    and classification, 48,
    51–52
  optical properties, 204
  quantitation, 33
  ultrasound imaging and,
    60–62
Plaque ablation
  comparison of lasers for, 204
  by pulsed laser, 203–214
    conditions for
      effectiveness, 213
    energy consumption,
      211–213
    long vs. short pulse
      modes, 203–206
    photothermal model,
      206–208
    selectivity vs. normal
      vessel wall, 210–211, 212
    stages, 206
    threshold characteristics
      of efficiency, 208–210

by ultrasound angioplasty
    mechanism, 291–292
  system in development,
    292–293
  in vitro studies and effect
    on arterial wall, 287–288
Plasminogen activators,
    outcome of
    post-thrombolytic
    PTCA and, 371
Platelet adhesion, activation,
    and aggregation, in
    thrombus formation, 550
Platelet-derived growth factor
  cellular and molecular events
    induced by, 539–540
  in restenosis, 498, 528
  in restenosis prevention,
    521–526
    blocking PDGF effects,
      522–524, 525
    future studies, 524–525
  in smooth muscle cell
    proliferation and
    migration, 514–515,
    516, 528, 530, 536–538
Platelet-derived growth factor
    antagonist, for
    restenosis prevention,
    561
Platelet-derived growth factor
    receptor, 521–524, 525,
    539, 540
Platelet inhibitors, in
    restenosis prevention,
    502
Popliteal artery occlusion,
    ultrasound
    recanalization for, 293
Popliteal region, laser
    angioplasty of, 246
Positron emission tomography
    (PET), myocardial
    viability assessed by,
    13–15
Pressure monitoring catheter,
    monorail-type, 121
Pressures, peripheral coronary,
    measured in PTCA
    long-wire technique, 98
Primary Angioplasty
    Recanalization (PAR)
    Registry, 363
Prostacyclin, for restenosis
    prevention, 560
Prostaglandin E1, for
    restenosis prevention,
    561
Proteoglycan synthesis, in
    wound healing, 499
PTCA (*see* Percutaneous
    transluminal coronary
    angioplasty)

PTCAS (*see* Percutaneous
    transluminal coronary
    angioscopy)
Pulmonary artery branch
    stenosis, interventional
    catheterization
    treatment, 636–638
  complications, 638
  restenosis, 638
  results, 637–638
  technique, 637
Pulmonary valve stenosis,
    interventional
    catheterization
    treatment, 625–628
  complications, 628
  results, 626–628
  technique, 625–626
Pulmonary vein stenosis,
    interventional
    catheterization
    treatment, 638–639

R

Radiography, digital, in blood
    flow assessment, 19
Radionuclide imaging (*see*
    Nuclear cardiology
    techniques)
Randomized Intervention
    Treatment of Angina
    (RITA), 137–138
Recanalization, differences in
    mechanisms, 504
Recatheterization, in
    valvotomy follow-up,
    601–605, 615–617
Renin-angiotensin system, in
    vascular wall,
    528–529
  therapeutic effort to inhibit,
    530
Reocclusion
  after lytic therapy, 370
  with PTCA vs. lytic therapy,
    369
Rescue angioplasty, 371–372
Restenosis
  angioscopy, atherectomy
    specimens, and
    autopsies in, 510
  in balloon aortic
    valvuloplasty, 579
  in balloon mitral valvotomy,
    601–602, 604, 606
    echocardiographic
      follow-up, 618–619
    hemodynamic follow-up,
      616–617
    Montreal Heart Institute
      experience, 616–617,
      621

cell biology
angiotensin II in
neointimal cell
proliferation, 527–533
paradigm based on,
495–508
in directional coronary
atherectomy, 167, 168
predictors, 62
in excimer laser coronary
angioplasty, 236
late restenosis, 229
extent of dissection and, 61
growth factors in, 497–498,
499–500
histology, 496–497
lumen diameter, 509
mechanisms, 509, 547,
549–550
testable hypotheses,
499–501
with Palmaz-Schatz
coronary stent,
328–329
prevention, 504
future directions,
515–517
by inhibition of vascular
smooth muscle cell
proliferation, 535–546
limitations of previous
trials, 501–502
local delivery of
therapeutic agents,
542–543
pharmacologic therapy (*see*
Pharmacologic therapy,
in restenosis
prevention)
platelet-derived growth
factor in, 521–526
potential therapies, 502
PTCA vs. laser balloon
angioplasty for,
267–268
in PTCA, 187–190, 316,
319, 547
risk factors, 548–549
in pulmonary branch
angioplasty, 638
as response to injury,
496–501, 521–522
with Rotablator, 144
stenting for, 304–305, 315,
316–317
stenting for failed
angioplasty and, 304
thrombosis and, congruent
risk factors, 509–510
time course, 495
in Wallstent experience,
335–336, 339,
341–342

Resting ^{201}TI imaging, 10
Retroperfusion, 462
Rheology of blood flow, in
arterial thrombosis,
510–511
Ridogrel, for restenosis
prevention, 561
Right coronary artery stenosis,
directional coronary
atherectomy for, 164,
165
RITA (Randomized
Intervention Treatment
of Angina), 137–138
Rotablator, 62 (*see also*
Percutaneous
transluminal rotary
ablation, with
Rotablator)
burr size, 146
design, 141–142
tip, 142
Rotational ablation, high-speed
(ROTA), 696, 702
Rotational thrombectomy,
percutaneous (*see*
Percutaneous rotational
thrombectomy)
Ruiz-Lau-up guidewire, 592
Rx catheter, 120
Rx perfusion balloon catheter,
473
Rx Perfusion catheter, 121

S

SAMI (Streptokinase
Angioplasty Myocardial
Infarction) trial, 361
Saphenous vein grafts
laser angioplasty and, 228
Palmaz-Schatz coronary
stent and, 327, 329
Scintigraphy
dipyridamole thallium, 9–10
exercise thallium, 6–9
in coronary angioplasty
patient, 10
resting thallium, 10
Serotonin antagonist, for
restenosis prevention,
561
Shock (*see* Cardiogenic shock)
Simpson Coronary
AtheroCath, 61,
158–159, 161–163,
164
Single photon emission
computed tomography
(SPECT) 201TI
scintigraphy, 7, 8, 9
Sliding rail balloon catheter
systems, 120

Monorail (*see* Monorail
system)
Smooth muscle cells
angiotensin II in
hypertrophy of,
529–530
growth factors stimulating
proliferation of,
514–515, 516,
521–522, 528,
536–538, 549
proliferation and migration
in arterial injury,
514–515, 516,
521–522
role of thrombus, 516
response to injury, 527–528,
535–536
in restenosis, 500, 501, 528
in restenosis prevention,
503, 528
inhibitory therapy,
535–546
Solid-state transducers, in
ultrasound imaging,
57
Solitaire catheter, 120
Spears USCI laser balloon
angioplasty catheter,
264
Spectral diagnosis, 183–186
Spectroscopy, fluorescence, in
laser angiosurgery II,
198–200
SPECT 201TI scintigraphy, 7,
8, 9
Speedflow catheter, 121
Speedy catheter, 127
Stack perfusion catheter, 461,
462, 471–472
autoperfusion angioplasty
with, 472–476
diagram, 472
specifications, 472
Starling principle, 651, 652
Stenosis
aortic (*see* Aortic stenosis)
branching, PTCA long-wire
technique for, 92, 93
critical ileofemoral,
cardiopulmonary bypass
support and, 439, 441
echocardiographic
applications
quantitation of severity,
67–68, 69, 70
reduction assessment in
balloon valvuloplasty,
72, 73
femoropopliteal, argon laser
angioplasty for, 256,
257, 258
mitral (*see* Mitral stenosis)

monorail system treatment,
116
Palmaz-Schatz coronary
stent and, 325, 326
of pulmonary artery branch,
interventional
catheterization
treatment, 636–638
of pulmonary valve,
interventional
catheterization
treatment, 625–628
of pulmonary vein,
interventional
catheterization
treatment, 638–639
residual, with PTCA vs. lytic
therapy, 368
restenosis (*see* Restenosis)
subaortic, interventional
catheterization
treatment, 632
treated with monorail
system
high-grade stenosis
without total
obstruction, 126
left circumflex artery
branching stenosis, 125
right coronary artery
stenosis, 118
tricuspid, interventional
catheterization
treatment, 632–633
in ultrasound angioplasty,
294–295, 296
Stenting
intracoronary, rationale and
advantages, 301
with monorail catheters,
127, 128–129
Stents
as bailout devices after failed
angioplasty, 302–304
experimental testing,
301–302
future directions, 305
heat-activated recoverable
temporary (*see* HARTS
device)
implantation, 302–303, 696
peripheral stents,
310–311
ultrasound imaging in,
62–63
nitinol, 349–350
Palmaz-Schatz (*see*
Palmaz-Schatz coronary
stent)
peripheral
initial experience in
human vessels, 309
results, 311–312

Stents *(cont.)*
technique of implantation, 310–311
technique of implantation and results, 310–312
for restenosis prevention, 304–305
self-expanding intravascular
animal experimentation, 308, 309, 310
coronary implants, implantation technique and results, 312–315
design and methods, 307–308, 316
discussion, 315–317
histologic analysis, 308–309, 311, 312
nonsurgical implantation, 307–318
Strecker, 38
types under investigation, 302
Wallstent (*see* Wallstent experience)
Stent thrombosis, 316
Steroids, for restenosis prevention, 565
Strecker stent, angioscopic view, 38
Streptokinase, 378–379
for acute myocardial infarction, 387, 389
arrhythmias after, 390
case examples, 392–406
historical experience, 359–360
protocol, 388
results, 400, 407
time to treatment and percentage of patients studied, 393
t-PA and ASCAP vs., 400–402
with angioplasty, 361
left ventricular function and, 381
mortality and, 381–383
in optimal thrombolytic regimen, 383–384
patency of infarct-related artery and, 380–381
Streptokinase Angioplasty Myocardial Infarction (SAMI) trial, 361
Stress response, with 201TI imaging, 6
ST segment changes
in balloon inflation, 459, 460
in thrombolyis in acute myocardial infarction, 401–403, 405

Stunned myocardium, 3–4, 479
in dog model, 5
Subaortic stenosis, interventional catheterization treatment, 630
Sulfinpyrazone, for restenosis prevention, 559
Superficial femoral artery
laser angioplasty of, 39, 245–250
sclerotic, observations, 37
Supported angioplasty, 425–433
autoperfusion (*see* Autoperfusion balloon angioplasty)
cardiopulmonary bypass support (*see* Percutaneous femorofemoral cardiopulmonary bypass support)
clinical practice, 430–432
factors defining patient risk, 425–426
hospital mortality, 430
left ventricular assist devices (*see* Left ventricular assist devices)
myocardial perfusion, 426–427
national registry, 429–430
options for risk groups, 431
results, 430–431
systemic circulatory support, 427–428
technique, 428–429
Surgical standby (*see* Percutaneous transluminal coronary angioplasty, surgical standby)

T

Tachycardia
antitachycardia pacing, 666
atrioventricular node reentrant, catheter ablation, 673, 676–677
ventricular (*see* Ventricular tachycardia)
TAMI (Thrombosis and Angioplasty in Myocardial Infarction), 360, 370–371
Technetium 99m myocardial perfusion agents, 11–12, 13
Technology
development, 1–3

clinical assessment, 2–3
medical-industrial interactions, 3
rationale, 1–2
new, 691–693
TEC (*see* Transluminal extraction-endarterectomy catheter)
Thallium 201 imaging
for detection of myocardial viability
dipyridamole thallium scintigraphy, 9–10
exercise thallium scintigraphy, 6–9, 10
experimental validation, 4–6
resting, 10
FDG imaging vs., 14
Thermal angioplasty (*see* Excimer laser coronary angioplasty; Laser angiosurgery; Microwave balloon angioplasty)
Thermal fusion of soft tissues, by laser balloon angioplasty, 264–265
Thermal perfusion balloon catheters, 475–476
Thermodilution coronary sinus catheter, for coronary blood flow measurement, 19–20
Thrombectomy, percutaneous rotational (*see* Percutaneous rotational thrombectomy)
Thrombin, in thrombosis, 512
Thrombin content of injured arteries, 513
Thromboembolism, pacing modes and, 657
Thrombogenicity, laser balloon angioplasty and, 267
Thrombolysis
in acute myocardial infarction, in community hospital, 387–411
case examples, 392–406
discussion, 399–402, 404, 406–408
indications, 387–388
management after, 398–399
procedure, 388–389, 390
procedure for IV streptokinase therapy, 388
results, 389–393
angioscopy after, 47–48

future directions, 516–517
by laser (*see* Laser thrombolysis)
objectives, 274
percutaneous rotational thrombectomy as alternative to, 171–176
PTCA vs., angioscopy in selecting, 42
strategy, 80
therapeutic goals, 513–514
Thrombolysis and Angioplasty in Myocardial Infarction (TAMI), 360, 370–371
Thrombolysis in Myocardial Infarction (TIMI), 360–361, 370, 371, 400
Thrombolytic therapy
for acute myocardial infarction
agents, 378–379 (*see also specific agents*)
best drug, dose, and heparin regimen, 383–384
clinical end points, 380–383
costs, 402, 404, 407
implications of randomized trials, 375–385
patient selection controversies, 375–378
results of recent trials, 407
in acute myocardial infarction
deficiencies, 360–362
PTCA vs. lytic therapy, 367–369
reasons for catheterization after, 409
angioplasty after, 370–371
Thrombosis
acute coronary, etiology and treatment, 273
after arterial injury, pathogenesis, 510–513
cellular proliferation and migration and, 514–515
closed-chest swine model, 174–175
in excimer laser coronary angioplasty, 236
restenosis and, congruent risk factors, 509–510
stent, 316
Thromboxane A2, for restenosis prevention, 559–560
Thrombus, 509, 511–512
dissolution by ultrasound angioplasty, 290–291

growth factors and, 515
intracardiac, detected by echocardiography, 69
left arterial, transesophageal echocardiography in assessment of, 590
microwave balloon angioplasty and, 284–285
prevention after angioplasty, 515–516
role in smooth muscle cell proliferation, 516
Ticlopidine, for restenosis prevention, 560
TIMI (Thrombosis in Myocardial Infarction), 360–361, 370, 371, 400
Tissue characterization, ultrasonic, 64
Tissue effects of laser balloon angioplasty, 264–265, 267
Tissue plasminogen activator (t-PA), 378, 379
for acute myocardial infarction
protocol, 390
results, 407
streptokinase and ASCAP vs., 400–402
left ventricular function and, 381
mortality and, 381–383
in optimal thrombolytic regimen, 383
patency of infarct-related artery and, 380–381
recombinant (rt-PA), thrombolytic therapy with, 360
t-PA (*see* Tissue plasminogen activator)
Transcatheter blood flow measurement, 19–26
Doppler catheter and guidewire, 20–21
impedance catheter and guidewire, 21–25
thermodilution coronary sinus catheter, 19–20
Transducers, in ultrasound imaging, 55–57
Transesophageal echocardiography, for valve assessment, 590–591
Transforming growth factor, in smooth muscle cell proliferation and migration, 514, 515, 516, 528, 530, 537–538

Transfusion catheters, in acute coronary occlusion, monorail system experience, 122–123
Transfusion requirement, in cardiopulmonary bypass support, 450, 451
Transluminal extraction-endarterectomy catheter, atherectomy with, 149–155, 695, 702
case selection criteria, 150–151
device description and illustration, 150, 151–152
historical perspective, 149–150
procedure, 150
results, 151–152, 152–154
Transthoracic echocardiography, transesophageal echocardiography vs., 590–591
Transvalvular left ventricular assist (*see* Hemopump)
Transvenous catheter ablation, of cardiac arrhythmias (*see* Arrhythmias, transvenous catheter ablation)
Tricuspid stenosis, interventional catheterization treatment, 632–633

U

Ultrasound angioplasty, 287–297
ablation mechanism, 291–292
ablation system in development, 292–293
clinical studies, 10, 293–295
for femoral artery occlusion, 294
method of percutaneous arterial recanalization, 293
peripheral, safety and limitations, 295–296
for popliteal artery occlusion, 293
in vitro and in vivo studies of thrombus dissolution, 290–291
in vitro studies of plaque ablation, 287–288
in vitro studies of vascular reactivity, 288–289

in vivo animal studies, 289–290
Ultrasound generator, Baxter-Edwards, 292
Ultrasound images, three-dimensional reconstruction of, 64, 65
Ultrasound imaging, intravascular
angioscopy vs., 59
anticipated developments, 63–64
catheter design and new advances, 55–57
clinical applications and technical advances, 55–66
guidance for catheter therapies, 59–63
image interpretation, 57–59
quantitation, 59
Ultrasound (*see also* Echocardiography)
diagnostic vs. therapeutic, 291
Doppler systems, catheter-based, 27
Urokinase, 378, 379

V

Valvotomy (*see* Percutaneous balloon mitral valvotomy; Percutaneous double-balloon mitral valvotomy)
Valvular regurgitation, detection by Doppler echocardiography, 68–69, 71, 72
Valvular stenosis (*see* Stenosis)
Valvuloplasty
aortic, 628–630 (*see also* Percutaneous balloon aortic valvuloplasty)
cardiopulmonary bypass support in, 484
catheter balloon (*see* Catheter balloon valvuloplasty)
mitral, 630–632
pulmonary, 625–628
subaortic, 630
tricuspid, 632–633
Vascular injury
restenosis as response to, 496
smooth muscle cell proliferation and migration in, 514–515, 516, 521–522

Vascular reactivity, to ultrasound angioplasty, 288–289
Vascular smooth muscle cells (*see* Smooth muscle cells)
Vascular system, excimer laser ablation in, 225
Vein grafts
insertion site stenosis of, balloon angioplasty and, 84, 86
saphenous
laser angioplasty and, 228
Palmaz-Schatz coronary stent and, 327, 329
Velocity measurements, in stenosis assessment, 68, 69
Ventricle, left (*see* Left ventricle)
Ventricular septal defect closure, 644, 645
Ventricular tachycardia
balloon inflation and, 460
catheter ablation
"chemical" ablation, 679–680
with high-energy shocks, 673
with radio frequency energy, 677–680, 682
Verapamil, for restenosis prevention, 563–564

W

Wallstent experience, 304, 333–347
discussion
early occlusion and late restenosis, 341–342
follow-up, 344–345
limitations of study, 343–344
relative risk analysis, 342–343
methods
angiographic follow-up, 335, 336, 337, 339
angiographic variables, 336, 337
implantations by vessel type and date of implantation, 334
indications for stenting, 334
quantitative coronary arteriography, 335
relative risk analysis, 336–337
restenosis, 335–336
statistical, 336–338

Wallstent experience *(cont.)*
  stent implantations by
    vessel type, 334
  study patients, 333–335,
    336
  results
    long-term follow-up,
      339–340, 341
    occlusion and restenosis
      rate, 337, 338–339

relative risk analysis, 339,
  340
Warfarin, for restenosis
  prevention, 558
Wiktor stent, 98
Wound healing process
  granulation phase, 497,
    498–499, 501
    restenosis prevention and,
      503

inflammatory phase,
  497–498, 501
  restenosis prevention and,
    502–503
matrix remodeling phase,
  497, 499
  restenosis prevention and,
    503
restenosis as manifestation
  of, 496

clinical implications of
  hypothesis, 503–504

X

Xenon chloride excimer laser,
  223–224 (*see also*
  Excimer laser coronary
  angioplasty)